Lee's *Synopsis of* **Anaesthesia**

Eleventh edition

In memory of John Alfred Lee (1906–1989)

To V. A., G. R. and J. D.

Among the experiments that may be tried on man, those that can only harm are forbidden; those that are innocent are permissible; those that are beneficial are obligatory – Claude Bernard (1813–1878).

A new scientific truth does not triumph because it convinces its opponents making them see the light, but rather because its opponents eventually die and a new generation grows up that is familiar with it. – Max Planck (1858–1947).

It is the duty of the anaesthetist to study the well-being of the patient as well as the convenience of the surgeon.

Eternal vigilance is the price of safety.

The duty of the anaesthetist towards his patient is to take care.

Primum non nocere – First of all, do no harm.

The proper dose of any drug is enough. – Dr J. H. Drysdale.

Knowledge is of two kinds; we know a subject ourselves or we know where we can get information about it. – Samuel Johnson (1709–1784).

When you breathe you inspire, when you do not you expire.

Worry enough, but not too much. – C. L. H.

Lee's
Synopsis of
Anaesthesia

R. S. Atkinson *OBE, MA, BChir, FRCAnaes*
Honorary Consulting Anaesthetist, Southend Hospital, UK

G. B. Rushman *MB, BS, FRCAnaes*
Consultant Anaesthetist, Southend Hospital, UK

and

N. J. H. Davies *MA, DM, MRCP, FRCAnaes*
Consultant Anaesthetist, Southampton General Hospital, UK

Eleventh edition

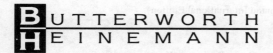

Butterworth-Heinemann Ltd
Linacre House, Jordan Hill, Oxford OX2 8DP

 PART OF REED INTERNATIONAL BOOKS

OXFORD LONDON BOSTON
MUNICH NEW DELHI SINGAPORE SYDNEY
TOKYO TORONTO WELLINGTON

By J. Alfred Lee

First Edition 1947
Second Edition 1950
Third Edition 1953
Reprinted with minor
  amendments 1955
Reprinted 1956
Reprinted 1957
Fourth Edition 1959
Reprinted 1960
Italian First Edition 1963

*By J. Alfred Lee
  and R. S. Atkinson*

Fifth Edition 1964
Spanish Edition 1966
Sixth Edition 1968
Seventh Edition 1973
French Edition 1975
Portuguese Edition 1976
German Edition 1977

By R. S. Atkinson, G. B. Rushman and J. Alfred Lee

Eighth Edition 1977
Reprinted 1979
Ninth Edition 1982
Tenth Edition 1987

Greek Edition 1979
Polish Edition 1981
Spanish Second Edition 1981
Italian Second Edition 1986
German Second Edition 1986

By R. S. Atkinson, G. B. Rushman and N. J. H. Davies

Eleventh Edition 1993

© Butterworth-Heinemann Ltd 1993

British Library Cataloguing in Publication Data
Atkinson, R. S.
  Lee's Synopsis of Anaesthesia. –
  11 Rev. ed
  I. Title
  617. 96

ISBN 0 7506 1449 8
ISBN 0 7506 1608 3 (Butterworth-Heinemann International Edition)

Composition by Genesis Typesetting, Laser Quay, Rochester, Kent
Printed in England by Clays Ltd, St Ives plc

Contents

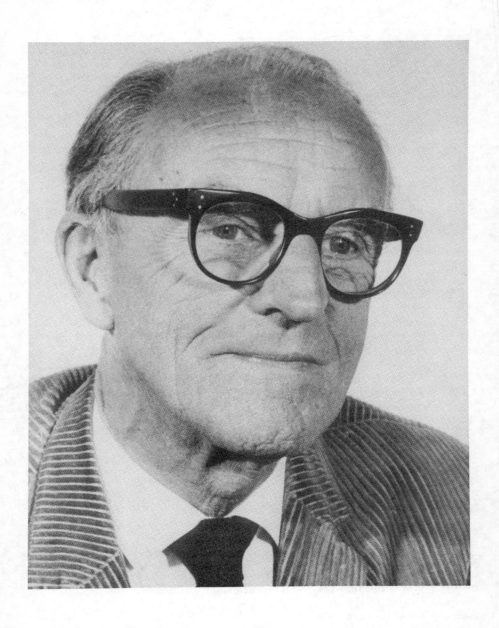

John Alfred Lee
(1906–1989)

Alfred Lee was born near Liverpool in 1906 and qualified from Newcastle upon Tyne, then a part of the University of Durham, in 1927. His early experience of anaesthesia was that expected of the House Surgeon of that time, usually an open-drop method and occasionally a primitive Boyles machine or a Clovers inhaler. After moving to Southend-on-Sea as a general practitioner, he continued to maintain an interest in anaesthesia and took up anaesthetic sessions at the hospital. In 1939, on the outbreak of hostilities, Alfred Lee became a wholetime specialist in the Emergency Medical Service, working at Runwell Hospital, near Southend. In 1948, the inauguration of the National Health Service enabled him to become a Consultant Anaesthetist, a post he held up to his retirement in 1971, when he became Honorary Consulting Anaesthetist. He continued his interest in anaesthesia and travelled extensively, attending many regional, national and international meetings right up to the month of his death in April 1989.

After the war years, there was a return of anaesthetists from the Services to civilian life. There were few texts on anaesthesia for them and Alfred Lee thought that something should be done about this. He approached John Wright and Sons Ltd of Bristol who asked him to submit some specimen chapters. The result was the publication of 'A Synopsis of Anaesthesia' in 1947. This first edition has since become a collectors item. It had 254 pages including the index and sold for a modest price. Alfred Lee was to participate in 11 editions over the next 40 years, some being translated into Italian, Spanish, French, Portuguese, German, Greek and Polish. He was also the author of many papers, wrote and edited a number of other texts and was for a time Assistant Editor and later Chairman of the Editorial Board of 'Anaesthesia'. His special interests included pre-operative care (he started an outpatient clinic for the pre-operative assessment of patients), postoperative care (Southend was the first non-specialist hospital to have a Postoperative Observation Ward adjacent to the theatres), regional analgesia (he advocated and taught extradural block long before it became common practice) and history (he was the first President of the History of Anaesthesia Society).

He was recognized widely as a teacher and clinician and lectured in Britain and abroad. He examined for the Final Fellowship Examination, was a member of the Board of Faculty of Anaesthetists, and President of the Association of Anaesthetists of Great Britain and Ireland. He was Joseph Clover lecturer in 1960. He served as President of the Section of Anaesthetics of the Royal Society of Medicine and in 1975 received the Hickman Medal. He was an Honorary Fellow of the Faculty of Anaesthetists of the Royal College of Surgeons in Ireland (1970), Gaston Labat Lecturer to the American Society of Regional Anesthesia (1985), Thomas Seldon Lecturer to the International Research Society (1985), and Koller Gold Medallist and Lecturer in Vienna (1984) to commemorate the centenary of local analgesia. This 11th edition is dedicated to his memory.

Preface to the eleventh edition

'The faintest ink is sometimes better than the strongest memory.'

John Alfred Lee published the first edition of *A Synopsis of Anaesthesia* in 1947 and it ran to 10 editions in his lifetime. He was active in the preparation of this 11th edition and it is a pleasure to record that he agreed to its being titled '*Lee's Synopsis of Anaesthesia*'. He also recognized that a new and younger co-author was needed if the 11th edition was to continue to reflect advances and changes in anaesthetic practice. He took part in early meetings to discuss the format of the 11th edition and had several meetings with Dr Nicholas Davies who had been recruited in this role. Dr Davies has brought to this volume the experience and breadth of vision of a younger man and the two remaining co-authors are grateful to him for accepting the invitation.

The 11th edition includes a digest of the increasing flood of specialist literature, with a concentration on the synoptic format. The chapters have been rearranged and many new ones added. There is an important new chapter on Safety in Anaesthetic Practice, which includes Audit, and new sections have been added to Cardiorespiratory Intensive Care, while the subject of Pain Management has been further developed. The history of anaesthesia is still an important part of this book as much of the information it contains is not readily available elsewhere. Once again we are indebted to Professor Ole Secher for his help. History has however been moved to the end of the text, followed by a new chapter describing many of the agents and techniques now discontinued or used only in developing countries.

Anaesthesia and intensive care are fast developing areas, and the role of the anaesthetist is extending. We have reflected this. The Synopsis remains however a practical book which gives advice to those confronted with unusual or difficult situations, structured information for those sitting examinations and an easy source of reference for established anaesthetists.

RSA
GBR

Preface to the eleventh edition

From the preface to the first edition

This book is not designed to take the place of larger textbooks of anaesthesia and analgesia. It is a summary of current teaching and practice, and it is hoped that it will serve the student, the resident anaesthetist, the practitioner and the candidate studying for the Diploma in Anaesthetics as a ready source of reference and a quick means of revision.

January 1947   JAL

Section 1
BASIC SCIENCES

Chapter 1

Physiology

This chapter outlines some aspects of interest to anaesthetists. The writings of Galen (130–199 AD), physician to the emperor Marcus Aurelius, probably mark the beginning of physiology as a separate subject from philosophy.

THE CELL

The body contains some 75×10^{12} cells, a third of which are red blood cells.

Cellular components

1. *Cell membrane.* This phospholipid bi-layer (about 7.5 nm thick) is semi-permeable, i.e. a barrier to the movement of large molecules and many water-soluble substances such as ions and glucose, but allowing free movement of water and urea. Proteins within the membrane form channels (*see below*) for diffusion or active transport, especially of ions, which maintain a membrane potential. Sugars attached to proteins and lipids on the outside of the cell act as receptors for some hormones, and take part in immune reactions. G-proteins allow information to pass from the receptor across the membrane to the intracellular effector.[1]

2. *Cytoplasm.* The fluid that bathes the organelles and nucleus.

3. *Nucleus.* Controls chemical reactions within the cell and cell reproduction. Its DNA content defines the physical characteristics of the individual.

4. *Nucleolus.* Concentrations of RNA within the nucleus.

5. *Structural proteins.* May be specialized, as in cilia, or the actin and myosin of skeletal muscle.

6. *Mitochondria.* Cytoplasmic organelles containing the enzymes for oxidative metabolism including the electron transport chain. They operate at a Po_2 of 0.13 to 0.4 kPa (1 to 3 mmHg). (Erythrocytes have neither mitochondria nor nuclei, thus do not reproduce and have non-aerobic metabolism.)

7. *Endoplasmic reticulum.* The site of all metabolic functions apart from those in mitochondria. Produces *peroxisomes* which contain oxidases for

detoxification. Substances to be secreted go to the *Golgi apparatus,* which also may form *lysosomes,* an intracellular digestive system to destroy unwanted material such as bacteria. Rough endoplasmic reticulum has RNA-containing *ribosomes* attached.

Cell membrane channels

The Nernst equation relates equilibrium membrane potential (around 70 mV) to ionic concentrations for an ion such as chloride that is not actively transported:

$$V = \frac{RT}{FZ} \times \ln \frac{[Cl^-]_{out}}{[Cl^-]_{in}}$$

where $[Cl^-]_{out}$ and $[Cl^-]_{in}$, the extra- and intra-cellular chloride concentrations are normally 125 and 9.0 mmol/l; R = gas constant; T = absolute temperature; F = Faraday constant; Z = valency.

$$\frac{RT}{F} = 26.5 \text{ at } 37°C$$

Sodium channels (0.3 × 0.5 nm) are voltage sensitive, open briefly in response to membrane depolarization and so propagate it further in excitable cells. Blocked by tetrodotoxin and reversibly blocked by local anaesthetics. Extracellular calcium ions stabilize the channels, and too low a concentration will cause tetany.

Potassium channels (0.3 × 0.3 nm) are also opened by membrane depolarization but more slowly than sodium channels. They are blocked by intracellular tetraethylammonium. The resultant outflow of potassium leads to repolarization and channel closure. Hodgkin and Huxley got Nobel prizes for their work on sodium and potassium channels.

Calcium channels

1. In cardiac muscle, calcium reaches the myofibrils, during depolarization, from the sarcoplasmic reticulum and from the extracellular fluid via the T-tubules. The latter route is more important and maintains the strength and duration of the contraction. The calcium binds to troponin and initiates contraction. Leaks of calcium into the cell during diastole cause slow depolarization.

2. In smooth muscle, the calcium ions entering the cell bind to a related protein, calmodulin.

The calcium channels in both these sites are 'slow' channels, and may be blocked by drugs (*see* Chapter 15).

3. In skeletal muscle, the opening of channels in sarcoplasmic reticulum causes calcium to be released onto troponin and contraction initiated.

4. Calcium channels in presynaptic terminals regulate transmitter release. Both calcium blockers and aminoglycoside antibiotics may potentiate non-depolarizing relaxants.

Chloride channels in the CNS are opened by gamma-aminobutyric acid (and glycine). The resultant chloride flux stabilizes the cell membrane. Facilitated by benzodiazepines. Barbiturates and other anaesthetics may open these channels and explain part of their mechanism of action.

Acetylcholine-sensitive channels (diameter 0.65 nm) are found at the neuromuscular junction. They are large proteins (MW 240 000), make the membrane permeable to all cations, especially sodium. Blocked by non-depolarizing relaxants. Circulating antibodies to these proteins have been demonstrated in patients with myasthenia gravis. (*See* Chapter 10.)

Cell respiration

Aerobic energy production takes place in mitochondria with the oxidation of glucose to water and carbon dioxide. The resultant energy is trapped in the high-energy third phosphate bond of adenosine triphosphate (ATP). There are two phases:

1. Anaerobic: glucose $\rightarrow$ pyruvate + 2 mol of ATP
2. Aerobic: pyruvate + $O_2 \rightarrow CO_2$ + water + 36 mol of ATP

The CO_2 originates from the glucose, whereas the respired O_2 is reduced to water. Thus O_2 consumption and CO_2 production are not necessarily equal. In hypoxia (or in cells such as erythrocytes, which have no mitochondria) pyruvate cannot be metabolized aerobically and is converted to lactic acid. The normal blood lactate/pyruvate ratio of 10 thus rises to 40 or more. Other anaerobic metabolites of pyruvate are also affected, e.g. the 3-hydroxy-butyrate/acetoacetate ratio rises from 2.7 to 10 or 15. (Note: lactic acidosis also occurs in alcohol intoxication, liver disease, and after fructose, sorbitol and xylitol infusion or biguanide administration.)

THE NERVOUS SYSTEM

Neurotransmitters

More than 30 have been proposed. They are either acetylcholine (ACh), amines, amino acids or peptides. In each case:

1. Synthesized in the presynaptic nerve terminal.
2. Released by the calcium influx in response to depolarization.
3. Action terminated by diffusion, a specific enzyme in the synaptic cleft, or re-uptake into the presynaptic terminal.
4. The relevant receptor can be stimulated *in vitro* by the neurotransmitter.
5. The postsynaptic receptor protein either opens an ion channel or activates cell metabolism.

Acetylcholine

Acetylcholine acts in at least four different sites:
1. Released in quanta by the terminal synaptic knobs of the motor axon in response to the calcium influx resulting from motor nerve stimuli. This causes depolarization of the membrane of the skeletal muscle motor end-plate. Blocked by: (a) non-depolarizing relaxants; (b) depolarizing relaxants, which

hold the end-plate membrane depolarized and therefore unable to react to ACh; (c) toxins, e.g. botulinus, aminoglycoside antibiotics; and (d) hypocalcaemia.

2. At parasympathetic nerve endings (muscarinic) causing smooth muscle contraction in the gut, urinary tract and bronchi, miosis, bradycardia and secretion from digestive glands. Blocked by drugs such as atropine, hyoscine and glycopyrrolate.

3. At sympathetic ganglia including the adrenal medulla (nicotinic action) and sympathetic nerve endings to sweat glands. Blocked by ganglion blockers, e.g. trimetaphan, at the ganglia and by atropine and hyoscine at the sweat glands.

4. In the central nervous system, especially motor cortex and basal ganglia. The inhibition by large doses of atropine and hyoscine (central anticholinergic syndrome) may be treated with physostigmine.

Amines

Adrenaline and noradrenaline. Act at sympathetic nerve endings (*see below* for autonomic nervous system), and in the CNS, especially the basal ganglia and hypothalamus.

Dopamine. Acts on receptors in the basal ganglia to influence skeletal muscles, and in the renal and mesenteric arteries causing vasodilatation and sodium excretion. In the hypothalamus it inhibits release of prolactin and other pituitary hormones. In the heart it stimulates β_1-receptors, and in large doses the α_1-receptors as well. Only its laevorotatory form crosses the blood-brain barrier. In the medulla it is involved with vomiting and blood pressure control. The subdivision of dopaminergic receptors is controversial. D_1-receptors stimulate adenyl cyclase, D_2-receptors may inhibit it. Butyrophenones, e.g. droperidol, some phenothiazines, metoclopramide and domperidone are dopaminergic blockers. *See* Chapter 29 for clinical uses.

5-Hydroxytryptamine.[2] An inhibitory transmitter in the brain stem and spinal cord. Three types of receptor have been identified. Hallucinogens stimulate $5-HT_2$ receptors. It may inhibit transmission of pain impulses in the dorsal horn.

Amino acids

Gamma-aminobutyric acid (GABA).[3] An inhibitory transmitter in the CNS. It acts on a chloride channel, the $GABA_A$ receptor to increase conductance and stabilize the membrane. Benzodiazepines facilitate this effect. The $GABA_B$ receptors in the spinal cord and cerebellum increase conductance in a potassium channel. The antispastic drug baclofen acts here and has been used to characterize the receptors.

Glycine. An inhibitory transmitter in the spinal cord. It acts in the same way as GABA, and is antagonized by strychnine and tetanus toxin. A strychnine-like effect may be the basis of the excitatory effects of methohexitone and propofol.[4]

Glutamate and aspartate. The major excitatory transmitters in the brain. Ketamine appears to bind to one of these receptors.

Polypeptides

Endogenous peptide opioid receptor ligands[5] stimulate specific receptors in the substantia gelatinosa, periaqueductal and periventricular areas and brainstem to regulate pain reception and responsiveness to environmental stimuli. They are subdivided into: opiomelanocortins (e.g. β-endorphin), enkephalins and dynorphins.

Opioid receptors are divided into mu (29%), kappa (37%) and delta (34%). Mu receptors are stimulated by morphine and blocked by naloxone, and some workers subdivide them into μ_1-receptors (analgesia) and μ_2-receptors (respiratory depression, pupillary constriction, constipation, addiction). Kappa receptors are stimulated by dynorphins (analgesia), and delta receptors by enkephalins. Other less well characterized receptors (epsilon and sigma) have been described.

Substance P. An 11-amino acid peptide which is a neurotransmitter for the pain pathway in the substantia gelatinosa of the dorsal horn of the spinal cord.

Many other peptides have been found at various sites throughout the CNS and may act as neurotransmitters.

Sleep

Sleep is a recurrent state of unconsciousness associated with a decreased response to external stimuli, from which the patient can readily be aroused. (Patient is from *pati,* Latin, to suffer or bear).

Two opposing states of sleep are described:[6]

1. Non-rapid eye movement (NREM) sleep has four stages where the EEG shows progressive slowing and an increase in amplitude. There are bursts of 10–14 Hz, 50 μV spindles. Heart and respiration rates are slow, motor tone is reduced. It lasts 60–90 min, followed by REM sleep lasting 30–60 min. The cycle is repetitive with great variation between individuals.

2. In REM (paradoxical) sleep there is a rapid low-voltage EEG like that in awake subjects with bursts of large phasic potentials originating in the pons. There is marked muscular relaxation, rises in respiratory and pulse rates and body temperature, increase in cerebral blood flow and tumescence of the penis. Dreams occur during REM sleep, which seems necessary for psychic well-being. Although depressed immediately after surgery, it may be intense from the second day onwards and coincide with periods of labile pulse and blood pressure and obstructive sleep apnoea.[7] It is inhibited by barbiturates, imipramine and monoamine oxidase inhibitors, but not by some benzodiazepines, e.g. flurazepam.

Sleep apnoea syndromes[8]

Central sleep apnoea occurs in patients with disease of the lungs, chest wall or nervous system, and be aggravated by premedication and anaesthesia. The great risk is hypoxia. *Ondine's Curse* is a particular example in which chemical drive to respiration is slight, and the patient depends on a state of wakefulness to stimulate breathing. Obstructive sleep apnoea[9] is common and may result from any cause of respiratory obstruction. It is again aggravated by depressant drugs. Marked oxygen desaturation, hypercapnia and cor pulmonale may occur. The *Pickwickian Syndrome*[10], in an obese male of snoring, daytime sleepiness and restless sleep, is an extreme example.

Action of Anaesthetic Agents on the Nervous System[11]

In clinical concentrations, there is no block of transmission in peripheral nerve fibres. Action is on specialized areas, such as synapses, and perhaps on fine unmyelinated terminals and specialized areas of the cell membrane, such as G-proteins.[1] Anaesthesia does not prevent the encoding of information into the brain's memory.[12]

Over the years various attempts have been made to account for the action of general anaesthetic agents. None of these theories is wholly satisfactory, but some of the most important are:

1. Absorption of anaesthetics by lipids, hence neurones are especially susceptible (H. H. Meyer (1853–1939) of Vienna[13] and C. E. Overton (1865–1933) of Zurich).[14] There is a positive correlation between potency and oil/gas partition coefficient.

2. Anaesthetics cause changes in cell metabolism of a physico-chemical nature, e.g. precipitation of colloids (Claude Bernard (1813–1878) of Paris),[15] changes in surface tension, permeability of cell membranes (e.g. chloride channels), viscosity, conformation of proteins, etc.

3. The inert gas effect. Ferguson[16] (1939) postulated that the narcotic potency of inert gases and vapours were inversely proportional to their vapour pressure. This is roughly true for the common anaesthetic agents, though it does not explain how the brain is affected.

4. The hydrate microcrystal theory of anaesthesia by non-hydrogen bonding agent:[17] the interaction of the molecules of the anaesthetic agent with water molecules in the brain, rather than with lipids. The anaesthetic molecule may act as a centre about which water molecules form crystals or clones. These might hinder the passage of ions through the cell membrane. However, anaesthetic agent potency correlates better with lipid solubility than with hydrate dissociation pressures.[18]

5. The multi-site expansion hypothesis.[19] The expansion of many molecular sites by anaesthetics can be reversed by high ambient pressures ('pressure reversal of anaesthesia').[20] This pressure reversal is seen in intact animals, but not observed in isolated neurones or synapses.

Cerebral blood flow

See Chapter 22, Neurosurgery.

The cerebrospinal fluid[21]

The term 'cerebrospinal fluid' (CSF) was first used in 1825 by the French physiologist F. Magendie (1783–1855).[22]

CSF pressure. Intracranial pressure is 100–150 mmH$_2$O above atmospheric, is closely related to venous rather than arterial pressure and originates from the secretory pressure of the choroid plexuses. The CSF pressure has to be sufficient to overcome the resistance to its absorption by the arachnoid villi. Intracranial pressure varies with the arterial pulse and with the intrathoracic pressure cycle of respiration. Large increases are seen on coughing, abdominal compression, etc. Intrathoracic pressure is transmitted to the intracranial veins via the jugular and vertebral veins. More prolonged elevation of pressure can be caused by faulty positioning on the operating table, such as by kinking the neck veins, though in time compensation occurs due to increased absorption of CSF. The CSF pressure falls with elevation of the head, but not below atmospheric. Obstructing the jugular veins increases intracranial venous pressure and so CSF pressure – Queckenstedt's test (Hans Queckenstedt, 1876–1918, of Rostock).[23] Changes in plasma osmolality affect CSF pressure.

Source. From the choroid plexuses of the third, fourth and lateral ventricles, largely by active secretion at about 0.4 ml/min. Sympathetic nervous system activity reduces CSF production. Some CSF comes from perivascular tissue water and ECF across the lining of the ventricles. About 500 ml can be secreted in 24 h if there is a free leak from the subarachnoid space.

Removal. Into the venous sinuses of the brain via the arachnoid villi, and into the lymph stream via the Pacchionian bodies (described by Antonius Pacchioni in 1705).

Physical characteristics. Clear and colourless with slight opalescence due to globulin. Specific gravity at 37°C 1003–1009 (average 1004.5). Viscosity averages 1.006 mPa.s the same as normal saline. Poor in cells, five or less lymphocytes per μl; more indicates meningeal irritation. CSF comprises about 8% of the intracranial contents. Volume of CSF 140 ml, of which half is cranial and half spinal. Only 15 ml is below T5.

Chemical characteristics. Protein low, 200–400 mg/l. Protein derived partly by filtration of plasma, partly from brain interstitial fluid and brain cells, and partly from cells in the meninges. An elevated protein in non-specific, but electrophoresis may be useful. Glucose 2.5–4.5 mmol/l, or 60–80% of blood level; sodium 135–147 mmol/l; chloride 110–125 mmol/l; urea 1.75–5.0 mmol/l. pH is 7.33, P_{CO_2} 50 mmHg and bicarbonate 25 mmol/l. Antibodies and white cells not found in CSF, hence risk of infection. After spinal analgesia both albumin and globulin increase.

Functions

1. Fluid cushion to protect the brain and spinal cord from trauma. Reduces effective weight of the brain.

2. By its absorption and formation, according to need, it can accommodate changes in volume of the other cranial contents.

3. It is closely related to the extracellular fluid that surrounds neurones, allows the exchange of metabolic products and may take the place of lymph.

Circulation of cerebrospinal fluid

Fluid formed by the choroid plexuses in the lateral ventricles passes through, on each side, the foramen of Monro (Alexander Monro (secundus) of

Edinburgh 1733–1817) to join that formed by choroid plexuses in the third ventricle; thence through aqueduct of Sylvius (1616–1672) to the fourth ventricle. Fluid leaves this for the subarachnoid space through the central foramen of Magendie (Francois Magendie 1783–1855 Parisian physiologist) and the lateral foramina of Luschka (Hubert von Luschka 1820–1875 German anatomist) and reaches the cisterna magna. It bathes the whole of the central nervous system and is absorbed into the venous sinuses through the arachnoidal villi. This circulation plays no part in spinal analgesia. There is evidence that CSF passes along spinal nerves in interaxonal channels within the subperineural space in both centrifugal and centripetal directions and that the entire central nervous system is surrounded by a membrane similar to and continuous with the pia-arachnoid.[24]

Ordinary doses of analgesic drugs injected into the spinal subarachnoid space do not reach the fourth ventricle, which contains in its floor the vasomotor and respiratory centres.

Identification of fluid following a suspected dural tap

1. Temperature. CSF is warm when it falls on to the skin.
2. It forms a cloudy precipitate when it falls into 2.5% thiopentone.[25]
3. The glucose contained in CSF will turn a test strip containing glucose oxidase, blue.[26]

Local analgesic solution, saline and water all give negative results.

The blood-brain barrier

Term coined by Ehrlich (Paul Ehrlich 1854–1915 of Steglitz and Frankfurt) in 1885. The barrier greatly slows uptake of some substances by the brain compared with other organs. There is no single anatomical structure that can be defined as the actual barrier. It develops during the early years of life.

Anaesthetic agents. Inhalation agents, thiobarbiturates, local analgesic drugs, etc. freely cross the barrier. When muscle relaxants are given i.v. they are found in the CSF in extremely low concentration. Physostigmine crosses the blood-brain barrier, neostigmine does not. Atropine and hyoscine cross it more readily than glycopyrronium.

Varieties of nerve fibre

There are three main types of nerve fibre:[27]

A Fibres. All medullated somatic nerve fibres of various diameters (2–20 μm). Rapid conduction. Skeletal motor fibres, touch, proprioceptor and some pain and thermal fibres. A fibres may be subdivided into α (70–120 m/s conduction velocity, 12–20 μm diameter), β (30–70 m/s, 5–12 μm), γ (15–30 m/s, 3–6 μm) and δ (12–30 m/s, 2–5 μm). Larger fibres develop more current at each node to stimulate the next node. The smallest fibres are most easily affected by drugs, and if the concentration of local analgesic is kept low enough, all the small fibres will be blocked without affecting the larger fibres. The largest fibres recover first from local analgesic drugs.[28]

B Fibres. Medullated autonomic fibres, i.e. preganglionic fibres or white rami. Diameter 1–3 μm. Conduction velocity 3–15 m/s.

C Fibres. Non-medullated fibres, both somatic and autonomic. All postganglionic sympathetic motor fibres (grey rami) and some preganglionic. Some afferents convey pain and heat sensation. Diameter less than 1 μm. Conduction velocity 0.5–2 m/s. Visceral afferents are C fibres. Compression blocks A fibres before C fibres, in contrast to the effects of local analgesics.

Pain is carried in C and Aδ fibres. The former conduct at 2 m/s, the latter at up to 30 m/s. The difference in velocity gives rise to the 'dual' appreciation of certain painful stimuli.

Afferent fibres have been classified separately[29] as: Ia and Ib, from muscle spindles and Golgi tendon organs (60–120 m/s); II, all other afferent myelinated fibres with conduction velocity greater than 30 m/s, somatic and autonomic; III, all afferent myelinated fibres with conduction velocity less than 30 m/s, somatic and autonomic; IV, all unmyelinated afferent fibres travelling in dorsal roots.

Anoxia lowers threshold of pain fibres. Stimulation of C fibres may cause a fall in blood pressure. Cold slows the rate of impulse conduction.

The Gate Control Theory of Pain[30]

This theory attempts to correlate physiological and psychological data. A schematic diagram (Fig. 1.1) assists in its understanding.

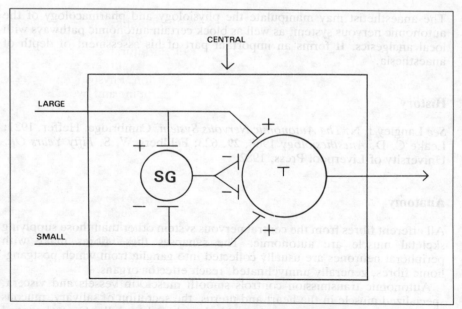

Fig. 1.1 The gate control theory of pain. T, target cells; SG, cells of substantia gelatinosa

It is postulated that both large fibres and small fibres act on target cells, the first central transmission cells and also on cells in the substantia gelatinosa. Some substantia gelatinosa (SG) cells have an inhibiting effect on the target cells (T) and so act as a modulator or 'gate' to the onward transmission of the pain impulses. The large fibres stimulate the SG cells and thus close the gate. Central control from the midbrain is also operative, acting on the inhibitory SG cells. Thus prior conditioning (emotions, memory, etc.), acupuncture or transcutaneous electrical neural stimulation (TENS) of the large fibres can modify the system by opening or closing the 'gate'. The theory, however, does not explain all the known facts.[31]

A careful distinction should be drawn between conscious feeling of pain and motor reaction to a painful stimulus. The integrity of the cerebral cortex is necessary for the full appreciation of pain. Motor reactions to painful stimuli may occur in decorticate animals and in lightly anaesthetized man.

Prostaglandins E_1 and E_2 sensitize the body to histamine, 5-HT, kinins and other pain-producing agents that act peripherally.[32] These can be reduced locally by aspirin, indomethacin and other prostaglandin synthetase inhibitors. Other prostaglandins act centrally to sensitize the body to pain. Paracetamol crosses the blood-brain barrier and reduces this activity. There is synergism between the actions of aspirin and paracetamol. Opiates also reduce appreciation of pain by occupying central enkephalin receptors, in addition to activity at kappa receptors in the dorsal horns of the spinal cord.

AUTONOMIC NERVOUS SYSTEM

The anaesthetist may manipulate the physiology and pharmacology of the autonomic nervous system, as well as block certain autonomic pathways with local analgesics. It forms an important part of his assessment of depth of anaesthesia.

History

See Langley J. N. *The Autonomic Nervous System.* Cambridge: Heffer, 1921; Leake C. D. *Anesthesiology* 1968, **29**, 623; Feldberg W. S. *Fifty Years On.* University of Liverpool Press, 1982.

Anatomy

All efferent fibres from the central nervous system other than those supplying skeletal muscle are autonomic. The synapses these fibres make with peripheral neurones are usually collected into ganglia from which postganglionic fibres, generally unmyelinated, reach effector organs.

Autonomic transmission controls smooth muscle in vessels and viscera, specialized muscle in the heart and uterus, the secretion of salivary, mucous and eccrine sweat glands, together with the adrenal medulla. Central control comes especially from the brain stem, hypothalamus and limbic system, but some degree of vasoconstriction is maintained even in tetraplegia.

Sympathetic outflow

Extends from spinal segments T1 to L2 or L3. In each segment the preganglionic cell bodies lie in the intermediolateral horn of the cord. Their axons leave with the anterior nerve roots, pass across the subarachnoid and extradural spaces, form part of the anterior primary ramus, and then as *white rami communicantes* join the corresponding paravertebral ganglion of the sympathetic chain. Here they may end in a synapse with a postganglionic cell body, or pass uninterrupted through the ganglion to synapse with a postganglionic cell in a collateral ganglion (abdomen) or other paravertebral ganglion (e.g. superior cervical ganglion). The postganglionic axon from the sympathetic chain may enter a sympathetic nerve (e.g. to the heart) or, as *grey rami communicantes* re-enter each spinal nerve for distribution. In the thoracic region each white ramus measures about 1 cm in length; this increases to 2–3 cm in the lumbar region. Each preganglionic axon diverges to 8 or 9 postganglionic neurones.

Sympathetic chain. This is composed of 3 cervical, 11 thoracic, 2–4 lumbar and 4 sacral ganglia. The chain receives white rami from T1 to L2 or 3, whereas from it every one of the spinal nerves receives a grey ramus communicans. The grey rami carry pilomotor and vasomotor fibres, and secretory fibres to sweat glands. They reach their destinations via spinal nerves and blood vessels. Synaptic transmission within sympathetic ganglia is cholinergic.

Craniosacral outflow (parasympathetic)

Preganglionic parasympathetic nerve fibres come from the midbrain, medulla and sacral cord. Their axons, which are medullated, synapse with postganglionic cells very near the organs they innervate. The postganglionic axons are non-medullated. The midbrain (or tectal) fibres come from the Edinger-Westphal nucleus of the 3rd nerve in the floor of the cerebral aqueduct, and end in the ciliary ganglion from which postganglionic fibres proceed as the short ciliary nerves to the sphincter pupillae and ciliary muscles, controlling the size of the pupil and canal of Schlemm. Bulbar outflow leaves in the 7th, 9th and 10th nerves, the 7th and 9th being responsible for secretion of saliva; the 10th nerve courses into the abdomen and innervates thoracic and abdominal visceral muscles and secretions.

The vagus (10th nerve) is not blocked by spinal analgesia. Stimulation of its afferent nerve endings, e.g. in the stomach during gastrectomy, results in discomfort to a conscious patient, helped by infiltration of local analgesic in the paraoesophageal tissues near the cardia.

Sacral fibres leave the cord in the cauda equina with the 2nd, 3rd, sometimes 4th, sacral nerves. After the anterior sacral rami have passed through the anterior sacral foramina the pelvic nerves or nervi erigentes, one on each side, are given off. They do not pass through the sacral sympathetic chain, but run direct to the hypogastric ganglia and thence to the pelvic viscera. Their postganglionic cell bodies are in the walls of the genitalia, bladder and rectum. Visceral afferents also travel with these nerves.

Distribution of vasomotor fibres

Head. Preganglionic sympathetic fibres from T1–3 pass to the stellate and superior cervical ganglia. Postganglionic fibres to (1) the vertebral nerve, a plexus around the vertebral and basilar arteries, (2) the internal carotid, external carotid, and middle meningeal arteries, (3) the cervical plexus, (4) the last four cranial nerves. Parasympathetic vasodilator nerves pass in the 7th nerve into the geniculate ganglion, enter the greater superficial petrosal nerve from which fibres travel with the internal carotid artery and its branches.

Arm. Preganglionic sympathetic fibres from T2–7 (some say T3–7, others T5–9) ascend in the sympathetic trunk to the middle cervical, stellate and 2nd and 3rd thoracic ganglia, pass via the axillary artery and brachial plexus to the arm vessels. There may be a small grey ramus, the nerve of Kuntz (1879–1957),[33] from the 2nd thoracic ganglion direct to the T1 spinal nerve and the lowest trunk of the brachial plexus, so bypassing the stellate ganglion. A similar nerve described by Kirgis and Kuntz connects the 2nd and 3rd thoracic nerves. So to block all vasoconstrictors of the arm there must be block of the 2nd and 3rd thoracic ganglia. If the stellate ganglion alone is blocked, Kuntz's nerve is missed; if brachial plexus alone is blocked, fibres going to the axillary artery escape.

Thorax. From T1–6 synapsing in the upper five thoracic ganglia and the three cervical ganglia. The heart is supplied by three cardiac nerves, postganglionic fibres from the cervical and at least the upper four thoracic ganglia. The lungs from T2–6 or 7 via the stellate and upper thoracic ganglia and the posterior pulmonary plexus, the oesophagus from T4–6. The thoracic and abdominal walls are supplied by the spinal nerves of the corresponding level.

Abdomen. Pass through T5 to L2 ganglia and form the three splanchnic nerves. Do not synapse until the coeliac ganglion (solar plexus), or the superior or inferior mesenteric ganglia, from which postganglionic fibres pass with arteries.

Leg. From T10 to L2 or 3 synapsing in L1–3 ganglia for the upper leg and in L4–5 for and L5 ganglia for the lower. The L3 ganglion is of practical importance as it sends a grey ramus to the L4 nerve and thence to the inner side of the foot via the femoral and saphenous nerves. Blockade of L2 and 3 ganglia stops sympathetic impulses to whole leg. Blockade of L1 ganglion on each side will cause impotence in the male.

Afferent side of the autonomic system

In a way that is analogous to somatic afferents, autonomic afferents carry pain impulses from the viscera and probably from the limbs,[34] with cell bodies in the posterior root ganglia of the spinal nerves. They travel with the corresponding efferent autonomic nerves and enter the cord between T1 and L3, except those from the bladder, rectum, prostate, cervix uteri and lower colon, which pass to the cord via nervi erigentes. For details of the nerve supply of the uterus *see* Chapter 22, Obstetrics.

Functions of autonomic system

The parasympathetic system produces localized effects and is anabolic. The cranial outflow supplies the heart and the gut with its outgrowths; it slows the heart, is motor and secretory to the alimentary canal and constrictor to the pupil. The sacral outflow is a mechanism for emptying, i.e. motor for bladder, rectum, and erection of penis.

The sympathetic outflow produces widespread effects. It causes secretion of catecholamines from the adrenal medulla, activates the body for defence and is catabolic. It constricts skin and splanchnic vessels and dilates muscle and coronary vessels; speeds the heart and increases its contractility; inhibits gut and bladder smooth muscle and constricts its sphincters; relaxes bronchial smooth muscle; dilates the pupil; and causes sweat gland secretion and piloerection.

At α_1-receptors adrenergic neurones cause skin, muscle, heart and splanchnic vasoconstriction, and mydriasis. Blocked by drugs such as prazosin and phenoxybenzamine. α_2-receptors are prejunctional, inhibit the release of noradrenaline, and are blocked by yohimbine. Central α_2-receptors cause a decrease in sympathetic activity, and are stimulated by clonidine. At β_1-receptors, adrenergic neurones cause cardiac stimulation and lipolysis. At β_2-receptors, vaso- and bronchodilatation, and glycogenolysis. Atenolol and metoprolol are β_1-blockers, propranolol is a mixed β_1- and β_2-blocker.

Autonomic function can be assessed by bedside tests of vagal (sinus arrhythmia, bradycardia on lying down or after Valsalva[35] manoeuvre) or sympathetic (blood pressure response to handgrip or standing) activity.[36]

Vaso-vagal syncope. A term used by Sir Thomas Lewis in 1932,[37] may occur in response to strong emotions, even fear of needles. Vagal outflow slows the heart and causes splanchnic vasodilatation. Skin vessels remain constricted, but blood pressure and heart rate fall greatly.

See also Tusiewicz K. In: *Anaesthesia Review 5*. (Kaufman L. ed.) Edinburgh: Churchill Livingstone, 1988, 54; Pincus D. and Magitsky L. *Int. Anesthesiol. Clin.* 1989, **27**, 219.

THE CARDIOVASCULAR SYSTEM

The electroccardiogram

History[38]

Augustus Desiré Waller (1856–1922), head of Physiology at St Mary's Hospital, London, first recorded in 1887 the electric current that precedes muscular contraction of the heart.[39] He was one of the first two physicians appointed to the National Heart Hospital, London. Development of the string galvanometer in 1901 by W. Einthoven (1860–1927), Professor of Physiology at Leiden where a demonstration of his work may be seen at the Boerhaave Museum,[40] led to clinical and experimental studies of the ECG. Sir Thomas Lewis (1881–1945) of University College Hospital, London published his pioneering book in 1911, *The Mechanism and Graphic Reproduction of the Heart Beat.* The cathode-ray oscilloscope was first used in ECG by Dock in 1929.[41] Auricular flutter was first described in 1910 by Wm Adam Jolly (1877–1939) and Wm Ritchie (1873–1945), both of London,[42] auricular fibrillation by Sir James Mackenzie (1853–1925) of Burnley and London in 1908,[43] pulsus alternans by Ludwig Traube (1818–1876) of Berlin in 1872[44] and gallop rhythm by Pierre C. E. Potain (1825–1901) of Paris three years later. Other pioneers of ECG were H. B. Williams in the USA and Karl Frederik Wenkebach (1864–1970) in Vienna.

Pioneers of the use of ECG in anaesthesia have included J. B. Heard and A. E. Strauss,[45] E. B. Krumbhaar,[46] and Michael Johnstone.[47] W. N. Rollason's book on the ECG was probably the first written by an anaesthetist.[48]

Standard leads

Bipolar leads. Record the potential differences produced by the heart beat between two limbs: I between the arms (left arm positive); II between right arm and left leg (positive); III between left arm and left leg (positive).

Unipolar leads. Record the potential difference between an exploring electrode and an indifferent electrode. There are three unipolar limb leads, described by Goldberg:[49] aVL from the left arm; aVR from the right arm; and aVF from the left leg. The letter 'a' refers to the augmentation (by about 50%) of the voltage that is obtained by using the other two limbs together as the indifferent electrode. Six unipolar chest leads complete the conventional ECG with the recording electrode placed thus: V_1 4th right interspace at sternal margin; V_2 4th left interspace at sternal margin; V_3 midway between V_2 and V_4; V_4 5th left interspace in midclavicular line; V_5 left anterior axillary line in horizontal line from V_4; V_6 left mid-axillary line in same horizontal line. The indifferent electrode is the three limb leads joined together.

The sensitivity is 1 mV/cm and the calibration also checks the square-wave response. The pen travels 1 cm in 0.4 s.

The normal waves and intervals obtained:

P wave: depolarization of the atria. Lasts less than 0.12 s. *P-R interval:* delay at the AV node. From beginning of P wave to beginning of QRS complex is not greater than 0.2 s. *QRS complex:* onset of ventricular depolarization. Not greater than 0.10 s. *S-T segment:* continued ventricular depolarization. *T wave:* ventricular repolarization. *Q-T interval:* from the beginning of the QRS complex to the end of the T wave. Normally about 0.4 s, but varies with heart rate. *U wave:* usually of low amplitude. May represent slow repolarization of the papillary muscles.

Chest leads

Introduced in 1932.[50] Popular in coronary and intensive care units because they can be used with little disturbance to the patient. Used mainly as monitors for abnormal rhythm and ST/T changes rather than for accurate diagnosis. Many different configurations have been described. CM5 is widely used (cardiac monitoring V_5), with the exploring positive left arm electrode in the V_5 position, negative right arm electrode over the manubrium and left leg lead to ground.

The cardiac output (*see also* Chapter 18)

Determined by:

1. Venous return (ventricular preload)

Venous filling of the heart during diastole depends on: (a) circulating blood volume; (b) venous tone, influenced by autonomic nerves, catecholamines, vasoactive drugs and anaesthetics; (c) inspiration, which results in a negative pressure in the thorax and diaphragmatic descent, which encourages the movement of blood from the abdomen towards the heart; (d) muscular activity (muscle pump); and (e) posture and gravity. The effect of venous return on cardiac output is summed up by Starling's (1866–1927) law of the heart.[51] 'The more the myocardial fibres are stretched during diastole, the more forcibly they will contract during subsequent systole, and therefore more blood will be expelled.'

End-diastolic volume of the ventricles is measured by e.g. echo-cardiography; central venous or right atrial pressure by manometry (Chapter 18), normally 5 mmHg (7 cmH$_2$O). It is usually the same as right ventricular end-diastolic pressure, and related to its volume, although this relationship is influenced by the compliance or stiffness of the ventricle. Similar considerations apply to the measurement of pulmonary capillary wedge pressure, an indirect measure of left atrial pressure, normally 10 mmHg. It may help to distinguish between blood loss or excessive venodilatation (low value) and heart failure (high value).

2. Myocardial contractility

Defined by the relationship between stroke volume or work (pressure × volume) and end-diastolic volume, i.e. the slope and position of the Starling curve. More than 80% of the O_2 consumption of the left ventricle is during isometric contraction, generating pressure, only a small fraction during the ejection of about 70 ml blood during systole, generating flow. Contractility is affected by: (a) sympathetic activity, which increases contractility, the inotropic effect; (b) positive inotrope drugs, e.g. digitalis, dobutamine; (c) negative inotrope drugs, e.g. lignocaine, thiopentone, halothane; (d) increased heart rate *per se* will increase contractility (Bowditch effect); and (e) abnormalities of myocardial metabolism caused by e.g. ischaemia, hypoxia, hypercapnia, acidaemia, cardiomyopathy.

ASSESSMENT OF MYOCARDIAL CONTRACTILITY

(a) Clinical: Blood pressure. Adequacy of organ perfusion especially skin, brain and kidneys. Raised venous pressure and peripheral oedema. Abnormal heart sounds. Pulmonary oedema.

(b) Non-invasive measurements: (1) Pre-ejection period (PEP). The total active electromechanical time (TAEMT) is from the Q wave of the ECG to the closure of the aortic valve (first component of the second heart sound). If the actual ejection time (measured with a force transducer over the carotid artery) is subtracted from this, the difference is the pre-ejection period, which correlates well with other measures of inotropy; (2) Echocardiography. Cavity sizes and wall motion, blood flow with Doppler techniques, circumferential velocity of shortening. The trans-oesophageal route is increasingly used;[52] and (3) Nuclear cardiology. Intravascular tracers such as technetium will assess myocardial function, and thallium will image coronary blood flow.

(c) Cardiac output measurement (*see* Chapter 18).

(d) Measurements made during cardiac catheterization: (1) ejection fraction (normally 60–75%).[53] The percentage of left ventricular diastolic volume that is ejected in systole and (2) left ventricular pressure measurements. Maximum rate of change of pressure (peak dP/dt), and the time taken to reach this value from the start of contraction. The shorter this time, the higher the contractility.

3. Cardiac rate

Slowed by the vagus, speeded by sympathetic action. May be less than 40 per minute in 25% of normal healthy students while asleep. Also slowed by raised blood pressure (baroreceptor reflex from the carotid sinus and aortic arch), raised intracranial pressure, hypothermia, myxoedema and nasopharyngeal stimulation or pressure on the eyeball. Bradycardia can be reversed by increasing the frequency and amplitude of IPPV or of voluntary respiration,[54] or by atropine. The Bainbridge reflex (1915) is a tachycardia in response to atrial stretch if the initial heart rate is slow, and is of little significance. If nicotine is injected into a coronary artery bradycardia and hypotension result (Bezold-Jarisch reflex). The normal heart slows on inspiration (sinus arrhythmia). This is a reflex from the lung stretch receptors to the medulla and vagus nerve. The heart rate assumes greater importance if stroke volume is limited, e.g. by aortic stenosis, and in infants.

4. Arterial blood pressure and peripheral vascular resistance

Ventricular afterload. The ventricular wall tension developed during systolic ejection. It is frequently and usefully equated with peripheral arterial resistance. When suddenly increased, the heart pumps less blood until either venous return and preload or myocardial contractility increase. If the ventricle is dilated the pressure within falls for a given wall tension, according to Laplace's law: pressure is proportional to the ratio of tension to radius.

Pulse pressure is the difference between systolic and diastolic blood pressures, normally 40 mmHg. Mean arterial pressure can be calculated as diastolic plus one third of the pulse pressure. It is displayed on automatic oscillotonometers and equals the cardiac output × peripheral resistance. The rate-pressure product is the product of systolic arterial pressure and pulse rate and gives a rough indication of cardiac work load and myocardial oxygen requirements. The limit above which myocardial ischaemia may occur in some patients is 12000. It correlates (poorly) with myocardial oxygen consumption during anaesthesia in many patients with coronary disease.[55]

For a discussion of a reduction of peripheral resistance by haemodilution *see* Messmer K. *et al. Eur. Surg. Res.* 1986, **18**, 254.

Blood volume

Normal adult blood volume is 75 ml/kg, but 10% less in the short obese subject and in the elderly.[56] About half the total blood volume is contained by the systemic venous system, and a fifth in the pulmonary vessels.

Coronary circulation

Normal coronary blood flow at rest is about 250 ml/min or 5% of the cardiac output; myocardial oxygen consumption is 40 ml/min or 15% of total body oxygen consumption. Blood flow and oxygen consumption are tightly correlated. The 'dominant' coronary artery is that which gives rise to the posterior interventricular branch (normally the right). There are extensive collaterals at all levels of the circulation. Blood flow through the coronary arteries varies throughout the cardiac cycle, about two-thirds occurring in diastole. The driving pressure can be taken as aortic pressure less ventricular diastolic pressure. The coronary sinus drains 90% of the blood from the left ventricle. Blood from the veins of Adam Christian Thebesius (1686–1732), German physician, drain directly into the ventricles or atria.

Coronary flow increases with oxygen consumption, as in exercise. Vagal stimulation has no direct effect on the coronary vessels. Sympathetic β stimulation causes vasodilatation, both directly and due to increased cardiac work, although α stimulation may have a slight vasoconstrictor effect. Angiotensin and vasopressin have a vasoconstrictor action. Dilators include adenosine, prostacyclin, nitroprusside and isoflurane. Although these drugs increase coronary flow more than oxygen consumption and so increase the coronary venous Po_2, they may theoretically 'steal' blood away from an area dependent on a collateral supply, and cause regional ischaemia in some patients.[57] The importance of this is most doubtful.

For the pharmacology of the coronary circulation *see* Sill J. C. *Can. J. Anaesth.* 1987, **34**, S2.

Cerebral circulation

See Chapter 22, Neurosurgery.

Capillary exchange

Capillaries are 5 μm in diameter at their arterial end where the pressure is 30 mmHg, and about 9 μm at the venous end where the pressure is 15 mmHg. Blood takes 1–2 s to pass through. Their walls are around 1 μm thick, and the structure varies widely in different organs. Exchange of fluid and bigger molecules occurs through the endothelial cell junctions, which typically allow the passage of molecules up to 10 nm in diameter, through 20–100 nm fenestrations in the cell body, or by vesicular transport. Fluid filtration depends on the balance between the pressure gradient across the capillary wall, which tends to drive fluid out, and the osmotic pressure gradient between the protein-rich plasma and the protein-poor interstitium which tends to drive fluid back in. For the whole body, up to 24 l/day of fluid leaks out at the arterial end, but most is reabsorbed at the venous end, with the remainder going into the lymphatics. Lymphatics have valves in the lumen and smooth muscle in the walls which pump fluid and protein out of the interstitium and maintain the pressure there slightly negative (about −6 mmHg). Lymph flow increases 10- to 50-fold before interstitial oedema occurs.

THE RESPIRATORY SYSTEM

The major function of the lungs is to exchange gases between blood and the atmosphere. The anaesthetist exploits this to administer anaesthetic agents, commonly controls respiration and corrects some of the disturbances in lung function that are caused by anaesthesia.

See also Symposium on the Lung. *Br. J. Anaesth.* 1990, **65**.

Anatomy

Larynx

The organ of voice, the sphincter between the pharynx and trachea. It extends from the root of the tongue to the trachea (Fig. 1.2) and lies opposite

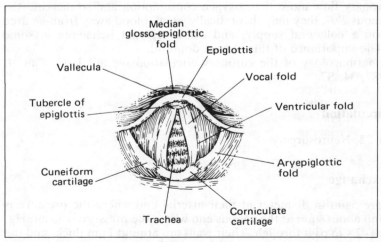

Fig. 1.2 A laryngoscopic view of the interior of the larynx. (From 'Gray's Anatomy', by kind permission of Professor T. B. Johnston)

C3–6 vertebrae; higher in children and females. The average length is 44 mm in males, 36 mm in females; transverse diameter 43 mm in males, 41 mm in females; anteroposterior diameter 36 mm in males and 26 mm in females. It is covered by the depressor muscles of the hyoid bone by the thyroid gland and by the cricothyroid muscles. Composed of the following cartilages, joined together by ligaments; thyroid, cricoid, two arytenoid, two corniculate (Santorini), two cuneiform (Wrisberg) and the epiglottis.

The cavity of the larynx extends from the superior laryngeal aperture to the lower border of the cricoid cartilage. The *piriform fossa* is a recess, on each side, bounded by the aryepiglottic fold medially and the thyroid cartilage and thyrohyoid membrane laterally. Beneath its mucosa lie twigs of the internal laryngeal nerve, which may be blocked by topical local analgesics. The depression between the dorsum of the tongue and the epiglottis is divided into two valleculae by the glosso-epiglottic fold. The epiglottis is not essential for swallowing, breathing, or phonation.

The superior laryngeal aperture is wider in front than behind, and slopes downwards and backwards. Bounded anteriorly by the epiglottis; laterally by the aryepiglottic folds containing the two small nodules on each side, cuneiform anteriorly and the corniculate posteriorly; and posteriorly by the arytenoids. This view is seen at laryngoscopy. The vestibule of the larynx is the superior part of the cavity of the larynx and extends from the aryepiglottic folds to the vestibular (ventricular) folds. Each of the latter is a ridge formed by the vestibular ligament and extends from the angle of the thyroid cartilage anteriorly, backwards along the side cavity of the larynx to the cuneiform cartilage. The vestibular folds are the false cords, the space between them is the rima vestibuli, whereas a depression on the side-wall of the larynx between the vestibular fold and the vocal fold (false and true cords) is the saccule of the larynx.

The vocal cords (folds) stretch from the thyroid cartilage anteriorly to the arytenoid cartilage of the corresponding side posteriorly. The space between the cords is the glottis. It is bounded in front by the intermembranous part of the cords (the vocal folds); behind, by the intercartilaginous part. The glottis is the narrowest part of the larynx in adults and measures about 2.3 cm from front to back in males, 1.7 cm in females. In children, the narrowest part is found just below the cords at the cricoid ring. The shape and width of the glottis vary with phonation and respiration and the tone of the muscles controlling it. When these are in spasm, the glottis is obliterated.

The mucosa of the upper part of the larynx is lined by squamous cells like the oropharynx; the part above the cords by ciliated epithelium; and the cords are covered by a thin layer of mucosa, closely adherent to them, and white in colour. The lower larynx is lined by ciliated epithelium with mucous glands and goblet cells.

MUSCLES

The extrinsic muscles are the thyrohyoid and the sternothyroid and the inferior constrictor of the pharynx. The first elevates, the second depresses the larynx while the third constricts the pharynx.

The intrinsic muscles: those that open and close the glottis: (1) The posterior (open) and lateral crico-arytenoids (close) and (2) the interarytenoid.

During inspiration, cords abduct. On expiration they return nearly to the midline. On phonation they actually touch.[58]

Those controlling the tension of the cords: (1) the cricothyroids are tensors of the cords; (2) the posterior crico-arytenoids; (3) the thyroarytenoids are relaxers of the cords; and (4) the vocales.

Those controlling the inlet of the larynx: (1) the aryepiglottics; and (2) the thyroepiglottics. In laryngeal spasm both the true and the false cords are adducted.

NERVE SUPPLY (FROM THE VAGUS)

All sensory nerve impulses from the larynx reach the nucleus solitarius in the medulla.

The *superior laryngeal branch* of the vagus arises near the base of the skull and divides into the *internal laryngeal nerve*, the sensory supply to both surfaces of the epiglottis and to the larynx down to the vocal cords, and the motor *external laryngeal nerve*, which supplies the cricothyroid muscle and the inferior constrictor of the pharynx, the division taking place slightly below and anterior to the greater cornu of the hyoid bone. The external laryngeal nerve may be injured during ligation of the superior thyroid vessels at thyroidectomy, causing temporary huskiness of voice. The *recurrent laryngeal branch* supplies the remaining intrinsic muscles and is sensory to the mucosa below the cords.

The recurrent laryngeal nerve carries abductor and adductor fibres, but if it is injured abductor paralysis is greater than adductor paralysis. With bilateral injury there is respiratory difficulty because the cords lie together and speech is difficult with a valve-like obstruction and inspiratory stridor. Complete paralysis of both recurrent nerves inactivates both abductor and adductor muscles. The tensing action of the cricothyroid muscles still maintains cords in adduction. Paralysis of one cord may be symptomless but paralysis of both is serious and may require surgery.

Paralysis of both recurrent and superior laryngeal nerves together produces the cadaveric position. In this, also seen when relaxants have had a full effect, the cords lie midway between abduction and adduction; they are not under tension because of cricothyroid paralysis.

Topical analgesia of the larynx may, by paralysing twigs from the external laryngeal nerves going to the cricothyroids, cause both a temporary alteration in the appearance of the cords and in the voice.

ARTERIAL SUPPLY

Laryngeal branches of the superior and inferior thyroid arteries which accompany the nerves.

See also Bartlett D. *Respiratory Functions of the Larynx. Physiol. Rev.* 1989, **69**, 33.

Trachea

Length about 10–11 cm, from the level of C6 to the carina and its division into the two main bronchi at T5. Anteriorly, this corresponds with the junction of the body and manubrium sterni, the angle of Louis. In children, carina is on a level with 3rd costal cartilage. The diameter of the trachea is about 1.2 cm, much smaller in the child, e.g. 3 mm in the neonate, or for an older child the diameter in millimetres corresponds to the age in years. Abnormal narrowing of the trachea in its middle third, making it difficult to introduce a tube of adequate size, has been reported.[59]

Tracheostomy should be performed below the first tracheal ring to avoid stenosis.

Blood supply. Upper two-thirds are supplied by the inferior thyroid artery and the lower one-third by the bronchial arteries. The arteries run circumferentially with few anastomoses in the long axis of the trachea.

Bronchial tree

RIGHT MAIN BRONCHUS

Shorter, wider and more in line with the trachea than the left main bronchus, hence a long tube or foreign body passes more easily into it. The right bronchus leaves the trachea at an angle of 25° from the vertical. It enters the right lung opposite T5. The upper lobe bronchus emerges just 2.5 cm from the carina.

Right upper lobe. Apical, posterior and anterior segments.
Right middle lobe. Lateral and medial segments.
Right lower lobe. Apical, medial basal (cardiac), anterior basal, lateral basal and posterior basal segments.

LEFT MAIN BRONCHUS

Narrower and longer than the right. Length before origin of upper lobe bronchus is 5 cm. It leaves the trachea at an angle of about 45° from the vertical and enters the lung opposite T6. The aorta arches over the left main bronchus.

Left upper lobe. Upper division bronchus: apical, posterior and anterior segments. Lingula (lower division) bronchus: superior and inferior segments.
Left lower lobe. Apical, anterior basal, lateral basal and posterior basal segments.

SMALLER BRONCHI

Subdivide progressively until the terminal bronchioles (the 16th generation) are reached. Beyond these are the primary lobules composed of respiratory bronchioles, alveolar ducts and alveolar sacs. Surface area of all the 300 million alveoli is 70 m^2, the size of a tennis court. The alveolar epithelial cells are mainly type I, but type II cells at the septal junctions secrete surfactant and act as precursors of the type I cells. The total thickness of the alveolar–capillary membrane is only 0.35 µm.

Cartilage is absent in bronchi less than 1 mm in diameter. Elastic tissue is distributed throughout the lung parenchyma and is responsible for passive expiration. Muscular fibres surround the airways down to the openings of the alveolar ducts.

Bronchial arteries from the thoracic aorta (one for the right two for the left lung) supply as far as the end of the terminal bronchioles. Distal to this, blood supply is from the pulmonary artery. There is some communication between the bronchial arteries and the pulmonary veins, but the bronchial veins drain into the systemic circulation.

Nerve supply. Each vagus passes to the back of the hilum and is joined by branches of the sympathetic, from T2 to 4 or 5 and also from the inferior and middle cervical ganglia, forming the anterior and posterior pulmonary plexuses. From there, fibres go to the main bronchi and the pulmonary artery, and their branches. Vagal activity causes bronchoconstriction and sympathetic activity bronchodilatation. The vagus also has afferent fibres.

Mucosa is ciliated epithelium. Each cell has some 200 cilia that have a wave-like motion resembling a cornfield in a breeze, beating upwards towards the mouth. The respiratory bronchioles are devoid of cilia, but above this level they are plentiful. Cilia are immersed in a layer of periciliary fluid, and their tips reach the mucus layer. They are not under nervous control. Mucociliary transport depends partly on the volume and pH of mucus.[60] It is depressed by general anaesthesia.

Lungs

Each lung is invaginated from the hilum into the closed sac of the pleura. If the thorax is laid open on both sides, a pressure of 7 mmHg in the trachea is necessary to keep the lungs from collapsing.

Handling of bioactive materials by the lungs

The whole cardiac output passes through the lung capillaries, and the vesicles in their endothelial cells have important metabolic functions. There is substantial pulmonary clearance of catecholamines and fentanyl, and production of prostaglandins, leukotrienes and thromboxanes.[61] The endothelium is the site of angiotensin converting enzyme, which also degrades bradykinin. Other non-respiratory functions include filtration of emboli and phagocytosis by macrophages.

Surfactant[62]

The alveoli are lined with a monomolecular layer of the phospholipid phosphatidyl choline, which is the major constituent of surfactant. 11% of surfactant is protein. Surfactant reduces surface tension, helps to stabilize the alveoli open and may help keep alveoli dry.[63] It is greatly reduced in the lungs of premature babies and contributes to the pathology of adult respiratory distress syndrome. It has been given as an aerosol to both groups of patients with some success.[64]

Physiology of respiration[65]

Respiration is the gaseous interchange between an organism and its environment. Oxygen is absorbed and carbon dioxide excreted. External respiration takes place in the lungs, internal respiration in the tissue cells.

Symbols used in respiratory physiology[66]

Primary symbols of physical quantities (large capitals): V = gas volume; P = gas pressure; F = fractional concentration of dry gas; D = diffusing capacity; R = respiratory exchange ratio; C = gas content in blood; Q = blood volume; S = saturation of haemoglobin with O_2. A dot above any symbol indicates a time derivative.

Secondary symbols for location of quantity. Gas phase (small capitals): I = inspired gas; E = expired gas; A = alveolar gas; T = tidal; D = dead space; B = barometric.

STPD = 0°C, 760 mmHg, dry; BTPS = body temperature and pressure, saturated with water vapour; ATPS = ambient temperature and pressure, saturated with water vapour.

Blood phase (small letters): a = arterial blood; v = venous blood; c = capillary blood; t = total; s = shunt. A dash above any symbol indicates a mean value; a prime (′) indicates end e.g. E′ = end-expiratory gas; c′ = end-capillary blood.

Abbreviations for lung volumes. VC = vital capacity; IC = inspiratory capacity; IRV = inspiratory reserve volume; ERV = expiratory reserve volume; FRC = functional residual capacity; RV = residual volume; TLC = total lung capacity; CV = closing volume. (Note that a capacity is always the sum of one or more volumes.)

f = respiratory frequency (breaths per unit time).

Examples of use of symbols: Pa_{O_2} = alveolar O_2 tension; D_{O_2} diffusing capacity for oxygen; $\dot{Q}c$ = blood flow through pulmonary capillaries; $\dot{V}_{O_2}$ = rate of O_2 consumption; FI_{O_2} fractional inspired oxygen concentration; P_B = barometric pressure; Ca_{O_2} arterial oxygen content.

Ventilation

The lung behaves as if it were suspended from the top of the thoracic cage. The alveoli near the top are more nearly at full stretch and so can receive less ventilation. There is a vertical gradient of ventilation, which increases further down the lung. This is also seen in the lateral position, where the lower lung receives more ventilation. During IPPV however, the situation is reversed because the paralysed diaphragm allows the abdominal contents to compress the lower lung.

Gas exchange in the lungs

Oxygen uptake at rest is normally 250 ml/min, and CO_2 production 200 ml/min. Values during anaesthesia are 10–15% lower. CO_2 diffuses from pulmonary arterial blood to alveolar gas, where the Pa_{CO_2} is determined by its rate of transfer and its dilution by alveolar ventilation. So if the inspired gas contains no CO_2 then Pa_{CO_2} is proportional to $\dot{V}_{CO_2}/\dot{V}_A$. It is independent of blood flow in the steady state. Therefore doubling alveolar ventilation will halve the alveolar P_{CO_2}. The half-time of this exponential process is that of washing out the body stores of CO_2, about 4 min. Halving ventilation will double P_{CO_2}, although the equilibrium in this case will be slower (up to 15 min) because of the limited metabolic production of CO_2. In apnoea, $Paco_2$ rises at 0.4–0.8 kPa/min (3–6 mmHg/min). Note that if ventilation is increased voluntarily, there will come a time (perhaps at about 60 l/min) when increased metabolism of the respiratory muscles offsets the extra CO_2 excretion.

Oxygen diffuses in the opposite direction, and the drop in partial pressure between inspired and alveolar gas is again proportional to $\dot{V}o_2/\dot{V}A$. After correcting for the fact that $\dot{V}o_2$ and $\dot{V}co_2$ are usually unequal (i.e. R is slightly less than 1.0), and thus expired volume is less than inspired volume, this relationship can be expressed as the alveolar air equation:

$$\text{Alveolar } Po_2 = Pio_2 - \frac{Paco_2}{R}[1 - Fio_2(1 - R)]$$

The term in square brackets can usually be taken as equal to 1.

There is little difference between alveolar and arterial Pco_2, but there may be a big difference for O_2, and the importance of this equation is that it allows the calculation of the A-a Po_2 gradient from arterial blood gas measurement. This answers the common clinical question: is the patient's arterial Po_2 appropriate for his Pco_2 and Fio_2?

Alveolar Po_2

The most important factors influencing this are those in the above equation: (a) *barometric pressure* P_B and *inspired oxygen concentration*, which together determine Pio_2. Saturated water-vapour pressure at body temperature (47 mmHg) must be subtracted from this Pio_2 for entry into the alveolar air equation. Thus with increasing altitude moist Pio_2 would become zero at 19.2 km (63 000 ft), where P_B is 47 mmHg and blood boils. Barometric pressure halves every 5.5 km (18 000 ft), and is 230 mmHg on the summit of Mount Everest: (b) *Arterial* Pco_2 and *respiratory quotient*. If R is 1, then the alveolar Po_2 drops by 1 mmHg for the same rise in $Paco_2$. Note that *alveolar ventilation* determines $Paco_2$, as described above, and so the relationship between Pao_2 and alveolar ventilation is also hyperbolic. As ventilation increases Pao_2 rises towards (but never reaches) Pio_2. At low levels of alveolar ventilation, small variation may produce large changes in Pao_2. *Metabolic rate* also determines $Paco_2$, which may be important in, for example, a shivering patient whose oxygen consumption may double. When not in a steady state (i.e. when the non-metabolic gases such as nitrogen or nitrous oxide are not in equilibrium), Pao_2 will also be influenced by: (c) *Cardiac output*. A drop in cardiac output causes Pao_2 to rise because less oxygen is absorbed. Mixed venous Po_2, however, falls to compensate: (d) *The second gas and Fink effect*. Increases Pao_2 during induction with nitrous oxide and decreases it in the earliest stages of recovery.

Alveolar − arterial (A − a) Po_2 difference

Normally about 10 mmHg, but may be over 30 mmHg in the elderly. There are 3 classic causes of a large A − a gradient.

(a) *Anatomical shunt*. The 'shunt equation' for calculating pulmonary shunt from oxygen content of blood and alveoli is:

$$\frac{\dot{Q}s}{\dot{Q}t} = \frac{Cc'o_2 - Cao_2}{Cc'o_2 - C\overline{v}o_2}$$

where $Cc'o_2$ is the O_2 content of end-capillary blood, where the Po_2 is taken to be the same as in alveolar gas. The bigger the shunt, the less effective is oxygen therapy at restoring the arterial Po_2 (Table 1.1).

Table 1.1

Per cent shunt	Per cent inspired O_2 needed to restore normal Pao_2
10	30
20	57
30	97
40	Not possible to restore to normal
50	Changes in inspired concentration have almost no effect on Pao_2

(b) *Diffusion barrier*. This is unusual, although equilibrium for O_2 across the alveolar-capillary membrane may not be reached if the membrane is thickened by disease, if the Pio_2 is low (e.g. high altitude), or if pulmonary capillary transit time is very much shorter than its normal value of 0.75 s (e.g. heavy exercise). Raising the inspired oxygen compensates for this. Diffusion is not a problem for CO_2 as it is 20 times as diffusible in aqueous media.

(c) *Ventilation-perfusion inequalities*. The blood flowing through high $\dot{V}/\dot{Q}$ areas with the higher Po_2 cannot compensate for that from low $\dot{V}/\dot{Q}$ areas because firstly, the shape of the haemoglobin dissociation curve means that the fall in saturation in low $\dot{V}/\dot{Q}$ areas is greater than the rise in high $\dot{V}/\dot{Q}$ areas and secondly, a greater proportion of pulmonary blood flow will pass through areas of low $\dot{V}/\dot{Q}$ ratio. Note that this is less of a problem for CO_2 because of its more linear dissociation curve, and an increase in ventilation will readily lower Pco_2. *Venous admixture* (sometimes confusingly called physiological shunt) is the proportion of mixed venous blood that would need to be mixed with end-capillary blood to produce the observed drop in Po_2, and includes effects due to (a), (b) and (c). There is a small venous admixture of 5% in normal subjects due to Thebesian veins, bronchial-to-pulmonary venous shunting and to normal $\dot{V}/\dot{Q}$ inequality. Values over 30% may be seen in congenital cardiac disease, gross obesity and a wide range of lung diseases.

Other factors influencing the magnitude of the A — a difference include: (d) actual value of Pao_2, as this determines position on the oxygen dissociation curve; (e) acid-base status, which can shift the curve; (f) cardiac output, by its effect on $P\overline{v}o_2$; (g) haemoglobin concentration: anaemia increases the A — a gradient; (h) alveolar ventilation: increased ventilation will increase the alveolar Po_2 and the A — a gradient.

Anaesthesia causes the appearance of atelectasis in the dependent part of the lung which increases shunt and areas of low $\dot{V}/\dot{Q}$ ratio. This widens the A – a Po_2 gradient. Inhibition of hypoxic pulmonary vasoconstriction by anaesthetic agents may make a minor contribution to this gradient.[67]

Oxygen carriage in blood

The oxygen dissociation curve of haemoglobin (Barcroft, 1872–1947, and Poulton, 1883–1939),[68] at 37°C, Pco_2 40 mmHg and pH 7.4, shows how the saturation of haemoglobin changes with Po_2 (Fig. 1.3). It shows that at a

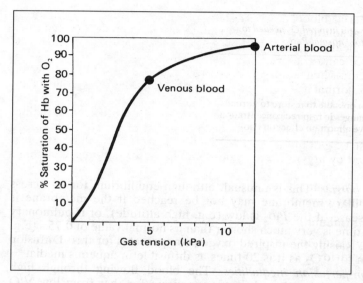

Fig. 1.3 The oxygen dissociation curve of haemoglobin

normal arterial value of 12–13.3 kPa (90–100 mmHg) haemoglobin is 97% saturated, at 8 kPa (60 mmHg) saturation is still 90%. Mixed venous blood has a Po_2 of 5.3 kPa (40 mmHg) and a saturation of 75%. The Pao_2 falls with increasing age.

Note that up to 1.6% carboxyhaemoglobin and 0.4% methaemoglobin is normal in non-smokers.

P_{50}

The oxygen tension needed for 50% saturation of haemoglobin, normally 3.5 kPa (26 mmHg), and is a way of describing any shift of the dissociation curve to the left or right. Such shifts occur with: (a) acidaemia (to the right) and alkalaemia (to the left), the Bohr effect (Christian Bohr 1855–1911, Copenhagen physiologist);[69] (b) Pco_2 (higher value shifts it to the right); (c) temperature (higher value shifts it to the right); (d) concentration of 2,3-diphosphoglycerate (2,3-DPG) in red cells (a decrease shifts it to the left, an increase to the right). 2,3-DPG concentration is increased by anaemia and chronic hypoxaemia, and decreased in stored blood (the 'Valtis-Kennedy' effect)[70] although restored within a few hours of transfusion. 2,3-DPG described in 1925.[71] It is formed in a shunt off the glycolytic pathway; (e) left-shift in CO poisoning; (f) left-shift with most abnormal haemoglobins; (g) right-shift in pregnancy;[72] (h) left-shift with hypophosphataemia; (i) Left-shift with ionic and non-ionic contrast media.[73]

Anaesthetics do not affect the P_{50}.

1 g of haemoglobin carries 1.34 ml of oxygen when fully saturated.[74] The theoretical value of 1.39 according to the iron content is seldom achieved.[75] In addition 0.0225 ml/dl/kPa (0.003 ml/dl/mmHg) oxygen is carried in physical solution.

So normal arterial blood has a oxygen content of 20 ml/dl (0.3 ml being carried in physical solution) and mixed venous blood 15 ml/dl. Oxygen must be breathed at nearly 3 atmospheres pressure before the arteriovenous content difference can be supplied by that in physical solution.

Cyanosis. Occurs when capillary blood has a reduced Hb level over 5 g/dl. If the Hb level is normal it is detected at arterial saturations of 85–90% (Pao_2 50–60 mmHg, 6.7–8.0 kPa), although there is much variation. If the Hb level is low it may not be detected however low the Pao_2. Best detected in the lips and buccal mucosa. The cyanosis produced by 5 g/dl of reduced Hb can be produced by just 1.5 g/dl of methaemoglobin or 0.5 g/dl of sulphaemoglobin. May be mimicked by argyria, from long-standing use of products containing silver.[76]

Oxygen flux. The rate of oxygen carriage in arterial blood[77] and can be calculated (ignoring physical solution) by:

$$\text{cardiac output (ml/min)} \times Sao_2 \times \text{Hb concentration (g/ml)} \times 1.34$$

It is normally about 1000 ml/min. Values below 400 ml/min are probably lethal if continued for a long time. Consciousness is likely to be lost in a normal person with a Pao_2 below 3.6 kPa (27 mmHg).

Carbon dioxide carriage in blood

Mixed venous Pco_2 is 6.1 kPa (46 mmHg), and CO_2 content 23.7 mmol/l (53 ml/dl). Arterial Pco_2 is 5.3 kPa (40 mmHg), and CO_2 content 21.9 mmol/l (49 ml/dl). Total body stores of CO_2 are 120 l. Carbon dioxide is carried in arterial blood in three forms:

1. As dissolved CO_2. Solubility at 37°C is 0.231 mmol/l/kPa (0.0308 mmol/l/mmHg), 23 times that of oxygen. This accounts for 5% of the total. It is very rapidly exchangeable.
2. As bicarbonate, mainly in plasma (90% of the total CO_2).
3. As carbamino compounds formed by the combination of CO_2 with NH_2 groups from haemoglobin in red cells. CO_2 combines on a negligible scale with plasma proteins. Reduced haemoglobin can take up more carbon dioxide in this way than oxyhaemoglobin. About 5–7% of CO_2 is carried in this way, depending on the haemoglobin saturation.

Haemoglobin is the main intracellular buffer for the H^+ ions produced with the bicarbonate. Reduced haemoglobin is a better buffer, and can carry more

CO_2 as carbamino compounds, which together account for the Haldane effect.[78]

The hydration of CO_2 to form carbonic acid is catalyzed by carbonic anhydrase in red cells, although an absence of this enzyme is quite compatible with life. The ratio of CO_2 to bicarbonate determines pH, and so ventilation plays a vital role in acid-base balance (see below).

Pulmonary circulation

Virtually the whole cardiac output passes through the lungs. Pulmonary arterial pressure is about one-sixth of systemic. The pulmonary blood volume is about 500 ml, but only 80 ml is in the capillaries.

Pulmonary vascular pressures. Affected by: (a) Posture. The lower pressures mean a greater influence of gravity. Blood flow is nearly zero at the lung apex and greatest at the bases in the erect position. This variation is greater than the similar variation in ventilation, so the ventilation-perfusion ratio is highest at the top of the lungs; (b) exercise results in increased pulmonary blood flow and moderate rise of pressure in the supine, but not in the erect position; (c) changes of up to 8 mmHg in intra-alveolar pressure cause equal changes in pulmonary arterial pressure, e.g. it falls during spontaneous inspiration; (d) hypoxia causes pulmonary vasoconstriction and hypertension. On a local level this tends to shunt blood away from hypoxic areas of lung, and improve ventilation-perfusion relationships. The response is greater to alveolar than pulmonary arterial hypoxia, is most active at a Po_2 of 30 mmHg, and is mediated by an unidentified local chemical. It is inhibited by volatile anaesthetic agents, but this is probably of little importance;[79] (e) acidaemia. A fall in pH of 0.1 increases pulmonary vascular resistance by 50%; (f) diseases, e.g. mitral valve disease, chronic lung disease, pulmonary embolus and left-to-right shunts all raise pulmonary arterial pressure; (g) autonomic system. α-stimulation causes weak vasoconstriction, whereas β-stimulation and parasympathetic activity cause vasodilatation; and (h) drugs. Vasoconstrictors: dopamine, 5-HT, histamine (H_1), PGE_2. Vasodilators: histamine (H_2), prostacyclin, PGE_1, bradykinin, atropine, opioids.

Regulation of respiration

Rhythmical breathing is controlled by the respiratory centre in the floor of the fourth ventricle (C. J. J. Legallois (1770–1814) in 1812[80] and Marie Jean Pierre Flourens (1794–1867), French physiologist). There are three main parts: (1) a medullary centre capable of initiating and maintaining sequences of respiration, though not of normal character; (2) an apneustic centre in the middle and lower pons, which if unopposed tends to produce inspiratory spasm or apneustic breathing; and (3) a pneumotaxic centre in the upper third of the pons that restrains the apneustic centre periodically. The centre is influenced from many sources: (a) from changes in arterial Pco_2.[81] The centre normally maintains the $Paco_2$ at 5.3 kPa. When it falls below 4–4.5 kPa, respiratory drive usually ceases, leading to apnoea. The effect of $Paco_2$ on the respiratory centre is modified by the CSF bicarbonate concentration, a reduction in which is the basis of acclimatization. A change in CSF pH is the primary stimulus. The respiratory centre takes about 30 s to respond to a change in Pa_{CO_2}; (b) by changes in body temperature; (c) by Hering-Breuer reflexes[82] (Hering, 1834–1918; Joseph Breuer, 1842–1925, Viennese general practitioner and psychiatrist); (d) by carotid body reflexes, largely hypoxia, shown to stimulate respiration by John Scott Haldane (1860-1936), Oxford physiologist, in 1905;[81] (e) by proprioceptive impulses from the whole body, which stimulate breathing on exercise; (f) by reflexes which modify respiration during talking, swallowing and inhaling pungent vapours (9th and 10th nerves); (g) by the hypothalamus and cerebral cortex; (8) pain.

There is a dose-dependent depression of the ventilatory response to CO_2 by anaesthetics. This is probably a central effect, although intercostal muscle activity is particularly depressed. Ether and nitrous oxide are much less depressant than the commonly used volatile agents. There is little difference in this respect between the latter.

Carotid and aortic reflexes and respiration[83]

Baroreceptors. Present in the carotid sinus (described by H. E. Hering[84] 1866–1948 in 1923) and in the aortic arch. Raising the blood pressure inhibits respiration (Corneille Heymans 1892–1968, Belgian physiologist).[85] Baroreceptors are also present in the great veins, right atrium and pulmonary artery, and increased pressure here may stimulate respiration. Such reflexes may cause the dyspnoea of heart failure and pulmonary embolism. Hypotension can cause the baroreceptors to initiate reflex bronchial dilatation.[86]

Peripheral chemoreceptors. Present in the carotid body[87] and aortic bodies.[88] The former are much more important, innervated from the glossopharangeal (IX) nerve and stimulate respiration when arterial Po_2 falls below about 8 kPa (60 mmHg), but not when O_2 content falls. Otherwise hypoxia directly depresses the respiratory centre.[89] The response is greater if the Pco_2 is raised acutely. The main cell in the carotid body is the glomus or type I cell, which secretes dopamine, although the mechanism of action is uncertain. They also respond to acidaemia, respiratory oscillations of Pco_2, hyperkalaemia (both of these may contribute to the exercise response) and to drugs such as doxapram and almitrine. However, patients who have lost both carotid bodies after bilateral carotid endarterectomies show a fairly normal response to mild exercise. Patients with severe chronic obstructive lung disease may be relatively unresponsive to their chronically raised Pa_{CO_2}, and be dependent on this hypoxic drive to breathing. If too much oxygen is given, severe hypoventilation may result.

There is a striking loss of chemoreceptor response to hypoxia with inhalational anaesthesia, which is seen at just 0.1 MAC. This affects respiratory control postoperatively, especially at altitude.[90]

Respiratory muscles

Inspiration. The diaphragm is by far the most important muscle of inspiration, although the external intercostals, pectoralis minor and the scalenes may all be active during quiet breathing. Sternomastoids, pectorals and extensors of the vertebral column may be used during active hyperventilation. The intercostals by themselves can maintain perfectly satisfactory ventilation. Anaesthesia causes rib-cage excursion to diminish and the end-expiratory tone in the diaphragm to be lost.

Expiration. Normally passive, but the muscles of the abdominal wall and perhaps the internal intercostals come into play when minute volume exceeds about 40 l/min. Anaesthesia causes phasic activity of the expiratory muscles that are normally silent.

Assessment of lung function

Simplest tests

1. *Match test.* Attempt to blow out a lighted paper match held 15 cm from the patient's wide open mouth. It is essential that the lips are not allowed to come together. Patients who can perform this test should maintain adequate ventilation after thoracic or abdominal surgery.

2. *Auscultation over the trachea during a forced expiration.* Breath sounds audible for more than 6 s denote airway obstruction. If the time is less than 5 s airway obstruction is most unlikely.

3. *Respiratory muscle strength.* The pressure generated at the mouth by a maximum attempt to breath in or out from an obstructed airway. Maximal inspiratory pressure (measured when near residual volume) is 100–125 cm H_2O, and maximal expiratory pressure (near total lung capacity) 150–200 cm H_2O.

Lung volumes that can be measured with a spirometer

The spirometer was invented in 1846 (Hutchinson, 1811–1861).[91]

1. *Tidal volume (V_T).* Volume of gas inspired or expired during each respiratory cycle (400–500 ml). Some remains in the dead space.

2. *Inspiratory reserve volume (IRV).* Maximum volume of gas that can be inspired from the normal end-inspiratory position (2500 ml).

3. *Expiratory reserve volume (ERV).* Maximum volume of gas that can be expired from the end-expiratory position (average 1200 ml).

4. *Inspiratory capacity (IC).* The maximum volume of gas that can be inspired from the end-expiratory level (average 3000 ml). The sum of (1) and (2) above.

5. *Vital capacity (VC).* Maximum amount of gas that can be expelled from the lungs following a maximal inspiration (average 4800 ml). The sum of (1), (2) and (3) above. If the expiration is performed as hard as possible (forced) it is the *forced vital capacity (FVC)*.

6. *Forced spirometry.* The *forced expiratory volume (FEV)* is the volume exhaled in a given time from the start of a forced expiration. The time chosen is usually 1 s (FEV_1). A normal individual can expire 75–80% of his FVC in 1 sec. Where there is obstruction to air flow (e.g. asthma, emphysema) FEV_1 is reduced to a much greater degree than FVC. In restrictive lung disease the FEV_1/FVC ratio may be high if airways are held open by fibrosis. These measurements can be made at the bedside with a dry spirometer, e.g. a Vitalograph. The concept of measuring the FEV as a fraction of VC was introduced in 1951.[92] FEV_1 first described by Ehrner.[93]

An elegant way of presenting this data is by plotting the instantaneous flow against volume of gas expired, the *flow-volume loop*. Different groups of lung diseases have characteristic shapes to this loop.

This is much easier for the patient than the seldom-performed *maximal breathing capacity (MBC)*: the maximum volume of air that can be breathed, measured for 15 s and expressed as l/min. Average values 120–170 l/min. Equals 35 x FEV_1.

7. *Peak expiratory flow rate.* The steepest part of the spirometer trace of a forced vital capacity estimation. It may be more conveniently measured with the Wright peak flow-meter.[94] Should be 500–600 l/min.

8. *Minute volume (VE).* Volume of air breathed out each minute. At rest 5 l/min.

Lung volumes that cannot be measured with a spirometer

1. *Residual volume (RV).* The volume of gas in the lungs after a maximal expiration (1200–1500 ml).

2. *Total lung capacity (TLC).* The volume of gas in the lung after a maximal inspiration (average 6000 ml). The sum of RV and VC.

3. *Functional residual capacity (FRC).*[95] The volume of gas in the lungs at the resting end-expiratory level. Varies according to posture. About 3000 ml standing up, but only 2000 ml supine. It is decreased during and after anaesthesia by about 18% (450 ml) due to cephalad movement of the diaphragm, decrease in rib-cage volume and possible shift of blood from the thorax.[96]

These volumes must be measured by gas dilution, body plethysmography or radiographic measurement.

Mechanical properties

1. *Compliance.* Volume change produced per unit pressure increment in l/cm H_2O. Normal values for a healthy young man are lung compliance 0.2 l/cm H_2O, chest wall compliance 0.2 l/cm H_2O, with a total compliance of 0.1 l/cm H_2O. Compliance depends on lung volume, which can be corrected by calculating *specific compliance*, i.e. compliance/FRC. *Elastance* is the reciprocal of compliance, measured in cm H_2O/l.

Static and dynamic compliance. Static compliance is measured when all airflow in the lung has ceased. Dynamic compliance is measured at zero air flow but during rhythmic respiration. This will decrease frequency of breathing increases mainly because of the differing time constants of different areas of lung. This may be an early sign of abnormalities of gas distribution, e.g. emphysema. (Time constant = resistance × compliance.)

2. *Airways resistance.* Pressure needed to generate a given inspiratory flow. Normal value less than 2.5 cm H_2O/l/s. Measured in the body plethysmograph, or by simultaneous measurements of flow and transpulmonary pressure during rapid breathing.

The *work of breathing* can be measured from the area enclosed by the curve on a plot of respired volume against transpulmonary pressure that represents one respiratory cycle. The normal metabolic cost of breathing is about

0.5–1.0 ml O_2 per l/min of ventilation at rest. With hyperventilation this may increase to 3–4 ml O_2 per l/min.

3. *Closing capacity (CC)*. The lung volume below which there is a detectable failure of ventilation in the dependent parts of the lung, caused by airway closure. If thhis occurs above the FRC there will be hypoventilation in these dependent areas, ventilation-perfusion inequality and an increased A − a Po_2 difference.

CC can be measured using a bolus of marker gas, such as helium, inspired at RV. After completing a full inspiration, the subject exhales his vital capacity slowly. Expired volume and helium concentrations are measured. CC is the lung volume at which there is a sharp rise in the alveolar plateau of helium concentration.

In normal subjects CC increases with age to approach the FRC. However, despite a period of intense interest in this measurement, the inter-subject variation has been so great that it has not fulfilled its promise as an early index of lung disease.

Measurements of gas exchange

Analysis of respired gases by Haldane (1860–1936) in 1896.[96]

1. *Dead space volume* (V_D)

Anatomical dead space ($V_{D_{anat}}$). Extends from the nostrils and mouth down to, but not including, the alveoli (about 2 ml/kg body weight).[97] Halved by tracheostomy or by endotracheal intubation. Increased by sitting up, extending the neck and protruding the jaw, old age and by increasing lung volume. Decreased by hypoventilation, which allows more time for gas mixing and exchange to occur. Measured by Fowler's method[98] which determines the volume expired before the alveolar plateau is reached, or by the Bohr equation which simply states that expired gas is a mixture of alveolar (CO_2-containing) and dead space (CO_2-free) gas:

$$\frac{V_{D_{anat}}}{V_T} = 1 - \frac{\text{mixed expired } Pco_2}{\text{alveolar (end-tidal) } Pco_2}$$

Physiological dead space ($V_{D_{phys}}$). A functional volume, which includes anatomical dead space plus *alveolar dead space*, i.e. alveoli that are ventilated but not perfused with blood and therefore play no part in gas exchange. Physiological dead space is estimated from another version of the Bohr equation: (modified by Enghoff)[99]

$$\frac{V_{D_{phys}}}{V_T} = 1 - \frac{\text{mixed expired } Pco_2}{\text{arterial } Pco_2}$$

The alveolar, and hence physiological dead, space are increased by lung disease (especially pulmonary embolism), anaesthesia, hypotension, IPPV and PEEP. Major contributions to dead space may be made by anaesthetic apparatus, masks, tubes, etc.

In normal patients $V_{D_{phys}}/V_T$ is less than 30% (i.e. ventilation is more than 70% efficient). With lung disease this may increase to 60–70%.

2. *Diffusing capacity* ($D_{L_{CO}}$). Carbon monoxide is used because its extremely high 'solubility' in blood (as a result of its avidity for haemoglobin)

means that its partial pressure in blood can be taken as zero, and so its transfer is limited only by diffusion. This is partly because of the alveolar-capillary membrane and partly to the finite rate of chemical combination with haemoglobin. These represent roughly equal barriers. Uptake of carbon monoxide is measured after a deep inspiration of 0.2% CO and a 10 s breathhold:

$D_{L_{CO}}$ = rate of CO transfer per mmHg pressure gradient

It is normally around 30 ml/min/mmHg. Commonly lowered in lung fibrosis and emphysema. In both diseases, the pulmonary capillary blood volume is reduced. Useful to correct for lung volume by dividing $D_{L_{CO}}$ by the gas dilution estimation that is obtained as part of this test, giving the K_{CO}. K stands for Krogh[100] (Marie Krogh, Copenhagen physiologist, as was her husband August Krogh).

ACID-BASE BALANCE

See also Astrup P. and Severinghaus J. W. *The History of Blood Gases, Acids and Bases*. Copenhagen: Munksgaard, 1987. The first measurement of blood gases was made in 1837.[101]

Hydrogen ion concentration and pH

An *acid* is a substance that can yield hydrogen ions (H^+ or protons) whereas a *base* tends to gain H^+. pH notation (p = Potenz or power) introduced by S. P. L. Sorensen (1868–1939),[102] Copenhagen physiologist, which expresses hydrogen ion concentration $[H^+]$ as its negative logarithm to the base 10. Normal pH in arterial blood 7.36–7.44, corresponding to $[H^+]$ of 36–44 nmol/l. The range compatible with life is roughly 20–160 nmol/l (pH 6.8–7.7). Hydrogen ions do not exist free in water, but as $(H_3O)^+$. pH of water is 7.0 at room temperature, 6.8 at 37°C. Both are electrochemically neutral, i.e. $[H^+] = [OH^-]$. Electrometric methods of determination measure ionic activity and not concentration.

pH units	$[H^+]$ nmol/l
7.0	100
7.2	63
7.4	40
7.6	25
7.8	16
8.0	10

Changes with temperature. pH of blood rises as its temperature falls, due to changes in the degree of ionization of the protein elements. The rise is 0.0147 pH units for each °C fall.[103]

Acidaemia and acidosis

In acidaemia, the arterial pH is below normal. In acidosis, there is a condition which would tend to cause acidaemia if uncorrected, although some compensatory mechanism may have restored the pH to normal. A similar definition exists for alkalaemia and alkalosis.

The bicarbonate buffer system

This is the most important buffer system in plasma. Carbonic acid exists in a state of equilibrium with hydrogen ions and bicarbonate ions:

$$H^+ + HCO_3^- \leftrightarrow H_2CO_3$$

By the law of mass action, at equilibrium:

$$[H^+][HCO_3^-] = \text{constant} \times [H_2CO_3]$$

or:

$$[H^+] = \text{constant} \times \frac{[H_2CO_3]}{[HCO_3^-]}$$

Carbonic acid comes from the hydration of CO_2 and its concentration is equivalent to solubility $\times$ Pco_2. If this is done, $[H^+]$ is in nmol/l, Pco_2 in mmHg and $[HCO_3^-]$ in mmol/l then the constant becomes 24 (180 if Pco_2 is in kPa):

$$[H+] = 24 \times \frac{Pco_2}{[HCO_3^-]}$$

This was derived by Henderson (1878–1942, Boston physiologist) and expressed in logarithmic form by Hasselbalch (1874–1962, Copenhagen biochemist) to give the *Henderson-Hasselbalch equation*:[104]

$$pH = pK + \log \frac{[HCO_3^-]}{[H_2CO_3]} = pK + \log \frac{[HCO_3^-]}{0.03 \times Pco_2 \text{ (mmHg)}}$$

pK varies with temperature and pH, but can be taken as 6.1. These relationships are often expressed graphically. Two factors are used as coordinates and iso-lines constructed for the third.

Other buffers

Haemoglobin is the most important buffer after the bicarbonate system. The histidine residues have pK's in the physiological range. Reduced haemoglobin is a stronger base than oxyhaemoglobin. Plasma proteins also act as buffers, but have only one-third the capacity of haemoglobin. Phosphates also act as buffers, have a better pK (6.8), but are present in low concentrations.

Metabolic or non-respiratory acidosis and alkalosis

This refers to acid-base disturbances caused by any substance other than carbon dioxide. Note that the lungs excrete 15 000 mmol of CO_2 per day, whereas other acidic products of metabolism are excreted by the kidney (about 100 mmol/day).

Metabolic acidosis

This may occur with: (1) diabetic keto-acidosis; (2) renal failure; (3) starvation; (4) infantile diarrhoea; (5) salicylate poisoning; (6) after severe muscular exercise; (7) any cause of poor tissue perfusion or hypoxia; (8) following cardiac arrest; (9) other causes of lactic acidosis; and (10) as compensation for respiratory alkalosis.

The clinical effects depend on the cause, but there is likely to be deep, gasping (Kussmaul) respiration, cardiac depression with an insensitivity to inotropes, poor peripheral perfusion with cold blue hands and feet, effects of hyperkalaemia seen on the ECG, dysrhythmias, impaired liver function, and perhaps impaired consciousness.

The body compensates by increased ventilation to lower P_{CO_2} and by increased renal excretion of H^+. Treatment should be directed to the primary cause of the acidosis, but may include administration of sodium bicarbonate.

Sodium bicarbonate is usually given as an 8.4% solution, which contains 1 mmol/ml. A useful empirical way of calculating the dose in mmol (or ml) is:

1/3 × Base deficit × Body weight in kg

Bicarbonate therapy can easily result in sodium overload, a metabolic alkalosis, and the left-shifted oxygen dissociation curve impairs oxygen delivery. It is often better to treat the primary cause, giving the body time to correct a modest metabolic acidosis itself.

Metabolic alkalosis

Often iatrogenic. Occurs following administration of excessive alkali, antacids or bicarbonate, and after loss of acid from the stomach, e.g. from vomiting or nasogastric aspiration, or from the kidney in hypokalaemia. The body compensates by increasing renal bicarbonate excretion and by a slight reduction in ventilation. Hypokalaemia may result.

Alkalosis is much more difficult to treat than acidosis, and is mainly of the primary cause. Potassium loss must be replaced, which may exceed 150 mmol/day. It is seldom necessary to give acids, but oral and i.v. ammonium chloride has been used.

Buffer base

The sum of all the buffer anions in the blood in mmol/l including the proteins.

Base excess

The amount of acid or base in mmol/l required for titration back to pH 7.4 at P_{CO_2} of 40 mmHg (5.3 kPa) at 37°C. By convention, an acid surplus (base deficit) is referred to as a negative base excess. Unlike buffer base it is independent of haemoglobin concentration. However the body *in vivo* is a worse buffer than blood *in vitro* because of the lower concentration of proteins in ECF, which can lead to inaccuracies if the above formula for correcting a base deficit is adhered to blindly.

Standard bicarbonate

This is the plasma concentration in blood with a Pco_2 of 40 mmHg (5.3 kPa), haemoglobin fully saturated, at 37°C. No information is obtained about respiratory acid-base balance. Normally 24 mmol/l. Measurements of bicarbonate included in the normal electrolytes are actually of total CO_2, whereas the blood gas analyser calculates it from the Henderson-Hasselbalch equation.

Respiratory acidosis and alkalosis

Caused by changes in arterial Pco_2, and hence carbonic acid. The ill effects of CO_2 excess in the context of anaesthesia were first emphasized by Waters.[105]

Respiratory acidosis. Hypercapnia or hypercarbia

ὑπὲρ (hyper = over) + καπνός (kapnos = smoke)
Causes in anaesthetic practice. (1) Ventilation impaired by respiratory obstruction, profound narcosis or relaxants; (2) severe bilateral lung disease, perhaps complicated by thoracotomy; (3) accidental administration of CO_2. This can raise the Pco_2 extremely quickly; (4) faulty CO_2 absorption due to defective soda lime or faulty system; (5) apnoeic insufflation oxygenation; (6) hyperpyrexia.

While every care should be taken to avoid hypercapnia, minor degrees may not be especially serious.

EFFECTS OF HYPERCAPNIA

1. Central nervous system. (a) Increased cerebral blood flow, cerebral blood volume and intracranial pressure; (b) muscle twitching and a characteristic flap of the hands; (c) progressive narcosis, deepening to coma as the $Paco_2$ rises from 12–16 towards 25 kPa.

The effects are related to the CSF pH, so patients with chronic hypercapnia can be quite alert despite a relatively high Pco_2.

2. Autonomic nervous system. (a) Sympathetic activation with a rise of circulating catecholamines; but with reduced sensitivity of the end organs to these catecholamines. Mild hypercapnia (up to $Paco_2$ 8–10 kPa) commonly causes dysrhythmias during anaesthesia. Sweating. (b) Parasympathetic activation (in general this is overshadowed by the sympathetic effect).

3. Respiratory system. (a) CO_2 stimulates breathing via the respiratory centre; (b) severe hypercapnia produces respiratory failure with its narcotic effect. Paradoxically at 'supercarbia' (Pco_2 around 50 kPa) the resumption of

breathing has been observed in dogs;[106] (c) Bohr effect:[69] the haemoglobin dissociation curve is shifted to the right.

4. Cardiovascular system.[107] (a) Depresses the heart directly, but this is overshadowed by reflex sympathetic stimulation and increased circulating catecholamines; (b) tachycardia; (c) multifocal ventricular extrasystoles, especially during halothane anaesthesia; (d) peripheral resistance usually rises slightly due to a central vasomotor effect (abolished by sympathetic block), although CO_2 has a peripheral vasodilatory effect; and (e) blood pressure usually rises.

5. Biochemical. (a) Compensatory metabolic alkalosis: secretion of acid urine with retention of bicarbonate; and (b) Hyperkalaemia.

6. Effects on action of drugs. (a) Changes of pH affect the ionization and protein binding of many drugs thereby altering the concentration of the active fraction (e.g. respiratory acidosis increases the dosage requirements of thiopentone); and (b) for effects on muscle relaxants *see* Chapter 10.

CARBON DIOXIDE WITHDRAWAL

Sudden fall of P_{CO_2} following a prolonged period of hypercapnia may itself produce untoward effects.

1. Hypotension and dysrhythmias, including ventricular fibrillation have been reported.[108] This has not been confirmed in some subsequent studies,[106] although sudden changes may occur in potassium and intracellular pH. The dissociation curve will move back to the left and may impede oxygen exchange at tissue level.

2. The sudden increase in CSF pH will reduce cerebral blood flow, and may lead to convulsions and death.[109]

3. Hypophosphataemia may occur, so repeated serum phosphate estimations may be needed.[110]

Respiratory alkalosis (hypocapnia)

This is caused by hyperventilation in response to hypoxia, lung disease or metabolic acidosis, or seen in some neurological disorders such as head injury. IPPV during anaesthesia can readily lower the P_{CO_2} to half its normal value.

EFFECTS OF RESPIRATORY ALKALOSIS

1. Central nervous system. (a) Reduction in cerebral blood flow, cerebral blood volume, intracranial pressure and cerebral venous P_{O_2}; (b) clouding of consciousness. A higher pain threshold has been observed in volunteers subjected to hyperventilation to a pH of 7.7.[111] Voluntary hyperventilation to lessen the pain of surgery was described by Bonwill in 1876;[112] and (c) tetany.

2. Cardiovascular system. Fall of blood pressure and cardiac output, with vasoconstriction.

3. Changes in the blood. (a) Hypokalaemia; (b) fall in ionized calcium, but slight increase in total plasma calcium; and (c) shift to the left of the oxygen dissociation curve.

4. Fetus. Reducing maternal P_{CO_2} by hyperventilation during anaesthesia for Caesarean section reduces fetal P_{CO_2} and increases fetal pH. Only with extreme hyperventilation (P_{CO_2} as low as 1.8 kPa) can fetal pH start to fall.

Fetal oxygenation can fall with a maternal Pco_2 below 2.2 kPa. Although both hypocapnia (to correct any fetal acidosis) and hypercapnia (to increase placental blood flow) have been recommended in the past, most clinicians currently aim for modest hyperventilation to bring the maternal Pco_2 to 4.0 kPa.[113]

5. Tetany. Not commonly associated with clinical anaesthesia.

6. Subsequent period of obligatory hypoventilation.

7. For effects on muscle relaxants see Chapter 10.

THE USE OF HYPERVENTILATION IN ANAESTHESIA

Before the wide use of end-tidal CO_2 measurement it was not uncommon for IPPV to reduce the $Paco_2$ to about 3 kPa (20–25 mmHg).

Advantages:

1. Full oxygenation is more likely.

2. A mild respiratory alkalosis is generally held to be safer than a respiratory acidosis.

3. The respiratory alkalosis itself may contribute to the anaesthetic state. There is a decrease in the discharge frequency from the reticular activating system. This is not caused by a decrease in cerebral blood flow because breathing 100% oxygen removes vasoconstriction in the retinal vessels (and so presumably in the other cerebral vessels) but does not decrease analgesia. The analgesic effect of hypocapnia is discussed by Gray.[111]

4. Cardiac effects of neostigmine minimized.

5. Hypocapnia is an important adjunct in techniques for induced hypotension.

Disadvantages:

1. If technique is faulty, undesirable sequelae may follow e.g. hypotension. Pco_2 cannot rise fast after a period of hypoventilation unless CO_2 is added to the inspired gases.

2. Cerebral vasoconstriction is undesirable if blood flow is borderline (e.g. cardiopulmonary bypass), and may lead to defects in subtle psychometric testing, even if there are no neurological abnormalities.[114] Increase in lactate/pyruvate ratio in CSF.

3. In obstetrics. Possible adverse effects on the fetus (*see* above and Chapter 22).

4. Other disadvantages include a reduction of cardiac output and depletion of extracellular potassium. After reversal of any relaxant, respiration often restarts at a $Paco_2$ below the preoperative value, provided that narcotics have not been given in excess. However, after a period of hyperventilation 5–10% CO_2 may need to be administered to raise Pco_2 above the apnoeic threshold.

THE KIDNEYS AND BODY FLUIDS

Body fluids

Total body water (TBW)

About 60% of body weight in men and 50% in women, but decreases with age. This decrease is due to a fall in the *intracellular fluid* (ICF). Thus in the standard 70 kg male, TBW is 42 litres, divided into 28 litres of ICF (2 litres of which are red blood cells), and 14 litres of *extracellular fluid* (ECF) (3 litres of which is blood plasma). The ECF in the interstitial space is in the form of a gel.

The volume and composition of the ICF is maintained by the integrity of the cell membrane and its Na^+/K^+ pump, whereas that of the ECF is maintained largely by the kidneys. The osmolality of the ECF is determined by adjustments in water balance, and the volume of the ECF by sodium balance.

ECF osmolality

Plasma osmolality is kept within a tight range of 275–300 mosmol/l by varying urine osmolality between 30 and 1400 mosmol/l. Any increase in osmolality stimulates osmoreceptor cells in the anterior hypothalamus, which cause thirst and the synthesis of vasopressin (antidiuretic hormone, ADH) in the supraoptic and paraventricular nuclei and its release from the posterior pituitary. Hypovolaemia, as detected by the intravascular volume receptors described below, is a lesser stimulus to ADH release. Trauma and surgery is a powerful stimulus to ADH release, when plasma levels can increase by a factor of 20–50.

ECF volume

The sensors of ECF volume are all intravascular: (a) baroreceptors in the carotid sinus and aortic arch; (b) receptors in the great veins and atria; (c) the renal arterioles in the juxtaglomerular (JG) apparatus. Note that these are all influenced by the autonomic nervous system. They control sodium excretion (and thus the volume of the whole ECF) by: (a) *Renin*. Released by the JG cells after a fall in renal perfusion pressure, an increased $[Na^+]$ in the tubular fluid of the macula densa or β-sympathetic stimulation. Cleaves the 10-amino acid peptide, *angiotensin I*, from a circulating glycoprotein made in the liver. Angiotensin I has two amino acids removed by angiotensin converting enzyme in the pulmonary endothelium to form *angiotensin II*. This has a circulating half-life of just 30 s, is a vasoconstrictor 50 times as potent as noradrenaline, and is the stimulus to the release of *aldosterone* from the zona glomerulosa of the adrenal cortex. Aldosterone acts on the distal tubules and collecting ducts to increase Na resorption. Surgery increases secretion of renin and aldosterone. (b) *Atrial Naturietic Peptide*. Released from granules in the myocardial cells of the atria, mainly the right, in response to atrial stretch. It is a 28-amino acid peptide which both acts as a vasodilator and increases renal blood flow, GFR and sodium excretion. *Intrarenal factors* also play a part. A sodium load causes an increased GFR, which itself promotes the proximal tubular resorption of sodium.

Kidney function

Renal blood flow

Normal renal blood flow is 1.2 l/min or nearly 25% of the cardiac output. Yet the weight of both kidneys is only 300 g, or 0.4% of body weight. Measured by clearance of para-aminohippuric acid (PAH), because it is about 90% extracted from the blood on one passage through the kidneys, although this method may be inaccurate under anaesthesia with low urine flows. The renal cortex receives 75% of the blood flow and the medulla 25%, but in haemorrhagic hypotension, blood is shunted towards the medulla.

Autoregulation of blood flow occurs between mean arterial pressures of about 80 to 180 mmHg. This is mediated locally by arteriolar smooth muscle and seems to be preserved under anaesthesia. Stimulation of the sympathetic supply (T4–L1) and high-dose dopamine constrict renal vessels by an α-effect. Low-dose dopamine (2 µg/kg/min) dilates renal vessels via dopaminergic receptors.

Renal oxygen consumption is high for its weight, 18 ml/min or 6 ml/min/ 100 g. Unlike most organs it varies with blood flow because this determines the amount of work needed for Na^+ resorption. The a–v O_2 content difference is therefore constant at 1–2 ml/dl.

Glomerular filtration

Measured from the *clearance*

$$\text{Clearance} = \frac{(\text{urine concentration} \times \text{urine flow})}{(\text{arterial plasma concentration})}$$

of a substance that is freely filtered by glomeruli, but then not resorbed nor excreted by the tubules, e.g. the fructose polymer, inulin. The clearance of endogenous creatinine is a useful but approximate alternative. Normal value is 125 ml/min, or 180 l/day. Molecules larger than 4–8 nm, depending on their charge, cannot be filtered. Albumin, for example, is just too big.

Tubular function

Most of the glomerular filtrate is reabsorbed by the tubules. Na^+ is actively reabsorbed throughout the tubule. Glucose is reabsorbed in the proximal tubule, but only up to a maximum rate, the 'transport maximum'. Thus there is threshold blood level of about 10 mmol/l below which there is no glycosuria. K^+ is secreted by the distal tubules, but reabsorbed more proximally. In the proximal tubule, H^+ is secreted by a Na^+–H^+ exchange mechanism, and is accompanied by HCO_3^- reabsorption. The H^+ is derived from the hydration of CO_2 and so depends on carbonic anhydrase. In the distal tubule and collecting ducts, H^+ is secreted by means of a proton pump, stimulated by aldosterone. There is a maximum H^+ gradient that can be generated here of about 1000 times the concentration in plasma, and urine cannot be acidified below a pH of about 4.5.

ELECTROLYTE BALANCE

Flame photometry pioneered in 1947.[115] Ion selective electrodes described in 1963.[116]

1. Sodium

Total body sodium is about 4000 mmol; nearly one-third of this is in bone. Typical dietary intake is 50–100 mmol/day, but can range from 1–400 mmol depending on dietary extreme. Urinary excretion can be varied over this range, but is usually about 90 mmol/l. Normal serum levels are 132–145 mmol/l of sodium and 98–106 mmol/l of chloride. Typical sodium concentrations in other body fluids: sweat 50, saliva 60, gastric juice 50, bile 145, small bowel 110, and large bowel, 50–75 mmol/l.

Sodium is 91% extracellular, being extruded from cells by the Na^+/K^+ pump and less able to enter the cell due to its larger hydrated ionic size than K^+. Sodium is the main determinant of ECF osmolality and its concentration is largely dictated by water balance. Sodium balance determines ECF volume.

Sodium depletion

Causes. Usually loss through vomiting, diarrhoea, intestinal fistulae or drainage, intestinal obstruction or thiazide diuretics.

Results. Lassitude, apathy, weakness, anorexia, headache, vomiting, postural hypotension. Poor peripheral tissue perfusion. Decreased ECF volume. Urine normal in amount, with ECF osmolality preserved at the expense of volume. Finally, coma and collapse. Blood urea rises. Urinary sodium less than 10–20 mmol/l. Hyponatraemia.

There is an acid–base disturbance if the loss of chloride and sodium ions is disproportionate. With continued loss of gastric juice there is a hypochloraemic alkalosis. With continued loss of fluid from the gut distal to the pylorus, there is a greater loss of sodium ions and an acidosis.

Treatment. Intravenous replacement with saline, either normal, twice normal (1.8%), or 30% (5 mol/l).

Sodium retention

May occur with water retention, as in oedema, or as disproportionate sodium retention causing hypernatraemia. Usually accompanied by hyperchloraemia. May be due to: (1) *Excessive intake* as in over-infusion of hypertonic saline or sodium bicarbonate at cardiac arrests, excessive oral intake as with high solute baby milk, or salt enemas; (2) *Inability to excrete* as in primary hyperaldosteronism, Cushing's syndrome, excessive steroid therapy, or essential hypernatraemia with some hypothalamic lesions.

Effects are: mild oedema, slight thirst, confusion, apathy, leading to coma. Treated by withholding sodium, frusemide and the gradual administration of hypotonic solutions.

The 'sick-cell syndrome'

There is evidence that in some severe pathological conditions, such as septic shock, disseminated malignancy and hepatic failure, the integrity of the cell membrane is diminished. This causes sodium to pass into cells and its serum concentration to fall. Total body sodium is normal. Potassium leaks out of the cells. Homeostatic responses are appropriate to this reduced sodium concentration. Hypertonic saline is of no value. Insulin and glucose has been used, but does not produce clinical improvement.

2. Potassium[117]

Potassium is largely intracellular (90%). Bone contains 8% of the total and only about 2% is in the ECF. Total body potassium is around 3200 mmol in a 70 kg man. Average dietary intake is 60–120 mmol/day. Normal concentrations: serum 3.5–5.0 mmol/l, urine about 60 mmol/l, intracellular space 150 mmol/l. An intravascular [K^+] electrode has been described.[118]

Potassium depletion

Causes. (a) Excessive loss from the gastrointestinal tract as a result of vomiting, diarrhoea, biliary fistula, etc. Diarrhoea contains 50–100 mmol/l, whereas gastric juice contains only 5–10 mmol/l. Hypokalaemia with vomiting is due to K^+ loss in the urine as the kidney tries to conserve hydrogen ions; (b) excessive loss in the urine as a result of diuretics, renal tubular disease, adrenal hyperactivity (Conn's or Cushing's syndrome, steroid therapy) and diabetic ketoacidosis; (c) inadequate replacement during long periods of intravenous fluid therapy; (d) hypokalaemia may also be caused by a shift into the cells, as in alkalosis, insulinoma or familial periodic paralysis; and (e) old age.

Results. Symptoms relate to disordered function of the three types of muscle. (a) Smooth muscle: constipation, nausea, distension and ileus; (b) skeletal muscle: hypotonia and weakness; (c) cardiac muscle: hypotension, sensitivity to digoxin, dysrhythmia and arrest. May impair renal tubular function (nephrogenic diabetes insipidus), and cause a metabolic alkalosis.

The diagnosis is confirmed by: (a) serum potassium, though this may be normal with intracellular depletion; (b) ECG changes: depression of ST segment, lowering, widening or inversion of T waves, prolongation of PR and QT intervals, appearance of U waves; and (c) response to treatment.

Management. Clinical judgement should be exercised before active treatment. Mild depletion may be treated with oral (150–200 mmol/day potassium chloride) or intravenous (KCl diluted to 40 mmol/l and given at no more than 40 mmol/h or 200 mmol/day. It is occasionally necessary to give it in higher concentration and faster, best done by infusion pump and under ECG control).

Proposed surgery may have to be delayed if the serum [K^+] is below 3.0 mmol/l, because of the risk of cardiac dysrhythmias, sensitivity to digoxin, muscle weakness and difficulty in reversing relaxants. In those with whole-body potassium deficiency, e.g. the elderly, patients with alkalosis, on long-term IPPV and those who have received diuretics, potassium replacement is best started at a serum [K^+] level of 3.5–4 mmol/l, and may require to be continued for several days. The addition of a potassium-sparing diuretic, e.g. amiloride, may be useful. The correction of hypokalaemia contributes to the correction of concurrent metabolic alkalosis and vice versa.

Hyperkalaemia

This is dangerous because of its effects on the heart. ECG abnormalities may occur at concentrations above 6–7 mmol/l, with a tall peaked T wave, absence of P wave, widening of QRS and finally a sine-wave pattern proceeding to ventricular fibrillation.

Causes. (a) Acute renal failure; (b) over-zealous intravenous replacement therapy, especially if urine output is low; (c) suxamethonium causes a rise in serum potassium of about 0.5–1.0 mmol/l in normal patients within 1–7 min of injection. The rise can exceed 2 mmol/l in patients with massive trauma, burns, tetanus and neurological lesions, e.g. stroke, cord transection, degenerative diseases of the pyramidal tracts, e.g. amyotrophic lateral sclerosis and Friedreich's ataxia, myopathies. Pretreatment with a non-depolarizing relaxant decreases this effect, but does not abolish it; (d) metabolic acidosis; (e) drugs:[119] potassium-sparing diuretics, ACE inhibitors, large doses of potassium salts of penicillin; (g) adrenal insufficiency; and (h) stored blood may contain 25 mmol/l.

Treatment. (a) Glucose (50 g) and insulin (10–20 units), which shift potassium into cells and lowers $[K^+]$ for 1–2 hours; (b) treatment of any acidosis with bicarbonate (100 mmol or more is needed); (c) calcium salts (10% gluconate 10–30 ml) oppose the action of K^+ on the heart and produce an immediate but short-lived improvement in the ECG; (d) calcium or sodium resonium cation exchange enemas; and (e) peritoneal or haemodialysis.

3. Calcium[120]

Normal serum level 2.1–2.6 mmol/l, just under half being ionized. Absorption in the small intestine encouraged by 1,25 dihydroxycholecalciferol, which is vitamin D_3 (cholecalciferol) that has been 25-hydroxylated in the liver and 1-hydroxylated in the proximal tubules of the kidney. Blood calcium is also raised by parathormone, which increases bone resorption, Ca resorption in the distal tubules and the production of 1,25 dihydroxycholecalciferol. These actions are balanced by calcitonin, which inhibits bone resorption and increases urinary Ca excretion.

In anaesthetic practice hypocalcaemia is seen after: (a) unintentional parathyroidectomy during thyroid surgery. Signs of tetany are those of Chvostek (facial muscle contraction on tapping the facial nerve at the angle of the jaw) and Trousseau (spasm causing wrist and thumb flexion and finger extension, perhaps induced by occluding the arm's circulation); (b) changes in pH (hyperventilation and alkalosis lowers serum ionized $[Ca^{2+}]$); (c) prolonged electrolyte losses through fistulae or during long-term intravenous therapy; and (d) transfusion with citrated blood. This is seldom important because citrate is normally rapidly metabolized in the liver and excreted by the kidneys, and any changes are small and transient.[121]

Hypercalcaemia is usually caused by excessive administration, malignancy or primary hyperparathyroidism.

Calcium measurements with an intravascular electrode have confirmed that calcium gluconate produces just as rapid rises in $[Ca^{2+}]$ as the chloride.[122]

Note that calcium chloride 10% contains about 1 mmol/ml Ca^{2+}, whereas the 10% gluconate contains just 0.22 mmol/ml. Hypocalcaemia produces lengthening of the QT interval. The recommended daily dietary intake is 20–30 mmol; or 0.5 mmol/g nitrogen for intravenous nutrition.

4. Phosphate

Total body phosphorus is 16–26 mol, 90% in bone. Normal serum phosphate level 0.8–1.45 mmol/l (higher in children). Parathormone promotes phosphaturia by inhibition of proximal tubular reabsorption. Hypophosphataemia is seen mainly during i.v. nutrition when the requirement is 0.5–0.75 mmol/kg/ day. It inhibits leucocyte function, and causes muscle weakness and osteomalacia. The oxygen dissociation curve shifts to the left. A raised phosphate is seen in hypoparathyroidism and renal failure.

5. Magnesium[123]

Normal serum magnesium 0.75–1.05 mmol/l. Fourth most plentiful cation. Total body magnesium is 1000 mmol, 99% of which is intracellular, 50% in bone and 20% in muscle. A cofactor in many biochemical reactions, and essential for normal function of cardiac, skeletal and smooth muscle and the neuromuscular junction. Recommended daily dietary intake is 12 mmol/day. Resorption in the loop of Henle is stimulated by parathormone. Levels may fall after use of diuretics (especially thiazides), electrolyte losses or prolonged intravenous therapy[124] in patients when the requirement is 1 mmol/g nitrogen. Lower levels often associated with hypocalcaemia, but can by itself cause paraesthesia, cramps, twitching, tetany, depression, weakness and resistant dysrhythmias. It may be given as magnesium chloride 0.5–1.0 mmol/kg/day.

A raised serum magnesium is rare and usually iatrogenic.[125] It causes pre- and postsynaptic neuromuscular blockade, CNS depression, absent brainstem reflexes, long PR interval and a wide QRS complex, cardiac arrest in diastole. Forced diuresis or dialysis may be needed.

Magnesium sulphate is used in North America for the treatment of toxaemia of pregnancy. It produces a useful combination of sedation, vasodilatation and a reduction in uterine tone.

6. Zinc

Recommended dietary intake 82–165 µmol/day. There are no body stores. Deficiency causes skin lesions around the mouth and at sites of trauma, inhibition of T-cell function, and may delay healing after prolonged illness.

References

1. Maze M. *Anesthesiology* 1990, **72**, 959.
2. Light A. R. et al. *Somatosensory Res.* 1983, **1**, 33.
3. Curtis D. R et al. *Brain Res.* 1977, **130**, 360.

4. Soar J. et al. *Br. J. Anaesth.* 1991, **66**, 398P.
5. Pleuvry B. J. *Br. J. Anaesth.* 1991, **66**, 370.
6. Aserinsky E. and Kleitman N. *Science* 1953, **118**, 273; Dement W. C. and Kleitman N. *Electroencephalogr. Clin. Neurophysiol.* 1957, **34**, 823.
7. Knill R. L. et al. *Anesthesiology* 1990, **73**, 52.
8. Stradling J. R. and Phillipson E. A. *Q. J. Med.* 1986, **58**, 3.
9. Hanning C. D. *Br. J. Anaesth.* 1989, **63**, 477; Hoffstein V. and Zamel N. *Br. J. Anaesth.* 1990, **65**, 139.
10. Gastaut H. et al. *Brain Res.* 1966, **1**, 167.
11. Halsey M. J. In *General Anaesthesia* (Nunn J. F. et al. ed.) London: Butterworths, 1989, 19; Kendig J. J. and Trudell J. R. In: *Scientific Foundations of Anaesthesia* (Scurr C. et al. ed.) Oxford: Heinemann, 1990, 314; Pocock G. and Richards C. D. *Br. J. Anaesth.* 1991, **66**, 116.
12. Griffiths D. and Jones J. G. *Br. J. Anaesth.* 1990, **65**, 603.
13. Meyer H. H. *Arch. Exp. Path. Pharmak.* 1899, **42**, 109.
14. Overton C. E. *Studien über Narkose.* Jena: G. Fischer, 1901. English translation published by Chapman and Hall (Lipnick R. L. ed.) 1990.
15. Bernard C. *Lecons sur les Anaesthésiques et sur l'Asphyxie.* Paris: Baillière, 1875.
16. Ferguson J. *Proc. R. Soc. B* 1939. **127**, 387.
17. Pauling L. *Science* 1961, **134**, 15; *Anesth. Analg.* 1964. **43**, 1 (reprinted in 'Classical File', *Surv. Anesthesiol.* 1970. **14**, 194).
18. Eger E. I. et al. *Anesthesiology* 1969, **30**, 129.
19. Halsey M. J. et al. *Br. J. Anaesth.* 1978, **50**, 1091.
20. Wann K. T. and Macdonald A. G. *Prog. Neurobiol.* 1988, **30**, 271.
21. Plum F. and Siesjö B. *Anesthesiology* 1975, **42**, 708; Bryce-Smith R. *Proc. R. Soc. Med.* 1976, **69**, 75.
22. Magendie F. *J. Physiol. Exp. Pathol.* 1825, **5**, 27.
23. Queckenstedt H. H. G. *Dt. Z. NervHeilk.* 1916, **55**, 325.
24. Steer J. L. and Horney F. D. *Can. Med. Ass. J.* 1968, **98**, 71.
25. Clatterberg J. *Anesthesiology* 1977, **46**, 309.
26. Berry A. *Anaesthesia* 1958, **13**, 100.
27. Erlanger J. and Gasser H. S. *Am. J. Physiol.* 1924, **70**, 624; 1929, **88**, 581 (reprinted in 'Classical File', *Surv. Anesthesiol. 1970*, **14**, 471). (For this work Erlanger and Gasser were awarded the Nobel Prize in 1944.)
28. Nathan P. W. and Sears T. A. *J. Physiol. (Lond.)* 1961, **157**, 565; **164**, 375; *Anaesthesia 1963*, **18**, 467.
29. Whitwam J. G. *Anaesthesia* 1976, **31**, 494.
30. Melzack R. and Wall P. D. *Science* 1965, **150**, 971 (reprinted in 'Classical File', *Surv. Anesthesiol.* 1972, **16**, 583).
31. Budd K. In: *Scientific Foundations of Anaesthesia* (Scurr C. et al. ed.) Oxford: Heinemann, 1990, 314.
32. Raja S. N. *Anesthesiology* 1988, **68**, 571.
33. Kuntz A. *The Autonomic Nervous System*, 2nd ed. Philadelphia: Lea & Febiger, 1934.
34. de Jong R. H. and Cullen S. C. *Anesthesiology* 1963, **24**, 628.
35. Valsalva, Antonia Maria (1666–1723) *De aure humana tractatus. Bononiae:* Typ. C. Pisarii, 1704.
36. Ewing D. J. In: *Autonomic Failure* (Bannister R. ed.) Oxford: OUP, 1983, 371.
37. Lewis T. *Br. Med. J.* 1932, **1**, 873.
38. Howell J. D. *Bull. Hist. Med.* 1984, **58**, 83; Comroe J. H. and Dripps R. D. *Science* 1976, **192**, 115.
39. Waller A. D. *J. Physiol. (Lond.)* 1887, **8**, 229; Besteman E. and Creese M. *Br. Heart J.* 1979, **42**, 61.
40. Einthoven Willem *Pflügers Arch.* 1903, **99**, 472 (translated in *Cardiac Classics* (Willius F. A. and Keys T. E., ed.) St Louis: Mosby, 1941, **2**, 722); Lancet 1912, **1**, 853.
41. Dock W. *Proc. Soc. Exp. Biol. Med.* 1929, **24**, 566.

42. Jolly W. A. and Ritchie W. R. *Heart* 1910, **2**, 177.
43. Mackenzie J. *Diseases of the Heart.* London: Oxford University Press, 1908.
44. Traube L. *Berlin Klin. Wochenschr.* 1872, **9**, 1, 185, 221.
45. Heard J. B. and Strauss A. E. *Am. J. Med. Sci.* 1918, **155**, 238.
46. Krumbhaar. B. *Am. J. Med. Sci.* 1918, **155**.
47. Johnstone M. MD Thesis, University of Belfast, 1948.
48. Rollason W. N. *Electrocardiography for the Anaesthetist.* Oxford: Blackwell, 1964.
49. Goldberger E. *Am. Heart J.* 1942, **23**, 483.
50. Wolferth C. C. and Wood F. C. *Am. J. Med. Sci.* 1932, **183**, 30; Wilson F. M. et al. *Am. Heart J.* 1934, **9**, 447.
51. Starling E. H. *The Linacre Lecture on the Law of the Heart* given at Cambridge in 1915. London: Longmans, Green & Co., 1918.
52. Chambers J. et al. *Br. Med. J.* 1988, **297**, 1071.
53. Robotham J. L. et al. *Anesthesiology* 1991, **74**, 172.
54. Brodsky M. et al. *Am. J. Cardiol.* 1977, **39**, 390.
55. Griffin R. M. In: *Anaesthesia Review 6* (Kaufman L. ed.) 1989, 75.
56. Albert S. N. *Blood Volume* Springfield, Ill.: Thomas, 1963.
57. Reiz S. et al. *Anesthesiology* 1983, **59**, 91.
58. *See also* Fink B. R. and Demarest R. J. *Laryngeal Biomechanics.* Cambridge, Mass.: Harvard University Press, 1978.
59. Stewart S. and Pinkerton H. H. *Br. J. Anaesth.* 1955, **27**, 492.
60. Sleigh M. A. et al. *Am. Rev. Respir. Dis.* 1988, **137**, 726; Widdicombe J. G. *Eur. Respir. J.* 1989, **2**, 107.
61. Bakhle Y. S. *Br. J. Anaesth.* 1990, **65**, 49.
62. Jones J. G. and Somerville I. D. In: *Anaesthesia Review 6.* (Kaufman L. ed.) 1989, 185.
63. Hills B. A. *Br. J. Anaesth.* 1990, **65**, 13.
64. Adults: Holm B. A. and Matalon S. *Anesth. Analg.* 1989, **69**, 805; Babies: Morley C. J. *Arch. Dis. Child.* 1991, **66**, 445.
65. *See also* Nunn J. F. *Applied Respiratory Physiology.* London: Butterworths, 3rd ed. 1987.
66. Pappenheimer I. R. et al. *Fed. Proc.* 1950, **9**, 602.
67. Hedenstierna G. *Br. J. Anaesth.* 1990, **64**, 507.
68. Barcroft J. and Poulton E. P. *J. Physiol.* 1913, **46**, 4; *Respiratory Function of the Blood.* Cambridge: Cambridge University Press, 1914.
69. Bohr C. *Skand. Arch. Physiol.* 1904, **16**, 402.
70. Valtis D. J. and Kennedy A. C. *Lancet* 1954, **1**, 119.
71. Greenwald G. *J. Biol. Chem. 1925*, **63**, 339.
72. Kambam J. R. et al. *Anesthesiology* 1986, **65**, 426.
73. Kim S.-J. et al. *Anesth. Analg.* 1990, **71**, 73.
74. Hüfner C. G. von *Arch. Anat. Physiol.* 1894, 130.
75. Gregory I. C. *J. Physiol.* 1974, **236**, 625.
76. Timmins A. C. and Morgan G. A. R. *Anaesthesia* 1988, **43**, 755.
77. Nunn J. F. and Freeman J. *Anaesthesia* 1964, **19**, 206.
78. Christiansen J. et al. *J. Physiol.* 1914, **48**, 244.
79. Eisenkraft J. B. *Br. J. Anaesth.* 1990, **65**, 63.
80. Legallois J. J. C. *Expérience sur le Principe de la Vie.* Paris, 1812.
81. Haldane J. S. and Priestley J. G. *J. Physiol. (Lond.)* 1905, **32**, 225.
82. Hering E. and Breuer J. *Akad. Wiss. Wien.* 1868, **57**, 672 (reprinted in 'Classical File', *Surv. Anesthesiol.* 1971, **15**, 595); and **58**, 909; *see also* Lee J. A. *Anaesthesia* 1968, **23**, 683.
83. Ward D. S. and Temp J. A. In: *Anaesthesia Review 8* (Kaufman L. ed.) 1991, 89.
84. Hering H. E. *Münch. Med. Wochenschr.* 1923, **70**, 1287.
85. Heymans C. *Le Sinus carotidien et les autres Zones vasosensibles réflexogènes.* Presse Université de France, 1929. (This work earned Heymans the Nobel prize in 1938.)
86. Daly M. de B. and Schweitzer A. *J. Physiol. (Lond.)* 1951, **113**, 442; Daly M. de B. and Angell James J. F. *Lancet* 1979, **1**, 764.

87. Heymans C. et al. *Archs Int. Pharmacodyn. Thér.* 1930, **39**, 400 (first described by H. W. L. Taube in 1743).
88. Heymans J. F. and Heymans C. *Archs Int. Pharmacodyn. Thér.* 1926, **32**, 9.
89. Neubauer J. A. et al. *J. Appl. Physiol.* 1990, **68**, 441.
90. Nunn J. F. *Br. J. Anaesth.* 1990, **65**, 54.
91. Hutchinson J. *Med. Chir. Trans.* 1846, **29**, 137.
92. Gaensler E. A. *Am. Rev. Tuberc. Pulm. Dis.* 1951, **64**, 256.
93. Ehrner C. *Acta Med. Scand.* 1960, **167**, suppl. 353.
94. Wright B. M. and McKerrow C. B. *Br. Med. J.* 1959, **2**, 1041: Wright B. M. *Br. Med. J.* 1978, **2**, 1627.
95. Wahba R. W. M. *Can. J. Anaesth.* 1991, **38**, 384.
96. Haldane J. S. *J. Physiol. (Lond.)* 1896, **13**, 419.
97. Radford E. P. *J. Appl Physiol.* 1955, **7**, 451.
98. Fowler W. S. *Am. J. Physiol.* 1948, **154**, 405.
99. Enghoff H. *Uppsala Lük För Förh.* 1938, **44**, 191.
100. Krogh M. *J. Physiol. (Lond.)* 1915, **49**, 271.
101. Magnus H. G. *Ann. Physiol. Chem. (Leipzig)* 1837, **17**, 583.
102. Sorensen S. P. L. *C. R. Trav. Lat. Carlsberg* 1909, **8**, 1.
103. Severinghaus J. W. *J. Appl. Physiol.* 1966, **21**, 1108.
104. Henderson L. J. *Am. J. Physiol.* 1908, **21**, 173 and 427; Hasselbalch K. A. *Biochem. Z.* 1916, **78**, 112 (see also 'Classical File', *Surv. Anesthesiol.* 1964, **8**, 486, 607).
105. Waters R. M. *New Orl. Med. Surg. J.* 1937, **90**, 219; *Can. Med. Assoc. J.* 1938, **38**, 240.
106. Graham G. R. et al. *Anaesthetist* 1960, **9**, 70.
107. Foëx P. In: *The Circulation in Anaesthesia* (Prys-Roberts C. ed.) Oxford: Blackwells, 1980.
108. Brown E. B. and Miller F. *Am. J. Physiol.* 1952, **169**, 56.
109. Cotev S. and Severinghaus J. W. *Anesth. Analg.* 1969, **48**, 42.
110. Storm T. L. *Br. Med. J.* 1984, **289**, 456.
111. Geddes I. C. and Gray T. C. *Lancet* 1959, **2**, 4; Robinson J. S. and Gray T. C. *Br. J. Anaesth.* 1961, **33**, 62.
112. Bonwill W. G. A. *Penna J. Dent. Science* 1876, **3**, 57 (reprinted in 'Classical File', *Surv. Anesthesiol.* 1964, **8**, 377).
113. Rampton A. J. et al. *Br. J. Anaesth.* 1988, **61**, 730.
114. Nevin M. et al. *Lancet* 1987, **ii**, 1493.
115. Hald P. M. *J. Biol. Chem.* 1947, **167**, 499.
116. Friedman S. M., Wong S-L. et al. *J. Appl. Physiol.* 1963, **18**, 950.
117. Vitez T. *Can. J. Anaesth.* 1987, **34**, S30.
118. Linton R. A. F. et al. *Crit. Care Med.* 1982, **10**, 337.
119. Rimmer J. M. et al. *Arch. Intern. Med.* 1987, **147**, 867.
120. Stevenson J. C. *Br. J. Hosp. Med.* 1984, **32**, 71.
121. Insalaco S. *J. Lab. Med.* 1984, **15**, 325.
122. Heining M. P. D. et al. *Anaesthesia* 1984, **39**, 1079.
123. Gambling D. R. et al. *Can. J. Anaesth.* 1988, **35**, 644; James M. F. M. In: *Lectures in Anaesthesiology 1988/1.* Zorab J. S. M. (ed.) Oxford: Blackwells, 1988, 63.
124. Zaloga G. P. and Chernow B. et al. *Chest* 1989, **95**, 257 and 391.
125. Ashton M. R. et al. *Br. Med. J.* 1990, **300**, 541.

Chapter 2

Pharmacology

PHARMACOKINETICS[1]

Pharmacokinetics embraces the absorption, distribution, protein binding, metabolism and excretion of drugs (what the body does to a drug).

Absorption

Oral. Easy, painless and often reliable. Affected by gastro-intestinal motility (mainly gastric emptying), administration of other drugs or food (metoclopramide may accelerate drug absorption) and the extent to which the liver metabolizes the absorbed drug ('first pass' effect). For example, some 75% of absorbed propranolol and even more of ketamine is destroyed by the first pass effect. However, some drugs are completely or largely inactivated in the gut, and others are unpalatable.

Sublingual. Useful for buprenorphine and nitrates. Absorption depends on the co-operation of the patient. Enters systemic circulation directly without first pass liver metabolism.

Intranasal. Absorbed into a good blood supply, but affected by colds and allergies (DDAVP, sufentanil).

Via the Lungs. Reliable, usually swift. *See* Chapter 11. Elimination of inhalational anaesthetics is guaranteed, which is not the case for parenteral drugs. May also be used at resuscitation for administration of adrenaline, isoprenaline, lignocaine, atropine, diazepam and naloxone.[2]

Rectal. Useful for some sedatives, premedicants and analgesics (diazepam, diclofenac), if the drug is retained long enough for absorption. About 50% may be absorbed into the systemic circulation and 50% into the portal vein, although the proportion is variable. A rate-limiting membrane is used.

Transcutaneous. Slow but reliable and painless (long-acting coronary vasodilators, hyoscine and fentanyl).

Eye-drops. Drugs such as β-blockers, anticholinesterases and catecholamines are absorbed via the nasolacrimal canal, not subject to first pass metabolism, and so can exert a significant systemic effect.

Injection. (Intradermal, subcutaneous, intramuscular, intravenous). Absorption not always reliable, e.g. ketamine is excellent, but diazepam worse than when given orally. Depends on the drug, its pH and the local blood flow. Intramuscular absorption is delayed in shock. It may be difficult to be sure if an injection is i.m. or s.c. if the patient is obese. Intramuscular injections may be painful (penicillin) or may damage other structures (e.g. sciatic nerve). Intravenous injection is accurate and certain. Blood levels rise rapidly. Osmolalities of drugs supplied for injection varies greatly, e.g. fentanyl is close to zero.[3]

Distribution

Drugs cross membranes by: (a) passive diffusion, especially of lipid-soluble drugs through lipid components, at a rate proportional to the concentration gradient and the ratio of membrane area to thickness. This is hampered by drug ionization, which in turn depends on local pH. Basic drugs tend to accumulate where the pH is lower and so ionization is favoured, and the converse for acidic drugs. This is 'ion-trapping'; (b) carrier transport by membrane proteins (L-dopa, some ions); and (c) passing through aqueous pores. Binding to proteins affects distribution.

pKa is the negative logarithm of the dissociation rate constant Ka, and is the pH at which a drug is 50% ionized, and at which changes in pH make the greatest difference to the proportion that is ionized.

Metabolism

Drug metabolism generally aims to increase polarity and water solubility to allow renal excretion.

Phase 1 Reactions. Mainly in the liver, catalysed by mixed function oxidase cytochrome P450. (a) *Oxidation*: halothane (to trifluoracetic acid), thiopentone (to pentobarbitone), alcohol, dopamine, benzodiazepines. (b) *Reduction*: reductive dehalogenation of halothane; chloral hydrate (to trichloroethane). (c) *Hydrolysis*: pethidine, lignocaine and (in the plasma) suxamethonium (to succinate and choline).

Phase 2 Reactions. Synthetic or conjugation reactions. Often the rate-limiting steps. *Glucuronide conjugation,* e.g. morphine, salicylates and bilirubin. *Sulphate conjugation*, e.g. isoprenaline and paracetamol. *Acetate conjugation*, e.g. isoniazid, some sulphonamides. *Amino acid conjugation*, e.g. salicylic acid with glycine or glutamine. Glycine conjugation of bromsulphthalein is used as a test of hepatic function. *Methylation*, e.g. adrenaline.

Phase 1 and phase 2 reactions may be impaired in neonates. Phase 1 reactions are particularly depressed in the elderly.

Enzyme inducers enhance the metabolism of drugs by causing increased synthesis and reduced elimination of both phase 1 and 2 enzymes. They may be drugs themselves (barbiturates, phenytoin, steroids, alcohol). Hypoxia is also an enzyme inducer. Induction may be dangerous (reduced effect of warfarin after starting phenytoin), cause prolonged action if the metabolites are active (diazepam), or cause toxicity if those metabolites are harmful (halothane). Inhibitors of hepatic enzymes include cimetidine, monoamine oxidase inhibitors, tolbutamide and toxic doses of alcohol.

Excretion

1. *In bile*. For example some antibiotics, muscle relaxants, pethidine. There is active excretion of water-soluble drugs or metabolites with a molecular weight above 350. Biliary excretion may reach saturation. Free drug may be liberated in the gut and reabsorbed, e.g. fentanyl (enterohepatic circulation). Some drugs (ketamine, lignocaine) have a high *intrinsic hepatic clearance*, and are almost completely removed from plasma in one hepatic circulation. Their clearance is therefore dependent on liver blood flow.

2. *In urine*. By glomerular filtration if the drug is not protein-bound, or active secretion by the proximal tubule. Both acidic and basic drugs have specific transport mechanisms in the proximal tubule, but they do not usually interfere with each other. Probenecid inhibits secretion of acidic drugs (penicillin). Thiazides inhibit urate secretion. Basic drugs cleared at the proximal tubule include dopamine, lignocaine, morphine and neostigmine. Distal tubular diffusion of the non-ionized forms of drugs promotes excretion of basic drugs if the urine is more acid, and of acidic drugs if the urine is more alkaline.

$$\text{Renal clearance} = \text{urine flow} \times \frac{\text{urine concentration}}{\text{plasma concentration}}$$

3. *In expired gas*. The common and efficient route for inhalation agents. Other drugs are partially eliminated by this route (alcohol and paraldehyde).

4. *In milk or saliva*. For example narcotic and hypnotic drugs.

Pharmacokinetic terminology

Compartmental models. A bolus of drug is distributed into one compartment (the plasma), which may communicate with other compartments (representing the rest of the body). A two-compartment model is adequate to describe the distribution of many drugs, although more compartments are likely to provide greater accuracy.

In *zero-order or non-linear* kinetics, the rate of elimination or distribution of a drug is independent of its concentration (alcohol, or at high concentrations of phenytoin or thiopentone when enzymes are saturated).

In *first-order or linear* kinetics, elimination (and the movement of the drug between compartments) is an exponential process, i.e. the rate of change is proportional to the absolute value. In the simplest one-compartment model, the decline of concentration C with time t is described by:

$$-dC/dt = kC$$

or:

$C = C_o.e^{-kt}$ where C_o is the initial concentration at zero time.

The *elimination rate constant* is k, and defines the fraction of drug that is eliminated in unit time. The *time constant* is the time taken for the concentration to decline to 1/e of its initial value, and equals 1/k. The *half-life* ($t_{1/2}$) is the time taken for the concentration to be halved, and equals $(\log_e 2)/k$ or 0.693/k.

In a multi-compartment model, decline of plasma concentration is multi-exponential. In the commonly-used two-compartment model, the bi-exponential decline is characterized by an initial rapid distribution phase, the α phase, distribution half-life $T_{1/2\alpha}$, followed by a slower elimination phase, the β phase, elimination half-life $T_{1/2\beta}$.

Volume of distribution (Vd) is the apparent volume of water into which a drug disperses after administration. It is calculated from the initial dilution by extrapolating the concentration-time curve back to time zero.

Volume of distribution at steady state (Vd_{ss}) is used for multi-compartment models. It is the apparent volume of water into which a drug disperses, measured by its dilution in a steady state, when the drug is being administered and there is no net loss or gain. It is the amount of drug in the body divided by its plasma concentration. If this volume equals plasma volume, it suggests that the drug remains in the vascular space. If smaller than plasma volume, binding to plasma proteins is likely; if larger than the whole body water, this implies uptake in fat or tissue proteins.

Clearance is the volume of plasma from which a drug is completely removed in unit time. It equals: $k \times Vd$ or $(0.693 \times Vd)/T_{1/2\beta}$

For a multi-compartment model it also may be calculated as:

$$\frac{\text{Total dose administered}}{\text{Area under the concentration–time curve}}$$

Thus drug half-life depends on the two independent variables, clearance and volume of distribution.

Extraction ratio of a drug by a particular organ is the fraction cleared at each pass, or its arteriovenous concentration difference divided by the arterial concentration. *Organ clearance* is organ blood flow × the extraction ratio. Total clearance is the sum of all individual organ clearances. Renal clearance can be measured separately to assess the contribution made by the kidneys to total body clearance.

PHARMACODYNAMICS

Pharmacodynamics concerns drug action (what a drug does to the body), which is affected by:

1. *Physico-chemical properties*, e.g. volatile anaesthetics, chelating agents and antacids.

2. *Enzyme inhibition*, e.g. aspirin, neostigmine, penicillin and monoamine oxidase inhibitors.

3. *Receptor action*, in which receptors specific for certain drugs or groups of drugs have a high affinity for small concentrations of agonists, and a variable degree of reversibility in response to changing drug concentration. The fraction of the receptors occupied is $[D]/(K_D+[D])$ where $[D]$ is drug concentration and K_D is the dissociation constant of the drug-receptor complex. This equation is analogous to the Michaelis-Menten equation for the interaction of an enzyme with its substrate. The dose-response curve is

thus hyperbolic, but the sigmoid log(dose)–response curve is often used as it displays a wide range of doses.

Receptors are usually large glycoproteins (MW 50000–500000) spanning the cell membrane, but can be intracellular. The glycosylation site is outside and binds the drug. Receptor activation may open or close ion channels (fast); may influence G proteins in the membrane that have a binding site for a guanine nucleotide, activate membrane enzymes, and produce 'second messengers' (e.g. cyclic AMP at β-receptors) to influence intracellular events (intermediate speed);[4] or affect DNA transcription, e.g. thyroid hormones, steroids, (slow).

Agonists and antagonists

Agonists combine with receptors to initiate a response. Competitive antagonists combine with, and block, receptors but produce no response. Non-competitive antagonists (e.g. high-dose phenoxybenzamine) have exceptionally strong receptor affinity. Partial agonists can produce a response, but always less than that caused by a full agonist. The ratio of its greatest response to that of a full agonist is its *intrinsic activity*. At low concentrations of a full agonist, when free receptors are plentiful, a partial agonist will augment the response, but will reduce the response at higher concentrations of the full agonist.

Some β-blockers (e.g. propranolol) have minimal agonist or 'intrinsic sympathomimetic' activity. Others have strong partial agonist activity (e.g. oxprenolol). The opioids also range from pure agonists (e.g. pethidine and fentanyl) through partial agonists (e.g. nalorphine and buprenorphine) to the almost pure antagonist, naloxone. Some opioids are agonists at one type of receptor but antagonists at another, e.g. nalbuphine and buprenorphine are mu agonists but kappa antagonists. The kappa activity of opioids may be *potentiated* by clonidine.

Efficacy is the maximum effect of an agonist. *Potency* is the dose required to produce a given effect, and allows comparison of the *dose equivalence* of different drugs.

Hysteresis is when the effect of a given plasma concentration is less when it is rising than when it is falling. It is due to relatively slow access from plasma to receptor, or slow kinetics of the receptor itself.

Chemotherapeutic index or ratio is the mean lethal dose divided by the mean effective dose, i.e. LD_{50}/ED_{50}, or kill/cure doses. *Tolerance* describes a decreasing response to a drug, despite a constant plasma level. It may be due to *down-regulation*, a change in receptor numbers, e.g. repeated exposure to adrenergic bronchodilators. Other causes include enzyme induction, or exhaustion of a transmitter, e.g. indirectly-acting sympathomimetics, sometimes called *tachyphylaxis*.

References

1. Hladky S. B. *Pharmacokinetics*. Manchester: Manchester University Press, 1990.
2. Greenbaum R. *Anaesthesia* 1987, **42**, 927; Editorial, *Lancet* 1988, **1**, 743.
3. Bretschneider H. *Anesth. Analg.* 1987, **66**, 361.
4. Maze M. *Anesthesiology* 1990, **72**, 959.

Chapter 3

Physics[1]

BEHAVIOUR OF GASES

Kinetic theory states that gas molecules are continually moving. Collisions with the walls of any enclosing space give rise to the pressure of the gas in the space. The more molecules, the greater the pressure. Temperature makes them move faster, have more vigorous and frequent collisions, and so increases pressure.

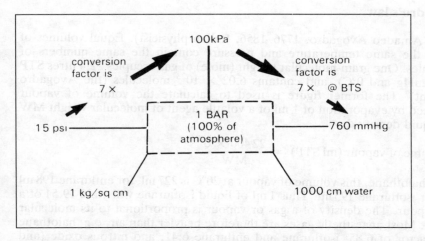

Fig. 3.1 Equivalent pressures in different units (a rough approximation). For exact values *see* Appendix

Pressure is force per unit area. 1 pascal = 1 newton per m². Standard atmospheric pressure is 760 mmHg = 1.033 kg/cm² = 14.7 lb/in² = 101.325 kPa = 1.01325 bar. 1 torr = 1 mmHg (Evangelista Torricelli, 1608–1647, Italian physicist).

Boyle's law

(1662; Robert Boyle, 1627–1691, English chemist). The volume V of a given quantity of gas varies inversely with the pressure P to which it is subjected, if the temperature remains constant.

Charles' law

(1787; Jacques Alexandre Cesar Charles, 1746–1823, French physicist). The volume of a given quantity of gas is proportional to its absolute temperature T, if its pressure remains constant. (T = Centigrade temperature + 273°.)

Boyle's and Charles' laws can be expressed as PV = nRT for ideal gases, where n is the number of moles of gas present and R is the molar gas constant.

Dalton's law of partial pressures

(1801; John Dalton, 1766–1844, Manchester chemist). The pressure of a component gas in a mixture of gases equals the pressure which that quantity of gas would produce were it alone. Thus the total pressure of a mixture of gases equals the sum of the individual partial pressures. The partial pressure of a gas in a mixture is its percentage by volume divided by the total gas pressure.

Avogadro's law

(1811; Amadeo Avogadro, 1776–1856, Italian physicist). Equal volumes of gas at the same temperature and pressure contain the same numbers of molecules. One gram-molecular weight (mole) of gas occupies 22.4 litres STP (760 mmHg and 0°C), and contains 6.02×10^{23} molecules (the Avogadro constant). The former figure is used to calculate the volume of vapour produced by evaporation of 1 ml of a volatile agent of molecular weight MW and liquid density d:

$$\text{Volume of vapour (ml STP)} = \frac{22\,400 \times d}{MW}$$

For halothane, this volume of vapour at 20°C is 227 ml, for enflurane 198 ml and for isoflurane 195 ml. Thus 1 ml of liquid isoflurane will yield 19.5 l of a 1% vapour. The density of a gas or vapour is proportional to its molecular weight. Most anaesthetic gases are therefore heavier than air, e.g. halothane by a factor of 6.85; isoflurane and enflurane 6.41; and nitrous oxide (and CO_2) 1.53. Water vapour is only 0.63 times the density of air. The figure for helium is 0.14.

Graham's law of diffusion of gases

(1831; Thomas Graham, 1805–1869, Scottish physician and chemist). The rate of diffusion of a gas varies inversely as the square root of its density or molecular weight.

Henry's law of solution of gases

(1803; William Henry, 1774–1836, English chemist).[2] If equilibrium is established between a gas and a liquid exposed to it, the partial pressure (or tension) of the gas in the liquid equals its partial pressure in the gas phase. Henry's law states that the amount of gas dissolved at any temperature is proportional to its partial pressure. The lower the temperature, the more can dissolve.

Solubility of gas in liquid

(1894; Wilhelm Ostwald, 1853–1932, Russian-German physical chemist. Nobel prize-winner, 1909). The *Ostwald coefficient* (λ) is the amount of gas which dissolves in unit volume of solvent, measured under the conditions of temperature and pressure at which solution takes place. The *Bunsen coefficient* (α) is the amount of gas at STP which dissolves in unit volume of solvent at a partial pressure of 760 mmHg. The two coefficents are related by:

$$\lambda = \frac{\alpha \times \text{absolute temperature of solvent}}{273}$$

and are identical at 0°C. The *partition coefficient* of a gas between two phases or solvents is the ratio of the amounts dissolved in equal volumes of each. If one phase is gas, it is the same as the Ostwald coefficient. It is useful in anaesthesia because it can be used to calculate distributions between any two solvents, whether liquid or solid (e.g. rubber). Solution in rubber may slow the build-up of concentration in a closed circuit.

Vapours

An 'ideal' gas, in which the only interactions between molecules are collisions, cannot be liquefied. This is not true for a real gas provided the temperature is low enough and the pressure high enough. Above its *critical temperature*, a gas cannot be liquefied, however high the pressure. The *critical pressure* is that needed to liquefy a gas at its critical temperature. A *vapour* is a gas below its critical temperature, although the two terms are often used imprecisely. At room temperature both CO_2 and nitrous oxide are vapours.

When a vapour is in equilibrium with its liquid, it is said to be *saturated*, and its pressure is the *saturated vapour pressure* (SVP). SVP increases non-linearly with temperature, and can be calculated from the Antoine equation.[3] The *boiling point* of a liquid is the temperature at which the saturated vapour pressure equals the ambient atmospheric pressure. *Relative humidity* is the actual water vapour pressure as a percentage of the SVP at a given temperature.

OSMOTIC PRESSURE

Osmosis is the migration of solvent (usually water) into a compartment where the concentration of solute is higher, across a membrane that is permeable to the solvent but not to the solute. The pressure required to prevent this migration is the osmotic pressure, measured as osmolarity (osmol/l of solution, e.g. plasma) or osmolality (osmol/kg of solvent). For dilute solutions in water these are nearly equal and often used interchangeably.

An osmole (osmol) of a substance is its molecular weight in grams divided by the number of freely moving particles each molecule liberates in solution. When an osmole of a substance is dissolved in one litre of water, it exerts an osmotic pressure of 22.4 atmospheres. Osmolarity and osmolality of solutions are measured by the degree to which the freezing point is depressed. A solution of strength of 1 osmol/l depresses the freezing point 1.86°C. The freezing point of human plasma is −0.54°C and the osmolarity 290 mosmol/l. An approximate plasma osmolarity may be calculated by adding the molar concentrations of glucose and urea to twice the sodium concentration.

FLUID FLOW

A Newtonian fluid (e.g. water) is one in which shear rate is proportional to shear stress. Thus the ratio of shear stress to shear rate (viscosity) is independent of flow rate. Blood is non-Newtonian: its viscosity increases at low shear rates.

Laminar flow through tubes

Poiseuille's (1799–1868) Law:[4] for laminar flow through tubes, the flow rate is directly proportional to the perfusion pressure, but proportional to the fourth power of the radius:

$$\dot{Q} \alpha \frac{\pi(P_1 - P_2)r^4}{8\eta l}$$

where $\dot{Q}$ = flow rate, P_1 and P_2 are the pressures at each end of the tube, r and l = radius and length of the tube, η = viscosity of the fluid.

Turbulent flow through tubes

Turbulent flow through a tube occurs when flow exceeds a critical value. Turbulence is facilitated by irregularities and corners in the tube. Conversion from laminar to turbulent flow increases resistance, which itself becomes roughly proportional to flow. The dimensionless Reynolds number[5] (Re) must exceed 2000 for turbulence to occur:

$$Re = \frac{\text{diameter} \times \text{density} \times \text{average velocity}}{\text{viscosity}}$$

Flow through orifices

An orifice is an opening whose length is much less than its diameter. It causes turbulence and the resistance to flow is related to gas density rather than viscosity. Helium–oxygen mixtures may be useful in upper airway obstruction (*see* Chapter 8). In rotameters, the gas flow around the bobbin is laminar at low flow rates, so viscosity is important. At higher flows, the annular aperture around the bobbin resembles an orifice, and density is important.

Venturi principle

Described in 1797 (Giovanni Battista Venturi, 1746–1822, Italian physicist). When a fluid flows through a tube of varying diameter, the pressure is lowest at the point of maximum velocity, because pressure energy drops as kinetic energy increases — Bernoulli's Law (Daniel Bernoulli, 1700-1782). With suitable flow and a 'venturi' cone-shaped tube, sub-atmospheric pressure can easily be produced. The injector replaces the smooth construction of a venturi tube with a nozzle through which fluid is injected at high velocity. Surrounding fluids are thus sucked in with the main stream. Examples of clinical application: (1) suction apparatus; (2) entrainment of air or oxygen, in oxygen therapy; (3) jet ventilation, e.g. by Sander's injector during bronchoscopy.

Measurement of gas flow

(1) Rotameter (e.g. anaesthetic flow-meters); (2) pneumotachograph; (3) thermal dilution; (4) electromagnetic; (5) mechanical (e.g. Wright's respirometer); (6) other anemometers (e.g. hot wire); (7) bubble flow-meter; and (8) doppler principle.

HEAT

One calorie raises the temperature of 1 g of water by 1°C, and equals 4.2 joule. The *specific heat* is the amount of heat energy required to raise 1 kg of a substance by 1°C.

The *latent heat* of vaporization is the quantity of heat required to change unit mass of a substance from liquid to vapour without change of temperature. The latent heat of melting is the quantity of heat required to change unit mass of a substance from solid to liquid without change of temperature.

Heat may be transferred by conduction, convection, radiation, evaporation or addition or subtraction of warm or cold fluids from a body. *Thermal conductivity* is the rate of heat transfer per unit area per unit temperature gradient. A 'black body' absorbs all incident radiation. Although the melanin in the skin of coloured people absorbs visible wavelengths, both white and coloured races absorb infra-red radiation. Therefore, for the purposes of heat balance, the skin of all patients acts like a black body radiator.

For temperature measurement *see* Chapter 18.

RADIATION

Marie (1867–1934) and Pierre (1859–1906) Curie isolated radium in 1898.[6] Wilhelm von Röntgen (1845–1923, Würzburg physicist) discovered X-radiation in 1895.[7]

Alpha particles are positively charged helium nuclei, beta particles are electrons. Beta particles have a lower mass, higher velocity and are more penetrative. Gamma and X-rays are part of the spectrum of electromagnetic radiation and are highly penetrative.

The bequerel (Bq) is the SI unit of radioactivity and is one nuclear transformation per second. 1 curie (the old unit) $= 3.7 \times 10^{10}$ Bq. The gray (Gy) is the SI unit of absorbed dose of ionizing radiation and is 1 J/kg. 1 Gy = 100 rad (Röntgen absorbed dose, the old unit). The sievert (Sv) is the SI unit of dose equivalent which allows for the relative effects of different types of radiation. It is approximately equal to 1 Gy or 100 rem (the old unit), and used for recommended limits of exposure for patients and health care workers. A chest radiograph results in a dose of about 0.25 mSv, a CT scan up to 20 mSv. The average environmental exposure in the UK is 1.9 mSv/year; maximum total body exposure for the public is 5 mSv/year (subject to an average dose limit of 1 mSv/year); maximum exposure for most organs of the body is 50 mSv/year; radiation workers are allowed to receive 10 times this amount; exposure to 10 Sv is always fatal.

ELECTRICITY

Charge is the amount of electricity associated with an object. *Current* is the flow of electrical charge. One coulomb is the charge transferred when 1 ampere (A) flows for 1 sec. *Static electricity* is the charge produced by rubbing two dissimilar materials together. It can produce sparks of intense heat when it discharges by contact with a conductor.

Potential difference (or electromotive force) is analogous to pressure difference. Two points in an electric circuit have a potential difference of 1 volt (V) if 1 J of energy is released when 1 coulomb of electricity is transferred.

Resistance to flow of electricity is measured in ohms. Ohm's law described in 1827 (Georg Ohm, 1787–1854, German physicist) states that 'the ratio of the potential difference between the ends of a conductor to the current flowing in it is always constant, provided that the physical conditions of the conductor such as temperature remain constant'. This ratio is the resistance (R):

$$R = \frac{E}{I}$$

where E = potential difference in volts, I = current in amps. If the resistance is 1 ohm then a potential difference of 1 V will result in the flow of 1 A. Resistances in series are additive, i.e. R = (R₁ + R₂); but if placed in parallel:

$$\frac{1}{R} = \frac{1}{R_1} + \frac{1}{R_2}$$

Electrical power is measured in watts (W) = J/sec. Watts = volts × amps.

A *capacitor* is a store for electric charge. Its capacitance (measured in farads) is the coulombs stored per volt potential difference. An *inductor* is a conductor that resists any change in current passing through it. A *transistor* is a controllable semi-conductor switching device that can allow accurate amplification of a signal. A *transducer* is a device that converts one form of energy to another, usually electrical.

Surgical diathermy[8]

First used by Harvey Cushing in neurosurgery.[9] Diathermy is a radio-frequency (0.3–3 MHz) power oscillation with the patient forming part of the circuit, producing intense heat (over 1000°C) at the small electrode which the surgeon uses in the wound, and only slight warmth in the area of the large 'earth-plate'. Modern transistor apparatus uses the higher frequencies and a continuous current for cutting, and uses the lower frequencies in 20 msec bursts for coagulation. The power used is 50–400 W and the current through the patient about 200–400 mA, but may be 2 A during urological resection. Fortunately, radiofrequency AC is very poor at causing ventricular fibrillation. Modern machines may be isolated from earth to help prevent mains electrocution.[10]

The apparatus may cause explosions, or interfere with monitors and cardiac pacemakers. Monitor interference may be reduced by using a completely different power point. Poor contact of the earth-plate with skin may cause burns. A broken earth-plate lead may cause the patient to earth himself to part of the operating table and thus acquire a burn. A sparking earth-plate lead may ignite a spirit-based skin preparation. Unintended use when the active electrode is touching the wrong part of the patient, or a surgeon or assistant, may cause a burn. Diathermy in the mouth has caused a tracheal tube to ignite. Intestinal gases may be flammable and opening a colostomy with diathermy has caused an explosion.[11] Bipolar diathermy, where the current just passes from one blade of a forceps to the other, uses less power and interferes least with monitors and pacemakers.

Electrocution

Mains frequency (50 Hz in UK, 60 Hz in USA) is particularly effective in producing ventricular fibrillation. Dry skin resistance may be 1 Mohms/cm², which can be reduced to 500 ohms by electrode jelly. 1 mA AC or 5 mA DC gives a tingling feeling in the skin, 15 mA AC or 75 mA DC causes muscle contraction, and over 70 mA AC or 300 mA DC may cause ventricular fibrillation (this current need only flow for less than 20 ms). As little as 44 µA may cause ventricular fibrillation if applied direct to the heart.[12] Direct current flowing through skin can destroy tissue giving a 'punched-out' open sore.

Execution by the electric chair uses a current of 5–10 A, *see* Jones G. R. N. *Lancet* 1990, **335**, 713.

Safety precautions

The patient should be isolated from earth if possible, perhaps incorporating a transformer in the power supply. He should be protected from the metal of the table, which is capacitively coupled to earth at diathermy frequencies. The current between any electrode and earth should not be more than 10 µA (for ECG, etc.). Diathermy should make an audible noise when activated, and the electrode sheathed when not in use. Earth-free solid-state or battery powered diathermy sets are preferred. With any monitoring or diathermy equipment, leakage current between mains supply and patient circuit must not exceed 0.1 mA; if it does, the mains should be automatically isolated with an alarm. Household earth leakage circuit breakers are not suitable for use with anaesthetic equipment. Correct wiring in mains plug: in Europe, brown = live, blue = neutral, green/yellow = earth. Electrical distribution boards may be hazardous.[13]

Vascular catheters should be filled with dextrose, not saline, and needle electrodes avoided where possible. For diathermy in the presence of a cardiac pacemaker, *see* Chapter 20.

Interference with monitors can be reduced by keeping patient impedance relatively low, keeping the source of the interference as far from the monitor as possible, screening the monitor and its leads and earthing the screen, using twisted leads in high-voltage lines, and rearranging the position of the monitor and its leads.

See also the excellent *Hospital Technical Memoranda.* HTM1 Antistatic precautions, rubber, plastic and fabrics; HTM2 Antistatic precautions, flooring in anaesthetizing areas; HTM22 Piped medical gases, medical compressed air and medical vacuum installations. The safety requirements of medical electrical equipment is contained in IEC document 601–1, and adopted in the UK as BS 5724 (1979).

FIRES AND EXPLOSIONS[1]

The risks involved with the use of flammable anaesthetic agents have diminished greatly as these agents are now infrequently used. Elaborate precautions needed to minimize the possibility of sparks in operating theatres are often unnecessary.

Certain anaesthetic gases and vapours, such as diethyl and divinyl ether, ethyl chloride and cyclopropane, form flammable mixtures with air or oxygen. Nitrous oxide also supports combustion strongly. Mixtures corresponding exactly with the chemical equation, so that combustion is complete (*stoichiometric*) are most easily ignited and generate the most powerful deflagrations. There are limits of flammability, when the mixture becomes too weak, or the oxygen content too low.

Detonations or explosions are usually associated with a high oxygen content in the mixture, and are produced by an exothermic chemical reaction. Before an explosion can occur, a source of heat sufficient to raise a liquid to its flash point, or a vapour to its ignition temperature, is required. This is called the 'activation energy'. Halothane, enflurane and isoflurane are non-flammable and non-explosive at room temperature in either air or oxygen at normal concentrations. In a 30%/70% O_2/N_2O mixture they can only be ignited at concentrations above 4.75%, 5.75% and 7.0% respectively, and so can be regarded as nearly non-flammable under clinical conditions.

Sources of ignition

Heat. From hot surfaces, wires, thermocautery. The minimal temperature that will ignite a flammable vapour in air is around 400–500°C.

Electric current. Either in normal use, e.g. diathermy, electric cautery, monitors, sparks from electric motors, switches etc.; or as a result of faulty short-circuits.

Static electricity. Electric charge may be produced by many objects made from non-conducting materials such as rubber, plastic, wool and artificial fibres.

Spontaneous ignition. A rapid pressure rise causes a gas to get hotter. Any oil or grease in contact with nitrous oxide or oxygen may ignite when a cylinder is opened. Lubricants must not be used on reducing valves and cylinders. Open cylinder valves slowly.

Alcohol-based skin preparation solutions are flammable, and can pool in skin creases. Flammable gases such as hydrogen and methane may be found in the bowel, and flammable materials may be produced by the decomposition of tissues and water as a result of diathermy or cautery. When diathermy is applied to the bladder, hydrogen is given off and may ignite. Lasers in or near the airway may ignite vapours and rubber or plastic equipment.

Some recommendations for prevention

1. Avoid flammable agents. Much medical electrical equipment used now is unsafe in their presence.

2. Electrical medical equipment used between 5 and 25 cm of any potential leak of flammable anaesthetic agents must be 'anaesthetic-proof' (AP), which is designated by a symbol of a green dot or band bearing the letters AP inside an inverted triangle. Equipment used within 5 cm of a potential leak, or used within the gas circuit, must be anaesthetic-proof category G equipment (APG).

3. Static sparks are more frequent when the air is dry and the barometric pressure high. Keep the relative humidity above 60%.

4. Conducting 'antistatic' rubber (incorporating carbon black during its manufacture) in contact with a conducting floor will effectively earth equipment in theatre. Overall resistance between different objects should be 0.1 to 10 Mohms. The resistance between two electrodes 600 mm apart in new floors should lie between 50 000 ohms and 2 Mohms. Resistance of antistatic rubber may increase with age. Footwear should have a resistance between 0.1 and 1 Mohms per shoe (if less than 0.1 Mohms there is a danger of accidental electrocution on contact with high voltages). Cotton is a suitable for clothing because its resistance drops markedly in normal moist room air. The resistance of the patient's breathing tubing should lie between 25 kohms and 1 Mohms per 1.5 m.

5. Rooms where explosive anaesthetics are used should ideally have 5–10 air changes per hour. Air inlets should be at least 2 m above floor level and air outlets at floor level.

References

1. *See also* Macintosh R. R., Mushin W. W. and Epstein H. G., *Physics for the Anaesthetist*. 4th ed. Oxford: Blackwell 1987; Moyle J. T. B. In: *Anaesthesia Review 6*. (Kaufman L. ed.) Edinburgh: Churchill Livingstone 1989, 257; Parbrook G. D. et al. *Basic Physics and Measurement in Anaesthesia*, 3rd ed. Guildford: Butterworth-Heinemann 1990.
2. Henry W. *Phil. Trans. R. Soc.* 1803. **93**, 29.
3. Rodgers R. C. and Hill G. E. *Br. J. Anaesth.* 1978, **50**, 415.
4. Poiseuille J. L. M. *C. R. Acad. Sci. Paris* 1840, **11**, 1041; Hagen A. *Ann. Phys. Leipzig* 1839, **46**, 423.
5. Reynolds O. *Phil. Trans.* 1883, **174**, 935.
6. Curie M. and Curie P. *C. R. Acad. Sci. Paris* 1898, **127**, 175, 1215.
7. von Röntgen W. C. *S. B. d. Phys. Med. Ges. zu Würzb.* 1895, 132.
8. Nagelschmidt F. *Münch. Med. Wochenschr.* 1909, **56**, 2575.
9. Cushing H. and Bovie W. T. *Surg. Gynecol. Obstet.* 1928, **47**, 751; Goldwyn R. M. *Ann. Plast. Surg.* 1979, **2**, 135.
10. Mackintosh I. P. and Zorab J. S. M. In: *Surgery for Anaesthetists* (Zorab J. S. M. ed.) Oxford: Blackwell 1988, 5.
11. Barrkman M. F. *Br. Med. J.* 1965, **1**, 1594.
12. Hull C. J. *Br. J. Anaesth.* 1978, **50**, 647.
13. Nieman M. et al. *Anaesthesia* 1988, **43**, 584.

Chapter 4

Computing, clinical trials and statistics

COMPUTERS

Microprocessors and computers have now pervaded the operating theatre, and have proved good servants for anaesthetists, but as yet poor masters. Some monitors (e.g. pulse oximeters) require observation; other equipment is more reliable and accurate, and demands less attention from its user (e.g. automatic blood pressure recorders). But paperwork has not lessened, and indeed has proliferated. Data storage can be corrupted by a trivial insult and needs careful backup. If complete reliance is placed on computers, a minor electronic problem can lead to major chaos.

Computers have been used in several areas of anaesthesia:

Equipment. (a) Most commonly in non-invasive monitors, such as oxygen saturation and blood pressure.[1] Artefact rejection is not always satisfactory; (b) to analyse a repetitive analogue signal such as the ECG, and measure rate or detect arrhythmias; (c) to present what otherwise would be a mass of data in a way that is accessible to the anaesthetist, such as the EEG;[2] (d) to control and automatically calibrate other monitors, e.g. neuromuscular transmission, gas concentrations. Sometimes it is possible to share (multiplex) an expensive monitor such as a mass spectrometer between several patients;[3] (e) to control and monitor the function of the anaesthetic machine itself. A sophisticated example, with many sensors, is from Utah;[4] (f) to enable the telemetry of data; and (g) to provide intelligent alarms for all monitors.

Automatic Administration of Drugs. When a drug is given to achieve a result that can be readily monitored, computer-controlled feed-back to syringe pumps is feasible. This may achieve the desired response faster and more smoothly, e.g. vasoactive drugs to control blood pressure,[5] muscle relaxants while monitoring the EMG,[6] insulin to regulate blood sugar, volatile agents to achieve an end-tidal value,[7] and opioids using a pharmacokinetic model to predict a plasma level.[8] A reliable monitor of depth of anaesthesia would provide a strong impetus to this work.

Anaesthetic Record. May be based on the automatic record[9] that can be generated from most monitors. Some data has to be entered manually, such as pre-operative assessment, techniques used, drug and fluid administration, complications and instructions to recovery staff. It is this interface between the anaesthetist and the computer that has been the weak link, especially in a crisis, although a keyboard, barcodes, touch-responsive screen, light pen and digitizing pad have all been tried. Voice synthesis and recognition may ultimately be more successful.[10]

These systems[11] are expensive, cannot reject artefacts and paperwork is still needed. Clinical judgement is still essential. There is lack of agreement over what constitutes a complete record. Their big advantage is that, unlike paper records, in which one record relates to one anaesthetic on one patient, automatic records are relational, i.e. for large-scale audit, the database can be accessed for operations, drugs, etc. on many patients. To be widely accepted they will have to show greater reliability or a reduction in the anaesthetist's workload. Some 11% of an anaesthetist's time may be consumed by keeping a manual record.[12] For the Data Protection Act, *see* Chapter 19.

Audit.[13] *See* Chapter 19.

Education and Research. To collect, analyse, present and store research data, especially in large-scale studies. In pharmacokinetic and physiological modelling.[14] Computer-based simulators[15] have been developed to teach all aspects of anaesthesia, from screen-based 'flight simulators',[16] the response to various critical incidents,[17] to a device such as CASE, a sophisticated simulator complete with mannequin, anaesthetic machine and monitors.[18] Computers are already used to mark examination papers, but simulators could form an important part of examinations. Full electronic retrieval of journals should soon be possible.[19]

Departmental Organization. Helping with the pre-anaesthetic interview,[20] scheduling operations and anaesthetists,[21] and billing.

Artificial Intelligence. This involves strategies and methods of using a database of facts and rules,[22] and may play a large part in future diagnosis and management of patients. A well-known system developed for anaesthetic management is ATTENDING.[23] The doctor needs confidence in the safety of such systems.[24]

CLINICAL TRIALS[25]

Clinical trials of new drugs offer considerable challenges. It is difficult to: (1) ensure similarity between two or more groups of patients, except for the factor under investigation; and (2) eliminate observer or operator bias. The fact that clinical trials are performed in a controlled environment limits the application of any knowledge gained to situations outside that environment.

Planning of trials

This must include consideration of:

1. The hypothesis to be tested should be simple. The *null hypothesis* form the basis of much statistical testing, i.e. that there is no difference between two treatments.

2. Control group. If the patient is not his own control, matching must consider sex, age, disease severity, etc. For instance, females are more prone to postoperative nausea than males.

3. Randomization[26] of the members of a group is often needed to eliminate bias. Tables of random numbers are available.

4. Accompaniments of anaesthesia, such as altered respiration, changes in cardiac output and posture may affect observations.

5. Dosage and route of administration of drugs. Results obtained in a clinical trial may not apply to different doses or routes.

6. Persons carrying out trials of a technique are often more skilled, e.g. local blocks.

7. The number of patients studied must be appropriate for the size of the effect that is sought. Too few may not reveal uncommon side-effects, especially if the operator is not looking for them. Too many is wasteful, may be unethical or deny advances in therapy to some patients. A statistician should be involved from the beginning.

There is a difference between statistically and clinically significant observations. If many patients have been required to demonstrate a statistically significant effect, the clinician must judge whether it is sufficient to affect clinical practice.

Investigation of a new drug

There are various stages of investigation before clinical release:

1. Chemical tests of purity and, where appropriate, tests for bacterial sterility.

2. In animals. Tests of activity, potency and side-effects: minimum lethal dose on large numbers of small animals, effects on cardiovascular, respiratory, central and autonomic nervous systems, hepatotoxicity, nephrotoxicity and teratogenicity. Wide species variation may mean that potential hazards to man are missed, or may hinder investigation of valuable therapeutic agents.

3. In humans. The use of healthy volunteers is limited to small numbers and it is not possible to investigate effects on disease. In the UK, the Committee on Safety of Medicines looks continuously at new drug submissions. Doctors wishing to conduct trials themselves can apply for the Committee's approval. It may be unethical to pay volunteers, or to use volunteers from prisons or mental institutions, especially with incentives of reduction in sentence. The use of placebos may not be ethical.

Clinical trials in patients should be planned to obtain the maximum amount of unbiased information, from the minimum number of patients, in the shortest time and with the least potential hazard and inconvenience. Protocols must be sanctioned by the appropriate ethical committee and rejected if badly designed. Patients should not be submitted to known hazards, and invasive measurements may not be justified. Informed consent should be obtained. A pilot study is usually wise.

Blind trials[27]

Designed to eliminate observer bias. A *single-blind* trial means the patient is unaware of the treatment he is receiving. In a *double-blind* trial, the observers are also unaware. Blindness may not be achieved because of some obvious difference in physical or pharmacological properties of substances under test, and observer bias is likely. Identical preparations of active drug and placebo should be prepared. The key to such a trial must be available in case of an emergency.

STATISTICS[27]

Defined as numerical facts systematically collected, on a given subject. A pioneer was W. Farr (1807–1883), who wrote the classic *Vital Statistics*.[28] He agreed with John Snow, following the cholera epidemic in Newcastle upon Tyne in 1853, that the disease was due to contaminated water (after first opposing the theory). *Descriptive* statistics are used to summarize data, *inferential* statistical tests are used to draw conclusions, e.g. whether results obtained from a small sample of patients apply to a large population.

Descriptive statistical terms

The *mean* is the sum of the observations divided by their number. The *median* is the observation which has half the number of observations lying above and half below it, on a distribution curve. The *mode* is the most frequent observation, the highest point on the curve. The *range* is the difference between the smallest and largest observation. It may be useful to divide the range into four *quartiles*, each containing an equal number of observations. The *normal* or Gaussian distribution is a symmetrical, bell-shaped curve, and *parametric* tests may be used to draw conclusions. Otherwise non-parametric tests should be used.

Variance is a measure of the scatter of observations around their mean. It is the sum of the squares of the differences between the individual observation and their mean, divided by their number:

$$\frac{\Sigma(\bar{x} - x)^2}{n}$$

Standard deviation (SD or sigma, σ) is the square root of the variance. For a normal distribution, 68% of data lies within 1 SD of the mean, 95% within 2 SD, and 99.7% within 3 SD. *Standard error of the mean* (SEM) is SD divided by the square root of n. These terms are used to describe the scatter of symmetric data, but if it is skewed then the range or quartiles may be better. More reliable estimates of variability in the general population are obtained by using $(n - 1)$ rather than n, especially when the sample size is small. The *coefficient of variation* is the SD as a percentage of the mean.

A *linear analogue scale*[29] may be used to assess, e.g. severity of pain. The patient is asked to mark a point on a line, where the scale ranges from zero (no pain at all) to a maximum, say 10 (the most that can be imagined).

Inferential tests

These test the data to calculate (for example) a *probability*, P, of the differences between two groups being due to chance. $P < 0.05$ means that the probability of an event occurring by chance is less than 5% (1 in 20), and is a commonly-chosen level of statistical significance. Such a result is not necessarily of clinical importance. A type I error is when the null hypothesis is wrongly rejected (no difference really existed), and a type II error when it is wrongly accepted (and a real difference exists between the groups).

Differences between means. With reasonably large numbers of observations (25–30) the *standard error of the difference between two means* may be taken to be the square root of the sum of the squares of the two individual standard errors of the separate means in the two samples. A difference of more than twice this SE may be accepted as significant, $P < 0.05$. With smaller numbers, the *t-test* is more appropriate.

Student's t test.[30] May be applied when the observations are 30 or less. A calculation of 't' is made, the observed difference between the sample means divided by the calculated standard error of the difference between the means. A table of t values is then used to read the P value. The distributions must be normal with similar variances.

Chi-squared test (χ^2). Tests for an association between different characteristics by comparing occurrences of data. The data is not normally distributed, but belongs to several discrete categories, e.g. numbers of patients who vomit after different drugs. It should not be used for small numbers (5 or less). χ^2 equals the sum of the squares of the difference between the observed number and the expected number, divided by the expected number. The value of χ^2 and the number of sub-groups contributing to it are used to enter tables of χ^2 which give the P value.

Sequential analysis. Can be applied when there is a simple investigation between two alternatives, e.g. comparing a single outcome of two drugs. Special charts of squared paper are used. Beginning in the bottom left-hand corner, a line of crosses can be made proceeding vertically if the first alternative occurs and horizontally if the second applies. If the drugs or procedures are carried out in matched pairs, the line of crosses will gradually extend across the graph. When the line crosses pre-drawn limits representing various P values, the result is significant at that level.

Correlation and regression. Regression analysis places a line of best fit through a group of points plotted with the independent variable on the x-axis (abscissa) and the dependent variable on the y-axis (ordinate). The regression or correlation coefficient (r) measures how scattered the data points are about this line. Values of 1 and −1 indicates a perfect fit to lines with a positive and negative slope respectively. Zero indicates no correlation.

Confidence intervals. It is common now to report the 95% confidence limits of data, rather than calculating P values, both for parametric[31] and non-parametric tests.[32]

References

1. Green M. et al. *Int. J. Clin. Monit. Comput.* 1984, **1**, 21.
2. Thomsen C. E. et al. *Br. J. Anaesth.* 1988, **63**, 36.

3. Gothard J. W. W. et al. *Anaesthesia* 1980, **35**, 890.
4. Loeb R. G. et al. *Anesthesiology* 1989, **70**, 999.
5. Meline L. J. et al. *Anesth. Analg.* 1985, **64**, 38.
6. Ritchie G. et al. *Ann. Biomed. Eng.* 1985, **13**, 3; Asbury A. J. and Linkens D. A. *Anaesthesia* 1986, **41**, 316.
7. Westenskow D. R. et al. and Zbinden A. M. et al. *Br. J. Anaesth.* 1986, **58**, 555 and 563.
8. Alvis J. M. et al. *Anesthesiology* 1985, **63**, 41; Ausems M. E. et al. *Br. J. Anaesth.* 1985, **57**, 1217.
9. Gravenstein J. S. et al. (ed.) *The Automated Anesthesia Record and Alarm Systems.* Boston: Butterworths, 1987; *Automated Anaesthetic Records* (Kenny G. N. C. ed.) *Clin. Anaesthesiol.* 1990, **4**(1).
10. Sarnat A. J. *Med. Instrum.* 1983, **17**, 25.
11. Block F. E. et al. *J. Clin. Monit.* 1985, **1**, 30; Karliczek G. F. et al. *Int. J. Clin. Monit. Comput.* 1987, **4**, 211.
12. McDonald J. S. et al. *Br. J. Anaesth.* 1990, **64**, 582.
13. Tyndall R. et al. *Computers in Medical Audit.* London: Royal Society of Medicine, 1990.
14. Philip J. H. *Int. J. Clin. Monit. Comput.* 1986, **3**, 165.
15. Gravenstein J. S. *Anesthesiology* 1988, **69**, 295; Good M. L. *Anaesthesia* 1990, **45**, 525.
16. Schwid H. *Comput. Biomed. Res.* 1987, **20**, 64.
17. Good M. L. et al. *J. Clin. Monit.* 1988, **4**, 140; Schwid H. A. and O'Donnell D. *Anesthesiology* 1990, **72**, 191.
18. Gaba D. M. and Deanda A. *Anesthesiology* 1988, **69**, 387.
19. Harris D. K. *Arch. Surg.* 1986, **121**, 1113.
20. Tompkins B. M. et al. *Anesth. Analg.* 1980, **59**, 3.
21. Ernst E. A. et al. *Anesth. Analg.* 1977, **56**, 831.
22. Shortcliffe E. H. *JAMA* 1987, **258**, 61; Greenes R. A. and Shortcliffe E. H. *JAMA* 1990, **263**, 1114.
23. Miller P. L. *Anesthesiology* 1983, **58**, 362; Miller P. L. *Int. J. Clin. Monit. Comput.* 1986, **2**, 135.
24. Brahams D. and Wyatt J. *Lancet* 1989, **ii**, 632.
25. Gore S. M. and Altman D. G. *Statistics in Practice* London: British Medical Association, 1982; Lunn J. N. (ed.) *Epidemiology in Anaesthesia.* London: Edward Arnold, 1986; *Clinical Trials* London: Medico-Pharmaceutical Forum, 1987.
26. Altman D. G. *Br. Med. J.* 1991, **302**, 1481.
27. Armitage P. and Berry G. *Statistical Methods in Medical Research* Oxford: Blackwells, 1987; Campbell M. J. and Machin D. *Medical Statistics: a commonsense approach* Chichester: John Wiley, 1989.
28. Farr W. *Vital Statistics.* London: Stanford, 1885.
29. Revill S. I. et al. *Anaesthesia* 1976, **31**, 1191.
30. Gosset W. S. *Biometrica* 1908, **6**, 1.
31. Gardner M. J. and Altman D. G. *Br. Med. J.* 1986, **292**, 746.
32. Campbell M. J. and Gardner M. J. *Br. Med. J.* 1988, **296**, 1454.

Section 2
GENERAL ANAESTHESIA

Chapter 5

Preanaesthetic assessment and premedication[1]

The patient about to undergo an operation should be assessed by an anaesthetist. In addition to taking an anaesthetic history, performing the relevant physical examination, and writing up the drugs for premedication, the anaesthetist should allow the patient to ask questions, state anxieties,[2] and be informed as to the likely plan of campaign leading up to the actual anaesthetic, and after the operation.

THE PREOPERATIVE CONSULTATION[3]

The notes and patient are checked for:
 (a) Medical history.
 (b) Current medication.
 (c) Previous anaesthetics, and their side-effects.
 (d) Current physical status.
 (e) Crowns and bridge-work on the front teeth.
 (f) A consent form, signed by patient and surgeon.
 (g) Any questions the patient may have.
 (h) Appropriate laboratory findings and availability of cross-matched blood, if required. (The patient is not accepted for anaesthesia in the absence of these.)
 Beware the 'I'll see them in the anaesthetic room' trap!
 Sedation and preoperative medication may then be prescribed.
 The incidence of medical disease in the surgical outpatient is high,[4] so that it is advantageous to see patients in the *anaesthetic outpatient clinic* at least a week before surgery. The patient should be referred to the clinic either routinely or:
 (1) when the operation is likely to be major;
 (2) when special techniques (e.g. controlled hypotension) are envisaged; and
 (3) in the presence of systemic disease (e.g. cardiovascular), which is likely to add to the risk of surgery.[5]

In the clinic, a history and examination can be undertaken and special investigations ordered. Treatment can be instituted as an outpatient to ensure the patient is as fit as possible before surgery. Autologous blood donation can be organized. When necessary, the patient can be followed up by repeated attendances at the clinic. Time of bed occupancy may thus be reduced.

Medical history

This can be facilitated by asking the patients to complete preoperative question check sheets (Fig. 5.1)

It should be noted that some patients do not tell doctors about their disabilities, e.g. muscle weakness (perhaps some denial process is responsible).

Important points to glean from the notes

1. Previous illnesses, operations and anaesthetics. Complications of previous administrations may be avoided on this occasion.

2. Drug therapy, e.g. corticosteroids, insulin, antihypertensive drugs, calcium antagonists, tranquillizers, digitalis, mono-amine oxidase inhibitors, tricyclic antidepressants, anticoagulants, oral contraceptives, barbiturates, diuretics. Drug allergies. Drug addiction.

3. Symptoms referable to the respiratory system. Respiratory reserve, cough, sputum, bronchospasm, ability to expel secretions. Smoking habits. Smoking should be discontinued prior to the anaesthetic.

4. Cardiovascular system. Previous myocardial infarction. Exercise tolerance. Anginal pain. Decompensation. Untreated hypertension is associated with increased risk to the surgical patient.[6]

5. Tendency to postanaesthetic vomiting. This will affect the choice of anaesthetic drugs.

6. Pregnancy. Non-urgent surgery should be postponed if pregnancy is suspected and menstrual history can often identify women at risk.

7. Alcohol intake. The alcoholic patient may suffer from cirrhosis of the liver, cardiomyopathy, diminished adrenocortical response to stress, electrolyte imbalance, hypoglycaemia, bone marrow depression, neuropathy and psychosis. The anaesthetist should look for signs and symptoms appropriate to these complications as well as to the alcohol withdrawal syndrome. (Perioperative infusion of alcohol, 8% in saline, has been suggested in such cases.)

Medical examination

1. *Assessment of pulmonary function.* Clinical and monitored signs of respiratory disease. Respiratory pattern and character, type of operation, presence of added sounds on auscultation, localizing signs, mediastinal shift, finger clubbing, cyanosis.

2. *Assessment and prediction of cardiac risk in non-cardiac surgery.*[7] Patients with serious heart disease are not always symptomatic. A diastolic

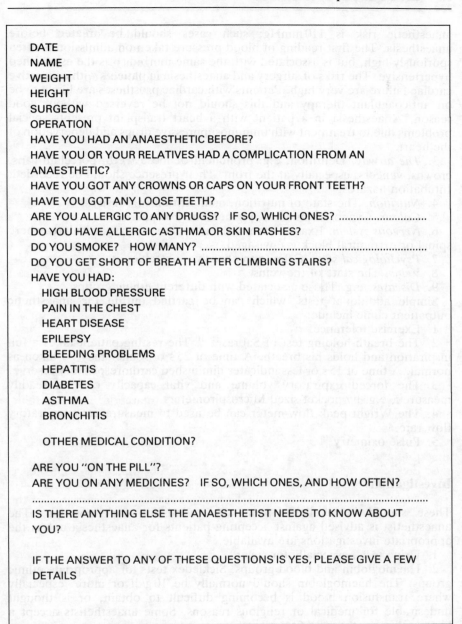

DATE
NAME
WEIGHT
HEIGHT
SURGEON
OPERATION
HAVE YOU HAD AN ANAESTHETIC BEFORE?
HAVE YOU OR YOUR RELATIVES HAD A COMPLICATION FROM AN
ANAESTHETIC?
HAVE YOU GOT ANY CROWNS OR CAPS ON YOUR FRONT TEETH?
HAVE YOU GOT ANY LOOSE TEETH?
ARE YOU ALLERGIC TO ANY DRUGS?   IF SO, WHICH ONES? ....
DO YOU HAVE ALLERGIC ASTHMA OR SKIN RASHES?
DO YOU SMOKE?   HOW MANY? ....
DO YOU GET SHORT OF BREATH AFTER CLIMBING STAIRS?
HAVE YOU HAD:
   HIGH BLOOD PRESSURE
   PAIN IN THE CHEST
   HEART DISEASE
   EPILEPSY
   BLEEDING PROBLEMS
   HEPATITIS
   DIABETES
   ASTHMA
   BRONCHITIS

   OTHER MEDICAL CONDITION?

ARE YOU "ON THE PILL"?
ARE YOU ON ANY MEDICINES?   IF SO, WHICH ONES, AND HOW OFTEN?
....
IS THERE ANYTHING ELSE THE ANAESTHETIST NEEDS TO KNOW ABOUT
YOU?

IF THE ANSWER TO ANY OF THESE QUESTIONS IS YES, PLEASE GIVE A FEW
DETAILS

Figure 5.1 Preanaesthetic check sheet

murmur is unequivocal evidence of heart disease. A systolic murmur with no interval between the murmur and the second heart sound is likely to be associated with organic disease. Presence of a thrill indicates organic disease.[8] Acute myocardial ischaemia may be present without obvious symptoms; this, and the previous silent coronary thrombosis, may cause inverted T waves on the ECG. The diastolic pressure above which hypertension is a major anaesthetic risk is 110 mmHg; such cases should be treated before anaesthesia. The first reading of blood pressure taken on admission is often spuriously high, but is associated with the same morbidity as the established hypertensive. The risks of surgery and anaesthesia in patients with congestive cardiac failure are very high. Patients with cardiac prostheses are likely to be on anticoagulant therapy and this should not be reversed without good reason. Anaesthesia in a patient with a heart transplant presents special problems due to treatment with immunosuppressive drugs and denervation of the heart.[9]

3. *The airway*. Dentition, e.g. prominent or loose teeth, porcelain caps, crowns, veneers, especially at the front. Their presence should be recorded. Intubation hazards.

4. *Nutrition*. The state of nutrition, malnutrition or obesity.

5. *Colour*. Cyanosis, jaundice, pigmentation or pallor.

6. *Nervous system*. Examination of the nervous system, particularly where spinal or extradural block is envisaged.

7. *Psychological state*. Calm, apprehensive, unstable, etc.

8. *Veins*. The state of the veins.

9. *Diseases*. e.g. Those associated with different ethnic groups.

Simple additional tests, which can be carried out in the anaesthetic outpatient clinic include:

1. Exercise tolerance.

2. The breath-holding test of Sabrasez.[10] The resting patient takes a full inspiration and holds his breath. A time of 25 s or longer may be taken as normal. A time of 15 s or less indicates diminished cardiorespiratory reserve.

3. The forced expiratory volume and vital capacity can be readily measured, e.g. by pocket-sized Microspirometers.

4. The Wright peak flow-meter can be used to measure peak expiratory flow rate.

5. Pulse oximetry.

Investigations

These should be available soon after admission for operation. The anaesthetist is advised against accepting patients for anaesthesia unless the appropriate investigations are available.

1. Urine tests, especially for sugar.

2. Haemoglobin and blood groups. Sickledex tests for appropriate ethnic groups. The haemoglobin should normally be 10 g/dl or more, especially where transfusion blood is becoming difficult to obtain, or is thought undesirable for medical or religious reasons. Some anaesthetists accept a lower value in otherwise fit patients.

3. Blood urea and electrolytes, especially for the elderly, those with cardiovascular disease and before major surgery. Hyperkalaemia and hypokalaemia are particularly important. Other biochemical screening tests are sometimes justified, eg Ca^{++}. Random blood sugar estimation above 11.1 mmol (200 mg/dl) is diagnostic of diabetes mellitus.[11]

4. Chest radiograph. In patients of retirement age, immigrants, or with a history or signs of chest disease, or following trauma. It may be useful as a

baseline for postoperative care. It does, however, carry a small risk of radiation damage. Routine chest radiography of patients not being operated on for chest or heart conditions has been questioned.[12]

5. Electrocardiogram. Essential in patients with cardiovascular disease or an abnormal pulse. Some authorities recommend routine ECG's on all elderly patients. Abnormalities are picked up increasingly as patients get older.

6. Other special investigations may be ordered where indicated.

In certain cases it is desirable to refer the patient to other departments for advice (e.g. diabetes, hypertension, cardiac failure, infections, and respiratory failure).

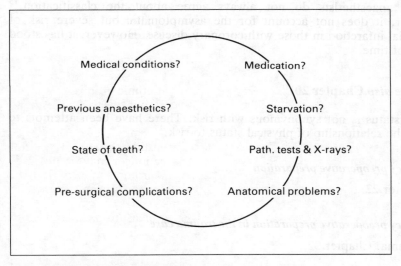

Figure 5.2 Simple questions for the preanaesthetic visit

Assessment of Physical Status (PS)

The American Society of Anesthesiologists classified patients into a number of grades according to their general condition.[13]

A.S.A. classification

ASA 1. The patient has no organic, physiological, biochemical or psychiatric disturbance. The pathological process for which operation is to be performed is localized and does not entail a systemic disturbance.

ASA 2. Mild to moderate systemic disturbance caused either by the condition to be treated surgically or by other pathophysiological processes. Mild organic heart disease, diabetes, mild hypertension, anaemia, old age, obesity, mild chronic bronchitis.

ASA 3. Limitation of life-style. Severe systemic disturbance or disease from whatever cause, even though it may not be possible to define the degree of disability with any finality, e.g. angina, healed myocardial infarction, severe diabetes, and cardiac failure.

ASA 4. Severe systemic disorders that are already life-threatening, and not always correctable by operation, e.g. marked cardiac insufficiency, persistent angina, active myocarditis, advanced pulmonary, renal, endocrine or hepatic insufficiency.

ASA 5. Moribund. Little chance of survival, but submitted to operation in desperation. Little, if any, anaesthesia is required.

If the operation is an emergency, the letter E is placed beside the numerical classification, and the patient is considered to be in poorer physical condition.

The ASA scheme is the most comprehensive system, but ignores the risk of the asymptomatic patient who, for example, may have severe coronary artery disease. It also ignores the inherent risks of a particular operation.

The system (which has now been revised)[14] has been criticized in that different anaesthetists do not always agree about the classification.[15] Moreover, it does not account for the asymptomatic but severe risk of myocardial infarction in those with coronary disease. However, it has stood the test of time.

Risk (*See also* Chapter 20)[16]

Physical status is not synonymous with risk. There have been attempts to analyse the relationship of physical status to risk.[17]

Emergency preoperative preparation

See chapter 22

Emergency preoperative preparation in the trauma case

See Trauma, Chapter 32.

Treatment of pre-existing diseases

Some forms of treatment may be instituted before operation.

Dental treatment. Refer the patient to the dental surgeon.

Smoking. Should be stopped 4–6 weeks before surgery to reduce postoperative pulmonary morbidity. Stopping for 12–24 hours benefits the cardiovascular system by withdrawing carbon monoxide and nicotine; stopping for a few days will benefit ciliary activity; stopping for 1–2 weeks will reduce sputum volume. If stopping smoking increases the risk of deep vein thrombosis, this can be prevented by anticoagulants.[18]

Smokers exhibit a variety of pulmonary disorders including airway obstruction and reduced lung compliance, diminished peak flow rate, increase in functional residual capacity, diminished diffusing capacity and reduced surfactant. Those who smoke one or more packets of cigarettes daily have chronic bronchitis. Elevated carboxyhaemoglobin levels are also found. In abdominal operations postoperative chest complications are six times more frequent in smokers than in nonsmokers. Smoking may interfere with wound healing, especially in plastic surgery.[19]

Malnutrition. In appropriate cases, high-protein diets, vitamins, etc. can be ordered. Intravenous feeding is justified pre-operatively in certain patients, e.g. those with carcinoma of the oesophagus. (*See* Chapter 34)

Obesity. This is the enemy of both surgeon and anaesthetist. Treated properly by a 1000-calorie diet, excellent results may be obtained, even in the few weeks at the anaesthetist's disposal. Walking for 1 hour expends 300 calories. It is important to give the patient a diet sheet that can readily be understood, to explain the purpose of the diet, and the need to attend the outpatient clinic at regular (fortnightly) intervals for weight check and for interview so that the anaesthetist can give appropriate encouragement or scolding. (*See also* Chapter 20). **Failure to lose weight is no reason to accept an unnecessarily fat patient for anaesthesia.**

Psychological factors.[20] Occasionally patients are terrified of anaesthesia, or may fear a particular anaesthetic technique (face-mask, spinal anaesthesia). A little time spent in discussion with these patients is invaluable and may in fact bring some patients into hospital who would otherwise default. It should rarely be necessary to force an unwelcome technique on a patient.

One other advantage of the thorough preoperative investigation of the patient is the assurance and confidence that the anaesthetist feels, should medicolegal proceedings be instituted by the patient after operation.

'It is the fate of those who toil at the lower employments of life, to be exposed to censure without hope of praise; to be disgraced by miscarriage or punished for neglect, where success would have been without applause, and diligence without reward' (Dr Samuel Johnson).[21]

Preoperative preparation of specific medical diseases is discussed in Chapters 20 & 21.

'Fit for Anaesthetic'

This is a vague concept but usually implies that the patient who is not unduly old, lives a normal life, is free from serious signs and symptoms of disease, is not receiving drug treatment for abnormalities, has reasonable exercise tolerance for his age, is not unduly overweight and appears emotionally stable. In the light of the more detailed ASA status analysis, the global concept of 'fit' is outmoded. (*See* 'Assessment of physical status', above). Physical status is close to, but not the same as 'risk'.

Cancelling cases

The paramount concern is the safety of the patient. More and more of the decisions about the patient's fitness for surgery are being left to the anaesthetist. This calls for skilful judgement. Occasionally, it may not be in the sick patient's interest to be cancelled, and calculated risks may have to be taken with agreement of the patient or relatives. Operations may be cancelled:

1. Because of inadequate preparation by the surgical team, e.g. Blood test results or blood transfusion not available at the preoperative visit. The anaesthetist should be sympathetic but inflexibly firm; and

2. Because of risk arising from the poor condition of the patient. The anaesthetist should ask 'Is there any way in which this patient can be

improved?' If so, the operation may be postponed. If not, the question becomes 'Is the risk of anaesthesia justified by the probable benefits of the operation?' If the answer is 'no', then 'Would a different type of anaesthesia be suitable' (e.g. regional analgesia or ketamine)? If the answer to this is negative, it may either be due to shortcomings in the patient's health, or shortage of facilities in the hospital, e.g. lack of intensive care, nursing shortage, etc.

The anaesthetist has a right to refuse a patient for anaesthesia, either temporarily or permanently. He also has a right to postpone an anaesthetic (even for an 'emergency' case) if he thinks that the patient's condition can be improved by a delay. CEPOD found that only one in 20 of all their 'out of hours' (night and weekend) cases were true emergencies and concluded that far too many patients are put at unnecessary risk by being operated on as emergencies.

In this situation, the anaesthetist may well be faced by an angry patient, an enraged surgeon, or both. He may be accused of work-dodging, cowardice or even incompetence. He will be asked for the results of many tests to justify his clinical judgement. When insulted, he should resist the temptation to insult in return. He should offer sympathy and constructive advice, e.g. referral to another unit with more facilities. It must be remembered that one is not refusing the patient an operation, but merely an anaesthetic in a particular set of circumstances. Subsequently, the patient may be offered to another anaesthetist (often of less experience) without any hint of the previous cancellation. It may be humbling to discover that another anaesthetist has 'got away with' the risk that one originally thought was unjustifiable.

The effects of pre-existing drug therapy

ANTI-HYPERTENSIVE DRUGS

Patients are normally kept on antihypertensive medication. The safety factor is the knowledge that these drugs have been given and their pharmacology is known. The restoration of normal blood volumes in the hypertensive patient by adequate antihypertensive therapy is the pathophysiological basis for this safety factor. Risk of precipitate falls of arterial pressure at induction of anaesthesia, does, however, still exist in the patient who says that he takes his antihypertensive medication, but does not in fact do so. Pre-induction volume loading goes some way to preventing these falls, and the avoidance of hypovolaemia during surgery is important. The patient is fully monitored during anaesthesia. Bradycardia, due to unopposed vagal action, is treated with atropine or glycopyrronium.

Patients receiving β-blocking drugs should not have the medication discontinued. There is evidence that halothane is a safe agent in these circumstances.[22]

ACE INHIBITORS

These are oral only and so may have to be withdrawn following abdominal surgery. They may be given on the day of operation, and resumed as soon as oral intake is restarted. Administration of ACE inhibitors may reduce the glomerular filtration rate in the presence of renal artery stenosis.

CALCIUM CHANNEL BLOCKERS. *See* Chapter 15

These should not be stopped prior to surgery without a very specific reason, because an exacerbation of angina may occur.

ANTIBIOTICS

Large parenteral doses (e.g. mega-doses poured into wound or peritoneum) of the aminoglycosides, neomycin, streptomycin and dihydrostreptomycin and the lincomycins can cause a neuromuscular block, which is potentiated by the volatile agents or depolarizing muscle relaxants. Other antibiotics which may cause a similar effect include kanamycin, tobramycin, polymyxin B, biomycin, bacitracin and colistin. Use of depolarizing muscle relaxants does not obviate this danger because there has been a report of this syndrome when suxamethonium had been used as the relaxant,[23] presumably due to the onset of dual block. This is not a common problem.

ANGINA PROPHYLAXIS DRUGS

Should be continued through the perioperative period. If the oral route is impossible, 'transdermal glyceryl trinitrate patch dressings' (Transiderm-Nitro, Deponit, Percutol) placed on the lateral chest wall, last about 24 h. Reapplication should be at a fresh site.

PSYCHOTROPIC DRUGS

Many psychotropic drugs potentiate the effects of anaesthetics. Extra-pyramidal effects (parkinsonism, akathesia, dystonia, dyskinesia) can occur, especially with butyrophenones. Dystonia may respond dramatically to injection of antiparkinsonism drugs such as benztropine, 1–2 mg i.v.

Grand mal epilepsy can be precipitated by tricyclic antidepressants, lithium and major tranquillizers, as well as by abrupt withdrawal of benzodiazepines. Major tranquillizers and tricyclic antidepressants have anticholinergic side-effects. Tricyclic antidepressants block the re-uptake of mono-amines into adrenergic nerve terminals so that circulating catecholamines are increased. Adrenaline is best avoided. Sinus tachycardia and ventricular dysrhythmias can occur. Conversely, sudden withdrawal of tricyclic antidepressant therapy can lead to malaise, fatigue, muscle pains, vomiting and diarrhoea.

Lithium toxicity (in the dehydrated patient) potentiates non-depolarizing relaxants.

MONO-AMINE OXIDASE INHIBITORS

These include phenelzine, iproniazid, tranylcypramine and isocarboxazid, which should be discontinued 2–3 weeks before elective surgery. The mode of action of this group of drugs is imperfectly understood and cannot be explained solely in terms of mono-amine oxidase inhibition. Reactions to pethidine, fentanyl, and phenoperidine and morphine have been reported in patients taking these drugs and deaths have occurred. Reactions include severe depression, coma, muscle twitching, hypotension, ataxia, ocular palsies, cerebral excitement and Cheyne-Stokes respiration. Relief has been obtained following administration of 25 mg of prednisolone hemisuccinate or chlorpromazine. Not all patients receiving treatment with MAOIs show adverse reactions. IV test doses of 5 mg, 10 mg, then 20 mg pethidine may be given and the effect on blood pressure and pulse rate observed.

Severe hypertensive effects and even death may occur when pressor drugs (e.g. the adrenaline in local analgesic solutions) are given to patients on MAOIs, but may be counteracted with phentolamine.

For postoperative analgesia in patients receiving mono-amine oxidase inhibitors, a combination of chlorpromazine and codeine has been used without ill effect. Regional blocks and non-steroidal anti-inflammatory drugs are also suitable.

PHENOTHIAZINE DERIVATIVES

These cause peripheral vasodilatation and a fall in blood pressure in some subjects, which may become severe during anaesthesia. Narcotics are potentiated. Other side-effects include liver dysfunction, anti-analgesia and pseudo-parkinsonism.

DISULPHIRAM (ANTABUSE)

Blocks the normal metabolism of alcohol causing an accumulation of acetaldehyde, which is responsible for the 'disulphiram reaction'. Used in the treatment of alcoholics. There may be a synergistic depressant effect with thiopentone.

LITHIUM CARBONATE AND ANAESTHESIA

(*See* Mogelnik S. and Ominsky A. J. *Anesth. Analg.* 1977, **56**, 462.) Lithium should be stopped 48–72h before a relaxant is given. It potentiates the non-depolarizing group of relaxants. In emergency cases, suxamethonium and regional blocks should be considered.

LEVODOPA

There is a slight risk of tachycardia and ventricular dysrhythmias with halothane, so it may be stopped on the day of operation only. Levodopa inhibits prolactin secretion and stimulates growth hormone production, which may make diabetic patients more liable to hyperglycaemia. The danger of stopping levodopa for longer than the day of operation is the reappearance of severe Parkinsonism, dysphagia and the risk of aspiration pneumonia. Butyrophenones antagonize the action of levodopa on dopaminergic receptors in the brain and should be used with caution.

STEROID THERAPY

Long-term steroid therapy calls for steroid replacement during anaesthesia (and subsequent starvation) with hydrocortisone, e.g. 100 mg, 6–12 hourly. Steroid creams and enemas also need to be considered.
See Chapter 20.

INSULIN

See Chapter 20, Diabetes.

THE CONTRACEPTIVE PILL

After major surgery, the relative risk of deep vein thrombosis in women taking oestrogen-containing combined oral contraceptive pills is about 2:1, compared with non-users.[24] Anaesthesia and the combined pill have additive effects because both reduce the activity of antithrombin III. The risk is greatest following hypotensive anaesthesia and major abdominal, orthopaedic and cancer operations.

Oestrogen-containing pills should, if possible, be discontinued four weeks before elective surgery and started again at the first period following an interval of two weeks after the operation providing that the patient is fully mobile. Should this not be possible because of unexpected surgery or other cause, prophylactic low dose heparin or dextan 70 should be considered. The risk increases with age, obesity, cigarette smoking, diabetes, hypertension and familial hyperlipidaemia. The risks associated with minor surgery or day-stay operations followed by full mobilization are not so great and oral contraceptives need not be discontinued, unless the surgery is on the legs, e.g. ligation of varicose veins. The 'progesterone-only' pill need not be discontinued before elective surgery.[25]

Patients on female sex hormone replacement therapy (HRT) probably do not require any special treatment.

THE DAY OF OPERATION

Food should be withheld for six hours and drink for four hours preceding operation. Excessive starvation and dehydration are to be avoided, especially in infants, who may suffer dangerous hypoglycaemia. (A drink two hours before anaesthesia in children is widely practised.)

Morphine premedication delays gastric emptying time, but diazepam, 10 mg does not. Gastric emptying time is increased after both atropine and glycopyrronium.

Lipstick, nail varnish and other cosmetics should be removed before the patient comes to theatre so that the anaesthetist can readily appreciate cyanosis, etc. Dentures, artificial limbs, artificial eyes, contact lenses, etc. should be removed before the journey to the theatre. Hearing aids may often be retained by the patient so that communication can be restarted in the postoperative ward.

The patient should not come to theatre with a full bladder. The appropriate blood test results are inspected and crossmatching may need to be confirmed.

An identification label is tied around the wrist or neck. This should state the name and case record number. The site of operation should be marked on the patient's skin with ink.

The completed consent form and ID band are inspected, and the patient asked to state his name and operation. More detailed consent forms may be required, e.g. for research procedures, sterilization, termination of pregnancy, and Jehovah's witnesses.

Emergency cases should be delayed if possible to allow the stomach to empty because gastric emptying may be considerably delayed after accidents, in labour and in the anxious patient. Resuscitative measures, such as intravenous infusion, may be required to improve the patient's condition, even at this late stage of the arrangements.

Premedication

"Empirical procedures, firmly entrenched in the habits of good doctors, seem to have a vigour and life, not to say immortality of their own" (H. K. Beecher).

History of premedication

In pre-anaesthetic days, both wine and opium were given to mitigate the terrors of surgery. The word itself first appeared in print in an article by the American editor-anaesthetist Frank Hoeffer McMechan (1873–1930) in 1920.[26]

The technique was employed only infrequently during the 50 years following the introduction of anaesthesia. It was recommended by Bellamy Gardner[27] and Dudley Buxton (1855–1931) of University College Hospital in the UK, and rules determining whether or not 'preliminary medication' should be used were published in 1911 in the USA,[28] while in 1914, it was stated that 'preliminary medication' was employed in 59% of hospitals in the USA.[29]

Papaveretum was prepared in 1909 by Hermann Sahli (1856–1933) of Berne and was marketed in Germany as Pantopon. Later, as Omnopon, it became popular in the UK.[30] Aspirin introduced into medicine in 1899 by Dreser. Pethidine, synthesized in 1939 by Schaumann and Eisleb in Germany during a search for an atropine substitute,[31] was first used in premedication by Schlungbaum[32] and in the USA in 1943.[33]

The term 'hypodermic' was first used in 1859.[34] Morphine introduced under the skin using a vaccination lancet, by G. V. Lafargue of St Emilion in 1836.[35]

(*See also* Duncum Barbara M. *The Development of Inhalation Anaesthesia.* London: Oxford University Press, 1947; Shearer W. *Br. J. Anaesth.* 1960, **32**, 554; 1961, **33**, 219.)

Reasons for administration of premedicants

1. Reduction of fear and anxiety.[36]
2. Reduction of saliva secretion.
3. Prevention of vagal reflexes, caused by surgical stimulation, (e.g. squint operations, stretching of anal sphincter), or associated with medication, (e.g. β-blockers).
4. As part of the anaesthetic technique, e.g. narcotic analgesics reduce the extrapyramidal movements sometimes seen after injection of methohexitone

or thiopentone; they also provide background analgesia during the operation, and give the anaesthetist information about how this patient responds to a given dose of any narcotic.

5. To produce amnesia. The incidence of amnesia is low with routine opiate premedication. Hyoscine causes amnesia in a small but significant group of patients. Benzodiazepines produce greater anterograde amnesia, and diazepam–hyoscine combinations cause complete amnesia in about 75% of patients. Oral lorazepam 2.5–5 mg is also associated with a high incidence of amnesia.

6. For specific therapeutic effects, e.g. transdermal glyceryl nitrate patches for angina patients, steroids, hyoscine[37], H_2 blockers, and potentially many other drugs.[38]

Drugs used for premedication

1. *Sedatives.* For example barbiturates, benzodiazepines, phenothiazines, etc. Patients in hot climates are more sensitive to sedative premedication than those living in temperate zones, due to their reduced BMR.

Sedative action is helped by the oral administration of a suitable hypnotic the night before operation, especially benzodiazepines.[36]

Clonidine (100 µg for adult males, 50 µg for adult females) has been used to decrease requirements of volatile anaesthetics[39] as has dexmedetomiclone.

Zopiclone 7.5 mg is a safe non-benzodiazepine alternative.[40] Chloral betaine may be useful in the elderly.

Sedative premedication does not lessen the need for kind, sympathetic care for patients at a time of great stress. For depressed patients, amitriptyline 25–50 mg is suitable, given by mouth the night before operation.

2. *Analgesics.* Narcotics usually produce a positively happy attitude, but at the price of some nausea in about 50% of patients (*see* Chapter 26). Hyoscine is commonly used as an antiemetic for this (as well as antisialogogue and sedative). Long-acting non-steroidal anti-inflammatory drugs (NSAIDs) give a useful background analgesia, upon which intraoperative and postoperative opiates develop an enhanced analgesic effect, without any more side-effects.[41] Ketoprofen, 100–200 mg, oral or rectal, and ibuprofen, 400 mg, are said to be equivalent to papaveretum 10 mg. Piroxicam dispersible 40 mg, will give 12–24 h useful analgesia (adult doses). Aspirin has been used in eclampsia.

3. *Opioids.* (Narcotics) *See* Chapter 26

4. *Neuroleptic Agents.* For example dehydrobenzperidol (droperidol) 0.02–0.1 mg/kg, I.M. or oral. Used for sedation and antiemesis. May cause hallucinations and dysphoria (*see below*).

5. *Anticholinergic agents.* Atropine, hyoscine and glycopyrronium (glycopyrrolate USP). Hyoscine has the great advantage that it is also a sedative, antiemetic and amnesic. It tends to produce less tachycardia than atropine. Glycopyrronium does not enter the brain, and lasts longer (*see below*).

6. *Oral antacids.* These are commonly prescribed for known risk cases and day-case patients, e.g. cimetidine 150 mg, ranitidine, 150 mg, famotidine, 40 mg, nizatidine 150 mg.[42] Cimetidine lasts longer than ranitidine.

7. *Drugs for specific effects.* For example salbutamol inhalation for

asthmatics and atenolol for hypertensives. Atenolol, 25 mg by mouth, the night before operation reduces the operative morbidity and mortality of hypertensive patients, including those who are hypertensive because of anxiety.

Beta blockers may be used to reduce anxiety.[36] GTN dermal patches are useful for the patient with coronary disease. Antibiotics may be given for infection prophylaxis.

In many hospitals, non-anaesthetic junior staff have a rather poor knowledge of the use of drugs employed by anaesthetists.[43]

The benzodiazepines

These are all good premedicants, can be given orally, and produce sedation, amnesia, and freedom from anxiety. The chief difference between them is their duration of action, and they can be used singly or in combination to produce a 'tailor-made' premedication for any type of surgery. They can be combined with oral analgesics to add background analgesia for the operation.

They do not affect cardiovascular stability, have only a minor effect on respiration, and they potentiate thiopentone.

Patients who are already regular takers of benzodiazepines will be resistant to the premedicant action of these drugs.

Temazepam (Euhypnos; Normison)[44] Short acting (4–8h). Adult dose 10–30 mg. Useful for night sedation or for premedication in all types of surgery, including day-stay. Temazepam is suitable for premedication in elderly patients undergoing minor surgery. Syrup is available for children, 2 mg/ml. Dose 0.5 mg/kg.

Midazolam (Hypnovel) Dose 5–7.5 mg i.v.[45] Has been used for night sedation before surgery (15 mg)[46] or as premedication.[47] It is also an induction agent in a dose of 0.3 mg/kg in the elderly,[48] especially combined with fentanyl[49]. Useful in mentally retarded patients.[50] In very common use as a sedative during regional analgesia.[51]

Lormetazepam. Duration 4 h, useful for premedication in the elderly. Dose 0.5–2mg.

Lorazepam. (Ativan) Dose 1.0–5.0 mg (0.03–0.1 mg/kg) orally or i.m., given 2 h preoperatively. Duration: 4–24 h with appreciable anterograde amnesia. More effective when given sublingually than when injected i.m. in premedication.[52] Abolishes the vasoconstriction which accompanies fear and attenuates the psychic sequelae of ketamine. Lorazepam reduces anxiety preoperatively more effectively than papaveretum. Particularly useful for elderly patients undergoing ophthalmic operations, where opiate-induced vomiting would be a hazard.

Diazepam. (Valium, Diazemuls, Atensine) Dose 10–20mg, orally or i.m. Duration 4–8 h. *See* Chapter 9 for further details. Combination with metoprolol greatly enhances its anxiolytic activity.[36]

Nitrazepam. (Mogadon, Remnos) Dose 5–10 mg. Duration 5–10 h. It does not induce microsomal activity and thus has no influence on the metabolism of other drugs. It may, however, be contra-indicated in severe chronic obstructive airways disease because it has been shown to produce a fall in ventilatory capacity and a worsening of ventilatory failure in such patients. The ageing brain becomes sensitive to it.

Flurazepam. (Dalmane) A useful hypnotic, without effect on REM sleep. Dose: 15–30 mg. Duration 5–10 h.

Flunitrazepam. (Rohypnol) Flunitrazepam 1 mg by mouth, has been recommended for premedication and as more effective than diazepam 10 mg or lorazepam 2.5 mg. Duration:4–8 h.

Flumazenil. The benzodiazepine antagonist, useful for reversing over-doses,[53] and after endoscopies where severe benzodiazepine sedation exists. Dose 0.1–0.5 mg. Duration about 30 minutes. Cardiovascular stability is reasonably well maintained.[54] It also reverses the helpful actions of benzodiazepines, e.g. anticonvulsant. It may not shorten recovery time after midazolam.[55] *See also* Chapter 9.

Butyrophenones

Haloperidol and Droperidol. These drugs have been used in premedication, because they produce mental detachment and are powerfully antiemetic. Large doses may cause extrapyramidal disturbances. They are best combined with phenoperidine or fentanyl. (*See* Chapter 9.)

Barbiturates and other drugs

For history of barbiturates, see Dundee J. W. and McIlroy P. D. A. *Anaesthesia* 1982, **37**, 726. Contra-indicated in porphyria.

Phenothiazine derivatives

Sedative, anxiolytic, antihypertensive, and antiemetic, these drugs are useful in combination with pethidine as premedicants. Dose chlorpromazine 25–50 mg; promethazine 12.5–50 mg – with or without pethidine. Patients with alcoholic liver disease are very sensitive to phenothiazines.

Trimeprazine tartrate. (Vallergan) Another valuable member of this group of drugs; available as a syrup for oral administration to children, although now largely superseded by benzodiazepines. Dose 3–4 mg/kg, 2 h pre-operatively.

Anticholinergic agents

ATROPINE SULPHATE

History. (From Atropos, the oldest of the Three Fates who severed the threads of life, which were spun by Clotho and mixed, those of good and evil fortune, by Lachesis). The alkaloid of the *Atropa belladonna* or deadly nightshade. Atropine was first suggested by E. A. Sharpey-Schaffer (1850–1935) Edinburgh physiologist in 1880 to reduce vagal tone during chloroform anaesthesia, and advocated by Dudley Buxton (1855–1935), London anaesthetist, 35 years later to inhibit secretions during ether anaesthesia. (*See also* Kessel J. *Anaesth. Intensive Care,* 1974, **2**, 77.) Not used in premedication before 1890, although it was given, as the extract, per rectum, in 1861 to control patients resistant to chloroform.[56]

The atropine group of alkaloids are esters formed by the union of an aromatic derivative of benzyl alcohol, tropic acid, with organic bases – tropine (atropine) and scopine (hyoscine). The tropic acid is the active radical. Atropine is the racemic mixture of dextro- and laevohyoscyamine, the laevo form being the more active; hyoscine is laevorotatory. First synthesized by Richard Willstaetter (1872–1942) in 1896 and again by Robert Robinson in 1917. Today it is usually prepared from the plant *Duboisia myoporoides*.

Uses. (1) To reduce secretions of saliva, especially in children, Down's syndrome, and when ether is used; (2) to prevent or reverse vagal bradycardia, which occurs with suxamethonium, short-acting opioids, anticholinergic drugs (e.g. neostigmine), halothane, high spinal block, β-blockade, surgical reflex stimuli (e.g. ECT, stretching sphincters, traction on gut) and to depress the oculocardiac reflex in ophthalmic and facial operations; and (3) to prevent or reverse gastro-intestinal hypermobility (e.g. due to neostigmine and during gastroscopies).

Action on autonomic nerves. Atropine has a blocking action on effector organs of structures supplied by the postganglionic cholinergic nerves, e.g. smooth muscles and secretory glands, acting on the effector cells, i.e. it competes with acetylcholine at the sites of its muscarinic activity. Atropine has no effect on either production or destruction of acetylcholine. Complete vagal block requires a dose of 3 mg. It is a parasympatholytic anticholinergic drug.

Action on central nervous system. Atropine stimulates the medulla and higher centres, and directly stimulates the respiratory centre. It causes auditory hyperacusis. Occasionally, restlessness and delirium are seen (central anticholinergic syndrome). All these limit its usefulness as a premedicant. In the elderly, prolonged sedation may result, which may be treated by physostigmine 1–2 mg i.v.[57]

The peak of its effect is 1 hour after hypodermic injection, wearing off rapidly.

Effects on eye. There is paralysis of the sphincter of the iris resulting in dilated pupils, although a dose of 0.5 mg intramuscularly does not greatly influence accommodation or size of pupil.[58] (The sphincter muscle is innervated from the third cranial nerve via the ciliary ganglion and short ciliary nerves.) Used as drops, 1% atropine does not appreciably raise the intraocular pressure in normal eyes. There is no contra-indication to the use of intramuscular or intravenous atropine in a patient with glaucoma, even of the narrow-angle type, because significant dilatation of the pupil does not occur. Topical atropine is, however, contra-indicated. Down's syndrome patients may show sensitivity to topically-applied atropine (to the eye); and hyoscine is perhaps better for injection.

Effects on respiratory system. Sweat, bronchial and salivary glands are paralysed, while bronchial muscle is relaxed, causing a slight increase in the anatomical and physiological dead space. Acts as a bronchodilator and reduces excessive bronchial secretion. Intramuscular injection 1 hour before anaesthesia suppresses salivation more efficiently than intravenous injection immediately before induction.

Action on circulatory system. Tachycardia, by peripheral vagal paralysis and its effect on the SA pacemaker. (Rate of heart sometimes slows initially (the Bezold-Jarisch reflex), due to action on the sino-auricular node, but this effect is not seen after intravenous injection of clinical doses.) This tachycardia, by shortening diastole, may decrease coronary filling time and increase myocardial oxygen consumption. It should be used with care in patients with coronary disease. Such tachycardia may also increase cardiac output, and thereby reduce a high CVP. Atropine tachycardia is less marked in the elderly.

Reflex bradycardia and neostigmine-induced bradycardia are prevented. In cases of gross tachycardia, e.g. in thyrotoxicosis, hyperpyrexia or heart disease, atropine is better avoided. Both atropine and hyoscine may cause dysrhythmias. Some cases of asystole can be reversed by atropine.

Atropine sometimes causes dilatation of the vessels of the face and a scarlatiniform rash.

Blood pressure not affected (unless depressed by bradycardia, when atropine raises it).

Action on alimentary canal. The tone and peristalsis of the gut and urinary tract are decreased. Like hyoscine and glycopyrronium, atropine lowers the opening pressure of the cardiac sphincter of the stomach and hence increases the chances of regurgitation.[59] (Metoclopramide has the opposite effect.)[60]

Effect on the fetus. Atropine crosses the placenta rapidly (as a tertiary amine) to reach the fetal circulation. It has been used as a test of placental insufficiency and in the diagnosis of fetal hypoxia. Atropine administered as premedication to the mother may protect the fetus and newborn from vagal reflexes occurring during birth and resuscitation.

Pharmacokinetics. Plasma half-life 2–3 hours, 50% is protein bound. Elimination is slow in children under two years of age and in the elderly. Excretion is partly by the kidneys, another part being destroyed in the body, with the formation of tropine and tropic acid. Atropine pharmacokinetics are affected by moderate haemorrhage and hypothyroidism.[61]

Dosage. Usual adult dose, 0.5–1 mg i.m. (in children 0.015 mg/kg) 1 hr. before operation. Before neostigmine, 1–2 mg. Oral adult dose 2 mg, (0.03 mg/kg in children), 90 min before operation.

Overdose of Atropine

Mad as a hatter (Central stimulation)
Hot as a hen (Inhibition of sweating)
Blind as a bat (Paralysis of accommodation)
Red as a beetroot (Facial vasodilation)
Dry as a bone (Salivary inhibition)

Given in adequate dosage of 1–1.5 mg intravenously, atropine blocks the muscarinic action of neostigmine on the heart, gut and salivary glands. Its cardiac effects come on more rapidly than its antisalivary effects. Atropine has a wide therapeutic ratio and doses up to 200 mg have been used in psychiatry.

Inhibition of sweating may lead to increase in temperature. It may therefore be avoided in pyrexial children.

Milk secretion is not affected, although the drug may be excreted into the milk.

Acts as a local analgesic, being half as potent as procaine.

It inhibits the muscarinic but not the nicotinic effects of acetylcholine. It raises the basal metabolic rate. Like morphine, may produce a skin weal after subcutaneous injection.

Effects of atropine on the eye, heart and salivary glands less marked in negroes than in caucasians,[62] who may therefore require larger dosage.

The cerebral toxic effects (the anticholinergic syndrome) can be blocked by physostigmine (*see below*).

HYOSCINE HYDROBROMIDE (Scopolamine)

History. The name 'scopolamine' is derived from *Scopolia carniolica*, the plant from which it was first isolated and named after Johannes Antonius Scopoli (1723–1788), a physician from Carniola, a province in Slovenia.[63]

Also derived from *Hyoscyamus niger* (henbane). Isolated in 1873.[64]

Originally used as a mixture of laevo- and dextro-alkaloids, and achieved a reputation for unreliability. When it was discovered that only the laevo form was pharmacologically active, this was prepared and sold in Germany under the name of Scopolamine, where it soon became widely used. A pioneer in the UK was Dudley Wilmot Buxton. In 1903, It became popular for preoperative medication because it dried secretions, was sedative, antiemetic and amnesic – a superb combination.

Used, together with morphine, before anaesthesia in 1900 by Schneiderlinn.[65] It is a better drying agent than atropine. Was used to produce amnesia in labour (twilight sleep).[66] Crosses the blood-brain barrier, as a tertiary amine.

Pharmacodynamics. Actions similar to atropine. Chief difference is that hyoscine is a central sedative, causing drowsiness, sleep, and amnesia in some patients. Occasionally it produces restlessness and excitement, which can be relieved by physostigmine, especially in geriatric patients and those with unrelieved pain. It decreases the intensity and duration of analgesia produced by opiates, pethidine and methadone. Physostigmine improves the quality but not the speed of recovery from nitrous oxide/enflurane anaesthesia.[67]

Hyoscine is a mild respiratory stimulant, whereas its actions on the iris, the salivary, sweat and bronchial glands are stronger than that of atropine. It is a moderately powerful antiemetic. Tachycardia may occur, as after atropine. Action on heart, intestine and bronchiolar muscle is weaker than that of atropine.

Dose – 0.3–0.6 mg. i.v. or i.m., and 1 mg by mouth. For paediatric dosage *see* Chapter 22 Paediatric surgery.

Combination of hyoscine 0.4 mg with pethidine 100 mg or papaveretum 20 mg forms a useful sedative before operation.

HYOSCINE BUTYLBROMIDE (Buscopan)

A useful drying agent given i.v. immediately before induction of anaesthesia. It increases heart rate and reduces secretions, but its action is rather short. Like propanthelene bromide, it inhibits peristalsis during gastroscopy. Can be absorbed from skin, e.g. posterior to the pinna.

Dose – 10–30 mg.

GLYCOPYRRONIUM BROMIDE (Robinul, glycopyrrolate, USP)

Synthesized by Franko and Lunsford[68] and first used in anaesthesia by Boawright C. F., Newell R. C. et al.[69] A quaternary ammonium compound with anticholinergic properties. It does not readily cross the placental or blood-brain[70] barriers, and does not cause central anticholinergic effects. Like atropine and hyoscine it reduces the tone of the lower oesophageal sphincter and so may contribute to regurgitation of gastric contents[71] (the opposite effect to metoclopramide). It suppresses gastric secretion better than atropine or hyoscine, and results in less tachycardia and dysrhythmia. It efficiently dries up salivary secretions, being five times more potent than atropine and longer lasting.

For ECT with methohexitone, atropine and glycopyrronium are identical in drying secretions, but glycopyrronium does not cause so much tachycardia. Both drugs are satisfactory when used prior to suxamethonium in preventing bradycardia. Associated with faster emergence from anaesthesia than when atropine has been used.

Dose – Premedication i.m. (adult) 0.2–0.4 mg; (child) 10 µg/kg. Intravenous use to protect against bradycardia (adult) 0.2 mg or 4–5 µg/kg; (child) 5–10 µg/kg. The full dose of 0.9 mg does not cause significant changes in heart rate.[72] In clinical doses it does not affect the pupil size. Not antiemetic.

Table 5.1 Comparison of anticholinergic drugs

Drug	Atropine	Hyoscine	Glycopyrronium
I.v. dose (µg/kg)	5–20	5–10	3–10
Onset time (i.v.)	1 min	1 min	1 min
Length of action	3 h	2 h	6 h
Effect on heart rate	++++	+++	++
Inhibition of salivation	+++	+++	+++
Rare side effects on CNS	'CACS'	'CACS'	NIL
Control of muscarinic effect of neostigmine	+++	+++	+++

The central anticholinergic syndrome (CACS)

Diagnosis. Patients, especially elderly ones, may, after treatment with anticholinergic drugs, show excitement, drowsiness or even coma. They may also suffer from thought impairment, disturbances of recent memory, hallucinations, ataxia or behavioural abnormalities. They may be slow to 'wake up properly' in the postoperative ward, are restless and show signs of the 'locked-in syndrome'.

Treatment. Physostigmine salicylate, an anticholinesterase drug with a tertiary amine, allowing it to cross the blood-brain barrier (neostigmine has a quaternary amine which prevents this), reverses the syndrome. *Dose.* 2 mg i.v. given cautiously, and repeated if necessary. The drug has also been used in the treatment of depressant effects on the central nervous system of ketamine, tricyclics, phenothiazines, droperidol and even halothane.[73]

In clinical doses it does not adequately reverse neuromuscular block,[74] while its cholinergic effects are minimal. It is derived from the Calabar bean.

References

1. *See also* Lee J. A. *Anaesthesia* 1949, **4**, 169; Atkinson R. S. In: *Preparation for Anaesthesia* (Stevens A. J. ed.). *Clin. Anesthesiol.* 1986, **4**, 445; Barash P. *Clinical Anaesthesia*. Philadelphia: Lippincott, 1989; Barash P. *Handbook of Clinical Anaesthesia*. Philadelphia: Lippincott, 1989.
2. McCleane G. J. and Cooper R. *Anaesthesia*. 1990, **45**, 153.
3. Heavey A. *Br. J. Hosp. Med.* 1988, **39**, 433–439
4. Cheng J. and Kay B. *Manual of Anesthesia and the Medically Compromised Patient*. Philadelphia: Lippincott, 1990; Kyei-Mensah K. and Thornton J. A. *Br. J. Anaesth.* 1974, **46**, 570.
5. Pedersen T. Eliasen K. and Henriksen E. *Acta Anaes. Scand.* 1990, **34**, 144; Mangano R. *Preoperative Cardiac Assessment*. Philadelphia: Lippincott, 1990.
6. Prys-Roberts C. In: *Medicine for Anaesthetists* (Vickers M. D. ed.). Oxford: Blackwell, 1977; (Brown B. R. ed.). *Anaesthesia and the Patient with Heart Disease* Philadelphia: Davis, 1980.
7. Foëx P. *Br. J. Anaesth.* 1978, **50**, 15; Mangano R. *Preoperative Cardiac Assessment*. Philadelphia: Lippincott, 1990.
8. Fleming P. R. *Br. J. Anaesth.* 1974, **46**, 555.
9. Kanter S. F. and Samuels S. I. *Anesthesiology* 1977, **46**, 65.
10. Sabrasez *Bordeaux Med. J.* 1902.
11. Alberti K. G. M. M. and Hockaday T. D. R. In *Oxford Textbook of Medicine*, 9.51 2nd ed, 1988, ed Wetherall D. J., Oxford Medical Publications, Oxford.
12. National Study by R. Coll. Radiol. *Lancet* 1979, **2**, 83; Denham M. et al. *Br. Med. J.* 1984, **288**, 1726. Other workers find it important: Tornebrandt K. and Fletcher R. *Anaesthesia* 1982, **37**, 901.
13. *Anesthesiology* 1963, **24**, 111; Owens W. D. et al. *Anesthesiology* 1978, **49**, 239; Editorial, *Anesthesiology* 1978, **49**, 233.
14. Keats A. S. *Anesthesiology* 1979, **51**, 179.
15. Owens W. D. et al. *Anesthesiology* 1978, **49**, 239.
16. Pedersen T., Eliasen K. et al. *Acta Anaesthesiol. Scand.* 1990, **34**, 144; Lunn J. N. *Anaesthesia* 1990, **45**, 1; Chopra V., Bovill J. G., et al. *Anaesthesia* 1990, **45**, 3.
17. Brown D. L. (ed.) *Risk and Outcome in Anaesthesia*. Philadelphia: Lippincott, 1988.
18. Pearce A. C. and Jones R. M. *Anesthesiology* 1984, **61**, 576; Cole P. and Saloojee Y. *Br. Med. J.* 1985, **291**, 142.
19. Nolan J. , Jenkins R. A. et al. *Plast.* Reconstr. Surg. 1985, **75**, 544; Rees T. D. et al. *Plast.* Reconstr. *Surg.* 1984, **73**, 911.
20. *See also* Maxwell H. In: *Preparation for Anaesthesia* (Stevens A. J. ed.). *Clin. Anesthesiol.* 1986, **4**, 473.
21. Mann G. V. *N. Engl. J. Med.* 1974, **291**, 178, 276; Smith L. H. Jr. *The Obese Patient*. Philadelphia and London: Saunders, 1976; Johnson S. Preface to *The Dictionary of the English Language*. 1755.
22. Roberts J. G. *Br. J. Anaesth.* 1976, **48**, 315.
23. Foldes F. F. et al. *JAMA* 1963, **183**, 672.
24. Stadel B. V. *N. Engl. J. Med.* 1981, **305**, 612 and 672.
25. Guillebaud J. *Br. Med. J.* 1985, **291**, 498; *British National Formulary* 1985, **10**, 260.
26. McMechan F. H. *Am. J. Surg.* 1920, Quarterly suppl. 34, 123; *Lancet* 1928, **2**, 1252.
27. Bellamy Gardner H. *Br. Med. J.* 1910, **2**, 766. ; Buxton W. D. *Proc. R. Soc. Med.* 1908–1909, **2**, 60.
28. Collins C. U. *JAMA* 1911, 26 March.
29. Gwathmey J. T. *Anesthesia*. New York and London: D. Appleton & Co., 1914, p. 847.
30. Leipoldt C. L. *Lancet* 1911, **1**, 368; Kerri Szanto M. *Can. Anaesth. Soc. J.* 1974, **23**, 239.
31. Schaumann O. and Eisleb O. *Dtsch. Med.* Wochenschr. 1939, **65**, 967.
32. Schlungbaum H. *Med. Klin.* 1939, **35**, 1259.

33. Rovenstine E. A. and Battermann R. I. *Anesthesiology* 1943, **4**, 126.
34. Hunter C. *Br. Med. J.* 1859, **19**.
35. Lafargue G. V. *C. R. Acad. Sci. Paris* 1836, **2**, 397.
36. Jakobsen C. J. et al. *Anaesthesia* 1990, **45**, 40.
37. Koski E. M. J. et al. *Br. J. Anaes.* 1990, **64**, 16.
38. Nimmo W. S. *Br. J. Anaesth.* 1990, **64**, 7.
39. Richards M. J., Skues M. A. et al. *Br. J. Anaesth.*, 1990, **65**, 157.
40. Editorial, *Lancet* 1990, **335**, 507.
41. Hodsman N. B. A, Burns J., et al. *Anaesthesia.* 1987, **42**, 1005.
42. Gallagher E. G. et al. *Anaesthesia* 1988, **43**, 1011–1014., Escolano F. et al. *Anaesthesia* 1989, **44**, 212; Dubin S. A. *Anesth. analg.* 1989, **69**, 680.
43. Carnie J. and Johnson R. A. *Anaesthesia* 1985, **40**, 1114.
44. Ratcliff A. et al. *Anaesthesia.* 1989, **44**, 812.
45. Mcateer E. J. et al. *Anaesthesia* 1984, **39**, 1177; Whitwam J. G., Al-Khudari B. et al. *Br. J. Anaesth.* 1983, **55**, 77.
46. Irjala J. et al. *Anaesthesia* 1989, **44**, 685.
47. Sjörall S. et al. *Anaesthesia* 1982, **37**, 924.
48. Dundee J. W. et al. *Anaesthesia* 1985, **40**, 441.
49. Ben-Shlomo I. et al. *Br. J. Anaesth* 1990, **64**, 45.
50. Tuel D. C. and Weis F. R. *Anesthesiology* 1990, **72**, 216.
51. Wilson E. et al. *Br. J. Anaesth.* 1990, **64**, 48.
52. Gale G. D. et al. *Br. J. Anaesth.* 1983, **55**, 761.
53. Pollard B. J. *Anaesthesia* 1989, **44**, 137–138.
54. Fisher G. C. et al. *Anaesthesia* 1989, **44**, 101.
55. Luger T. G. *Br J. Anaesth* 1990, **64**, 53.
56. Pithra J. *Medical Times, Lond.* 1861, **2**, 121.
57. Smith D. S. et al. *Anesthesiology* 1979, **51**, 343.
58. Cozantis D. A. *Anaesthesia* 1975, **34**, 236.
59. Mirakhur R. K. et al. *Anaesthesia* 1979, **34**, 453.
60. Brock-Utne J. G. et al. *Anaesthesia* 1976, **31**, 1186.
61. Smallridge RC, Chernow B, Critical care medicine, 1989, **17**, 1254.
62. Garde J. F. et al. *Anesth. Analg.* 1978, **57**, 572.
63. Soban D. In *Progress in Anaesthesiology.* (eds Boulton T. B. et al.) Amsterdam: Excerpta Medica Foundation, 1970, 193.
64. Ladenburg A. *Ann. Chem. Pharmac.* 1881, **206**, 274.
65. Schneiderlinn J. *Aertz. Mitt. a. Baden* 1900, **54**, 104.
66. Gauss C. J. *Arch. Gynaek.* 1906, **78**, 579.
67. Kesecioglu J. et al. *Acta Anaes. Scand.* 1991, **35**, 278.
68. Franko B. V. and Lunsford C. D. *J. Med. Pharm. Chem.* 1960, **11**, 523.
69. Boawright C. F. et al. *Am. Acad. Ophthal. Otolaryngol.* 1970, **74**, 1139.
70. Proakis A. G. and Harris G. B. *Anesthesiology* 1978, **48**, 339.
71. Brock-Utne J. G. et al. *Can. Anaesth. Soc. J.* 1978, **25**, 144; Brock-Utne J. G. *Anaesthesia* 1976, **31**, 1186.
72. Salem M. G. and Ahearn R. S. *J. R. Soc. Med.* 1986, **79**, 19.
73. Hill G. E. et al. *Can. Anaesth. Soc. J.* 1977, **24**, 707.
74. Baraka A. *Br. J. Anaesth.* 1978, **50**, 1075.

Chapter 6

Anaesthetic equipment

'We shape our tools, and thereafter our tools shape us'

There is value in standardization of equipment within a unit, but there is also a good argument for a variety of equipment to meet the varying requirements of individual patients and for training purposes.

Evaluation of medical anaesthetic equipment

British Standard 5724 – Part 1 (1979 & 1989) – safety
    Part 2 – specifications
    Part 3 – performance
European equivalent is IEC 601.
The European Medical Device Directives (in force in 1993)
    A. Implantable Active Devices, e.g. pacemakers
    B. Medical Devices Class 1. heart valves
        Class 2. Powered nonimplantable devices, e.g. anaesthetic equipment
    C. In-Vitro diagnostics
The accredited mark is 'CE' 'Horizontal standards' concern electrical safety, sterilization, biocompatibility. 'Vertical standards' concern clinical investigation protocols and standards specific to a given device.

ANAESTHETIC MACHINES

Apparatus for administration of inhalation anaesthesia

For the origins of the plenum system of vaporization of volatile agents, *see* Boulton T. B. Classical File, *Surv. Anesthesiol.* 1985, **29**, 191. The Junker's Inhaler (Junker F. A, 1828–1901) *Med. Times & Gaz.* 1867, **2**, 590; and *ibid*, 1868, **1**, 171) using air blown over chloroform with a hand pump, was an early example. It was founded on B. W. Richardson's ether spray, used for the production of analgesia by the use of cold. Dates of introduction of some machines: Frederick Hewitt (1857–1916) of London, 1898; Charles Teter of Cleveland 1902; Elmer Isaac McKesson (1881–1935) of Toledo, physiologist, anaesthetist and manufacturer, 1910; Walter R. Boothby (1880–1953) of the Mayo Clinic, 1910; Frederick J. Cotton (1869–1938) of Boston, 1910; James Tayloe Gwathmey (1863–1944) of New York, 1914; Karl Connell (1873–1941) New York anaesthetist, 1911; Richard von Forregger (1873–1960), New York manufacturer, 1914; Henry Edmund Gaskin Boyle (1875–1941) London anaesthetist, 1917.

Anaesthetic machines may provide continuous or intermittent flow. The intermittent flow apparatus may be plenum (machine powered) or 'draw-over' (patient powered).

The 'Boyle machine'[1]

Gases are delivered from pipelines or cylinders via a reducing valve, which reduces the pressure to the flow-meters where flow is controlled by a needle valve. Two or more vaporizers are usually provided and increasing amounts of the gases can be diverted through them. Gases then pass into a Magill attachment (Mapleson-A) or alternative system.

The original Boyle machine of 1917 was an adaptation of the American Gwathmey apparatus,[2] and that of Marshall in London. It was built by the firm, Coxeters, under the personal direction of Lord George Wellesley (a great grandson of the first Duke of Wellington). In its original form, it housed two nitrous oxide and two oxygen cylinders in a wooden box and used a water-sight flow-meter and an ether vaporizer. It had a pressure gauge on the oxygen cylinders, fine-adjustment reducing valves and a spirit flame to warm these and prevent obstruction of gas flow from freezing of water vapour, an impurity in early gas supplies. A Cattlin bag, a three-way stopcock and a face-mask completed the apparatus. A portable form was designed for use with the British Army in France. Subsequent modifications were:

1920. Addition of vaporizing bottle to flow-meters.
1926. Addition of second vaporizing bottle and bypass controls.
1927. Addition of third water-sight feed tube for carbon dioxide.
1930. Addition of plunger device to Boyles bottle.
1931. Dry bobbin type of flow-meter displaced water-sight feed.
1937. Rotameters displaced dry bobbin flow-meters.

The modern Boyle's apparatus bears little resemblance to the original model. For a description of the modern machine *see* Ward C. S. *Anaesthetic Equipment*. 2nd ed. London: Baillière, 1985; Henville J. D. Recent developments in anaesthetic machines and ventilators, in *Anaesthetic Review*–1 (Kaufman L. ed.) London: Churchill Livingstone, 1982.

Cylinders

UK colours and pressures when full at 15°C: oxygen (white shoulders/black body) – 137 bar; nitrous oxide (blue) – 54 bar; carbon dioxide (grey) – 50 bar; Air (grey body/black and white quartered shoulders) – 137 bar; entonox (blue body/white and blue quartered shoulders) – 137 bar; and cyclopropane (orange) – 5 bar;

Cylinders are made of molybdenum steel. They are checked at intervals by the manufacturer for defects by subjecting them to tests: (1) *Tensile test:* this is carried out on at least 1 out of every 100 cylinders manufactured. Strips are cut and stretched – the 'yield point' should not be less than 15 tons/in^2; (2) *Flattening, impact and bend tests*: also carried out on at least 1 out of every 100 cylinders made; (3) *Hydraulic or pressure test:* usually a water-jacket test. The filling ratio of a cylinder is the ratio of weight of gas in the cylinder to weight of water the cylinder could hold. Nitrous oxide cylinders are filled to a filling ratio of 0.75. Great care is taken that the gas is free from water vapour, otherwise when the cylinder is opened, temperature falls and water vapour would freeze and block the exit valve. Cylinder outlet valves use the pin-index system (British Standard 1319, 1955) so arranged that it is impossible to connect cylinders to wrong yokes,[3] and the yokes connected to flow meters via non-interchangeable screw-threaded connectors (NIST). Before connection to the yoke, the cylinder valve is turned on briefly to flush out inflammable dust. After connection, the cylinder valve is slowly opened 2.5 turns. Machine backflow check valves prevent transfilling of cylinders.

Calculation of cylinder contents: Nitrous oxide by weight (1.87 g/l of gas); critical temperature 36.5°C, critical pressure 72 bar. (Note that nitrogen impurity exists in nitrous oxide cylinders, especially at first opening).[4] Oxygen and air content calculated by pressure gauges.

Table 6.1 Cylinder sizes[5]

OXYGEN (black body/white shoulder in UK)

Size	Capacity (l)	Weight (Kg)	Valve type
C	170	2	pin index
D	340	3.4	pin index
E	680	5.4	pin index
F	1360	14.5	bullnose

NITROUS OXIDE (blue in UK)

Size	Capacity (l)	Weight (Kg) Cylinder	Gas	Valve type
C	450	2	0.85	pin index
D	900	3.4	1.7	pin index
E	1800	5.4	3.4	pin index
F	2600	14.5	6.8	wheel

Piped gas supplies[6]

Oxygen (white, 4 bar), nitrous oxide (blue, 4 bar), Entonox (oxygen and nitrous oxide mixture in equal volumes), compressed air (black, 7 bar for instrument use, 4 bar – medical quality) and vacuum (yellow) may be supplied by pipe-lines (UK colours). Banks of supply cylinders are housed in a ventilated fireproof room and automatically switch (with warning lights), to the reserve bank when the running bank is near exhaustion. The machine to pipeline connections are 'tug-tested' to ensure security.

Liquid oxygen supply[8]

Oxygen is stored in a thermally insulated vessel at a pressure of about 1200 kPa and at a temperature lower than the critical temperature (minus 119°C). Evaporation requires heat. Fresh supplies of liquid oxygen are pumped from a tanker into a storage vessel, which rests on a weighing balance so that a dial measures the mass of liquid. Reserve banks of oxygen cylinders are kept in case of failure of supply. Liquid oxygen stores are housed away from main buildings because of the fire hazard.

Accidents have occurred due to the wrong connection of pipe-lines to anaesthetic apparatus. The union between hoses and the anaesthetic machine should be permanent.[9] The routine pre-anaesthetic drill will detect any such fault. Hoses are colour coded and when repairs are necessary a complete hose assembly is provided. A 'permit to work' system[10] requires in the UK a certificate in six parts to be signed as appropriate and is used when the action of one group of workers could directly or indirectly expose others to hazard. Three levels of hazard are identified: high, when work involves cutting an in-service pipe-line, with danger of cross-connection or pollution; medium, work on a terminal unit where more than one gas is supplied, with danger of cross-connection; and low, where only one gas is involved. Hazards include mechanical, electrical failures, and failures of correct interaction between anaesthetist and machine. There must be enough light shining on the machine (and the patient) to see everything clearly.

Pressure and contents gauges

These indicate the cylinder contents in the case of oxygen and carbon dioxide. In the case of nitrous oxide they read 'full' until the last liquid is vaporized, when the pressure declines with the last 1/2 h use of the contents. The BS 4272 (1968) gives a scale marked '0; 1/4; 1/2; 3/4; full'.

The preanaesthetic machine checklist

The following procedure has been recommended.[11] At the start the apparatus is disconnected from all piped medical gases and the oxygen and nitrous oxide cylinders turned off.

1. Check that full cylinders are properly attached to their yokes and all turned off.

2. Open the O_2 and N_2O flow-meter valves 2–3 full turns and ensure all others closed. No flow occurs.

3. Turn on O_2 cylinder. Check O_2 gauge for adequate content. O_2 flow-meter should register a flow. Adjust to test flow 4 l/min. *If any N_2O flow registers, reject machine.*

4. Turn on N_2O cylinder and check that N_2O rotameter registers a flow. *If O_2 flow changes, reject machine.*

5. Set the O_2 failure device in operation if not automatic.

6. Turn off O_2 cylinder. Check that O_2 bobbin falls completely to bottom of tube. Check that O_2 failure device works. *If O_2 flow-meter registers any flow when N_2O only turned on, reject machine.*

7. Insert O_2 pipe-line probe into supply connection, with 'tug test'. This cancels operation of O_2 failure alarm. Check the O_2 flow-meter. Set at 4 l/min. An oxygen analyser confirms the nature of the gas.

8. Turn off N_2O cylinder. *If O_2 bobbin demonstrates any fall when N_2O turned off, reject machine.*

9. Insert N_2O probe into pipe-line connection, with tug test. *If any change in position of O_2 bobbin, reject machine.*

10. The circuit system outlet is occluded to ensure that pressure relief valve on back bar is operative.

The oxygen flush is operated.

The contents, closure, backbar locking, and control knob function of vaporisers are checked and also any electrical devices, e.g. monitors. The circuit systems are checked for leaks and loose connections by occluding the outlet while gas flows. The bobbins dip slightly, and the pressure relief valve opens. This test should not be performed if there is no pressure relief valve.

The whistle discriminator[12] enables the nature of a gas issuing from a pipeline to be determined. With nitrous oxide, the note falls one-and-a-half tones from the oxygen note.

Pressure reducing valves (pressure regulators)

Reducing valves were first used in association with the oxygen-hydrogen blow lamp in 1816 and the 'lime-light' of 1826 and (a) give safe working pressures; (b) prevent equipment damage; (c) maintain constant pressure within the machine; and (d) allow delicate control of gas flows. There is no pressure regulator on the cyclopropane lines. The classic reducing valve was the Adams valve (named after an employee of Messrs Coxeter, the manufacturers). A toggle mechanism occludes the orifice when pressure rises. Dust filters are incorporated. The Medishield 5 valve reduces to 810 kPa and the M valve to 405 kPa. The McKesson valve to 465 kPa. In the US, regulating valves vary from these values.

Flow restrictors

Pipe-line gas supplies at 405 kPa (about 4 atmospheres) are commonly transferred to the flow-meters without interposition of a reducing valve. Sudden pressure surges are prevented by the use of a flow restrictor, which is a constriction in the low-pressure circuit upstream to the flow-meter. The fine-adjustment control would require recalibration if the pipe-line pressure changed markedly. Flow restrictors are also used downstream of vaporizers to prevent back-pressure effects.

Flow-meters

Theory

Flow rate through a tube is proportional to the fourth power of the radius. With a given pressure difference across an orifice, flow rate of gas is proportional to the square of the diameter of the orifice. Flow rate along a tube depends on the viscosity of a gas. Flow rate through an orifice depends on density and varies as the reciprocal of the square root of the density.

Types of flow-meter

These may be divided into variable orifice and fixed orifice types.

VARIABLE-ORIFICE METERS (FIXED-PRESSURE DIFFERENCE)

1. The rotameter. The type used today in most modern machines. As a gas-measuring device it was patented in Germany in 1908 by Karl Küppers of Aachen, and used in anaesthesia by Maximilian Neu,[13] an obstetrician gynaecologist of Heidelburg, in 1910; Magill suggested its use independently in 1932 and used it a few years later. R. Salt developed it further in 1937.

Gas is led to the base of a finely wrought glass tube, slightly smaller on cross-section at bottom than at top. A light metal float (bobbin) rides the gas jet; notches in its edge cause it to rotate. As the bobbin rises with increased flow, the size of the annulus between it and the glass tube increases. Height of top of float gives rate of flow, the gas escaping between the rim of the metal float and the walls of the glass tube. The glass tubes must be vertical, and clean, and the float rotate freely. A wire stop keeps the float in sight at the top. The calibration of the glass tubes takes into account both the density and the viscosity of the gases passing through them. Viscosity is important at low flows because gas flow round the bobbin approximates to tubular flow (diameter of orifice less than length), but density is important at high flows (diameter of orifice greater than length). Consequently, a rotameter calibrated for carbon dioxide will not read true for cyclopropane, because although their densities are similar (44:42) their viscosities are different (1:0.6). The needle valve control knob carries the name of the gas and is colour coded. The oxygen control knob commonly protrudes further out than the others to assist recognition.

The needle valve may be upstream of the rotameter (UK), or downstream (USA), which maintains a more constant pressure in the rotameter tube.

The rotameter bank may have the oxygen on the left (UK) or right (parts of USA). In either case, the flow across the top of the rotameter block is from right to left, which diminishes the risk from leaks at the top of the oxygen rotameter.

2. The Heidbrink meter. A black inverted float is free to rise within a metal tube with a varying taper. The upper end projects into a glass tube. It is accurate for low flows and also accommodates high flows.

3. Connell meter. A pair of stainless-steel balls move within a tapered glass tube on an inclined plane (historical interest).

FIXED-ORIFICE METERS (VARIABLE-PRESSURE DIFFERENCE)

Pressure differentials across an orifice vary with changes in flow. Pressure varies as the square of flow rate.

1. *Pressure gauge meter.* The pressure build-up proximal to the constriction is measured utilizing a Bourdon pressure gauge, which is then calibrated for flow (used on some air cylinders).

2. *Water depression meter.* Pressure on two sides of the fixed orifice is measured by means of a water manometer.

Inaccuracies and dangers of rotameters

1. Static electricity and dirt can cause as much as 35% inaccuracy. It can cause sticking of the bobbin, especially when low flows are used.

2. Cracked flow-meter tubes with consequent leaks may result in delivery of a hypoxic mixture.

It is safer to place the oxygen flow-meter last in the flow-meter bank. An internal arrangement at the top of the rotameters allows this to be achieved even with the oxygen rotameter on the left, and the bank on the left side of the machine.

3. A defect in the top sealing washer of a rotameter can cause fatal deprivation of oxygen.[14]

4. The rotameter tube must be vertical.

5. The small bobbin of a cyclopropane or carbon dioxide flow-meter can become jammed at the top of the tube so that the anaesthetist is unaware that gas is flowing.

6. Back-pressure (*see below*).

Effect of barometric pressure

Flow-meters are calibrated for use at sea level. They become inaccurate at high altitudes or in hyperbaric chambers.

Flow-meters also become inaccurate when a restriction at the outlet causes a pressure build-up. This may occur when some humidifiers, nebulizers, etc. are in use. Flow is then greater than indicated with variable-orifice-type flow-meters. In the fixed-orifice type, a large flow may be indicated even when there is complete occlusion of the outlet. These inaccuracies can be corrected by placing the control valve distal to the orifice. In the pressure-compensated flow-meter, pressure in the flow-meter itself is the same as that in the supply line. The flow-meter is calibrated in terms of litres the gas will occupy after discharge to atmospheric pressure.[15]

A simple flow-meter has been described for unusual gases.[15]

Oxygen flush (bypass)

The control should not be able to be left on accidentally, or it will dilute anaesthetics and allow awareness. The flowrate is more than 35 l/min.

Vaporizers

These may be draw-over (*see* Chapter 36) or machine gas driven – 'plenum' (variable bypass and measured-flow).

Both variable bypass (tec-type; 'tec' = 'temperature compensated') and measured-flow (kettle-type) vaporizers when fully turned off can leak anaesthetic vapours into the circuit.[16]

Some machines inject liquid agent into the gas stream in exact amounts controlled by feedback from vapour analysers further down the stream, and the required percentage dialled in by the operator. This is analogous to fuel injection.

A wide variety of vaporizers are now available. In general they are designed for use with a particular agent (sometimes, e.g. 'Selectatec', with lockouts preventing use of more than one at a time) or in a particular situation (e.g. 'Triservice' type). Some are designed to prevent spillage if not kept vertical (e.g. Mk 4 Fluotec).

Hook-on mountings, e.g. 'Selectatec', can cause major leaks of anaesthetic gas if not locked on properly.

Concentration distal to vaporizer depends on:

1. SVP of the inhalation agent (isoflurane 250; enflurane 184; halothane 240). The higher the SVP, the greater the concentration delivered. The gas diverted through the vapour chamber becomes fully saturated with the volatile agent.

2. Temperature (by raising the SVP). The heat for vaporizing the agent comes from the liquid agent itself, which cools as a result. (*See* Compensation, below.)

3. The 'splitting ratio', i.e. the proportion of the total flow that is diverted to the vaporizing chamber.

4. The surface area of the vapour chamber, including wick.

5. Flow characteristics through the vapour chamber.

6. The amount of liquid in the vapour chamber (concentration falls when nearly empty)

Compensation devices to stabilize the delivered concentrations

Efforts are made to overcome change of concentration with ambient temperature, rate of evaporation and the degree of heat-gain from the vaporizer jacket or the surroundings by:

1. Automatic variation of the outlet port of the vaporizing chamber with temperature. The use of bimetallic (zinc-copper or zinc-brass) bars or a thermosensitive capsule, or both.

2. By bubbling the gas through the agent as in the 'copper kettle' to provide a saturated vapour that can be diluted to obtain the desired concentration. (The vapour chamber of a 'tec' type also produces a saturated vapour, due to the large surface area.)

3. To maintain the liquid at constant temperature. The use of a waterbath or calcium chloride crystals to provide extra heat (e.g. in EMO).

Many vaporizers have interlocks to prevent more than one being on at one time. Some have spill-proof devices to prevent liquid loss if placed in non-vertical positions. Keyed filling ports, which only connect with specific filler tubes of specific bottles of specific agents, are common. Vaporizers are serviced at regular intervals e.g. yearly.

The problem posed by desflurane is that its boiling point is near to room temperature, and it might have to be kept in cooled vaporizers or in warmed cylinders.[17] While sevoflurane can be vaporized, a 'Trilene interlock' may be needed to prevent it being used with soda lime.

Oxygen failure warning (alarm) devices

The ideal warning device should: (1) not depend on the pressure of any gas other than the oxygen itself; (2) an alarm system should not utilize battery or mains power; (3) the signal should be audible and of sufficient length, volume and character; (4) there should be a warning of impending failure, and a further warning that failure has occurred; (5) when it comes into operation: (*a*) other gases should cease to flow; (*b*) the breathing system should open to the atmosphere; and (*c*) inspired oxygen concentration should be at least equal to that of air, and build-up of carbon dioxide should not occur; and (6) it should be impossible to resume anaesthesia until the oxygen supply has been restored.

Pressure relief valves

These prevent damage to the machine, should the outlet become obstructed (flow restrictors are satisfactory only as a means of smoothing surges of pressure). Pressure relief valves are combined non-return and pressure relief valves and are usually fitted at the end of the back bar, downstream from the vaporizers. They are set to operate at 30–40 kPa (300–400 cm H_2O). (BS4272 Part 1 1968.)

Pressure limiting valves

These aim to prevent damage to the patient's airways. They have a much lower opening pressure (e.g. 4 kPa) than pressure relief valves. Such valves may be built into the breathing systems. In addition, the 2 litre rubber reservoir bag, when distended with pressure, seldom reaches pressures above 5 kPa[18] before it splits although plastic disposable bags used in the USA can develop high pressures.[19] A pressure limiting reservoir bag used in conjunction with a pressure limiting valve has been described.[20] Unfortunately, a steady pressure of 4 kPa (30 mmHg) at the alveoli will stop the pulmonary circulation (PA systolic pressure = 25 mmHg), so this hazard is not prevented by these valves.

Expiratory valves

These are one-way, spring-loaded, fully adjustable valves. When open, they should have minimal resistance to expiration (1–5 mmHg). During spontaneous breathing they should always be fully opened (when the 'opening pressure' is 1–5 mmHg) because their setting determines the mean pressure in the anaesthetic circuit and in the patient's respiratory tract. During manual IPPV, they are usually nearly closed with a small leak. During ventilator IPPV, they are usually completely closed. Heidbrink-type expiratory valves should be sterilized by autoclaving because antiseptic solutions may produce corrosion, stickiness and consequent increased resistance to opening pressure. Partial closure of the valve during spontaneous respiration produces a crude form of PEEP.

The widespread use of electronics in anaesthetic machines, with or without built-in monitoring, provides a high level of sophistication but at the price of vulnerability to mains failure.

Intermittent flow machines

For example McKesson, are of historical interest. BS 4272 Part 1 (1968) defines their standards. Many of them could deliver continuous flow.

Portable anaesthetic machines

Triservice, Portablease, Fluoxair. Many of these use a low-resistance draw-over vaporizer and an inflating bellows with one way valves and facilities for oxygen enrichment.

Factors affecting carbon dioxide elimination

1. Fresh gas flow rate.
2. Apparatus deadspace,[21] both static and dynamic.
3. Leaks in the anaesthetic system (especially ventilators).
4. Waveform and settings of the ventilator.
5. Design of the systems.
6. Patient's alveolar ventilation (patient's respiratory drive and performance; patient's respiratory waveform).

Reservoir bags

These are usually made of antistatic rubber (black because of the carbon content) and should be large enough to supply the patient's inspiratory volume (e.g. 2 l for an adult). They also act as an excellent visual monitor of spontaneous respiration. (*See also* Pressure limiting valves, above.) In paediatric anaesthesia a smaller bag gives a better indication of tidal excursion.

(For assessment of expiratory valves and reservoir bags, *see* Mostafa S. M. and Hall I. D. *Anaesthesia* 1985, **40**, 55.)

Face masks

These should be easy to clean and sterilize after each patient, and be anti-static. They should provide a good fit with the patient's face and add minimal dead space. The dead space of a face mask may be considerable (7–198 ml) and this may equal or exceed the anatomical dead space of an average adult. In children and infants it is possible for the mask and attachments to double or treble the dead space. The Rendell-Baker-Souchek facemask and partitioned adaptor greatly reduce this dead space. Flavoured masks are available, e.g. chocolate, raspberry, cherry etc. The face mask connectors also add to the dead space (Ruben valve: 9 ml; angle connection and expiratory valve: 28–30 ml). A disposable face mask is available. An airtight seal between a face mask and the edentulous patient can often be improved by retention of dentures.

'Brain' laryngeal masks[22]

An easy alternative where face-masks are unsatisfactory (e.g. in bearded patients) and intubation is difficult or impossible[23]. They are normally inserted blind to behind the larynx. In difficult cases this is facilitated by extension of the head, insertion with the aperture facing backwards, then rotation to the forwards position within the pharynx. Malposition may be caused by the mask being: (a) not in far enough; (b) too far in – within the oesophagus; and (c) having pushed the epiglottis down between it and the glottis.[24] Repositioning is straightforward. Several sizes are available: sizes 1, 2 and 2½ suitable for children and sizes 2, 3 and 4 for adults. The cuff of size 3 takes about 20 ml, size 4 about 30 ml. Although designed for spontaneous respiration, they have been used for gentle IPPV,[25] but they do not protect the airway from aspiration pneumonia,[26] and therefore are not appropriate for Caesarean section.[27] They may be lubricated with lignocaine gel to reduce coughing. The depression of pharyngeal reflexes by propofol is particularly advantageous in assisting their insertion immediately after induction.

The pilot balloon has been exploded off during sterilization, and entered the pipe of the laryngeal mask.[28]

Entonox apparatus

The premixed gases are supplied from the cylinder via a two-stage valve. The first stage is a simple, reducing valve which decreases pressure to about 1350 kPa (200 lb/in^2). The second incorporates a tilting valve, which opens to the negative pressure of inspiration but is closed when the positive pressure of expiration pushes down a sensing diaphragm. Little inspiratory effort is needed to produce a high flow rate. Gas cannot flow when pressure in the cylinder falls below 1350 kPa (200 lb/in^2) so that a proportion of gas is wasted. This is a safety factor should separation of the premixed gases have occurred, because since residual gas is likely then to be rich in nitrous oxide. The apparatus is compact and portable, weighing 6.1 kg with a full 500-litre cylinder. BS 4272 Part 2 (1968) defines their standards.

Premixed gases can also be used with a calibrated flow-meter and the Magill circuit.

ANAESTHETIC GAS DELIVERY SYSTEMS

These use rubber or plastic pipe. Rubber pipe is made antistatic by addition of carbon, which is responsible for its black colour. Corrugations make the pipes kink-proof. Connections are made with 8.5 (paediatric), 15, 22, or 30 (exhaust) millimetre tapers, with or without locking rings. There is inevitably resistance to flow and deadspace in such tubular systems.[29] Some rebreathing is almost inevitable, and the patient compensates for this by physical and perhaps physiological means. Attempts to reduce rebreathing usually employ either valves or large gas flows. It can be assessed by capnography.[30]

Semi-closed methods

These methods may allow some degree of rebreathing and may or may not be used in conjunction with carbon dioxide absorption. If the Magill attachment (Mapleson System A) is used,[31] effective carbon dioxide elimination requires spontaneous respiration, an expiratory valve of minimal resistance and a total gas flow greater than the alveolar ventilation (approximately 70% of the respiratory minute volume of the patient). There is no rebreathing if the fresh gas supply is more than 5 l/min for a 70-kg patient. Studies of the effect of fresh gas flows lower than alveolar ventilation indicate that with mild rebreathing the system acts as simple added dead space, but with gross rebreathing the entire system acts as a mixing device. Variations in tidal volume can be significant.

Classification

Mapleson made a theoretical study of several variations of the Magill attachment. He classified them as shown in Fig. 6.1.

Mapleson system A

The most satisfactory with spontaneous respiration (e.g. Magill system). A flow of about 5 l/min is required (in young healthy patients) to flush carbon dioxide from the system. In *assisted* or *controlled respiration*, the expiratory valve must be partly closed. The Magill system is efficient with regard to carbon dioxide disposal in both spontaneous and controlled ventilation with gas flows of 5–6 l/min.

The advancing cone front of laminar flow[32] may explain how some hypoventilating patients, breathing spontaneously under anaesthesia with small tidal volumes (e.g. 100 ml), may ventilate reasonably effectively. The gas in the centre of a tube may reach the end of the tube preferentially. This only occurs with laminar flow. Furthermore, the higher the patient's alveolar CO_2 the more CO_2 is excreted at each breath.

Variations of the Mapleson A system

THE LACK SYSTEM[33]

The patient breathes through concentric tubes. The outer tube is inspiratory, the large inner tube is expiratory; the valve is situated near the anaesthetic apparatus. The commercial version has an inspiratory limb capacity of 500 ml and resistance to respiration is acceptable. The Lack system, unlike the Bain,

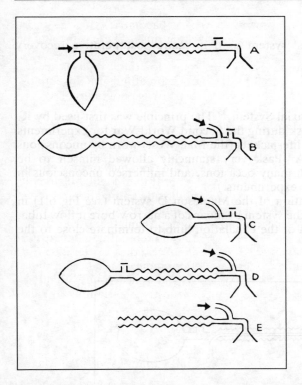

Figure 6.1 The Mapleson classification of anaesthetic systems.

does not readily permit the use of mechanical ventilators. It can be easily adapted for use with scavenging systems. The Lack Parallel system has two tubes side by side.

MILLER PREFERENTIAL FLOW SYSTEM

Similar to the Lack but has no valves.

ENCLOSED AFFERENT RESERVOIR[34]

The inspiratory reservoir bag is inside a rigid bottle (to which the expired gases pass via a one-way valve, before being vented). It is equally efficient during spontaneous respiration or IPPV.

Mapleson B

Not in common clinical use.

Mapleson C

For example, the 'Water's' system used in many postoperative recovery wards.

Mapleson D

For example, the Bain Co-axial System.[35] The principle was first used by R. R. Macintosh and E. A. Pask during the Second World War for experiments on the buoyant qualities of life-jackets (the Mae West) worn by unconscious subjects.[36] (The late E. A. Pask very staunchly allowed himself to be anaesthetized with ether on many occasions, and immersed unconscious in choppy water, during these experiments.)

The system is a modification of the Mapleson D system (*see* Fig 6.1) in which the fresh gases enter the system by means of a narrow-bore inflow tube, which lies within the lumen of the exhalation limb to terminate close to the patient end (Fig. 6. 2).

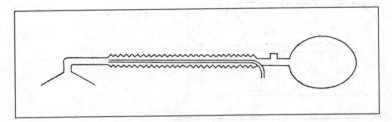

Figure 6.2 The Bain System.

Advantages. The system carries a single tube to the patient. It is light in weight, can be used in all age groups, is adaptable to all types of anaesthetic procedures and can be used with spontaneous respiration and IPPV. (The Bain expiratory valve is normally closed for mechanical IPPV, the expired gases exiting via the ventilator.) It is controlled entirely from the machine end of the system. Scavenging of expired gases is facilitated. The Penlon co-axial system is a modification in which the inner tube is made of antistatic material; the outer tube is transparent to facilitate inspection. The Penlon co-axial valve is used to fit the system to the outlet of the anaesthetic apparatus. Hazard can occur if the inner tube becomes broken or dislodged because considerable dead space may then occur. This is tested for in the pre-anaesthetic checklist by occluding the exit port of the inner tube with the little finger while gas is flowing from the machine, and noting the drop in flow-meter bobbins (only if the machine has a pressure release valve).

With IPPV a fresh gas flow of 70 ml/kg (5 l/min for a man of 70 kg) produces normocapnia, and 100 ml/kg mild hypocapnia. $Paco_2$ is related to fresh gas flow in patients weighing more than 40 kg. Below this, more carbon dioxide is produced per unit of body weight and a minimal flow of 3.5 l/min has been recommended for patients weighing less than 50 kg. A flow of about 3 l/min is used with small children and infants.

With spontaneous respiration, recommended fresh gas flow rates have varied from three times the minute volume to between 90 and 160 ml/kg. The differences probably reflect the respiratory depression caused by premedication, the depth of anaesthesia and the ratio of inspiration to expiration. In view of the higher gas flows required during spontaneous respiration, the Mapleson A (Magill) system is then more economical than the Bain.

Variations of the Bain include the Mera F-type with twin hoses.

Recommended fresh gas flows for use with spontaneous respiration are: Lack, 70; Magill, 70; and Bain, 100 ml/kg/min. These flows should be increased by about 10% for each degree Centigrade above 37°C.[37] Routine capnography enables fresh gas flows to be adjusted for individual patients. In particular, the elderly produce far less CO_2 and require much less fresh gas. (Note that capnograph sampling from the patient end of a Bain system may give false results because of the jet of fresh gas impinging on the sampling port.)

Mapleson E

For example, the Ayre's T-piece[38] (*see* also Chapter 22 Paediatric) Advocated primarily for use in infants and young children. In order to prevent dilution of inspired gases with air on the one hand, or rebreathing with carbon dioxide accumulation on the other, it is recommended that the total fresh gas flow should be about twice the minute volume of the patient, and the volume of the reservoir tube equal to about a third of the tidal volume. Classically modified by Jackson Rees who added a bag for monitoring and IPPV.[39] Gases can be scavenged.

Variations of the T-piece technique to avoid expiratory resistance include the use of a Y-piece, the provision of a hole in the adaptor of the tracheal tube, lifting up the diaphragm of any expiratory valve with a safety-pin. The main advantage of the T-piece technique is the absence of resistance to expiration, a factor of crucial importance in small children.

Efficiency of systems with spontaneous respiration:

A > D, E > C > B

Efficiency of systems with IPPV:

D, E > B > C > A

The Hafnia systems

These are modifications of Mapleson A, B, C and D systems, using suction directly from the system to prevent atmospheric pollution. The expiratory valve is replaced by a suction port and an ejector flow-meter.

The Burchett and Bennett Co-axial Breathing System

This combines the benefits of the Mapleson A, D and E systems.

The Humphrey System (ADE system)[29]

A single lever changes from one system to the other. This combines the Mapleson A, D and E principles.

Rebreathing and deadspace[40]

The patient's dead space is increased by most anaesthetic apparatus, and efforts are made to reduce this to a minimum, by adequate fresh gas flows (70% of MV for Magill system; ranging to 200% of MV for T-piece). Rebreathing of some alveolar gas occurs with most anaesthetic breathing systems (especially the Bain), but in practice does not greatly raise the patient's $Paco_2$, because a reasonably lightly anaesthetized person can compensate for this to some extent.

Non-rebreathing valves

Advantages are. (1) No possibility of rebreathing provided the dead space of the valve itself is small; (2) can be used for spontaneous or controlled respiration; and (3) can be used to measure minute volume, if the flow-meters are accurate.

Disadvantages. (1) Wasteful; (2) variations of minute volume during spontaneous respiration require frequent adjustment of the flow-meters to prevent collapse or distension of the reservoir bag; (3) valves may stick; and (4) some valves are noisy.

Some *examples* of non-rebreathing valves:

1. The Ruben valve. A bobbin moves against a spring to act as a unidirectional valve and an outlet valve prevents admission of atmospheric air. Dead space 9 ml. Low resistance. The resuscitation version has no outlet valve so that a patient breathing spontaneously will inhale air from the atmosphere.

2. The Ambu valves. The bobbin of the Ruben valve is replaced by one or two silicone rubber flaps. The valve can be dismantled easily for cleaning and sterilization. It is possible to reassemble the valve incorrectly with consequent risk of hypoxia. It can be used with a self-inflating bag. The valve with one flap is only suitable for IPPV. The valve with two rubber flaps is suitable for IPPV or spontaneous respiration. It has a very low dead space.

The ideal valve should have no forward leak, no back leak, low resistance, minimal dead space, minimal opening pressure without sticking, light weight, transparency, easy cleaning and sterilizing, reliability and durability, and a single expiratory port for collecting and measuring exhaled air.

Insufflation techniques

Tracheal insufflation via a small catheter, used by Elsberg of New York in 1910 and by Magill and C. Langton Hewer, of London in 1923, still occasionally finds a use in upper airway manipulations.

Rebreathing with carbon dioxide absorption – closed systems, low-flow systems

History

Introduced by John Snow in 1850,[41] used by Franz Kuhn (1866–1929), of Kassel, in 1906 in Germany.[42] A closed-circuit system for use by coal miners was described by Theodore Schwann (1810–1882), known for his nerve cells, and professor in the University of Liege, in 1877.[43] Revised by Dennis Jackson (1878–1930) of Cincinnati in 1915 for work on animals (after working on problems of ventilation in submarines, during the First World War);[44] and by Waters in 1920 in clinical anaesthesia.[45] The circle or two-phase system was devised by Brian Sword (1889–1956) of North Carolina,[46] in 1926. W. B. Primrose (1892–1977), of Glasgow, used caustic soda solution as an absorber in 1931,[47] while Dräger patented an apparatus with a closed system in 1926.[48]

The closed, circle, or low-flow system

Founded on the principle that if sufficient oxygen is added to supply body's basal needs and carbon dioxide is absorbed, the same mixture of gases can be rebreathed repeatedly. Adult basal oxygen consumption varies between 200 and 400 ml/min. The system may be completely closed, or it may have a leak, when used with slightly larger flows. There is a rubber reservoir bag in the system. The system may be 'to-and-fro' or 'circle'.

Administration of the volatile agent:

1. *By vaporiser.* The vaporizer may be *outside* the breathing circuit (VOC) in the fresh gas supply line, or the vaporizer may be *inside* the breathing circuit (VIC) when the patient's inspirations or expirations go through the vaporizer, which must then be of 'low resistance' type. (The plenum types are completely unsuitable for VIC use.) In this case the vaporizer increases the vapour tension with each breath and is potentially very dangerous.

2. *By direct injection of liquid agent into the system.* Carefully calculated amounts of liquid volatile agent have been injected at one-minute intervals into the expiratory limb of the circle system. (Not a technique for the beginner.) Computer–controlled servo injection systems acting on feedback from in-circuit vapour analysers are used for the more expensive agents, e.g. desflurane.

Initially, larger flows are used to fill the system with the desired mixture of anaesthetics and oxygen, then, after two minutes, the gas flows are reduced.

Soda-lime

Used to absorb the carbon dioxide. A mixture of 90% calcium hydroxide with 5% sodium hydroxide and 1% potassium hydroxide, with silicates to prevent powdering. It is essential for effective absorption that moisture (14–19%) be incorporated within the granule. The hydroxides combine with carbon dioxide in the presence of water to form carbonates. Soda-lime granules are size 4–8 mesh to minimize resistance to breathing and to allow plenty of surface for absorption (4 mesh is 4 quarter-inch openings per inch; 8 mesh 8 eighth-inch openings per inch). Air space in the charged canister should equal the patient's tidal volume. Nearly half the volume in a properly packed canister consists of intergranular space. The chemical change involved in absorption results in water and the carbonates of the respective metals, and heat production, the heat of neutralization. (Sevoflurane and trichloroethylene should not be used with soda-lime because they may be decomposed in this heat.) Soda-lime can absorb about 20% of its own weight of CO_2. Storing soda-lime in its container does not interfere with its efficiency.

Durasorb is an improved soda-lime, with a prolonged effective life, which does not overheat. Its pink colour turns to white when it becomes inactive.

Baralyme (barium hydroxide lime, USP) is 80% calcium hydroxide with 20% barium octohydrate. It is said to be less caustic, and to produce less heat than soda-lime. No silica is necessary to produce hardness. It contains mimoza Z and ethyl violet as indicator; the pink granules change to purple when exhausted. Used in space craft.

The highest permissible concentration of carbon dioxide in an anaesthetic system is 0.2%. The soda-lime must be fresh and tidal exchange must be adequate for efficient CO_2 elimination. Vertical position of the canister prevents 'channelling' of gas flow down the edges, but even so, the centre of the canister tends to be used preferentially, resulting in loss of efficiency, which is not evident to the naked eye because the visible soda-lime has not yet changed colour. In practice this is rarely a problem because most systems have a huge excess of efficiency.

Signs of exhaustion of soda-lime.
(1) Change of colour of granules;
(2) monitoring: rise in measured $ETCO_2$ on the capnograph;
(3) clinically: rise in blood pressure followed eventually by a fall;
(4) rise in pulse rate;
(5) deepening of spontaneous respiration; and
(6) increased oozing from wound and perhaps sweating.

The 1 lb canister will last about 6 h intermittently, 2 h continuously. In practice it is unwise to wait until the soda-lime is completely exhausted. Fresh absorbent should always be used if there is any doubt of its efficiency.
Temperature during absorption. This arises from the heat of the chemical reaction of neutralization, which is exothermic. The temperature within the canister may reach 60°C in that part of the canister where active absorption is occurring.

Monitoring the low-flow system

Inspired oxygen and end tidal CO_2, anaesthetic agent, tidal volume, respiratory rate, airway pressure, basal oxygen consumption.

Applications

(1) Economy in use of gases; (2) less pollution of theatre atmosphere; and (3) humidification and warming of inspired gas.

Disadvantages

(1) Hypoxia may occur because the circuit gases have a different concentration to the added fresh gases. Circuit oxygen concentration is monitored; (2) hypercapnia may occur. Circuit CO_2 concentration should be monitored; (3) even small leaks have a disastrous effect on circuit gas concentrations. Tight fit of mask to patient may cause trauma; (4) greater risk of disconnections, due to greater complexity of pipework; (5) alkaline dust may pass to patient; (6) resistance to breathing and dead space may be high; (7) increased carbon dioxide content of inspired gas, because absorption is far

from perfect; (8) dilution of gases in reservoir bag by nitrogen in the circuit in the early part of the administration; and (9) volatile agents may be adsorbed to soda-lime, lowering the initial concentration and 'hanging over' to subsequent patients.

Apparatus

1. The Waters 'to-and-fro' single-phase system (Fig. 6.3).[49] Gases pass through the canister during both inspiration and expiration. Fresh gases are led to the patient close to the mask.

2. The circle or two-phase system. An inspiratory and expiratory tube are used, with valves to ensure a one-way flow of gases; breathing in two phases and low dead space. The soda-lime can be by-passed and the canister can be easily removed for recharging. Fresh gases must not enter just before the expiratory valve, or they will be wasted and hypoxia may occur. A pop-off valve must not be placed between patient and inspiratory valve.

Circle absorption and fresh gas flow. At higher flows the system behaves like a semi-closed system and soda-lime is unnecessary. With basal flows, rebreathing is total and expired carbon dioxide is removed by soda-lime. At fresh gas flows of 1–2 l/min, the circuit concentration of volatile agents is about half the fresh gas concentration. At fresh gas flows of 3–4 l/min, circuit volatile concentrations are about equal to the fresh gas concentrations. Circuit gas concentrations are monitored. The fresh gas flow-rates required for rebreathing systems have been studied using a mathematical model.[50] With a flow-rate of 7 l/min, nitrogen elimination is complete in 5 min for practical purposes. With the flow reduced to 500 ml/min, the nitrogen concentration in the system is still 20% after 1 h. With an inflow of 500 ml/min

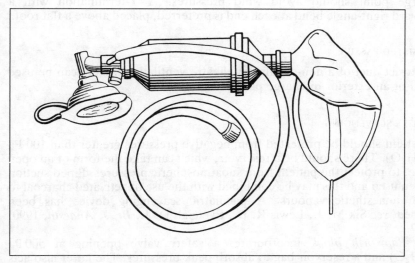

Figure 6.3 The Waters 'to-and-fro' carbon dioxide absorber. (British Oxygen Company Ltd.)

Entonox, F_{IO_2}, falls to dangerously low levels, but at 1000 ml/min F_{IO_2} remains at about 40% (assuming an oxygen consumption of 225 ml/min).

A low flow regime of 1000 ml/min nitrous oxide and 600 ml/min oxygen will provide an F_{IO_2} between 35 and 25% over a range of oxygen consumption between 150 and 300 ml/min. Nitrous oxide uptake declines exponentially from 462 ml/min to 110 ml/min after 2 hours.

Mechanical dead space

Mechanical dead space is the addition to dead space, which is produced by the anaesthetic apparatus.[51] It increases the P_{aco_2}, but, provided F_{IO_2} is generous, may not affect P_{ao_2}. It may be used deliberately to keep the P_{aco_2} normal during hyperventilation intended to prevent alveolar collapse.

Mechanical dead space in a circle absorber is space between face and beginning of double corrugated tubing. Cope's modification of Waters's absorber is designed to minimize dead space when anaesthetizing children.

Scavenging systems

Collection of effluent gases from anaesthetic systems requires the use of a collecting valve and the use of tubing to duct the waste to atmosphere. Scavenging systems may be classified as:

(1) PASSIVE

The total flow resistance should not exceed 50 Pa ($0.5 \, cmH_2O$) at 30 l/min and copper pipes of 28–35 mm outer diameter are thought to be satisfactory. The discharge point should avoid wind pressures. A T-termination with a downward right-angle bend at each end is preferred, placed above a flat roof.

(2) ASSISTED PASSIVE

The extract duct of a non-circulatory theatre ventilation system can be used instead of an exterior discharge point.

(3) ACTIVE SCAVENGING

The patient should be protected from negative pressures greater than 100 Pa (1 cm H_2O). There should be a reservoir, which can take the form of an open T-piece, to protect the patient from subatmospheric pressures. Piped suction has been used and this may be combined with the use of activated charcoal to remove anaesthetic vapours. A paediatric scavenging device has been described, *see* Sik M. J., Lewis R. B., Eveleigh D. J., *Br. J. Anaesth*, 1990, **64**; 117.

The Papworth block incorporates a safety valve opening at 500 Pa (5 cmH_2O) and a reservoir bag to absorb peak pressures. The latter also acts as a monitor of the system.

The Cardiff Aldasorber contains activated charcoal, which removes anaesthetic vapours but not nitrous oxide. Its duration of active use is gauged by the gain in weight due to adsorbed agent.

Monitoring inhaled gases and vapours (see also *Chapter 18*)

Oxygen. (1) Polarographic, reliable; (2) the fuel cell analyser. Can be affected by water vapour and needs replacing every year or so; and (3) paramagnetic. Requires removal of a gas sample from the system for analysis.
Carbon dioxide. Infra-red absorption. Most of these require removal of a gas sample from the system for analysis, but at least one has the infra-red cell in the anaesthetic system. Reliable and robust.
Volatile agents. (1) Infra-red absorption, as for carbon dioxide, but with gas-specific spectra; (2) Drager Narkotest; silicone rubber lengthens in the presence of halothane, related to its concentration; and (3) change in frequency of a quartz crystal oscillator (The Engstrom Emma). Affected by water vapour, which usually raises the reading by 0.3–0.5%.

MECHANICAL VENTILATORS

See also Chapter 12.[52]
Some points to consider when acquiring a ventilator for theatre or ITV:
Physical characteristics. Valve resistance important where SIMV, pressure support and CPAP are used.
Triggering. There is a tendency to place the trigger sensor nearer to the patient to get a faster response and higher sensitivity, especially where tachypnoea (commonly) exists.
Safety and reliability. Automatic alarm for disconnection requires automatic oxygen flow if gas supply fails, automatic battery backup if mains fail, and automatic ventilation if apnoea occurs. Partial ventilatory support features, which are now added to the range of IMV, CPAP, and SIMV, now include MMV, with extremely rapid response times for use in severe tachypnoea.
Pressure Support (PS). With various rise times, and ability to combine with SIMV. Features desirable in CPAP include (1) the inspiratory flow must always exceed that of the patient, e.g. 60 l/min; (2) minimal effort is needed to trigger the system; (3) minimal resistance in expiration; (4) the provision of full alarms and automatic override in CPAP; and (5) gas usage is economical. Built-in monitoring of airway resistance, calculation of auto-PEEP, and peak inspiratory pressure are important for assessing the patient's progress.
Built in monitoring. Spo_2 and $ETco_2$ may be included in the ventilator itself, but a higher number of monitoring functions included in one machine means more disruption when one of them fails and the machine is removed for service. Do_2 and Vo_2 are valuable.

ACCIDENTAL DISCONNECTION

Constant vigilance is required. Ill-fitting tapers should be discarded. Minor leaks may have serious consequences and disconnection monitors (signalling if 10 cm water pressure is not reached at least every 20 s; and if airway pressure exceeds 50 cm. water during IPPV) are required. *See also* Chapter 14.

MAINTAINING THE AIRWAY

To maintain a patent airway in an anaesthetized patient, it is usually necessary to displace the mandible anteriorly (holding up the jaw) by pressure just superior to the angle of the mandible. Some pressure may be required and both skill and experience are necessary for success. The patient's head is extended to 25° beyond the horizontal, which tends to lift the epiglottis out of the way. If this method fails, a pharyngeal airway is inserted, but this may cause coughing in light anaesthesia. With the head extended, the tongue will sit in front of the curved shaft of the airway, leaving the end clear in the laryngopharynx. Airway obstruction is usually caused by the tongue but the epiglottis may also be responsible.

Many airways have been designed but most anaesthetists use the Guedel pharyngeal airway in rubber or plastic.[53] Every attempt is made to avoid the use of these in patients with frontal crowns, caps, veneers, or very loose teeth, because a powerful bite will put great pressure (0.25 metric tonne) on these and may dislodge them (*see* Chapter 14); in these patients, the use of a rubber or plastic nasopharyngeal airway is appropriate but also carries risk of nasal haemorrhage.

ALTERNATIVE AIRWAYS

1. Brain laryngeal mask (*see above*).
2. Postpalatal and postglossal variants (rather disappointing).
3. Tracheal tube.

LARYNGOSCOPES (*See* Chapter 11)

TRACHEAL TUBES AND CONNECTIONS

See Chapter 11. These tubes are of rubber or plastic. A red additive/preservative gives the rubber tubes their characteristic colour. The markings indicate the maker; the inside diameter in millimetres; the outside diameter in millimetres; 'oral' or 'nasal' design (the pilot tube of a nasal cuff tube enters the shaft of the tube much nearer to the connector); single- or multiple use; code of the implantation test ('I.T.'); and the markings of the number of centimetres from the tip.

See Thompson P. W. *Ann. R. Coll. Surg.* 1983, **65**, 14, and for the history of the development of standards in the development of anaesthetic equipment, Rendell-Baker J. in *Anaesthesia, Essays on its History.* (Rupreht J. and van Lieburg M. I. ed.) Berlin: Springer-Verlag, 1985, 159; Ward C. S. *Anaesthetic Equipment.* 2nd ed. Eastbourne: Ballière Saunders, 1985.

Transducers. Calibration and care *See* Chapter 18

Computers on the anaesthetic machine *See* Chapters 4 and 18

Monitors *See* Chapter 18.

Automated record keeping *See* Chapters 4, 18 and 19

Syringe pumps[54]

These are usually electrically driven by mains, battery or both with a motor turning a leadscrew. Alerts are frequently provided for power failure, empty syringe and occlusion of delivery pipe. Battery backup is particularly important in patient transfer situations.

Ideal properties include: reliability, electrical safety, accuracy, ease of use, robustness, ability to use a variety of syringe types and sizes and clear displays and instructions.

RS232 or similar interface for computer control.[55]

Applications include control of diabetes, pain relief, total intravenous anaesthesia, cardiovascular support[56], relaxants and sedation in intensive care.

Equipment for developing countries[57]

Low capital and revenue cost have high priority. Cylinders have relatively little place. Monitoring is primarily clinical, as instrumental monitoring is highly vulnerable, not least to frequent power failures. Syringe drivers have proved too complex.

1. Draw over anaesthesia (*see* Chapter 36) with self-inflating manual ventilation bags. The Ambu E and Laerdal IVA valves play an important part in these systems.

2. Open ether with Schimmelbusch mask (*see* Chapter 36)

3. Intravenous techniques – ketamine, propofol, benzodiazepines, opioids.

4. Oxygen concentrators.[58]

5. Low-cost volatile agents – trichloroethylene (available in France), halothane, ether.

6. A simple electric ventilator is available, with battery backup. (Manley Medical Engineering Ltd., Copley House, Parsonage Lane, Farnham Common, Slough, SL2 3PA.)

For further information: ECHO, Ullswater Crescent, Surrey, CR5 2HR (081-660 2220).

CARE AND STERILIZATION OF EQUIPMENT

Disinfection is the killing of non-sporing micro-organisms. Sterilization is the killing of all micro-organisms including viruses, fungi and their spores, if any.

Methods of sterilization

1. Heat sterilization

Moist heat. Moisture increases cellular permeability and heat coagulates protein. Boiling (100°C) for 15 min kills bacteria, but spores may escape destruction. Increased pressure makes it possible to produce higher temperature. In the modern autoclave, air is exhausted and replaced by steam at 134°C and 32 lb/in pressure for 3½ min. To remove moisture, the steam is evacuated and replaced by sterile air. The cycle takes about 10 min. Useful for metal objects and fabrics. This will kill all living organisms provided the material treated is properly wrapped to allow penetration. Deterioration of rubber and plastics is hastened by this method and exposure for 15 min to a temperature of 121°C may be substituted. Sharp instruments become dulled. Low-temperature (73°C) steam sterilization (290 mmHg pressure) takes just over 2 h; if formaldehyde is added, spores are also killed, which is a method for materials harmed by steam at higher temperatures.

Dry heat. 160°C for an hour. Useful for powders, greases, oils and glass syringes.

2. Chemical sterilization

Useful for objects that will not withstand heat, e.g. endoscopes. Chemicals kill by coagulation or alkylation of proteins. Non-sporing bacteria, viruses, the tubercle bacillus and spores are resistant to destruction (in ascending order). Chemicals only act on exposed surfaces, some react with metals, some impregnate materials (e.g. rubber) and remain as a source of irritation. Rubber and plastics are particularly subject to destruction by strong chemicals.

Formaldehyde. Can be used for endoscopic equipment, catheters, etc. Residual formaldehyde persists after prolonged airing and may harm the skin or bring tears to the endoscopist's eye.

Ethylene oxide (C_2H_4O). A colourless gas and a good bactericidal agent, although very toxic to inhale. It has good penetrability and few materials are harmed. It is effective against all organisms, but is slow (8–12 h). The gas is explosive at concentrations in excess of 3% in air, and it is necessary to use a

10% mixture with carbon dioxide at a relative humidi of 30–50%. A good method of sterilizing complicated and delicate apparatus (e.g. pump oxygenators, Ruben's valves, plastic tubing, Teflon prostheses, catheters, etc.), although the method is expensive and time consuming. The accepted method of removing adsorbed ethylene oxide by allowing 7 days shelf-life is inadequate, and the pulling of 6 post-sterilization vacuums is advised. Even this, however, is not accepted by all authorities. Ethylene oxide has also been used for sterilization of artificial ventilators after prolonged use in dirty cases and at least 4 hours flushing with air is recommended on completion of the process. The preferred method of sterilization of respiratory equipment.

The cylinders containing the mixture are identified by aluminium paint; the shoulder is red and below it is a circular band of yellow paint.

LIQUIDS

Phenol (1–5%). First prepared in 1821 by F. F. Runge (1795–1867) of Breslau and employed by Joseph Lister (1827–1912) of Glasgow in 1865. Used to clean surfaces of apparatus. Should not be used on equipment that comes into contact with the patient. Does not kill spores.

Iodine (0.5–2% in alcohol). May irritate or burn the skin. Povidone-iodine (Betadine) is less irritant.

Ethyl Alcohol (70–80%). Is more efficient than absolute alcohol. Isopropyl alcohol, 50–70%, can also be used.

Hexachlorophene (pHisoHex) (50–70%). One of the few antiseptics that does not lose its properties in the presence of soap.

Chlorhexidine (Hibitane). A 0.1% aqueous solution for 20 min for sterilization of endotracheal tubes and other anaesthetic equipment; 0.5% in 50% ethyl alcohol for skin sterilization (30 s).

Glutaraldehyde (Cidex). Commonly used for endoscopes. Used as a 2% solution made alkaline by the addition of 0.3% sodium carbonate. This will kill bacteria in 15 min and spores in 3 h. Users wear gloves, and if the room is not very well ventilated, gasmasks.

Hypochlorites (e.g. Milton). Used for hepatitis B virus.

Liquid disinfectants must make contact with all the inside area of the immersed tubing, which must then be dried in a heated ultrafiltered drying chamber. Improper cold sterilization is potentially hazardous.

3. Gamma rays (ionizing radiation)

Lethal dose for bacteria is 2.5 megarads. Usually obtained from a cobalt-60 source. Tubes, catheters, etc. can be sterilized in a transparent plastic envelope. *(See* Rainey H. B. *Anaesth. Intensive Care* 1974, **2**, 48.)

4. Ultraviolet Light

Has been used to kill organisms by submitting the whole operation area to the light. Patients and staff must be protected from sunburn. All skin must be covered and plain spectacles worn with an eyeshade.

5. Filtration

Filters are used to prevent the entry of organisms (e.g. into ventilators). They will remove all particles down to a diameter of 0.5μ with a 99.99% efficiency. The filters themselves can be autoclaved. The Millipore filter is commonly used for repeated injections via indwelling epidural catheters.

Anaesthetic vapours in the concentrations generally produced in anaesthetic equipment cause a reduction in viability of such organisms as *Escherichia coli.*

Tracheal tubes, suction catheters, airways

The use of presterilized disposable articles is now common. Where this is not possible they may be washed with soap and water and well rinsed. A suitable brush should be used to clear the inside of tubes and airways. They may then be sterilized by boiling, although this tends to soften the rubber tracheal tubes. Portex tubes should be boiled with a stylet *in situ* so that they retain their curvature. Armoured latex tubes should be handled with care since they may be compressed by Chealte's forceps, when hot. Alternatively, tubes may be soaked in a solution of 0.1% chlorhexidine (Hibitane). They should be stored in dust-free containers.

Expensive apparatus, such as endobronchial tubes, must be handled carefully to prevent deterioration. Gamma-radiation sterilization is satisfactory.

Another method is to place all suitable equipment in a domestic dishwater in which temperatures of 70°C are reached. A commercially supplied detergent, providing 33 ppm of available chlorine, is used. Although this does not guarantee absolute sterility, the method kills those pathogenic organisms with which anaesthetic equipment is likely to be contaminated, except spores and some viruses.

Face-masks

These may deteriorate with repeated boiling. It has been found that thorough washing in soap and water and then placing in a bowl of water between 60 and 70°C for 2 min, followed by rinsing under running tap-water at the same temperature for 2 min, will reduce the number of pathogens present to a very small number.

Laryngoscope blades

(1) May be boiled or autoclaved, provided they are detachable; (2) stand in 5% phenol for 30 min; (3) formalin oven; and (4) simple treatment between cases is to wipe with 70% alcohol or 0.1% chlorhexidine in 70% alcohol.

The Macintosh spray should not be boiled because the rubber of the internal tube swells slightly. A jet is then delivered instead of a fine spray.

Rebreathing tubes, reservoir bags

Repeated boiling destroys the antistatic properties of rubber. It is common practice, therefore, to wash, rinse and allow the tubing to dry between cases. It may be boiled once a week for 10 min, or after particularly contaminated cases. Corrugated tubing, face-masks and reservoir bags can be pasteurized (75°C for 10 min). Only vegetative organisms need be killed because spores are relatively unimportant. Disposable plastic corrugated tubing is in common use. Organisms present may be *Streptococcus pyogenes, Staphylococcus aureus* and *Pseudomonas pyocyanea.*

Waters' canisters

These should be sterilized daily, or after each anaesthetic where the patient is suffering from tuberculosis or upper respiratory tract infection.

Circle absorbers

These can be sterilized by gamma radiation, formaldehyde vapour or ethylene oxide. Alternatively, they should be frequently dismantled, cleaned and disinfected with spirit. Another approach is to prevent entry of organisms by using a filter on the expiratory limb of the circuit. Bacterial contamination of anaesthetic gases delivered from anaesthetic systems is not a large problem if ordinary hygienic measures are observed.

Ventilators

Proper sterilization is essential when they are used in intensive therapy units. The methods available include: (1) autoclaving; (2) internal irrigation with antiseptics, provided the circuit is watertight; (3) ultrasonic nebulization with alcohol, although this presents a flammability hazard; (4) ultrasonic nebulization with hydrogen peroxide; (5) use of disposable patient-breathing circuits; (6) use of a bacterial filter to prevent entry of organisms, although these must be heated to prevent clogging by condensation.

Humidifiers

These provide an ideal environment for bacterial growth. Prevented by use of 60°C running temperature for 'pasteurization'. Copper sponges have also been advocated because the metal has an antibacterial effect.

Contamination with tubercle bacilli

This may be expected after anaesthesia in the presence of open pulmonary tuberculosis. The tracheal tubes, suction catheters, rebreathing tubing, etc.

should be disposable, but if not they may be placed immediately in an antiseptic solution (e.g. 0.1% chlorhexidine for 1 h). They can then be cleaned and scrubbed with soap and water with less danger to personnel. After this they can be sterilized by boiling or autoclaving. Boiling for 3 min will kill tubercle bacilli.

The to-and-fro system is preferable to the circle absorber in the presence of tuberculosis because it is more easily cleaned and sterilized.

Hepatitis B and C

See Chapter 17. The virus is not destroyed by boiling but by pasteurization at 60°C for 10 h. It is killed by autoclaving and gamma radiation. Of the chemical disinfectants, the best results are obtained with hypochlorite.

Syringes and needles

Plastic, disposable, presterilized syringes and needles are now generally used.

Disposable syringes are made from polystyrene or polypropylene. Plunger grommets are attacked by paraldehyde and some X-ray contrast media. In emergency, some disposable syringes can be sterilized by boiling for 5 min in distilled water.

Instruments for local blocks

In the absence of gamma-radiation sterilized disposable sets, special packs can be made up for each type of procedure, containing needles, syringes, cotton drapes, swabs and dishes. These, and ampoules of local analgesic solutions, such as lignocaine, amethocaine hydrochloride and bupivacaine (and adrenaline), can be autoclaved once at 160°C for 20 min at 20 psi. Some double-wrapped bupivacaine ampoules have been sterilized by ethylene oxide, others by steam autoclaving.

Disposable sets are also available for intradural or extradural block, gamma-radiation sterilized.

Tests for sterility

The inclusion of heat sensitive tape or a Browne's tube in the set is a safeguard. If the appropriate temperature has been reached, there is a change in colour. Indicator tape is more commonly used.

Tests for sterility in mass-produced preparations (e.g. intravenous fluids) are not easy to perform. *Product control* presents problems due to cultural, technical and statistical difficulties. There is no single medium that will allow growth of every organism. Sampling can also result in contamination so that false-positive results are obtained. Samples tested may not subsequently be available for use. *Process control*, by examination of the effect on a challenge organism, offers an alternative approach, although with its own problems.

References

1. Boyle H. E. G. *Br. Med. J.* 1917, **2**, 653; Hadfield C. F. *Br. J. Anaesth.* 1950, **22**, 107; Hewer C. Langton *Anaesthesia* 1967, **22**, 357; Obituary of Boyle, *Anaesthesia* 1967, **22**, 710; Watt O. M. *Anaesthesia* 1968, **23**, 103; Bryn T. K. *The Development of Anaesthetic Apparatus*. Oxford: Blackwell, 1975; Hewer C. L. *Anaesthesia* 1977, **32**, 908.
2. Gwathmey J. T. *Anesthesia*. New York: Appleton, 1914, p. 174.
3. Rawstron R. E., McNiell T. D. *Brit. J. Anaesth.* 1962, **34**; 591 and 670
4. Snowdon S. L., Head-Rapson H. G. *Anaesthesia*, 1991, **45**; 1084.
5. Howell R. S. C. In: *Anaesthesia Review* (Kaufman L, ed), 7th ed, Churchill Livinstone, 87.
6. *Health Technical Memorandum* No. 22 (and Supplement). London: DHSS, 1977.
8. Bancroft M. L. et al. *Anesthesiology* 1980, **52**, 504.
9. *Health Equipment Information* 1975, **61**, 38 and 75.
10. *Hospital Technical Memorandum* No. 22 (HTM 22, DHSS, 1972); Elton V. *Health and Safety Executive* 1976, **29**, 4.
11. *Checklist for anaesthetic machines. A Recommended procedure based on the use of an oxygen Analyser*. 1990, Association of Anaesthetists of Great Britain and Ireland, 9, Bedford Square, London WC1B 3RA.
12. Wright B. M. *Lancet* 1977, **2**, 1008; Footerman D. S. *Anaesthesia* 1983, **38**, 672.
13. Neu M. *Münch. Med. Wochenschr.* 1910, **57**, 1873.
14. Gupta B. L. and Varshneya A. K. *Br. J. Anaesth.* 1975, **47**, 805.
15. Farquhar I. and Eldridge P. *Br. J. Anaesth.*, 1990, **64**; 113.
16. Cook T. L. et al. *Anesth. Analg.* 1977, **65**, 793.
17. Miller E. D., Greene N. M. *Anesth Analg.* 1990, **70**, 1; Jones R. M., Cashman J. M. et al. *Anesth. Analg.* 1990, **70**, 3.
18. Johnstone R. E. and Smith T. C. *Anesthesiology* 1973, **38**, 192.
19. Parmley J. B. et al. *Anesth. Analg.* 1972, **51**, 888.
20. Newton N. I. and Adams A. P. *Anaesthesia* 1978, **33**, 689.
21. Macfie A. G. *Anaesthesia* 1990, **45**, 145.
22. Brain A. I. J. *Br. J. Anaesth.* 1983, **55**, 801–5.
23. Calder I., Ordman A. J., et al. *Anaesthesia* 1990, **45**, 137.
24. Payne J. *Anaesthesia* 1989, **44**, 865.
25. Hammond J. E. *Anaesthesia* 1989, **44**, 616.
26. Griffin R. and Hatcher I. S. *Anaesthesia* 1990, **45**, 1039.
27. Freeman R. and Baxendale B. *Anaesthesia* 1990, **45**, 1094.
28. Conacher I. D. *Anaesthesia* 1991, **46**, 164; *See also* Cyna A. M., MacLeod D. M. et al. *Anaesthesia* 1990, **45**, 167.
29. Criswell J. et al. *Anaesthesia* 1990, **45**, 113.
30. Miller D. M. *Br. J. Anaesth* 1990, **64**, 251.
31. Magill I. W. *Proc. R. Soc. Med.* 1929, **22**, 83 and 1967, **60**, 16.
32. Rohrer F. *Pflüg. Arch. Ges. Physiol.* 1915, **162**, 225.
33. Lack J. A. *Anaesthesia* 1976, **31**, 259; Lack J. A. *Anaesthesia* 1976, **31**, 576; Lack J. A. and Davies R. J. *Anaesthesia* 1976, **31**, 951, and addendum, 1253.
34. Voss T. J. V. *Anaesth. Intensive. Care* 1985, **1**, 98.
35. Bain J. A. and Spoerel W. E. *Can. Anaesth. Soc. J.* 1972, **19**, 426.
36. Macintosh R. R. and Mushin W. W. *Medical Times* 1945, **73**, 53; Macintosh R. R. and Pask E. A. *Br. J. Indust. Med.* 1957, **14**, 168.
37. Radford E. P. *J. Appl. Physiol.* 1955, **7**, 451.
38. Ayre T. P. *Lancet* 1937, **1**, 561; *Curr. Res. Anesth. Analg.* 1937, **16**, 330; *Br. J. Surg.* 1937, **35**, 131 (reprinted in 'Classical File', *Surv. Anesthesiol.* 1967, **11**, 400); *Br. J. Anaesth.* 1956, **28**, 520; *Anaesthesia* 1967, **22**, 359.
39. Rees G. J. *Br. J. Anaesth.* 1960, **32**, 132.
40. Macfie A. G. *Anaesthesia* 1990, **45**, 145.
41. Snow J. *Lond. Med. Gaz.* 1851, **12**, 622.

42. Kuhn F. *Dtsch. Zeit. Chir.* 1906, **81**, 63.
43. Reinhold H. in: *Anaesthesia. Essays on its History* (Rupreht J. and van Lieburg M. J., ed.). Berlin: Springer-Verlag, 1985.
44. Jackson D. E. *J. Lab. Clin. Med.* 1915, **1**, 1 (reprinted in 'Classical File', *Surv. Anesthesiol.* 1965, **98**, 9).
45. Waters R. M. *Curr. Res. Anesth. Analg.* 1924, **3**, 20.
46. Sword B. C. *Curr. Res. Anesth. Analg.* 1930, **9**, 198 (reprinted in 'Classical File', *Surv. Anesthesiol.* 1981, **25**, 65).
47. Primrose W. B. *Br. Med. J.* 1934, **1**, 478; **2**, 339.
48. Waters R. M. *Anesthesiology* 1943, **4**, 596; and Patterson R. W. In: *Anaesthesia; Essays on its History* (Rupreht J. and van Lieburg M. J., ed.) Berlin: Springer-Verlag, 1985, 74 and 167.
49. Waters R. M. *Curr. Res. Anesth. Analg.* 1926, **5**, 160; *Ann. Surg.* 1936, **38**, 103; *Proc. R. Soc. Med.* 1936, **30**, 11.
50. Holmes C. McK. and Spears G. F. S. *Anaesthesia* 1977, **32**, 846.
51. Macfie A. G. *Anaesthesia* 1990, **45**, 145.
52. Fernandez R. et al. *Intensive Care World* 1990, **7**, 32.
53. Guedel A. E. *JAMA* 1933, **100**, 1862 (reprinted in 'Classical File', *Surv. Anesthesiol.* 1966, **10**, 515).
54. Stokes D. N. et al. *Anaesthesia* 1991, **45**, 1062.
55. Tackley R. M. et al. *Br. J. Anaesth.* 1989, **62**, 46.
56. Colvin J. R. and Kenny G. N. C. *Anaesthesia* 1989, **44** 37.
57. Nordberg E. M. *Br. Med. J.* 1984, **289**, 92.
58. Fenton P. M. *Anaesthesia* 1989, **44**, 498–503.

Chapter 7

Inhalation anaesthesia

The uptake of anaesthetic gases and vapours[1]

Anaesthetic gases and vapours can be assumed to be inert and their uptake, therefore, determined by physical principles. Uptake can be divided into two phases:

The pulmonary phase. Inhalation of gas or vapour to establish an alveolar concentration and diffusion across the pulmonary membrane to reach pulmonary and hence arterial blood.

The circulatory phase. Transfer to the brain and other organs by the circulation. The brain concentration is ultimately proportional to the alveolar partial pressure. We can therefore speak of the *minimum alveolar concentration* of an anaesthetic agent that will produce general anaesthesia.[2] Strictly speaking, tension rather than concentration is the important factor. Minimal alveolar concentration (MAC) will vary with altitude, whereas minimal alveolar pressure (MAP) would be reasonably constant.[3]

The pulmonary phase

Diffusion across the pulmonary membrane is rarely a limiting factor. In health, arterial tension will be virtually equal to alveolar tension. We may consider some of the factors that regulate alveolar tension:

Inhaled concentration. The inspired concentration (or tension) of the anaesthetic agent determines the alveolar and arterial tensions at equilibrium. Increasing the inspired concentration will speed up the rate of induction, provided that breath holding, laryngospasm or coughing is not induced.

Alveolar ventilation. The anaesthetic agent in inspired gases is immediately diluted by the functional residual air. It takes many breaths before the alveolar concentration approximates to inspired concentration. In a non-rebreathing system, equilibration takes about 3 min in a healthy subject, or longer with a very soluble agent. Equilibration is hastened by increasing alveolar ventilation. Induction is therefore speeded by taking deeper breaths and slowed down when there is rebreathing, respiratory depression or respiratory obstruction, even in one lung or part of a lung.

Blood/gas partition coefficient. The partition coefficient of a substance is the ratio, at equilibrium, of its concentration on the two sides of a diffusing membrane or interface. Alveolar concentration of anaesthetic agent is less than inspired concentration because of diffusion of molecules from the alveoli to the pulmonary blood, especially with agents of higher solubility. Approximate figures for the coefficient are:

Anaesthetic agent	Blood/gas coefficient
Xenon	0.14
Nitrous oxide	0.47
Desflurane	0.42
Sevoflurane	0.6
Isoflurane	1.4
Enflurane	1.9
Halothane	2.4

When blood solubility is high, alveolar concentration does not equilibrate with inhaled concentration. Induction is slow because alveolar tension, and hence arterial tension, remains low. It may be speeded by increasing alveolar ventilation. When blood solubility is low, alveolar concentration soon equilibrates with inhaled concentration. Induction is rapid and is not materially affected by taking deeper breaths.

In other words, with a low blood/gas partition coefficient, a change in inhaled concentration is soon reflected as a change in arterial tension. When the coefficient is high changes in inhaled concentration are not rapidly reflected in the arterial blood. This coefficient is a most important physical characteristic in determination of the clinical usefulness of a drug.

Partial pressure of anaesthetic agent in blood returning to the lungs. The tension in mixed venous blood, and hence in pulmonary arterial blood, depends on the redistribution of the agent in the circulatory phase. A high tension in pulmonary arterial blood will raise alveolar concentration. This occurs when redistribution to other tissues is slowed (e.g. in shock) and as total body saturation occurs.

Pulmonary blood flow. Pulmonary blood flow carries away the anaesthetic agent from the lungs. It is equivalent to cardiac output, except in some cases of congenital heart disease, pulmonary haemangioma, etc. A higher pulmonary blood flow will slow induction, especially for the more soluble agents.

Ventilation–perfusion relationships. Gross disturbances delay the uptake of anaesthetic agents.

The second gas effect. The uptake of one agent may be accelerated if given in association with a high concentration of another agent (e.g. halothane and nitrous oxide). The rapid absorption of the second gas has the effect of increasing the alveolar concentration of the first agent.

The concentration effect. Uptake of vapour from the alveoli lets more fresh gas be brought into the lungs and increases alveolar concentration more rapidly. This effect is most marked at high inspired concentrations (i.e. for nitrous oxide) when the volume of vapour absorbed is high.

The effect of anaesthetic apparatus. Both the volume of the system, and the solubility of vapours in rubber components and soda-lime, buffer the rise of initial concentration, especially in low-flow closed systems.

The circulatory phase

Cardiac output. Under basal conditions about 70% of the cardiac output goes to the brain, heart, liver and kidney, which comprise about 7% of the total body weight. About 14% of the cardiac output goes to the brain, which comprises about 2.2% of the total body weight. During induction, therefore, a relatively high proportion of the inspired gas goes to the brain.

Cerebral blood flow. Cerebral blood flow is maintained even in shock states up to the moribund stage (BP less than 40 mmHg) and takes a greater proportion of cardiac output, increasing the effect of inhaled anaesthetics. Addition of CO_2 to inspired gases may speed induction by increasing cerebral blood flow (as well as ventilation). Many of these factors also apply to the uptake and distribution of intravenous anaesthetic agents.

Secondary saturation of body tissues.[4] The brain receives initially a high proportion of anaesthetic agent. But as time goes on there is redistribution of the agent as it comes into equilibrium with the body tissues as a whole. Relatively large amounts of anaesthetic agent must be given during induction because of the recirculation of the agent to tissues other than the brain. As these depots becomes saturated, smaller amounts of anaesthetic are required to maintain anaesthesia (law of diminishing resistance of Gill[5]).

The rate of saturation of non-nervous tissues depends on:

1. The tissue blood flow. The *vessel-rich group* includes heart, kidney, liver and endocrine glands which, with the brain, receive 75% of the cardiac output. *Muscles and skin* less than 20% of the cardiac output under resting conditions. There is a *vessel-poor group* of tissues including bone, ligament and cartilage, which makes up a quarter of the body mass but has little influence on redistribution. *Fatty tissues* have a much lower perfusion than muscles at rest but a far greater capacity for uptake of anaesthetic agents. This may slow induction and recovery in obese subjects.

2. The tissue/blood partition coefficient for the anaesthetic agent, which varies but little between the different body tissues with the exception of fat.

3. Time constants. These depend on the above two factors. The time constant is the time taken for the tissue to become equilibrated. It is short when perfusion is high and lengthened when solubility is great. Average values include: for nitrous oxide 1·3 min in the vessel-rich group, 30 min in muscle and 100 min in fat; for halothane the respective figures are 3.3, 106 and 2720 min.[1]

Minimum Alveolar Concentration (MAC)

The minimum alveolar concentration of an anaesthetic agent to produce lack of reflex response to skin incision in 50% of subjects. Studies in man give the following results (vol%): halothane, 0.76; isoflurane, 1.15; enflurane 1.68; sevoflurane, 2; desflurane, 6; nitrous oxide, 101. Minimum blood concentration (MBC) is another expression of potency. Another measure of potency is the AD_{95} (anaesthetic dose 95) or MAC_{95}, which is the alveolar concentration of the agent to produce lack of reflex response to surgery in 95% of subjects (one standard deviation from MAC_{50}). This figure is much more relevant to clinical anaesthesia and values are approximately 1.5 times those for MAC_{50}, (*see above*). When mixtures of agents are used their separate MAC fractions are simply additive in producing the total anaesthetic effect on the subject.

Physical Factors

1. *The saturated vapour pressure*. When this is low, it is not possible to make a high concentration available for inhalation. If it approximates to ambient pressure, special vaporizers may be required.

2. *Blood/gas partition coefficient*. When this is low, changes in inhaled concentration are quickly reflected as changes in alveolar and hence blood concentration. Anaesthesia can be deepened quickly and the agent is more useful. *See also* above.

3. *Irritability*. Alveolar equilibration is delayed when an irritant agent produces breath-holding or laryngospasm, or when it produces marked respiratory depression.

Clinical applications

Factors that increase the speed of induction of inhalation anaesthesia include:
1. Inhaled concentration of gas or vapour.
2. Hyperventilation, voluntary or controlled, to increase alveolar ventilation.
3. Presence of poor circulation to the non-vital organs. Shock, dehydration, old age, wasting of body tissues.
4. High gas flow systems aid in speed of equilibration of alveolar gases with the anaesthetic mixture. Thus non-rebreathing methods allow for faster induction than low flow systems.

Factors that decrease the speed of induction include:
1. Respiratory obstruction, laryngospasm, bronchial secretions and lung disease.
2. Respiratory depression: (*a*) due to premedication; (*b*) due to use of intravenous barbiturates for induction of anaesthesia; and (*c*) due to the inhalation agent itself.
3. Increased circulation to non-vital organs. In anxiety, thyrotoxicosis, obesity, children and young persons. Where the muscle and fat mass is large. In robust subjects.

Recovery from anaesthesia

Recovery is the period from the cessation of the administration of anaesthesia until the patient is awake and with protective reflexes. Recovery from inhalation anaesthesia involves all the factors mentioned concerning the uptake of the anaesthetic agent. It is in fact a re-equilibration of the body with atmospheric air, and excretion/metabolism of inhalation agents.

Recovery is more rapid when secondary saturation of the body tissues has not had time to occur. Tension of the agent in the arterial blood and brain falls rapidly because equilibration is occurring both with alveolar air and body tissues. For example, a child given an inhalation induction in the anaesthetic room will rapidly lighten if allowed to breathe room air during transfer to the operating theatre (primary saturation) but recovery is slow after more prolonged anaesthesia. Hyperventilation aids elimination of gases and vapours and hypoventilation vice versa. Recovery from anaesthesia can be monitored by the cerebral function monitor. The central cholinergic syndrome may impede recovery of consciousness and can be controlled by physostigmine 1–2 mg i.v. There is also evidence that physostigmine improves the quality of recovery from nitrous oxide/enflurane anaesthesia[6]; Some aspects of mental ability may be impaired for up to 48 hours after surgery.[7]

There is often divergence between subjective and objective estimates of recovery. Delayed recovery from anaesthesia may be due to non-anaesthetic factors.[8]

Clinical signs of anaesthesia

Since the early days of anaesthesia, it has been apparent that the anaesthetist must rely on a series of physical signs to indicate the onset of anaesthesia and to determine its depth. This was appreciated by the early anaesthetists, including John Snow (who described 'five stages of narcotism')[9] and Francis Plomley,[10] but it was not until Arthur Eames Guedel,[11] then of Indianapolis, developed his classic table of the signs of anaesthesia with division, into stages and planes, using open ether, that a detailed system became generally accepted. The stages of ether anaesthesia were based on: (1) a progressive increase of muscular paralysis (eyeball muscles, intercostals, diaphragm); and (2) a progressive abolition of reflex response. (For details *see* earlier editions of this Synopsis.)

These signs have now been superceded by the newer agents and techniques, and especially by the widespread use of muscle relaxants and intermittent positive pressure ventilation. Some points, however, remain valid, e.g. excitement may occur in very light planes of anaesthesia, eyeball movements occur in light anaesthesia as does lacrimation. Autonomic responses can still occur in the presence of full muscular relaxation, and stress responses occur (*see* Chapter 22).

Balanced anaesthesia

The concept of balanced anaesthesia started in 1911 when George Washington Crile (1864–1943) of Cleveland, Ohio, taught that psychic stimuli must be obliterated by light general anaesthesia, whereas the noxious impulses due to surgery must be blocked by local analgesia – the so-called theory of anoci-association.[12] In 1926 John S. Lundy (1894–1972) of the Mayo Clinic introduced the term 'balanced anaesthesia' for a combination of agents such as premedication, regional analgesia and general anaesthesia.[13]

The triad of anaesthesia

Rees and Gray of Liverpool divided anaesthesia into three basic components: (1) narcosis; (2) analgesia; and (3) relaxation. Gray renamed the triad:

(1) narcosis; (2) reflex suppression; and (3) relaxation. With selective drugs, it is possible to vary one component of the triad without affecting the others.

Anaesthesia (or analgesia) is a process of modification of the normal physiological reflex response to the stimuli provided by surgery (and anaesthesia). The triad of anaesthesia may be considered as: (1) inhibition of the afferent part of the reflex system; (2) depression of the central synaptic mechanisms of coordination; and (3) block of the efferent part of the reflex arc. It is valid to include attenuation of the stress response with these three (producing the 'quadrant of anaesthesia')

Inhalation anaesthetic agents

The *ideal inhalational agent*[14] does not exist, but desirable properties include: (1) a stable molecule, not broken down by light, soda-lime, not requiring preservatives, and long shelf life; (2) non-flammable in air, oxygen or nitrous oxide; (3) potent enough to allow use with high concentrations of oxygen; saturated vapour pressure high enough to allow easy vaporization; (4) low solubility in blood to allow rapid induction and recovery as well as rapid response to changes in inhaled concentration; (5) pleasant and non-irritating to inhale; (6) devoid of organ-specific toxicity; (7) lack of toxic effect when inhaled in low doses by theatre staff; (8) should not undergo metabolism in the body; (9) minimal cardiovascular and respiratory side-effects; (10) should provide some analgesia; (11) CNS effects should be readily reversible and be without stimulant activity; (12) no sensitization of the heart to catecholamines; (13) no interactions with other drugs; and (14) cheap to manufacture.

Nitrous oxide

Gas[15] first prepared by Priestley (1733–1804) in 1772. Anaesthetic properties suggested by Sir Humphry Davy (1778–1829) in 1799. In 1808, P. C. Barton (1786–1808), of Philadelphia, again described the exhilarating effects of nitrous oxide. Both he and the distinguished surgeon Willard Parker (1800–1884) of New York may have influenced Colton who demonstrated its effects to Horace Wells (1815–1848), dentist of Hartford, in 1844, who in turn used it in dentistry and had one of his own teeth painlessly extracted by John M. Riggs on 11 December. After an unsuccessful demonstration before John Collins Warren (1778–1856) the surgeon and the students at the Massachusetts General Hospital, Wells continued to use it in his practice, but its use was temporarily forgotten and it was overshadowed by ether. Gardner Quincy Colton (1814–1898, a pupil of Parker) revived its use in 1867–1868 and this time the American dental profession showed considerable interest. In 1863 he established himself in practice in New York City and there founded the Colton Dental Association. T. W. Evans (1823–1897), US dentist working in Paris, introduced it to his colleagues in London in 1868,[16] having learnt its use the previous year from Colton at the International Congress of Medicine in Paris. Later in the same year, the gas was supplied compressed into cylinders and became available two years later as liquefied N_2O. Edmund Andrews (1824–1904)[17] of Chicago, combined it with oxygen, to give longer anaesthesia, in 1868. In 1878 Paul Bert (1830–1886), of France, administered it in a hyperbaric chamber.[18] In 1868 J. T. Clover (1825–1882), London anaesthetist, successfully demonstrated its use at the Radcliffe Infirmary, Oxford,[19] and proved it to be a true anaesthetic, not a means of causing asphyxia. Bert was an early user of Edmund Andrew's nitrous oxide – oxygen mixture to prolong anaesthesia and to avoid asphyxia.[20] First apparatus for the sequential use of nitrous oxide and ether described by Clover.[21] Early users of the nitrous oxide, oxygen, chloroform ether sequence were F. J. Cotton (1869–1938); W. M. Boothby (1880–1953) of Boston; J. T. Gwathmey (1863–1944) of New York City; Geoffrey Marshall (1887–1982) and H. E. G. Boyle (1875–1941) of London (*see also* Boulton T. B. 'Classical File', *Surv. Anesthesiol.* 1985, **29**, 201). A reducing valve was described in 1873[21a] Sir F. Hewitt (1857–1916)[22] and E. I. McKesson (1881–1935), an early pioneer of careful notekeeping in anaesthesia,[23] were pioneers in its use, and today it is very widely used in anaesthesia. The book *Nitrous oxide–Oxygen Anesthesia* by F. W. Clement (1892–1970) appeared in 1939. The book *Untoward Effects of Nitrous Oxide Anaesthesia* by C. B. Courville, Los Angeles neuropathologist, appeared in 1939. It dealt with acute asphyxia caused by McKesson's technique of secondary saturation.[24] In 1956 H. C. A. Lassen, Copenhagen physician, reported that very prolonged nitrous-oxide–oxygen anaesthesia could cause bone-marrow aplasia.[25] May cause macrocytic anaemia by inhibiting vitamin B_{12}. (*See also Under the Influence*, Smith W. D. A. London: Macmillan, 1982 and Frost F. A. M. in: *Nitrous Oxide* (Eger E. L. ed.) London: Arnold, 1985, Ch. 1.)

MANUFACTURE

By heating ammonium nitrate, as a solid or as an aqueous solution of 83% ammonium nitrate to 240°C. At higher temperatures the percentage of impurities increases. The issuing gas is collected, purified and compressed into metal cylinders at $50\,kPa \times 100$ (750 lb/in^2). The cylinders are painted French blue (in Britain) and common sizes are 200 gal (907 litres) and 400 gal (1814 litres).

$$NH_4NO_3 \rightarrow 2H_2O + N_2O$$

Nitric oxide (NO) and nitrogen dioxide (NO_2) are produced as impurities so that the gases evolved must be washed with water and caustic soda, in turn, before being passed through activated alumina to remove water vapour. At various stages, monitors are used to detect the presence of higher oxides of nitrogen. As a further check, regular random sampling of cylinders is carried out.

The amount present in the cylinder can only be ascertained by weighing, because the gas is in liquid form and the gas pressure above the liquid level remains reasonably constant as long as any liquid remains. In fact some fall in pressure occurs due to fall in temperature as the liquid nitrous oxide evaporates using latent heat.[26] Up to four-fifths of the contents of a full cylinder is in the liquid state, so, in use, cylinders must have their valves elevated above the horizontal. Just before exhaustion of the cylinder, when all the liquid is vaporized, the pressure quickly drops to zero. Cylinders are filled to a filling ratio (ratio of weight of nitrous oxide to weight of water the cylinder could hold) of 0.75 in temperate and 0.67 in tropical climates. The cylinder weights, full and empty, are stamped on it; 100 gallons of nitrous oxide weigh 850 g or 30 oz (1 US gallon = ⅝ Imperial gallon; 1 cubic foot = 6¼ Imperial gallons; 1 Imperial gallon = 4½ litres).

PHYSICAL PROPERTIES

Sweet smelling, non-irritating, colourless gas; the only inorganic gas in common use possessing anaesthetic properties. Boiling point −88.5°C. Molecular weight 44. Critical pressure 72.5 atmospheres. Critical temperature 36.5°C. Specific gravity 1.5, that is, 1½ times heavier than air. Density at 15°C and 1 atmosphere is 1.875 g/l. Velocity of sound in nitrous oxide is 262 m/sec (compared with 317 oxygen) and a suitable whistle can be used to differentiate the two gases; change from oxygen to nitrous oxide causes the pitch to fall one-and-a-half tones.[26] Neither flammable nor explosive, but supports the combustion of other agents, even in the absence of oxygen, if a high temperature (above 450°C) is supplied to initiate decomposition into nitrogen and oxygen. The oil/water solubility ratio is 3.2. Water will take up 100 vol%, while blood plasma dissolves 45 vol%. Nitrous oxide is fifteen times more soluble than oxygen. The partition coefficient is 0.47 between blood and gas, 1.0 between brain and blood, and 3.0 between fat and blood.

Nitrous oxide is eliminated unchanged from the body, mostly via the lungs. It is stable and is unaffected by soda-lime.

For estimation of blood nitrous oxide levels *see* Saloojee Y. and Cole P. *Anaesthesia* 1978, **33**, 779; *see also* White D. C. in: *Recent Advances 16* (Adams A. P. and Atkinson R. S., ed.) Churchill Livingstone, 1989; and Eger E. I. '*Nitrous Oxide*' New York: Elsevier, 1985

IMPURITIES IN NITROUS OXIDE

Two cases of poisoning in the UK were reported in detail by Clutton-Brock.[27] Investigation showed that a batch of nitrous oxide had become contaminated with nitric oxide (NO) and nitrogen dioxide (NO_2). Both these substances are toxic. One patient died.

The clinical features are: (1) cyanosis (methaemoglobinaemia); (2) respiratory difficulty; and (3) circulatory failure. Higher oxides of nitrogen can cause distress above 100 ppm, but clinical features may be delayed for several hours.

A crude test for contamination[28] is to put a piece of moistened starch-iodide paper into a large syringe and then fill this with the suspected nitrous oxide mixed with 25% oxygen and wait for 10 min. If the gas is contaminated by over 300 ppm, the starch iodide will turn blue.

See also a series of papers on the subject, *Br. J. Anaesth.* 1967, **39**, 343 et seq. and Editorial, *Lancet* 1967, **2**, 930.

MODE OF ACTION

Nitrous oxide is a potent analgesic but a weak anaesthetic (MAC = 105 vol%). Anaesthesia is induced relatively rapidly because of its low blood/gas partition coefficient.

Table 7.1 Physical properties of some inhalation anaesthetics

Anaesthetic	Molecular weight	Boiling point (°C)	Vapour pressure @ 20°C (mmHg)	Liquid density	Oil/water solubility	MAC	Blood/gas coefficient
Nitrous oxide N_2O	44	-89	5200	1.2	2.2	104	0.47
Halothane $CF_3CHClBr$	197	50	243	1.87	220	0.75	2.3
Enflurane CHF_2-O-CF_2CHFCl	184	56.5	174.5	1.52	120.1	1.68	1.9
Isoflurane $CHF_2-O-CHCl-CF_3$	184	48.5	238	1.50	120.1	1.15	1.4
Sevoflurane $(CF_3)_2CH-O-CH_2F$	200	58.5	162	–	53.0	2.0	0.6
Desflurane $CF_3CHF-O-CHF_2$	168	23.5	673	–	19.0	6.0	0.4

It may cause the release of encephalin in the central nervous system. Endorphins may be involved in nitrous oxide analgesia and depletion of endorphin stores may lessen this effect.[29] There is evidence of reversal of analgesia by naloxone.[30]

Tolerance has been demonstrated in volunteers to the analgesic effects.[31] This can develop in 2 hours, and might be of significance in awareness during nitrous oxide/relaxant anaesthesia. Augmentation of sensory evoked potentials has been demonstrated during recovery from nitrous oxide and may be significant in the aetiology of postoperative excitatory phenomena.[32]

SIDE-EFFECTS OF NITROUS OXIDE

Nitrous oxide is usually regarded as a non-toxic anaesthetic agent, provided that it is administered with a sufficient concentration of oxygen. Undesirable effects may, however, sometimes occur:

1. Nitrous oxide in the alveolar gases will equilibrate with blood, tissue and gas-containing spaces within the body more rapidly than nitrogen diffuses out into alveolar gas. There is a thirty-five-fold difference in the blood/gas partition coefficients of the two gases (nitrous oxide 0.47, nitrogen 0.013) and for every molecule of nitrogen removed from air spaces, 35 molecules of nitrous oxide will pass in. There is thus an increase in the volume of the gas space when that space is compliant (pneumothorax, gut, air embolus) and an increase in pressure when the space cannot expand (sinuses, the middle ear, in pneumo-encephalography). In surgery for retinal detachment where sulphur hexafluoride is used, nitrous oxide can diffuse in and cause a considerable rise in intraocular pressure. It should be discontinued preferably 15 minutes before injection of the bubble or at least at the same time[33]. Postoperative hearing loss has been attributed to changes in middle-ear mechanics and rupture of the ear drums.[34] The increased middle-ear pressure may cause problems in otological surgery (e.g. myringoplasty) and should nitrous oxide be undesirable, oxygen or oxygen-enriched air may be used as

the carrier gas.[35]. Gas, while in the gut, may become metabolized by anaerobic organisms through a reductive pathway.

2. Nitrous oxide inactivates the vitamin B_{12} component (i.e. cobalamin) of the enzyme methionine synthetase. The onset of inhibition has been studied in the rodent,[36] but is thought to be much slower in man.[37] Significant falls in plasma methionine concentrations during routine minor and intermediate surgery have not been demonstrated,[38] a period of at least 8 hours of nitrous oxide anaesthesia probably being needed to demonstrate a fall.[39] Recovery of the enzyme system is slow so that changes may be observed in the postoperative period.

Nitrous oxide interferes with folate metabolism and impairs DNA synthesis following prolonged inhalation.[40] Bone-marrow aplasia and fatal agranulocytosis[25,41] have followed prolonged administration of nitrous oxide in the treatment of poliomyelitis and tetanus. Exposure of patients to nitrous oxide for periods up to 6 hours or longer may result in megaloblastic anaemia,[42] but there is evidence that a biochemical change can be detected after 1 to 2 hours.[43] Occupational exposure to nitrous oxide may result in myeloneuropathy, resembling subacute combined degeneration of the cord, the result of axonal degeneration. This emphasizes the need for the avoidance of pollution of the atmosphere of the operating room[44]. Estimation of the urinary nitrous oxide is a simple and accurate method of biological monitoring of exposure to the gas in the atmosphere.[45] Recent work may be reassuring.[46] (*See also* Sharer N. M. and Nunn J. F. *Br. J. Anaesth.* 1983, **55**, 693; Amos R. J. and Amess J. A. et al. *Br. J. Anaesth.* 1984, **56**, 103; Sweeney B. and Bingham R. M. et al. *Br. Med. J. 1985*, **291**, 567; Nunn J. F., *Br. J. Anaesth.*, 1987, **59**, 3; White D. C. in: *Recent Advances in Anaesthesia and Analgesia-16* (Atkinson R. S. and Adams A. P. ed.) Edinburgh: Churchill Livingstone, 1989)

3. Although teratogenic changes have been observed in pregnant rats exposed to nitrous oxide for prolonged periods, there is no evidence of harm to the fetus in humans.[47]

4. Nitrous oxide has minimal effects on respiration. Tidal volume may decrease slightly and respiratory rate increase without change in $Paco_2$. Hypoxic drive is blunted. The effect on cardiac muscle is depressant, but this is more than compensated for by an increase in catecholamines, which is more marked under hyperbaric conditions.[48]

DIFFUSION HYPOXIA[49]

Immediately after nitrous oxide anaesthesia, hypoxia may occur, because nitrous oxide diffuses out into alveolar gas faster than nitrogen (from room air) can diffuse in. The dilution of alveolar oxygen results in diffusion hypoxia, and may be harmful in certain patients. The remedy is to add oxygen to inspired air during the first 10–15 min after anaesthesia.

NITROUS OXIDE IN ANAESTHESIA

Advantages include the analgesic properties, non-irritant properties, low blood solubility, accuracy of administration, and additive effects allowing lower doses of volatile agents. Nitrous oxide also speeds induction with volatile agents (second gas effect).

Nitrous oxide is a weak anaesthetic agent, and smooth anaesthesia with the sole agent is difficult to obtain consistently, even for short operations; it is used as an adjuvant and as a gaseous vehicle for the administration of more potent volatile agents. Nitrous oxide–oxygen mixtures are usually administered after premedication, intravenous induction and with a volatile or intravenous supplement. Muscle relaxants may be used not only to provide full muscular relaxation, but also to obtund reflex movements. Under these circumstances it is possible to have very light planes of anaesthesia in a totally paralysed patient. Factors that may be considered are:

1. Reports of awareness[50] (*see also* Chapter 14). These would seem to be more common where sedative premedication has been omitted and other adjuvants used in minimal dosage (e.g. in Caesarean section).

2. Recollection of incidents occurring during operation when the patient is later subjected to hypnosis, though this does not necessarily indicate awareness at the time.

3. The EEG: cerebral function monitor[51] or evoked potentials may have a place in determining the level of consciousness when intravenous agents are administered, but further work is required to assess its usefulness in inhalation anaesthesia.

4. The aware, paralysed, terrified patient may show sympathetic activity, e.g. dilatation of pupil, rapid bounding pulse.

It is common practice to prevent awareness by including a volatile agent in the inhaled gas mixture.

Factors causing unplanned awareness during operation.[52] These include: (1) induction. The risk is increased when ultra-short-acting intravenous agents are used for induction prior to intubation under full paralysis; (2) ventilators may mix air or oxygen with the anaesthetic gases due to faulty adjustment or leaks; (3) faults in the anaesthetic machine, e.g. oxygen bypass left on or failure of N_2O supply; and (4) with closed systems it takes time to build up adequate alveolar tension of an agent. High flow-rates of N_2O during induction help to prevent awareness as also does the administration of premedication.

PREMIXED NITROUS OXIDE/OXYGEN

Premixed nitrous oxide/oxygen (80:20) at a maximum cylinder pressure of $47\,kPa \times 100$ ($700\,lb/in^2$) was used in the US in 1945.[53] Certain mixtures of nitrous oxide and oxygen will remain in the gaseous phase at pressures and temperatures at which nitrous oxide by itself would normally be a liquid (Poynting effect). *Entonox* (50:50 mixture) is sold commercially.[54] The top is painted white and the body French blue. If such cylinders are exposed to cold ($-7°C$), some of the nitrous oxides separates as a liquid and may lead to delivery of uneven mixtures, too much oxygen at the beginning and too much nitrous oxide at the end of the cylinder life. Cooling caused by expansion of gases while in use is not likely to result in this. Danger of separation can be avoided by immersing the cylinder in water at 52°C and inverting it three times, or by keeping it in a room at or above a temperature of 10°C for 2 h before use. Uses of *Entonox* include the relief of pain from dressing surgical wounds, chest physiotherapy, removal or changing of thoracotomy drains and coronary infarction. The apparatus can be used in ambulances, for IPPV in the intensive therapy unit for a limited time, where it provides good analgesia without marked cardiovascular depression, and in dental anaesthesia and obstetric analgesia. The English National Board for Midwifery permit its use by midwives on their own responsibility.

Premixed 50% nitrous oxide and 50% oxygen can also be supplied by pipeline and this has been shown to be safe and practical.[55]

NITROUS OXIDE AND ANALGESIA

Nitrous oxide is a good analgesic agent, a 25% concentration in oxygen being compared favourably with morphine for relief of postoperative pain while having little general effect on consciousness. Psychomotor performance is not affected at concentrations of nitrous oxide below 8–12%.[56] The use of nitrous oxide in obstetrics is discussed in Chapter 22.

Nitrous oxide is a very useful agent, which has been in use for over 145 years. Some workers think that its undesirable properties outweigh its benefits. The case is well argued, both for and against in *Nitrous Oxide* (Eger E. I. ed.) London: Arnold, 1985.

Xenon

Isolated in 1898 by William Ramsey (1852–1916), Nobel prizeman in chemistry 1904. First used in 1951. Radioactive xenon used in cerebral blood-flow studies. One study[57] suggests that xenon compares favourably with nitrous oxide in terms of haemodynamic, neurohumoral and anti-nociceptive properties.

Volatile agents

Halothane *(Fluothane)*

2,bromo-2-chloro-1,1,1,trifluoroethane

HISTORY

Synthesized in the laboratories of Imperial Chemical Industries near Manchester by C. W. Suckling in 1951[58] and studied pharmacologically by James Raventós (1905–1983)[59] in succeeding years. Used clinically in 1956 by M. Johnstone[60] of Manchester followed by Bryce-Smith and O'Brien[61] of Oxford.

PHYSICAL PROPERTIES

A colourless liquid volatile anaesthetic with molecular weight 197, specific gravity 1.87, boiling point 50°C, saturated vapour pressure at 20°C 243 mmHg.

Minimal alveolar concentration for anaesthesia 0.75 vol%. Has a characteristic odour. Oil/water solubility coefficient 220. Blood/gas partition coefficient 2.4 (which is low); fat/blood 60.0; brain/blood 2.6. Decomposed by light (stabilized by 0.01% thymol), but is stable when stored in amber-coloured bottles. It can be used safely with soda-lime. The vapour is absorbed by rubber (rubber/gas partition coefficient at 20°C is 120). In the presence of moisture it attacks tin, brass and aluminium in vaporizers and circuits. Non-flammable and non-explosive when its vapour is mixed with oxygen in any concentration (or under hyperbaric conditions) used clinically. May be decomposed by an open flame liberating bromine.

PHARMACODYNAMICS

A potent anaesthetic agent. Vapour is pleasant to smell and is non-irritant. For induction of anaesthesia, 2–4% vapour is necessary; for maintenance, 0.5–2%.

Cardiovascular system. Arterial pressure falls, though not invariably. Cardiac output falls as a result of depression of the myocardium.[62] Dilatation of the smooth muscles of blood vessels (including the coronary arteries), sympathetic ganglionic blockade and central vasomotor depression contribute to a fall in arterial pressure. Cardiac output may fall as a result of bradycardia caused by halothane, an effect reversed by atropine. Treatment with beta-blocking drugs does not contra-indicate careful halothane anaesthesia. [63]

Dysrhythmias. (1) Increased myocardial excitability, ventricular extra-systoles, ventricular tachycardia and even ventricular fibrillation. Factors that increase the likelihood of ventricular dysrhythmias include carbon dioxide retention, sensory stimulation in light anaesthesia, and the injection of drugs with a beta-stimulant effect. Cardiac arrest has been reported following adrenaline infiltration during halothane anaesthesia. Other workers have used the combination without incident. Intravenous infusions of adrenaline or noradrenaline during halothane anaesthesia at rates of more than 10 µg/min have been found to provoke dysrhythmias.[64] It has been recommended[65] that adrenaline infiltration may be safely used in a dosage of 10 ml of l in 100 000 concentration in a 10-min period or 30 ml/h, provided ventilation is adequate. (2) Bradycardia, which may result in hypotension. Nodal rhythm; rarely of serious import. Dysrhythmias may be treated by the withdrawal of halothane, substituting another drug and by ensuring that arterial tensions of oxygen and carbon dioxide are within normal limits.

Central nervous system. Halothane is a potent anaesthetic, but not a good analgesic at low concentrations. It increases cerebral blood flow and raises the CSF pressure.

Respiratory system. Halothane is a respiratory depressant. Respiratory rate is increased and depth decreased. Bronchial relaxation may be due to blockage of reflex pathways causing bronchoconstriction, rather than to depression of bronchial muscular tone. Not a bronchial irritant; pharyngeal and laryngeal reflexes depressed early, and secretions not stimulated. Control of respiration is facilitated by halothane but care is necessary to prevent rapid uptake as a result of increased alveolar ventilation with consequent hypotension due to myocardial depression.

Muscular system. Moderate relaxation is produced by anaesthetic concentrations and the masseters are relaxed early, making laryngoscopy relatively easy.

The uterus. Halothane may cause uterine atony and post-partum haemorrhage if used in obstetrics. This makes it potentially dangerous as an anaesthetic agent for operative delivery, although it is an excellent anaesthetic for external version. Many anaesthetists find it useful in operative delivery if used in low concentration (0.5%).

Halothane, even in concentrations as low as 0.5% may produce increase in blood loss during therapeutic abortion,[66] even when oxytocin is administered. Uterine muscle may behave differently in late pregnancy as compared with the earlier trimesters.

The liver.[67] Massive hepatic necrosis following halothane anaesthesia was reported in 1958,[68] though widespread attention was not drawn to the problem until 1963. Subclinical 'halothane-hepatitis' may also occur.[69]

Theories of liver toxicity mechanisms include:

1. *Toxic reaction to a metabolite.* Up to half of halothane in body tissue may be degraded.[70] Biotransformation is complex, but the products of the reductive metabolic pathways are more dangerous than those arising from oxidative metabolism.

Patients who suffer from hypoxaemia during or after operation may be at risk and this includes those of middle age, especially females, and the obese.

2. *Hypersensitivity reactions.* The anaesthetist should be wary of repeated administration within 3 months (UK Committee on Safety of Medicines recommendation), but there are other views.[71] There may be hypersensitivity reactions to halothane.[72] Patients at particular risk may include those with a tendency to develop organ-specific auto-immune disease. There is evidence that covalent binding to plasma proteins may be important. A specific test for halothane auto-immune antibodies is positive in a high proportion of those with serious halothane-induced hepatitis.[73]

3. *Genetic factors.* These may be of importance.

The jaundice, which may be associated with halothane anaesthesia, is hepatocellular. Biochemical changes include elevation of aminotransferases.

Histology may be able to exclude other causes of jaundice following liver biopsy, but it is difficult to differentiate between virus A and drug hepatitis.

Animal experiments show a correlation between cytochrome P450 enzymes and liver damage. Lipid peroxidation occurs in man after administration of clinical concentrations of halothane for 2 h. The importance of these investigations is not fully understood and more work remains to be done.

In a full and comprehensive survey carried out in 1985,[74] the conclusions reached were that:

1. Halothane could be given to children repeatedly because the risk factor is very small, but this has been contested.[75]

2. Pre-existing liver disease, provided that it is not due to a previous halothane administration, is no contra-indication, although acute liver dysfunction from any cause may well contra-indicate any form of surgery and anaesthesia.

3. Severe liver damage is unlikely to follow a single administration of halothane.

4. Repeated administration to adults, particularly obese, middle-aged women, at intervals less than say 12 weeks, may cause acute liver damage. There are no means of predicting this, and the exact 'safe interval' is not known. However, where there is a strong clinical indication, it may be safer to use repeated halothane than one of the alternatives.[76]

5. If a repeated halothane administration is contemplated, the reasons for

the anaesthestist's choice should, for medicolegal reasons be charted, while the records of the earlier administration should if possible be scrutinized for any problems that may have arisen. Should these have been present, then no second administration should be undertaken.

Other causes of postoperative jaundice include the effect of drugs (such as phenothiazines, monoamine oxidase inhibitors, intravenous tetracycline), blood transfusion, shock, benign postoperative cholestasis, septic cholangitis, coincidental virus hepatitis.[77] Hepatitis B antigen[78] should be excluded. Stress and starvation may produce overt jaundice in subjects with Gilbert's syndrome[79] (familial unconjugated hyperbilirubinaemia) but the serum transaminases remain normal.

Metabolism of halothane.[80] Up to 20% of the halothane taken up by the body is metabolized. Evidence in humans that enzymatic metabolizm occurs include the appearance of bromide, chloride, trifluoracetylethanolamide, chlorobromodifluoroethylene, and trifluoroacetic acid in the urine. Trifluoroacetic acid is relatively non-toxic and is the main oxidative metabolite. Metabolites are slowly cleared from the body for as long as 3 weeks. The products of reductive metabolism may be more significant.

Use with muscle relaxants. Non-depolarizing relaxants are potentiated. The ganglionic-blocking effect of tubocurarine is potentiated and hypotension may result.

Temperature. Induction of anaesthesia with halothane is soon followed by a drop of up to 1°C in oesophageal temperature, together with a rise of up to 4°C in skin temperature. This is thought to be caused by redistribution between core and peripheral tissues. Later, skin temperature may fall as peripheral vasodilatation aids heat loss.

Shivering. Shivering and tremor have frequently been reported during the immediate postoperative period following halothane anaesthesia. It may be associated with a generalized increase in muscle tone, clonic or tonic. There may sometimes be an association between shivering and temperature falls during anaesthesia, and it has been suggested that the former can be prevented by delivering warmed humidified gases to patients during surgery.[81] Opioids have been recommended in management.

INDICATIONS

The introduction of halothane revolutionized anaesthetic practice because of its potency and lack of irritation. It remains a useful agent for producing smooth induction in children and in difficult adults (e.g. those with a degree of respiratory obstruction).

Enflurane (*Ethrane*, *Alyrane*)

HISTORY

The first clinical account on enflurane appeared in 1966.[82] Developed by Ross Terrell in the USA in 1963.

PHYSICAL PROPERTIES

This is 1,1,2-trifluoro-2-chloroethyl difluoromethyl ether (CHF_2-O-CF_2CHFCl) with molecular weight 184, boiling point 56.5; SVP 175 mmHg;

MAC 1.68 in oxygen, 1.28 in 70% nitrous oxide; partition coefficients at 37°C blood/gas 1.91; oil/gas 98.5; water/gas 0.78. Concentrations above 4.25% are flammable in 20% oxygen in nitrous oxide. Stable with soda-lime and metals. Contains no preservative.

PHARMACODYNAMICS

The central nervous system. EEG changes of an epileptiform nature may occur, which are more common during hypocapnia and may persist for several weeks.[83] Cerebral blood flow increased.

The cardiovascular system. As depth of anaesthesia is increased, there is a reversible fall in arterial pressure as a result of myocardial depression. Serious dysrhythmias are uncommon. Relatively safe when adrenaline infiltration is used; up to three times the dose permitted with halothane is reported to be safe.[84]

The respiratory system. Pulmonary ventilation depressed; tidal volume decreased, perhaps with a rise in respiratory rate. Salivary and bronchial secretions not increased. May cause occasional sighing respiration.

Muscular relaxation. Produces moderate relaxation. The activity of non-depolarizing relaxants is enhanced;[85] activity of suxamethonium not altered.

PHARMACOKINETICS

Elimination mostly via the lungs. About 3% is metabolized in the body and the fluoride ion excreted by the kidney, although not in clinically significant amounts.

USE IN OBSTETRICS

Has been used successfully (1.0%) in anaesthesia for Caesarean section without causing depression of the fetus.[86]

CLINICAL USES

Less potent than halothane and therefore a higher concentration is required for equivalent effect. Levels of anaesthesia can be changed quickly. Recovery is smooth and reasonably rapid, with shivering, nausea and vomiting infrequent. For induction in spontaneously breathing patients: up to 5%, for maintenance 1.5–3%.

CONTRA-INDICATIONS

Renal failure, because of possible harmful effect of the fluoride ion. Epilepsy may indicate caution because of the effect on the EEG.

Isoflurane (*Forane, Aerrane, Nederane*)

[$CHF_2.OCHCl.CF_3$] An isomer of enflurane.

HISTORY

Isoflurane is a fluorinated methyl ethyl ether synthesized by Ross Terrell in 1965. The same worker had synthesized enflurane in 1963.[87] Used in clinical anaesthesia by Dobkin et al., 1971[88] and Stevens et al.[89]

PHYSICAL PROPERTIES

A colourless volatile liquid with properties outlined in *Table 7.1*. The saturated vapour pressure is similar to that of halothane. Theoretically it could be used in the same vaporizer as halothane, although this is not recommended on safety grounds. Induction and recovery are rapid, partly because the blood/gas partition coefficient is lower (1.4) than that of halothane or enflurane, but also because the fat solubility is only about half that of halothane. MAC is 1.15 in oxygen and 0.66 in 70% nitrous oxide. Isoflurane is stable and no preservatives are necessary to prevent its decomposition. It does not react with metal in breathing systems. BP 48.5°C.

PHARMACODYNAMICS

Cardiovascular system. Isoflurane is a myocardial depressant[90] but it has less effect on the heart muscle than either halothane or enflurane. Systemic arterial blood pressure falls during isoflurane anaesthesia,[91] primarily as a result of a fall in systemic vascular resistance.[92] Isoflurane anaesthesia is associated with a stable cardiac rhythm and the myocardium is not sensitized to catecholamines.[93] Heart rate may increase, especially in young patients.

Coronary steal. Isoflurane has been shown to be a powerful coronary vasodilator in patients with coronary artery disease, the end-tidal concentration being 1%[94]. Coronary steal theoretically may occur if healthy myocardium receives increased blood flow at the expense of myocardium supplied by a stenosed vessel. It has been pointed out that normally coronary blood flow is related to myocardial oxygen demand so closely that coronary a-v oxygen content difference remains stable. If autoregulation is impaired by a potent coronary vasodilator, blood flow is elevated inappropriately relative to oxygen demand. No harm results if arteries are normal. Isoflurane is a mild negative inotropic agent *in vitro*.[95] Others have shown that isoflurane with nitrous oxide improves the tolerance to pacing induced myocardial ischaemia in patients with significant coronary artery disease[96]. Work in swine[97] suggests that isoflurane may be safer than halothane in the presence of critical coronary stenosis, whereas in dogs[98] isoflurane caused steal, but halothane did not.

Respiration. Like halothane and enflurane, isoflurane causes a decrease in tidal volume and increase in respiratory rate.[99] In terms of respiratory depression, it occupies a position intermediate between halothane and enflurane. Isoflurane depresses the respiratory response to hypoxaemia and hypercapnia. The incidence of coughing and laryngospasm during induction is greater than with halothane[100] because the vapour is mildly irritant.

Central nervous system. Low concentrations do not cause any increase in cerebral blood flow, provided that the Pa_{CO_2} is normal.[101] Therefore it has some superiority over halothane and enflurane in neurosurgical anaesthesia.

However, larger concentrations do increase cerebral blood flow. At 2 MAC it can make the EEG isoelectric and so may offer some protection against the cerebral effect of hypoxia.[102] It has no protective effect on the development of post-traumatic cerebral oedema.[103]

Muscle tone. Like halothane and enflurane, isoflurane relaxes muscles, often satisfactory for abdominal surgery, but at the expense of cardiorespiratory depression. It potentiates non-depolarising relaxants.

The reproductive system. The effect on the pregnant uterus is similar to that of halothane and enflurane and is dose related. In a concentration of 0.75% it is suitable for Caesarean section.

Liver. Repeated isoflurane administration has failed to produce measurable changes in liver function.[104]

PHARMACOKINETICS

Only about 0.2% of inhaled isoflurane can be recovered as urinary metabolites.[105] Serum fluoride after 3 MAC hours exposure amounts to only about 5% of the levels associated with renal toxicity.[106] The likelihood of renal or hepatic toxicity following isoflurane anaesthesia is thought to be very low.

INDICATIONS

Of the various inhalation agents available, isoflurane has the advantage of providing stability of cardiac rhythm and lack of sensitization of the heart to exogenous and endogenous adrenaline. Rapid recovery is an advantage in the daystay patient. The drug has a stable molecule and is unlikely to be toxic to the vital organs. It produces hypotension with less cardiac depressant action than halothane. For maintenance with spontaneous breathing 1–2.5% is usually needed.

(*See also* Eger E. I. *Anesthesiology* 1981, **55**, 559 and Jones R. M. In: *Recent Advances in Anaesthesia and Analgesia* – *15* (Atkinson R. S. and Adams A. P. ed.) Edinburgh: Churchill Livingstone, 1985.)

Choice of volatile agent

Of the three volatile agents currently available in the UK, halothane, enflurane and isoflurane, personal choice may be influenced by a number of factors: (1) repeat anaesthetics using halothane may carry a risk of liver toxicity, although this is low and repeated administration may be justified in circumstances where halothane is particularly advantageous; (2) halothane is the least irritant to inhale while being the most potent. It may therefore be the best agent when rapid smooth induction is required, e.g. in children, in the presence of respiratory obstruction; (3) halothane is the agent most likely to cause ventricular dysrhythmias in the presence of hypercapnia or adrenaline; (4) isoflurane causes the least direct myocardial depression and the most peripheral dilatation of vessels. It may be the best agent to use when myocardial depression is unwanted, although the possibility of steal may be considered disadvantageous; (5) enflurane occupies a mid position in terms of effects on the cardiovascular system. Disadvantages include a lack of potency, which may prolong induction, possible deleterious effects on diseased kidneys caused by the fluoride ion, and possible epileptogenic effects in susceptible individuals. Enflurane is the most difficult to use without nitrous oxide because of its lack of potency; (6) in terms of cost halothane is cheaper than enflurane, which is cheaper than isoflurane. All three are stable in the presence of soda-lime and can be used in rebreathing systems; (7) isoflurane is commonly used in neurosurgery because it shows the least tendency to increase cerebral blood flow and may offer some protection to the brain against hypoxia; and (8) the lower solubility of isoflurane may result in quicker recovery and it may, therefore, be useful in day surgery.

Newer anaesthetic agents

Two newer agents, which are not yet commercially available in the UK, are desflurane and sevoflurane.

Desflurane

$(CF_3.CHF.O.CHF_2)$
This fluorinated methyl ethyl ether is a promising agent. Developed in the USA[107]. First reports in the UK followed administration to volunteers at Guy's Hospital.[108]

PHYSICAL CHARACTERISTICS

Molecular Weight 168. Saturated vapour pressure at 20°C 673 mmHg. Blood-gas partition coefficient 0.4. MAC in oxygen 6.0%. No preservative required. Stable in soda-lime.

VAPORIZER

Because of the low boiling point (23.5°C) standard tec vaporizers are unsatisfactory and special vaporizers are being developed.

CARDIO-RESPIRATORY EFFECTS

These are similar to those of isoflurane. Some fall in arterial pressure and some depression of respiration is to be expected. The myocardium is not sensitized to catecholamines.

ADVANTAGES OF DESFLURANE

(1) Because of the low blood/gas partition coefficient, induction, change of depth of anaesthesia and recovery will be rapid. The vapour is not unpleasant to inhale. Solubility in body tissues is low so that in a closed breathing system the concentration of vapour in the system will approach that in the basal flow more rapidly than in the case of other agents. It may well find a role in day

case surgery.[109] (2) The molecule is stable in soda-lime and biotransformation is negligible.[110] There are unlikely to be hepatorenal toxic effects.

DISADVANTAGES

Desflurane will be expensive, although this is to some degree offset by its use in a closed system. The MAC of 6% means that it is less potent than some other agents.

Sevoflurane

First used in North America in 1971.[111] MAC is 2%. The low solubility in blood (0.6) was an attractive feature. There are, however, a number of drawbacks. Sevoflurane is less stable in soda-lime than the commonly used volatile agents. It disappears into soda-lime at appreciable quantities at higher temperatures (6.5% degradation at 22°C and up to 57.4% at 54°C.[112] There is also some breakdown in the body, but fluoride concentrations are not greater than those seen after enflurane anaesthesia.[113] Animal work suggests that its effect on the cardiovascular system is similar to that of isoflurane.[114]

(*See also*, Jones R. M. *Br. J. Anaesth.*, 1990, **65**, 527; Wrigley S. R. and Jones R. M. *Curr. Opin. Anaesthesiol.* 1991, **4**, 534; Ewart I. A. and Jones R. M. *Curr. Anaesth. Crit. Care*, 1991, **2**, 243).

Environmental effects

There is growing interest in the possible effects of gaseous and volatile anaesthetic agents on the environment. Nitrous oxide, possibly the worst offender, can photodissociate or react with atomic oxygen in the stratosphere to produce nitric oxide, which contributes to the destruction of ozone. Chlorine-containing molecules are probably more destructive than those with fluorine.[115] Anaesthesia contributes at most 0.01% to the total atmospheric burden of chlorine-containing compounds and will have a negligible impact on global warming.[116]

References

1. *See also* Kety S. S. *Anesthesiology* 1950, **11**, 517; Eger E. J. *Anesthetic Uptake and Action.* Baltimore: Williams & Wilkins, 1974; Hull C. in: *Scientific Foundations of Anaesthesia.* (Scurr C., Feldman S. and Soni N. ed.), Oxford: Heinemann, 1990, 572.
2. Merkel G. and Eger E. I. *Anesthesiology* 1963, **24**, 346 (reprinted in 'Classical File', *Surv. Anesthesiol.* 1974, **18**, 594); Eger E. I. et al. *Anesthesiology* 1956, **26**, 271.
3. Fink B. R. *Anesthesiology* 1971, **34**, 403.
4. McKesson E. I. *Can. Med. Assoc. J.* 1921, **11**, 130 (reprinted in 'Classical File', *Surv. Anesthesiol.* 1968, **12**, 435).
5. Gill R. *The Chloroform Problem.* Edinburgh: Blackwood, 1906, Vol. 2.
6. Kesecioglu J and Rupreht J. *Acta Anaesthesiol. Scand.* 1991, **35**, in press.
7. Herbert M. et al. *Br. Med. J.* 1983, **286**, 1539.
8. Fraser A. C. L. and Goat V. A. *Anaesthesia* 1983, **38**, 128.

9. Snow J. *Anesthesiology* 1950, **11**, 517; Eger E. J. *Anesthetic* London, 1847.
10. Plomley F. *Lancet* 1847, p. 134 (30 January) (reprinted in 'Classical File', *Surv. Anesthesiol.* 1970, **14**, 88).
11. Guedel A. E. *Inhalation Anesthesia* 1937 and 2nd ed. London: Macmillan, 1951.
12. Crile G. W. *Lancet* 1913, **2**, 7; *Surg. Gynecol. Obstet.* 1911, **13**, 170; *Ann. Surg.* 1908, **47**, 866; *Boston Med. Surg. J.* 1910, **163**, 893 (reprinted in 'Classical File', *Surv. Anesthesiol.* 1966, **10**, 291).
13. Lundy J. S. *Minnesota Med.* 1926, **9**, 399 (Reprinted in 'Classical File', *Surv. Anesthesiol.* 1981, **25**, 272.)
14. Heijke S. and Smith G. *Br. J. Anaesth.* 1990, **64**, 3; Jones R. M. In: *Anaesthesia.* (Nimmo W. S. and Smith G., ed.) Oxford: Blackwell, 1989, 34; Jones R. M. *Br. J. Anaesth.* 1990, **65**, 527.
15. *Gas*, a word invented by the Flemish chemist Johannes Baptiste van Helmont (1577–1644) from the Greek work *Khos* = chaos.
16. Evans T. W. *Br. J. Dent. Sci.* 1868, **2**, 196.
17. Andrews E. A. *Chicago Med. Examiner* 1868, **19**, 656 (reprinted in 'Classical File', *Surv. Anesthesiol.* 1963, **7**, 74).
18. Bert P. *C. r. Soc. Biol. Paris* 1878, **87**, 728; 1879, **89**, 132.
19. Clover J. T. *Br. Med. J.* 1868, **2**, 201.
20. Bert P. *C. r. Acad. Sci. Paris* 1883, **96**, 1271.
21. Clover J. T. *Br. Med. J.* 1876, **2**, 74.
21a. Hele W. *Trans Odont Soc*, 1873, **5**, 95.
22. Hewitt F. *Lancet* 1885, **1**, 840.
23. McKesson E. I. *Am. J. Surg.* (Anesth. Suppl.) 1916, **7**, February.
24. Courville C. B. *Medicine* 1936, **15**, 129 (reprinted in 'Classical File', *Surv. Anesthesiol.* 1958, **2**, 523, 660) McKesson E.I. *Can Med Ass J*, 1921, **11**, 130.
25. Lassen H. C. A. *Lancet* 1956, **1**, 525.
26. Wright B. M. *Lancet* 1977, **2**, 1008.
27. Clutton-Brock J. *Br. J. Anaesth.* 1967, **39**, 388.
28. Kain M. L. et al. *Br. J. Anaesth.* 1967, **39**, 425.
29. Rupreht J. et al. *8th World Congress WSFA, Manila*, 1984, **2**, A386.
30. Yang J. C. et al. *Anesthesiology* 1980, **52**, 414.
31. Rupreht J. et al. *Acta Anaesthesiol. Scand* 1985, **29**, 635.
32. Rupreht J. and Shimoji K. et al. *J. Neurosurg. Anesthesiol.* 1989, **1**, 91.
33. Stinson T. N. and Donlon J. V. *Anesthesiology* 1982, **56**, 385.
34. Owen W. D. et al. *Anesth. Anal.* 1978, **57**, 283.
35. Mann M. S. et al. *Anaesthesia* 1985, **40**, 8.
36. Deacon R. et al. *Eur. J. Biochem.* 1980, **104**, 419; Koblin D. D. et al. *Anesthesiology* 1981, **54**, 318.
37. Koblin D. D. et al. *Anesth. Analg.* 1982, **61**, 75.
38. Nunn J. F. et al. *Br. J. Anaesth.* 1986, **58**, 1.
39. Amess J. A. L. et al. *Lancet* 1978, **2**, 339; Amos R. J. et al. *Lancet* 1982, **2**, 835.
40. Bank R. G. S. and Henderson R. J. *J. Chem. Soc. (A)* 1968, 2886.
41. Annotation, *Lancet* 1978; **2**, 613.
42. Nunn J. F. and Chanarin J. *Br. J. Anaesth.* 1978, **50**, 1089.
43. Hill G. E. et al. *Br. J. Anaesth.* 1978, 50, 555.
44. Layzer R. B. *Lancet* 1978, **2**, 1227.
45. Sonander H. et al. *Br. J. Anaesth.* 1983, **55**, 1225.
46. Reagan J. O. et al. *Anesth. Analg.* 1987, **66**, 5146; Tyson G. et al. *ibid*, **66**, 5182.
47. Konieczko K., Chapple J. C. and Nunn J. F. *Br. J. Anaesth.* 1987, **59**, 449.
48. Hornbein T. F. et al. *Anesth. Analg.* 1982, **61**, 553
49. Fink B. R. *Anesthesiology* 1955, **16**, 511; Fink B. R. et al. *Fed. Proc.* 1954, **13**, 354.
50. Hutchinson R. *Br. J. Anaesth.* 1961, **33**, 463; Utting J. F. *Anaesth. Intensive Care* 1975, **3**, 334; Editorial, *Br. Med. J.* 1980, **1**, 811.
51. Maynard M. et al. *Br. Med. J.* 1969, **4**, 545; Dubois M. et al. *Anaesthesia* 1978, **33**, 157.

52. Waters D. J. *Br. J. Anaesth.* 1968, **40**, 259.
53. Barach A. L. and Rovenstine E. A. *Anesthesiology* 1945, **6**, 449.
54. Hill D. W. *Physics Applied to Anaesthesia.* 3rd ed. London: Butterworths, 1976, 44.
55. MacGregor, W. G. et al. *Anaesthesia* 1972, **27**, 14.
56. Allison R. H. *Br. J. Anaesth.* 1979, **51**, 177.
57. Boomsma F., Rupreht J. and Veld A. J. *Anaesthesia* 1990, **45**, 273–278.
58. Suckling C. W. *Br. J. Anaesth.* 1957, **29**, 466.
59. Raventós J. *Br. J. Pharmacol.* 1956, **11**, 394 (reprinted in 'Classical File', *Surv. Anesthesiol.* 1966, **10**, 183).
60. Johnstone M. *Br. J. Anaesth.* 1956, **28**, 392.
61. Bryce-Smith R. and O'Brien H. D. *Br. Med. J.* 1956, **2**, 969; *Proc. R. Soc. Med.* 1957, **30**, 193.
62. Prys-Roberts C. et al. *Br. J. Anaesth.* 1972, **44**, 634; Prys-Roberts C. et al. *Br. J. Anaesth.* 1974, **16**, 105.
63. Roberts J. G. *Br. J. Anaesth.* 1976, **48**, 315.
64. Andersen N. and Johansen S. H. *Anesthesiology* 1963, **24**, 51.
65. Katz R. L. *Anesthesiology* 1962, **23**, 597.
66. Grant I. S. *Br. J. Anaesth.* 1980, **52**, 711.
67. Neuberger J. and Williams R. *Br. Med. J.* 1984, **289**, 1136.
68. Virtue R. W. and Payne K. W. *Anesthesiology* 1958, **19**, 562.
69. Lecky J. N. and Cohen P. S. *Anesthesiology* 1970, **33**, 371.
70. Carpenter R. L. et al. *Anesthesiology*, 1986, **65**, 201.
71. Spence A. A. *Br. J. Anaesth.* 1987, **59**, 529.
72. Neuberger J. et al. *Br. J. Anaesth.* 1983, **55**, 15.
73. Kenna J. G. et al. *Br. J. Anaesth.* 1987, **59**, 1286.
74. Stock J. C. L. and Strunin L. *Anesthesiology* 1985, **63**, 424.
75. Kenna J. G. et al. *Br. Med. J.* 1987, **294**, 1209.
76. Adams A. P. et al. *Br. Med. J.* 1986, **293**, 1023.
77. Johnstone M. *Br. J. Anaesth.* 1964, **36**, 718; Hart S. M. and Fitzgerald P. G. *Br. J. Anaesth.* 1975, **47**, 1321.
78. Blumberg B. S. et al. *Ann. Intern. Med.* 1967, **66**, 924.
79. Gilbert A. and Lereboullet P. *Semaine médicale, Paris* 1901, **71**, 241; Quinn N. W. and Gollan J. L. *Br. J. Oral Surg.* 1975, **12**, 285.
80. Geddes I. C. *Br. J. Anaesth.* 1972, **44**, 953; Cousins M. J. et al. *Anesth. Analg. 1987*, **66**, 299.
81. Pflug A. E. et al. *Can. Anaesth. Soc. J.* 1978, **25**, 43.
82. Virtue R. W. et al. *Can. Anaesth. Soc. J.* 1966, **12**, 233 (reprinted in 'Classical File', *Surv. Anesthesiol.* 1977, **21**, 210).
83. Julien R. M. and Kavan E. M. *J. Pharmacol. Exp. Ther.* 1972, **123**, 393; Grant I. S. *Anaesthesia* 1986, **41**, 1024; Nicoll J. M. V. *Anaesthesia* 1986, **41**, 927.
84. Reisner L. S. and Lippmann M. *Anesth. Analg.* 1975, **64**, 468; Johnston R. R. et al. *Anesth. Analg.* 1976, **55**, 709.
85. Lebowitz M. H. et al. *Anesthesiology* 1970, **19**, 355.
86. Coleman A. J. and Downing J. W. *Anesthesiology* 1975, **43**, 354.
87. Vircha J. F. *Anesthesiology* 1971, **21**, 4.
88. Dobkin A. B. et al. *Can. Anaesth. Soc. J.* 1971, **18**, 264.
89. Stevens D. J. et al. *Can. Anaesth. Soc. J.* 1971, **18**, 500.
90. Beaupre P. N. et al. *Anesthesiology* 1983, **59**, A59.
91. Wade J. G. and Stevens W. C. *Anesth. Analg. (Cleve.)* 1981, **60**, 666.
92. Eger E. I. *Anesthesiology* 1981, **55**, 559.
93. Johnson R. R. et al. *Anesth. Analg. (Cleve.)* 1976, **55**, 707.
94. Reiz S., Balfors E. and Sorensen M. B. et al. *Anesthesiology*, 1983, **59**, 91–97.
95. Merin R. G., Lowenstein E. and Gelman S. *Anesthesiology* 1986, **64**, 137; Moffat E. A. et al. *Anesth Analg* 1986, **65**, 53.

96. Tarnow J., Markschies-Horning A. and Schulte-Sasse U. *Anesthesiology* 1986, **64**, 147.
97. Roberts S. L., Gilbert M. and Tinker J. H. *Anesth. Analg* 1987, **66**, 485.
98. Buffington C. W. and Levine A. *Anesthesiology 1986,* **65**, A6.
99. Calverley R. K. et al. *Anesth. Analg. (Cleve.)* 1978, **57**, 610; Fourcode H. E. et al. *Anesthesiology* 1971, **35**, 26.
100. Friesen R. H. and Lichter J. L. *Anesth. Analg. (Cleve.)* 1983, **62**, 411; Pandit V. A. et al. *Anesthesiology* 1971, **35**, A445.
101. Wade J. G. and Stevens W. C. *Anesth. Analg. (Cleve.)* 1981, **60**, 666; Eger E. I. *Anesthesiology* 1981, **55**, 559.
102. Newberg L. A. and Michenfelder J. D. *Anesthesiology* 1983, **59**, 29.
103. Smith A. L. and Marque J. J. *Anesthesiology* 1976, **45**, 64.
104. Jones R. M. et al. *Anaesthesia*, 1991, **46**, 686.
105. Holaday D. A. et al. *Anesthesiology* 1975, **43**, 325.
106. Mazze R. I. et al. *Anesthesiology* 1974, **40**, 536.
107. Eger E. I. *Anesth. Analg.* 1987, **66**, 983.
108. Jones R. M. et al. *Br. J. Anaesth.* 1990, **64**, 11.
109. Jones R. M. et al. *Br. J. Anaesth.* 1990, **64**, 482.
110. Wrigley S. R. et al. *Anaesthsia* 1991, **46**, 615.
111. Wallin R. F. and Napoli M. D. *Fed. Proc.* 1971, **30**, 442.
112. Strum D. P., Johnson B. H. and Eger E. I. *Anesthesiology* 1987, **67**, 779.
113. Jones R. M. *Br. J. Anaesth.* 1990, **65**, 527.
114. Bernard J. M., Wouters P. F. et al. *Anesthesiology* 1990, **72**, 659.
115. Logan M. and Farmer J. G. *Br. J. Anaesth.* 1990, **63**, 645.
116. Brown A. C., Canosa-Mas C. E. et al. *Nature* 1989, **341**, 635; *Lancet*, 1989, **ii**, 279.

Chapter 8

Gases used in association with anaesthesia[1]

Oxygen [O_2]

History

John Mayow[2] (1643–1679) of Oxford showed that a component of air was used up by a burning candle or a live mouse. Joseph Priestley[3] (1733–1804) discovered 'dephlogisticated air' in 1772, as did Carl Wilhelm Scheele (1742–1786) in 1771. Antoine Laurant Lavoisier (1743–1794) and Pierre Simon Laplace[4] (1749–1827) coined the term 'oxygène' (oxy = acid; gene = producer) in 1779, and were the first to compare the heat produced by respiration in animals and by the combustion of carbon. They showed a relationship between oxygen used and carbon dioxide produced. Justus von Liebig[5] (1803–1873), Darmstadt chemist, in 1851 showed that carbohydrates and fats were substrates and not carbon itself. Thomas Beddoes (1760–1808) used oxygen in medical treatment in 1794 at Bristol. Barth compressed the gas into cylinders in 1868.

Modern use of oxygen was popularized in 1917 by J. S. Haldane (1860–1936) during the First World War,[6] and by Yandell Henderson, the New Haven physiologist (1873–1944).

Preparation

Priestley prepared oxygen by heating red mercuric oxide. In the 1850s a French chemist, Boussingault, discovered that at a temperature of about 1000°C barium monoxide would absorb oxygen from air forming barium dioxide and release it at a higher temperature. This process was patented by his pupils the Brin brothers in the 1880s. Their company eventually became British Oxygen.

Medical and industrial oxygen is now manufactured by the fractional distillation of liquid air (nitrogen comes off first), patented by Carl Linde of Germany. Boiling point of oxygen −183°C; of nitrogen −195°C. Oxygen cylinders are painted black with white shoulders in the UK (International Standards Organization), blue in some European countries and green in the USA. The cylinders contain gaseous oxygen compressed to 137 bar. Also supplied as a liquid at about −183°C in insulated tanks at a pressure of around 10.5 bar. One ml of liquid oxygen gives 842 ml of gas at 15°C. Pipeline pressure is 4.1 bar.

The oxygen concentrator[7] produces oxygen from ambient air by preferential absorption of nitrogen on zeolites (crystalline aluminosilicates). It behaves like a molecular sieve with a pore size of 0.5 nm. The resultant gas contains 6% of harmless impurities, mostly argon. It is suitable for use in hospitals, remote areas, developing countries and in the military. Small machines producing about 2 l/min are cheaper than cylinders for domestic use.[8]

Properties

Molecular weight 32. Solubility in water 0.024 ml/ml at 37°C, 0.031 at 20°C, 0.049 at 0°C. Boiling point −183°C. Critical temperature −118.4°C. Critical pressure 50.8 bar. Specific gravity 1105 (air is 1000). Density 1.35 kg/m^3 at 15°C. Electric sparks convert it into ozone (O_3).

When compressed, oxygen may ignite grease or oil (as in a diesel engine). It encourages fires, although not itself flammable. Oxygen (and nitrous oxide) cylinders should be turned on momentarily before being fitted to the machine to allow any dirt in the valve to escape. They should be turned on slowly after fitting to prevent sudden surges of pressure in the reducing value and contents gauge.

Air

Atmospheric air contains 78.08% nitrogen, 20.95% oxygen, 0.93% argon, 0.03% carbon dioxide, plus traces of neon, helium, krypton, hydrogen and xenon in descending order of abundance. Medical air is supplied in the UK in grey cylinders with black and white shoulder quadrants, compressed to 137 bar. In many hospitals it is also supplied by pipeline at 4 bar. It is used as a respired gas and to drive ventilators. It also drives surgical drills, etc. but these need a pressure of 7 bar or above. It has less impurities than industrial compressed air, no water and less than 0.5 mg/m^3 of oil mist. It is not bacteriologically sterile.[9]

Carbon Dioxide [CO_2]

Discovered by Jean Baptiste von Helmont (1597–1644) and isolated by Joseph Black (1728–1799) in 1757 who showed that it was produced by respiration, combustion and fermentation. Used to produce 'suspended animation' and surgical anaesthesia in animals in 1824 by Henry Hill Hickman (1800–1830).[10] 30% CO_2 was used by Ralph Waters (1883–1979) to render humans unconscious in 1928.[11] The stimulating effect on respiration was shown by Herman and Escher in 1870,[12] and became used by anaesthetists for this purpose soon after the work of Haggard and Yandell Henderson[13] in the USA (1921) who recommended 5% CO_2 in oxygen (to overcome collapse due to anaesthesia) and John Scott Haldane (1860–1936) in Britain.[14] It remains widely used although tragedies continue to occur with accidental overdosage.[15]

The ill effects of inadequate ventilation were thought to be caused by hypoxia until Ralph Waters, then in private practice in Sioux City, Iowa, pointed out the possibility of CO_2 excess.[16] He realized that the respired CO_2 could be controlled, at least in anaesthetized animals, following the work of D. E. Jackson, a Cincinnati pharmacologist.[17] John Snow was, of course, an even earlier pioneer of CO_2 absorption.[18] Waters' first reason for the use of CO_2 absorption was economy and convenience; even more important when he started to use cyclopropane. Only later did he stress the possible harm produced by excessive CO_2.[19] After relaxants were introduced and IPPV became commonplace, hypocapnia was readily produced. This was thought to be harmless or possibly beneficial,[20] but today most anaesthetists try to achieve a $Paco_2$ that is at or only just below normal levels. If this is difficult (e.g. in the elderly), up to 5% CO_2 may be added to the inspired gases.

Properties

Colourless gas, pungent odour in high concentration. Molecular weight 44. Boiling point $-78.5°C$. Solubility in water $0.88\,ml/ml$ at $20°C$. Critical temperature $31°C$. Critical pressure $73.8\,bar$. Specific gravity 1520 (air is 1000). Density $1.87\,kg/m^3$ at $15°C$.

Preparation and storage

In Britain obtained from four sources: (1) from fermentation in the brewing of beer; (2) by-product of manufacture of hydrogen in petroleum refining; (3) from the combustion of other fuels; and (4) by heating magnesium and calcium carbonate in the presence of their oxides. Only a small fraction of the CO_2 manufactured is used for medicinal purposes.

It is stored in grey cylinders at $50\,bar$ (or for industrial use in refrigerated tanks). Solid CO_2 is stored and transported in insulated containers. The filling ratio in cylinders is 0.75 in temperate climates and 0.67 in the tropics. The liquid phase disappears when about 83% of the gas has been discharged.

Oxygen–CO_2 premixed cylinders are available in various combinations. Such cylinders are black with grey/white shoulder quadrants and filled to a pressure of 137 atmospheres.

Effects on respiratory system. See Chapter 1

Inspired air contains 0.03%, mixed expired gas 3.5–4% and alveolar gas 5.6%. Breathing 5% CO_2 in air or oxygen is tolerable, but higher amounts cause dyspnoea, headaches, etc. Above 10% the narcotic effect becomes more marked, and at 30% there is an isoelectric EEG and coma. Muscle twitching, a flap of the hands and fits may occur before coma supervenes. At 40% breathing is depressed.

Variation in $Paco_2$ between 2 and $12.7\,kPa$ probably does not alter the MAC of halothane,[21] but CO_2 narcosis occurs in patients with respiratory failure whose $Paco_2$ exceeds $12–16\,kPa$[22] and is closely related to the pH falling to between 6.8 and 7.1 in the cerebrospinal fluid. Any 'inert gas' effect of CO_2 is small. CO_2 has been extensively used to anaesthetize small laboratory animals.

Hypercapnia by itself depresses the heart, but this is masked by a rise in plasma catecholamines. Multifocal ventricular extrasystoles may occur. For effects on cerebral blood flow *see* Chapter 22, Neurosurgery.

Clinical uses

1. To hasten inhalational induction especially with agents of high solubility. Adding 5% CO_2 for no longer than 5 min stimulates respiration and helps to overcome laryngeal spasm and breath-holding. It will also speed elimination of such agents at the end of surgery (*see* Chapter 7).
2. To widen the glottis and facilitate blind intubation.
3. Added to inspired gases to prevent hypocapnia during passive hyperventilation in anaesthesia; or to facilitate the onset of respiration after passive hyperventilation, following complete reversal of relaxant drugs.
4. As a cerebral vasodilator in studies of cerebral blood flow.
5. Added to the oxygenator gas mixture during hypothermic cardiopulmonary bypass in order to maintain $Paco_2$ and pH when these values are corrected to body temperature. This approach is losing ground to the alpha-stat method, which allows hypocapnia and alkalosis to occur at low temperatures. *See* Chapter 22, Cardiothoracic.
6. To insufflate the abdomen for laparoscopy.
7. For cryoprobes.

Contra-indications

1. Carbon dioxide administration is a potential source of great danger.[23] The attachment of a CO_2 cylinder to the anaesthetic machine only at the specific request of the anaesthetist, maximum flow limits and the wider use of capnography should help prevent tragedies. CO_2 rotameters are not always fitted to anaesthetic machines.
2. In respiratory failure or obstruction, treatment with CO_2 has no place and is likely to be harmful.

Water vapour

Water has a high specific heat ($4.2 \, kJ/kg/°C$, ten times that of copper). Inspired air is warmed to body temperature and fully saturated with water vapour by the time it reaches the trachea. If the trachea is intubated, this process has to take place in the tracheobronchial tree. Air saturated with water vapour at 15, 20 and 37°C has partial pressures of water vapour of 12, 18 and 47 mmHg and water contents of 13, 19 and 50 mg/l respectively.

Helium (He)

Isolated by Sir W. Ramsey (1852–1916) (British chemist and Nobel prizewinner in 1904 for his work on the inert gases) in 1895.

Preparation

From natural gas, some gas wells in Poland, Texas and New Mexico contain about 1%. Natural gas from the North sea contains only 0.01–0.03%. Air contains 0.0005%. Helium cylinders are brown, helium-oxygen cylinders brown with brown/white shoulder quadrants. The pressure in a full cylinder is 137 bar.

Properties

Inert, colourless, odourless gas. Molecular weight 4. Boiling point −269°C. Solubility in water 0.0088 ml/ml at 20°C. Critical temperature −268°C. Specific gravity 178 (air is 1000). Critical pressure 2.3 bar. Density 0.17 kg/m^3 at 15°C. Second lightest gas (to hydrogen).

A mixture of 21% oxygen and 79% helium has a specific gravity of 341 (air is 1000). Its low density enables this gas mixture to flow through an orifice three times as fast as air, for the same pressure gradient. Thus patients with upper airway obstruction will benefit. Because its viscosity is very similar to oxygen, it will make no difference to the laminar flow in smaller airways, but the lower Reynolds number for helium mixtures will encourage laminar flow.

Helium's low solubility has led to its use in the measurement of lung volumes by gas dilution. Like nitrogen, it will also help prevent alveolar collapse. Its diffusibility and low solubility make it less likely than nitrogen to be responsible for decompression sickness. It has a high thermal capacity, which encourages loss of body heat.

If fed through a nitrous oxide flow-meter, the reading must be multiplied by 3.3 to get the approximate flow rate. It diffuses through rubber.

References

1. *See also* Howell R. S. C. In: *Anaesthesia Reviews 7 & 8.* (Kaufman L. ed.) Edinburgh: Churchill Livingstone, 1990 & 1991, 87 & 195 respectively.
2. Mayow J. *Tractactus Quinque Medicophysici, No.2.* Oxford: 1674.
3. Priestley J. *Phil. Trans.* 1772, **52**, 147; *Experiments and Observations on Different Kinds of Air,* vol. 2, sect. III-V, 29–103 (reprinted in Classical File, *Surv. Anesthesiol.* 1976, **20**, 81).
4. Lavoisier A-L. and Laplace P. S. *Mém. Prés. Acad. Sci. Paris* 1780, **103**, 566.
5. von Liebig J. *Letters on Chemistry.* 3rd ed. 1851.
6. Haldane J. S. *Br. Med. J.* 1917, **1**, 181.
7. O'Sullivan J. *Br. J. Pharmaceut. Pract.* 1988, **10**, 395.
8. Howard P. *Oxygen Therapy* Bristol: Wright, 1987.
9. Bjerring P. and Oberg B. *Anaesthesia* 1986, **41**, 148.
10. Thompson C. J. S. *Br. Med. J.* 1912, **1**, 843.
11. Leake C. D. and Waters R. M. *Anesth. Analg. Curr. Res.* 1929, **8**, 17.
12. Herman L. and Escher T. *Pflügers Arch. Ges. Physiol.* 1870, **3**, 3.
13. Henderson Y. *Br. Med. J.* 1925. **2**, 1170.
14. Haldane J. S. and Smith J. L. *J. Path. Bact.* 1893, **1**, 168.
15. Razis P. *Anaesthesia* 1989, **44**, 348.
16. Waters R. M. *Curr. Res. Anesth. Analg.* 1924, **3**, 20; Waters R. M. et al. *Curr. Res. Anesth. Analg.* 1931, **10**, 10.
17. Jackson D. E. *J. Lab. Clin. Med.* 1915, **1**, 1.

18. Foregger R. *Anesthesiology* 1960, **21**, 20.
19. Waters R. M. *Can. Med. Assoc. J.* 1927, **17**, 1500; Waters R. M. et al. *Curr. Res. Anesth. Analg.* 1931, **10**, 10.
20. Geddes I. C. and Gray T. C. *Lancet* 1959, 24.
21. Eisele J. H. et al. *Anesthesiology* 1967, **28**, 856.
22. Westlake E. K. et al. *Q. J. Med.* 1955, **24**, 155.
23. Nunn J. F. *Br. J. Anaesth.* 1990, **65**, 155.

Chapter 9

Intravenous anaesthetic agents

The ideal intravenous agent reliably and pleasantly induces full anaesthesia within one arm–brain circulation time, is free from side-effects and completely wears off in a few minutes. It must be capable of infusion to maintain anaesthesia without problems.

Intravenous anaesthetic agents may be used for: (1) the induction of anaesthesia; (2) as the sole agent for operations (TIVA); (3) to supplement volatile anaesthesia or regional analgesia; and (4) for sedation.

The injection of a potent drug into the bloodstream cannot be readily withdrawn, whereas inhalation agents can be more easily eliminated.

History

Johann Sigmund (1623–1688), a German Physician, injected opium intravenously, to produce unconsciousness in 1665. Pierre-Cyprien Oré (1828–1891)[1], professor of Physiology at Bordeaux, used chloral hydrate intravenously in 1872 in a patient suffering from tetanus. The hypodermic syringe and needle were not, as popularly supposed, invented by the Frenchman, Charles Gabriel Pravaz (1791–1853) of Lyon.[2] Francis Rynd (1801–1861) of Dublin in 1845[3] used a trocar and cannula with morphine for the treatment of trigeminal neuralgia; he did not use a syringe. Alexander Wood (1817–1884)[4] of Edinburgh was the true founder of hypodermic medication. He used a Ferguson syringe. The Record syringe of metal and glass was introduced around 1906 in Berlin, and the French Luer followed it.[5] The first needle to remain patent, for multiple injections was described by Torsten Gordh in 1945. (Syringe from Greek *Syrinx* = a tube or pipe.)

Intravenous hedonal was studied by Nicolas P. Krawkow[6] (1865–1924) and used clinically by Serge Federov (1869–1936) at St Petersburg, Russia, and in 1912 by Max Page in London; in 1909 Burckhardt (1872–1922) of Nüernberg gave chloroform and ether by the intravenous route.

Barbituric acid synthesized by Adolf v. Baeyer (1835–1917) of Munich in 1864 but its narcotic effects not discovered. Later, also in Munich, barbiturate was synthesized by Emil Fischer (1852–1918) and Joseph Friederich von Mering (1849–1908) in 1903:[7] this was diethyl barbituric acid or Veronal. Phenobarbitone was discovered in 1912. Somnifaine was the first barbiturate to be given intravenously; it is a combination of diethyl and diallyl barbituric acids, and was used in France by Bardet in 1924.[8]

H. Noel and Henry Souttar (1875–1964), surgeons, used intravenous paraldehyde in 1913.[9] Intravenous morphine and hyoscine were employed for 'twilight sleep' in 1916.[10]

In 1927 Bumm introduced Pernocton[11] while Zerfas of Indianapolis, USA, used sodium amytal intravenously two years[12] later. This was soon followed by Nembutal (pentobarbitone).[13] Magill was the first to demonstrate this clinically in Britain[14] and John Silas Lundy[15] (1890–1974) of the Mayo Clinic in the USA in 1931.

Martin Kirschner (1879–1942) of Heidelberg gave Avertin (bromethol) intravenously in 1929.[16]

Hexobarbitone was the first drug to make intravenous anaesthesia popular and was used by Helmut Weese (1897–1954), professor of pharmacology at Dusseldorf and later director of pharmacology at Bayer (Wuppertal-Elberfeld), the true father of intravenous anaesthesia, and Walter Scharpff in 1932,[17] having been synthesized by Kropp and Taub in Elberfeld. It was first given in Great Britain in 1933 by Ronald Jarman (1898–1973) and L. Abel in London.[18]

Pentothal sodium (thiopentone) was synthesized in 1932 by Ernest Henry Volwiler and Donalee Tabern[19] and introduced into clinical practice by Lundy of the Mayo Clinic on 18 June 1934,[20] and by Waters of Madison on 3 March 1934,[21] the former being the more influential. First used in Great Britain by Jarman and Abel in 1935.[22]

Its fate in the body and distribution described by Brodie in 1950.[23] Methohexitone, a methyl barbiturate, first used by Stoelting in 1957.[24]

Thiopentone was originally employed as the sole anaesthetic and this led to many deaths, e.g. at Pearl Harbour on 9 December 1941[25] from cardiovascular depression in otherwise resistant young men.

Intermittent doses along with nitrous oxide and oxygen, first described by Geoffrey Stephen William Organe (1908–1986) and Broad in 1938.[26]

Thiopentone and methohexitone are the most useful barbiturates for intravenous anaesthesia. (*See also* The 50th Anniversary of the Use of Thiopentone, Editorial, Papper E. M. *Anaesthesia* 1984, **39**, 517; Editorial, Dundee J. W. *Br. J. Anaesth, 1984,* **56**, 211.

Intravenous ether was used in animals by Nikolai Ivanovitch Pirogoff (1810–1881) in Russia in 1847, a year after Morton's use of ether by inhalation. Used in surgery by Ludwig Burckhardt (1872–1922), Nuremberg surgeon, in 1909. A 2.5–5% solution in normal saline or glucose 5% was used.

Many intravenous anaesthetic agents have been tried but have not survived. Examples include hydroxydione in 1955; propanidid in 1956; gamma-hydroxy-butyric acid in 1960 and alphaxalone/alphadolone (Althesin) in 1971. Propofol has become established as a serious rival to thiopentone (*see* below).

Technique of intravenous injection

Good illumination and a sharp needle are essential for successful intravenous injection. The Y-cannula is most convenient and comes in several sizes, 16–27G. The easiest and most accessible vein should be chosen. Emla cream provides skin analgesia, which is especially helpful in children and it takes about an hour to work. 27, or even 29 G needles are useful in infants and those with tiny veins, e.g. addicts.

Suitable sites are:

(1) the forearm;

(2) the back of the hand.[27] Less risk of arterial puncture, but haematomas here are very noticable;

(3) anterior to the elbow-joint. Less painful, but risk of brachial artery puncture;

(4) anterior to the wrist joint. Useful in chubby babies;

(5) the internal saphenous vein, anterior to the medial malleolus – the skin overlying this is tough and sensitive;

(6) the external jugular vein. Ideal in horses, etc;

(7) subclavian vein – by supraclavicular puncture;

(8) a scalp vein in infants; and

(9) the femoral vein, medial to the artery, if all else fails.

When the arm is chosen, the veins are made as prominent as possible by the use of a venous tourniquet, such as a length of rubber tubing around the arm secured by means of artery forceps. Applied near the site of injection, the tourniquet steadies the vein proximally, while the anaesthetist's finger, by stretching the skin, steadies it distally. This is very important in thin old people whose veins, although prominent, very readily slip about beneath the skin and may be displaced from the point of the needle.

The artery must not be occluded in addition to the vein; the presence of arterial pulsation is a most useful guide to the position of an artery and hence to avoidance of intra-arterial injection.

Soaking the whole arm in hot water to produce hyperaemia or light general anaesthesia by causing venodilatation, makes injection easier (and pleasanter). If Emla (eutectic mixture of local anaesthetics) cream containing 5% lignocaine and 5% prilocaine is rubbed into the skin and left on as a dressing for 1 hour, the subsequent puncture of the skin is rendered painless.[28]

When the skin has been well cleaned with an antiseptic (thought by many workers to be a waste of time and effort), the needle is inserted so that it comes to lie between the skin and the vein wall. The point is now advanced and the vein wall is pierced at a different level from the skin puncture. This tends to prevent transfixion of the vein and lessens haematoma formation when the needle is withdrawn. With the needle point within the lumen of the vein it should, if possible, be advanced for a short distance to prevent slipping out.

A few drops of lignocaine can be injected into the dermis with an intradermal needle before the larger needle is inserted, if necessary, to dilate the vein and reduce pain caused by the larger needle. Otherwise the tip of the needle is pressed on to the skin to blanch it, for 10 sec, before the needle is advanced through the skin, or the needle is inserted immediately after a sharp local slap or a cough.

With the needle in the vein, the aspiration test is performed and injection can commence. After withdrawal of the needle, oozing should be checked by firm pressure for several minutes and elevation of the limb, if necessary. For technique of setting up an intravenous drip *see* Chapter 17. Nitroglycerin ointment may aid venepuncture by increasing skin vasodilatation.[32]

BARBITURATES

Thiopentone sodium BP

Thiopental USP (*Pentothal; Trapanal; Penthiobarbital; Intraval; Nesdonal; Farmotal*).

This is sodium ethyl (1-methyl butyl) thiobarbiturate. It is the sulphur analogue of pentobarbitone. Introduced commercially as Pentothal sodium in 1935.

Thiopentone is a yellow amorphous powder with odour resembling H_2S. It is soluble in water and alcohol and forms a 2.5 or 5% solution in distilled water of pH 10.5, which is highly alkaline (pH of blood 7.4). To prevent formation of free acid by carbon dioxide from the atmosphere, 6% anhydrous sodium carbonate is added to the powder, which is prepared in an atmosphere of nitrogen. In solution thiopentone is not very stable, but can be left for 24–48 h or longer without harm resulting on subsequent injection, provided the solution remains clear. A solution that is cloudy should be discarded. The oil/water coefficient is 4.7.

Thiopentone is supplied in ampoules, with sterile distilled water sufficient to make a 2.5% solution. Anaesthesia with thiopentone should never be undertaken lightly because of its side-effects. Average dose 4–7 mg/kg i.v.

Pharmacodynamics

The central nervous system. Like other barbiturates, it causes sedation, hypnosis, anaesthesia and respiratory depression, depending on the dose and rate of injection. There is an anticonvulsant action.[29] The cerebral cortex and ascending reticular-activating system are depressed before the medullary centres. Cerebral blood flow and CSF pressure are reduced, and intracranial pressure falls. Cerebral oxygen consumption is reduced. Thiopentone in doses insufficient to cause unconsciousness is antanalgesic, and this sensitivity to pain lasts into the postoperative period.

There is a reasonably consistent correlation between depth of anaesthesia and EEG pattern, although not with plasma barbiturate levels.

In monkeys, thiopentone in doses greater than would be required for anaesthesia may, if given soon after acute global brain ischaemia (e.g. after cardiac standstill), reduce the degree of cerebral damage. Relevance to human patients is still controversial.

Acute tolerance.[30] There is a relationship between the induction dose of thiopentone and the blood thiopentone level at which patients awake from anaesthesia. With larger induction doses the patient wakes at a higher blood level. A high initial concentration of thiopentone in the brain may result in an increased acute tolerance to supplementary doses. The greater the initial dose, the greater will be the increments of drug required to maintain surgical anaesthesia. For these reasons it is difficult to correlate blood levels with depth of anaesthesia, but about 7 µg/ml is an average level.

pH effect. Thiopentone has a pK value of 7.6. Acidosis reduces the thiopentone concentration in the plasma of experimental animals by up to 40%, with return to control levels on return of pH to normal.

Protein binding. About 87% of the thiopentone in peripheral blood is bound to plasma proteins, chiefly albumin,[31] and so is inactivated. This bound percentage decreases in old age. The tissues are in equilibrium only with the unbound fraction. pH changes may affect the ratio of bound to unbound thiopentone,[32] maximum binding occurring at pH 8. The degree of binding also varies according to the concentration of thiopentone, being greatest when the concentration is low. Thiopentone enters red blood cells in a concentration about 40% of that found in plasma.

Respiratory system. Depression of the respiratory centre, depending on the dose and rate of injection, antagonized by surgical stimuli and potentiated by opioids. The sensitivity of the respiratory centre to CO_2 is reduced. A deep breath or two, or a yawn, may precede the depression, which is a reduced depth rather than a reduced rate of respiration. It is because of the hypoxia produced by this depressant action that thiopentone may be dangerous from the respiratory viewpoint. Transient apnoeas are common and treated by gentle manual IPPV.

Cardiovascular system. Myocardial contractility is reduced, but this is compensated by tachycardia. Myocardial oxygen consumption may be increased by this. *Peripheral vascular resistance* (PVR or SVR) is slightly reduced, leading to pooling of blood in the periphery, causing reduction in cardiac output, particularly in hypovolaemia and untreated hypertension. The drug is especially dangerous when the heart can not compensate for changes in vascular haemodynamics, e.g. β-blockade, constrictive pericarditis, tight valvular stenosis, complete heart block. *Hypotension*, depending on rate and amount of drug injected. Hypotension is probably caused by dilatation of the vascular bed especially in skin and muscle, perhaps due to depression of the vasomotor centre; the effect usually passes off within minutes. Blood pressure falls are likely to be greater in hypertensive or hypovolaemic patients and in those with cardiac or adrenocortical insufficiency.

Rapid injection of too much thiopentone may have a catastrophic effect on the circulatory system.

Larynx. Increased sensitivity to stimuli. Laryngeal spasm may occur.

Eyes. Pupils first dilate, then contract. Sensitivity to light remains until the patient is deep enough to permit incision of the skin, and at this stage the eyeballs are usually centrally placed. Thiopentone reduces intraocular tension. Loss of eyelash reflex is a sign of induction of anaesthesia.

Pregnant uterus. Thiopentone has no effect on its tone, and so is a poor agent used alone for external version. It readily passes the placental barrier, achieving its maximal concentration in fetal blood very soon after its injection into the mother.

Kidney. Specific effects are unimportant. A powerful stimulator of ADH.

Pharmacokinetics

After a single small dose of thiopentone, its level in the plasma falls rapidly and the patient regains consciousness as a result of redistribution of the drug to viscera, lean body mass (muscles, etc.) and fat during the first 10 min after intravenous injection. After a single large dose, or repeated small doses, however, the resulting equilibrium plasma level may be high enough to cause anaesthesia and because of the slow metabolism of thiopentone, anaesthesia is prolonged. Anaesthesia depends not only on the concentration of the drug, but also on the length of time of exposure of tissues to the drug. It rapidly crosses the blood–brain barrier because of its low degree of ionization and its high lipid solubility. It is the unionized part that crosses the barrier and its concentration in the cerebrospinal fluid approaches that in the plasma in 15 min. Equilibrium between plasma and brain is established 1 min after intravenous injection. The initial high uptake of thiopentone by the brain, due to its high lipid solubility and non-ionization, accounts for the rapidity of the onset of anaesthesia. There is a small decrease in plasma potassium following injection. Distribution follows a bi- or tri-exponential model, first phase 2–4 min., second phase 40–50 min. Thiopentone metabolism begins after 15 min. Elimination half-life is 9 h. The liver is the principal site of breakdown and this may be a more important factor, than generally supposed, in the early recovery from its effects (hepatic extraction ratio 0.15). Between 10 and 15% of the drug in the body is metabolized each hour; muscular tissue may help in its detoxification as may the kidneys. The degree of liver dysfunction must be considerable before a patient shows diminished tolerance to thiopentone, and tolerance is decreased only to intermittent doses given over a long period. The products of thiopentone breakdown are removed via the kidneys, but renal disease is not a contra-indication to its use, although a uraemic patient will require smaller amounts than a normal patient. A high blood urea prolongs thiopentone narcosis. Eliminated more rapidly in the young than in the old, who require smaller doses.

Miscellaneous effects. It passes into the breast milk shortly after injection. There is a positive relationship between the induction dose and the plasma urea and the plasma haemoglobin levels, both due to plasma binding of the drug. Barbiturates induce the secretion of enzymes from the liver that metabolize warfarin and related anticoagulants. In some patients a localized muscular spasm is seen following injection. It usually takes the form of pronation of the forearm receiving the injection, which can be lessened by narcotic analgesics.

Skin rashes have been very occasionally reported following its use. Anaphylactic response has been described and is rare. This is the classic anaphylactic reaction type 1 sensitivity mediated by immunoglobulin E (*see below*).

Causes muscular necrosis if injected into muscular tissue. It is a poor relaxer of the muscles but following a rapid induction dose, examinations under anaesthesia are usually possible (e.g. gynaecology); manipulations of the spine or joints can be carried out if dosage is sufficient.

Course of anaesthesia

At the time of operation, the stomach and bladder should be empty. When an intravenous anaesthetic is given the following should be at hand in case of need: (1) a laryngoscope; (2) tracheal tubes; (3) oxygen; (4) a mask and reservoir bag; (5) a tilting table; (6) suction apparatus; and (7) suitable syringes and needles, e.g. the Y-can, and the normal resuscitation equipment.

The first injection should be 4–8 ml of 2.5% solution and it can be made quite rapidly in fit subjects; more slowly in others. The concentration of the drug reaching the brain in arterial blood immediately after injection is determined by the rate of injection. Just after the onset of unconsciousness, there is often a deep breath, followed by a period of respiratory depression. During this period no further injection should be made. Consciousness is lost in one arm–brain circulation time, but maximum depth of anaethesia occurs some 30–60 s later. With normal breathing re-established, the patient inhales an appropriate anaesthetic mixture, e.g. nitrous oxide, oxygen and isoflurane, with or without an intravenous narcotic analgesic. Further small increments of thiopentone may be given to smooth out equilibration with the inhalation agents.

The criteria of depth are: (1) the activity of respiration in relation to surgical stimuli; and (2) reflex movements of the patient in relation to such stimuli. When stimuli are severe, depth may have to be increased, e.g. when skin is incised or sutured.

Doses of thiopentone required vary from 3–5 mg/kg. Seldom should a larger dose be injected. A small dose results in a short period of narcosis, but larger doses may be followed by prolonged sleep. Additional doses within 36 h cause cumulation.

Control of the airway is of primary importance in anaesthesia. Frequently a pharyngeal, nasopharyngeal airway or laryngeal mask is necessary, but these should only be used if the airway becomes obstructed without them, because they may stimulate pharyngeal reflexes, which upset the smooth course of the anaesthesia. They may also cause laryngospasm.

Respiratory obstruction caused by the tongue falling back, or respiratory depression may occur. The remedy for this is to secure a free airway and to ventilate the lungs with an appropriate anaesthetic gas mixture. The surgeon should, if necessary, be asked to wait until control of the airway is regained. The intravenous injection of a short-acting relaxant, e.g. suxamethonium, will also abolish spasm of the larynx temporarily. Patients vary greatly in the amounts of drug they require to abolish reflex response to stimuli. Males need more than females; the fat need more than the thin; the young need more than the old.

Recovery from anaesthesia

The patient is laid on the side to prevent respiratory obstruction. Oxygen is administered. Rate of recovery is influenced by the amount of premedication and the amount of thiopentone injected. During the immediate postoperative period, the airway and the tidal exchange must be carefully watched. The return of normal mental faculties does not accompany apparent return of full consciousness. Day cases should always be accompanied after thiopentone anaesthesia and must not drive a car to their home or engage in responsible activity for 24 h.

Complications of thiopentone anaesthesia

LOCAL COMPLICATIONS

1. Perivenous injection. This may cause pain, redness and swelling; haematoma formation; bruising; and rarely ulceration (due to alkalinity of the solution). It may lead to median nerve injury if injection is made into the medial side of the antecubital fossa. Should solution be deposited outside the vein, 10 ml of 1% lignocaine with hyalase 1000 units can be injected into the area. This dilutes the thiopentone solution and, by promoting vasodilatation, aids absorption.

2. *Intra-arterial injection.* This may follow misplacement of the needle or accidental injection into an arterial cannula. Warning of the possibility of this was first pointed out in 1943.[33] When it occurs the patient usually, but not always, feels severe burning pain down the arm and hand. It can be avoided by ensuring that the artery is not occluded by the tourniquet before injection and by injecting 2 ml of solution, and inquiring if pain is experienced by the patient. Only if this is absent should the main injection proceed. This mishap may be dangerous and has led to necrosis of the hand. Sudden death from this cause has been reported. Accidental intra-arterial injection into arteries around the ankle and back of hand may occur. *Immediate signs* may include:

(*a*) a white hand with cyanosed fingers due to arterial spasm, which may be accompanied or followed by arterial thrombosis; (*b*) patches of skin discoloration; and (*c*) onset of unconsciousness may be delayed.

Late signs may include:

(*a*) ulcers or blisters; and (*b*) oedema of forearm and hand. Oedematous areas may recover, the cause of such cases being spasm rather than thrombosis. Gangrene following the intra-arterial injection of 2.5% solution is extremely rare.[34]

Anatomy. Division of the brachial artery above the elbow joint occurs in 10% of patients. When division is high, the ulnar artery reaches the forearm by running superficial to the flexor muscles and may run: (*a*) below the deep fascia all the way down; (*b*) below the deep fascia proximally, later becoming subcutaneous; or (*c*) subcutaneous near the elbow, later becoming deep to the deep fascia. It is this abnormal ulnar artery in its superficial position immediately deep to the median cubital vein, and without the protection of the aponeurotic tendon of the biceps, which may be accidentally punctured and used for injection.

When the brachial artery divides above the elbow, the common interosseous branch of the ulnar artery is usually given off from the radial artery, so if the ulnar artery is punctured, its deep common interosseous branch is usually not involved.

Some of the adverse effects of the intra-arterial injection of drugs are due to the thrombosis of the small arteries supplying nerves, and so interfering with their conduction of motor impulses.

The pH of 2.5% solution of thiopentone in water is 10.8 (pH of blood is 7.4). It is thus a strong alkaline irritant.

Pathology (*a*) The changes in pH of thiopentone, which occur when it is mixed with blood in an artery, result in precipitation of solid crystals of thiopentone (as well as haemoglobin), which are swept along and eventually block small vascular channels at arteriolar and capillary levels. The crystals remain in the small vessels and their irritant properties cause a local release of noradrenaline with subsequent vascular spasm. Therefore, the more drug is injected, the greater will be the effect – an argument in favour of the use of dilute solution; (*b*) the essential lesion is arterial thrombosis, and it may not become complete for 5 days; and (*c*) endothelial damage may be a factor.

Management. When thiopentone has been injected into the lumen of an artery during induction of anaesthesia the suggested lines of treatment are as follows: (*a*) Leave needle in the lumen of the artery and immediately inject 500 units of heparin down this needle; it reverses the alkalinity of the thiopentone and prevents thrombosis; (*b*) Dilution of injected thiopentone with saline; (*c*) Relief of arterial spasm and pain by injection of papaverine 40–80 mg in 10–20 ml of saline; or tolazoline (Priscol) 5 ml of 1% solution, or as a continuous drip; or phenoxybenzamine, 0.5 mg or as a drip 50–200 μg/min; or urokinase;[36] or by immediate brachial plexus or stellate ganglion block;

(*d*) Continue anaesthesia as an effective method of securing vasodilatation, using halothane; and (*e*) Later treatment of such symptoms as may arise.

If possible abandon the proposed operation and institute systemic anticoagulant therapy with heparin.[35]

The oral, longer-acting anticoagulants may be necessary for the following 2 weeks.

3. Thrombophlebitis. This may occur in spite of a clean, aseptic venepuncture and is due to chemical irritation of the vein wall. It may follow the injection or be postponed for 7–10 days. It should be treated by heat and rest.

4. Injury to nerves, especially the median, following injection into the medial side of the antecubital fossa. Accidental injection into the median nerve is likely to produce an intense shooting pain in the distribution of the nerve, together with sudden flexion of the wrist and thumb. The area should be generously infiltrated with a local analgesic solution and in severe cases, a neurological opinion sought.

5. Broken needle. As the fracture usually occurs between the hub and the shaft, at least 0.5 cm of shaft should always be outside tissues.

6. Autoerythrocyte sensitization syndrome. The painful bruising syndrome.[37]

7. Contamination of the solution with glass spicules (not confined to thiopentone); suggested use of a filter.

GENERAL COMPLICATIONS

1. Respiratory depression. For treatment, *see above.* Apnoea during intravenous anaesthesia may be due to: (*a*) relative over-dose of drug; (*b*) respiratory obstruction above the glottis, e.g. the tongue falling back.

2. Circulatory collapse. This is usually caused by a relative over-dose causing vasodilatation and myocardial depression. *Treatment:* raise the legs, give oxygen by IPPV and infuse fluids intravenously.

3. Laryngeal spasm. This may result from: (*a*) Direct local stimulation by an airway, saliva, blood, etc.; (*b*) Stimulation of some remote area, e.g. anal sphincter, cervix uteri, etc. (Brewer–Luckhardt reflexes); and (*c*) Part of a general anoxic spasm.

Thiopentone predisposes to laryngeal spasm. Oxygen should be administered under pressure. Intravenous injection of 20–30 mg of suxamethonium may be required to relax the spasm.

4. *Coughing*. Depth should be gradually increased. Nitrous–oxide–oxygen, volatile or analgesic agents may be required in resistant cases. Hiccup occasionally seen.

5. *Postoperative vertigo, euphoria and disorientation*. Because of the possibility of this condition, outpatients should be accompanied home and not allowed to drive a car or to cook.

6. *True cutaneous allergy*. Can occur either in the form of a scarlatiniform rash or as true angioneurotic oedema. Photosensitivity to thiopentone in patients recently exposed to sunlight has been reported.

7. *Severe anaphylactic reactions (allergy)*. *See* Chapter 14. These reactions, although rare, are dangerous. They may take the form of cutaneous manifestations (rashes, weals, flushes, oedema), cardiovascular collapse (hypotension, tachycardia), bronchospasm, laryngospasm and muscle rigidity or abdominal pain.

Advantages and disadvantages of thiopentone anaesthesia

The advantages are: (1) ease and rapidity of induction; (2) absence of stage of delirium; (3) rapid recovery (with correct dosage) and relative freedom from vomiting and postoperative discomfort, etc.; and (4) ability to increase depth rapidly.

The disadvantages are: (1) respiratory depression; (2) tendency to laryngeal spasm; and (3) circulatory depression in poor-risk patients.

Indications

These are legion, almost every operation in surgery having been performed under intravenous barbiturate anaesthesia. It is specially useful: (1) for induction of general anaesthesia; and (2) for controlling convulsions during general or local anaesthesia, eclampsia, epilepsy, tetanus, etc.

Contraindications

1. Porphyria,[38] which may be congenital or appear as acute attacks of abdominal pain somewhat resembling lead poisoning, with the passage of urine that assumes a dark reddish colour after being left exposed to daylight for some hours. Barbiturates may precipitate lower motor neurone paralysis and perhaps death, and are absolutely contra-indicated. If suspected, the urine should be tested for porphyrins. It has been suggested that not all patients with porphyria are sensitive to barbiturates. *See also* Chapter 20.

2. A history of thiopentone anaphylaxis, which has a high mortality.

Relative contra-indications

In the following procedures and types of case, special care is needed, and oxygen or nitrous oxide with oxygen should be given in addition.

1. Shocked, debilitated, severely anaemic and uraemic cases: small doses are required. The drug causes vasodilatation and reduces cardiac output. The administration of pure oxygen is useful in all such patients before anaesthesia is induced. It also aids the removal of nitrogen from the lungs and allows

nitrous oxide to exert its analgesic effects more quickly, thereby reducing the need for thiopentone.

There may be a dose of the drug small enough for induction of anaesthesia with safety in even the most decrepit patient, but in the gravely ill, other methods have some advantages.

2. Children under one year: because while their respiratory centres are easily depressed, their upper respiratory passages are relatively small, these factors predisposing to hypoxia. Many workers disagree. Children do not like needles.

3. Patients with gross dyspnoea due to cardiac or respiratory disease. Thiopentone should be used with extreme caution, if at all, in cases of constriction pericarditis, tight valvular stenosis and complete heart block. There is sudden perfusion of the drug into coronary vessels in right-to-left shunt.

4. Patients with respiratory obstruction or status asthmaticus.

5. Operations in which the return of reflexes immediately after operation is desirable. It is difficult to have a patient adequately anaesthetized one minute and coughing the next, e.g. in tonsillectomy.

6. Cases of acute intestinal obstruction. Regurgitation may follow loss of consciousness, and aspiration of stomach contents may cause dangerous laryngeal spasm unless proper care is taken to prevent it.

7. Patients with acute inflammation about the mouth, jaw and neck. Several deaths have occurred under thiopentone anaesthesia in such patients. A likely cause of death is interference with the airway associated with spasticity of the jaw due to inflammatory oedema.

8. Obstetrics: for external version, thiopentone is a poor relaxant; for delivery, no more than an induction dose should be used (250 mg).

9. In any severely ill patient, the drug should be used cautiously in minimal dosage.

10. Cases of dystrophia myotonica. *See* Chapter 20. The patients react normally to non-depolarizing relaxants, but abnormally to thiopentone,[39] similarly to most respiratory depressants and prolonged apnoea may follow injection of more than 100 mg.

11. Alcoholics taking disulfiram (Antabuse) and patients suffering from poisoning with dinitro-orthocresol, a weed killer (barbiturates and DNC have a synergistic depressant effect on cellular respiration).

12. Hypokalaemic familial periodic paralysis. *See* Chapter 20.

13. Huntington's chorea. *See* Chapter 20.

14. Patients with difficult veins. There is no excuse for subjecting a patient to the painful experience of multiple needle punctures in an effort to provide a pleasant induction of anaesthesia.

15. Thermally injured children between the ages of 6 and 16 who have recovered from their injuries require about 60% more thiopentone than similar normal children and an induction dose of 7–8 mg/kg may be required.

Methohexitone

(*Brietal; Brevital; Methohexital USP; Sombulex*)
    First described by Chernish S. M. et al. in 1956[40] and used clinically by Stoelting in 1957 in the USA and by Dundee and Moore in 1961 in the UK.[41]

This is a methylated oxybarbiturate with the chemical name sodium 1-methyl-5-allyl-5-(1-methyl-2-pentynyl) barbiturate. To each 500 mg of powdered drug is added 30 mg of sodium carbonate. When used in 1% solution the pH is 11.1. While it is two and three times as potent as thiopentone, complete recovery is quicker. Less irritating than thiopentone solution when injected into tissues, but intra-arterial methohexitone is as irritant and dangerous as thiopentone in the same concentration, but the 1% solution as commonly used is less dangerous than 2.5% thiopentone. Pain on intravenous injection, which can be abolished by 1 mg/ml lignocaine. Causes less cardiovascular depression than thiopentone (also due to myocardial depression and vasodilatation). Tremor, coughing and hiccups occur (reduced by opioids, e.g. fentanyl, 0.1 mg i.v. but fentanyl has been known to cause a cough).[42]

Methohexitone has been found to cause abnormal spike discharges in epileptic subjects. It does not suppress epileptic manifestations, and may be implicated in the aetiology of fits during anaesthesia. Can cause anaphylactic, histaminoid reactions. The drug is redistributed and then detoxicated in the liver (hepatic extraction ratio 0.5).

Induction of anaesthesia results in a slight fall in the plasma potassium level. Dosage of the 1% solution is about 1 mg/kg for induction (50–120 mg) (similar in volume to 2.5% thiopentone) and this is usually followed by nitrous oxide and oxygen. The aqueous solution is stable for at least 6 weeks at room temperature.

Pharmacokinetics

It has a terminal half-life of 97 min. Total body plasma clearance four times greater than that of thiopentone. Thus it may be preferable to thiopentone when a rapid recovery is required, especially after large or repeated doses.

Intramuscular methohexitone

This is reported to give satisfactory pre-anaesthetic sedation in about 85% of paediatric cases. The dose recommended is 6.6 mg/kg in 2% solution given into the upper and outer quadrant of the buttock. Sleep usually comes on in under 10 min. Abscesses and sloughs are rare. Has also been given per rectum, 15–20 mg/kg.

NON BARBITURATES

Etomidate (*Hypnomidate*)

This is a carboxylated imidazole (ethyl-1-(α-methyl-benzyl) medazole-5-carboxylate) ($C_{14}H_{16}N_2O_2$). It was synthesized and studied by Janssen and co-workers in 1971 and used in man by Alfred Doenicke of Munich and colleagues in 1973. It is a white crystalline powder, soluble in a wide range of solvents including water, ethanol and propylene glycol. The commercial preparation is presented in 10-ml ampoules containing 2 mg/ml of the drug dissolved in water with 35% propylene glycol. The pH is 8.1.

Pharmacodynamics

Etomidate is used as an intravenous induction agent. Its great advantage is that it does not usually depress arterial pressure. Recovery is rapid. Most patients wake following a single induction dose in 6–8 min and the quality of recovery is good. Repeated doses are not cumulative.

The incidence of pain at the site of injection is high, occurring in a quarter to a half of patients. It can be reduced by fast injection, by use of a large vein in the antecubital fossa and by the addition of 0.1% lignocaine.

Muscle movements associated with induction are commoner than after thiopentone. The incidence is decreased when narcotic analgesics are used in premedication and increased by even mild reflex stimulation. It potentiates both types of muscle relaxants.[43]

Central nervous system. The EEG changes are similar to those seen in association with thiopentone. The muscle movements frequently seen during induction with etomidate are not associated with epileptiform discharges. The origin of these movements therefore probably lies in deep cerebral structures or the brain stem.

Etomidate is a good hypnotic but it does not prevent movement as a result of surgical stimulation. Autonomic responses are not blocked.

Cerebral blood flow is reduced. Intraocular pressure is reduced in premedicated patients.

Cardiovascular system. There is no overt depression of the cardiovascular system,[44] making it the induction agent of choice for patients with poor cardiac function or hypertension.

Respiratory system. Respiratory rate slows and tidal volume rises for a brief period following induction. Respiration may then be shallow, but apnoea is likely to be brief and is less common than after thiopentone. Coughing and hiccup are uncommon.

Alimentary system. Nausea and vomiting occur more commonly than following other intravenous induction agents.[45]

Metabolism. No significant effects have been described in terms of liver function or plasma electrolytes.

Pharmacokinetics

In the blood etomidate distributes equally between red blood cells and plasma; the protein binding is 76.5%. Only 2.5% of the injected dose remains in the circulation 2 min after administration, at which time peak concentrations are found in the brain and major organs. The drug is thought to be metabolized rapidly in the liver by esterases and the decomposition products excreted in urine and bile.

Clinical use

Cardiovascular stability and rapid recovery are features that commend its use as an induction agent in sick and shocked patients. Anaesthesia is then continued using other agents. A single shot dose by itself is unsatisfactory owing to the pronounced muscle movements often seen; use of adjuvant agents then may hinder recovery. Dose 0.3 mg/kg. Etomidate may, very rarely, cause an anaphylactoid reaction.[46]

Etomidate infusion suppresses the secretion of cortisol and aldosterone for up to 22 h following its termination and is not recommended. An increased mortality was associated with etomidate infusion in the ITU.[47]

The drug also causes a depression of the normal increase in plasma cortisol concentration that occurs during surgery.[48]

A single injection of etomidate is reported to cause a significant reduction in secretion of cortisol[49] but there is doubt whether this has clinical importance.[50]

Propofol

2, 6 di-isopropylphenol (*Diprivan*)

First reported use in 1977.[51] The original product was dissolved in Cremophor EL.[52] Diprivan is a 1% formulation in an oil and water emulsion containing 10% soya bean oil, 1.2% egg phosphatide and 2.25% glycerol.

The induction dose is 1–2.5 mg/kg. The effective blood concentration (EC_{90}) is 3.4 μg/ml with 67% N_2O.[53]

Resistance to the anaesthetic effects of propofol is occasionally encountered. Such patients may require either strong premedication with opioids, or 50% increase of propofol dosage, both for induction and infusion. Quality of anaesthesia is good but myoclonic movements have been observed[54] (as with many intravenous agents other than thiopentone), *see* Side-effects below. Emergence is more rapid than with thiopentone, without hangover (assessed by the Steward Score), although a central anticholinergic type of response has been reported.[55]

Pharmacokinetics

Rapid distribution (T1/2α 2–8 min), and elimination (T1/2β 56–109 min) as glucuronide, with renal excretion[56] mainly on a biexponential model, (or 3-compartment open model with central elimination).[57] Highly lipophilic. ED_{95} is 3 μg/ml. Post-anaesthesia performance of mental, manual and mechanical tasks is back to normal within 1–2 h. Cumulation in a third compartment is extremely slight, and takes many hours or days to develop. Clearance of propofol is said to be dependent on hepatic blood flow,[58] but clinical equilibration with the recommended infusion dose is slower in fat patients than in the lean. Faster distribution in pregnancy.[59]

Pharmacodynamics

Dose-related surgical anaesthesia. Respiratory depression, dose-related, at blood concentrations above 10 μg/ml. Anticonvulsant activity (a 'propofol withdrawal syndrome' of minor twitches has been proposed after prolonged use as a sedative),[60] despite the reports of myoclonic movements associated with its use[54].

Cardiovascular effects

1. Arterial hypotension,[61] usually preventable by vascular volume loading or by head-down tilt. This hypotension is greatest in untreated hypertensives.[62] Systolic pressure reductions of 50% have been seen with 2 mg/kg boluses of propofol.[63] It must be used with caution in the hypovolaemic patient and in those anaesthetized in postures other than the supine horizontal.[64]

2. Reduction of systemic vascular resistance of up to 30% in man on bolus doses of 2 mg/kg is responsible for the hypotension.

3. Slight myocardial depression.[65] The left ventricular dP/dt falls at propofol concentrations above 10 μg/ml (overdose range). At anaesthetic concentrations, cardiac output rises slightly, with a reduction of cardiac work and MVO_2,[66] due to reduction of afterload. There is no evidence of myocardial regional oxygenation imbalance. Many workers have found no evidence of myocardial depression in man or dogs.

4. Slight bradycardia (*see* Doze V. A., Westphal L. M., White P. F., *Anesth. Analg.* 1986, **65**, 1189) about 10 bpm on average, is probably due to central vagal activity. The atrial – His interval lengthens about 10% from 80 ms. The sinus node recovery time (SNRT) lengthens about 20% from 1000 ms. Very rarely, A-V block develops, so premedication with an anticholinergic drug may be desirable, especially in β-blocked and Ca-antagonized patients. Glycopyrronium is very suitable for preventing any such bradycardia.

5. Variable reductions in blood catecholamines.

6. In the Sick Sinus syndrome, propofol may be associated with brief periods of atrial flutter.

7. Hypertrophic obstructive cardiomyopathy (HOCM). Propofol 1 mg/kg given slowly over 4 min with an opioid, has given good cardiovascular stability and increased cardiac output.

Side-effects

Nausea and vomiting 1–2% (less than with almost any other technique). Pain on injection, more so in small peripheral veins. Pain reduced by mixing with local analgesics or diluting the drug with an equal volume of saline, or cooling the drug.[67]

Cerebral side-effects. Propofol reduces the duration of the fit in electroconvulsive therapy, but 'fits' have been reported to be associated with its use. The Committee on Safety of Medicines recommend care with its use in epileptics. Myotonic effects: these have been classified as (1) minor, i.e. twitches of hands and feet and (2) major, resembling a convulsion, or opisthotonus. These effects have not endangered life and are short-lived except in patients with dystrophia myotonica.[68] A central anticholinergic type of response has been reported.[55]

Interactions

The duration of action of concomitant alfentanil is prolonged to a half-life of 75 min.[57] Interaction with fentanyl is more complex.[69]

Clinical use

1. As an induction agent. It is an excellent induction agent for day case anaesthesia. (*see* Wetcher P. L. *Anesthesia for Ambulatory Surgery*, 2nd Ed. Philadelphia: Lippincott, 1990.) Because of its rapid recovery, it reduces pressure on postoperative facilities, enabling a higher throughput.

2. As an infusion for maintenance of anaesthesia (TIVA). The maintenance infusion rate (MIR) is initially 10 mg/kg/h, falling to 8 mg/kg/h after some minutes and then to 6 mg/kg/h. (*See* Roberts F. L., Dixon J. et al. *Anaesthesia* 1988, **43**(suppl), 14.) Computerised controls have been developed for this. For management of TIVA, *see below*.

3. For control of status epilepticus.[70]

4. For sedation in critically ill patients[71] and head injuries, 1 to 5 mg/kg/h, with rapid offset, and very slight accumulation.

Table 9.1 Comparison of some intravenous anaesthetic agents

Anaesthetic	Induction dose (mg/kg)	Repeat dose (mg/kg)	Duration (min)
Propofol	1–3	0.5	2
Thiopentone	5	2	5
Methohexitone	1.5	0.5	3
Etomidate	0.2	0.1	2

THE BENZODIAZEPINES (*see also* Chapter 5)

History

In the mid-1950s work on the existing tranquillizers was extended; these included chlorpromazine, reserpine and meprobamate. The benzheptodiazepines had been studied in Cracow, Poland in the 1930s[73] and elsewhere. Chlordiazepoxide was prepared in 1960 and named Librium, the pharmacology having been elucidated by Randall. First used clinically in 1961. First reported as an intravenous anaesthetic in the UK in 1966 (diazepam). The group includes chlordiazepoxide, diazepam, nitrazepam (Mogadon), temazepam (Normison), midazolam (Hypnovel), oxazepam, 1965 (Serenid D), Medazepam (Nobrium), chlorazepate (Transcene), lorazepam, 1977 (Ativan), flunitrazepam (Rohypnol) flurazepam, 1970 (Dalmane), triazolam, lormetazepam, and loprazolam.

The benzodiazepines differ from the barbiturates in four respects: (1) habituation unusual; (2) withdrawal effects may occur; (3) no significant enzyme induction; and (4) REM sleep not greatly inhibited.

The benzodiazepines are depressors of the limbic system and are classed as minor tranquillizers. They depress emotional response and alertness, are anticonvulsant from their centrally-acting muscle relaxant effects. GABA (the neurotransmitter) release is facilitated and they may depress noradrenaline secretion. Biotransformation to active metabolites may occur. Continuous infusion may be used.

Diazepam

Used for premedication and sedation. A lipid-soluble base, dissolved in propylene glycol, Cremophor EL, or soya bean oil/water emulsion (Diazemuls), which is less painful on injection.

Pharmacodynamics

Central nervous system. The actions of benzodiazepines on the central nervous system are mediated by facilitation of the inhibition of synaptic transmission by gamma-aminobutyric acid (GABA). Relieves tension and anxiety. Causes drowsiness and controls convulsions. Not analgesic. Its effects summate with those of other sedatives including alcohol. Can be safely given to patients receiving mono-amine oxidase inhibitors. Thought to depress the limbic system and the amygdala where fear, anxiety and aggression are generated. Cortex not depressed. Causes anterograde amnesia (about 10 min after intravenous injection, sometimes much longer after oral doses). Used to control drug-induced dyskinesias. Does not cause nausea or vomiting. Does not increase cerebral blood flow and can be used in patients with head injury.

Respiratory system. Causes a slight depression of breathing, usually not serious.

Cardiovascular system. Myocardial depression and hypotension not common, but can cause collapse.

Muscular system. Potentiates non-depolarizing relaxants and reduces the amount of relaxation caused by suxamethonium. Relieves muscle spasm and spasticity.

Pharmacokinetics

98% bound to plasma proteins. Rapid redistribution to muscle and fat, with T1/2β of 4 h (much longer in preterm neonates – 40–400 h).[74] The major active metabolite is desmethyldiazepam with an elimination half-life of 24 hours.

There is considerable enterohepatic recirculation. Allergy to diazepam has been reported. Benzodiazepines are potentiated and prolonged by inhibition of their metabolism by cimetidine. Excretion of metabolites is mostly in the gut and urine.

Benzodiazepine receptors related to the GABA/chloride channels have been demonstrated in man and may be found in the brain cortex, spinal cord and other tissues. (*See also* Whitwam J. G. *Anaesthesia* 1983, **38**, 93.)

Clinical uses

Dose of diazepam: 0.1–0.3 mg/kg oral or i.m. These doses given intravenously produce sedation to anaesthesia. In children, diazepam has been given per rectum 0.75 mg/kg, maximum dose 20 mg. There is great variation of response to this drug.

Also used: (1) as an adjunct to light intravenous anaesthesia, e.g. in conservative dentistry; (2) as the sole anaesthetic in cardioversion; (3) before bronchoscopy under local analgesia; (4) to control postoperative restlessness; (5) as an anticonvulsant in status epilepticus; (6) to control drug-induced dyskinesia; (7) in the treatment of tetanus; (8) in the treatment of eclampsia (but diazepam crosses the placental barrier); (9) for cardiac catheterization; (10) to reduce hallucinations after ketamine; and (11) for fibre-endoscopy of stomach, etc. (to control secretions, atropine must be given first). rapid injection can cause apnoea.

Diazepam should not be mixed with other drugs and should be injected into large veins to reduce the incidence of thrombophlebitis.

Diazepam is available in the form of tablets, syrup and ampoules for injection (5 mg/ml in polyethylene glycol). Also as rectal suppository, 5 and 10 mg.

Following intravenous injection there is a small fall in plasma potassium. Car driving should be prohibited for 10–12 h after a significant dose of diazepam.

Midazolam[75] (*Hypnovel*)

This is a water-soluble benzodiazepine which can be used for induction of anaesthesia, and sedation. The duration of action is slightly shorter than diazepam and it does not irritate veins.

Pharmacokinetics

95% bound to plasma albumin. Distributed as two-compartment model. $T1/2\beta$ 1.45 h.[76] Metabolized by hepatic P450 to 1- and 4-hydroxymethyl midazolam. Severe accumulation occurs in hepatic failure.

Pharmacodynamics

Onset of action in 1–2 mins, duration 1–2 h. Sedation dose 0.05–0.1 mg/kg, anaesthetic induction dose 0.15–0.3 mg/kg. Infusion rate for sedation 2–5 µg/kg/min. Transient apnoea has been observed with a dosage of 0.15 mg/kg which is not sufficient to induce anaesthesia reliably in unpremedicated subjects. Anterograde amnesia and drowsiness are common. It can be used with fentanyl as a cardiovascular-stable anaesthetic, reversible by flumazenil.[77] Cardiovascular stability is good, with 10% falls of arterial pressure in 10% of subjects, and some tachycardias.

(*See also* Sear J. W. *Anaesthesia* 1983, **38**, Suppl. 10; Gamble J. A. S. et al. *Anaesthesia* 1981, **36**, 868.)

Lorazepam (*Ativan*)

May be given orally or by injection. Long duration of action. Has an elimination half-life of 12 h and has no pharmacologically active metabolites. Produces sedation, drowsiness and amnesia. Useful for premedication. Oral dose 1–5 mg or may be given intramuscularly, dose 2–4 mg. The great advantage of lorazepam is the lack of nausea and vomiting in ophthalmic cases, and the length of action.

Antagonists

Flumazenil is the specific antagonist at GABA controlled chloride channels. Adult dose 0.1–0.5 mg, given slowly i.v. or i.m. Onset 1–5 min; Duration 1–3 h. Side-effects: these mainly arise from reversal of benzodiazepine effects, e.g. appearance or reappearance of convulsions, return of anxiety and respiratory responsiveness.[78] Successfully reverses benzodiazepine-fentanyl anaesthesia[79]

NEUROLEPT ANALGESIA

This describes the state of a patient following the administration of an analgesic, such as phenoperidine or fentanyl, and a sedative such as haloperidol and droperidol. Thalamonal (Innovar) is a premix of 50:1 droperidol and fentanyl, each ml contains droperidol 2.5 mg and 0.05 mg fentanyl.

The term 'neurolepsis' was coined by Delay in 1959.[82] and 'neurolept analgesia' was introduced by J. A. De Castro and Mundeleer of Brussels in the same year.[83]

A development of the artificial hibernation, neurovegetative block, ataralgesia concepts. Neuroleptic agents and phenothiazines used in anaesthesia are chemically based on methyl ethylamine and are related to gamma-hydroxybutyric acid (GABA).

SHORT-ACTING NARCOTIC ANALGESICS (OPIOIDS)

Note: for other opioids, *see* Chapter 26.

Phenoperidine hydrochloride (*Operidine*) and Fentanyl citrate (*Phentanyl; Sublimaze*)

These are chemically related to pethidine but are much more potent. Like it, they produce all the effects of opioids, such as intense analgesia, respiratory depression, which precedes the analgesia, miosis, nausea and vomiting, which outlasts the analgesia, bradycardia, various effects on smooth muscle depending on the dose used, and addiction. Adult doses: phenoperidine 1–2 mg, fentanyl 0.025–0.1 mg. Respiratory depression is managed by IPPV, or antagonized by naloxone. Infusion dose of fentanyl to prevent postoperative stress response 4–10 µg/kg/h.[84]

Onset: respiratory depression in 30–60 s, analgesia in 5–10 mins.

Duration: 30–60 min. Fentanyl undergoes enterohepatic recirculation with rebound effects at 3–5 h after injection.[85] (These effects do not exceed the initial ones, but delayed respiratory depression following apparent recovery of respiratory activity after fentanyl has been reported.) Phenoperidine is metabolized and excreted in the urine in equal amounts; fentanyl is mostly destroyed in the liver and about 10% excreted in the urine. Should be used carefully in patients who have been taking mono-amine oxidase inhibitors within 14 days. Bolus fentanyl can cause a cough.[86] Large doses of fentanyl may result in muscular rigidity, making IPPV difficult, but a relaxant will overcome this effect. Fentanyl is highly lipophilic and is rapidly absorbed from the epidural and other fatty spaces giving blood levels similar to the intravenous route.[87]

Alfentanil (*Rapifen*)

First used in 1981.

Adult dose for supplementary analgesia without apnoea: 5–10 µg/kg; dose for suppressing the 'stress response': 50–100 µg/kg. Infusion dose: 0.5–1 µg/kg/min (30–60 µg/kg/h) if no other opioids have been given.

Onset: 30–60 s.

Duration: 5–10 min, doubled by propofol.

Pharmacokinetics[88]

90% bound to plasma proteins, only moderately lipid-soluble, biexponential decay,[89] T1/2α 5 min, T1/2β 95 min (63 min in children), hepatic extraction ratio 0.4–0.7.

Particularly suitable as a supplement to anaesthesia in short procedures and in day case surgery. May also be used in repeated dosage or continuous infusion in major surgery.

To prevent metabolic and endocrine responses to surgery, high doses are necessary before the start of the operation, not after it has begun.

Sufentanil

Dose for supplementary analgesia: 0.1 µg/kg; dose for suppressing 'stress response': 5–20 µg/kg; infusion dose: 0.01 µg/kg/min.

Onset: 1–4 min[90]

Duration: 30–60 min.

Pharmacokinetics

Highly lipophilic, 90% bound to plasma glycoprotein and albumin; biexponential decay, T1/2β 164 min, (53–55 min in children.)[91] Metabolized by O-demethylation and N-dealkylation.

Pharmacodynamics

Intense analgesia with good cardiovascular stability even at 'stress response inhibiting doses'.[92]

A powerful respiratory depressant.[93] (For effects on cerebral circulation and metabolism, *see* Milde L. M., Milde J. H., Gallagher W. J. *Anesthesia and Analg* 1990, **70**, 138.)

Clinical uses of short-acting opioids

1. As analgesics.
2. To produce apnoea when it is desired to institute or maintain mechanical ventilation in the intensive therapy unit, e.g. chest injuries.
3. To attenuate 'stress responses' during surgery. Doses of 50 µg/kg of fentanyl have been used with oxygen, with or without diazepam for cardiac surgery; also by continuous infusion.
4. To produce neurolept analgesia.

BUTYROPHENONES

Droperidol (*Dehydrobenzperidol; Droleptan; Inapsine*)

Pharmacodynamics

One of the butyrophenone series of drugs, which causes mental detachment, absence of voluntary movements (catatonia) and a specific inhibitory effect on the chemoreceptor trigger zone controlling nausea and vomiting. A weak α-adrenergic receptor blocking action (sometimes causing hypotension). The butyrophenones compete with GABA at postsynaptic receptor sites. They have similar actions to the phenothiazines and are dopaminergic antagonists.

Pharmacokinetics

Dose: 0.1 mg/kg.
Onset: 3–20 min after i.v. injection.
Duration: up to 12 h. Large doses may cause extrapyramidal dyskinesia, which can be overcome by anti-parkinsonism agents (other than levodopa), atropine, diazepam or promethazine.

Haloperidol (*Serenace*)

Antiemetic dose: 0.05 mg/kg.
Onset: 10 min.
Duration: 24–48 h.
Haloperidol crosses the placenta.

Uses of neurolept analgesia

1. As premedication, 0.5–2 ml of Thalamonal. Occasionally unpleasant subjective sensations and muscular dyskinesia are experienced.
2. Sedation for burns dressings, needle punctures, sutures and other minor traumas, and for diagnostic procedures, e.g. aortography, angiocardiography, fibreoptic gastroscopy, bronchoscopy and oesophagoscopy, and regional analgesia.
3. In certain neurosurgical operations when the patient's conscious co-operation is required during surgery, e.g. in stereotactic surgery and anterolateral tractotomy. It reduces the cerebrospinal fluid pressure in normal patients and those with space-occupying lesions. No significant effect on cerebral blood flow or oxygen consumption. May raise intracranial pressure in head injury or cerebral tumour.
4. As a supplement to thiopentone, relaxant and nitrous oxide – oxygen anaesthesia. IPPV is commonly employed. Droperidol, 5–20 mg, is followed by incremental doses of fentanyl until apnoea occurs. Nitrous oxide, oxygen and relaxants are then administered and the trachea intubated. Naloxone may be needed at the end of the operation. Impending awareness is indicated by movement, sweating, a rise in blood pressure or pulse rate, and oesophageal contractility.[94]
5. During bypass in cardiovascular surgery.
6. In the intensive therapy unit to facilitate intubation and IPPV.
Car driving should be forbidden during the 24 h following the use of neurolept analgesia.

THE PHENOTHIAZINE DERIVATIVES

This group of drugs includes, among hundreds of others:

Promethazine hydrochloride, BP (*Phenergan; Atosil*)

(N-(2-dimethylamino-*n*-propyl)-phenothiazine hydrochloride). It is thought to stabilize cell membranes and the coverings of the endoplasmic reticulum. First used in anaesthesia in the 'lytic cocktail'.

Pharmacodynamics

(*a*) Promethazine is a powerful hypnotic in its own right and potentiates barbiturates and narcotic analgesics, possibly by an influence on liver cells.

(*b*) Powerful antagonism to histamine by its effect on H_1 receptors.

(*c*) It is a potent depressant of upper respiratory tract reflexes and is a bronchodilator.

(*d*) It has slight atropine-like activity.

(*e*) It is said to increase sensitivity to pain.

(*f*) It antagonises 5-hydroxytryptamine. Promethazine is particularly useful as a premedication, especially in asthmatics.

It is supplied as 2.5% solution and as tablets, 25 mg, and elixir, 5 mg–5 ml. Dose for premedication 25–50 mg i.m. *See* Chapter 5.

Trimeprazine tartrate BPC (*Vallergan*)

See Chapter 5.

Promazine hydrochloride, BP USP (*Sparine*)

A useful antiemetic. Average dose 25–50 mg.

Prochlorperazine maleate, BP USP (*Stemetil; Compazine*)

Excellent antiemetic, dose 12.5–25 mg. Has been used to control vertigo after inner and middle-ear operations.

Chlorpromazine Hydrochloride, BP (*Largactil, Megaphen, Hibernal*)

See 10th ed, of Synopsis of Anaesthesia.

DISSOCIATIVE ANAESTHESIA

Ketamine (*ketalar; Ketaject*)

Ketamine is 2-*o*-chlorophenyl-2-methylaminocyclohexanone hydrochloride. It is a white crystalline substance with a characteristic smell. Readily soluble in water, pH 3.5–4.1 in 10% solution. Supplied in 1, 5 and 10% solutions. Forms a precipitate with barbiturates.

History

A related compound, phencyclidine (Sernyl) was synthesized by Victor Maddox of Detroit, investigated by Chen of Ann Arbor[95] and was used in anaesthesia, but was withdrawn because of the high incidence of hallucinations, although it is still used in animals.

Ketamine was synthesized by Stevens of Detroit and tested on volunteers from a state prison in Michigan in 1964. It was used in anaesthesia in 1965 by Domino and Corssen.[96] It proved a promising new agent, particularly for use in developing countries or in the field situation. Since then considerable interest has developed in this compound, which has certain properties not shared by other agents. (*See* Corssen G. In: *Anaesthesia; Essays on its History* (Rupreht J. et al. ed.) Berlin: Springer-Verlag, 1985, 92.)

Pharmacodynamics

Ketamine is rapidly absorbed after oral, intramuscular or intravenous administration. The injection of a therapeutic dose of ketamine produces a state of *dissociative anaesthesia*. The sleep produced is somewhat different from that of conventional anaesthesia. It occurs within minutes of intramuscular or intravenous injection and lasts for up to 15 min. Analgesia is a marked feature.

Cardiovascular system. Systolic and diastolic blood pressures are raised and pulse rate increases. There is evidence that ketamine is a direct myocardial stimulant because the rise in blood pressure can be prevented by administration of verapamil, a calcium antagonist. Ketamine causes pulmonary vasconstriction and undesirable strain on the right heart in some cases of valvular heart disease. Ketamine may act by increasing the availability of calcium across cell membranes. The chronotropic effect is not blocked by verapamil. There is a rise in plasma noradrenaline, which can be reduced by prior administration of droperidol. Premedication with propranolol or atropine does not prevent rise of blood pressure and increase of pulse rate when ketamine is used. There is an antidysrhythmia effect. Ketamine prevents reflex adrenergic responses of peripheral blood vessels to surgical stimuli.

Respiratory system. Respiration is not depressed, except by large doses, and is usually mildly stimulated. Airway obstruction occurs under deep ketamine anaesthesia. The prevention of aspiration under ketamine cannot be guaranteed.

Alimentary system. Has analgesic effects when taken by mouth.[97] Nausea and vomiting occur and require prophylaxis. Salivation may be troublesome unless prevented by hyoscine.

Ocular. Some rise of intraocular pressure may occur, but this is transient and ketamine has been recommended for tonometry in children. Eye movements and nystagmus may occur.

Skin. Transient erythema has been reported in 15% of patients, but is of little consequence.

Cerebral. Increases cerebral blood flow and intracranial pressure with marked regional variations.[98] Dreaming, hallucinations and delirium occur. Phonation may take place in light ketamine anaesthesia.

Limbs. Non-purposeful movements are seen in light ketamine anaesthesia.

Pharmacokinetics

It is converted to water-soluble norketamine by N-demethylation and hydroxylation of the cyclohexanone ring. These are excreted in the urine. T1/2β 153 min.[99] Vd 2.3 l/kg.

Clinical uses

Dosage: 1–2 mg/kg, i.v. and supplementary doses of 0.5 mg/kg, or 10 mg/kg i.m. Intravenous infusion rate: 40 µg/kg/min. There is a small amount of cumulation.

Onset: 1 min (i.v.) and 10 min (i.m.) (shorter in children).

Ketamine is a rapidly acting parenteral anaesthetic causing sedation, profound analgesia, catalepsy, some increase in striated muscle tone, mild cardiovascular stimulation, but only slight diminution of pharyngolaryngeal reflexes. Not very efficient as an obtundor of visceral pain. It increases salivation so that atropine should always be used. Intravenous injection should take 60–120 s. Has been employed: (1) as the sole agent for minor operations; (2) as an induction agent before general anaesthesia; (3) when airway control is difficult; (4) for certain neurological radiodiagnostic and therapeutic procedures in children to abolish movement; (5) when maintenance of blood pressure is important, e.g. in states of shock and in some poor-risk patients and in the elderly; (6) in open heart surgery; (7) for manipulations; (8) for dressing of burns, skin debridement, skin grafts, etc.; (9) for dealing with mass casualties; (10) in developing countries or when anaesthetists are unavailable; (11) when intramuscular injection is more convenient than intravenous; (12) subanaesthetic doses are used to produce analgesia;[100] (13) for induction of anaesthesia in small children. A 0.1% solution in 5% dextrose has been given as a slow i.v. drip for postoperative pain relief and for analgesia in patients in the intensive care unit; and (14) for use in TIVA, see Restale J. et al. *Anaesthesia* 1988, **43**, 46.

(For pharmacokinetic effects of ketamine infusions, *see* Idvall J. et al. *Br. J. Anaesth.* 1979, **51**, 1167.)

Duration: 3–10 min (i.v.) and 10–30 min (i.m.).

Adverse reactions

1. Hypertension, tachycardia and rashes.
2. Dreams. Vivid unpleasant dreams occur, and occasionally true hallucinations. The incidence of these emergence phenomena increases with age, being about 5% under 5 years of age, and 50% in adulthood. They can be reduced by: (a) leaving the patient without stimulation in the recovery period; (b) use of opiate and hyoscine premedication; (c) injection of droperidol (2.5–7.5 mg, i.m. or i.v.) towards the end of surgery; and (d) small amounts of diazepam, lorazepam or thiopentone. These dreams occur during and following surgery not seen with l-ketamine. 4-aminopyridine, 0.3 mg/kg, aids recovery from ketamine (and diazepam) unconsciousness.[101]

Used in Bier's technique for intravenous regional analgesia, ketamine produces analgesia in the arm, unfortunately followed by unconsciousness a few minutes after release of the tourniquet[102] and extradurally, 4 mg in 10 ml of 5% dextrose in water when it is reported to give good pain relief after operation without side-effects.[103]

Ketamine produces only transient hormonal changes, which are minor in comparison with those superimposed by surgery. Ketamine analgesia is partially reversed by naloxone.[104]

Ketamine has been used for intradural analgesia in war surgery.[105] It can also be given orally. (*See also* Ketamine; its pharmacology and therapeutic uses. White P. F. et al. *Anesthesiology* 1982, **56**, 119.)

TOTAL INTRAVENOUS ANAESTHESIA (TIVA OR INFUSION ANAESTHESIA)

(*See also* Sear J. W. In: *Recent Advances in Anaesthesia and Analgesia – 16* (Atkinson R. S. and Adams A. P. eds.) Edinburgh: Churchill Livingstone, 1989.)

This technique may be used for general anaesthesia or sedation during regional blockade. It may be used alone or in combination with gaseous anaesthetics. The following agents have been used: barbiturates, etomidate, propofol, ketamine, GABA, and narcotic analgesics.

Total intravenous anaesthesia implies that the patient is kept unconcious and free from harmful reflex responses entirely by the use of agents administered intravenously with the addition of muscle relaxant drugs to provide relaxation, prevent motor responses and allow IPPV. The lungs are ventilated with air and oxygen enriched air.

Some methods used include:

1. Anaesthesia is induced using midazolam 0.07 mg/kg followed 2 min later by ketamine 1.0 mg/kg and vecuronium 0.1 mg/kg and then the infusion rate of ml/h calculated as half the patients body weight in kg,[72] using a mixture of ketamine 200 mg, midazolam 5 mg, and vecuronium 12 mg in 50 ml saline.
2. Propofol infusion has also been used with alfentanil.[80]
3. Computerised infusion systems have been developed.[81]

Precautions need with TIVA[106]

1. Machine check before use
2. Battery backup is important, for failure of mains supply
3. Empty syringe warning is important
4. Blocked delivery pipe warning is important
5. Full resuscitation equipment required
6. The delivery pipe/i.v. cannula – union should be 'pull- detachable' to prevent the cannula from being pulled out
7. The i.v. cannula should be kept in sight to monitor this
8. Caution about using mixtures of i.v. agents – they may interact or have different lengths of action
9. A proper syringe refill system for use during the anaesthetic must be organized before starting.

10. Respiratory monitoring is essential, e.g. with mask and bag system using air or oxygen/nitrous oxide as the fresh gas.

11. Awareness may be a problem when relaxants are used, as with a 'volatile' technique. *See* Chapter 14.

Monitoring depth during total intravenous anaesthesia

1. The pattern of movement of the bag on the breathing system.

2. The isolated arm technique.[107] A response to asking for a squeeze of the anaesthetists hand implies wakefulness.

3. Lower oesophageal contractions (spontaneous–SLOC; provoked–PLOC).[108] Rather variable, reduced by atropine, and affected by surgical stimulus[109]

4. Frontalis EMG.[110] Effective even in the presence of moderate vecuronium block.[111]

5. The EEG (*see* 'Awareness', Chapter 14). The changes are somewhat specific to each individual agent, but has been used to automatically control propofol infusion.[112] Analysis methods include median frequency, spectral array, spectral edge, spectral bands, and direct frequency measurement.

6. Sensory evoked potentials (SEP). Commonly the auditory evoked response (AER) is used. The microvolt waveform generated at a postaural electrode by auditory clicks is flattened ('amplitude') and slowed ('latency') by adequate anaesthesia.[113] An AER index is generated by computer, scores below 100 indicate reasonable anaesthesia. Computers can be used to predict infusion rates.[114]

SEDATION TECHNIQUES – 'SEDOANALGESIA'

This is a combination of regional analgesia and light sedation, perhaps aided by some forms of sensory deprivation, e.g. ear muffs, eye shades, etc. Most of the agents in this Chapter have been mentioned as having sedative actions. Because of the side-effects of all these drugs, and the need to monitor and control the patient's physiology during surgery, these techniques need as much care from the anaesthetist as a full general anaesthetic. (*See also* Sedation Techniques Willatts S. M. and Kong K. M. In *Recent advances in Anaesthesia – 16* (Atkinson R. S. and Adams A. P. eds), Edinburgh: Churchill Livingstone, 1989.

Adverse drug reactions, *see* Chapter 14. They may be due to 'non-anaesthetic' drugs.[115] Perianaesthetic rashes are not uncommon.[116]

References

1. Oré P. C. *Bull. Soc. Chirurg.* 1872, **1**, 400; *see also* Sabathié M. and Delperier A. *Progress in Anaesthesiology.* Amsterdam: Excerpta Medica, 1970, 841.

2. Pravaz C. G. *C. R. Seances Acad. Sci.* 1853. **36**, 88

3. Rynd F. *Dublin Med. Press* 1845, **13**, 167.
4. Wood A. *Edin. Med. Surg. J.* 1855. **82**, 265.
5. Howard-Jones N. J. *J. Hist. Med.* 1947, **2**, 201.
6. Krawkow N. F. *Arch. Ex. Path. Phearmak.* 1908, Suppl., 317.
7. Fischer E. and von Mering J. *Ther. d. Gegenw.* 1903, **5**, 97
8. Bardet D. *Bull. Gen. Therap.* 1921 **1**, 27; Fredet P. and Perlis R. *Bull. et Mém. Soc. Nat. de Chir* 1924 **50** 789.
9. Noel H. and Souttar H. S. *Ann. Surg.* 1913, **57**, 64.
10. Bredenfeld E. *Z. Ex. Path. Ther.* 1916, **18**, 80.
11. Bumm R. *Klin. Wochenschr.* 1927, **6**, 725.
12. Zerfas L. G. and McCallum J. T. C. *J. Ind. Med. Assoc.* 1929, **22**, 47.
13. Fitch R. H. et al. *Am. J. Surg.* 1930, n.s. **9**, 110.
14. Magill I. W. *Lancet*, 1931, **1**, 74.
15. Lundy J. S. *Surg. Clin. North Am.* 1931, **11**, 909.
16. Kirschner M. *Chirurg.* 1929, **1**, 673; Macintosh R. R. et al. *Lancet*, 1941, **2**, 10: Thornton H. L. et al. *Anesthesiology* 1945, **6**, 583.
17. Weese H. and Scharpff W. *Dtsch. Med. Wochenschr.* 1932, **58**, 1205.
18. Jarman R. and Abel L. *Lancet*, 1933, **2**, 18.
19. Tabern D. L. and Volwiler E. H. *J. Am. Chem. Soc.* 1935, **57**, 1961
20. Lundy J. S. and Tovell R. M. *North West Med.* 1935, **33**, 308; Lundy J. S. *Proc. Staff Meet. Mayo Clin.* 1935, **10**, 536 (reprinted in 'Classical File', *Surv. Anesthesiol.* 1958, **2**, 231): Corssen G. In: *Anaesthesia; Essays on its History* (Rupreht J. et al. ed.) Berlin: Springer Verlag, 1985, 88.
21. Pratt T. W. et al. *Am. J. Surg.* 1936, **31**, 464.
22. Jarman R. and Abel L. *Lancet*, 1936, **1**, 422.
23. Brodie B. B. et al. *J. Pharmacol. Exp. Ther.* 1950, **98**, 85 (reprinted in 'Classical File'. *Surv. Anesthesiol.* 1965, **9**, 391).
24. Stoelting V. K. *Anesth. Analg. Curr. Res.* 1957, **36**, 49.
25. Halford F. J. *Anesthesiology* 1943, **4**, 67.
26. Organe G. S. W. et al. *Lancet*, 1938, **2**, 1170.
27. Nitescu P. et al. *Acta Anaesthesiol Scand.* 1990, **34**, 120.
28. Gunawardene R. D. and Davenport H. T. *Anaesthesia* 1990, **45**, 52.
29. Lawson S, Gent J. P. and Goodchild C. S. *Br. J. Anaesth.* 1990, **64**, 59.
30. Dundee J. W. et al. *Br. J. Anaesth.* l956, **28**, 344; Mark L. C., Papper, E. M. et al. *New Eng. J. Med.* 1949, **49**, 1546.
31. Sorbo S. et al. *Anesthesiology*, 1984, **61**, 666.
32. Brodie B. B. et al. *J. Pharmac. Exp. Ther.* 1950, **98**, 85 (reprinted in 'Classical File', *Surv. Anesthesiol.* 1965, **9**, 391).
33. Macintosh R. R. and Heyworth P. S. A. *Lancet*, 1943, **2**, 571.
34. Dundee J. W. *Anesthesiology* 1983, **59**, 154.
35. Lazarus H. M. et al. *J. Surg. Res.* 1977, **22**, 46.
36. Corser G. et al. *Anaesthesia* 1985, **40**, 51.
37. Hales P. *Anaesth. Intensive Care* 1981, **9**, 390.
38. Dundee J. W. and Riding J. E. *Anaesthesia* 1955, **10**, 55; Dundee J. W. et al. *Anesth. Analg. Curr. Res.* 1962, **41**, 567; Bush G. H. *Proc. R. Soc. Med.* 1968, **61**, 171.
39. Dundee J. W. *Curr. Res. Anesth. Analg.* 1952, **31**, 257; Lodge A. B. *Br. Med. J.* 1958, **1**, 1043; McClelland R. M. A. *Br. J. Anaesth.* 1960, **32**, 81.
40. Chernish S. M. et al. *Fed. Proc.* 1956, **15**, 409.
41. Dundee J. W. and Moore J. *Anaesthesia* 1961, **16**, 50.
42. Bohrer H., Fleischer F. and Werning P. *Anaesthesia* 1990, **45**, 18
43. Fragen R. J. et al. *Br. J. Anaesth.* 1983, **55**, 433.
44. Rifat K. et al. *Can. Anaesth. Soc. J.* 1976, **23**, 492.
45. Holdcroft A. et al. *Br. J. Anaesth.* 1976, **48**, 199.
46. Sold M. J. *Anaesthesia* 1985, **40**, 1014.
47. Ledingham I. McA. and Watt I. *Lancet* 1983, **1**, 1270.

48. Moore R. A. and Allen M. C. *Anaesthesia* 1985. **40**, 124.
49. Yeoman P. M. et al. *Br. J. Anaesth.* 1984, **56**, 1291P.
50. Duthrie D. J. R. et al. *Br. J. Anaesth.* 1985, **57**, 156; Byrne A. J. and Yeoman P. M. *Br. J. Anaesth.* 1985, **57**, 1264.
51. Kay B. and Rolly G. *Acta Anaesthiol. Belg.* 1977, **28**, 303.
52. Rogers K. M. et al. *Br. J. Anaesth.* 1980, **52**, 407; Kay B. and Stephenson D. K. *Anaesthesia* 1980, **35**, 1182; Rutter D. V. et al. *Anaesthesia* 1980, **35**, 1188; Kay B. *Anaesthesia* 1981, **36**, 863; Major E. et al. *Br. J. Anaesth.* 1981, **53**, 267.
53. Spelina K. R. et al. *Br. J. Anaesth.* 1986, **58**, 1050.
54. Committee on Safety of Medicines. *Current problems No 20*, August 1987; Saunders and Harris, *Anaesthesia*, 1990, **45**, 552; Mather S. J. and Edwards N. D., Biswas A. *ibid*, 1096.
55. Saunders and Harris *Anaesthesia* 1990, **45**, 552; Mather S. J. and Edwards N. D., Biswas A. *ibid*, 1096.
56. Simons P. J. et al. *Postgrad. Med. J.* 1985, (suppl 3) **64**, (abstract)
57. Gepts E, et al. *Anaesthesia* 1988, **43**, (suppl) 8.
58. Cockshott I. D., Briggs L. P. *Br. J. Anaesth.* 1987, **59**, 1102.
59. Gin T. and Gregory M. A. *Br. J. Anaesth.* 1990, **64**, 148.
60. Lawson S. et al. *Brit. J. Anaesth.* 1990, **64**, 59; Au J. et al. *Anaesthesia.* 1991, **46**, 238; Imray J. McG. and Hay A. *Anaesthesia* 1991, **46**; 704.
61. Mackenzie N. and Grant I. S. *Br. J. Anaesth.* 1985, **57**, 725; Grounds R. M. and Twigley A. J. et al. *Anaesthesia* 1985, **40**, 735; Patrick M. R. et al. *Postgrad. Med. J.* 1985, **61**(suppl 3); 23.
62. Grounds R. M. et al. *Anaesthesia* 1985, **40**, 735.
63. Monk C. R. and Coates D. P. et al. *Br. J. Anaesth.* 1987, **59**, 954.
64. Fahey L. T. et al. *Anaesthesia* 1985, **40**, 939.
65. Sear J. W. et al. *Anaesthesia* 1988, **43**(suppl), 17; Youngberg J. A., Texidor M. S. and Smith D. E. *Anesth. Analg.* 1987, **66**, 1891.
66. Vermeyen K. M. et al. *Br. J. Anaes.* 1987, **59**, 1115.
67. McCirrick A. and Hunter S. *Anaesthesia* 1990, **45**, 443; Marsch S. C. U. and Schlaefer H. G. *Anesth. Analg.* 1990, **70**, 127.
68. Speedy H. *Br. J. Anaesth.* 1990, **64**, 110.
69. Dixon J. et al. *Br. J Anaesth.* 1990, **64**, 142.
70. Mackenzie S. J. et al. *Anaesthesia* 1991, **45**, 1043.
71. Aitkenhead A. R. et al. *Lancet* 1989, **ii**, 704.
72. Restall J. et al. *Anaesthesia* 1988, **43**, 46; Bailie R. et al. *Anaesthesia* 1989, **44**, 60.
73. Dziewonski K. and Sternbach L. H. *Chem. Abst.* 1936. **30**, 2971.
74. Morselli P. L. et al. *Handbook of Clinical Pharmacokinetics* (Gimaldi M. and Prescott L. ed.) New York: Adis Health Science Press, 1983.
75. Conner J. T. et al. *Anesth. Analg. (Cleve.)* 1978, **57**, 1; Fragen R. J. et al. *Anesthesiology* 1978, **49**, 41; Reeves J. G. et al. *Can. Anaesth. Soc. J.* 1979, **26**, 42; Forster A. et al. *Br. J. Anaesth.* 1980, **52**, 907.
76. Salonen M. et al. *Anesth. Analg.* 1987, **66**, 625.
77. Kaukinen S., Kataja J. and Kaukinen L. *Can. J. Anaesth.* 1990, **37**, 40.
78. Bernstein K. J. *Anesth. Analg.* 1990, **70**, 122
79. Kaukinen S., Kataja J. and Kaukinen L. *Can J. Anaesth.* 1990, **37**, 40.
80. Brown B. L. et al. *Brit. J. Anaesth.* 1990, **64**, 396P: Marsh B. et al. *Brit. J. Anaesth.* 1991, **67**, 41; Raftery S. et al. *Brit. J. Anaesth.* 1991, **97**, 218P.
81. Schuttler J. et al. *Anaesthesia* 1988, **43**, Suppl. 2; White M. and Kenny G. N. C. *Anaesthesia* 1990, **45**, 204; Kenny G. N. C. and White M. *Anaesthesia* 1990, **45**, 692; Skipsey I. G. et al. *Brit. J. Anaesth.* 1991, **67**, 218P.
82. Delay J. *Psychopharmacological Frontiers*. Boston: Little, Brown & Co., 1959.
83. De Castro J. and Mundeleer P. *Anesth. Anal. Paris*, 1959, **16**, 1022.
84. Hickey P. R. and Hansen D. D. *Anesth. Analg.* 1985, **64**, 1137.
85. Dundee J. W. *Anaesthesia* 1961, **16**, 61.
86. Bohrer H., Fleischer F. and Werning P. *Anaesthesia* 1990, **45**, 18.

87. Loper K. A. et al. *Anesth. Analg.* 1990, **70**, 72.
88. Robbins G. R. and Wyands J. E. et al. *Can. J. Anaesth.* 1990, **37**, 52.
89. Roure P. et al. *Br. J. Anaesth.* 1987, **59**, 1437–1440.
90. Hickey P. R. and Hansen D. D. *Anesth. Analg.* 1984, **63**, 117.
91. Davis P. J. et al. *Anesth. Analg.* 1987, **66**, 203.
92. Moore R. A. et al. *Anesthesiology* 1985, **62**, 725.
93. Bailey P. L. and James B. et al. *Anesth. Analg.* 1990, **70**, 8.
94. Thomas D. I. and Aitkenhead A. R. *Br. J. Anaesth.* 1990, **64**, 306.
95. Chen G. et al. *J. Pharmacol. Exp. Ther.* 1966, **152**, 332.
96. Domino E. F. et al. *Clin. Pharmacol. Ther.* 1965, **6.** 279; Corssen G. and Domino E. F. *Anesth. Analg. Curr. Res.* 1966, **45**, 29.
97. Morgan A. J. and Dutkiewicz T. W. S. *Anaesthesia* 1983. **38**, 293.
98. Hougaard K. et al. *Anesthesiology* 1974, **41**, 562.
99. Grant I. S., Nimmo W. S. et al. *Br. J. Anaesth.* 1983, **55**, 1107–1111.
100. Sher M. H. *Anaesth. Intensive Care.* 1980, **8**, 359; Currie M. A. and Currie A. L. *Ann. R. Coll. Surg.* 1984, **66.** 424.
101. Agoston S. et al. *Br. J. Anaesth.* 1980, **52**, 312.
102. Amiot J. F. et al. *Anaesthesia* 1985, **40**, 899.
103. Islas J. A. et al. *Anesth. Analg. (Cleve.)* 1985, **64**, 1161.
104. Finck A. D. and Ngai S. H. *Anesthesiology* 1982, **56**, 291.
105. Bion J. F. *Anaesthesia* 1984, **39**, 1023.
106. Donenfeld R. F. *Anesth. Analg.* 1990, **70**, 116.
107. Russell I. F. *Br. J. Anaesth.* 1986, **58**, 965.
108. Evans J. M. et al. *Br. J. Anaesth.* 1987, **59**, 1346; Aitkenhead A. R. et al. *Anesthesiology* 1987, **67**, A671.
109. Thomas D. I. and Aitkenhead A. R. *Br. J. Anaesth.* 1990, **64**, 306.
110. Edmonds H. L. and Paloheimo M. *Int. J. Clin. Monit. Comput.* 1985, **1**, 201.
111. Edmonds H. L. et al. *Anesthesiology* 1985, **63**, A324.
112. Schwilden H. et al. *Br. J. Anaesth.* 1989, **62**, 290.
113. Heneghan C. P. H. et al. *Br. J. Anaesth.* 1987, **59**, 277; Thornton C. et al. *Br. J. Anaesth.* 1989, **63**, 113, 411.
114. Harrison M. J. *Br J. Anaesth.* 1990, **64**, 283, 287.
115. Parker S. D., Curry C. S. and Hirshman C. A. *Anesth. Analg.* 1990, **70**, 220.
116. Desmueles H. *Anesth. Analg.* 1990, **70**, 216.

Chapter 10

Muscle relaxants

It is usual to classify muscle relaxants used in anaesthesia as: (1) non-depolarizing agents, e.g. tubocurarine, atracurium, vecuronium, pancuronium and alcuronium (tachycurares), and (2) depolarizing agents, e.g. decamethonium and suxamethonium (leptocurares). Under certain circumstances the depolarizing drugs can exert a non-depolarizing effect, the so-called dual or biphasic block.

Muscular relaxation can also be produced centrally by deep general anaesthesia or peripherally by local nerve block. Most relaxants in clinical use are highly ionized and therefore are confined to the extracellular fluid.

History

1596 Sir Walter Raleigh (1552–1618) mentioned the arrow poison in his book *Discovery of the Large, Rich, and Beautiful Empire of Guiana*. It is possible that the poison he described was not curare at all.[1]

1811–1812 Sir Benjamin Collins Brody (1783–1862)[2] experimented with curare (*Phil. Trans.* 1811, **101**, 194; 1812, **102**, 205). He was the first to show that artificial respiration could maintain life in curarized animals.

1825 Curare brought to Europe by Charles Waterton (1782–1865) – *Wanderings in South America*. He described a classic experiment in which he kept a curarized she-ass alive by artificial ventilation with a bellows through a tracheostomy.[3]

1850 Claude Bernard (1813–1878),[4] The great French physiologist, stimulated by Francois Magendie (1783–1855), showed that curare acts by paralysing the myoneural junction. This led to his discovery of the concept of the motor end-plate. George Harley (1829–1896), of ACE anaesthetic mixture fame, showed that curare (wourali) was an efficient antidote to strychnine poisoning and also to tetanus.[5]

1858 Lewis Albert Sayer (1820–1900) used curare to treat tetanus in New York.[6]

1862 Curare used by Chisholm, in the American Civil War.

1872 Curare used by Herman Askan Demme (1802–1867) in the treatment of tetanus.

1894 R. Boehm (1844–1926), the German pharmacologist, separated curare into 'pot', 'gourd' and 'tube' curare according to the method used for storing it by the South American Indians. In 1897 he isolated highly active extracts from calabash curare.[7]

1912 Curare used by Arthur Läwen (1876–1958) of Konigsberg[8] in an effort to reduce the amount of ether employed in abdominal surgery with IPPV.

1914 Physiological actions of acetylcholine described by Dale (1875–1968).[9] Twenty-five years later he showed that acetylcholine is responsible for neuromuscular transmission, an effect blocked by curare.[10]

1934 First therapeutic use of curare in the UK (the treatment of tetanus) at Cambridge by Cole.[11]

1935 King (1887–1956)[12] of London, working in Sir Henry Dale's laboratory, isolated *d*-tubocurarine chloride from the crude drug and established its chemical structure and Ranyard West used it in the treatment of tetanus.[13]

1938 Richard C. Gill (1902–1958), American explorer, drew attention to it in his book *White Water and Blue Magic*, 1940, New York.

1939 Abraham Elting Bennett[14] of Omaha (Neb) employed curare to modify metrazol-induced convulsive therapy. Later used by H. Palmer,[15] of Hill End Hospital, Hertfordshire. Curare came to anaesthesia via psychiatry (electroplexy). Bennett arranged for crude curare to be given by Gill to McIntyre of the University of Nebraska who first standardized the drug.

1942 Harold R. Griffith (1894–1985) and Enid Johnson (now of Nova Scotia) used curare (the commercial preparation Intocostrin, prepared by Horace Holaday) at the suggestion of Dr Lewis Wright of E. M. Squibb Co.,[16] deliberately to give relaxation during surgery on 23 January in Montreal, Canada. A famous day in the history of anaesthesia.[17] Messrs Squibb obtained their supply of curare from R. C. Gill who brought it back from an expedition to Ecuador.

1943 Extraction of tubocurarine from *Chondrodendron tomentosum* by Wintersteiner[18] and Dutcher of Boston – the source of the drug as used today. First publication of Stuart Chester Cullen (1909–1979) of Iowa City[19] When given a sample of the preparation 'Intocostrin', Cullen first tried it on animals, and producing apnoea, was not able easily to ventilate them artificially, and so did not proceed to use it on humans. Griffith was also given a sample, but as he was familiar with the management of apnoea due to cyclopropane with IPPV the apnoea caused by curare was not a problem. Thus he rightly claimed priority for the introduction of relaxants into anaesthetic practice.

1944 Earliest mention of the use of curare with unsupplemented nitrous oxide and oxygen by Ralph Milton Waters (1883–1979) of Madison, in abdominal surgery;[20] also by Harroun in thoracic surgery.[21]

1945 First reported use in Britain of curare (Intocostrin) by Barnett Mallinson.[22]

1946 1946 T. C. Gray (1913–) and John Halton (1904–1969) of Liverpool established the position of curare in Britain.[23]

1947 Bovet described gallamine triethiodide.[24] This was used clinically in France by Huguenard and Boué in 1948[25] and by William Woolf Mushin (1910–   ) in 1949 in Britain.[26] Influential article describing use of gas, oxygen, pethidine and curare by William B. Neff.[27]

1948 Decamethonium described by Barlow and Ing[28] and by William Drummond Macdonald Paton (1917) and Eleanor Zaimis (1915–1982).[29] Used clinically by Geoffrey Organe (1908–1989) in 1949.[30]

1949 Daniel Bovet of the Pasteur Institute, Paris later moving to Rome, and others introduced suxamethonium.

1951 Suxamethonium first used in anaesthesia by Otto von Dardel, in Stockholm[31] and by Otto Mayerhofer (1920–) in Vienna.[32] Cyril Fredrick Scurr (1920–) introduced it into Britain.[33]

1954 Sensational article by Henry Knowel Beecher (1907–1976) and D. P. Todd (1918–) suggesting that the use of relaxants increased deaths due to anaesthesia nearly sixfold.[34] This has, of course, been completely disproved.

1956 W. D. M. Paton made the distinction between depolarizing and non-depolarizing relaxants.[35]

1958 A new relaxant from *strychnos toxifera* later named alcuronium, described.[36]

1961 Alcuronium first used.[37]

1967 Pancuronium (Pavulon) described clinically,[38] following pharmacological investigations in 1966.[39]

1968 Pancuronium introduced by Burkett W. R. et al.[40]

1970 Correct structure of tubocurarine molecule worked out.[41]

1979 Vecuronium introduced by Durant et al.[42]

1980 First clinical use of vecuronium (Norcuron).[43]

1981 Atracurium described by Hughes and Payne.[44]

(*See* Cullen S. C. *Anesthesiology* 1947, **8**, 479; Robbins B. H. and Lundy J. S. *Anesthesiology* 1947, **8**, 252; McIntyre A. R. *Curare: Its History, Nature and Clinical Use.* Chicago: Univ. of Chicago Press, 1947; Thomas K. B. *Curare. Its History and Usage.* London: Pitman, 1964; Stovner J. In: *Muscle Relaxants* (Katz L. ed.). Amsterdam: Excerpta Medica, 1975, Chap. 10; Betcher A. M. *Anesth. Anal. 1977,* **56**, 305; Crul J. F. *Acta Anaesthesiol. Scand.* 1982, **26**, 409; Humble R. M. The Gill Merritt Expedition. *Anesthesiology* 1982, **57**, 519; Suxamethonium, the development of a modern drug from 1906 to the present day. Dorkin H. R. *Med. Hist.* 1982, **26**, 145.)

The physiology of the neuromuscular junction

It was shown by Sir Henry Dale (1875–1968), in 1934, that acetylcholine is responsible for neuromuscular transmission, an effect blocked by curare,[45] and, in 1936, that a motor nerve liberates acetylcholine from the dense projections in the nerve terminal at the myoneural junction on the arrival of a nerve impulse.[46] Acetylcholine crosses the junctional cleft and becomes fixed at lipoprotein receptors on the junctional folds of the end-plate membrane and permits entry of sodium, which causes a sudden depolarization with exit of potassium from the muscle fibre. The depolarization passes along the membrane of the muscle fibre and is the final stimulus for causing the contraction of the contractile part of the muscle fibre. The released acetylcholine is meanwhile hydrolysed by acetylcholinesterase in the region of the motor end-plate, so that when the excited muscle fibre has come out of its refractory state, it will not become excited again by a depolarized end-plate unless a new nerve impulse has arrived and released a new supply of acetylcholine.

Depolarization causes Ca^{++} to enter the nerve terminal. Increased permeability of the special sodium (Na^+) channels in the neuromuscular junction to Na^+ is the trigger that leads to the propagating action potential. Na^+ enters the fibre, then K^+ leaves, as the action potential proceeds. A change of resting potential of 20 mV is adequate to initiate this process. Fresh acetylcholine (ACh) is synthesized in the axoplasm of the nerve terminal from choline obtained from the ECF and is transferred to vesicles ready for use. This process may be defective in the shocked, acidotic or toxaemic patient, making reversal of relaxants impossible. ACh exists in the nerve terminals in two forms – storage and releasable. ACh release is a self-potentiating process, leading to greater release and giving access to the storage granules for further and subsequent release. Relaxant drugs act on the postjunctional receptors of the neuromuscular junction, and also the prejunctional receptors on the last part of the nerve fibre, where they prevent this self-potentiating release of ACh, causing the characteristic 'fade' seen on neuromuscular monitoring during partial relaxation. (*See also* 'Neuromuscular Blockade Monitoring', Pearce A. C. In: '*Recent Advances in Anaesthesia and Analgesia – 16*', (Atkinson R. S. and Adams A. P. ed.) Edinburgh: Churchill Livingstone, 1989.)

ACh release and receptor stimulation in response to a nerve action potential is far greater than that required to elicit a single muscle fibre contraction. This large 'safety factor' means that up to 70–80% of the receptors can be occupied before surgical relaxation develops, and, conversely, reversal can be clinically adequate, even though many receptors are still blocked. Postoperative introduction of drugs that interact with relaxants may cause paralysis to redevelop.[47]

There are (at least) three receptors at the neuromuscular junction (two in the muscle and one in the nerve ending), which respond to ACh, by opening an ion channel: prejunctional, postjunctional and extrajunctional.

1. The postjunctional receptors

These are 8–9 nm in diameter with a central pit. The mouth of these special sodium channels is surrounded by five protein moieties, two of which (α) are cholinoceptors, which respond to ACh or depolarizing relaxants, causing the other three subunits to rotate to a new conformation with opening of the channel. Na^+ and Ca^{++} move into the muscle and K^+ moves out.[48] Non-depolarizing blockers bind to α units, preventing access of ACh, blocking the channel closed. (Depolarizing relaxants block the channel open, with initial stimulation, e.g. muscle fasiculations.) There are several hundred thousand receptors in each neuromuscular junction. Other drugs blocking these receptors are: local analgesics, aminoglycoside and polymyxin antibiotics, barbiturates, procainamide, quinidine and disopyramide. Other reactions in postjunctional receptor channels: (*a*) desensitization, occurring within the receptor molecule, agonist binding failing to cause an opening reaction. Caused by agonists (carbachol, suxamethonium, decamethonium), barbiturates, ACh esterase inhibitors (neostigmine, edrophonium, pyridostigmine, DFP), Ca^{++} channel blockers (verapamil), local analgesics, phenothiazines, phencyclidine, volatile anaesthetics, aminoglycoside antibiotics, substance P, alcohol. (*b*) Physical channel blockade. This prevents normal flow of ions through the tube and thus depolarization. May be caused by local analgesics (on the Na^+ channel of nerve), and Ca^{++} antagonists (on the Ca^{++} channels of heart and blood vessels). This blockade can occur in two modes, blocked when open and blocked when closed. Physical blockage by a molecule of an open channel (by cationic drugs only) relies on the channel being open in the first place, and the development of this is proportional to the frequency of channel opening. Physical blockade of a closed channel may be caused by hexamethonium, tricyclic drugs, and naloxone. Muscle relaxants, e.g. decamethonium and suxamethonium, have been known to cause physical channel blockade. (*c*) Blockade of the intracellular mechanism, e.g. by entry of decamethonium, dantrolene (Dantrium).

Phase 2 block involves the above mechanisms at different subphases (*see below*).

2. Prejunctional receptors

These control an ion channel that is specific for Na^+ (which is essential for synthesis and mobilization of transmitter). They are blocked by curare, resulting in 'fade' and exhaustion. They are blocked by aminoglycoside and polymyxin antibiotics.[49] The action of polymyxin here is due to competition with Ca^{++},[50] does not produce 'fade', can be reversed by Ca^{++} administration, and is made worse by neostigmine. Corticosteroids, barbiturates, anticonvulsants, antidysrhythmics, β-blockers, and lithium may also cause this effect, potentiating muscle relaxants.

Prejunctional block caused by relaxants is quite different from that due to Mg^{++} or aminoglycoside and polymyxin antibiotics.

3. Extrajunctional receptors

These appear all over the surface of the muscle fibre, when the muscle is denervated or deprived of nerve stimulation, by injury, burn, stroke or even disuse.[51] They are similar to, but more responsive than, junctional receptors to depolarizing agents, and less responsive to non-depolarizing agents.[52] When these receptors are present in large numbers, suxamethonium causes substantial flow of ions across the membrane producing hyperkalaemia, which is difficult to suppress by prior non-depolarizing drugs. (Tubocurarine can act as an agonist on these receptors.[53]) They are present before birth and in infancy, without causing problems for the anaesthetist.

α-adrenergic receptors have also been found on the nerve terminals. They may be involved in the improved muscle performance seen when adrenaline levels are high.

Characteristics of muscle

A skeletal muscle fibre is a very long cell, and may run the whole length of the muscle. There are many myofibrils in each cell, with neuromuscular junctions extending throughout the length of the muscle. The external ocular muscles are different, having multineuronal innervation of fibres and a tonic response to suxamethonium.

The features of a drug that determine its performance as a muscle relaxant include:

1. Its electrostatic characteristics (particularly the position and number of its quaternary nitrogen groups). An interonium distance of 11 Å, as in pancuronium, was thought to be an effective spatial arrangement, allowing the second nitrogen to repel incoming ACh electrostatically. That a bond is formed between a non-depolarizing relaxant and a neuromuscular postjunctional cholinoceptor is shown by the fact that the effect of tubocurarine is not proportional to its plasma concentration, but continues after decline of this level. (However, depolarizing relaxants do show the 'washout phenomenon'.) The high level of ionization of relaxants means that they are confined to the extracellular space, and undergo no renal tubular reabsorption.

2. Its steric nature, i.e. the way it fits the neuromuscular receptors. Receptor occupancy varies between one relaxant and another, and the steeper the occupancy/concentration profile, the more rapid is a drug's onset and wear-off characteristic. Atracurium is faster than tubocurarine. For clinical relaxation, the human diaphragm requires 90% receptor occupancy, whereas the tibialis anterior needs only 20%. An average value is around 70%. Adductor pollicis may thus still be completely paralysed, even after the patient has resumed normal respiration. This is significant, because adductor pollicis is often used for monitoring.

3. The balance between its hydrophilic and hydrophobic characteristics.

4. Its optical isomerism (e.g. l-tubocurarine is ineffective).

CHARACTERISTICS OF NON-DEPOLARIZING NEUROMUSCULAR BLOCKERS

1. Do not cause muscular fasciculation.
2. Mostly mono- or bis-quaternary salts with interonium distances of 7–14 Å, and high electrostatic characteristics, i.e. very hydrophilic.
3. Relatively slow onset (1–5 min).
4. Reversed by neostigmine and other anticholinesterases.
5. Effects reduced by adrenaline and acetylcholine. Also by suxamethonium (but not in myasthenics).
6. The relaxed muscle is still responsive to other stimuli (mechanical and electrical).
7. In partial paralysis, neuromuscular monitoring shows: (*a*) 'fade'; (*b*) post-tetanic facilitation, followed by exhaustion; and (*c*) depression of muscle twitch.
8. Potentiated by volatile agents, and Mg^{++}.[54]
9. Slow dissociation constant at receptors.
10. Mild cooling antagonizes their effects.
11. Greater cooling (below about 33°C) potentiates them.
12. Repeated tetanic bursts cause their effect to wear off.
13. Acidosis increases duration and degree of non-depolarizing block.[55]

Characteristics of depolarizing (phase 1) blocking drugs

1. Cause muscular fasciculation (but not in myasthenic man and in some other species). Extra-ocular muscles exhibit a tonic response.
2. The depolarized muscle fibres are unresponsive to other stimuli. The Na^+ channels are blocked open.
3. Repolarization is interfered with. The resting membrane potential is held up until phase 2 block develops, when it returns to $-70\,mV$.
4. Not reversed by neostigmine and other anticholinesterases.
5. In partial paralysis, the neuromuscular monitoring shows: (*a*) depression of muscle twitch; (*b*) no 'fade', but a well sustained response; and (*c*) no post-tetanic facilitation (*see below*).
6. Potentiated by isoflurane, enflurane, acetylcholine, respiratory alkalosis, hypothermia and Mg^{++}.[54]
7. Antagonized by ether, halothane, acidosis, and non-depolarizing relaxants.
8. Fast dissociation constant at receptors. There is little or no bond between drug and receptor.
9. Repeated or continuous use leads to 'phase 2 block' (*see below*).

Neuromuscular monitoring with or without the electromyogram (EMG)[56]

(*See also* Neuromuscular Blockade Monitoring, Pearce A. C. In: '*Recent Advances in Anaesthesia and Analgesia* (Atkinson R. S. and Adams A. P. ed.) Edinburgh: Churchill Livingstone, 1989).

The electric stimulus is a rectangular pulse of 0.2 ms of supramaximal intensity (100–200 mV, transcutaneous). The ulnar nerve at elbow or wrist is a convenient site, while avoiding the twin dangers of: (1) having the stimulating electrodes too close to the recording electrodes; and (2) directly stimulating the long flexors of the forearm. If an EMG is not available, a useful measure can be made by watching or feeling the fingers and thumb or by using an ECG, with electrodes on the thenar and hypothenar eminences and the back of the hand. For a tetanic burst, 50 Hz is adequate. A negative response to stimulation may mean that (1) the neuromuscular junction is blocked; (2) the stimulator is not working; or (3) the ulnar nerve is not in its usual position.

The neuromuscular transmission monitor compares well with the old force transducers.[57] Paraesthesia after neuromuscular twitch monitoring has been described postoperatively.[58]

Response to electrical stimulation

First use of nerve stimulator to assess neuromuscular transmission in man in 1949.[59] Electrical responses to nerve stimulation recorded on EMG in 1952.[60] Mechanical responses first recorded in the same year.[61] In the absence of complete paralysis caused by *non-depolarizing* block the single twitch and tetanic stimulation lead to a successive fade in the response. Following a tetanic stimulus, a single-twitch stimulus causes an increased response, i.e. Post-tetanic facilitation (thought to be due to release of increased quanta of acetylcholine for a few seconds). Post-tetanic facilitation is followed by a period of post-tetanic exhaustion due to depletion of readily available acetylcholine.

In contrast, with *depolarizing agents* there is a well-sustained response to successive stimuli following both a single-twitch stimulus and fast tetanic stimuli. There is no post-tetanic facilitation.

Train-of-Four Stimulation.[62] Four stimuli are given in succession, and the resulting contractions give as much information as a tetanic burst, and may be repeated more frequently. It is less painful than tetanic stimulation. The ratio of the amplitude of the fourth evoked response to that of the first is used as a measure of neuromuscular transmission and compares well with clinical tests of recovery.[63] The fourth is eliminated at about 75% depression of the control, the third at 80% and the second at 90%. Absence of all four indicates complete block.

A T_4/T_1 ratio > 60% is equivalent to being able to raise the head from the bed and having normal respiratory function tests.[64] A T_4/T_1 ratio > 75% is equal to being able to cough properly, open the eyes and protrude the tongue on command.

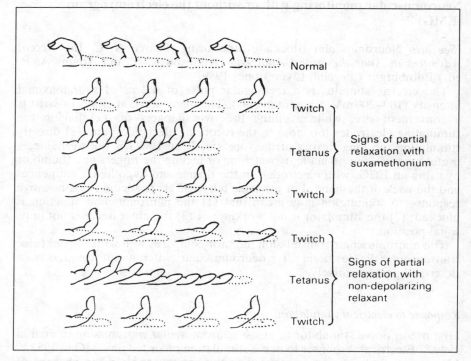

Figure 10.1 Finger twitch response to ulnar nerve stimulation

Post-tetanic count (PTC) is a method of evaluating an intense non-depolarizing neuromuscular block. The number of single twitch responses to nerve stimuli at 1 Hz following a 5-sec tetanus at 50 Hz is an indication of recovery from a relaxant, when the 'train-of-four' stimulation shows nothing.[65] Commonly, 1–5 twitch responses occur.

Double burst stimulation (DBS) (see also Engbaek J. et al. *Br. J. Anaesth.* 1989, **62**, 274). More sensitive than 'train-to-four' for manual detection of small degrees of non-depolarizing block. Two short 50 Hz bursts, separated by 750 ms, each burst containing three stimuli. At T_4/T_1 ratio of 0.5, the second burst shows a 50% reduction in force (estimated manually).

(For monitoring in tetraparesis, *see* Monitoring of curarization in patients with tetraparesis. Fiacchino F., Bricchi M. and Lasio G. *Anaesthesia* 1990, **45**, 128.)

Electromyography has been made easy and practical for the anaesthetist.[66]

Dantrolene, an agent used for the treatment of malignant hyperpyrexia, is a muscle relaxant, acting on the sarcoplasmic reticulum, reducing calcium flux.

Non-depolarizing relaxants[67]

Pharmacokinetics
Poorly bound to plasma proteins, and excepting atracurium, eliminated unchanged by the kidneys, and to a smaller extent in the bile (except gallamine). Biliary excretion increases in renal failure. The drugs are concentrated in the kidneys, liver and cartilage. Early hepatic uptake lowers the plasma concentration of these drugs (except gallamine and atracurium). These pharmacokinetics are altered in liver disease, increasing the terminal elimination half-life ($T\frac{1}{2}_\beta$) by about 50%.[68]

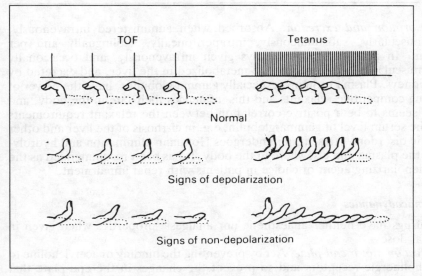

Figure 10.2 Finger twitch response to 'train-of-four' and tetanic stimulation of ulnar nerve.

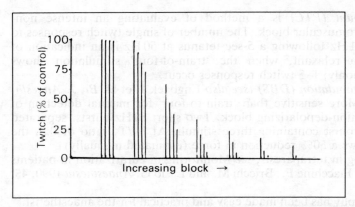

Figure 10.3 Measured responses to 'train-of-four' stimuli during progressive non-deplorazing relaxation. At 80% block (reasonable abdominal relaxation), T_4 disappears. At 90% block (excellent abdominal relaxation) T_2 has disappeared.

Table 10.1 Pharmacokinetic data

	Distribution volume (l/kg)	Clearance (ml/kg/min)	Effective blood concentration (mg/l)
Alcuronium	0.37	1.3	0.8
Atracurium	0.16	5.0	1.3
Gallamine	0.23	1.2	10.0
Metocurine	0.45	1.2	0.6
Pancuronium	0.28	1.8	0.3
Pipecuronium	1.20	14.0	–
Tubocurarine	0.45	3.0	1.0
Vecuronium	0.35	5.0	0.2

Absorption and excretion. Absorbed when administered intravenously, intramuscularly, subcutaneously, intraperitoneally, sublingually and per rectum. In practice, nearly always given intravenously, and occasionally intramuscularly. Most of them are metabolized in the liver, and excreted by the kidneys. Plasma proteins, especially gamma-globulins, have the power of binding competitive relaxants and this influences their fate in the body, and there seems to be a positive correlation between the relaxant requirements and the serum level of gamma-globulin, e.g. in cirrhosis of the liver and other hepatic disorders. Atracurium undergoes Hofmann elimination and hydrolysis in the plasma and elsewhere in the body. It has been recommended as the non-depolarizing agent of choice in patients with renal impairment.[69]

Pharmacodynamics

The drugs have neither anaesthetic nor analgesic properties when given in clinical doses.

Effect on motor end-plate. Act by preventing the binding of acetylcholine to the cholinergic receptors and so prevent the changes in the end-plate that cause muscular tone and contraction. Therapeutic doses produce the following effects in sequence: ptosis, imbalance of extra-ocular muscles with diplopia (which rarely may last several days), relaxation of muscles of the face, jaw, neck and limbs, and, finally, abdominal wall and diaphragm.

Effects on respiration. Paralysis of the muscles of respiration causing apnoea; the diaphragm, being less sensitive than other muscles, is usually the last one to be paralysed.

Effects on circulation. There may be hypotension[70] with tubocurarine, hypertension with pancuronium, tachycardia with gallamine and skin flushing with atracurium.

Synergy of relaxants. This is potentiation of one by another, when used together.[56, 71] For example, one-fifth of the usual dose of tubocurarine or pancuronium will double the effect of atracurium.

Histamine release.[56] Any of these drugs may release histamine at the first injection. Tubocurarine is the most likely to do so, and vecuronium probably the least likely. A second injection on the same day will not do so (owing to the great rapidity with which the histamine release develops tachyphylaxis). Development of true allergy with antibody formation, may of course occur in days or weeks following exposure to any drug.

Gastro-intestinal system. The cardiac sphincter is probably not relaxed completely and still has an opening pressure of 25 cm of water.

Clinical use

Following induction of anaesthesia the relaxant is injected intravenously. The patient's lungs are gently inflated with nitrous oxide, oxygen and volatile agent. Care must be taken not to inflate the stomach. After 1–3 min, when the effect of the muscle-relaxant drug is maximal, intubation of the trachea is carried out. IPPV is maintained, and additional doses of muscle relaxant are given as required.

During thiopentone–gas–oxygen–relaxant anaesthesia the following clinical signs often indicate the need for more relaxant: (1) hiccup, caused by contraction of the periphery of the diaphragm; (2) rigidity of the abdominal wall; (3) increased resistance to inflation of the lung (in the absence of respiratory obstruction), i.e. decreased compliance; (4) bucking or coughing on the tracheal tube; and (5) as indicated by neuromuscular monitoring.

Analgesic supplements may be required if: (1) the patient moves his skeletal muscles in response to the surgical stimulus, e.g. face, limb or neck muscles, especially swallowing or frowning; (2) rise of blood pressure and pulse; (3) sweating, unexplained by other causes, occurs; and (4) there is reflex response to surgical stimuli, e.g. hiccups. Many anaesthetists routinely administer an intravenous or inhalation supplement to prevent possible awareness.

Whenever muscle relaxants are used, it is of paramount importance to see that the patient is breathing reasonably deeply before leaving the operating table. A relatively large number of patients may have a defect in neuromuscular transmission on their arrival in the postoperative room. Respiratory depression at the end of the operation should be treated either by IPPV until the tidal volume becomes normal or, more usually, by administration of neostigmine with atropine. The use of a nerve stimulator to monitor the proper recovery of the neuromuscular junction is employed.

CLINICAL SIGNS OF INCOMPLETE REVERSAL

(1) Shallow respiration; (2) Jerky respiration; (3) 'Tracheal tug', and 'see-saw' respiration, where, as the abdomen moves out, the chest moves in; (4) Cyanosis; (5) A restless, frightened, struggling patient, who says that he cannot breathe; (6) Diplopia; (7) Inability to raise head or extrude tongue.

MANAGEMENT OF INCOMPLETE REVERSAL

1. IPPV is given with a mask and oxygen, while the degree of incomplete reversal is assessed.

2. If mild (T_4/T_1 ratio > 50%, respiration is almost adequate) more neostigmine or other anticholinesterase is given.

3. If severe (T_4/T_1 ratio < 50%, respiration is obviously inadequate) the patient is sedated (e.g. with diazepam) intubated and IPPV continued with a ventilator for at least an hour, acid-base status is determined and corrected. The serum electrolytes are estimated and normalized. Re-assessment is performed using a nerve stimulator.

4. Alternative diagnoses are considered, which include overdose of inhalation agents, opioids; antibiotics or barbiturates, renal failure, botulism, myasthenia gravis, myasthenic syndrome, adrenal failure, hypothermia, renal failure, overdose of relaxant.

Infants and children tolerate muscle relaxants well if the dosage is suitably adjusted to their general condition and body weight (*see* Chapter 22).

Choice of non-depolarizing relaxant.

Anaesthetists use the relaxants with which they are familiar. However, the following suggestion for preferred relaxants may help the tyro:

In renal failure – vecuronium or atracurium; in myasthenia gravis – if relaxants are essential, one-tenth of the normal dose of atracurium; in hepatic failure – atracurium; in arterial surgery, to maintain arterial pressure – pancuronium; to deliberately reduce blood pressure – tubocurarine; in obstetrics – any relaxant except gallamine; in short cases – vecuronium; and for 'crash induction' without using suxamethonium – atracurium or vecuronium.

Occasionally some residual paresis of the muscles of accommodation persists for 24 hours after operation, making reading difficult.

The drugs must be used with special care if given to the same patient on two occasions within 24 hours, because a cumulative effect may occur.

Atracurium besylate[56] (*Tracrium*)

First used in 1980.[72]

PHARMACY

Mol Wt 1243. pH of solution 3.5, stored at 4°C in refrigerator.

PHARMACOKINETICS

1. Absorption: from i.m. and i.v. routes.
2. Distribution: throughout ECF. No effective crossing of the placenta.[73]
3. Metabolism: Hofmann degradation and alkaline ester hydrolysis in the plasma and elsewhere in the body (producing a monoquarternary alcohol at first). (A. W. von Hofmann (1818–1892) German chemist who made his discovery in 1848.)[74] Elimination half-life for atracurium is 20 min. The resulting tertiary amine, laudanosine,[75] has slow renal elimination, crosses the blood-brain barrier and increases the MAC of halothane by 30% in high concentrations (unlikely to be found in clinical situations). Mean half-life for the monoquarternary alcohol is 39 min, that for laudanosine is 234 min.

PHARMACODYNAMICS

1. Bolus dose average 0.5 mg/kg. Infusion average 0.5 mg/kg/h. Potentiated by enflurane and isoflurane, less so by halothane.[76]
Infants are slightly more resistant than adults.[77] Dose for premature neonates is 0.3 mg/kg
2. Speed of onset 1–2 min. This can be halved by the 'Priming technique', where 0.1 mg/kg is injected 3–5 min before the main dose (unpleasant for patient).
3. Duration 20–40 min, even in anephric patients,[78] the elderly and severely ill.[79] Duration doubled at 25°C.[80]
4. Quality of reversal with neostigmine or edrophonium is extremely good.[81]
5. Side-effects (no vagolytic effects on the heart. This may allow bradycardia to occur.)[82] Angioneurotic oedema has occurred.[83] Histamine release[56] does not occur when the drug is injected slowly over 75 s,[84] or when less than 0.6 mg/kg is injected.
The clinical signs sometimes following atracurium (e.g. flushing of the skin, maculopapular, pruritic rash, suggestive of mediator release from mast cells in the presence of IgE) do not correlate with plasma histamine levels,[85] nor with complement C_3 conversion.[86] These effects are however abolished by pretreatment with i.v. cimetidine 4 mg/kg and chlorpheniramine 0.1 mg/kg or phenylhydramine 0.3 mg/kg.[87] Intraocular pressure no change, or a fall.[88] Intracranial pressure – unaltered.
Suitable in anephric patients (the relaxant of choice).[89] Suitable in patients with atypical cholinesterase.[90] Suitable in intermediate cases – (a relaxant of choice).[91] Long cases – suitable with intermittent injection or continuous infusion.[92] Infusion rate 0.5 mg/kg/h with cessation at 15 min before the estimated end of the operation (e.g. at closure of the peritoneum in an abdominal case). Simple neuromuscular monitoring is desirable but not essential. Caesarean section – suitable.[93] With tourniquets – suitable.[94] Organophosphorus poisoning – suitable.[95] Myasthenia gravis – suitable.[96]

Vecuronium bromide[56] (*Norcuron*)

First used in 1979 in France.[42, 43]

CHEMICAL BASIS

It has rings A and D. The D ring is similar to pancuronium. The A ring is modified by a tertiary nitrogen at 2B, giving less stability in solution, a shorter time-course and lack of cumulation *in vivo*.[97] The solution (pH 4) is stable for 24 h at 25°C. Mol Wt 638.

PHARMACOKINETICS

Absorption – from i.m. or i.v. route:
    Distribution – throughout the ECF. The lipophilic effect of the single quaternary nitrogen enhances rapid uptake into hepatocytes. No effective crossing of the placenta.
    Metabolism – theoretically in the liver with excretion in the urine.

PHARMACODYNAMICS

Bolus dose average 0.1 mg/kg (adults, infants and elderly). Infusion 0.2 mg/kg/hr. Potentiated (but not much extended) most by enflurane, >isoflurane >halothane. Potentiated and prolonged by previous suxamethonium. Time of onset 1–2 min (can be shortened by preloading with a small dose, 6 min before the main dose).[98] Duration 10–20 min (much longer with higher doses), not influenced by renal failure. Side-effects – no effect on vascular system in clinical doses. (*See also Clinics in Anesthesiology*. 1985, **3**, 347.)

Tubocurarine chloride BP (*Tubarine*)

Source from bark, leaves and vines of *Chondrodendron Tomentosum* growing near upper reaches of the Amazon. Has long been used by Amazonian Indians as poison for the heads of their arrows. They transport it in bamboo tubes, hence the name tubocurarine. It is a monoquaternary alkaloid, an isoquinoline derivative.

PHARMACOKINETICS

Dose – 0.5 mg/kg
    Onset: 3 min after i.v. injection; 10 min after i.m. injection.
    Duration: about 40 min, prolonged by volatile anaesthetics, shortened by alkalosis. Cumulation occurs.
    Distribution: to extracellular fluid, muscles, liver, kidney, and cartilage. It is retained in spleen, heart and lungs in an inactive state. It is bound to serum albumin.

PHARMACODYNAMICS

Non-depolarizing block with pre- and post-junctional components. Reversal by anticholinesterases is satisfactory, except in acidosis, hypokalaemia or overdose.

SIDE-EFFECTS

Respiration. Paralysis of muscles of respiration, rarely bronchospasm, notably in asthmatic patients.

Histamine release. Occurs but circulatory collapse is rare.

Circulation. Hypotension due to ganglion blockade, potentiated by halothane and reversed by calcium. Allergic circulatory collapse due to histamine release has been reported, but is rare; anaphylactoid response has occurred.[99] There is an antifibrillatory action on the ventricles and a decreased likelihood of dysrhythmia. The drug is strongly concentrated in heart muscle.

OTHER FEATURES

Small amounts cross the placenta, not affecting the baby in clinical dose. Patients with liver disease may require more tubocurarine than usual.

Potency enhanced by inhalation agents, 1.5–2 times (enflurane > isoflurane > halothane), and by previous injection of suxamethonium.[100]

Gallamine triethiodide BP (*Flaxedil*)

PHARMACODYNAMICS AND PHARMACOKINETICS

Shows an atropine-like vagal blocking effect on the post-ganglionic nerve endings of the heart, which results in tachycardia, even with small doses, e.g. 20 mg. This outlasts the relaxant effect. It often causes a slight rise in blood pressure, and this with the tachycardia may result in more bleeding.[101] Allergic reactions have been reported following its use.[102] It passes the placental barrier. About 80% is excreted by the kidneys, and so it should not be used in patients with renal disease.

Dose: 1–2 mg/kg.

Alcuronium chloride, diallyl nortoxiferine (*Alloferin*)

This is a medium to long-acting non-depolarizing relaxant. Deteriorates on exposure to air and sunlight and therefore is supplied in coloured ampoules. Does not cross the placenta in significant amounts.[103] It is bound to serum albumin. Should be avoided in renal failure.[104] Anaphylactoid reactions have been reported.[105] After the distribution phase (20 min) it is metabolized very slowly.

Dose: 0.3 mg/kg.

Duration: 20–60 min.

Pancuronium bromide (*Pavulon*)

First described in 1967.[106]

PHARMACODYNAMICS

A bis-quaternary amino-steroid, devoid of hormonal activity, first synthesized by Savage and Hewett in 1964 and used clinically in 1967.[38, 39] An insignificant proportion of it crosses the placental barrier. It causes noradrenaline release, and 30% is excreted by the kidney, 25% excreted in bile (one-third of this as hydroxylated drug). It should be avoided in renal failure.[107] Does not cross the blood-brain barrier. It becomes strongly bound to gamma-globulin and moderately bound to serum albumin, so less than 13% of the dose is unbound and active.[108] Not cumulative. Sometimes it causes stimulation of the myocardium[109] with rise in pulse rate and blood pressure and block of vagal muscarinic receptors.[110] It can release histamine from the tissues. In total biliary obstruction the drug should be used with care.[111] Safe in patients susceptible to malignant hyperpyrexia.[112]

Dose: 0.05–0.1 mg/kg.
Duration: 20–30 min.

Mivacurium chloride[113] (Mivacron)

A benzylisoquinolinium compound. This is a short-acting muscle relaxant, metabolized by plasma cholinesterase, with a duration of action approximately twice that of suxamethonium. The products of hydrolysis are eliminated in the bile and urine. Onset time is reported as 3.5 min with a duration of 10–15 min. Major cardiovascular side-effects have not been reported, although there may be some histamine release, some fall of arterial pressure and some fall in heart rate. The duration of action may be prolonged when plasma cholinesterase is low. Dose: 0.15–0.25 mg/kg.

Doxacurium

Dose: 0.03 mg/kg.
Peak onset: 4–6 mins,[114]
Duration: 1 h.
Side-effects: vascular effects are minor.[115]

Pipecuronium (Arduan)

Dose: 0.05 mg/kg.[116]
Chemistry. A steroid analogue of pancuronium with quaternary nitrogen at the 2 and 16 positions and longer interonium distance.
Pharmacy. 4 mg powder/ampoule, solution stable 24 h at 4°C.
Pharmacokinetics. Two-compartment model. Concentrated in kidney, liver and spleen; 85% is excreted by the kidneys.[117] Does not cross the placenta. Cumulation occurs. Potentiated by enflurane. Similar to pancuronium.[118]
Pharmacodynamics. Reversibly inhibits serum cholinesterase. Onset in 3 min. Duration 1–2 h.
Side-effects. Very little on circulation.

Antagonists to non-depolarizing relaxants (Anticholinesterase drugs)

Neostigmine

HISTORY

Neostigmine methylsulphate (Prostigmine) was synthesized by Aeschlimann and Reinert in 1931.[119] It is twice as powerful as physostigmine (isolated in

1864 from the calabar bean by Sir T. R. Fraser (1841–1920), Scottish pharmacologist who also showed that atropine counteracts its effects, *Trans. R. Soc.* Edinburgh 1866/67, **24**, 715, and discovered the drug strophanthin), the anticurare action of which was discovered by Jacob Pal (1863–1936) in 1900,[120] and used in animal experimentation in 1909.[121]

It prevents the normal hydrolysis of acetylcholine and so allows it to accumulate.

PHARMACOKINETICS

Neostigmine is partly broken down by serum cholinesterase and partly excreted unchanged by the kidneys. Renal failure reduces the clearance its drugs by up to four times.[122] Binds to the esteratic subsite of cholinesterase with its carbonate group.

Neostigmine is also a depolarizer and can cause on its own a depolarizing type of block[123] due to build-up of acetylcholine. Phase 2 block can eventually result. The amount needed to cause paralysis by persistent depolarization is much greater, normally, than that required to antagonize a clinical dose of non-depolarizing relaxant. It does not always reverse block due to: (1) aminoglycoside antibiotics and (2) phase 2 block following suxamethonium.

When injected into a conscious patient it may cause muscular fasciculations and severe colic. In addition, it is a direct stimulant of cholinergic effector cells. It has nicotinic effects and has a direct stimulant action on muscle. In small doses it stimulates and in larger doses it depresses autonomic ganglia. It also has muscarinic properties (from *Amantia muscaria*), which are blocked by atropine, e.g. bradycardia, intestinal peristalsis and spasm, bronchial and salivary secretion and bronchospasm, stimulation of the sweat glands, contraction of the pupil and contraction of the bladder. Dose is 2.5–5 mg,[124] with atropine 1.5 mg or glycopyrronium 0.5 mg. Renal excretion accounts for 50% of its clearance.[125] Duration: 2 hours.

Edrophonium (*Tensilon*)

Edrophonium has, like neostigmine, anticholinesterase, depolarizing and direct stimulating actions on the motor end-plate. It may cause fasciculation; quicker in onset, but small doses (10 mg) are not as long lasting as neostigmine, consequently recurarization may follow (although this is not seen following repeated injection of 20 mg at 3-min intervals).[126] Dose is 10–70 mg. It is rapidly metabolized, in small doses (10 mg) but not in large doses (70 mg)[127] when its pharmacokinetics are similar to pyridostigmine and neostigmine.[128] Its pattern of reversal suggests that it acts at prejunctional receptors.

Pyridostigmine[129] (*Mestinon; Regonol*)

Used in treatment of myasthenia gravis. Its duration of action (6 h) makes it especially suitable for reversal of relaxants in cases of renal failure where the excretion of the relaxant may be delayed.[130] Dose: 10 mg. It is capable of penetrating the blood-brain barrier.

Physostigmine salicylate[131] (*Antilirium*)

An alkaloid obtained from the West African calabar bean. An anticholinesterase with a tertiary amine structure that can cross the blood-brain barrier. Used to treat the anticholinergic syndrome (*see* Chapter 14) produced by atropine, hyoscine and other related alkaloids. It does not adequately antagonize neuromuscular block in doses up to 4 mg.

Clinical uses of neostigmine

In the average case, towards the end of the operation, $Paco_2$ should be normalized. Atropine and neostigmine are given. If 5 mg of neostigmine does not reverse the block, as assessed by nerve stimulator, the following factors should be considered: (1) has enough time been allowed since the last dose of relaxant? Twitch height using a nerve stimulator may take up to 15 min to recover, or up to 30 min when height is initially less than 20% of control; (2) has too much relaxant been given, e.g. in renal failure and elderly patients? (3) what is the acid-base and electrolyte status? (4) what is the temperature? (5) is the patient receiving other drugs that might make antagonism difficult, e.g. aminoglycosides? and (6) has excretion of the relaxant been impeded?

Breathing can be stimulated by moving the tube within the trachea and by application of a suction catheter to the carina. CO_2, 5%, can also be given. IPPV must be carried out until the patient can ventilate himself adequately. Low blood pressure and poor tissue perfusion may retard reversal.

Clinical signs of adequate relaxant reversal by neostigmine:[132] (1) return of normal tidal exchange measured either by an anemometer or by the flow-meters of the anaesthetic machine using a Ruben or other non-rebreathing valve; (2) ability to cough; (3) ability to open eyes and keep them open; (4) presence of tone in the masseters; (5) ability to raise the head from the pillow or to lift arm;[133] and (6) return of full muscular activity shown after electrical nerve stimulation.

Failure to breathe after full reversal may be caused by low CO_2 levels, opioid depression, breath-holding, other causes of respiratory depression (e.g. cerebral).

It is of fundamental importance that the anaesthetist should not leave the patient until he is able to ventilate himself adequately and his muscular power has returned. If this is not so, IPPV should be continued.

For paediatric dosage *see* Chapter 22.

Depolarizing relaxants

Suxamethonium chloride, Succinylcholine (*Scoline; Anectine; Curaryl*)

HISTORY

Prepared in 1906 by Reid Hunt (1870–1948) and Taveau of Boston.[134] In 1949 Bovet and his colleagues[135] and J. C. Castillo and Edwin de Beer[136] described the paralysing action of the *bis*-choline esters of succinic acid, showing that they produced muscular paralysis of short duration and rapid onset. Used in anaesthesia in 1951.[137] Prolonged apnoea found to be associated with an abnormal cholinesterase value by James G. Bourne of London and his colleagues in 1952.[138] The hereditary nature of this abnormality was shown in 1953[139] (*see also* Dorkin, Huw R. *Med. Hist.* 1982, **26**, 145).

CHEMISTRY

The dicholine ester of succinic acid. The active part of the molecule is the cation, formed by the succinic radical with a quaternary ammonium group at each end of the molecular chain. If these end-groups contain three methyl groups (CH_3), the substance is a suxamethonium compound; if two methyl and one ethyl (C_2H_5), then it is an ethonium compound – hence suxamethonium and suxethonium. Solutions deteriorate in hot environments.

DOSE

1 mg/kg (2–3 mg/kg neonates less than 10 weeks of age). Onset in 10–30 sec. Duration of bolus 1–5 min. Average dose for intubation 25–100 mg. By infusion 4–10 mg/min as 0.1% solution.

Pharmacy

Hydrolysis occurs at room temperature. The drug should be stored at 4°C.

PHARMACOKINETICS[140]

   Absorption. i.m., i.v., or s.c.
   Distribution. Throughout the ECF, and slightly across the placenta.
   Metabolism. First order pharmacokinetic elimination by hydrolysis to succinyl monocholine, then to choline and succinic acid by plasma cholinesterase. (EC 3.1.1.8.) Dibucaine number (DN) 75–85. This is the percentage inhibition of cholinesterase by 10^{-5} molar solution of dibucaine. The 'Fluoride number' is the percentage inhibition of cholinesterase by 5×10^{-5} molar sodium fluoride. Urea inhibition has also been used. Plasma cholinesterase is found in plasma but not in red cells; also in the liver, brain, kidneys and pancreas. It also hydrolyses ester-linked local analgesics and other drugs. Plasma cholinesterase is a lipoprotein synthesized in the liver. Failure of its action, due to abnormality or deficiency, prolongs the action of suxamethonium. Of the population 94% are normal E^uE^u genotypes with normal enzyme activity and a DN of 75–85. Three abnormal genes exist: E^a (atypical) homozygotes comprise 0.03% of the population; E^f (fluoride-resistant) homozygotes comprise 0.0003% of the population; E^s (silent) homozygotes comprise 0.001% of the population. Normal serum cholinesterase level about 80 units/ml.

ABNORMALITIES OF SUXAMETHONIUM METABOLISM.[141]

   1. *Abnormal plasma cholinesterase (inherited)*[142]
      1.1 Atypical cholinesterase – Mendelian recessive E^aE^a homozygotes (1 per 3000 of population) have 1–2 h apnoea, during which phase 2 block develops (DN 16–25). Heterozygotes (1 per 25 of population) have little or no disturbance (DN 50–65), with apnoeas up to 10 min.

1.2 Fluoride-resistant. Homozygotes have 1 h apnoea, with phase 2 block (DN 16–25). Heterozygotes have 10 min apnoea (DN 50–65).

1.3 Silent gene.

All the possible combinations of heterozygotes exist (1 in 25 of the population, with apnoeas around 10 min).[143]

2. Plasma cholinesterase deficiency.

2.1 Acquired. After X-ray therapy, after organophosphorus poisoning, in hyperpyrexia, in cardiac failure, in hepatic failure, uraemia, hypoproteinaemia due to malnutrition or plasmapheresis, e.g. in lupus erythematosus, myasthenia gravis, Goodpasture's syndrome, and Rh incompatibility,[144] in trophoblastic disease,[145] pregnancy, puerperium, the newborn (50% of adult levels), myxoedema, asthma, obesity and following treatment with: cyclophosphamide, ecothiopate, procainamide, quinidine, phenothiazines, ketamine, trimetaphan, pancuronium, MAOIs, oral contraceptives (20–30% reduction) and metrifonate (antibilharzial drug).[142]

2.2 Congenital. Presents unexpected danger to the patient. Hydrolysis proceeds only at the rate of 5% per hour. Inherited absence due to the silent gene E^S.[146] Homozygotes have 1–2 h apnoea, and phase 2 block develops in the course of this. Heterozygotes have normal DN and FN[147] but only half the normal plasma cholinesterase activity.[142]

3. Plasma cholinesterase antagonism. By anticholinesterases (eg. neostigmine), and tacrine.

4. Plasma cholinesterase excess. The result is shortening of the duration of activity of the drug.

4.1 Acquired. In obesity, toxic goitre, nephrosis, depression, psoriasis, and alcoholism.

4.2 Congenital. The C_5 variant.

PHARMACODYNAMICS

Muscular system.

Phase 1 block preceded by muscle fasciculation (see above), potentiated by isoflurane, anticholinesterases, magnesium and lithium.

Phase 2 block accompanies the prolonged action of suxamethonium, whether due to infusion or to abnormal cholinesterase activity. This development is slightly potentiated by enflurane and rather less so by halothane.[148] The development has 4 phases:[149]

Phase A – depolarizing block which may last 30–50 min.

Phase B – non-depolarizing block develops quite quickly.

Phase C – A plateau 30-min period of no change.

Phase D – A 'wearing-off phase' up to 2 h long.

In infants, phase 2 block may not be associated with prolonged paralysis.[150]

Reversal – phase 2 block has been reversed by neostigmine and other anticholinesterases, but the results are not consistent, thus this approach is not in routine use. A test dose of edrophonium can be used as a pointer to the likely response.[151]

SIDE-EFFECTS

Prolonged apnoea. This was first reported in 1952.[152] After a single dose of suxamethonium the commonest causes are:

1. Atypical serum cholinesterase. Homozygotes for the atypical gene show this. A heparinized sample of blood and a full clinical history will be required. Over 25% of patients with suxamethonium apnoea have normal enzymes.[153]

2. Dehydration and electrolyte imbalance leading to the development of dual block at a very early stage.

3. An overdose of the relaxant drug, i.e. total of more than 1 g in an infusion.

4. A low serum cholinesterase level in the blood. This seldom causes prolonged apnoea if 50 mg is not exceeded, a dose adequate for most patients requiring a single injection, e.g. for intubation or ECT. It is unlikely to be the cause of apnoea prolonged beyond 20–30 min, if the serum cholinesterase level is more than 25 units. Apnoea due to a low cholinesterase value may be reversed by a blood transfusion because even stored blood contains 30 units/ml of cholinesterase and retains 80% of its cholinesterase activity after storage for 25 days at 6°C. 0.5 l of fresh blood restores the serum cholinesterase level by 10 units/ml; 0.5 l of stored blood restores it by 5 units/ml. Fresh frozen plasma is also useful because it contains 36–40 units/ml. Cholinesterase activity can be measured in patients who have undergone plasmapheresis and in whom the use of suxamethonium is contemplated.[154]

5. An excessive formation of succinyl monocholine. In 1952 it was pointed out that the hydrolysis of succinylcholine takes place in two stages, succinyl monocholine being the intermediate product.[155] This has between 5% and 20% the relaxing effect of the parent compound,[156] but because it is hydrolysed rather slowly by both acetyl and serum cholinesterase, it may accumulate in the bloodstream, but only if relatively large amounts of suxamethonium (more than 0.5 g) have been used, e.g. as drip infusion.

6. Phase 2 block (dual block), a phenomenon described by Zaimis[157] in 1953.

Other causes of prolonged apnoea

1. Central depression of the respiratory centre by a narcotic analgesic, thiopentone, or volatile anaesthetics.

2. Hypocapnia. In this case respiration will recommence if the carbon dioxide level is allowed to rise above 6 kPa (42 mmHg).

3. Hypercapnia. Very high carbon dioxide levels (> 13 kPa) can paralyse the respiratory centre and cause apnoea.

4. Depression of the lung stretch receptor mechanism during controlled respiration. This will usually yield to the addition of carbon dioxide to the inspired gas for short periods.

5. Reflex laryngeal apnoea. Due to the presence of a tracheal tube. Removal of the tube or deflation of the cuff leads to restoration of spontaneous respiration.

6. Head injury and acute rise of intracranial pressure.

7. There are some gravely ill patients who breathe again only with difficulty once they become apnoeic. In such patients it may be wise not to abolish voluntary respiration at all.

8. Metabolic acidosis can cause a clinical picture similar to that of myoneural block. The cause of prolonged apnoea is not always fully understood.[158]

Differential diagnosis between hypopnoea caused by central depression and that caused by peripheral paralysis when nerve stimulator is not available
    1. *Central Depression*. Breathing slow, reasonably deep. No tracheal tug; no pause at end of inspiration.
    2. *Peripheral Paralysis* (myoneural block). Breathing jerky, shallow and of normal rate. Pause after inspiration and again after expiration (Morton's rectangular breathing).[159] Tracheal tug.

Management of unexpectedly prolonged apnoea after suxamethonium
    1. IPPV and sedation are maintained until monitoring shows the block to have worn off.
    2. A blood sample is taken for cholinesterase analysis.
    3. Fresh frozen plasma or cholase may be administered to correct the deficiency.
    4. Near relatives are screened and if positive, issued with warning cards or bangles.

Management of known or suspected suxamethonium sensitive patients
    1. Suxamethonium is avoided if possible.
    2. If suxamethonium is indicated for the anaesthetic sequence (e.g. for ECT), it may be given to documented heterozygotes only, in very small test doses, e.g. 0.05–0.1 mg/kg, when it produces a normal response.[161] A normal dose of 1 mg/kg, when given to a heterozygote, produces apnoea for 10 min, and very rarely up to an hour.
    3. In homozygotes, a rapid-onset, short-acting non-depolarizing drug may be used (e.g. mivacurium).
    Hyperkalaemia. Potassium is released from muscles following suxamethonium injection, causing a rise of serum potassium of 0.2–0.4 mmol/1. Much greater hyperkalaemia occurs after burns (3 weeks–3 months), tetanus and spinal cord injuries. Also in patients with upper and lower motor neurone lesions, congenital cerebral palsy, Duchenne's muscular dystrophy, wasting secondary to chronic arterial insufficiency, and severe intra-abdominal infection. This great release is the result of extrajunctional receptor stimulation (*see above*).
    Raised intraocular pressure. (This may be important in the presence of a perforating eye injury.) Suxamethonium, 1 mg/kg, raises the pressure by an average of 7 mmHg, partly as a result of tonic contraction of the extraocular muscles, with return to normal pressure in 10 minutes, caused by absorption of aqueous humour (the extraocular muscles may remain contracted for 30 min, upsetting the calculations used in squint correction). The lens is left nearer the corneal endothelium, with greater risk of damage during lens extraction and implants. Some workers view its use in severe glaucoma with reserve.
    Muscle pains. These were first observed in 1950.[162] The pain is influenced by age, sex and physical fitness. It is suggested that uncoordinated muscle contractions that precede paralysis are the cause of the pain[163] but this is probably not so.[164] Pains are more frequent in women and middle-aged patients than in those at the extremes of age and in men. The incidence is

reduced during pregnancy.[165] The longer the interval between the injection of an intravenous barbiturate and the suxamethonium, the more intense the postoperative discomfort. Pains may be delayed until the third or fourth postoperative day. Post-suxamethonium sore throat may be a muscle-produced pain and not due to trauma.[166]

Pain is less frequent in patients who are muscularly 'fit' than in the 'unfit' and when the injection is given slowly.

Prevention of muscle pains
1. Pre-curarization,[167] the i.v. injection of a small dose of a non-depolarizing relaxant (e.g. tubocurarine, 3–5 mg[168] or gallamine, 5–20 mg) 3 min before the suxamethonium. Larger doses (tubocurarine, 10 mg or gallamine, 60 mg) given 1 min before the suxamethonium are said to be equally effective and to cause no problems with either intubation or prolonged apnoea. Muscle fasciculations may also be reduced by i.v. injection of suxamethonium, 10 mg, and injection of the rest of the dose after a 1-min interval,[169] or when it is given in a drip at a rate of less than 2 mg per sec.[170]
2. Intravenous injection of lignocaine 2–6 mg/kg following thiopentone and 3 min before the relaxant.[171] This also prolongs apnoea. Intravenous lignocaine may cause significant sinus bradycardia or even asystole.[172] It restricts increase in serum potassium and decrease in serum calcium.[173]

It is suggested that the muscle-spindle injury – as shown by the creatinine phosphokinase level[171] – is produced by suxamethonium given intermittently, especially if the patient is receiving halothane. This may result in myoglobinuria which may, among other things, give a positive Haemostix reaction in urine. Visible fasciculations are not constantly related to the severity of any subsequent symptoms.[171, 174].

These muscle pains may not be prevented by atracurium.[175] A rise in myoglobin can be detected in some patients who receive suxamethonium; this can be prevented by the prior injection of a non-depolarizing relaxant.[176]

Effect in malignant hyperpyrexia. Suxamethonium is one of the drugs most commonly implicated in this condition. Incidence 1:100 000 adult anaesthetics. It then causes muscle rigidity, not relaxation. *See* Chapter 14. Suxamethonium is best avoided in children with Duchenne muscular dystrophy because of the risk of malignant hyperpyrexia.[177]

Dystrophia Myotonica. Suxamethonium exacerbates this with body rigidity preventing respiration and intubation.

Cardiovascular system. Bradycardia and cardiac arrest may occur on the second, or even the first injection. Prevented by prior atropine or gallamine. Cardiac arrest due to hyperkalaemia may occur when suxamethonium is given to patients with existing hyperkalaemia, 3-week old burns, crush injuries, widespread denervation, or tetanus. The treatment is standard CPR with lignocaine to prevent dysrhythmias, and measures to reduce serum potassium.

Suxamethonium may cause a rise in blood pressure, perhaps due to ganglion stimulation, a nicotinic response.

Central nervous system. Muscarinic effects may occur.

Alimentary system. Muscarinic effects, salivation and gastric secretion. Increase in intragastric pressure to more than 20 mmHg, due to severe muscle fasciculation. The cricopharyngeal sphincter loses its tone.

Placental barrier. Small amounts of this highly polarized drug do in fact reach the fetus, but are without effect on the baby. Excellent for operative obstetrics and Caesarean section.

Histamine release. True anaphylaxis without previous exposure, has been reported, with bronchospasm, hypotension, acute circulatory collapse,[178] pharyngeal and facial oedema, and a positive transfer (Prausnitz–Kustner) reaction.

PREVENTION OF SOME SIDE-EFFECTS

(Except perhaps rise of intraocular pressure)

1. Self-taming by 10 mg suxamethonium injected a minute before induction of anaesthesia (unpleasant for the patient).

2. Precurarization 3 min before induction of anaesthesia; gallamine 20 mg, tubocurarine 3 mg, vecuronium 0.5 mg,[179] or other non-depolarizing drug. *See also* under 'muscle pains'.

Use of different relaxants in the same patient

The effects of different non-depolarizing relaxants are additive. In general, depolarizers should not be used after non-depolarizers. Only if the effects of the first drug have worn off should one of the other group be used.

Some factors influencing neuromuscular block

In disease

1. *Myasthenia gravis and myasthenic syndrome* (*see* Chapter 20).
2. *Liver and kidney disease.*
3. *Electrolyte imbalance.* Particularly changes in potassium.
4. *Connective tissue diseases* may show increased sensitivity to non-depolarizing relaxants.
5. *Dystrophia myotonica. See above.*
6. *Hypothermia* potentiates the effects of depolarizing relaxants and tends to diminish the activity of non-depolarizing relaxants. The action of atracurium may be prolonged, perhaps as a result of slowing of the Hofmann elimination process.[179]
7. *Repeated plasmapheresis* may lead to progressive depletion of serum cholinesterase.[180]

Effect of drugs

1. *Aminoglycoside antibiotics.* Neomycin (first reported by Pridgen J. E. *Surgery* 1956, **40**, 571), streptomycin, kanamycin, gentamicin, tobramycin, bacitracin, colimycin, polymixin, clindamycin and colistimethate, if given parenterally or intraperitoneally, may cause a non-depolarizing block that will be potentiated by non-depolarizing relaxants. It is not always reversed by

neostigmine. Tetracycline and penicillin show no neuromuscular blocking activity.

2. Ecothiopate eye drops are an anticholinesterase used in the treatment of glaucoma. Apnoea from an intubating dose of suxamethonium may be prolonged. The effects of ecothiopate drops may last for 3 weeks.

3. Aprotinin (Trasylol). Slightly reduces the serum cholinesterase activity of the blood, but unless its level is already very low from other causes, prolonged apnoea is very unlikely.

4. Metriphonate, used in the treatment of urinary schistosomiasis, reduces serum cholinesterase.[181]

5. Lithium Salts. Lithium was introduced for the control of mania in 1949.[182] Now used for the treatment of manic-depressive states. A raised blood lithium level potentiates the effects of anaesthesia and relaxants and it is suggested that at least two doses should be omitted before anaesthesia.[183] Delayed onset and prolongation of suxamethonium block may result.[184] Potent diuretics may increase its toxicity.[185] Pre-operative dehydration is to be avoided because as this may cause lithium toxicity.[186]

References

1. Carman J. A. *Anaesthesia* 1968, **23**, 706.
2. Holmes T. *Brody* London: T. Fischer Unwin, 1898.
3. Reprinted in 'Classical File', *Surv. Anesthesiol.* 1978, **22**, 98; McDowall G. *Anaesth. Intensive Care* 1982, **10**, 4; Symposium on Charles Waterton, *Br. J. Anaesth.* 1983, **55**, 221; Maltby J. R. In: *Anaesthesia; Essays on its History* (Rupreht J. van, Lieburg M. J. et al. ed.), Chapter 2.4. Berlin: Springer-Verlag, 1985.
4. Bernard C. *C. R. Soc. Biol. Paris* 1851, **2**, 195; *Leçon sur les Effets des Substances Toxiques et Médicamenteuses.* Paris: Baillière, 1851.
5. Paton A. *Practitioner* 1979, **223**, 849.
6. Sayer L. A. *N. Y. J. Med.* 1858, **4**, 250.
7. Boehm R. *Arch. Pharm.* 1897, **235**, 660.
8. Läwen A. *Beitr. Klin. Chir.* 1912, **80**, 168.
9. Dale H. H. *J. Pharmacol. Exp. Ther.* 1914, **6**, 147.
10. Dale H. H. *Br. Med. J.* 1934, **1**, 835.
11. Cole L. *Lancet* 1934, **2**, 475.
12. King H. *J. Chem. Soc.* 1935, **57**, 1381; *Nature* 1935, **135**, 469.
13. West R. *Lancet* 1936, **1**, 12.
14. Bennett A. E. *JAMA* 1940, **114**, 322; Bennett A. E. et al. *JAMA* 1940, **114**, 1791; Bennett A. E. *Am. J. Psychiatry* 1941, **97**, 1014.
15. Palmer H. *J. Ment. Sci.* 1946, **92**, 411.
16. Betcher A. M. *Anesth. Analg. (Cleve.)* 1977, **56**, 305.
17. Griffith H. R. and Johnson G. E. *Anesthesiology* 1942, **3**, 418 (reprinted in 'Classical File', *Surv. Anesthesiol.* 1957, **1**, 174).
18. Wintersteiner O. and Dutcher J. D. *Science* 1943, **97**, 467.
19. Cullen S. C. *Surgery* 1943, **14**, 261.
20. Waters R. *Anesthesiology* 1944, **5**, 618.
21. Harroun P. et al. *Anesthesiology* 1946, **7**, 24.
22. Mallinson F. B. *Lancet* 1945, **2**, 75.
23. Gray T. C. and Halton J. A. *Proc. R. Soc. Med.* 1946, **39**, 400 (reprinted in 'Classical File', *Surv. Anesthesiol.* 1974, **18**, 500.) Gray T. C. *Br. J. Anaesth.* 1983, **55**, 227.
24. Bovet D. et al. *C. R. Séances Acad. Sci.* 1947. **225**, 74.
25. Huguenard P. and Boué A. *C. R. Acad. Sci.* **17**, 1948.

26. Mushin W. W. et al. *Lancet* 1949, **1**, 726.
27. Neff W. B. et al. *Calif. Med.* 1947, **66**, 67.
28. Barlow R. B. and Ing H. R. *Nature* 1948, **161**, 718; *Br. J. Pharmacol.* 1948, **3**, 298 (reprinted in 'Classical File', *Surv. Anesthesiol.* 1961. **5**, 213).
29. Paton W. D. M. and Zaimis E. J. *Nature* 1948, **162**, 810.
30. Organe G. S. W. et al. *Lancet* 1949, **1**, 21.
31. von Dardel O. and Thesleff S. *Nord. Med.* 1951, **46**, 1308; *Acta Chir. Scand.* 1952, **103**, 321 (translated in 'Classical File', *Surv. Anesthesiol.* 1967, **11**, 176).
32. Brücke H. et al. *Wien. Klin. Wochenschr.* 1951, **47**, 885; Mayerhofer O. *Br. Med. J.* 1952, **2**, 1332.
33. Scurr C. F. *Br. Med. J.* 1951, **2**, 831.
34. Beecher H. K. and Todd D. P. *Ann. Surg.* 1954, **140**, 2 (reprinted in 'Classical File', *Surv. Anesthesiol.* 1971, **15**, 394, 496).
35. Paton W. D. A. *Br. J. Anaesth.* 1956, **28**, 470.
36. Bernauer K. et al. *Helv. Chem. Acta* 1958, **41**, 2293.
37. Hugin W. and Kissling P. *Schweiz. Med. Wochenschr.* 1961, **91**, 445; Seegar R. et al. *Anaesthesist* 1962, **11**, 37; Lund L. and Stovner J. *Acta Anaesthesiol. Scand.* 1962, **6**, 85.
38. Baird W. L. M. and Reid A. M. *Br. J. Anaesth.* 1967, **37**, 775; Crul J. F. *Proc. 4th* World Congr. Anaesth. Amsterdam: Excerpta Medica, 1968, p. 418.
39. Burkett W. R. and Bonta K. L. *Fed. Proc.* 1966, **25**, 718.
40. Burkett W. R. et al *Br. J. Pharmacol.* 1968, **32**, 671.
41. Everett A. J. et al. *J. Chem. Soc. Sect. D.*, Chem. Commun. 1020.
42. Durant N. N. et al. *J. Pharm. Pharmacol.* 1979, **31**, 831.
43. Crul J. F. and Booij L. H. D. J. *Br. J. Anaesth.* 1980, **52**, 495.
44. Hughes R. and Payne J. P. *Br. J. Anaesth.* 1981, **53**, 45.
45. Dale H. *Br. Med. J.* 1934, **1**, 835.
46. Dale H. et al. *J. Physiol.* 1936, **86**, 353.
47. Standaert F. G. *Clin. Anesthesiol.* 1985, **3**, 243.
48. Guy H. R. *Biophysical J.* 1984, **35**, 249.
49. Marshall I. G. and Henderson F. *Clin. Anesthesiol.* 1985, **3**, 261.
50. Singh Y. N. L. *Br. J. Anaesth.* 1982, **54**, 1295.
51. Stya M. and Axelrod D. *J. Neurosci.* 1984, **4**, 70.
52. Azar I. *Anesthesiology* 1984, **61**, 173.
53. Trautmann A. *Nature* 1982, **298**, 272.
54. Sinatra R. S. et al. *Anesth Analg. (Cleve.)* 1985, **64**, 1220.
55. Funk D. I. *Acta Anaesthesiol. Scand.* 1980, **24**, 119.
56. Jones R. M. *Anaesthesia* 1985, **40**, 964.
57. Windsor J. P. W. et al. *Anaesthesia* 1985, **40**, 146.
58. Sia R. L. and Straatman N. J. A. *Anaesthesia* 1985, **40**, 167.
59. Grob A. et al. *Bull. Johns Hopkins Hosp.* 1949, **84**, 279.
60. Churchill-Davidson H. C. and Richardson A. T. *Proc. R. Soc. Med.* 1952, **45**, 179.
61. Thesleff S. *Acta Physiol. Scand.* 1952, **25**, 348.
62. Roberts D. V. and Wilson A. *Br. J. Pharmacol.* 1968, **34**, 229; Ali H. H. et al. *Br. J. Anaesth.* 1970,**42**, 967; Lee C. M. *Anesth. Analg. Curr. Res.* 1975, **54**, 649; Zeh D. W. and Katz R. L. *Anesth. Analg. Curr. Res.* 1978, **57**, 13; Ali H. H. and Savarese J. J. *Anesthesiology.* 1976, **45**, 216.
63. Miller R. D. *Anesthesiology* 1976, **44**, 318.
64. Ali H. H. et al. *Br. J. Anaesth.* 1971, **43**, 473; Ali H. H. et al. *Br. J. Anaesth.* 1975, **47**, 570.
65. Viby-Mogensen J. et al. *Anesthesiology* 1981, **55**, 458.
66. Lam H. S. et al. *Br. J. Anaesth.* 1981, **53**, 1351.
67. Norman J. *Clin. Anesthesiol.* 1985, **3**, 273.
68. Duvaldestin P. et al. *Clin. Anesthesiol.* 1985, **3**, 293.
69. Miller R. D. *Can. Anaesth. Soc. J.* 1979, **26**, 83.
70. Coleman A. J. et al. *Anaesthesia* 1972, **27**, 415.
71. Wong K. C. *Fed. Proc.* 1969, **28**, 420; Jones R. M. *Anaesthesia* 1985, **40**, 964.

72. Stenlake J. B. In: *Advances in Pharmacology and Therapeutics* (Stoclet J. P. ed.) Oxford: Pergamon, 1980; Hughes R. and Chapple D. J. *Br. J. Anaesth.* 1980, **52**, 238P; Kreig N. and Crul J. F. et al. *Br. J. Anaesth.* 1980, **52**, 783; Hughes R. and Chapple D. J. *Br. J. Anaesth.* 1981, **53**, 31; Payne J. P. and Hughes R. *Br. J. Anaesth.* 1981, **53**, 45.
73. Skarpa P. et al. *Br. J. Anaesth.* 1983, **55**, 275; Flynn P. J. et al. *Br. J. Anaesth.* 1984, **56**, 599.
74. Evans D. H. *Anesthesiology* 1985, **63**, 118.
75. Chapple D. J. and Miller A. A. *Br. J. Anaesth.* 1987, **59**, 218.
76. Sokoll M. D. et al. *Anesthesiology* 1983, **58**, 450.
77. Brandom B. W. et al. *Anesthesiology* 1983, **58**, A440.
78. Hunter J. M. et al. *Br. J. Anaesth.* 1982, **54**, 1251.
79. Rowlands D. E. *Br. J. Anaesth.* 1983, **55**, 123and 125.
80. Flynn P. J. et al. *Br. J. Anaesth.* 1984, **56**, 967.
81. Jones R. M. et al. *Br. J. Anaesth.* 1984, **56**, 453.
82. Bellis D. J., Day S. and Barnes P. K. *Anaesthesia* 1990, **45**, 118.
83. Srivastava S. *Br. J. Anaesth.* 1984, **56**, 932.
84. Scott R. P. F. et al. *Br. J. Anaesth.* 1985, **57**, 550.
85. Barnes P. K. et al. *Br. J. Anaesth.* 1984, **56**, 795P.
86. Madden A. P. et al. *Br. J. Anaesth.* 1985, **57**, 541.
87. Aldrete J. A. *Br. J. Anaesth.* 1985, **57**, 929.
88. Maharaj R. J. et al. *Br. J. Anaesth.* 1984, **56**, 459.
89. Hunter J. M. et al. *Br. J. Anaesth.* 1984, **56**, 941.
90. Baraka A. et al. *Br. J. Anaesth.* 1984, **56**, 930.
91. Pearce A. C. et al. *Br. J. Anaesth.* 1984, **56**, 973.
92. Eager B. M. et al. *Br. J. Anaesth.* 1984, **56**, 447.
93. Flynn P. J. *Br. J. Anaesth.* 1984, **56**, 599.
94. Suppan P. *Br. J. Anaesth.* 1984, **56**, 931.
95. Baraka A. et al. *Br. J. Anaesth.* 1984, **56**, 673.
96. MacDonald A. M. et al. *Br. J. Anaesth.* 1984, **56**, 651; Bell C. F. et al. *Anaesthesia* 1984, **39**, 961.
97. Buzello W. and Noldge G. *Br. J. Anaesth.* 1982, **54**, 1151.
98. Gergis S. D. et al. *Br. J. Anaesth.* 1983, **55**, 835.
99. Baldwin A. and Churcher M. D. *Anaesthesia* 1979, **34**, 339.
100. d'Hollander A. A. et al. *Br. J. Anaesth.* 1983, **55**, 13.
101. Casele F. E. and Farman J. V. *Br. J. Anaesth.* 1970, **42**, 65.
102. Walmsley D. A. *Lancet* 1959, **2**, 237; Evans P. J. D. and McKinnon I. *Anaesth. Intensive Care* 1977, **5**, 239; Fisher M. McD. *Anaesth. Intensive Care* 1978, **6**, 62.
103. Booth P. N. et al. *Anaesthesia* 1977, **32**, 320.
104. Havill J. H. et al. *Anaesth. Intensive Care* 1978, **6**, 234.
105. Fisher M. M. et al. *Anaesth. Intensive Care* 1978, **6**, 125; Pusey J. M. et al. *Anaesthesia* 1987, **42**, 164.
106. Baird W. L. M. and Reid A. M. *Br. J. Anaesth.* 1967, **39**, 775 (reprinted in 'Classical File', *Surv. Anesthesiol.* 1981, **25**, 133).
107. Havill J. H. et al. *Anaesth. Intensive Care* 1978, **6**, 234.
108. Thompson J. N. *Anaesthesia* 1976, **31**, 219.
109. Coleman A. J. et al. *Anaesthesia* 1972, **27**, 415; Seed R. F. and Chamberlain J. H. *Br. J. Anaesth.* 1977, **49**, 401.
110. Pratila M. G. and Pratilas V. *Anesthesiology* 1978, **49**, 338; Smith G. et al. *Br. J. Anaesth.* 1970, **42**, 923.
111. Somagyi A. A. et al. *Br. J. Anaesth.* 1977, **49**, 1103.
112. Cain P. A. and Ellis F. R. *Br. J. Anaesth.* 1977, **49**, 941.
113. Savarese J. J. et al. *Anesthesiology* 1988, **68**, 723; Stoops C. M. et al. *Anesth. Analg.* 1989, **68**, 333; Caldwell J. E. et al. *Br. J. Anaesth.* 1989, **63**, 393; Ali H. H. et al. *Br. J. Anaesth.* 1988, **61**, 541; Ostergaard D. et al. *Acta Anaesth. Scand.* 1989, **33**, A165; Phillips B. J. and Hunter J. M. *Br. J. Anaesth.* 1992, **68**, 492.
114. Basta S. J. et al. *Anesthesiology* 1988, **69**, 478; Scott R. P. F. and Norman J. *Br. J. Anaesth.* 1988, **61**, 505P.

115. Murray D. J. et al. *Anesthesiology* 1988, **69**, 472; Bracey B. J. et al. *Can Anaesth. Soc. J.* 1989, **36**, S117.
116. Agoston S. and Richardson F. J. *Clin Anesthesiol.* 1985, **3**, 361.
117. Caldwell J. E. et al. *Anesthesiology* 1988, **70**, 784.
118. Caldwell J. E. et al. *Br. J. Anaesth.* 1988, **61**, 693; Stanley J. C. et al. *Br. J. Anaesth.* 1988, **61**, 505P.
119. Aeschlimann J. A. and Reinart M. *J. Pharmacol.* 1931, **43**, 413.
120. Pal J. *Zbl. Physiol.* 1900, **14**, 255.
121. Meltzer S. J. and Auer J. *J. Exp. Med.* 1909, **2**, 622.
122. Cronnelly R. *Clin Anesthesiol.* 1985, **3**, 315.
123. Payne J. P. et al. *Br. J. Anaesth.* 1980, **52**, 69.
124. Viby-Mogensen J. et al. *Anesthesiology* 1979, **50**, 539.
125. Cronnelly R. et al. *Anesthesiology* 1979, **51**, 222.
126. Bevan D. R. *Anaesthesia* 1979, **34**, 614.
127. Morris R. B. et al. *Anesthesiology* 1981, **54**, 399; Cronnelly R. et al. *Anesthesiology* 1982, **57**, 261.
128. Cronnelly R. et al. *Clin Pharmacol. Ther.* 1980, **28**, 78.
129. Long G. et al. *Anaesth. Intensive Care* 1981, **9**, 144.
130. Miller R. D. and Cullen D. J. *Br. J. Anaesth.* 1976, **48**, 253.
131. Baraka A. *Br. J. Anaesth.* 1978, **50**, 1025.
132. Miller R. D. *Can. Anaesth. Soc. J.* 1979, **26**, 83.
133. Bar Z. G. *Anaesthesia* 1985, **40**, 630.
134. Hunt R. and Taveau R. de M *Br. Med. J.* 1906, **2**, 1788.
135. Bovet D et al. *R. C. 1st Sup. Sanot.* 1940, **12**, 107.
136. Castillo J. C. and de Beer E. J. *J. Pharmacol.* 1950, **99**, 458 (reprinted in 'Classical File'. *Surv. Anesthesiol.* 1964, **8**, April).
137. Von Dardel O. and Thesleff S. *Nord. Med.* 1951, **46**, 1308.
138. Bourne J. G. et al. *Lancet* 1952, **1**, 1225.
139. Forbat A. et al. *Lancet* 1953, **1**, 1067.
140. Cook D. R. et al. *Clin. Pharmacol. Ther.* 1976, **20**, 493.
141. Motulsky A. G. In: *Pharmacogenetics* (Steinberg I. and Bearn D. ed.) New York: Grune & Stratton, 1964.
142. Viby-Mogensen. *Cholinesterase and Succinylcholine.* Kobenhavn: Laegeforenningens Forlag, 1982.
143. Owen H. and Hunter A. R. *Br. J. Anaesth.* 1983, **55**, 349.
144. Evans R. T. et al. *Anaesthesia* 1980, **35**, 198.
145. Davies J. M. et al. *Anaesthesia* 1983, **38**, 1074.
146. Dean D. and Emmanuel E. R. *Anaesth. Intensive Care* 1983, **11**, 259.
147. Henderson R. S. and Holmes C. McK *Anaesth. Intensive Care* 1976, **4**, 351.
148. Hilgenberg J. C. and Stoetling R. K. *Anesth. Analg. (Cleve.)* 1981, **60**, 192.
149. Viby-Mogensen J. *Anesthesiology* 1981, **55**, 429.
150. Sutherland G. A. et al. *Can. Anaesth. Soc. J.* 1983, **30**, 342.
151. Donati F. and Bevan D. R. *Anaesth. Analg. (Cleve.)* 1985, **64**, 773.
152. Harper J. K. *Br. Med. J.* 1952, **1**, 861; Hewer C. L. *Br. Med. J.* 1952, **1**, 971; Love S. H. S. *Anaesthesia* 1952, **7**, 113.
153. Viby-Mogensen J. and Hanel H. K. *Acta Anaesthiol. Scand.* 1978, **22**, 371.
154. Wood G. J. and Hall J. M. *Br. J. Anaesth.* 1978, **50**, 945; Evans R. T. et al. *Anaesthesia* 1980, **35**, 198.
155. Whittaker J. P. and Wijesundera S. *Biochem. J.* 1952, **52**, 475.
156. Lehmann H. and Silk E. *Br. Med. J.* 1953, **1**, 767.
157. Zaimis E. *J. Physiol.* 1953, **122**, 238.
158. Bauld H. W. et al. *Br. J. Anaesth.* 1974, **46**, 273.
159. Morton H. J. V. *Proc. R. Soc. Med.* 1945, **38**, 441.
160. Vickers M. D. *Br. J. Anaesth.* 1963, **35**, 528.
161. Cass N. M. et al. *Anaesth. Intensive Care* 1982, **10**, 25.

162. Bourne J. G. et al. *Lancet* 1952, **1**, 1225; von Dardel O. and Thesleff S. *Acta Chir. Scand.* 1952, **103**, 321; Churchill-Davidson H. C. *Br. Med. J.* 1954, **1**, 74.
163. Waters D. J. and Mapleson W. W. *Anaesthesia* 1971, **26**, 127.
164. Verma R. S. *Anaesthesia* 1982, **37**, 688.
165. Datta S. and Crocker J. S. *Br. J. Anaesth.* 1977, **49**, 625.
166. Capan L. M. et al. *Anesthesiology* 1983, **59**, 202.
167. Cullen D. J. et al. *Anesthesiology* 1971, **35**, 527; Freund F. G. and Rubin A. P. *Anesthesiology* 1972, **36**, 185.
168. Wig J. and Bali I. M. *Can. Anaesth. Soc. J.* 1979, **26**, 94.
169. Baraka A. *Anesthesiology* 1977, **46**, 292; Verma R. S. and Reader M. S. *Anesthesiology* 1983, **59**, 487.
170. Feingold A. and Velasquez J. L. *Br. J. Anaesth.* 1979, **51**, 241.
171. Wikinski R. et al. *Anesthesiology* 1965, **26**, 3.
172. Demczuk R. J. *Anesthesiology* 1984, **60**, 69.
173. Chatterji S et al. *Anaesthesia* 1983, **38**, 867.
174. Collier C. B. *Anaesth. Intensive Care* 1980, **8**, 26.
175. Budd A. *Anaesthesia* 1985, **40**, 642.
176. Laurence A. S. *Anaesthesia* 1985, **40**, 854.
177. Rosemberg H and Heiman-Patterson T *Anesthesiology* 1983, **59**, 362.
178. Youngman P. R. and Wilson J. D. *Lancet* 1983, **2**, 597.
179. Ferres C. J. et al. *Br. J. Anaesth.* 1983, **55**, 735.
180. Paterson J. L. et al. *Br. Med. J.* 1979, **2**, 580.
181. James M. F. M. *Br. Med. J.* 1978, **1**, 442.
182. Cade J. F. J. *Med. J. Aust.* 1949, **2**, 349.
183. Havdala H. S. et al. *Anesthesiology* 1979, **50**, 534.
184. Hill G. E. et al. *Anesthesiology* 1977, **46**, 122.
185. Oh T. E. *Anaesth. Intensive Care* 1977, **5**, 60.
186. Schou M. *Br. Med. J.* 1981, **283**, 1253.

Chapter 11

Tracheal intubation

History

Tracheal insufflation in animals was described by Andreas Vesalius (1514–1564) of Padua in 1555,[1] and by Robert Hooke (1635–1703) in 1667.[2] C. Kite of Gravesend described oral and nasal intubation for resuscitation of the apparently drowned in 1788.[3] Pierre Joseph Desault (1744–1795) and his pupil Marie F-X Biehat (1771–1802) were early intubators for laryngeal obstruction. Intubation through a tracheostomy was performed in 1858 by John Snow to anaesthetize animals. Friederich Trendelenburg (1844–1924) of Rostock used the method in man in 1871, occluding the trachea by an inflatable cuff.[4]

William MacEwen (1848–1924) of Glasgow in 1878 passed a tube from the mouth into the trachea, using his fingers as a guide in the conscious patient;[5] through it he gave chloroform and air for removal of a carcinoma of the mouth after first using it for the relief of obstruction in laryngeal diphtheria. Historically, tracheostomy was preferred to intubation because it was supposed that a laryngeal tube would not be tolerated. These early attempts were all made to prevent aspiration pneumonia in surgery of the upper air passages. Karl Maydl (1853–1903) of Prague employed the tube of J. P. O'Dwyer (1841–1898) of Cleveland,[6] designed for the treatment of laryngeal diphtheria, in anaesthesia.[7]

Franz Kuhn of Kassel (1866–1929)[8] extended the technique in 1901 by using a flexible metal tube introduced on a curved guide through the mouth, palpating the epiglottis with the fingers of his left hand. His preference was for inhalation anaesthesia, the patient breathing to and fro through the tube.[9]

In 1907, Barthélemy and Dufour of Nancy, France, blew chloroform vapour and air from a Vernon Harcourt (1834–1919) inhaler[10] and a rubber catheter, guided into the trachea by touch – the first use of insufflation endotracheal anaesthesia.[11] Samuel James Meltzer (1851–1920) and his son-in-law John Auer (1875–1948), physiologists at the Rockefeller Institute, New York City, furthered insufflation endotracheal anaesthesia in animals in 1909.[12] They blew anaesthetic vapour through a narrow tube placed near the carina, the gases returning either through a second tube or around the insufflation tube. The neurosurgeon Charles Albert Elsberg (1871–1948) of New York and others[13] applied the technique to man in the same year, while in 1912 Robert Kelly (1879–1944) of Liverpool brought the method to Britain.[14]

Indirect laryngoscopy with a mirror was pioneered by M. Garcia (1805–1906), a teacher of singing in London.[15] Alfred Kirstein (1863–1922) of Berlin[16] and Gustav Killian (1860–1921) of Freiburg, the original bronchoscopist[17] pioneered direct laryngoscopy in 1895 and 1912 respectively. Chevalier Jackson (1865–1958) of Philadelphia did his first bronchoscopy in 1899, and published a book in 1907[18] which popularized direct laryngoscopy.

Largely as a result of their experiences after the First World War as anaesthetists to Sir Harold Gillies (1882–1960), the plastic surgeon at the Queen's Hospital for Facial and Jaw Injuries at Sidcup (1919), Edgar Stanley Rowbotham (1890–1979) and Ivan Whiteside Magill[19] (1888–1986) used first insufflation through one (later two) narrow gum-elastic tubes passed via a laryngoscope (one insufflating warm ether vapour from a Shipway apparatus[20] with an electric motor, the other carrying it away), and then inhalation endotracheal methods, breathing in and out through a single tube.[21] Magill published his results of blind nasal intubation with a wide-bore rubber tube during the years following 1928.[22] The first blind nasal intubation was performed by Stanley Rowbotham.[23] Inflatable cuffs have been used for many years (e.g. Dorrance)[24] but were reintroduced by Ralph Milton Waters and Arthur E. Guedel in 1928.[25] A pilot balloon was described in 1893 by Victor Eisenmenger (1864–1932),[26] by Green in 1906[27] and reintroduced by Langton Hewer in 1939.[28]

Before the days of muscle relaxants, blind nasal intubation was popular because it was quicker than oral intubation under direct-vision and deep inhalational anaesthesia. The use of muscle relaxants to facilitate intubation was pioneered by Bourne.[29]

(*See also* Gillespie N. A. In: *Endotracheal Anesthesia* 2nd ed. (Bamforth B. J. and Siebeckar K. L. ed.) University of Wisconsin Press, 1943; *Endotracheal Anaesthesia: its Historical Development* Waters R. M. and Guedel A. E. *Anesth. Analg. Curr. Res.* 1933, **12**, 196 (Reprinted in 'Classical File', *Surv. Anesthesiol.* 1984, **28,** 76); Sir Ivan Magill's Contributions to Anaesthesia, Bowes J. B. and Zorab J. S. M. In: *Anaesthesia: Essays on its History* (Rupreht J. et al. ed.) Heidelberg: Springer-Verlag, 1985.)

Apparatus

Tubes

Traditional tubes for either nasal or oral intubation were Magill tubes of mineralized rubber. The red colour was due to the preservative. Oral tubes had thicker walls. The tube number was the internal diameter in millimetres. Most tubes now are made of semi-rigid material, usually PVC (polyvinyl chloride), e.g. Portex. If boiled and left to cool on a curved wire stylet they permanently assume that curve. The toxicity of the PVC is tested by implantation in rabbit muscle (I.T. = 'implantation tested') or by cell culture. Z79 is the committee in the US that approves anaesthetic equipment. Red rubber, silicone and PVC are all flammable in concentrations of oxygen and nitrous oxide that are used clinically.[30] Plastic tubes may fracture after exposure to temperatures of around −20°C and rubber is less susceptible to this cold stress.[31]

There are many tubes for special purposes. The *Cole tube* has a shoulder to prevent endobronchial intubation and is widely used with a T-piece proximal end for neonatal resuscitation but liable to cause laryngeal damage if used for a longer time.[32] A *microlaryngeal tube* is a 5.0 mm tube with an adult-sized cuff for microlaryngeal surgery. The *Oxford* is an inverted L-shaped tube[33] which conforms to the passage from mouth to trachea to prevent kinks even when the head is fully flexed. Its internal diameter is the same throughout but the thickness of the part which lies in the mouth and pharynx, is twice that of the distal part. It has a posterior bevel. *Wire-reinforced* silicone rubber tubes also resist kinking and are available down to 2.5 mm. *Preformed* nasal and oral tubes, such as the RAE (Ring, Adair, Elwyn)[34] pattern, are widely used in faciomaxillary surgery.

Cleaning. Disposable tubes, sterilized by gamma-rays, are used in many hospitals. Red rubber tubes should be cleaned with soapy water outside and inside with a test-tube brush. Heating to 80°C for 10 min (pasteurization) will kill potentially harmful vegetative organisms but does not kill spores. Rubber tubes can be autoclaved up to six times without much deterioration.

Laryngoscopes

The prototype is that of Chevalier Jackson (1865–1958),[35] later modified by Magill,[36] Paluel J. Flagg (1886–1970) of New York;[37] Miller[38] and Robert Macintosh of Oxford (1897–1989).[39] Magill's laryngoscope was modelled on that of William Hill,[40] laryngologist to St Mary's Hospital, London. The light was originally powered from the electric mains, but is now supplied from a 3-volt battery in the handle or by a fibreoptic cable. The *Magill* blade is U-shaped on cross-section and designed to lift the epiglottis forward. The *Macintosh* instrument's blade is shorter, curved and Z-shaped on cross-section. Its tip enters the vallecula, lifts the base of the tongue and with it, the epiglottis, so that the cords can be visualized. Most of the epiglottis is supplied by the internal branch of the superior laryngeal nerve. A version made of acetyl co-polymer can be boiled but not autoclaved.

While the blade of each instrument is designed to be inserted into the right side of the patient's mouth, moving the tongue over to the left, there is a blade available for the *left side*.[41] Full-size blades can be used for quite small children, but neonates and babies may require special straight blades, e.g. the *Oxford* infant blade.[42] These can be fitted with a channel for oxygen administration during intubation.

The *Polio* laryngoscope can be used on patients in iron-lung respirators, its Macintosh-type blade makes an angle of approximately 135° with the handle. Other blades may help with a difficult intubation.[43] The *Bullard* intubating laryngoscope is useful when the neck is immobile and mouth opening restricted. It has fibreoptics, suction and intubation channels, and is made in adult and paediatric versions.[44]

Intubating forceps

Magill's instrument, made in two sizes, is commonly used. A modification with an antero-posterior grip has been described.[45] First used to introduce gum-elastic catheters for insufflation anaesthesia.

Connectors

15 mm connectors are made for all tube sizes, and 8.5 mm connectors for 6.0 mm tubes and below. There are a variety of other connectors which may provide a port for suction, e.g. Magill, Cobb. There is a higher resistance to gas flow through right-angled connectors because turbulence may occur. A flexible catheter mount ends in a 22 mm taper connector (BS 3849) for attachment to the breathing circuit.

Inflatable cuffs[46]

Cuffs prevent leakage between the endotracheal tube and the trachea. They are used in IPPV and to prevent aspiration of gastric contents, blood and mucus, especially in cases of intestinal obstruction and in operations on the upper airways. Available on tubes down to about 5.0 mm. The integrity of the cuff should be tested before use. The tube to the pilot balloon enters the shaft of a nasal tube much nearer its proximal end than for an orotracheal tube.

The traditional cuff is 2–3 cm long and of the low-volume high-pressure type. Used to ensure airtight tracheal anaesthesia, instead of pharyngeal gauze packing.[47] Tracheal wall pressure is likely to be less than cuff pressure, but may be nearly equal if the cuff is floppy,[48] and high cuff pressure may damage tracheal mucosa. Cuffs should not be inflated more than is needed to prevent audible leakage of gas when the reservoir bag is compressed.[49] Low-pressure high-volume cuffs have some advantages, but they too may injure the tracheal epithelium. Cuff pressure may be monitored and should not exceed 30 cmH$_2$O or 22 mmHg.[50] The rise in pressure that occurs as nitrous oxide diffuses into the cuff may be minimized by inflation with normal saline, filling the cuff with anaesthetic gas mixtures,[51] or the use of a pressure limiting device or a foam-filled cuff.

Lubricants

A greasy or water-soluble lubricant applied to the tube, with or without local analgesic (e.g. 2–4% lignocaine), may reduce trauma but not necessarily the incidence of sore throat. There may be significant systemic absorption of lignocaine.[52]

Topical analgesia

Cocaine was first used to suppress the laryngeal reflex in general anaesthesia by Rosenberg in 1895[53] and by Magill, to aid intubation, in 1928.[54] Analgesic solution should be sprayed onto the superior laryngeal aperture, the cords and the mucosa of the larynx and trachea. Lignocaine 3 mg/kg or 5 ml of 4% solution for a 70 kg man should not be exceeded. Many sprays have been described, e.g. the Forrester[55] or metered-dose aerosols. They can become a source of infection.

Indications for tracheal intubation

Experienced opinions vary: some workers intubate almost every patient and others are much more conservative. Tracheal intubation should not be used without a real indication. The duration of an operation is not of itself an indication. There are no absolute contra-indications. The main indications are:

(1) *To maintain airway* if otherwise difficult because of anatomy, position of patient, operation site, or liability to laryngeal spasm (e.g. haemorrhoidectomy, etc.). A clear airway is particularly important if hypotension is induced.

(2) *To allow IPPV.* (*a*) If relaxation is needed, e.g. many abdominal operations; (*b*) in thoracic operations where suction can also be easily carried out; (*c*) to minimize the dose of volatile agent and/or allow large doses of narcotics: ventilation with a facemask may result in gastric distension; and (*d*) in paediatric anaesthesia where respiration is easily embarrassed and enthusiasts intubate almost invariably. Intubation halves the anatomic dead space.

(3) *To prevent aspiration or allow bronchial suction* of stomach contents or blood and debris from operations on the head and upper airways.

Orotracheal intubation

Technique under direct-vision

The condition of the teeth and any anatomic factors that may cause difficulties should be assessed. A small pillow should usually be placed under the occiput to flex the neck and extend the atlanto-occipital joint.[22] This straightens the path from the upper incisors to the larynx. Loose, filled or capped teeth, especially upper incisors, may be protected from the laryngoscope blade by a guard. General anaesthesia is induced by an intravenous or inhalational agent. Hypoxia is less likely for up to 4 min of apnoea if pure oxygen has been breathed for the previous 3 min. A little more intravenous agent or the introduction of a volatile agent may be needed before the injection of suxamethonium 1–1.5 mg/kg or while waiting for a non-depolarizing relaxant to take effect. Relaxation must be profound. Alternatively deep inhalational anaesthesia must be established (in the second plane or below, with complete suppression of reflexes). Less harm is done by getting the patient a little too deep than by using force in a patient with active reflexes and rigid neck muscles. Absence of reflexes and adequate muscular relaxation are necessary for laryngoscopy in all but expert hands.

The suppression of laryngeal reflexes by propofol has encouraged some to use this (2.5 mg/kg), perhaps preceded by alfentanil 30 μg/kg[56] or lignocaine 1.5 mg/kg,[57] to allow intubation with no muscle relaxant. This is not recommended for the inexperienced.

USING THE CURVED BLADE (MACINTOSH)

The curved blade may be the easier to use if the patient has a full set of teeth, and may cause less stretching of the faucial pillars and less bruising than a straight blade. It should be inserted towards the right side of the patient's mouth to prevent the tongue blocking the view of the larynx. The blade tip is passed along the tongue in front of the epiglottis to the vallecula and is used to lift the base of the epiglottis forwards to reveal the cords. Backward pressure on the thyroid cartilage by an assistant may help bring the cords into view. A curved tube is easier to insert than a straight one. A stylet may be used.

USING THE STRAIGHT BLADE (MAGILL)

The lubricated blade is gently inserted at the right side of the mouth and progressively advanced. When the epiglottis is seen it is elevated by the tip of the blade, care being taken not to scratch the posterior pharyngeal wall. The tongue and epiglottis are now lifted forwards, i.e. in the direction of the ceiling, to expose the pallid cords. The upper teeth must not be used as a fulcrum.

DIFFICULTIES

Not always easy to predict and sometimes falsely predicted when intubation proves quite easy.[58] Grading of difficulty has been proposed according to the amount of the larynx exposed at laryngoscopy.[59] The incidence of reported difficulties varies from as high as 1 in 8 to a more realistic 1 in 300 adult patients.[60] They may be anticipated in those with: (a) a short muscular neck with a full set of teeth; (b) a receding lower jaw; (c) a long high-arched palate and narrow mouth, as in Marfan's syndrome; (d) protruding upper incisors ('rabbit teeth'). Their absence usually makes intubation easy; (e) patients in whom the tongue obscures the faucial pillars, uvula and soft palate when the mouth is opened wide and the tongue protruded;[61] (f) a distance between the lower border of the chin and the thyroid notch of less than 6 cm;[62] (g) difficulty in opening the jaw, e.g. surgical wiring, arthritis of the temporomandibular joints; (h) very large breasts or gross obesity; (i) limited neck extension, e.g. cervical spondylosis, fusion of the atlanto-occipital joint and calcification of interspinous ligaments,[63] burns contractures at the front of the neck, bony spicules on the spinous processes of the cervical vertebrae, use of hard collars in neck injuries; (j) cicatricial conditions of the mouth; (k) trismus; (l) a calcified stylohyoid ligament causes difficulty in lifting the epiglottis from the posterior pharyngeal wall and may be accompanied by a skin crease over the hyoid bone;[64] (m) tumours of the mouth or larynx, laryngocele (pathological enlargement of the saccule of the larynx),[65] epiglottic cyst;[66] (n) hypertrophy of the posterior one-third of the tongue; (o) achondroplasia, where there may be a kyphosis between C2 and C3;[67] (p) subglottic stenosis, following previous prolonged intubation or tracheostomy; (q) acromegaly (*see* Chapter 20); (r) trauma to the head and neck; (s) in children, such syndromes as Pierre Robin and Treacher Collins; and (t) in late pregnancy.

Various radiological predictors of difficulty have also been suggested, e.g. (1) Increased distance between the mental symphysis and the lower alveolar margin, which requires wide depression of the lower jaw during intubation; (2) a ratio of effective mandibular length to its posterior depth that is less than 3.6;[63] and (3) reduction in the radiological distance between the occiput and the posterior tubercle of C1 or the C1–C2 intergap.[68] Attempts to extend the head on the neck will then result in anterior bowing of the cervical spine and anterior displacement of the larynx. Sagittal magnetic resonance images of the upper airways may be valuable in specialized cases.[69]

It may be unwise to abolish spontaneous respiration in some of these patients before intubation without checking that manual ventilation is possible using a facemask. Leaks around a facemask may prevent manual ventilation in patients with facial deformities. Even a beard may present difficulty. Some equipment should be available wherever anaesthesia is given: two laryngoscopes with assorted blades, Magill forceps, gum-elastic bougies, malleable stylets, oro- and naso-pharyngeal airways, various sizes of tracheal tubes, suction apparatus, and an emergency kit for transtracheal ventilation.[70] More specialized, less frequently used equipment is conveniently kept together centrally.

Many of the anatomic difficulties listed above will still be present after any operation, and will add to the dangers of removing any tracheal tube until the patient can maintain the airway and breathing. Difficulties and solutions should be recorded in the notes.

(*See also* Latto I. P. and Rosen M. *Difficulties in Tracheal Intubation.* Eastbourne: Baillière Tindall, 1985.)

IMMEDIATE COMPLICATIONS

(1) Kinking, biting or swallowing[71] of the tube causing obstruction; (2) disconnection of anaesthetic circuit from the tube; (3) blockage of tube by blood, mucus, etc. This may need sucking out; (4) accidental extubation; (5) obstruction by the inflated cuff, especially if a weak portion herniates over the tip of the tube; (6) obstruction by apposition of the bevel of the tube against the tracheal wall; and (7) intubation of the right bronchus if tube is too long. Average distance between central incisors and carina is 27 cm in an adult male and 23 cm in a female. The tip of the tube moves about 4 cm caudal as the neck moves from full extension to full flexion.[72] In the newborn, 5 cm separates the gums from the cords, and a similar distance separates the cords from the carina. Diagnosed by low oxygen saturations, absence of air entry into left lung, and jerky breathing or bucking.

IS THE TUBE CORRECTLY PLACED IN THE TRACHEA?

It is easy to intubate the oesophagus. The anaesthetist can only be certain that the tube has been correctly placed in the trachea if (a) he has watched it pass through the cords and can still see it in front of the arytenoids, or (b) if tracheal rings can be seen when a fibreoptic bronchoscope is passed down the tube,[73] or (c) if CO_2 is present and continues to be present in the expired gas. Stomach gas may contain CO_2 after facemask ventilation, although ventilation of the stomach reduces the level of CO_2 after a few breaths.[74] If capnography is not available, a disposable colorimetric CO_2 detector has been described.[75]

Other tests of tube placement, which require some familiarity, include (a) the oesophageal detector device, which exploits the rigidity of the tracheal wall compared with the oesophagus and does not allow the distal end of the tube to be blocked when suction is applied;[76] (b) auscultation for air entry over the trachea and the absence of a gurgle over the epigastrium when the reservoir bag is squeezed; (c) palpating the tube in the larynx through the mouth or at the front of the neck; and (d) the use of a lighted stylet down the tube whose light shines through the front of the neck.

The feel and movements of the reservoir bag, auscultation of the chest and observation of its movements may all be unreliable. Bag movement can seem just like respiratory movement even when the tube is in the oesophagus. Oximetry is not a particularly useful early warning sign of oesophageal intubation, especially if preoxygenation has taken place.[74] The results of unrecognised oesophageal intubation can be brain damage or death.[77] *If the clinical state of the patient should deteriorate after intubation or if there is any doubt whatsoever about tube placement, the tube should be removed and the patient ventilated by facemask.* A facemask may even be used with the open tube in place if the anaesthetist is unwilling to remove it. *'When in doubt, take it out'.*

The anaesthetist must also be convinced that all parts of each lung are being ventilated, by auscultation over the trachea, each upper zone and each axilla. Causes of diminished air entry into one lung are endobronchial placement of tube, pneumothorax, bronchial obstruction by gastric contents, blood, secretions, tumour, etc.

Technique of blind orotracheal intubation

This is very occasionally necessary when abnormal anatomy precludes the use of a laryngoscope or when the nasal route is undesirable. There are three methods. The patient should be deeply anaesthetized.

1. An assistant draws the tongue forwards while the anaesthetist stands facing the patient and on his left, passes two fingers of his left hand over the dorsum of the tongue and hooks the epiglottis forwards. The tube, which must be fully curved, is guided by these two fingers into the glottis. Curved introducers may help, as used by Franz Kuhn in 1901.[9]

2. The anaesthetist stands in his usual place at the head of the table and inserts his left thumb into the patient's mouth and his fingers on the patient's chin. The tip of the thumb makes contact with the back of the tongue. This gives good control of the forward and backward movement of the lower jaw. The tube is guided into the glottis with the right hand.

3. The tube, which must not be too fully curved, can be passed 'blind' through a prop held in the mouth, with the head in full extension.

Nasal intubation

Indications

(1) When an oral tube is in the surgeon's way, e.g. in dental extraction and operations on the tongue; and (2) in the presence of crowns or other dental work vulnerable to damage by a laryngoscope.

Some workers of experience find no use for this technique, concerned for the dangers of epistaxis and avulsion of nasal polyps, which may then enter the lungs. Others point to the dangers of the use of the laryngoscope with risks of dental damage, etc. and inhalation of tooth fragments. The main indication for blind intubation is in the patient in whom direct laryngoscopy is likely to be difficult, or has failed. The anaesthetist will not succeed with blind intubation in these cases unless he is practised in the technique.

Technique for blind nasal intubation

Distance between nares and carina averages 32 cm in males and 27 cm in females, i.e. 4 to 5 cm further than from incisors to carina. Extreme gentleness should prevail. It is a knack, only acquired by practice. The experienced worker employs tubes of the size, shape and consistency to suit his individual technique.

1. The nares should be examined for patency by listening to the patient's breathing with each naris occluded. Nasal polypi should be excluded. The nasal mucosa can be shrunk by 4% cocaine spray, which is relatively toxic, 1% adrenaline in oil, or 3% lignocaine and 0.25% phenylephrine.[78]

2. Select the largest size of tube which should pass atraumatically through the larger naris: for a big man up to 10, for a small woman between 5 and 7. The position of the patient's head depends on the curve of the tube: the greater the curve, the more flexed should be the head. Magill advised the position adopted 'when sniffing the morning air', the head on a single pillow, with slight extension of the atlanto-occipital joint.

3. The anaesthetist may attempt intubation with the patient apnoeic after muscle relaxation, or under deep inhalational anaesthesia with CO_2 added to stimulate respiration and widen the glottis on inspiration. Some find blind intubation easier in the paralysed patient because reflex laryngospasm does not occur.[79]

4. The tube, with its concavity directed to the patient's feet, is inserted into the naris directly backwards, not upwards. Movement of the bevel by rotation of the tube may assist, either at this stage or when the tube enters the nasopharynx from the nose.

5. If the patient is breathing spontaneously, the opposite nostril is occluded so that all breathing is taking place through the tube. The jaw should be slightly elevated to lift the epiglottis from the posterior pharyngeal wall. If the right naris is used the head should be inclined slightly to the right, and vice versa. The anaesthetist should listen carefully to the respiration. The breath sounds conducted through the tube become maximal when its tip is immediately above the glottis. If the tube does not enter the larynx, its direction may be adjusted by rotation of the tube, rotation of the neck or digital movement of the larynx to meet the advancing tube. Should the tube enter the oesophagus it can be partially withdrawn and its tip directed anteriorly by increased extension of the neck or by using a tube with a larger curvature. Occasionally the tip of the tube impinges on the anterior commissure of the larynx, when it will often enter the larynx if the neck is flexed or a tube of lesser curvature is used. As the tube passes the cords a slight snap is often noticeable and there may be some coughing or breath-holding in the lightly anaesthetized patient, even when muscle relaxant drugs have been employed. In the patient who is not paralysed the tube may enter the trachea during the explosive cough which may follow spasm of the cords. In the case of failure to intubate through one naris, success may be achieved through the other, or with a tube of different curvature.

6. Normal free breath sounds at the proximal end of a tube of reasonable length show that it is in the trachea. If the tube can be inserted fully and no breath sounds heard, it is probably in the oesophagus. Normal breathing through the tube, while the lower jaw is pushed backwards, suggests successful intubation. Capnography confirms this.

DIFFICULTIES

If unsuccessful, blind intubation should not be persisted in or trauma may result. Tubes, which must be supple and rather soft, should always be handled daintily and not forcibly rammed down the patient's throat. Difficulty may be encountered if the tube is not sufficiently curved. A radius of curvature of 10 cm is suitable. The tube may get stuck in the vallecula, between the base of the tongue and the epiglottis, when rotation of the tube should allow it to slip down the lateral wall of the pharynx. It may also get stuck in a pyriform fossa, lateral to the correct position. This is likely where the nose is asymmetric, and is overcome by rotating the tube, by moving the larynx laterally to meet the tube or by rotating the patient's head. Soft, worn-out tubes may curl up in the pharynx. It is particularly important to select a tube with a curvature appropriate for a patient whose neck is fixed.

If blind intubation fails, the tip of the tube can be guided into the trachea by the Magill intubating forceps,[45] or a wire hook in the oropharynx to guide the tube backwards or forwards.

A prominent arch of the atlas vertebra may cause obstruction and perhaps its overlying mucosa to be torn. To overcome this a small suction catheter may be threaded through the endotracheal tube and tension kept on it as it is delivered through the mouth, thus displacing the tip of the tube and overcoming obstruction.

Epistaxis, though messy, seldom interferes with the anaesthesia or causes postoperative discomfort. Partial obstruction of a nasotracheal tube by an avulsed piece of turbinate may occur.[80] The tube may be compressed by nasal spurs and a deviated septum. The opposite naris or orotracheal intubation may have to be used. Nasal intubation has been followed by bacteraemia in 12% of children[81] and in 17–21% of adults.[82] The significance of these findings in patients at risk of developing endocarditis is not known.

Technique for direct-vision nasal intubation

Needed when a nasotracheal tube is desirable and if blind intubation fails. The laryngoscope is inserted after the tube tip has been inserted as far as the hypopharynx. The tube is guided between the cords, either by slight movement of the tube or with the aid of intubation forceps. If the tube is too curved or the head too extended it may impinge against the anterior commissure of the larynx. This can often be remedied by keeping the tube pressed against the anterior commissure, withdrawing the laryngoscope, flexing the head and pushing the tube home 'blind'.

Failed intubation

Persistent attempts at intubation of a difficult case is often unproductive and can even be disastrous. It may be better to admit defeat at a relatively early stage. A plan of management must be adopted that ensures *oxygenation of the patient without aspiration*. This 'failed intubation drill' is most commonly needed in obstetric anaesthesia but is an important part of every anaesthetist's training. Difficulty with tracheal intubation is one of the most important factors leading to deaths attributed to anaesthesia.

Tunstall's drill for the patient at high risk of aspiration:[83] call for senior help; keep cricoid pressure applied; tilt the patient head down in the left lateral position; suck pharynx if needed; ventilate gently with 100% oxygen by facemask (it may be necessary to use an airway or even to release cricoid pressure to do this); pass a gastric tube to empty stomach and instill 20 ml 0.3 M sodium citrate; and remove gastric tube. Then either establish spontaneously breathing inhalational anaesthesia if the operation is urgent (all operations were conducted in this way before the 1930s), or wait for the patient to recover when alternative methods of intubation may be considered (*see* below) or regional analgesia[84] used. Not all workers agree with turning of the patient into the lateral position which may be impractical and make ventilation difficult, and with the passage of a gastric tube, which may itself provoke vomiting.[70]

Spontaneously breathing anaesthesia may be aided by (a) nasopharyngeal airways, which may be bilateral;[85] (b) laryngeal mask airway, which does not prevent aspiration, but has been easy to insert in patients who are very difficult to intubate;[86] (c) oesophageal obturator airway, used mainly outside hospital;[87] and (d) oesophageal gastric tube airway, passed into the oesophagus and its cuff inflated with 35 ml of air. Displaces the larynx forward and provides an airway. Designed for resuscitation.[88]

Many techniques have been described to aid intubation in the difficult patient. (a) It is often easier to pass a malleable 60 cm, 15 FG gum-elastic bougie, with its tip curved anteriorly, into the trachea and use it as an introducer.[89] The correct placement of the bougie in the trachea can be confirmed by the fact that its whole length cannot be inserted into the lungs, whereas it can into the oesophagus. Passage of the tube over the bougie may be helped by keeping the laryngoscope in the mouth, and by rotating the tube 90° anti-clockwise before the bevel reaches the larynx.[90] (b) A size 3 or 4 laryngeal mask airway will allow a 6.0 mm tube (or an introducer for a bigger tube) to be introduced blindly though it.[91] (c) Difficulties due to gross obesity may be overcome with a polio laryngoscope. (d) The use of a rigid bronchoscope to introduce a cuffed tracheal tube threaded over it, may facilitate a difficult intubation, especially if mouth opening is poor.[92] (e) A lighted stylet inside the tube, which shines through the skin at the front of the neck, may help find the trachea.[93] (f) An epidural catheter or a guide wire may be passed retrogradely through the cricothyroid membrane up to the pharynx and out through the mouth or nose, and used as an introducer for a tracheal tube.[94] (g) Fibreoptic laryngoscopy (*see below*).

Transtracheal ventilation may be life-saving. A 14G intravenous cannula or needle is thrust into the larynx through the cricothyroid membrane and connected to a modified bronchoscope injector with an oxygen pressure of up to 4 bar.[95] The emergency oxygen flush may be a more readily available source of high pressure oxygen. A standard resuscitation bag may provide adequate ventilation through a 12G cannula, and a 4.0 mm mini-tracheostomy tube or other commercial cricothyrotomy kits should allow relatively easy ventilation. (Dilatation and passage of a 6.0 mm airway will allow adequate spontaneous breathing.) Various improvised connectors have also been used: e.g. a tracheal tube adaptor thrust into the barrel of a syringe or into part of a drip set, or by the sharp end of a drip chamber being inserted into the trachea, the other end connected to a source of oxygen.[96] With all these methods there must be a clear expiratory pathway to prevent dangerously high airway pressures, if necessary through a second needle or cannula in the cricothyroid membrane.[97] If ventilation is satisfactory then intravenous anaesthesia may be used. If percutaneous transtracheal ventilation fails, tracheostomy may be needed.

See Davies J. M. *Can. J. Anaesth.* 1989, **36,** 668; King T. A. and Adams A. P. *Br. J. Anaesth.* 1990, **65**, 400; Wright E. M. and Major E. In: *Recent Advances in Anaesthesia and Analgesia 17.* (Atkinson R. S. and Adams A. P. ed.) Edinburgh: Churchill Livingstone, 1992.

Fibreoptic laryngoscopy

A fibreoptic instrument was first used to aid nasal intubation in 1967.[98] The fibreoptic bronchosope was introduced in 1968[99] and used for intubation in 1972.[100] Training in its use should be available.[101]

It is the method of choice for the intubation of an awake patient under topical analgesia, perhaps supplemented with sedation, but can also be used in anaesthetized patients either breathing spontaneously, with controlled ventilation, or with percutaneous transtracheal jet ventilation.[102] Most find the technique more difficult in the anaesthetized patient, and for oral intubation rather than nasal, although oropharyngeal airways may be adapted to allow fibreoptic laryngoscopy while breathing anaesthetic gases. The instrument is used as an introducer. A 3.0 mm tube may be passed over the smallest laryngoscope, but babies may also be managed by using the suction channel to pass a guide wire into the trachea as an introducer. The use of an armoured tube will ensure that it does not compress the fibrescope after insertion, making its withdrawal from the tube impossible.

Possible indications for awake intubation, apart from difficulty in intubation by other methods: (1) full stomach; (2) upper airway obstruction; and (3) bronchopleural fistula. The following methods of local analgesia may be used: (a) atropine or hyoscine premedication; (b) sucking an amethocaine 60 mg lozenge; (c) cocaine applied to the nasal mucosa; (d) spraying the mouth, pharynx, cords and trachea through the laryngoscope; (e) bilateral superior laryngeal nerve block, either percutaneously[103] or via the pyriform fossae with Krause's forceps; (f) transtracheal injection of 2–4% lignocaine 2 ml; (g) inhalation of lignocaine via a nebulizer.[104] Diazepam 5–10 mg, midazolam 2–7.5 mg and fentanyl 50–150 µg i.v. are useful adjuncts. Even when doses of lignocaine greater than those recommended are used, plasma levels are not toxic, but peak levels may not be reached for up to 1 hour after administration.

See also Murrin K. R. In: *Difficulties in Tracheal Intubation* (Latto I. P. and Rosen M. ed.) Eastbourne: Baillière Tindall, 1985, 90; Ovassapian A. *Fiberoptic Airway Endoscopy in Anesthesia and Critical Care.* New York: Raven Press, 1990.

Extubation

Extubation normally causes a rise in blood pressure and pulse rate, which can result in myocardial ischaemia in patients with coronary disease. Lessened by lignocaine, 60 mg down the tube[105] or 1 mg/kg i.v.[106] a few minutes before extubation, which will also help prevent coughing.

Laryngeal spasm is sometimes seen after extubation. Pharyngeal secretions should be removed by suction and the patient allowed to breathe 100% oxygen before extubation. The airway must then be watched carefully. It may be more safely managed in the lateral head-down position. Spasm has been prevented or treated by: (a) giving oxygen at positive pressure via a facemask; (b) small dose of suxamethonium and ventilation with oxygen; (c) ensuring full reversal of any non-depolarizing relaxant; (d) doxapram 1.5 mg/kg;[107] (e) incremental doses of diazepam 0.5–1 mg;[108] (f) topical analgesia; (g) physostigmine 0.04 mg/kg;[109] and (h) lignocaine i.v.[110] Re-intubation may be required.

Laryngeal spasm may result in acute pulmonary oedema, as may other causes of upper airway obstruction,[111] possibly due to low alveolar pressures encouraging fluid transudation.

Difficulty in extubation is unusual, but may be caused by the cuff failing to deflate or becoming distorted, or the tube accidentally becoming sutured in place. Airway obstruction after extubation may be caused by a haematoma in the neck.

Suction

Hypoxia and atelectasis may occur during bronchial suction, which may be minimized by continuing IPPV, jet ventilation or preoxygenation.[112] Catheter sizes are expressed in FG (French Gauge). Division by 3 gives the approximate external diameter in millimetres. Lengths vary between 38 and 61 cm. If its external diameter is not more than half the internal diameter of the tracheal tube, a significant negative pressure will not develop in the lungs during suction.[113]

Anaesthetic agents in relation to tracheal intubation

Induction agents. Intubation with intravenous agents alone is not recommended. Laryngeal reflexes are usually active and laryngeal spasm and coughing often occurs. This problem is least likely after propofol. Induction is usually followed by a muscle relaxant or progression to deep inhalation anaesthesia with spontaneous respiration. In the latter case, any agent may be used, although respiratory and cardiovascular depression will occur. Halothane is still popular in children.

Suxamethonium. Its speed of onset and profound relaxation makes intubation quick, easy and atraumatic. A suitable dose is up to 1–1.5 mg/kg. Works in less than 1 min, while its effect, including apnoea, seldom lasts more than a few minutes. Can be given intramuscularly 3 mg/kg if veins are difficult, e.g. in infants.

Non-depolarizing relaxants. Vecuronium or atracurium take up to 90 sec to produce relaxation adequate for intubation, during which time gentle facemask ventilation is applied. Ways of trying to shorten this time include: (1) giving the relaxant shortly before the induction agent (if venous access is secure); and (2) 'priming' with a tenth of the ED_{95} (e.g. vecuronium 5 µg/kg, atracurium 25 µg/kg) 4 min before induction and the main dose; some give double this or more; the improvement is slight.[114] Doubt has been cast on the safety of either approach, and suxamethonium remains the quickest way of achieving suitable conditions for intubation.

Relaxants should never be given unless the anaesthetist is confident of his ability to ventilate the lungs using a facemask.

Endotracheal absorption of drugs[115]

Adrenaline,[116] isoprenaline, lignocaine, atropine,[117] diazepam and naloxone[118] are quickly absorbed if given down a tracheal tube. This route is endorsed by the Resuscitation Council[119] and the American Heart Association,[120] although the doses and volumes have not been established. The latter recommend the same dose as would be used intravenously, but the former suggest twice that amount. Probably best given diluted in 10 ml normal saline through a catheter placed at the tip of the tube, and distributed throughout the lungs by a few large breaths. It may be easier in some settings (e.g. outside hospital), but does not have such a reliable therapeutic effect as the intravenous route.[121]

Reflex responses to laryngoscopy and intubation[122]

During light general anaesthesia, direct laryngoscopy and intubation, uncomplicated by hypoxia, hypercapnia or cough, cause an increase in heart rate and arterial pressure, and dysrhythmia in up to 90% of patients because of afferent stimulation of the vagus and a sympatho-adrenal response.[123] Hypertensive subjects show an exaggerated response. Endorphin release also occurs on intubation.[124] These reflexes are of little significance in healthy patients, but of concern in patients with, for example, coronary artery disease, raised intracranial pressure or intracranial aneurysm. Sudden death has been reported.[125] There is no influence of the type of laryngoscope blade used.[126] The responses are less under deep general anaesthesia, adequate topical analgesia, and with smooth blind nasal intubation. Results using fibreoptic intubation are conflicting.[127]

These responses may be minimized by: (a) fentanyl at conventional doses of 2–6 µg/kg,[128] or high doses of up to 50 µg/kg; (b) alfentanil 10–40 µg/kg;[129] (c) lignocaine 1–1.5 mg/kg given i.v. or by inhalation. This is not always effective, and is best given 4 min before laryngoscopy;[130] (d) vasodilators such as sodium nitroprusside 1–2 µg/kg, isosorbide dinitrate 80 µg/kg[131] or α-blockers; (e) premedication with clonidine 5 µg/kg;[132] (f) esmolol 150 mg;[133] (g) induction with propofol;[134] (h) verapamil 0.1 mg/kg i.v.,[135] nifedipine 10 mg sublingually a few minutes before induction[136] or diltiazem 0.2–0.3 mg/kg 1 min before laryngoscopy;[137] or (i) enalapril 5 mg orally 4 h preoperatively, or captopril 12.5–25 mg sublingually 25 min preoperatively.[138]

Intraocular and intracranial pressures may rise at tracheal intubation especially if suxamethonium is employed. Two-fold increases in ICP have been seen in patients with brain tumours, prevented by pre-treatment with metocurine.[139] Non-depolarizing relaxants are not associated with this problem unless histamine is released.[140]

Complications after intubation

1. Direct trauma

To the lips, teeth, gums, eyes, nose, uvula, throat and larynx, resulting in hoarseness, dysphagia, sore throat,[141] etc. Sore throat may also result purely from suxamethonium muscle pain.[142] Teeth are commonly damaged,[143] and a guard may be helpful.[144] If a tooth is knocked out, it must be found and prevented from disappearing into the trachea. If a radiograph shows it to be in a bronchus, it should be removed bronchoscopically. It should be handled only by the crown and placed in saline because reimplantation may be possible.

Nasal intubation may dislodge nasal polyps, cause epistaxis, damage turbinates,[145] or cause ulceration of turbinates if intubation is prolonged.[146] Tears in the mucosa of the pharynx, oesophagus,[147] larynx or trachea may result in extensive surgical and mediastinal emphysema. Retropharyngeal abscess has been reported.[148]

A haematoma may form in the cords, especially the left, or in the supraglottic region, which may result in dysphonia and dysphagia but usually clears up in a few days. It bears no constant relationship to the difficulty of intubation. The arytenoids may be dislocated,[149] or more serious damage done to the laryngeal muscles and ligaments. Permanent alteration of the voice was once reported in 3% of patients after intubation.[150] Subtle voice changes can be quantified by laryngeal acoustics.[151]

2. Nerve injuries

Recurrent laryngeal nerve palsy has been reported following intubation and results in a paralysed cord.[152] Idiopathic palsy of the recurrent nerve, a transient cranial mononeuropathy can occur with a reasonable chance of good recovery.[153] The law of F. Semon (1849–1921) states that in a disorder of the laryngeal motor nerves, the abductors of the cords are the first and occasionally the only muscles affected.[154] Bilateral cord paralysis, perhaps due to pressure of the inflated cuff on the laminae of the thyroid cartilage and the recurrent nerves[155] may result in increasing airway obstruction, which requires facemask CPAP or re-intubation.

Lingual nerve palsy due to acute compression or stretching in its course from the medial surface of the mandible to the underside of the tongue has occurred, especially on the right. The prognosis is good.[156]

3. *Fracture-subluxation of the cervical spine*

Careless movement of the head can result in serious injury, particularly if there are fractures, malformations or abnormal fragility of the cervical spine, and if muscle tone has been abolished by relaxants. It may be wise to ask the surgeon to hold the head in a safe position during intubation.[157]

4. *Infections*

Sinusitis and otitis media may result from nasotracheal intubation. If the base of the skull is fractured, infection may spread to the brain. Intubation may cause the bronchial tree to become contaminated, and mucociliary clearance is impaired by breathing dry gases.

5. *Tracheal rupture during anaesthesia*[158]

In both adults and neonates, and not necessarily associated with trauma.

6. *Ignition of the tube during laser surgery* (*see* Chapter 22)

7. *Acute glottic oedema*

This is rare, but may follow prolonged intubation or short-term intubation with a tube that is too large and allowed to move within the larynx, e.g. on coughing, or in a patient with acute laryngitis. More serious in children because of the small larynx and loose submucosal tissue in the subglottic region.

Presents up to several hours after extubation with hoarseness, cough, choking, restlessness, stridor, ashy grey pallor, and the signs of upper airway obstruction, i.e. inspiratory indrawing at the suprasternal notch, epigastrium, intercostal spaces or around the clavicles.

Sedation is contra-indicated. Humidification and nebulized racemic adrenaline may be useful. Re-intubation with a smaller tube may be needed, or even tracheostomy.

8. *Ulceration and granuloma formation in the larynx*[159]

Rarely, a contact ulcer may form in the mucosa over the prominent tip of the vocal process of one or both arytenoids in the posterior third of the rima glottidis, or in the subglottis of children. A contact ulcer is not necessarily due to intubation trauma but may be caused by movement of the cords against the tube as it lies in the larynx. These movements are not always abolished by anaesthesia. Ulceration is more common after lengthy intubation, but can occur after intubation for routine surgery, usually of the head and neck in women. The ulcer may proceed to the formation of a granuloma, which can become pedunculated and obstruct the airway. Granulomas on the vocal processes may become adherent across the midline, forming a fibrous band.[160] In the trachea, tracheomalacia, fibrosis and stenosis may result.

If hoarseness persists for more that a week postoperatively, laryngoscopy should be performed. A contact ulcer will heal if the voice is completely rested. A granuloma may need to be excised.

The laryngeal mask airway[161]

This airway is a cuffed mask designed to fit closely over the laryngeal aperture. It is made in five sizes: size 1 for babies up to 6.5 kg, size 2 for children between 6.5 and 25 kg, size 2½ for children from 20–30 kg, sizes 3 and 4 for small and large adults. Before use, the cuff should be fully deflated and lubricant applied to the back of the mask. After induction of anaesthesia with propofol, which depresses laryngeal reflexes, or the establishment of sufficiently deep inhalational anaesthesia, it is introduced blindly into the hypopharynx. If difficult, insertion may be easier with the aperture facing backwards, and the mask then rotated when in the pharynx. It is best not inserted immediately after only thiopentone because laryngeal reflexes are still active. Muscle relaxants are not needed. The cuff is inflated with about 2–4 ml (size 1), 10 ml (size 2), 14 ml (size 2½) 20 ml (size 3) and 30 ml (size 4) of air, when the front of the neck is seen to swell. It forms a seal around the larynx, and allows spontaneous ventilation or IPPV without intubation of the trachea or oesophagus. If the epiglottis is folded downwards by the tip of the mask on insertion, the airway may be obstructed. *The seal does not always prevent aspiration of stomach contents,*[162] indeed, the opening of the oesophagus may be included within the cuff. Gastric distension may occur if used for IPPV with airway pressures over about 2 kPa. A bite-block is useful. It is best removed when protective reflexes have fully returned, and the patient has started to swallow. Suction is usually not needed.

The airway provides a relatively secure, hands-free airway in place of a facemask or tracheal intubation for routine anaesthesia in both adults and children,[163] although a careful watch for obstruction must be kept. It is valuable in many operations, especially those on the head and neck, or where the airway may give difficulties, e.g. radiotherapy[164] and dental extractions[165] in children. It causes only a small rise in heart rate and blood pressure, comparable with those seen after insertion of an oropharyngeal airway.[166] It may be easy to insert in those patients in whom laryngoscopy and tracheal intubation is difficult, and has even been used for emergency Caesarean section when intubation proved impossible.[86] In the latter case a cuffed tube in the oesophagus may help prevent regurgitation and aspiration. Both adult sizes will allow a 6 mm cuffed endotracheal tube to be passed through it blindly into the trachea.[91] The laryngeal mask airway may have a role in airway management by paramedical staff.[167] It is autoclaved after use.

See also Brodrick P. M. et al. *Anaesthesia* 1989, **44**, 238; Maltby J. R. et al. *Can. J. Anaesth.* 1990, **37**, 509.

Tracheal intubation in infants and children

Induction with a volatile agent, especially halothane (with or without nitrous oxide), or an intravenous agent may be used. If relaxants are needed and venepuncture is difficult, suxamethonium 3 mg/kg can be injected i.m. In *neonates,* awake intubation is sometimes preferred because it avoids hypoxia caused by spasm or obstruction, but anterior fontanelle pressure can rise three-fold and this may put a pre-term baby at risk of intraventricular haemorrhage.[168] The head and shoulders of the baby must be held firmly by an experienced assistant and the larynx pushed backwards. The tip of a straight laryngoscope blade is inserted at the right side of the mouth, pushes the tongue to the left, and is placed deep (posterior) to the epiglottis to lift it forwards. At birth, the trachea is 4 cm long and 6 mm wide.

The *child's* larynx differs from the adult: (a) it is well anterior and higher. the rima glottidis is opposite the C3–4 interspace in the infant, in adults one space lower; (b) the epiglottis is relatively longer and V-shaped, instead of flat as in the adult. It makes an angle of 45° with the anterior pharyngeal wall whereas in adults it lies closer to the base of the tongue; (c) the narrowest part of the larynx is at the level of the cricoid cartilage, which is not distensible, as are the cords, which form the narrowest part in adults. A tracheal tube may be passed through the glottis, but be held up at the cricoid causing trauma and oedema. If this occurs, a smaller tube should be substituted; (d) a child's laryngeal reflexes are very active; and (e) the morbidity from long-term intubation, even up to 6 weeks or more, is small.[169]

Less flexion of the cervical spine for laryngoscopy is needed than in adults,[170] and in infants it is not necessary to have the head on a pillow. A well-developed occiput may make intubation more difficult. Uncuffed tubes are normally used below the age of about 10 years.

Length of trachea (cm) is age divided by 4 plus 4. In children measurements have not confirmed that the main bronchi leave the trachea in a manner different to that in adults.[171]

Size of tubes

In the neonate an orotracheal tube should be 10–11 cm long. Length (cm) of orotracheal tube in older children is age divided by 2 plus 12. Nasotracheal tubes are 3 cm longer, or may be calculated (in cm) from 3 times the internal diameter (mm) plus 2.[172] For neonates internal diameter of tube is 2.5–3.0 mm; 3.0–3.5 mm for 1 to 3 months; 3.5–4.0 mm up to 1 year; 4.0–4.5 mm up to 2 years; 4.5–5.0 mm up to 4 years; 5.5 up to 6 years; 6.0 up to 8 years; 6.5 up to 10 years; 7.0 up to 12 years. A rough guide is to use a tube that is the size of the distal phalanx of the patient's little finger. Formulae for internal diameter: up to 6 years, age divided by 3 plus 3.5; over 6 years, age divided by 4 plus 4.5. Smaller sizes should be readily available in case of the occasional subglottic stenosis. This is more common in the presence of imperforate anus.[173] In small children and infants it is important to confirm by auscultation that the tracheal tube is not too long and reached either main bronchus. For resistance to breathing in tracheal tubes in infants, *see* Hatch D. J. *Anaesthesia* 1978, **50**, 959.

References

1. Wedley J. R. *Br. J. Clin. Equip.* 1979, **4**, 49.
2. Hooke R. *Phil. Trans. R. Soc.* 1667, **2**, 539.
3. Davison M. H. A. *Br. J. Anaesth.* 1951, **23**, 238.
4. Trendelenburg F. *Arch. Klin. Chir.* 1871, **12**, 121.
5. MacEwen W. *Br. Med. J.* 1880, **2**, 122 (reprinted in 'Classical File', *Surv. Anaesthesiol.* 1969, **13**, 105).

6. O'Dwyer J. *Med. Rec.* 1887, **32**, 557.
7. Maydl K. *Wien. Med. Wochenschr.* 1893, **43**, 102.
8. Zinganell K. *Anaesthetist* 1974, **23**, 308; Sweeney B. *Anaesthesia* 1985, **40**, 1000.
9. Kuhn F. *Zbl. Chir.* 1901, **28**, 1281.
10. Harcourt V. *Br. Med. J.* 18 July 1903.
11. Barthélemy and Dufour, *Presse Méd.* 1907, **15**, 475.
12. Meltzer S. J. and Auer J. *J. Exp. Med.* 1909, **11**, 622.
13. Elsberg C. A. *N. Y. Med. Rec.* 1910, **77**, 493; *Ann. Surg.* 1910, **52**, 23.
14. Kelly R. E. *Br. Med. J.* 1912, **2**, 617, 1121.
15. Garcia M. *Proc. R. Soc. Lond.* 1855, **7**, 399.
16. Kirstein A. *Allg. Med. ZentZtg* 1895, **34**, 110; *Lancet* 1895, **1**, 1132; Hirsch N. P. et al. *Anaesthesia* 1986, **41**, 42.
17. Zollner F. *Arch. Otolaryngol.* 1965, **82**, 656.
18. Jackson C. *Tracheobronchoscopy, Esophagoscopy and Gastroscopy.* St Louis: Mosby, 1907.
19. Magill I. W. *Lancet* 1923, **2**, 228; Magill I. W. *Anaesthesia* 1975, **30**, 476; Condon H. A. and Gilchrist E. *Anaesthesia* 1986, **41**, 46.
20. Shipway F. *Lancet* 1916, **1**, 70.
21. Rowbotham E. S. and Magill I. W. *Proc. R. Soc. Med.* 1921, **14**, 17; Magill I. W. *Proc. R. Soc. Med.* 1929, **22**, 83 (reprinted in 'Classical File', *Surv. Anesthesiol.* 1978, **33**, 580).
22. Magill I. W. *Br. Med. J.* 1930, **2**, 817.
23. Rowbotham E. S. *Br. Med. J.* 1920. **2**, 590.
24. Dorrance G. M. *Surg. Gynecol. Obstet.* 1910, **11**, 160.
25. Guedel A. E. and Waters R. M. *Curr. Res. Anesth. Analg.* 1928, **7**, 238 (reprinted in 'Classical File', *Surv. Anesthesiol.* 1984, **28**, 71).
26. Eisenmenger C. *Wien. Med. Wochenschr.* 1893, **43**, 199.
27. Green N. W. *Surg. Gynecol. Obstet.* 1906, **2**, 512.
28. Hewer C. L. *Recent Advances in Anaesthesia and Analgesia.* 3rd ed. London: Churchill, 1939, 115.
29. Bourne J. G. *Br. Med. J.* 1947, **2**, 654.
30. Wolf G. L. and Simpson J. I. *Anesthesiology* 1987, **67**, 236.
31. Dahlgren B.-E. et al. *Anaesthesia* 1988, **43**, 683.
32. Cole F. *Anesthesiology* 1945, **6**, 87; Mitchell M. D. and Bailey C. M. *Br. Med. J.* 1990, **301**, 602.
33. Alsop A. F. *Anaesthesia* 1955, **10**, 401.
34. Ring W. H. et al. *Anesth. Analg.* 1975, **54**, 273.
35. Jackson C. *Surg. Gynecol. Obstet.* 1013, **17**, 507.
36. Magill I. W. *Lancet* 1926, **1**, 500.
37. Flagg P. J. *Arch. Otolaryngol.* 1928, **8**, 716.
38. Miller R. A. *Anesthesiology* 1941, **2**, 317.
39. Macintosh R. R. *Lancet* 1932 **1**, 205; Boulton T. B. 'Classical File' *Surv. Anesthesiol.* 1983, **27**, 396; Jephcott A. *Anaesthesia* 1984, **39**, 474.
40. Hill W. *Br. Med. J.* 1909, 16 October.
41. Pope E. S. *Anaesthesia* 1960, **15**, 326.
42. Bryce-Smith R. *Br. Med. J.* 1952, **1**, 217.
43. McIntyre J. W. R. *Can. J. Anaesth.* 1989, **36**, 94.
44. Borland L. M. and Casselbrant M. *Anesth. Analg.* 1990, **70**, 105.
45. Magill I. W. *Br. Med. J.* 1920, **2**, 670; Libermann H. *Anaesth. Intensive Care* 1978, **6**, 162.
46. Latto I. P. In: *Difficulties in Tracheal Intubation* (Latto I. P. and Rosen M. ed.) Eastbourne: Baillière Tindall, 1985, 48.
47. Guedel A. E. and Waters R. M. *Curr. Res. Anesth. Analg.* 1928, **7**, 238.
48. Black A. M. S. and Seegobin R. D. *Anaesthesia* 1981, **36**, 498.
49. Guedel A. E. and Waters R. M. *Ann. Otol. Rhinol. Lar.* 1931, **40**, 1139.
50. Seegobin R. D. and Van Hassalt G. L. *Br. Med. J.* 1984, **288**, 965.
51. Reader J. C. et al. *Anaesthesia* 1985, **40**, 444.

52. Sellers W. F. S. and Dye A. *Anaesthesia* 1985, **40**, 483.
53. Rosenberg P. *Berl. Klin. Wochenschr.* 1895, **32**, 14.
54. Magill I. W. *Proc. R. Soc. Med.* 1929, **22**, 83.
55. Forrester A. C. *Br. J. Anaesth.* 1974, **46**, 413.
56. Saarnivaara L. and Klemola U-M. *Acta Anaesthesiol. Scand.* 1991, **35**, 19.
57. Mulholland D. and Carlisle R. J. T. *Anaesthesia* 1991, **46**, 312.
58. Wilson M. E. et al. *Br. J. Anaesth.* 1988, **61**, 211.
59. Cormack R. S. and Lehane J. *Anaesthesia* 1984, **39**, 1105.
60. Williams K. N. et al. *Br. J. Anaesth.* 1991, **66**, 38.
61. Mallampati S. R. et al. *Can. Anaesth. Soc. J.* 1985, **32**, 429; Samsoon G. L. T. and Young J. R. B. *Anaesthesia* 1987, **42**, 487.
62. McIntyre J. W. R. *Can. J. Anaesth.* 1987, **34**, 204.
63. White A. and Kander P. L. *Br. J. Anaesth.* 1975, **47**, 468.
64. Kinyemi O. O. and Elegbe E. O. *Can. Anaesth. Soc. J.* 1981, **28**, 80.
65. Divekar V. M. et al. *Can. Anaesth. Soc. J.* 1979, **26**, 141.
66. Kloss J. and Petty C. *Anesthesiology* 1975, **43**, 380.
67. Berkowitz I. D. et al. *Anesthesiology* 1990, **73**, 739.
68. Nichol H. C. and Zuck D. *Br. J. Anaesth.* 1983, **55**, 141.
69. Schneider M. et al. *Acta Anesthesiol. Scand.* 1989, **33**, 429.
70. Rosen M. In: *Difficulties in Tracheal Intubation.* (Latto I. P. and Rosen M. ed.) Eastbourne: Baillière Tindall, 1985, 152.
71. Hoffman S. et al. *Anesth. Analg.* 1984, **63**, 487.
72. Conrardy P. A. et al. *Crit. Care Med.* 1976, **4**, 8.
73. Birmingham P. K. et al. *Anesth. Analg.* 1986, **65**, 886.
74. Guggenberger H. et al. *Acta Anaesthesiol. Scand.* 1989, **33**, 112.
75. O'Flaherty D. and Adams A. P. *Anaesthesia* 1990, **45**, 653.
76. Williams K. N. and Nunn J. F. *Anaesthesia* 1989, **44**, 412.
77. Green R. A. In: *Anaesthesia Review 4.* London: Churchill Livingstone, 1987, 147; Utting J. E. *Br. J. Anaesth.* 1987, **59**, 877.
78. Gross J. B. et al. *Anesth. Analg. (Cleve.)* 1984, **63**, 915.
79. Maltby J. R. et al. *Anesthesiology* 1988, **69**, 946.
80. Boysen K. *Anaesthesia* 1985, **40**, 1024.
81. Berry F. A. et al. *Pediatrics* 1973, **51**, 476.
82. McShane A. J. and Hone R. *Br. Med. J.* 1986, **292**, 26 and 410.
83. Tunstall M. E. *Anaesthesia* 1976, **31**, 850; Tunstall M. E. and Sheikh A. *Clin. Anaesthesiol.* 1986, **4**, 171.
84. Lyons G. *Anaesthesia* 1985, **40**, 759.
85. Elam J. O. et al. *Anesth. Analg. Curr. Res.* 1969, **48**, 307.
86. Chadwick I. S. and Vohra A. *Anaesthesia* 1989, **44**, 261; Reynolds F. *Anaesthesia* 1989, **44**, 870; McClune S. et al. *Anaesthesia* 1990, **45**, 227.
87. Werman H. A. et al. *Am. J. Emerg. Med.* 1987, **5**, 79.
88. Tunstall M. E. and Geddes C. *Br. J. Anaesth.* 1984, **56**, 659.
89. Macintosh R. R. *Br. Med. J.* 1949, **1**, 28.
90. Dogra S. et al. *Anaesthesia* 1990, **45**, 774.
91. Heath M. L. and Allagain J. *Anaesthesia* 1991, **46**, 545.
92. Rigg D. and Dwyer B. *Anaesth. Intensive Care* 1985, **13**, 431.
93. Ainsworth Q. P. and Howells T. H. *Br. J. Anaesth.* 1989, **62**, 494.
94. Harmer M. and Vaughan R. S. *Anaesthesia* 1980, **35**, 921.
95. Spoerel W. E. et al. *Br. J. Anaesth.* 1971, **43**, 932; Layman P. R. *Anaesthesia* 1983, **38**, 478.
96. Debenham T. R. *Anaesthesia* 1985, **40**, 599.
97. Craft T. M. et al. *Br. J. Anaesth.* 1990, **64**, 524.
98. Murphy P. *Anaesthesia* 1967, **22**, 489.
99. Ikeda S. *Keio J. Med.* 1968, **17**, 1.
100. Taylor P. A. and Towey R. M. *Br. J. Anaesth.* 1972, **44**, 611; Conyers A. B. et al. *Can. Anaesth. Soc. J.* 1972, **19**, 654.

101. Vaughan R. S. *Br. J. Anaesth.* 1991, **66**, 538.
102. McLellan I. et al. *Can. J. Anaesth.* 1988, **35**, 404.
103. Gotta A. W. and Sullivan C. A. *Br. J. Anaesth.* 1981, **53**, 1055.
104. Palva T. et al. *J. Oto-Rhino-Laryngol.* 1975, **37**, 306.
105. Bidwai A. V. et al. *Can. Anaesth. Soc. J.* 1978, **25**, 416.
106. Bidwai A. V. et al. *Anesthesiology* 1979, **51**, 171.
107. Owen H. *Anaesthesia* 1982, **37**, 1112.
108. Thind G. S. *Anaesthesia* 1983, **38**, 393.
109. Rupreht J. and Dworacek B. *Anaesthesia* 1983, **38**, 394.
110. Gefke K. et al. *Acta Anaesthesiol. Scand.* 1983, **27**, 111.
111. Lang S. A. et al. *Can. J. Anaesth.* 1990, **37**, 210.
112. Selsby D. and Jones J. G. *Br. J. Anaesth.* 1990, **64**, 621.
113. Rosen M. and Hillard E. K. *Anesth. Analg.* 1962, **41**, 50.
114. Donati F. *Can. J. Anaesth.* 1988, **35**, 1.
115. Greenbaum R. *Anaesthesia* 1987, **42**, 927; Editorial. *Lancet* 1988, **1**, 743.
116. Chernow B. et al. *Anesth. Analg.* 1984, **63**, 829.
117. Greenberg M. I. et al. *Ann. Emerg. Med.* 1982, **11**, 546.
118. Berlot G. et al. *Anaesthesia* 1985, **40**, 819.
119. Resuscitation Council (UK). *Resuscitation for the Citizen.* 1984.
120. American Heart Association. *JAMA* 1986, **255**, 2933.
121. Quinton D. N. et al. *Lancet* 1987, **1**, 828.
122. Thomson I. R. *Can. J. Anaesth.* 1989, **39**, 367.
123. Reid L. C. and Brace D. E. *Surg. Gynecol. Obstet.* 1940, **70**, 157.
124. Lehtinen A.-M. *Br. J. Anaesth.* 1984, **56**, 247.
125. Gibbs J. M. *N. Z. Med. J.* 1967, **66**, 456.
126. Cozanitis D. A. et al. *Can. Anaesth. Soc. J.* 1984, **31**, 155.
127. Finfer S. R. et al. *Anaesth. Intensive Care* 1989, **17**, 44; Smith J. E. et al. *Br. J. Anaesth.* 1991, **66**, 546; Schaefer H.-G. *Br. J. Anaesth.* 1991, **66**, 608.
128. Van Aken H. et al. *Anesthesiology* 1988, **68**, 157.
129. Crawford D. C. et al. *Br. J. Anaesth.* 1987, **39**, 707.
130. Laurito C. E. et al. *Anesth. Analg.* 1988, **67**, 389; Wilson I. G. et al. *Anaesthesia* 1991, **46**, 177.
131. Hatano Y. et al. *Acta Anesthesiol. Scand.* 1989, **33**, 214.
132. Ghignone M. et al *Anesthesiology* 1986, **64**, 36.
133. Helfman S. M. et al. *Anesth. Analg.* 1991, **72**, 482.
134. Harris C. E. et al. *Anaesthesia* 1988, **43**, (Suppl) 32.
135. Nishikawa T. and Namiki A. *Acta Anesthesiol. Scand.* 1989, **33**, 232.
136. Indu B. et al. *Can. J. Anaesth.* 1989, **36**, 269.
137. Mikawa K. et al. *Anaesthesia* 1990, **45**, 289.
138. McCarthy G. J. et al. *Anaesthesia* 1990, **45**, 243.
139. Stirt J. A. et al. *Anesthesiology* 1987, **67**, 50.
140. Michenfelder J. D. *Anesthesia and the Brain.* New York: Churchill Livingstone, 1988, 145.
141. Loeser F. A. et al. *Can. Anaesth. Soc. J.* 1980, **27**, 56.
142. Caplan I. M. et al. *Anesthesiology* 1984, **59**, 202.
143. Clokie C. et al. *Can. J. Anaesth.* 1989, **36**, 675.
144. Boswell D. E. et al. *J. Med. Defence Union* 1990, **6**, 14.
145. Scammon F. L. and Babin R. W. *Anesthesiology* 1983, **59**, 352.
146. Sherry K. M. *Anesthesiology* 1983, **59**, 148.
147. O'Neill J. et al. *Anesthesiology* 1984, **60**, 482.
148. Majumdar B. et al. *Anaesthesia* 1982, **37**, 67.
149. Frink E. J. and Pattison B. D. *Anesthesiology* 1989, **70**, 358.
150. Kark A. E. et al. *Br. Med. J.* 1984, **289**, 1412.
151. Priebe H-J. et al. *Anesth. Analg.* 1988, **67**, 219.
152. Hahn F. W. et al. *Arch. Otolaryngol.* 1970, **92**, 226; Ellis P. D. M. *Anesthesiology* 1977, **46**, 374.

153. Blau J. N. and Kepadia R. *Br. Med. J.* 1972, **4**, 259.
154. Semon F. *Arch. Laryngol.* 1881, **2**, 197.
155. Gibbin K. P. and Eggiston M. J. *Br. J. Anaesth.* 1981, **53**, 1091.
156. Loughman E. *Anaesth. Intensive Care* 1983, **11**, 171.
157. Stauffer J. L. et al. *Am. J. Med.* 1981, **70**, 65.
158. Smith B. A. C. and Hopkinson R. B. *Anaesthesia* 1984, **39**, 894; Correspondence, *Anaesthesia* 1985, **40**, 211 and 212; Gaukroger P. B. and Anderson G. *Anaesth. Intensive Care* 1986, **14**, 199.
159. Keane W. M. et al. *Ann. Otol. Rhinol. Laryngol.* 1982, **91**, 584; Balestrieri F. *Otolarnygol. Clin. North Am.* 1982, **15**, 567.
160. Ruiz K. et al. *J. Roy. Soc. Med.* 1990, **83**, 806.
161. Brain A. I. J. *Br. J. Anaesth.* 1983, **55**, 801; Brain A. I. J. et al. *Anaesthesia* 1985, **40**, 356; Brain A. I. J. *The Intavent laryngeal mask instruction manual.* Henley-on-Thames: Intavent International, 1990.
162. Payne J. *Anaesthesia* 1989, **44**, 865; Griffin R. M. and Hatcher I. S. *Anaesthesia* 1990, **45**, 1039.
163. Mason D. G. and Bingham R. M. *Anaesthesia* 1990, **45**, 760.
164. Grebenik C. R. et al. *Anesthesiology* 1990, **72**, 474.
165. Bailie R. et al. *Anaesthesia* 1991, **46**, 358.
166. Braude N. et al. *Anaesthesia* 1989, **44**, 551; Hickey S. et al. *Anaesthesia* 1990, **45**, 629.
167. Davies P. R. F. et al. *Lancet* 1990, **336**, 977.
168. Friesen R. H. et al. *Anesth. Analg.* 1987, **66**, 874.
169. Black A. E. et al. *Br. J. Anaesth.* 1990, **65**, 461.
170. Westhorpe R. N. *Anaesth. Intensive Care* 1987, **15**, 384.
171. Kubota, Y. et al., *Anesthesiology*, 1986, **64**, 374.
172. Yates A. P. et al. *Br. J. Anaesth.* 1987, **59**, 524.
173. Inkster J. S. In: *Recent Advances in Anaesthesia and Analgesia – 12* (Hewer C. L. and Atkinson R. S. ed.) Edinburgh: Churchill Livingstone, 1976, 61.

Chapter 12

Artificial ventilation of the lungs

History

This was introduced by Arthur E. Guedel (1883–1956) and David Treweek of Los Angeles in 1934,[1] using ether. Starting off in Stage 3, Plane 2, they quickly increased the ether concentration and produced hyperventilation by bag pressure (assisted respiration) in a closed circuit with the soda-lime canister in operation. They therefore caused a depression of the respiratory centre, hypocapnia and apnoea followed in about 4 min, the so-called 'ether apnoea'. Waters in 1936 first used the term 'controlled respiration'. It is now usually obtained by the use of muscle relaxants or narcotic analgesics.

Artificial ventilation of the lungs was used for the treatment of emphysema in 1951,[2] and in the intensive therapy unit dates from the poliomyelitis epidemic in Copenhagen in 1952.[3] (For history, *see also* Price J. L *Med. Hist. 1962*, **6**, 67.) Rudolf Matas (1860–1957), surgeon of New Orleans, used intralaryngeal intubation with a modified Joseph P. O'Dwyer's (1871–1897) tube in 1902.[4] An early ventilator was described by Janeway in 1913.[5] The Stockholm surgeon, Clarence Crafoord[6] (1899–1984) reported on his spiropulsator in 1940 (the Frenkner spiropulsator was made with the help of P. Frenkner, an ENT surgeon, and Andersson, an engineer in Stockholm; it was driven by compressed air), and in the following year Nosworthy's classic paper appeared.[7] The first British ventilator in commercial production was manufactured by Blease. (*See also* Woolam C. H. M. *Anaesthesia* 1976, **31**, 537, 666; Mushin W. W. et al. *Automatic Ventilation of the Lungs*, 3rd. ed. Oxford: Blackwell, 1980.)

Many accidents have occurred because of disconnection or failure of mechanical ventilators during anaesthesia. The use of disconnection alarms is therefore recommended. For many years IPPV was always carried out by manual compression of the reservoir bag and this technique should not be entirely discarded today.[8]

Apnoea can be produced during anaesthesia by:

1. Use of a muscle relaxant drug to paralyse the respiratory muscles, which is also often given at induction to facilitate tracheal intubation.

2. Depressing the respiratory centre with barbiturates, narcotic analgesics, volatile agents or a combination of these – a pharmacological method.

3. Hyperventilation to reduce $Paco_2$ and physiological stimulus to respiration.

4. A combination of the above methods.

Physiology

In positive-pressure breathing, inspiratory, intrapulmonary and intrapleural pressures are positive instead of negative, as during normal breathing. These effects are greater when the chest wall is intact than during thoracotomy.

Intrapleural pressure. During spontaneous respiration, the pressure is $-5\,cmH_2O$ at end of expiration, and during inspiration it is $-10\,cmH_2O$. In IPPV, pressure rises during inspiration from $-5\,cmH_2O$ to $+3\,cmH_2O$ and falls to $-5\,cmH_2O$ during expiration.

Damage to lungs. Rupture is unlikely, because during coughing and straining pressure may rise to $100\,cmH_2O$. It is difficult to increase pressure above $50\,cmH_2O$ by bag pressure.

Compliance. Anaesthesia, with or without IPPV, produces about a 50% reduction in lung compliance.

Dead space. There is an increase in the ratio of physiological dead space to tidal volume (V_D/V_T). This may reach values of 0.4–0.7 in ventilated anaesthetized subjects, compared to a value of less than 0.3 for spontaneous respiration. The ratio increases with: (1) lung pathology; (2) age; and (3) increasing respiratory frequency. Mechanical dead space may be deliberately added in certain intensive-care situations to produce normal $Paco_2$ during hyperventilation.

Respiratory alkalosis may be caused. This tends to increase the affinity of haemoglobin for oxygen, to cause cerebral vasoconstriction and to decrease cardiac output. Blood pressure is likely to fall, especially when the patient was previously in hypercapnia. Over-ventilation raises the pain threshold, possibly by depressing the ascending reticular formation. Hypocapnia during anaesthesia may not be as benign as was once thought. This has been shown by an increase in postoperative reaction time. Hypocapnia, by causing vasoconstriction in normal brain tissue, directs blood flow into nearby pathological areas, which have vasodilatation due to local tissue acidosis (inverse steal). Intracranial and intraocular pressure is reduced. There may also be a reduced blood flow to the placenta.

Cardiovascular changes. First described by André F. Cournand.[9] (1) Abolition of thoracic pump. At the end of positive-pressure inspiration, right atrial pressure is raised and hence venous return and cardiac output are decreased. This is compensated for by a rise in the peripheral venous pressure, which re-establishes venous return to its former level – due to venoconstriction; (2) cardiac tamponade; not clinically important; and (3) retention of sodium and pulmonary oedema may be caused by long-term IPPV.

Oxygen consumption is reduced because of abolition of respiratory work.

Technique

Tracheal intubation is usually employed. A cuffed tube facilitates easy control of ventilation. Laryngeal masks have been used for short periods but are not generally recommended for IPPV.

Seldom should a pressure of $40\,cmH_2O$ be exceeded – even though during a severe bout of coughing an intrabronchial pressure of $100\,cmH_2O$ has been recorded. Rupture of the lung and its sequelae, pneumothorax, mediastinal emphysema, pulmonary interstitial emphysema and subcutaneous emphysema, are unlikely if due care is taken.

1. Muscle relaxants. The respiratory muscles are usually paralysed by the intravenous injection of a muscle relaxant drug in a dosage sufficient to allow IPPV to be undertaken. Often not needed in intensive care.

2. Intravenous agents. Background respiratory depression with narcotic analgesic drugs facilitates IPPV. Occasionally large doses are employed to produce 'narcotic-induced apnoea'.

3. Inhalation agents. Those with a respiratory depressant action can be used in a similar manner, provided cardiovascular depression is avoided.

Continuous positive airway pressure (CPAP)

This is a term generally used when positive pressure is applied to the airway of a patient who is breathing spontaneously. It has been advocated in a variety of clinical conditions, including respiratory distress of the newborn, following cardiac surgery, etc. It is sometimes valuable during weaning from IPPV. In general the effects of CPAP are similar to those of PEEP.

Positive end-expiratory pressure (PEEP)[10]

In clinical practice it has been found useful in situations where the arterial oxygen tension remains low despite high inspired oxygen concentration. It has been found useful during conditions such as fat embolism and respiratory distress of the newborn. It has proved possible to use PEEP without harmful effects on the cardiac output, although hypovolaemia should be corrected.

The importance of PEEP in intensive care situations is recognized, but there appears to be no place for it during anaesthesia for routine surgical operations. The FRC falls during anaesthesia whether respiration is spontaneous or artificial, but PEEP does not necessarily correct any disturbance of blood gases.

The possible harmful effects of PEEP include:

1. Reduction of cardiac output secondary to decreased venous return to the heart.[11] Any advantage gained by increasing Pao_2 may be offset if reduced cardiac output diminishes the overall oxygen delivery to the tissues. A Swan-Ganz catheter will allow measurement of mixed venous oxygen tension, cardiac output, oxygen consumption and delivery.

2. The increased airway pressure can result in pneumothorax and even air embolism and pneumoperitoneum.[12] Chest radiography may be needed.

3. Renal function may be impaired.[13] Increased output of antidiuretic hormone may be stimulated with reduced urine output and water retention.

4. Rise in cerebral venous and intracranial pressures in parallel with increase in mean intrathoracic pressure.

Indications for PEEP. Cannot be rigidly defined, but may include:

1. In respiratory distress syndrome of both adults and the newborn.

2. A trial of PEEP may be considered whenever PaO_2 cannot be elevated to acceptable levels (say 7 kPa or 50 mmHg) with an F_{IO_2} of 0.5. PEEP may raise Pao_2 with less danger of oxygen toxicity to the lungs than if higher

inspired oxygen concentrations are used. Monitoring of blood gases is essential.

Special care is necessary when PEEP is applied in:
1. Hypovolaemia.
2. Chronic bronchitis, emphysema and bronchospasm.
3. The presence of fractured ribs because of the increased danger of pneumothorax. It is safer with a chest drain in place.
4. Autonomic neuropathy, e.g. in diabetes mellitus.

Intermittent mandatory ventilation (IMV)[14]

This technique has been advocated during weaning from mechanical ventilation. The patient is allowed to breathe spontaneously, but the ventilation is augmented mechanically according to a pre-set minute volume. This can be achieved on servo-ventilators by decreasing the frequency progressively to every second or every fifth breath. It differs from the triggering devices used on earlier ventilators in that the patient cannot activate the mechanical ventilator at a high respiratory rate and the method can be used with volume-cycled as well as pressure-cycled apparatus.

IMV may assist weaning from mechanical ventilation. Synchronized IMV (SIMV) allows the mandatory ventilation to be synchronized with the patient's own inspiratory effort, and is sometimes more effective. Some patients require the additional help to inspiration given by a small positive pressure applied to the airway (pressure support).

Use of IPPV in anaesthesia

When muscle relaxants are used, controlled breathing is usually necessary in order to provide a proper interchange of gases. In thoracic surgery controlled respiration prevents paradoxical breathing, and mediastinal flap. In abdominal operations it allows good relaxation with control of the patient's oxygenation and carbon dioxide elimination. It allows surgery without deep anaesthesia and thus many anaesthetists use it during operations when muscle relaxation is not necessary. It may reduce the amount of thiopentone and relaxant required during the operation, thus contributing to the speedy recovery of consciousness and muscle tone.[15]

High-frequency positive pressure ventilation (HFPPV)[16]

Three types of high-frequency low tidal volume ventilation have been used: high-frequency positive pressure ventilation (HFPPV) 1–2 c/s; high-frequency jet ventilation (HFJV), up to 7 c/s; and high-frequency oscillatory ventilation (HFOV), 5–40 c/s.[17] HFPPV may be delivered using a conventional ventilator circuit, HFJV is given with Venturi equipment, whereas HFOV uses high-frequency solenoid valves.

The technique can be applied using a narrow-bore insufflation tube down the centre of a tracheal tube, in the management of anaesthesia for resection of tracheal stenosis;[18] the tracheal tube is placed proximal to the stenosis and the insufflation tube advanced distal to it so that ventilation can be maintained while the ends of the trachea are freely mobilized. The method has also been used in the care of neonates with the respiratory distress syndrome[19] and also for microlaryngeal laser surgery.[19a]

HFPPV has applications in the management of acute respiratory failure, although its role is controversial. It has been reported to cause improved oxygenation in infants,[20] and adults,[21] though controlled trials relating to survival are not available. Patients with large air leaks due to bronchopleural fistula may do well.[22]

See also Smith B. E. *Br. J. Anaesth.* 1990, **65**, 735.

For the history of ventilation at high respiratory frequencies, *see* Smith R. B. *Anaesthesia* 1982, **37**, 1011.

Ventilators

(For history of ventilators *see* Bendixen H. H. *Acta Anaesthesiol. Scand.* 1982, **26**, 279.)

Manually operated ventilators[23]

There are several simple contrivances that have been developed for ventilation of the lungs. They are portable and suitable for emergency or short-term use. Manual ventilators are useful during transfer of intensive care patients around the hospital. Desirable design features are reviewed by Gray A. J. G. *Br. J. Hosp. Med.* 1981, **25**, 173. (1) a reservoir bag with mask or tracheal tube, provided there is a source of oxygen or compressed air; (2) the Ambu Bag and the Laerdal Bag. The shape is automatically restored after compression and air is drawn in from the atmosphere. Oxygen enrichment of the air can be obtained if the bag is connected to an oxygen supply, but this is not significant unless a reservoir tube is also used[24]; (3) the Oxford Inflating Bellows[25]; (4) The Cardiff Inflating Bellows[26]; (5) the Cardiff Infant Inflating Bag.[27]

Automatic ventilators

For a full description of many of these machines available *see* Mushin W. W. et al. *Automatic Ventilation of the Lungs*, 3rd ed. Oxford: Blackwell, 1980. Some general principles only will be noted here.

Desirable features of an ideal ventilator

The ideal ventilator is compact, portable, robust, simple to operate and economical to purchase, use and maintain. Provision should be made for: (1) a maximum inspiratory flow-rate up to 80 l/min. A tidal volume between 50 and 1500 ml at frequencies between 10 and 50/min. The I:E ratio should be variable; (2) positive pressure during expiration, when desired. There should be continuous monitoring of airway pressure and expired minute volume; (3) use with air, oxygen-enriched mixtures or anaesthetic gases and vapours; (4) humidification of the inspired air; (5) nebulization of drugs; (6) easy to clean and sterilize. Additional systems include use of bacterial filters or disposable tubing; (7) use with non-rebreathing or closed circuit; (8) adaptation for paediatric use; (9) monitoring of oxygen percentage in gases delivered to the patient, or use of a blender so that desired concentration can be set; (10) a warning system and provision for manual ventilation in an emergency. Abnormal pressure build-up, circuit disconnection or power failure should activate warning devices; (11) prevention of gas loss in ventilator tubing due to expansion of the corrugated tube and to the compression of the gas in these tubes. The tubes behave in a similar manner to the respiratory airways and may produce an increase in total dead space. The volume of gas losses may amount to 140 ml/breath. To obviate these factors non-expanding tubes can be used or tidal volume measured at the catheter mount. A spirometer at the ventilator end of the expiratory limb may include gas losses in measured tidal volume. Gas loss is particularly important when volume preset ventilators are used. A dynamic method for measuring the internal compliance of ventilators has been described;[28] and (12) provision of the facility of intermittent mandatory ventilation or mandatory minute volume (*see above*).

Characteristics of ventilators

Pressure preset – build up to a preset pressure. Small leaks are automatically compensated for. Large leaks may cause the machine to stop if the preset pressure is not reached.

Volume preset – deliver a set volume of gas. Pressure will build up to overcome an obstruction. A safety blow-off is necessary, usually about 30 cmH$_2$O.

Cycling. This refers to the mechanism that brings about the change from the inspiratory to the expiratory phase. (The change from expiration to inspiration is usually controlled by a timing mechanism.) Machines may be *pressure cycled*, *volume cycled*, or *time cycled*. In the strict sense, time cycled refers to machines with an auxiliary timing mechanism, but in the wider sense it applies to any machine in which the duration of inspiration and expiration is set by the operator.

Wave Form

1. Pressure generators. A rapid inflationary stroke to produce a square wave form. Prolongation of inspiratory phase much above 1 s does not increase filling of lungs.

2. Flow generators. Triangular wave form. Inflation pressure increases steadily throughout inspiratory phase.

Type of activation

1. Electrical. Mains or battery.

2. Compressed gas. By pipeline or a compressor can be used.

Notes on some ventilators

Many models are now in production and it is impossible to describe them all (*see also* Chapter 6).

1. The Manley Ventilators.[29] A simple minute volume divider which is operated by the gas flow delivered to it. The tidal volume is set, and the machine delivers the minute volume supplied to it at an appropriate rate at a maximal inspiratory pressure of 35 cmH$_2$O. Pressure can be varied. Newer

modifications include the Brompton Manley[30] and the Manley Pulmovent. The Manley Servovent is a high powered versatile apparatus, volume cycled flow generator and volume preset.

2. Cape Ventilator.[31] A popular and robust apparatus which has stood the test of time. It was volume cycled.

3. Nuffield Anaesthetic Ventilator.[32] Small and compact; convenient for use with Bain anaesthetic system. Powered by compressed gas.

4. Servo-ventilators.[33] The electronic circuits of these ventilators allow control of the various facets of IPPV by operation of simple controls. These include rate, inspiratory pressure, wave form, sighing, triggering, control of oxygen concentration and provision for intermittent mandatory ventilation. The models in production provide autoclavable patient circuits and are generally powered by compressed air or other gas. These and other electronic ventilators are designed for use in intensive therapy units.

5. Bag in bottle ventilators. Popular for use with circle systems, but need a separate driving gas supply. The design of the bellows must ensure that inward gas leaks do not occur.

6. A number of ventilators have been developed for use in infants and children, providing small tidal volumes and minimal dead space. Examples include the Bourns, Loosco Amsterdam, and Sheffield.

7. Some small and compact ventilators have been designed for emergency use and use during transport of patients, e.g. the MinEpac Emergency Ventilator.[34]

References

1. Guedel A. F. and Treweek D. M. *Curr. Res. Anesth. Analg.* 1934, **13**, 263 (reprinted in 'Classical File', *Surv. Anesthesiol.* 1970, **14**, 405).
2. Boutourline-Young H. J. and Whittenberger J. L. *J. Clin. Invest.* 1951, **30**, 838.
3. Lassen H. C. A. *Lancet* 1953, **1**, 37 (reprinted in 'Classical File', *Surv. Anesthesiol.* 1978, **22**, 398); Ibsen B. *Proc. R. Soc. Med.* 1954, **47**, 52.
4. Matas R. *Am. Med.* 1902, **3**, 97.
5. Janeway H. H. *Ann. Surg.* 1913, **58**, 927.
6. Andersson E. et al. *Acta Otolaryngol.* 1940, **28**, 95.
7. Nosworthy M. D. *Proc. R. Soc. Med.* 1941, **34**, 497.
8. Gilbertson A. A. *Anaesthesia* 1982, **37**, 987.
9. Cournand A. et al. *Am. J. Physiol.* 1948, **152**, 161.
10. Cheney F. W. et al. *Anesthesiology* 1967, **28**, 670.
11. Courmand A. et al. *Am. J. Physiol.* 1948, **152**, 162; Morgan B. C. et al. *Anesthesiology* 196, **27**, 584.
12. Summers B. *Br. Med. J. 1979*, **1**, 1528.
13. Hale S. V. et al. *Anesthesiology* 1974, **41**, 452.
14. *See also* Downs J. B. et al. *Chest* 1973, **64**, 331; Downs J. B. et al. *Anesth. Analg (Cleve.)* 1974, **53**, 437; Desautels D. and Bartlett J. L. *Respiratory Care* 1974, **19**, 187; Lawler P. G. and Nunn J. F. *Anaesthesia* 1977, **32**, 138.
15. Gray T. C. and Jackson-Rees G. *Br. Med. J. 1952*, **2**, 891.
16. *See also* Gioia F. R. and Rogers M. C. In: *Recent Advances in Anaesthesia and Analgesia – 15.* (Atkinson R. S. and Adams A. P. ed.) Edinburgh: Churchill Livingstone, 1985; Annotation, *Lancet*, 1986, **1**, 477.
17. McEvoy R. D. *Anaesth. Intensive Care* 1985, **13**, 178.
18. Eriksson I. et al. *Acta Anaesthesiol. Scand.* 1975, **19**, 113.

19. Heijmann K. and Sjostrand U. *Opuscular medica* 1974, **19**, 235.
19a. Dhara S. S. and Butler P. J. *Anaesthesia* 1992, **47**, 421.
20. Frantz I. D. et al. *Paediatrics* 1983, **71**, 483.
21. Schuster D. P. et al. *Chest* 1981, **80**, 682.
22. Turnbull A. D. et al. *Ann. Thorac. Surg.* 1980, **32**, 468.
23. *See also* Harber T. and Lucas B. G. B. *Ann. R. Coll. Surg. Eng.* 1980, **62**, 291.
24. Birt R. C. *Anaesthesia* 1965, **20**, 323.
25. Macintosh R. R. *Br. Med. J.* 1953, **2**, 201; Macintosh R. R. and Mushin W. W. *Br. Med. J.* 1955, **2**, 202.
26. Hillard E. K. and Mushin W. W. *Br. Med. J.* 1960, **2**, 729.
27. Mushin W. W. and Hillard E. K. *Br. Med. J.* 1967, **1**, 416.
28. Loh L. and Chakrabarti M. K. *Anaesthesia* 1971, **26**, 414.
29. Manley R. W. *Anaesthesia* 1961, **16**, 317.
30. English I. C. W. and Manley R. E. W. *Anaesthesia* 1970, **25**, 541.
31. Waine T. E. and Fox D. E. R. *Br. J. Anaesth.* 1962, **34**, 410.
32. Adams A. P. and Henville J. D. *Anaesthesia* 1977, **32**, 34.
33. Ingelstedt S. et al. *Acta Anaesthesiol. Scand.* 1972, Suppl. 47.
34. Burchell G. B. *Anaesthesia* 1967, **22**, 647.

Chapter 13

Production of ischaemia during operations

Bleeding is due to cutting blood vessels!

Some patients bleed very little with a normal blood pressure and the relationship between BP and bleeding is not as clear as was once thought. It has even been suggested that a reduction of arterial pressure by 20–40 mmHg is sufficient to reduce bleeding.

History of induced ischaemia during operations

In former times, chloroform was used in an effort (often very successful) to reduce bleeding.

Controlled arteriotomy followed by autotransfusion.[1] This is haemorrhagic hypotension (shock), and is associated with reduced oxygen availability and metabolic acidosis. It is no longer employed.

High intradural spinal analgesia by Griffiths and Gillies in 1948.[2]

High extradural spinal analgesia by Bromage in 1951.[3]

Ganglion-blocking agents. Demonstration of the ganglion-blocking effects of hexamethonium and also of pentamethonium, used to reverse the actions of decamethonium,[4] clinical hypotension shown to follow pentamethonium.[5] Hexamethonium preferred to pentamethonium by Hunter.[6] Pentolinium used by Enderby.[7] Trimetaphan used by Sarnoff[8] and by Magill and others.[9] Phenactropinium reported on by Robertson and others.[10]

Vasodilators. Sodium nitroprusside was used to control hypertensive crises in 1929[11] and to reduce bleeding during anaesthesia in 1962;[12] used in Britain in 1968.[13]

The influence of the head-up posture on the production of hypotension was early demonstrated by Enderby and was named 'postural ischaemia' by Sir Henry Dale after watching Enderby at work in 1949 (see *Hypotensive Anaesthesia* (Enderby G. E. H. ed.) Edinburgh: Churchill Livingstone, 1985). The term 'physiological trespass' was coined by John Gillies of Edinburgh.[14] The plastic surgeon Sir Archibald McIndoe gave it his influential support in its early days. Halothane was advocated for hypotension in 1960.[15] Propranolol was used to control the tachycardia sometimes seen.[16]

The rubber bandage or tourniquet was introduced in 1869 by Esmarch.[17]

Increased bleeding during anaesthesia

Anaesthetic causes

The production of unconsciousness results in the release of vasomotor tone at the periphery and while those vessels supplying the skin and muscles dilate, those going to the kidney and splanchnic area constrict.

Bleeding may be made worse by: (1) respiratory obstruction; (2) hypercapnia; (3) coughing during induction and maintenance, especially in surgery involving the head and neck. This raises the intrathoracic pressure, venous pressure, and hence causes venous oozing; (4) resistance in the anaesthetic system, including a tight expiratory valve causing a rise in intrathoracic pressure during expiration; and (5) unnecessary production of tachycardia by atropine and other vagolytic drugs.

Non-anaesthetic causes

(1) Venous congestion secondary to: (*a*) posture; (*b*) heart disease; (*c*) lung disease; (*d*) overtransfusion; (2) the hyperaemia of acute and chronic inflammation; (3) conditions causing a rise in the basal metabolic rate; (4) operations involving vascular tissues, e.g. muscle or gland; (5) a rise in blood pressure. This does not always increase bleeding; (6) bleeding associated with systemic disease such as deficiency of clotting factors, e.g. idiopathic cytopaenic purpura, liver disease, disseminated intravascular coagulopathy, haemophilia (*see also* Chapter 20); (7) haemorrhagic tendency due to treatment: (*a*) massive blood transfusion; (*b*) citrate intoxication; (*c*) incompatible blood transfusion: remedy – stop transfusion and give massive doses of steroids (*see also Chapter 17*); (*d*) previous administration of anticoagulants; and (*e*) trauma to the blood in extracorporeal circulation; (8) there is no certain relationship between the degree of bleeding and the fall in blood pressure. Some patients bleed when the blood pressure is very low; and (9) bleeding caused by drugs other than anticoagulants, e.g. aspirin.

A clinical haematologist should be involved at an early stage.

Ischaemia during operation

In addition to the total ischaemia produced in the limbs by tourniquets (*see below*), relative ischaemia may be produced by:

1. Reduction of *venous* bleeding by elevating the part to be operated on, e.g. head-up in mastoid or facial surgery, Trendelenberg position in varicose vein surgery.

2. Reduction of *capillary* bleeding by local injection of vasoconstrictors e.g. adrenaline, vasopressin, etc.

3. Reduction of *arterial* bleeding by (a) reducing pulse rate; (b) reducing arterial pressure; and (c) reducing $Paco_2$, by IPPV.

A comprehensive ischaemic technique may use all three of these approaches.

The production of adequate ischaemia does not always demand a reduction of arterial pressure.

Reduction of arterial pressure

Produced by:

A. REDUCTION OF CARDIAC OUTPUT

1. Reduction of cardiac output by producing bradycardia with beta blockade, short-acting opioids, halothane, etc.
2. Reduction of cardiac output by myocardial depression, e.g. by beta-blockade, halothane, enflurane.
3. Reduction of cardiac output by reducing venous return with vasodilators and head-up position, by spinal blockade, and by application of negative pressure to the lower limbs after moderate hypotension has been induced by a ganglionic blocking agent.[18] Some workers have used PEEP to reduce venous return.

B. REDUCTION OF PERIPHERAL VASCULAR RESISTANCE BY DRUGS

1. Volatile agents, especially isoflurane.
2. Nitroprusside and nitrites (*see below*).
3. Ganglionic blocking drugs (*see below*).

C. REDUCTION OF PERIPHERAL RESISTANCE BY SPINAL BLOCKADE

See Chapter 25.

The 'normal' blood pressure during sleep is often little above 80 mmHg.[19] Blood pressure should be monitored frequently by the most accurate method available. A systolic pressure of 60–80 mmHg usually gives adequate ischaemia for most operations.

Ganglionic blocking agents

Pharmacodynamics

Ganglion blocking agents may cause: (1) low arterial pressure with postural sensitivity; (2) release of autonomic tone by paralysis of ganglia at the preganglionic synapses of both sympathetic and parasympathetic systems, the former predominating; (3) non-depolarizing myoneural block increased; (4) respiratory depression; and (5) dilated pupils.

Hypotension and decreased haemorrhage may be due to: (1) the effects of gravity on blood distribution when the arterial pressure is low; (2) the effects of gravity on venous blood, causing it to pool in the distended veins of the lower and dependent parts of the body; and (3) the reduced cardiac output consequent on the reduced venous return to the heart. As both sympathetic and parasympathetic ganglia are blocked, hypotension depends on the original balance of these two. Where there is great parasympathetic tone, its release will cause tachycardia, so that hypotension will not be maximal. Tachycardia may also be due to the hypotension stimulating the baroceptor mechanism, an example of Marey's law. Myocardial ischaemia may occur, but a reduction in peripheral resistance requires less myocardial work and oxygen consumption.

The drugs pass the placental barrier but do not cause ill effects in the fetus.

Renal blood flow. Glomerular filtration decreases with the fall in blood pressure and ceases at about 50–70 mmHg. Renal perfusion sufficient to meet the metabolic needs of the kidney does not suffer until the pressure is much lower, and as the pressure rises, function returns.

The liver. Little harm appears to result from reasonable hypotension.

Cerebral blood flow. Opinions vary about this, some investigators finding a reduced cerebral blood flow, others finding it well maintained due to decreased cerebrovascular resistance,[20] but this is influenced by blood gas homeostasis, blood viscosity, CSF pressure and body temperature as well as by the diameter of the vessels. In cerebral atheroma, the vessels cannot dilate to decrease vascular resistance and ischaemia may therefore occur in such patients.

Coronary blood flow. The state of the coronary vessels is important in the development of cardiac ischaemia when hypotension occurs, but low arterial pressure reduces cardiac work and the demand of the myocardium for oxygen so that myocardial perfusion remains adequate.[21] There is no evidence that hypotensive anaesthesia causes any permanent damage to the myocardium[22] seen on electrocardiographic evidence, although marked T or ST wave alterations would indicate acute ischaemia.

Lung changes. The physiological dead space (adequate ventilation of underperfused alveoli) is increased by hypotension under IPPV as it also is by the head-up position, by haemorrhage, and by the rise in the mean intrathoracic pressure associated with IPPV. Hypoventilation is to be avoided. Full oxygenation should always be maintained.

Pharmacokinetics. The drugs are not metabolized in the body, but are excreted via the renal glomeruli, 50% in 2 hours and 90% within 24 hours after intravenous injection. Renal failure may delay excretion and cause accumulation of the drugs. If the blood pressure drops below 50–70 mmHg glomerular filtration ceases and excretion will no longer take place.

Trimetaphan camsylate, BP (*Arfonad*)

This compound, a thiophanium derivative, was described by Randall and others[23] in 1949. First used in the UK by Magill, Scurr and Wyman in 1953.[24] It is a ganglion-blocking agent and has a direct dilator effect on peripheral vessels. It liberates histamine. During anaesthesia it can be given as an intravenous drip in a strength of 0.1% (1 mg/ml) at a rate of 0.1–5 mg/min. The drug can be given by repeated single injections of 2.5–10 mg of a 1% solution. It inhibits serum cholinesterase. Recovery is usually moderately rapid.

Trimetaphan causes more hypotension in arteriosclerotic patients than in those with normal blood pressure, and may cause a fall in body temperature after long operations. It may, however, result in tachyphylaxis, tachycardia and rather prolonged hypotension. It potentiates non-depolarizing neuromuscular block.[25] Partially excreted by the kidneys after destruction by cholinesterase, although the exact mechanism is in dispute. The maximum dose should not exceed 1 g.

Vasodilators

Sodium nitroprusside[26]

PHYSICAL AND CHEMICAL PROPERTIES

The commercial preparation (Nipride) is freeze-dried and presented as 50 mg dry powder in a sealed ampoule. Dissolved in 500 ml 5% dextrose for clinical use (100 or 200 µg/ml). Such solutions are unstable and must be protected from light (10% decrease in potency in 3 hours, 50% in 48 hours in bright light).[27] Appearance of blue colour suggests undue breakdown and such solutions should be discarded.

The solution should be prepared immediately before use.

PHARMACODYNAMICS

The action is a direct one on smooth muscle of blood vessels to produce relaxation and hence vasodilatation. The mode of action probably involves sulphydryl (SH) groups bound to smooth-muscle membrane.[28] There is a greater effect on arterial than on venous vessels.[29] Cardiac output is usually maintained, and here there is a major difference from the effect of other drugs. Tissue perfusion is unlikely to be compromised. Moderate tachycardia is frequent, probably caused by stimulation of baroreceptor reflexes. Renal blood flow is increased. It is a cerebral vasodilator, which tends to maintain cerebral blood flow as the blood pressure drops.

PHARMACOKINETICS

Sodium nitroprusside is rapidly broken down in the blood stream, probably both in the plasma and in the red cells, with the production of nitric oxide (NO) and hydrocyanic acid, which is then conjugated with thiosulphate to form thiocyanate. Overdosage leads to accumulation of free cyanide ions, so that dosage must be strictly controlled. Thiocyanate levels can be measured as a monitor of toxicity during prolonged administration of nitroprusside, although it rises too slowly to be a useful index of overdose during short-term infusions. Thiocyanate is excreted in the urine. A small amount of cyanide is excreted after combination with vitamin B_{12} to form cyanocobalamin, but this is not clinically important.

Toxic reactions. There have been some case reports of cardiovascular collapse and severe metabolic acidosis after administration of large doses of sodium nitroprusside in resistant patients. It is likely that such patients have suffered acute cyanide poisoning, the metabolic acidosis being a result of histotoxic hypoxia.[30] It has been suggested that the minimal lethal dose of nitroprusside for short-term infusions is about 200–300 mg, whereas a dose of more than 20 mg is rarely necessary.[31] Nitroprusside should be avoided when normal cyanide metabolism is inhibited as in liver or renal failure, Lebers optic atrophy[32] and tobacco amblyopia.

Treatment of overdose[31]. Fluid replacement should be adequate. If severe metabolic acidosis is confirmed, 25 ml 50% sodium thiosulphate[33] should be given intravenously over 3–5 min. If there is no improvement 20 ml (300 mg) of cobalt edetate is recommended at 1 ml/sec.[34]

CLINICAL USE

A separate intravenous infusion should be set up containing 100 or 200 µg/ml in 5% dextrose. The maximum safe dose should be calculated as 1.5 mg/kg and never exceeded. An electronic drip controller or 'Dial a Flow' should be used and T-piece or two-way tap systems avoided.

An initial infusion rate of 37.5 µg/min is recommended in the healthy adult. Response is usually seen within 30 s and thereafter arterial pressure changes determine the infusion rate; 10 µg/kg/min should not be exceeded. Arterial pressure begins to rise within one minute of the cessation of the infusion and is normally complete within 5–10 min. Blood pressure must be monitored closely throughout the operation, using a Dinamap or direct arterial method.

It has been suggested that the anaesthetic technique used should incorporate IPPV with a muscle relaxant and an inspired oxygen concentration of at least 33%.

The container of the drip solution should be protected from light by an opaque cover because the degradation products may result in toxicity.[35]

The return of normal blood pressure should take place within a few minutes of turning off the drip and, rarely, fluid loading or a pressor agent must be used.

INDICATIONS

(1) Neurosurgery. Cerebral aneurysms and arteriovenous malformations. (2) Phaeochromocytoma. (3) The surgery of scoliosis. (4) Aortic surgery. (5) Cardiopulmonary bypass, to decrease after-load in the immediate post-bypass period. (6) Intensive care. During long-term use plasma thiocyanate levels may be monitored to avoid overdose. Levels should not exceed 1.7 mmol/l (10 mg%). Acute hypertensive crises. Cardiogenic shock to reduce cardiac work. Management of ergot overdosage.[36]

Glyceryl trinitrate (Nitroglycerin; Nitrostat)

First used for the treatment of angina by William Murrell (1853–1912) of London, in 1879.[37] The raw material of dynamite. This has been used intravenously at a rate of about 20 µg/min. Its action is similar to that of nitroprusside, but it is claimed that the course of hypotension is smoother with fewer peaks and troughs of arterial pressure.

The unopened ampoules of 0.5% solution are reasonably stable but unused contents must be discarded once opened. It is rapidly destroyed in the liver. In the blood-stream methaemoglobin accumulates but this is of scant clinical importance.

PHARMACODYNAMICS

It produces relaxation of the smooth muscle in vessel walls, especially in veins. In reasonable dosage it improves coronary perfusion. Intracranial pressure rises.

Its solutions are absorbed by polyvinyl chloride containers and tubing so that polythene or glass must be used.

CLINICAL USE

Many workers employ a 0.01% solution with an initial drip rate of 10 μg/min. Hypotensive effects come on more slowly and last much longer than when sodium nitroprusside is infused. A power-driven infusion pump should be used for its administration. (*See also* Verner I. R. in: *Hypotensive Anaesthesia* (Enderby G. E. H. ed.) Edinburgh: Churchill Livingstone, 1985, 138.)

The purine, adenosine, has been successfully used to provide controllable and safe hypotension.[38]

Potentiation of hypotension

Volatile agents

All volatile agents potentiate hypotensive drugs. Isoflurane is especially useful because of its predominantly vasodilator properties. Its cardiovascular effects are more benign than those of halothane or enflurane and has emerged as a safe and controllable technique, given in the closed system with mildly hypocapnic IPPV, high oxygen tensions, and careful agent monitoring. For surgery of the upper body, head-up tilt increases its effectiveness. Like other volatile agents, it is more controllable in the sense that it can be removed from the body simply by reducing the inhaled percentage. It preserves cerebral and coronary perfusion, even in severe hypotension. However, occasionally it completely fails to produce an ischaemic operating field (this, after all, is the aim of the whole technique!), and a change to another agent is indicated.

β-Blockers

Used to produce bradycardia, normally with volatile agents and IPPV.[39]

1. Propranolol. A β_1- and β_2-blocker, 0.035 mg/kg i.v., repeated until the pulse rate is at the required rate; onset in one circulation time, duration about 45 min (ideal for many cases because it is wearing off as the operation finishes). Dangerous bronchospasm may occur in the asthmatic patient.

2. Metoprolol. A cardioselective β-blocker. Dose: 0.1 mg/kg, onset in one circulation time, duration 1–1.5 h. It is also satisfactory when used with halothane.[40]

The injections of β-blockers should be slow and given following the induction of anaesthesia and before the injection of the hypotensive agent.

Labetalol

It reduces arterial pressure by reducing cardiac output and heart rate, and decreasing peripheral resistance. First used in anaesthesia by Scott et al. in 1976.[41] α- and β-receptors are blocked so that hypotension is produced, without tachycardia, in association with halothane anaesthesia; dose: 5–25 mg i.v. Smaller doses are required when halothane is also administered, and even smaller doses when IPPV is employed.[41] Larger doses, up to 2 mg/kg have been given in association with a nitrous oxide, oxygen, relaxant, narcotic analgesic technique. Should marked bradycardia occur, atropine may be given, and this may result in a rise of arterial pressure. 10 mg of labetalol is equivalent to 2 mg of propranolol at β_1-receptors, 0.75 mg of propranolol at β_2-receptors, and 2 mg of phentolamine at α_1-receptors.[42] The half-life of labetalol given intravenously is between 3.5 and 6.3 hours, depending on the dose administered.[43] Deep planes of halothane anaesthesia may cause profound hypotension and bradycardia, but reversal is rapid when the concentration is reduced. Given with care, a useful agent in young and fit patients.

Clinical use of the ischaemic technique

The technique is simple, but must be meticulous. Both the airway and the patient's ventilation must be faultless, and adequate anaesthesia provided. Tracheal intubation and IPPV is usually employed (*see below*). A large-bore intravenous infusion is set up. If head-up tilt is required, a calculation is made to assess the cerebral arterial pressure, from the height above the arterial pressure measuring point. For monitoring, *see below*.

It must be remembered that adequate ischaemia does not always demand arterial hypotension, and that to induce severe hypotension in the pursuit of ischaemia, or at the request of a surgeon, may be indefensible. Greater difficulty in producing an ischaemic field of operation may be found:

1. where there is inflammation;
2. in young adult women; and
3. unexpectedly in any patient.

Failure to produce good ischaemia with ganglionic blocking agents may be due to: (1) incomplete block of sympathetic ganglia; (2) increased cardiac output due to tachycardia; or (3) presence of injected or endogenous noradrenaline or adrenaline in the circulation.

When the arterial pressure becomes unstable, with risk of severe hypotension, volume-loading the circulation with 0.5–1 l of colloid restores stability without compromising the ischaemic field.

A 'hypotension drill' must be worked out to cope with unexpected severe falls of systolic pressure, e.g. <60 mmHg.

1. Run the intravenous drip at full speed;
2. reduce the volatile agent, or vasodilator infusion;
3. inject atropine if bradycardia has become severe (<40 bpm);
4. inject ephedrine, 10 mg. i.v. repeated as necessary;
5. level the operating table, if head-up;
6. increase $F_{I}O_2$.

A preoperatively labile arterial pressure is an indication that small dosage of hypotensive agents will probably be adequate; other such indications for small dosage are increasing age and low metabolic rate. Arteriosclerotic patients require a small dose and little posture to get a profound effect, whereas young, fit patients, besides often developing tachycardia, require a steeper head-up tilt and higher initial dosage of antihypertensive drugs.

Posture

Gravity acting on the tilted patient results in blood pooling in the dilated (capacitance) veins, and this leads to decreased venous return and hypotension.

Posture is also used to make the operation site ischaemic. The blood pressure is said to be reduced 20 mmHg for each 2.5 cm of vertical height above heart level, so that when the head is tilted 25° upwards, the cerebral blood pressure is likely to be about 16 mmHg less than the blood pressure at heart level. Many, but not all, experienced workers consider it reasonably safe in normal patients to allow a 25° head-up tilt with a brachial arterial blood pressure of 60–70 mmHg.

Intermittent positive-pressure ventilation

This is usually employed with a high inspired oxygen concentration. Increased airway pressure is transmitted to the great veins and so venous return to the heart is decreased; this lowers the blood pressure further, depending on the pressure in the reservoir bag. Positive end-expiratory pressure (PEEP) is used as a supplement by some workers.

There are workers of experience in the production of hypotensive anaesthesia who allow their patients to breathe spontaneously.[44]

Monitoring induced arterial hypotension

The arterial pressure is monitored continuously if the pressure is low or unstable, or at 1-min intervals where adequate ischaemia has been produced without greatly lowering the pressure. Spo_2, capnography, and agent concentration are important.

Limits of safety

The usual monitor default limit of 50 BPM is satisfactory; a systolic pressure of half the preoperative level is normally a safe lower limit.

Towards the end of the operation the blood pressure is allowed to rise slowly, and no patient should leave the table unless his systolic pressure is 100 mmHg or more, except in exceptional circumstances, e.g. after some neurosurgical operations. Arterial pressure monitoring continues throughout the postoperative period.

The results in successful cases are: (1) an ischaemic field of operation; (2) easier surgical dissection; (3) reduction of amount of ligatured or cauterized tissue and consequent reduction in infection; and (4) decreased oozing beneath skin flaps, less postoperative oedema and hence better healing.

Enormous experience with the employment of hypotensive anaesthesia together with great professional skill has led Enderby to state that a systolic pressure of 60 mmHg at head level, can be produced in the majority of patients without complications.[45] For safe use, the technique demands expertise and experience.

Cerebral, coronary, renal and hepatic blood-flow during moderate induced hypotension is well preserved, as a result of autoregulation.

Prevention of postoperative 'afterdrop' of arterial pressure is achieved by levelling the table, and volume loading the patient with 0.5–1 l intravenously. Ephedrine, 30 mg i.m. can also be given.

Hypotension in children

This may be necessary in paediatric practice for operations such as resection of coarctation of the aorta, and scoliosis surgery.[46] Sodium nitroprusside is safe in a dose up to 10 µg/kg/min. High dosage can cause fatal cyanide intoxication.

The dangers of 'the hypotensive technique'

Many workers think that the technique should be confined to those cases where it makes the impossible possible. It should not be used to make the possible easy. Other workers employ it more liberally. Its advantages to the patient must be weighed against the increased risks. These are cerebral and coronary thrombosis, renal and hepatic ischaemia, reactionary haemorrhage, ileus, cerebral ischaemia, arterial thrombosis (e.g. the carotid, central retinal artery and limb arteries), and massive atelectasis.

Indications

These may include the following:

(1) neurosurgery, especially in operations for vascular tumours and aneurysms;

(2) peripheral vascular surgery, e.g. coarctation of the aorta to reduce bleeding from enlarged vessels in the chest wall;

(3) operations associated with voluminous haemorrhage, e.g. total cystectomy, abdominoperineal resection of the rectum, panhysterectomy and pelvic exenteration;

(4) plastic surgery and operations on the nose and lacrimal apparatus;[47]

(5) microsurgery (e.g. middle ear);

(6) when a patient's abnormal blood group makes transfusion difficult;

(7) pelvic floor repair operations;

(8) prostatectomy;

(9) to reduce uncontrollable bleeding during operation;

(10) intensive care;

(11) operations behind the eye because intraocular pressure is reduced; and

(12) to reduce blood-loss in operations on *Jehovah's witnesses*, a sect originating near Pittsburg in 1872, who proscribe blood transfusion. Autotransfusion is acceptable to some of them and was first performed in 1886.[48] For clean surgery, a Bentley recirculator is useful.[49]

Contra-indications

These vary in the practice of different workers. The following conditions may increase the danger: (1) respiratory inadequacy from any cause, especially obstructive airways disease; (2) bronchospasm and asthma; (3) diabetes, because ganglionic blocking agents increase the patient's response to insulin, and hypoglycaemia may result; (4) cerebral and coronary vascular disease and atheroma; (5) previous steroid therapy; (6) where there is poor renal or hepatic function; (7) in Addison's disease; (8) in pregnancy; (9) *when the technical skills and experience of the anaesthetist are not of a high order*; and (10) when the surgeon is not accustomed to working under hypotensive conditions.

Discussion

It would seem that in expert and experienced hands, induced hypotension in normal patients with the blood pressure reduced to 70–80 mmHg and even with 25° head-up tilt is reasonably safe. What is certain is that the technique can be lethal if its details are not fully understood and if it is not conducted impeccably.

The anaesthetist is warned against production of hypotension at the request of the surgeon where this may affect the safety of the patient.

Induced hypotension should only be employed if the anaesthetist and surgeon are in full agreement as to its desirability and are both experienced in its use.

(*See also* Enderby G. E. H. ed. *Hypotensive Anaesthesia* Edinburgh: Churchill Livingstone, 1985.)

Tourniquets

Tourniquets are used during operations on limbs. Care must be taken that they are properly applied. Pneumatic tourniquets using a Bourdon-type pressure gauge are not always well maintained with the risk of unduly high pressures causing nerve damage. Three hours is the absolute maximum. Application of tourniquets to the lower limbs raises the central venous pressure.

References

1. Gardner W. J. *JAMA* 1946, **132**, 572 (reprinted in 'Classical File', *Surv. Anesthesiol.* 1969, **13**, 220).
2. Koster H. *Am. J. Surg.* 1928, **5**, 554; Vehrs G. R. *NW. Med. Seattle* 1931, **30**, 256, 322; Griffiths, M. W. C. and Gillies J. *Anaesthesia* 1948, **3**, 134 (reprinted in 'Classical File', *Surv. Anesthesiol.* 1980, **24**, 342).
3. Bromage P. R. *Anaesthesia* 1951, **6**, 26.

4. Paton W. D. M. and Zaimis E. J. *Nature* 1948, **162**, 810.
5. Organe G. S. W. et al. *Lancet* 1949, **1**, 21.
6. Hunter A. R. *Lancet* 1950, **1**, 251; Shackleton R. P. W. *Br. Med. J.* 1951, **1**, 1054; Wyman J. B. *Proc. R. Soc. Med.* 1953, **46**, 605.
7. Enderby G. E. H. *Lancet* 1950, **1**, 1145; Enderby G. E. H. and Pelmore J. F. *Lancet* 1951, **1**, 663; Enderby G. E. H. *Lancet* 1954, **2**, 1097.
8. Sarnoff S. J. et al. *Circulation* 1952, **6**, 63.
9. Magill I. W. et al. *Lancet* 1953, **1**, 219.
10. Robertson J. D. et al. *Br. J. Anaesth.* 1957, **29**, 342.
11. Johnson C. C. *Arch. Int. Pharmacodyn. Thér.* 1929, **35**, 480.
12. Moraca P. et al. *Anesthesiology* 1962, **23**, 193.
13. Jones G. O. M. and Cole P. *Br. J. Anaesth.* 1968, **40**, 804.
14. Gillies J. *Ann. R. Coll. Surg.* 1950, **7**, 204.
15. Enderby G. E. H. *Anaesthesia* 1960, **15**, 25.
16. Hellewell J. and Potts M. W. *Br. J. Anaesth.* 1966, **38**, 794; Johnstone M. *Br. J. Anaesth.* 1966, **38**, 516.
17. Esmarch J. F. A. von *Der erste Verband auf dem Schlachtfelde.* Kiel: Schwers'sche Buchhandlung, 1869.
18. Saunders J. W. *Lancet* 1952, **1**, 1286.
19. Richardson D. W. et al. *Clin Sci.* 1964 **26**, 445.
20. Slack W. K. et al. *Lancet* 1963 **1**, 1082; Eckenhoff J. E. et al *J. Appl. Physiol.* 1963 **18**, 1130; Eckenhoff J. E. *Lancet* 1964, **2**, 711.
21. Hickey R. H. et al. *Anesthesiology* 1983, **59**, 226.
22. Rollason W. N. and Cumming A. R. R. *Anaesthesia* 1956, **11**, 319; Rollason W. H. and Hough C. M. *Br. J. Anaesth.* 1960, **32**, 276, 286; Simpson P. et al. *Anaesthesia* 1976, **32**, 1172.
23. Randall L. O. et al. *J. Pharmacol. Exp. Ther.* 1949, **97**, 48.
24. Magill I. W. et al. *Lancet* 1953, **1**, 219.
25. Sklar G. S. and Lanks K. W. *Anesthesiology* 1977, **47**, 31; Graham C. W. and Walts L. F. *Anaesthesia* 1979, **34**, 1005.
26. *See also* Verner I. F. In: *Hypotensive Anaesthesia* (Enderby G. E. H. ed.) Edinburgh: Churchill Livingstone, 1985.
27. Vesey C. J. and Battistoni G. A. *J. Clin. Pharm.* 1977, **2**, 105.
28. Needleman P. et al. *J. Pharmacol. Exp. Ther.* 1973, **187**, 324.
29. Wildsmith J. A. W. et al. *Br. J. Anaesth.* 1973, **45**, 71; Styles M. et al. *Anesthesiology* 1973, **38**, 173.
30. Cole P. V. *Anaesthesia* 1978, **33**, 473.
31. *See also* Vesey C. J. et al. *Br. J. Anaesth.* 1976, **48**, 651; Cole P. V. In: *Recent Advances in Anaesthesia and Anaglesia 13* – (Hewer C. L. and Atkinson R. S. ed.) Edinburgh: Churchill Livingstone, 1979.
32. Leber T. *Arch. Ophthalmol.* 1871, **17**, 249.
33. Michenfelder J. D. and Tinker J. H. *Anesthesiology* 1977, **47**, 441.
34. Bryson D. D. *Lancet*, 1978, **1**, 92.
35. Arnold W. P. and Longnecker D. E. *Anesthesiology* 1984, **61**, 254.
36. Carliner N. H. et al. *JAMA* 1974, **227**, 308.
37. Murrell W. *Lancet* 1879, **2**, 80.
38. Sollevi A. et al. *Anesthesiology* 1984, **61**, 400.
39. Hellewell J. and Potts M. W. *Br. J. Anaesth.* 1966, **38**, 794; Rollason W. N. *Br. J. Anaesth.* 1967, **39**, 183; Hewitt P. B. et al. *Anaesthesia* 1967, **22**, 82.
40. Jakobsen C.-J. et al. *Br. J. Anaesth.* 1986, **58**, 261.
41. Scott D. B. et al. *Br. J. Clin. Pharmacol.* 1976, Suppl. 817.
42. Green D. W. et al. In: *Hypotensive Anaesthesia* (Enderby G. E. H. ed.) Edinburgh: Churchill Livingstone, 1985.
43. Kanto J. et al. *Int. J. Clin. Pharmacol. Ther. Toxicol.* 1980, **18**, 191.
44. MacRae W. R. et al. *Anaesthesia* 1981, **36**, 312.

45. Enderby G. E. H. (ed.) *Hypotensive Anaesthesia.* Edinburgh: Churchill Livingstone, 1985, 267.
46. Schofield N. McC. In: *Anaesthesia for Orthopaedic Patients* (Loach A. ed.) London: Arnold, 1983.
47. MacRae W. R. et al. *Anaesthesia* 1981, **36**, 307; Boyd C. H. *Anaesthesia* 1982, **37**, 1146.
48. Duncan J. *Br. Med. J.* 1886, **1**, 192.
49. Clarke J. M. F. *Br. J. Hosp. Med.* 1982, **27**, 497.

Chapter 14

Accidents, complications and sequelae of anaesthesia[1]

There is an irreducible minimum of complications, sequelae and mortality resulting from surgical operation and the anaesthesia that goes with it. This does not imply negligence or blame, they are simply consequences of surgery and anaesthesia. A vast amount of research effort is undertaken to find ways of reducing these consequences.

RESPIRATORY DIFFICULTIES DURING OPERATION

Respiratory obstruction

The signs are: (1) inadequate tidal exchange; (2) retraction of the chest wall and of the supraclavicular, infraclavicular and suprasternal spaces; (3) excessive abdominal movement; (4) use of accessory muscles of respiration; (5) noisy breathing (unless obstruction is absolute and complete); (6) cyanosis; and (7) the natural heave of the chest and abdomen becomes replaced by an indrawing of the upper chest and an outpushing of the abdomen because of strong diaphragmatic action.

It must be remedied in all cases, after its cause has been diagnosed. It may be due to:

1. Obstruction at the lips. Especially in edentulous patients. Remedy is use of an oro- or nasopharyngeal airway.

2. Obstruction by the tongue. First mentioned by Hall in 1856.[2] Due to approximation of the tongue to the posterior pharyngeal wall (swallowing the tongue). It may be especially dangerous in the recovery phase. Much less likely to occur if the patient is nursed in the lateral position. The jaw is lifted up and forwards, a manoeuvre first described in 1874.[3] At the same time the atlanto-occipital joint (the head) is extended on the vertebral column. The genioglossus on each side is important in holding the tongue away from the posterior pharyngeal wall. There is phasic activity synchronous with breathing, and tone is maximal during inspiration. It is the abolition of this tone during anaesthesia that is a major contributor to obstruction. Once the atonic tongue falls into the pharynx, obliterating the pharyngeal lumen, the suction created by inspiration pulls the tongue further back, making the obstruction worse.[4] A pharyngeal airway (size 3 for men, size 2 for women, on average) is inserted and usually restores the airway.[5] If that fails, suxamethonium is injected intravenously and the patient ventilated via tracheal tube. A nasopharyngeal tube may overcome this obstruction. Changes in the position of the soft palate may be important.[6] The whole subject has been reviewed recently.[7]

3. *Obstruction above the glottis.* This may be due to a swab, a tooth, a foreign body, saliva, vomitus, blood or oedema. The obstructing material must be removed by the fingers, gravity, swabbing or suction. Very rarely, dislocation of the epiglottis, or cysts or tumours of the epiglottis are encountered. Treatment as for tongue obstruction.

4. *Obstruction at the glottis.* This is due to: (*a*) laryngeal spasm; (*b*) sphincter-like closure of the aryepiglottic folds; (*c*) approximation of the ventricular ligaments or false cords; (*d*) impaction of the epiglottis into the larynx. The remedy is visual disimpaction via a laryngoscope after ensuring proper relaxation; (*e*) occasionally in patients who have had a large dose of relaxant that is incompletely reversed, and have been intubated, respiratory obstruction develops after extubation because the relaxed cords, instead of becoming abducted during inspiration, become sucked in by the air-stream; and (*f*) foreign bodies, e.g. teeth, vomitus; laryngoscopy or bronchoscopy required.

Peripheral stimulation causing partial or complete spasm suggests the need for deeper anaesthesia. Such stimuli occur when the cervix uteri or anal sphincter are stretched, or when the coeliac plexus or its connections are stimulated.[8] Temporary cessation of surgical stimuli may be necessary occasionally. Complete spasm leading to increasing cyanosis and hypoxia is a potentially dangerous situation. It may resolve spontaneously, and oxygen is then given to restore arterial oxygen tension rapidly.

The condition may call for active treatment. If this is considered necessary, a short-acting muscle relaxant such as suxamethonium may be given i.v. or i.m. provided that means for artificial ventilation of the lungs are available. A small dose of non-depolarizing relaxant is often sufficient to abolish partial laryngeal spasm and may even result in increased tidal exchange. The passage of a tracheal tube between the cords ensures that the condition will not recur. It is a wise precaution always to have some suxamethonium within sight at induction of any anaesthetic.

If the patient is *in extremis*, a very large intravenous cannula (e.g. size 12G) can be inserted into the larynx through the cricothyroid membrane and oxygen given by jet technique[9] or insufflation of air, 2–3 l/min. Mini-tracheostomy sets are available commercially. As a 'last-ditch' airway, the spike of a 'giving-set', which enters the infusion bottle, can be thrust percutaneously into the trachea through a small incision and connected to an oxygen supply line.[10] Tracheostomy is needed only on the rarest occasions.

5. *Bronchospasm.* It is upon the patency of the bronchiolar lumen and the quiescence of the bronchial reflexes that smooth anaesthesia largely depends (Nosworthy).[11] Intubation makes bronchospasm worse but may become necessary. Irritability is greatest at the carina. Acute infection increases sensitivity. A tendency to asthma strongly predisposes to bronchospasm and wheezing. Pulmonary oedema also interferes with ventilation.

Management. (1) Diagnosis of cause; inadequate depth of anaesthesia, asthmatic tendency of patient, acute anaphylactic reaction. It should be differentiated from blockage of the tracheal tube and from laryngospasm. (2) Prevention by smooth induction and maintaining anaesthesia at suitable depth; spraying larynx and trachea with lignocaine; administration of bronchodilator drugs with premedication; aminophylline suppositories. (3) Bronchodilatation; salbutamol 4 µg/kg over 1 min i.v., or aminophylline 250–300 mg i.v. slowly. An adrenaline infusion 1–10 µg/min may be considered. Corticosteroids, e.g. hydrocortisone, 100 mg i.v. may be given but will not have an immediate action.

6. *Faults of apparatus.* (1) Misplacement or kinking of the tracheal tube; (2) obstruction of the tracheal tube or connections.

Management. All the anaesthetic apparatus is removed, including the tracheal tube. Sometimes capnography helps to confirm that the tracheal tube is correctly placed in the trachea. The lungs may be ventilated with oxygen by face-mask until the situation is restored. In the last resort, the lungs should be ventilated with air, using a mask and self-inflating bag.

Coughing

Occurs most commonly due to inadequate depth of anaesthesia when volatile agents are used and when patient has chemical (e.g. due to heavy smoking) or infective inflammation of the upper airways.

Coughing may cause trouble during anaesthesia with thiopentone; this is best controlled by deepening anaesthesia or use of a muscle relaxant. Coughing may be due to irritation of the larynx from regurgitated gastric material, from the use of artificial airways or from saliva.

Sleep apnoea

This is an absence of inflow of air into the nose and mouth occurring for at least 10 s, and repeated more than 30 times during a 7-hour period of sleep. It may be central, obstructive or mixed. Important in the postoperative period.

Respiratory arrest

Due to obstruction of the airway or to peripheral or central respiratory depression. Ondine's curse (named from the water sprite in German mythology who killed her victims by stopping respiration) a term first used in connection with anaesthesia by Severinghaus,[12] is primary alveolar hypoventilation (unexplained apnoea). It may follow surgery of the cervical cord.[13] Failure of automatic control of respiration for up to 10 s may occur in normal REM sleep.

Hiccup

This is a state of intermittent spasm of the diaphragm, accompanied by sudden closure of the glottis.

Causes. Stimulation of sensory nerve endings of phrenic, which are connected with the coeliac and other intra-abdominal autonomic plexuses. The vagus may also act as part of the afferent arc of the reflex. Thus, through these pathways, hiccup may arise from impulses in any abdominal or thoracic viscus. May occur before surgery.

Central stimulation of the medulla may be causal in, for example, alcoholic intoxication, uraemia, encephalitis.

Treatment

1. During anaesthesia: (*a*) deepening of anaesthesia by any method; (*b*) administration of muscle relaxant in relatively large doses; or (*c*) nasopharyngeal stimulation by use of suction catheter or pouring ice-cold saline into nares with cuffed tube in position.[14]

2. Before or after anaesthesia: block of phrenic nerves – either unilateral or bilateral has been tried in intractable hiccup – 10 ml of 0.5% bupivacaine is suitable; injection is made at a depth of 1–2 cm along a line extending 5 cm laterally from a point 2 cm above the sternoclavicular joint. Unfortunately, even bilateral division of the phrenic nerves may fail to cure hiccup, because of the associated spasm of the intercostal and accessory respiratory muscles.

RESPIRATORY COMPLICATIONS AFTER OPERATION

Postoperative chest complications have interested physicians and surgeons for many years. For history of this subject, see earlier editions of this Synopsis.

Retention of sputum

Causes

Poor expulsive mechanism after operation due to: (1) pain; (2) reduced movement of diaphragm, which may be due to residual myoneural block or to pain; (3) sedatives; (4) a tight binder or dressing; and (5) prolonged inhalation of cold, dry anaesthetic gas mixtures, which decrease ciliary activity.[15]

Atelectasis

Diagnosis. (1) Rapid breathing, 30–60/min; (2) rapid heart rate; (3) dilatation of alae nasi and slight cyanosis; (4) restricted movements of affected side of chest; (5) diminution of breath sounds and perhaps decreased resonance are almost normal after abdominal operations; (6) dependent part of lungs usually involved; and (7) radiographic appearance may resemble that of bronchopneumonia. Elevation of one or other side of diaphragm very common after upper abdominal operations, in absence of clinical atelectasis.

Massive collapse causes pain in the chest of sudden onset, dyspnoea, cyanosis, fever, tachycardia and mediastinal shift. Untreated atelectasis will lead to inequalities of ventilation/perfusion, hypoxaemia and infection.

Treatment. Physiotherapy and encouragement of coughing, with appropriate use of analgesics (e.g. narcotic analgesics, Entonox). When problems are anticipated, continuous extradural block or other regional technique is helpful. If sputum cannot be removed, other measures must be considered such as aspiration of sputum via a tracheal tube or bronchoscope, or mini-tracheostomy. Postoperative doxapram has been recommended.[15]

Factors influencing sputum retention and atelectasis

Site of operation. Most common after upper abdominal operations, especially if oblique or transverse incisions are not used.[16] Fairly common following operations for hernia. Of non-abdominal operations, thyroidectomy is most often followed by chest complications.
Dental sepsis.
Obesity.
Smoking.
Pre-existing lung disease.

Aspiration pneumonitis

Aspiration of stomach contents may occur before, during or after operation. Mendelson described the acid aspiration syndrome of late pregnancy in 1946[17] (*see* Chapter 22). Trouble may occur after aspiration of stomach contents of any pH, and solid material may cause obstruction. Aspiration pnemonitis is due to the damage to the respiratory epithelium and the vascular endothelium, resulting in leakage of fluid into the alveoli and interstitial spaces, increase of water in the lungs, reduced pulmonary compliance and acute pulmonary oedema. The clinical signs may be delayed.

Diagnosis

(1) Cyanosis, unrelieved by oxygen therapy; (2) tachypnoea; (3) tachycardia; (4) wheezing; (6) chest radiograph shows shadows; and (7) cardiovascular failure may supervene.

Management

(1) Tracheal lavage; (2) oxygen administration; (3) antibiotics; (4) bronchodilator drugs; (5) hydrocortisone may be given; and (6) chest physiotherapy. Severe cases may need bronchoscopy and/or IPPV.

Lung abscess

When foreign material is introduced into the trachea, it gravitates into the dependent apex of the lower lobe with the patient lying supine, and into the dependent upper lobe with the patient on the side: these are the commonest sites of abscess. Onset may be mild, after a latent period of 2–10 days, simulating early bronchopneumonia. The earliest X-ray sign is a patch of consolidation; later, a fluid level may be seen. Treatment is by postural drainage and antibiotics.

Surgical emphysema during anaesthesia

This was first reported in 1912[18] during insufflation endotracheal anaesthesia. Surgical emphysema may commence as a pulmonary interstitial emphysema due to overdistension of the alveoli. The gas tracks along the sheaths of the vessels to the hilum-mediastinal emphysema, from which it may spread: (1) to the neck; (2) to the abdomen; (3) behind the peritoneum; and (4) into the pleura (tension pneumothorax). Tension pneumothorax should be looked for if surgical emphysema appears. Mediastinal emphysema often causes a crushing sound when the stethoscope is applied to the left border of the heart – Hamman's sign.[19] Radiologically, there may be a small air space running parallel to the left or right border of the heart.

Pneumothorax

Most commonly occurs due to accidental opening of the pleural cavity during operations such as cervical sympathectomy, rib resection and nephrectomy. During the operation, the lungs should be inflated to expel air as the hole is closed. Pneumothorax can also occur as a complication of anaesthetic techniques such as intercostal or brachial plexus blocks or IPPV, especially if PEEP is used. It can arise as a complication of surgical emphysema, and also during laparoscopy.

Hypoxaemia after general anaesthesia

The Pao_2 decreases after general anaesthesia, even when respiratory function appears to be normal. It is influenced by the site of operation, smoking, age, the presence of cardiorespiratory disease and obesity. The Pao_2 falls with age. The hypoxaemia is caused by mismatching of ventilation/perfusion, and often corrected by oxygen administration, which may have to be continued for some days.

Extradural block may give some protection from postoperative chest complications but it is more effective after upper than after lower abdominal surgery. Extradural narcotics or local analgesics are often of value in the postoperative period.

PULMONARY EMBOLISM

Deep venous thrombosis in the legs and pelvis is more common in the elderly, the immobilized, patients on oral contraceptives, those with carcinoma, and patients after certain operations, e.g. pelvic surgery, hip surgery and varicose veins. The clinical presentation may be very varied: unexplained fever, faintness, dyspnoea, substernal discomfort, pleural pain and haemoptysis. Onset may coincide with getting up or straining at stool. Sudden onset of chest pain from second to fourteenth day after operation. Usually during second week. Pulmonary embolism may be small and ephemeral or large and fatal.

Signs

The following may be present: tachycardia, rise in CVP, hypotension, cyanosis, gallop rhythm, pleural rub, and signs of consolidation. *Radiographs of chest* may show linear shadows and an effusion. Pulmonary oligaemia indicates the embolus is large. *ECG* may show an S wave in limb Lead I, a Q wave in Lead III and T wave inversion in Lead III; these represent right heart strain. A perfusion scan is sometimes undertaken to confirm the diagnosis.

Non-fatal pulmonary embolism is common, but often undiagnosed. It may be confused with pneumonia, atelectasis, pleurisy, asthma or myocardial infarction. If the embolus is massive, there is profound shock and cardiac arrest may occur. Small emboli are often overlooked.

Treatment

The small embolus is not treated as such, but anticoagulants prevent the deep venous thrombosis extending. Venography and ligation of veins may be appropriate. For the large embolus, streptokinase therapy may be of benefit. For the massive embolus, resuscitative measures are needed and Trendelenburg's operation of embolectomy has been successful.[20]

Pulmonary embolism associated with operation

Characterized by increasing cyanosis and hypotension with adequate ventilation. The classic causes are: (1) hypernephroma; (2) liquor amni (in obstetric patients); and (3) detachment of a venous clot in the leg, following the application of an Esmarch bandage,[21] or a change of position of the patient.

Prevention of pulmonary embolism

This largely consists in the prevention, diagnosis and treatment of deep venous thrombosis (DVT). Most thrombi occur in the calf veins, but it is only when they extend into the iliofemoral veins or originate in pelvic veins that pulmonary embolism is likely. DVT usually starts during or very soon after operation. There is reduced fibrinolytic activity and increased platelet adhesiveness after operation.

Prevention of deep venous thrombosis

Anaesthesia may influence the incidence of deep venous thrombosis[22] Regional methods have some advantages.

Preventative measures include: (1) early ambulation; (2) elevation of the legs during operation; (3) intermittent pneumatic compression of the calf, replacing the normal calf-muscle pump effect; (4) knee-high elastic supports; (5) a heel cushion for use on the operating table, preventing pressure on calf veins; (6) low-dose subcutaneous heparin *(see below)*; and (7) infusion of 500–1000 ml (7–15 ml/kg) of dextran 70 has been shown to be effective in reducing the incidence of postoperative pulmonary embolism in gynaecological, general surgical and orthopaedic operations.[23] It can be continued postoperatively, 500 ml/day.[24]

Low-dose heparin or elastic supports are commonly used. Although low-dose heparin does not seem to increase intra-operative bleeding, the use of regional blocks should only be undertaken where there is a clear advantage. The avoidance of oral contraceptives containing oestrogen for 4 weeks before major surgery will reduce the incidence of DVT.

Postoperative care includes frequent movements of the ankles, feet and toes, and early ambulation.

Heparin

First discovered in 1916 by a medical student in Baltimore.[25] Calcium heparin 5000 units can be given subcutaneously 2 h before operation and 8-hourly after operation for 7–10 days,[26] to prevent venous thrombosis. Can also be given in ultra-low dosage.[27] Low molecular weight heparin has also been recommended.[28] A single daily injection of low molecular weight heparin fraction (1850 APIT units) provides effective prevention against postoperative major pulmonary embolism.[29] *(See also* Chapter 15.)

CARDIOVASCULAR SYSTEM

Cardiac dysrhythmias

When associated with anaesthesia and operation, were first reported in 1920.[30] May be associated with: (1) pre-existing cardiac pathology; (2) hypercapnia, hypoxaemia, toxaemia, drugs, etc.; (3) electrolyte imbalance or dehydration; or (4) myocardial ischaemia or infarction.

The following may occur:

1. Sinus tachycardia. The underlying cause should be treated.
2. Bradycardia. Usually responds to small dose of atropine (0.1 mg increments) and reduction of concentration or withdrawal of causative agent (e.g. halothane).
3. Atrial or ventricular premature contractions. Usually benign and require no specific treatment other than correction of hypercapnia if present and reduction in concentration of inhalation agent.
4. Paroxysmal supraventricular tachycardia. May be terminated by use of vagotonic manoeuvres.
5. Ventricular tachycardia. This can be important because it can result in impairment of cardiac output and may proceed to ventricular fibrillation. In the very ill patient cardioversion may be considered. Management includes use of verapamil.

6. Nodal rhythm. Common with inhalation anaesthetics; responds to intravenous atropine but seldom of serious significance.

7. Atrial fibrillation. Digoxin is the drug of choice for controlling the ventricular rate, but may carry a risk when given intravenously. Beta-adrenoceptor blocking agents may be used when digoxin is failing to control ventricular rate.

8. Cardiac arrest. *See* Chapter 31.

(*See also* Wendon J. and Bihari D. J., The Management of Acute Arrhythmias, In: *Recent Advances in Anaesthesia and Analgesia – 17* (Atkinson R. S. and Adams A. P. ed.) Edinburgh: Churchill Livingstone, 1991.

Hypertension in the immediate postoperative period

Possible causes are: (1) pain or full bladder; (2) hypercapnia; (3) emergence delirium; (4) unsuspected phaeochromocytoma (extremely rare); or (5) after coronary artery bypass grafting. A history of hypertension should be taken into consideration.

Air embolism

This was first reported in 1821 by Magendie,[31] and by Barlow in 1830.[32]

Causes

1. Surgical. Operations involving injury to veins in the neck, thorax, breast and pelvis; operations on the brain and cord in the sitting position; operations on the heart; and uterine curettage and insufflation. Gas embolism may complicate irrigation of semi-closed cavities with hydrogen peroxide (e.g. the mastoid).

2. Diagnostic and therapeutic injection of gas. Into peritoneal cavity, pleural cavity, large joints, urinary bladder, tissue spaces, e.g. the perinephric area and nasal antra, uterus and tubes.

3. Accidental entrance of air. During intravenous techniques.

Factors of importance. (1) the volume of air; (2) the speed of injection; (3) the pressure in the veins; (4) posture; and (5) general condition of patient.

Signs and symptoms

If air enters the veins in any quantity it will cause a hissing sound in the wound and it will go to the right heart and lung, causing an air-lock obstruction in the pulmonary artery. This may result in a loud precordial murmur, the so-called 'mill-wheel murmur'. It has been suggested that this term should be replaced by 'squelching gum-boot murmur' because the sound of the mill-wheel is unfamiliar to most modern anaesthetists.[33] There will also be sudden cyanosis, hypotension, engorged neck veins, tachycardia, irregular gasping respiration, progressing through tachypnoea and hypopnoea and followed by cardiac arrest. Early diagnosis can be made if: (1) an oesophageal stethoscope is in place;[34] (2) a Doppler ultrasonic flow detector is on the precordium;[35] and (3) monitoring of end tidal CO_2; it will fall abruptly if blood does not reach the lungs.

Treatment

(1) Prevent further entrance of air into the circulation, if necessary by compressing veins to raise venous pressure locally; (2) adjust position so that the entry site is below the heart, and if possible flood the wound with saline; (3) place the patient on the left side so that bubbles are carried away from the mouth of the pulmonary artery;[36] (4) give pure oxygen and stop administration of nitrous oxide; which is more soluble in blood than nitrogen and so will increase the size of the emboli. If the lung is damaged, IPPV will require great care; (5) insertion of a catheter to aspirate directly from the right heart; and (6) compression in a hyperbaric chamber is valuable in air embolism in divers.

For air embolism in neurosurgery, *see* Chapter 22.

POSTURE[37]

Trendelenburg position[38]

Friedrich Trendelenburg (1844–1924) first used his tilt in 1880 when Professor of Surgery at Rostock to facilitate urological operations. This was popularized by his pupil Willy Meyer in 1884 in the US. Trendelenburg later occupied the surgical chairs at Bonn and Leipzig. He described a tracheotomy tube with inflatable cuff in 1869.

Experimental work has shown that tilting into a steep Trendelenburg position in young patients under light anaesthesia has no effect on the gas tension of arterial blood, and none on the pH, minute volume and respiratory rate.[39] In short stout patients, especially if there is an abdominal mass, pressure on the diaphragm from the bowel may produce cyanosis and dyspnoea, and reduction of vital capacity by 15% unless IPPV is carried out. Except in very short operations, IPPV is preferable to spontaneous ventilation. Cyanosis also occurs in the face and neck of plethoric patients in this position, as a result of stagnant hypoxia due to gravity even in the presence of adequate ventilation.

If the arm is abducted, the elbow should be slightly flexed and pronated to prevent pull on the brachial plexus, and the head turned to the side of the arm, but every care should be taken to avoid this position of arm abduction with the head-down tilt.

Trendelenburg position may, however, have a harmful effect on the cardiovascular system, especially in shock where it can cause a fall in arterial pressure and cerebral perfusion. Prolonged head-down tilt can cause cerebral oedema and retinal detachment. Increased venous return can always be improved by raising the legs with the patient horizontal.

Steep Trendelenburg position is now rarely necessary. Some degree of tilt may, however, be preferable to deepening the level of anaesthesia or the injection of an extra dose of muscle relaxant in certain patients.

Prone position

The functional residual capacity is greater than in the supine position. A pillow should be placed under each shoulder and another under the pelvis, so that breathing is not unduly interfered with and so that all pressure is completely removed from the abdomen and its large venous channels. A cuffed tracheal tube is a wise precaution in case regurgitation of stomach contents should occur. Fat subjects tolerate this position badly. The unconscious patient when moved can easily suffer skeletal injury. Retinal arterial occlusion and blindness from pressure on the eye have been reported.[40]

Lithotomy position

When the lithotomy position is required, both legs should be moved together to avoid strain on the pelvic ligaments. If the patient is arranged while supine, so that the anterior superior iliac spines are on a level with the break in the table, he will be in a good lithotomy position when the legs are supported on the stirrups. The knee should be outside any metal supports.

Lateral position

This handicaps the patient's breathing. A bridge makes it still worse, so it should be used as little as possible and for a short time only; it may be associated with hypotension. In the lateral position with the patient breathing spontaneously, both ventilation and perfusion are concentrated in the lower lung, while IPPV diverts ventilation to the upper lung, thus increasing mismatch.

Supine position

Pressure on and stretching of nerves of the arm must be avoided by care of the arms. Legs should be flat on the table, not crossed one over the other. The tendo Achillis must not rest on the unpadded edge of the table. A soft pad, raising heels from the table, avoids pressure on the calf veins, and so may lessen the incidence of thrombosis occurring at this site.

Postoperative backache is not infrequent after operations performed in the supine position. It can often be prevented by the use of an inflatable wedge, as a lumbar support.[41]

Effect of changes of position of head and neck

A patient with a decreased cardiac output, carotid artery occlusive disease, etc. may be deprived of cerebral blood supply by changes in position altering the relationships of the vertebral vessels to surrounding bony structures as by rotation of the head, hyperextension of the neck at the atlanto-occipital joint to maintain a clear airway. This can be tested for at the pre-operative examination. Full extension may result in a faint.

Moving the patient

Anaesthetized patients tolerate moving badly; this is especially so when the blood pressure is low. All movements should be smooth and gentle, not jerky and rough.

Position in bed

The patient should lie in the semi-prone position until the reflexes return. This is maintained by a pillow between the bed and the chest; the lower arm is placed behind the trunk; the upper knee is flexed. This helps to maintain a free airway by causing the tongue to fall away from the posterior pharyngeal wall; it also helps to prevent aspiration of vomitus into the air passages. The patient should not be placed in a head-up position until it is quite certain that the cardiovascular system is able to maintain an adequate circulation to the brain. Otherwise syncopal reactions and even death may occur.

VOMITING AND REGURGITATION

The anaesthetist is faced with the problem of the aspiration of material from the alimentary canal into the air passages during induction, maintenance and immediately after anaesthesia.

Vomiting

The expulsion through the mouth of material from the alimentary tract by muscular action. The act of vomiting is preceded by salivation, rapid breathing, pallor, sweating, tachycardia and severe discomfort.

The vomiting centre is closely related to the respiratory and vasomotor centres and the salivary and vestibular nuclei, in the dorsolateral border of lateral reticular formation. The chemoreceptor trigger zone lies superficial to the true vomiting centre in the area postrema of the 4th ventricle. It has many dopamine receptors.

A pressure of $40\,cmH_2O$ is needed to lift the contents of the stomach into the mouth in the upright position. While the glottis goes into spasm during the expulsive phase, it soon relaxes, so that aspiration of stomach contents into the bronchial tree is almost bound to happen in the unconscious supine patient. It is more likely in very light anaesthesia, when the base of the tongue or pharynx is stimulated by airways, etc. and during recovery.

Vomiting is undesirable because: (1) it is unpleasant; (2) aspiration may result; (3) it may harm the eye, skin flaps or other areas, recently operated on; and (4) it may raise intraocular and intra-abdominal pressure.

Regurgitation

Being a passive act, regurgitation may be silent and unheralded, and so even more potentially dangerous than vomiting. The major mechanism preventing regurgitation is the barrier pressure; i.e. the difference between intragastric pressure and the pressure exerted by the lower oesophageal sphincter. Predisposing factors include: (1) the head-down position if the cardia is inefficient; (2) a stomach full of fluid; and (3) an indwelling stomach or oesophageal tube.

The cardiac sphincter

This is both a sphincter and a valve. It remains closed because of: (1) the presence of an anatomical muscular sphincter; (2) folds of thickened mucosa in the oesophagus; (3) the angle at which the oesophagus meets the fundus of the stomach; and (4) the pinch-cock action of the crus of the diaphragm (in two-thirds of patients the right crus only).

Its activity is controlled reflexly (vagus and sympathetic nerves). Its integrity is affected and it is made incompetent by: (1) anatomical abnormality, e.g. hiatus hernia; (2) the presence of a stomach tube; (3) passage of anaesthetic gas from above during attempts at IPPV; (4) attempts at active respiration in the presence of respiratory obstruction; and (5) intravenous atropine or hyoscine – this effect may be antagonized by metoclopramide, which itself increases the tone; dosage: 10 mg i.v. and by domperidone 10 mg before induction;[42] this agent is said to have fewer side-effects than metoclopramide, but on i.v. injection has caused cardiac standstill.[43]

The cricopharyngeal sphincter

This is at the upper end of the oesophagus at the level of C6 and is composed of striated muscle (the rest of the oesophagus has smooth muscle). Its action is both voluntary and reflex. Its integrity is affected by both anaesthetics and relaxants. It acts as a sphincter normally but as a valve when paralysed, when it tends to obstruct the passage of fluids from the pharynx to the oesophagus, but not in the reverse direction.

A classic paper on vomiting during anaesthesia was that by Morton and Wylie.[44] Attention was drawn to vomiting and regurgitation as major contributors to deaths associated with anaesthesia.[45]

The hydrodynamics of regurgitation

The normal intragastric pressure is $5–7\,cmH_2O$ and double this in advanced pregnancy. This is well below the pressure required for reflux through the cardia. Even when the stomach is distended the pressure is unlikely to be greater than $18\,cmH_2O$ unless there is contraction of the abdominal muscles.

Measurements of intragastric pressure during the fasciculation following injection of suxamethonium are usually not greatly increased, but in about 12% of patients a rise greater than $19\,cmH_2O$ occurs.

Dangers of aspiration of stomach contents

1. Laryngeal spasm, bronchopneumonia, atelectasis and lung abscess can all occur.

2. Reflex chemical trauma to bronchial and alveolar mucosa – acute exudative pneumonitis or Mendelson's syndrome,[17] a syndrome following the aspiration of acid gastric contents. Greatest risk is when a volume of more than 25 ml with a pH of less than 2.5 is aspirated. Although this is particularly likely to occur in obstetric patients, it is not confined to them. Following immediately, or after an interval of a few hours, the patient shows cyanosis, dyspnoea, bronchospasm, hypotension and tachycardia. There are rhonchi and rales in the chest with a characteristic radiographic appearance, viz. irregular mottled densities. There are no signs of massive atelectasis or mediastinal shift. Severe cases may progress to acute pulmonary oedema with rapid death, or the patient may succumb to pulmonary complication some days later.

3. Cardiac inhibition from reflexes originating in the bronchi, due to acid contamination.

Prevention of acid aspiration

(1) Ensure an empty stomach by: (*a*) pre-operative starvation; (*b*) emptying via a gastric tube; (*c*) use of metoclopramide 10 mg i.v. or i.m. to hasten gastric emptying; and (*d*) induction of vomiting by apomorphine, 0.5 mg increments until vomiting occurs. This is unpleasant.

(2) Inhibition of secretion of acid gastric juice by H_2 antagonists, e.g. ranitidine, 150 mg orally the night before and on the morning of operation;[46] cimetidine, 300 mg i.v. 2 h before induction.[47] A dose of 400 mg by mouth may have a similar effect. Famotidine 40 mg, and nizatidine 150 mg, are similar.[48]

(3) Neutralization of gastric contents by antacids, e.g. sodium citrate (15–30 ml of 0.33M solution). Its efficacy may be improved by turning the patient to promote mixing.

(4) Rapid sequence induction of anaesthesia. Pure oxygen is given for at least 3 min, followed by i.v. thiopentone 2–4 mg/kg, immediately followed by suxamethonium 1.0–1.5 mg/kg. Pretreatment with a non-depolarizer may be unwise.[49] The tube is inserted, its cuff immediately blown up. When suxamethonium is contra-indicated, a generous dose of non-depolarizing

relaxant has been advocated. When i.v. induction is contra-indicated, inhalational induction may be substituted.

(5) Cricoid pressure is used to prevent regurgitation by occlusion of the oesophagus by backward pressure on the cricoid as recommended by Sellick.[50] It should be applied as the patient loses consciousness. The tips of the first two fingers and thumb of an assistant are placed on the cricoid cartilage and pressed on to the vertebral column with moderate pressure. The neck is extended and the other hand placed behind the neck to steady it. This method must not be used during active vomiting because it may lead to oesophageal rupture. It also distorts the appearance of the glottis. Cricoid pressure, to be safe, must ensure that the onset of unconsciousness, the achievement of full muscular relaxation and the application of firm cricoid pressure are timed to occur simultaneously.[51] Personnel must be properly trained in its use.[52]

(6) Use a regional block technique, and allow the patient to remain awake and with full protective reflexes.

(7) Awake intubation of the trachea. Topical analgesia of the upper airways and fibreoptic endoscopy will enable a tube to be inserted into the trachea in the conscious patient.

There is no foolproof method of prevention of aspiration of gastric contents into the lungs however experienced the anaesthetist. Heavy sedation may result in aspiration of stomach contents in the ward before or after operation.

Treatment of acid aspiration

Prevent further aspiration by tilting the head downwards or turning the patient on one side. Use suction and give oxygen. Tracheal suction may be sufficient in mild cases, whereas in others suction through a bronchoscope will be required. Give bronchodilators, antibiotics and physiotherapy. Hydrocortisone[53] can be given. IPPV may be required.

Postoperative nausea and vomiting

Vomiting may be central from causes acting on the brain stem and higher centres; peripheral, from causes acting on the gut; and vestibular. It can be influenced by one or more of the following factors:

1. Anaesthetic agent and technique. Narcotic analgesics cause postoperative nausea and vomiting in some patients. Volatile inhalation agents may increase the incidence. Nitrous oxide and oxygen cause vomiting in about 15% of patients in an outpatient department. Children are more prone to vomit than adults. Intradural and extradural block usually cause less vomiting than inhalation of a volatile anaesthetic. Hypoxia predisposes to vomiting. Prolonged time of operation and depth of anaesthesia are unfavourable factors.

2. Type of patient. Some patients are ready vomiters, e.g. in travelling. Suggestion, and the example of surrounding patients, are important factors. Suitable pre-operative reassurance is important. More frequent in women than in men, and in the young than in the old.

3. *Condition of stomach.* Vomiting is likely unless the stomach is empty.

4. *Type of operation.* Vomiting is frequent after gynaecological surgery and laparotomy.

Treatment and prevention[54]

This consists largely in preventing the causal factors whenever possible, e.g. by avoiding narcotics. The following drugs may be used:

1. *Phenothiazines.* Act as dopamine antagonists on the chemoreceptor trigger zone, e.g. prochlorperazine (Stemetil) 12.5 mg i.m.; promethazine (Phenergan) 25 mg. The latter has antanalgesic effects, so is not the best agent for use in labour.

2. *Antihistamine agents.* For example cyclizine hydrochloride (Marzine) 50 mg i.m.[55] It can be given by suppository. It has been added to morphine in an effort to prevent nausea and vomiting, 15 mg to morphine 10 mg (Cyclimorph), but if given i.v. may cause collapse.

3. *Dopamine antagonists.* (*a*) Metoclopramide 10 mg acts both centrally and peripherally. It speeds gastric emptying time and increases the tone of the lower oesophageal sphincter. Will not relieve sea-sickness; and (*b*) domperidone 10 mg crosses the blood-brain barrier very slowly and so does not usually cause neurological or psychological side-effects.

4. *Butyrophenone derivatives.* For example droperidol (Droleptan) 1–5 mg. These drugs have a specific effect on the chemoreceptor trigger zone.

5. *Anticholinergic agents.* Hyoscine 0.4–0.6 mg. They inhibit the muscarinic activity of acetylcholine on the gut and may have a central action.

6. *$5HT_3$ antagonists.* Ondansetron has been used for the management of nausea and vomiting associated with chemotherapy, radiotherapy and surgery.

7. *Clonidine.* May have a place in reducing opioid-induced nausea (*see* Chapter 26)

8. *Acupuncture.* The P6 acupuncture point is 5 cm proximal to the wrist crease, between the tendons of the palmaris longus and the flexor carpi radialis of the right forearm, 1 cm below the skin, i.e. on 'the pericardial meridian'.[56]

NEUROLOGICAL COMPLICATIONS AND SEQUELAE

Convulsions[57]

Several types of abnormal muscular action may occur during anaesthesia: (1) clonus – usually occurring in light anaesthesia and disappearing when anaesthesia is deepened. Commonly seen in the legs and may be stopped by raising thighs, leaving legs unsupported or by injecting a small dose of muscle relaxant; (2) epilepsy – intubation may be required to ensure oxygenation; (3) convulsions due to hypoxia; (4) convulsions due to local analgesic drugs, e.g. lignocaine, bupivacaine. Treat with intravenous thiopentone and oxygen inhalations and/or suxamethonium. Diazepam may also be used; (5) tremor associated with the intravenous injection of barbiturate, usually a pronator spasm of the arm receiving the injection. Muscle movements are more common with the newer intravenous induction agents, e.g. etomidate; (6) enflurane and methohexitone cause increased activity on EEG, and epileptiform seizures have been reported; and (7) propofol has been reported to cause convulsions.[58]

Severe myoclonus (wrongly called shivering) after halothane may be mistaken for a convulsion.

Delayed recovery from anaesthesia

This may be due to: (1) *drugs used during operation* in relative overdosage, e.g. phenothiazine derivatives, narcotic analgesics, thiopentone, volatile agents. Unconsciousness associated with prolonged apnoea; (2) *disturbances of physiology resulting from anaesthesia,* e.g. hypercapnia, a hypoxic episode during anaesthesia, electrolyte and acid-base disturbances, fainting (especially in the dental chair), induced hypotension, hypothermia in infants; (3) *disturbances resulting from surgery*, e.g. shock, metabolic acidosis, fat embolism, air embolism, operative trauma in brain surgery; (4) *incidental disease*, e.g. cerebral embolism, thrombosis or haemorrhage, cardiac infarction, thrombosis or haemorrhage occurring during operation, myxoedema, hypopituitarism, hypoglycaemia, hyperglycaemic coma with ketosis, adrenal deficiency, uraemia, liver failure, an occult and undiagnosed meningioma.[59] The patient may have been unconscious before operation or may be moribund; (5) *drugs given before operation*, e.g. mono-amine oxidase inhibitors (with pethidine during operation), sedatives; (6) *the central anticholinergic syndrome*, may be treated with physostigmine salicylate, 1–2 mg (*see* Chapter 5); and (7) *early postoperative septicaemia*.

Peripheral nerve injuries[60]

First recognized by Budinger[61] (1894) as being due to malposition of the patient with consequent stretching and compression of nerves.

Aetiology

1. Stretching and compression of nerves may occur as a result of muscle relaxation, which allows adoption of unphysiological positions. This is combined with abolition of pain and discomfort that would otherwise act as a warning.

2. Injection of substances into or around nerves. Irritation may be chemical, as a result of direct needle trauma, or due to bacterial contamination or haematoma.

3. Use of tourniquets, if excessive pressure is allowed over a nerve trunk.[62] (The pneumatic tourniquet was introduced by Harvey Cushing of Boston to minimize bleeding from the scalp.[63]) It is essential to check the accuracy of the anaeroid gauge against a mercury column.[64] Pressure for upper-limb ischaemia need only exceed arterial blood pressure by 50–75 mmHg.

4. As a result of hypotension, causing ischaemia.

5. Toxicity due to degradation products of anaesthetic agents (e.g. sevoflurane).

6. Hypothermia, when minimal pressure may cause injury.

Specific neuropathies

1. Brachial plexus. Stretching can occur as a result of: (*a*) extension and lateral flexion of head to opposite side; (*b*) abduction, external rotation and extension of the arm; (*c*) suspension of the arm from a bar when the patient is in lateral position; (*d*) extreme abduction of the arms above the head with the patient supine; and (*e*) suspension by wrists to prevent slipping of patient in Trendelenburg position.

Compression can occur: (*a*) when shoulder braces are used with Trendelenburg position. If placed too medially the clavicle may be depressed so that the plexus has to traverse a longer and more devious course; (*b*) with the arm abducted and Trendelenburg position the plexus may be depressed and stretched over the head of the humerus. Shoulder braces, placed too laterally, may further depress the head of the humerus and with it the plexus; and (*c*) the plexus may be deviated posteriorly by the tendon of pectoralis minor or by the tip of the coracoid process in the obese patient undergoing cholecystectomy with gallbladder bridge inserted.

Various *congenital anomalies* may render plexus more vulnerable, e.g. hypertrophy of scalenus anterior or scalenus media, cervical rib, anomalous derivation of the plexus and abnormal slope of the shoulder.

The entire plexus may be injured or the upper roots only. It is less common for the lower roots to be affected alone. Involvement may be restricted to one cord.

To avoid stretching the plexus, the following measures should be taken: (*a*) shoulder braces must be padded and must make contact with acromion as far laterally as possible, but they are better avoided, the patient being supported on a non-slip mattress (Langton Hewer[65]); (*b*) arm-board must be built-up with pads to prevent backward displacement of arm; (*c*) hyperextension and external rotation of elbow must be avoided; (*d*) intravenous injections should be given with the arm at the patient's side or folded across the chest. Prognosis is good, but recovery may take months. The deltoid, biceps and brachialis are the muscles usually affected.

2. Radial nerve. Can be injured due to stretching if the arm is allowed to sag over the side of the table. Can be compressed by use of a vertical screen support. Wrist-drop results.

3. Ulnar nerve. Can occur if the elbow is allowed to fall over the sharp edge of the table so that the nerve is compressed against the medial epicondyle of the humerus. Injury has also been reported as a result of acute flexion of the elbow when the arm is placed in front of the chest. The nerve is stretched around the medial epicondyle of the humerus. Weakness of ulnar side of fist results and later 'claw hand'. Relatively minor trauma to the ulnar nerve may cause severe disability.[66]

4. Median nerve. May be damaged as a result of technically perfect intravenous injections in the cubital fossa, as a result of direct needle trauma or extravasation of drugs. Results in inability to oppose thumb and little finger.

5. *Lateral popliteal nerve.* Compression between the head of the fibula and a lithotomy pole badly placed damages the nerve and may result in foot-drop. This is the most frequently damaged nerve in the lower limb.

6. *Saphenous nerve.* Compression can occur between lithotomy pole and medial tibial condyle, when the leg is suspended lateral to the pole. Sensory loss results along the medial side of the calf.

7. *Sciatic nerve.* Can be traumatized by intramuscular injections in the buttock. It may be damaged in emaciated patients, lying on a hard table with opposite buttock elevated, as for hip-pinning. Paralysis of all muscles below knee, and perhaps of hamstrings results, with sensory loss.

8. *Pudendal nerve.* Can be compressed against a poorly padded perineal post during hip-pinning with traction to legs. The nerve is pressed against the ischial tuberosity. Result is loss of perineal sensation and faecal incontinence.

9. *Femoral nerve.* Can be damaged by use of a self-retaining retractor during lower laparotomy. Result is loss of flexion of hip and loss of extension of knee. Sensation is lost over the anterior thigh and anteromedial aspect of the calf.

Damage to nerves may be caused by a tourniquet (*tourner* = to turn) or compression bandage.[67]

10. *Supra-orbital nerve.* Can occur due to compression by a metal endotracheal connector or tight head-harness. Result is photophobia, numbness of the forehead and pain in the eye.

11. *Facial nerve.* Can be compressed between fingers and ascending ramus of mandible.[68] Result is facial paralysis. *Buccal branch* has been injured by tight harness. Result is paralysis of orbicularis oris.

12. *Abducens nerve with other cranial nerves.* Can follow spinal analgesia. *See* Chapter 25.

13. *Trigeminal nerve.* Toxic damage has followed use of trichloroethylene with soda-lime.

(*See also* Britt B. A. and Gordon R. A. *Can. Anaesth. Soc. J.* 1964, **11**, 514.)

Postanaesthetic excitement

Most common in children; after operations for cataract and in the strong and fit. Made worse by premedication with sedative but non-analgesic drugs, operations causing great pain or a full bladder. Analgesics should be given in adequate dosage for pain. Psychic abnormalities may be the cause.

Paralysis following intra- or extradural analgesia

See Chapter 25.

Neurological complications following general anaesthesia

Neurological complications can follow general as well as spinal analgesia, e.g. diplopia following thiopentone, curare and cyclopropane;[69] ascending spinal paralysis under nitrous oxide – oxygen, ether and gallamine;[70] peroneal nerve palsy and meningitis have been reported.[71]

Postoperative convulsions.[57] Possible causes include: hypoxia, cerebral oedema, alkalaemia, embolus (blood clot, fat or air), local analgesics, hyperpyrexia, hypoglycaemia, hypocalcaemia due to massive blood transfusion, cerebrovascular accident, uraemia or eclampsia.

Postoperative headache. Common. For management of migraine attacks *see* Fell R. H. *Anaesthesia* 1980, **35**, 1006.

AWARENESS OF SURGERY DURING GENERAL ANAESTHESIA[72]

Unexpected awareness under general anaesthesia is a continuous spectrum from the slightest brief sensation of hearing something, to being wide awake and conscious of all one's surroundings, very similar to patterns of awareness during sleep in bed at night.

It is possible that surgical stimuli actually lighten the level of anaesthesia, again analogous to sensory stimuli during ordinary sleep.

Risk of awareness under general anaesthesia is a problem.[73] The incidence of awareness with recall has been reported as between 0.2 and 0.9%[74] Some patients, anaesthetized with nitrous oxide – oxygen, IPPV and muscle relaxants, have reported awareness during anaesthesia.[75] Patients lightly anaesthetized for obstetric, dental, orthopaedic and cardiac operations can sometimes remember conversations that have taken place during the operation.[76] However, Artusio had shown long ago that stage 2 ether anaesthesia abolished awareness of sounds, vision and pain.[77]

Causes for unwanted awareness[78]

Faulty technique – 70% (including nitrous oxide/oxygen/opioid technique).
Failure to check equipment – 20%
Justified risks – 2.5%
Faulty equipment – 2.5%

Auditory awareness is the most common, closely followed by awareness of intubation (2 minutes after the induction agent being given). It may be reasonable to warn patients of possible auditory awareness in some situations, e.g. early part of Caesarean section. They need to be reassured that there will be no pain.

Physiology of awareness during over-light anaesthesia[79]

Awareness during anaesthesia is not an all-or-nothing feature, but a spectrum, ranging from unconsciousness with some movement to strong stimuli, through auditory awareness and awareness of pain, to full consciousness of the surroundings. Awareness, for example while surgery proceeds under local analgesia, or endoscopy under sedation is considered acceptable, even desirable. What is undesirable is unexpected or painful awareness that is remembered.

(1) Conscious awareness without amnesia, e.g. pain or conversations overheard and remembered – especially aroused by single-modality sensory input, of which auditory is by far the commonest). Meaningful sounds (whose input is directed to the dominant cerebral hemisphere), are a good example. They are more easily remembered afterwards.

(2) Conscious awareness with amnesia, e.g. obedience to spoken command during surgery that is not remembered.

(3) Subconscious awareness,[80] e.g. purposeful limb movements but no response to spoken command, which is more often caused by multiple-source or multi-channelled sensory input, or by sensory input from the non-dominant side of the body to the non-dominant cerebral hemisphere. Subconscious awareness is not usually remembered afterwards, but may be exposed later by hypnosis.[81] It is not known whether subconscious awareness matters, but it has been shown to influence postoperative behaviour[82] and even speed of convalescence.[83]

(4) Pseudo-awareness, e.g. where a patient becomes conscious of sounds and other sensations in the postoperative room, which are wrongly assumed to be occurring during surgery.

Initial reception of stimuli into a 'preconscious' cerebral process has been postulated. Subsequent routing into consciousness or subconsciousness depends on the nature of the stimulus (e.g. pain and hearing are more likey to enter consciousness),[84] and on the prevailing drug therapy, e.g. sedatives. Consciousness may be located in the dominant cerebral hemisphere, which is more susceptible to anaesthetics. The hippocampus may also be involved in the establishing of memory[85] mediated by N-methyl D aspartate, and blocked by aminophosphonovaleric acid.[86]

Measurement of consciousness and unconsciousness

(1) Cerebral metabolism studies, using a bloodflow marker (labelled iodo-antipyrine) for rCBF, and a local metabolism marker (labelled deoxyglucose) for rCMRGlucose. Thiopentone is found to reduce rCMRGlucose throughout the brain, with greatest effect on the visual and auditory pathways.[87] Halothane also causes widespread reduction of CMRGlucose,[88] in contrast to etomidate[89] and fentanyl.[90]

(2) Nuclear Magnetic Resonance (NMR).[91]

(3) Positron Emission Tomography (PET). Shows which parts of the brain are active at the time, using short half-life tracers, carbon 11 and 15, fluorine 18 and oxygen 15. This gives rCBF, $rCMRO_2$, rOER (oxygen extraction ratio), and rCBV for even small localized areas of brain.[92]

(4) Near infra-red absorption spectrophotometry. This gives global Hbo_2, HbR, total Hb, CBV, Svo_2 and oxidized mitochondrial cytochrome.

(5) Electroencephalogram (EEG).[93] The dominant frequency (zero crossing method)[94] is reduced to 5 Hz by anaesthetic concentrations of halothane and isoflurane, and 2 Hz by thiopentone. It remains at alpha frequencies (7.5–13 Hz) under enflurane and ketamine. Further analysis of EEG by spectral edge frequency analysis shows reductions of dominant

frequency of 8 Hz/MAC for halothane, 12 Hz/ED for thiopentone and 25 Hz/MAC for enflurane.[95] These changes lag behind the clinically-estimated changes of depth of anaesthesia.[96] Induction SEFs less than 15 Hz are associated with greatly reduced changes of arterial pressure in response to intubation.[97] 'Cerebral Function Monitoring' shows a reduction of amplitude with nitrous oxide,[98] and a rise in amplitude with thiopentone.

(6) Auditory,[99] visual, or somatosensory evoked potentials,[100] have shown anaesthesia-related changes, but are prone to interference unless relaxants are used. The volatile agents affect the latencies of waves III (superior olive) and V (inferior colliculus), but etomidate,[101] propofol[102] and fentanyl[103] do not.

(7) Frontalis electromyogram (EMG). There is reduction of tonic frontalis EMG activity with deepening anaesthesia[104] and an increase with strong stimuli, e.g. skin incision and intubation.

(8) Lower oesophageal contractions. These decrease in rate and pressure from several times a minute during consciousness to quietness at about 2 MAC, but are only an approximate guide to awareness.[105]

(9) Memory analysis, e.g. speaking words that the patient could not possibly already know, while 'unconscious'; then, after awakening, testing for familiarity with these words.[106]

Clinical detection of awareness

(1) In the unparalysed patient – movement, phonation.

(2) In the paralysed patient – sweating, reactive pupils, hypertension, tachycardia and lacrimation. These show a poor correlation with purposeful and verbal reactions to surgery, although sweating has been found to relate somewhat to awareness.[107] If consciousness is located in the dominant cerebral hemisphere,[108] then autonomic signs of light anaesthesia would not be expected to reliably demonstrate awareness, because their cerebral location is different. The connection between cerebral cortical and autonomic function in conscious man is not well maintained during adequate anaesthesia.

The 'isolated arm technique',[109] enables an otherwise paralysed patient to respond by squeezing the anaesthetists hand if awareness develops.

Prevention of awareness

Intravenous analgesics (e.g. fentanyl, alfentanil) may help to obtund pain (which is seldom the complaint), but **may not prevent awareness**.[110] Unexpected awareness under nitrous oxide – oxygen – opioid anaesthesia is very difficult to defend.

The most effective anaesthetics for preventing awareness are thiopentone and volatile agents, e.g. one MAC. Although the MAC_{95} values are determined for reflex responses to stimuli, they are also reliable guides for preventing awareness. The benzodiazepines, e.g. diazepam, temazepam and lorazepam, are also effective and may be conveniently used as premedicants. They have the particular advantage of reducing auditory sensitivity. (It is worth noting that atropine increases auditory sensitivity, and makes the risk of auditory awareness worse. However, hyoscine reduces awareness and recall, especially of abstract words,[111] less so for meaningful phrases.) Ear plugs for the patient and headphones playing soothing music have an important role. Some accidental awareness might be avoided if vapour analysers were installed in the breathing system.

Discontinuation of anaesthesia during surgery

When anaesthesia must be discontinued to save the patient's life during surgery. Diazepam may be used to depress hearing and memory formation.[112] Lorazepam reduces recall of ordinary events for long periods after dosage, but even so, meaningful words and painful experiences may be remembered.[113] Short-acting opioids may be used for analgesia here, but may further compromise cardiovascular stability.

Management of awareness

(1) Use a full dose of thiopentone to regain anaesthesia immediately; (2) talk to the patient reassuringly, explaining what is happening; (3) after the operation, talk to the patient again; and (4) later – arrange suitable psychological counselling to treat trauma that may have occurred.

When a patient complains of operative awareness some time later, listen, tend towards believing them (don't disbelieve them), arrange suitable psychological counselling.

EXTRAPYRAMIDAL SIDE-EFFECTS

Caused by phenothiazines, butyrophenone derivatives, metoclopramide,[114] large doses of methyldopa and rauwolfia alkaloids, levodopa.

Signs and symptoms

Acute dystonia, painless spasmodic contractions; akathesia, uncontrolled restlessness; pseudoparkinsonism; persistent tardive dyskinesia, grimacing, pulling faces, etc.

Treatment

Withdraw drug. For acute dystonic states, benztropine 2 mg i.v, procyclidine (Kemadrin) 10 mg i.v. (this may cause the anticholinergic side-effects of dry mouth, blurred vision and constipation) or diazepam 10 mg i.v.

MALIGNANT HYPERPYREXIA (MALIGNANT HYPERTHERMIA)

First put on a scientific basis by Denborough et al. in 1962.[115]

Definition

A specific condition in which heat production exceeds heat loss in the body to cause a rise of temperature of at least 2°C/h. First described in 1960 in Australia.

It is inherited as autosomal dominant with incomplete penetrance and generation skipping, possibly due to a defect in the gene responsible for calcium channels on chromosome 19. It is characterized by cyanosis, mottled rash, muscle rigidity (after suxamethonium), hypercapnia, hyperventilation, dysrhythmias and pyrexia (a relatively late sign). Exhaustion and cardiac failure cause death in 70%. The condition can be diagnosed quite early on by the recognition of an abnormally high end-tidal CO_2 as measured by capnography or by mass spectrometry.[116]

Pathophysiology

Drug administration, particularly anaesthetics but also mono-amine oxidase inhibitors, phenothiazines, amide local analgesics (lignocaine) and tricyclic antidepressants. The most commonly implicated agents are suxamethonium and halothane. Most others have rarely been implicated.[117]

Incidence

About 1 in 100 000 unselected population. Age distribution: 19 months to 70 years. It becomes more severe after puberty. The affected patient is commonly a young athletic male. In Denmark there was one case of fulminant hyperpyrexia in 250 000 anaesthetics but there was suspicion of it in 1:16 000 patients who received all types of anaesthetics and in 1:4200 when both suxamethonium and a potent inhalation agent were employed. Of those who received suxamethonium, 1:12 000 developed spasm of the masseters.[118]

Biochemistry

The primary lesion is in the skeletal musculature, probably in the sarcoplasmic reticulum, which contains an intergral enzyme system controlling movement of calcium ions.[119] There is also a suggestion that massive uncoupling of oxidative phosphorylation in the mitochondria could account for the rapid rise in temperature. The site of action of dantrolene[120] remains to be positively identified. The following parameters may be monitored: hypoxia, hypercapnia, hyperkalaemia, respiratory and metabolic acidosis, hypocalcaemia, hypomagnesaemia, hyperphosphataemia, diffuse intravascular coagulation, haemolysis, raised creatine phosphokinase (e.g. 80 000 units) and transaminases. Heat production is up to 2000 kJ/h.

Conditions with which it is particularly associated

Arthrogryposis multiplex congenita, osteogenesis imperfecta, congenital ptosis and strabismus, hernias, kyphoscoliosis, cleft palate and 'malignant hyperpyrexia myopathy', Duchenne progressive muscular dystrophy. Suxamethonium is avoided because of cardiac effects and risk of malignant hyperpyrexia.[121]

Management

(1) The anaesthetic mixture is withdrawn and the patient hyperventilated with oxygen. The severity of the condition is dose related, so early cessation of the anaesthetic is of the utmost importance; (2) the patient is cooled with ice, wet sheets, fan, cold water, gastric and peritoneal lavage; (3) blood-gas estimation, serum electrolytes, temperature measurement. Acidosis is corrected with bicarbonate; (4) glucose 50% 1 litre and insulin 100 units is infused; (5) diuresis is promoted; (6) dantrolene 1–10 mg/kg is injected i.v.; (7) dexamethasone 20 mg or another steroid is given i.v.; and (8) procaine 100 mg may be given i.v. up to 30 mg/kg.

An emergency pack for this condition may be kept in the theatre refrigerator. It contains procaine, isoprenaline, dopamine, methylprednisolone, 8.4% sodium bicarbonate, 50% glucose, dantrolene and insulin.

Prognosis

Is worse with late identification, increased dose of halothane or suxamethonium in attempt to abolish rigidity, temperature greater than 44°C, high level of rigidity (which persists after death). Successful treatment brings about reversal of effects in ½–1 h. Reappearance of symptoms some hours after successful treatment has occurred.[122]

Management of subsequent anaesthesia in a known case

In patients known to have malignant hyperpyrexia, a nitrous oxide – oxygen – opioid – non-depolarizing relaxant technique is recommended.[123]

Preoperative oral dantrolene is given for 24 h, 4 mg/kg divided into three or four doses. The following agents are considered safe: thiopentone, opiates, diazepam, pancuronium, vercuronium and probably nitrous oxide. Some doubt exists about phenothiazines. Lignocaine and atropine should be avoided. Bupivacaine may be safe.[124] Procaine is allowable. A vaporizer-free anaesthetic machine with new hoses is used. Full monitoring, cooling and treatment facilities are to hand. Pancuronium, if used, is not reversed with neostigmine and atropine, but IPPV is maintained until it wears off.

Investigation of patient and relatives

Muscle biopsy with measured exposure *in vitro* (Univ. Dept of Anaesthesia; University of Leeds; Malignant Hyperthermia Unit). Affected persons may wear bracelets with the name of the disease stamped on.

Dantrolene

Dantrolene is a muscle relaxant acting by uncoupling excitation – contraction sequence by reduction of calcium release from the sarcoplasmic reticulum. Dose: 1 mg/kg, i.v., repeated if necessary up to 10 mg/kg. Overdose effects may be seen in amounts above 4 mg/kg, i.e. weakness. Supplied in an ampoule containing dantrolene 20 mg, mannitol, 13 g, buffered to a pH of approximately 9.5 with sodium bicarbonate. Reversal, if necessary, by germine monoacetate 0.5 mg/kg and transiently by neostigmine 0.04 mg/kg. 4-aminopyridine may produce a slow, incomplete reversal.[125]

    (See also Ellis F. R. and Heffron J. J. A. In: *Recent Advances in Anaesthesia and Analgesia – 15* (Atkinson R. S. and Adams A. P. ed.) Edinburgh: Churchill Livingstone, 1985.)

SWEATING

Eccrine sweat glands are widespread and concentrated in the skin of the palms, soles, axillae and face. They are under sympathetic cholinergic neuronal control. Apocrine glands are confined to the axillae, perineum, buttocks and external genitals. The anaesthetist usually notices sweating on the forehead or face. Causes: (1) patient is too hot; (2) hypercapnia; (3) light anaesthesia; (4) shock; and (5) anxiety and high nervous tone.

    Treatment. If excessive, infusion of normal saline, after correction of the cause. Sweating is not necessarily a call for deeper anaesthesia.

ACCIDENTAL HYPOTHERMIA

This may occur during long operations, e.g. vascular surgery with massive blood transfusion, and can be minimized by operating in a warm theatre and the use of a warming blanket. The critical theatre temperature is about 21°C or 70°F (*see* Holdcroft A. *Body Temperature Control.* London: Baillière Saunders, 1980). Intravenous fluids should be warmed.

    Accidental hypothermia can also occur in the newborn, the aged, and secondary to such conditions as myxoedema, hypopituitarism, adrenal failure, drug overdose, apparent drowning and as a result of coma, immobility or exposure.

Management may include: (1) active rewarming, using a radiant heat cradle, warm water-bath at 37°C; (2) metal foil reflective space blankets; (3) cardiac output support; (4) correction of hypoxia with oxygen and IPPV if necessary; (5) steroids; and (6) glucose.

Physiological effects of hypothermia

Cardiovascular system

Dysrhythmias occur at temperatures below 30°C; spontaneous ventricular fibrillation may be seen, but is not likely above 28°C. Factors in its causation may include: (*a*) hyperkalaemia; (*b*) sudden pH and $Paco_2$ changes; and (*d*) citrate intoxication from tranfused blood.

Bradycardia not caused by vagal overactivity is progressive. The blood pressure falls with temperature drop. Stroke volume is little affected and coronary blood flow is well maintained. ECG changes include lengthening of the QRS complex and prolongation of the PR interval. Elevation of the ST segment with T-wave depression may occur. The J wave is a small positive wave on the downstroke of the R, which may appear at about 30°C. Vasoconstriction of skin vessels occurs.

Respiratory system

Measurements of human cerebral oxygen consumption indicate that at 30°C it is 39% and at 28°C 35% of normal.[126] The oxygen dissociation curve is shifted to the left so that liberation of oxygen to the tissues is hindered; although more oxygen is dissolved in plasma there is reduced availability of oxygen to the tissues due to: (*a*) depressed respiration; (*b*) decreased cardiac output; (*c*) vasoconstriction; (*d*) increased blood viscosity; and (*e*) arteriovenous shunts. Tissue oxygenation may be improved by controlled ventilation.

Acid–base balance

Acidosis tends to be a feature of hypothermia. Factors that may produce acidosis include: (*a*) increased solubility of carbon dioxide; (*b*) respiratory insufficiency; (*c*) increase in formation of lactic acid as a result of a metabolic deficit during circulatory arrest, hypoxia, shivering, surgical trauma or anaesthesia; (*d*) decreased breakdown of lactic acid due to impaired liver function; and (*e*) depression of renal function prevents correction of acidosis.

Measurement of pH presents some difficulties. Laboratory estimations are carried out at 37°C so a correction factor must be added of 0.0147 pH unit/1°C fall in temperature.[127] Direct $Paco_2$ measurement presents similar problems, the equation for correction being: $Pco_{2(t)} = Pco_{2(37)} \times 10^{0.019(t-37)}$.

Base excess measurements require no temperature correction.

Central nervous system

The cerebral cortex can tolerate the acute hypoxia due to complete circulatory arrest for 5–10 min at a temperature of 28°C and of 50 min at 15°C.

There is a reduction in cerebral blood flow, brain volume and intracranial pressure. Consciousness is usually lost between 28°C and 30°C. At 20°C cardiac arrest for 20 min or less is unlikely to do serious harm to the brain.[128]

Metabolism

With each fall of 1°C the metabolism is reduced 6–7%. The functions of the liver and kidneys are depressed during hypothermia so that drugs must be given in small amounts. Utilization of glucose is depressed, and continued intravenous infusion of glucose solution may result in a high blood-glucose level, not affected by insulin. Metabolism of substances like heparin, lactic acid and citrate is inhibited. The typical ECG change of QT prolongation is an indication for the administration of calcium gluconate or chloride. Renal blood flow, glomerular filtration and selective reabsorption are diminished. Below 30°C there is a secretion of dilute urine.

Electrolytes

There may be a rise in serum potassium. The cold heart is more sensitive to potassium, so small changes are of significance.

The neuromuscular junction

The duration and magnitude of block by depolarizing drugs are increased. The effect of non-depolarizing drugs is reduced. These changes are reversed on rewarming. *See also* Chapter 10.

The blood

Clotting mechanisms are depressed, platelet count falls rapidly,[129] and 'sludging' may occur in capillaries at very low temperatures. Viscosity is increased. As the metabolic demand for oxygen decreases, the saturation in venous blood rises. Oxygen is more soluble in plasma at low temperatures.

Rewarming

This must be undertaken with care as there is a danger of burning the patient if rewarming is overzealous. Rewarming can be expedited by use of a mattress with circulating fluid, by the use of warm blankets, warm water or warm air if care is taken. A temperature higher than 40°C should not be used.

Measurement of body temperature

See Chapter 18.

Temperature changes in shock

Temperature gradients between core and extremities develop during shock and these can be measured with sensitive electric thermometers, e.g. between oesophagus or rectum and the pad of the big toe. It has been suggested that a toe temperature of less than 27°C indicates a cardiac output of half normal.

MISCELLANEOUS COMPLICATIONS

Ophthalmological complications

1. *Corneal abrasion.* Prevented by tulle gras, adhesive tape sealing the lids or drops of castor oil or artificial tears into the conjunctival sac before anaesthesia. It can be diagnosed if a drop of 0.5% amethocaine is put into the eye, followed by fluorescein, when the abraded cornea will take up the stain. Treatment consists of a firm pad and bandage.

2. *Acute glaucoma* (closed angle) in susceptible patients who will complain of pain in and around the eye of a different nature to that due to foreign bodies or abrasions. On examination the eye is red, the cornea cloudy and the pupil dilated on the affected side. There may be nausea and vomiting. Treatment in emergency: acetazolamide 500 mg or a drip of 10% mannitol intravenously; physostigmine or pilocarpine drops, 1%, into the conjunctival sac. Skilled ophthalmic help needed urgently.

3. *Vitreous haemorrhage.* This has followed hypotensive techniques.

4. *Retinal infarction* from pressure of an anaesthetic mask on the eyeball. The blindness may be transient.

5. *Retinal emboli.*

6. *Transient blindness.* Due to spasm of basilar arteries,[130] or glycine absorption after transurethral surgery.

7. *Ocular displacement.* This has occurred during IPPV in the head-down position; due to increased venous pressure.

Spontaneous rupture of tympanic membrane

This has been reported in a previously fit patient receiving nitrous oxide and oxygen.[131]

Minor sequelae[132]

These are often the cause of considerable discomfort to the patient. They include trauma to lips, gums and teeth, sore throat, corneal, pharyngeal or laryngeal abrasions, superficial phlebothrombosis and simple ecchymosis following intravenous injections, backache following lithotomy position, nausea and vomiting and an occipital bald spot following pressure during prolonged surgery and for which a special pillow may be preventive. They occur in a disappointingly high proportion of patients and are only to be avoided by greater care in the handling of the unconscious. Minor sequelae following day-case surgery can cause considerable distress to an otherwise healthy subject.

Adverse drug reactions

Adverse reactions to anaesthetic contribute significantly to anaesthetic morbidity and to a smaller degree to anaesthetic mortality. It has been suggested that up to 100 deaths a year are directly associated with idiosyncracy or hypersensitivity rather than to errors of judgement.[133]

Clinical Manifestations. These may take the form of: (*a*) cardiovascular collapse (severe falls of arterial pressure, associated pallor, absent pulse); (*b*) bronchospasm, which may be associated with laryngospasm, muscle rigidity and abdominal pain; (*c*) oedema, which may involve the airway; (*d*) cutaneous manifestations, including flushing, rashes and weals; and (*e*) tachycardia and arrhythmias, including ventricular tachycardia may occur.

Clinical Management. (*a*) Withdraw all anaesthetic agents and administer oxygen; (*b*) give intravenous adrenaline in a bolus dose of 0.1 mg, which can be repeated; (*c*) rapid intravenous infusion of fluids, at least 1–2 litres likely to be required (up to 25% of plasma volume may have been lost); and (*d*) consider need for IPPV, bronchodilators (e.g. aminophylline 250 mg by infusion or salbutamol 0.25–0.5 mg), antihistamines (e.g. chlorpheniramine 10–20 mg i.v.), and steroids.

Recommendations[134] have been made concerning assessment at the time of the reaction, subsequent assessment and communication of the conclusions to the patient. The following procedure has been suggested:[135]

1. As soon as possible blood samples are taken into duplicate EDTA tubes and repeated sampling made at 1, 3, 6, 12 and 24 hours subsequently. It has also been suggested that blood samples be taken at 30, 60 and 90 min for estimation of tryptase released by mast cells.

2. The anaesthetist telephones the referral immunology laboratory, discusses the case, makes correct documentation and confirms correct sampling.

3. One set of samples is analysed at the base hospital for complete blood profiles and differential counts.

4. Plasma is separated from other samples and stored at −20°C before dispatch to the immunology laboratory with documentation.

5. The anaesthetist provides a full clinical account and also sends a 'yellow card' adverse reaction notification to the Committee on Safety of Medicines.

6. The immunology laboratory analyses the samples and arranges skin tests at a suitable time.

7. The immunology laboratory reaches a conclusion on the basis of the clinical history and haematological profile regarding the probable mechanism and causative agent.

8. These conclusions are communicated in writing to the anaesthetist and the patient's general practitioner. Safe drug combinations or alternatives are suggested.

9. The situation is explained to the patient who at all times carries a warning card.

A National Adverse Anaesthetic Reactions Advisory Service (NAARAS) was established offering advice and expertise to clinicians but has been disbanded. This was based at the Royal Hallamshire Hospital, Sheffield and two reports of its work were published.[136]

The Radioallergosorbent test (RAST). Radioactive iodine labelled anti-IgE antibodies bind to IgE antibodies that have reacted with polymer-coupled allergens. The radioactivity of the washed solid phase is directly proportional to IgE antibody of the serum under test. However, because of the lack of proper conjugates of many drugs and their metabolites the RAST procedure cannot be applied to many agents.

When a reaction occurs it is necessary to establish whether it is due to the technique or the drug. To incriminate the drug it is necessary to establish that mast cell degranulation has occurred. It is interesting to note that RAST IgE antibodies to suxamethonium are more widespread than would be expected in the general population and have a female bias. It is doubtful whether histamine release plays any role in the severe reaction. More work remains to be done, but at the present time it is more likely that skin testing is the most helpful diagnostic test although a battery of RAST tests may in the end prove superior.

See also Fisher M. *Curr. Anaesth. Crit. Care* 1991, **2**, 182.

HAZARDS TO MEDICAL AND NURSING STAFF[137]

There have been a number of surveys suggesting that the anaesthetist and other theatre staff are exposed to hazard as a result of their occupation. Anaesthetists are thought to be more prone to coronary artery disease and suicide than people in other occupations. Other hazards include liability to renal calculi, exposure to radiation (although the average exposure has been calculated as 13 mR/week against a maximum allowable exposure of 100), muscular and ligamentous strains as a result of lifting patients, the possibility of exposure to HIV-infection and hepatitis B antigen (*see below*), and fatigue (which may result in slow reaction time in an emergency and inability to form judgements). Many individual anaesthetists work long hours. Chronic intermittent exposure to nitrous oxide may interfere with vitamin B_{12} metabolism[138] and rarely causes polyneuropathy.[139]

Reproduction

Interest has been aroused in the possible effects of working conditions in operating theatres in respect to increased rates of spontaneous abortion,[140] an increased incidence of congenital abnormalities in children born, and in a higher than normal proportion of female to male births in the wives of male anaesthetists.[141] Mutagenic changes are unlikely in operating theatre personnel and there is no proof of any causal relationship between the data obtained[142] and any anaesthetic agent present in the atmosphere of operating rooms, but there is general agreement that all reasonable steps should be taken to reduce contamination. More recent work tends to be reassuring.[143]

Malignant disease

The finding of an increased incidence of malignancy in the lymphoid and reticular systems in anaesthetists has not been confirmed by a more recent study[144] and it does not appear that British anaesthetists suffer from cancer more than the general population.[141]

Measures to reduce pollution

1. Room ventilation. The air-conditioning systems of modern theatres are designed to prevent bacterial contamination and are ineffective in removing anaesthetic waste. The pattern of air flow in any operating room depends on many factors, which vary at different times.[145]

2. Disposal of waste gases to outside air. For active scavenging an appropriate device is essential to prevent negative pressure being transmitted to the patient circuit. It should be noted that tubing used in scavenging systems has no anti-static properties.

3. The use of low-flow (e.g. 1 l/min) rebreathing systems or completely closed systems reduces the amount of anaesthetic agent discharged into room air and reduces cost.

4. Total intravenous anaesthesia with avoidance of inhalation agents. *See* Chapter 9.

5. The use of regional analgesia combined with intravenous sedation.

6. Special problems exist in dental anaesthesia in the outpatient department,[146] but an effective gas collecting and disposal system has been described.[147] The design of pharyngeal and oral packs is also important.

7. Filling of vaporizers causes discharge of significant amounts of a volatile liquid to the atmosphere. It may be wise to charge vaporizers at the end of the day when few people are in the room, rather than at the beginning of a list.

Trace concentrations and performance[148]

Many studies have been made on the effects of trace concentration of anaesthetic agents on the anaesthetist, although much of the experimental evidence is based on amounts higher than the 600 ppm nitrous oxide and 10 ppm halothane commonly found. It is doubtful whether contamination of this degree has any effect on the anaesthetist's performance. The aim of scavenging is to reduce concentrations to about 30 ppm for nitrous oxide and 1 ppm for halothane.

The hazards to theatre personnel from blood of hepatitis B carriers

Anaesthetists should be protected by immunization. Hepatitis B antigen (HBAg), Australia antigen, serum hepatitis (SH) antigen, was first described by Blumberg in 1965 (for which he received the Nobel prize).[149] The incidence of the carrier state is about 0.2% in UK, 5% in the eastern Mediterranean countries and 10% in those of southeast Asia. The carrier state in a patient is an indication for very careful safeguards and not a contra-indication to surgical or obstetric care. The virus is transmitted not only by shed blood and body secretions but also by close physical contact. Patients with the antigen in their bloodstream range from those with jaundice (serum B hepatitis) to symptomless carriers, but all are potentially infective. If adequate hygienic measures are scrupulously observed by all contacts there need be no danger during surgical, obstetrical or medical investigation and treatment, nor need a carrier give up the practice of medicine.

Patients under high suspicion of being hepatitis B carriers include the following: (1) all patients with liver disease, both acute and chronic; (2) patients undergoing haemodialysis or who have received a renal transplant; (3) all patients suffering from leukaemia, reticuloses, polyarteritis nodosa or polymyositis; (4) patients being treated by radiotherapy or immunosuppressive drugs; (5) immigrants or visitors from countries with a high background of carriers; (6) patients who have been transfused in, or have recently returned from, areas with a high background of incidence; (7) patients who have ever received blood from paid donors; (8) inmates of prisons or institutions for the mentally defective; (9) drug addicts, prostitutes and homosexuals; and (10) those with tattoos.

Carriers can be divided into two groups:[150] (1) simple carriers who have anti-HBe and a low level of HBsAg in their blood; and (2) super-carriers who are HbsAg positive have higher titres of HBsAg and DNA polymerase in their blood and tend to have mildly raised serum liver transaminase levels. These latter are more infective. A super-carrier may convert to a simple carrier, perhaps after several years. To be certain of the carrier state, two or more blood specimens should be tested over a period of months.

The virus is killed by autoclaving and by ionizing radiation and probably does not survive immersion for at least 3 h in a hypochlorite-detergent mixture (e.g. Domestos or Chloros 10% with an ionic detergent), which corrodes metal, or in 10% formaldehyde, which does not. Glutaraldehyde is also effective.

Prevention of infection spread from carriers presenting for operation requires most diligent care to be taken:

1. Before operation. Prevention of contamination of nurses, assistants and porters, the anaesthetic trolley and its coverings, dressings, suction tubes and swabs. Disposables should be disinfected and incinerated. The number of individuals handling the patient must be kept to a minimum and all must be protected by gowns, gloves and overshoes. Buckets containing plastic bags partially filled with hypochlorite-detergent can receive swabs, used syringes, needles, gloves and overshoes, which are then discarded.

2. During operation. Theatre linen, if possible, should be burnt, if not it should be disinfected as above. Instruments must be disinfected before they are cleaned and autoclaved. Biopsy specimens and blood, etc. must be sent to the laboratory in sealed containers suitably labelled.

3. After operation. In the theatre, where possible everything should be washed down with hypochlorite-detergent and instruments soaked in 10% formaldehyde. Used syringes and needles must be disinfected for at least 3 hours and, in plastic bags, sent for destruction. Particular care must be taken to render needles harmless. Face-masks, tracheal tubes, reservoir bags, sucker tubing, etc. should be disinfected, then destroyed. Laryngoscope blades must be soaked for at least 3 hours in 10% formaldehyde. The anaesthetic machine should be well washed down with the recommended antiseptic solution and the ventilator decontaminated with formaldehyde. Infusion apparatus must be destroyed and not sent back to the blood bank. When possible, patients likely to be high risk should be placed at the end of the list.

Patients found to be 'Australia antigen positive' (surface antigen HBsAg) should be tested for 'e' antigen (HBeAg) and its antibody (anti-HBe).

Patients positive for HBeAg should be regarded as infectious and all precautions taken to avoid contamination with the patient's blood. The patient who is HBsAg positive but HBeAg negative may require further investigation but is non-infectious for practical purposes, although not acceptable as a blood donor.

Anyone at special risk, as after a prick from a needle contaminated with infected blood, may require an intramuscular injection of 500 mg of anti-HBAg serum (immunoglobulin).

AIDS

Anaesthetists and other workers in theatres should take sensible precautions against the possibility of inadvertent contamination with the human immunodeficiency virus. This includes wearing of gloves during venipuncture, setting up of drips and tracheal intubation and extubation, which is becoming standard practice in many countries.[151] Reasons why anaesthetists do not wear gloves have been analysed in a survey and shown to be largely invalid.[152]

(*See also* Lee K. G. and Soni N. *Anaesthesia* 1986, **41**, 1011; *AIDS and HIV infection*. A statement by the Royal College of Surgeons of England, 1992; *HIV Infection: Hazards to Patients and Health Care Workers During Invasive Procedures*. The Royal College of Pathologists, 1992.)

Addiction and the anaesthetist

Anaesthetists are an at risk group because of the relatively easy access they have to addictive drugs. Anaesthetists who have been addicted to opioid drugs should be advised to change to another specialty.

Suicides in anaesthetists in training

The incidence is rather high but there is no evidence that it has any relationship to the training or professional life style of the young doctor.[153]

References

1. Chopra V., Bovill J. G. and Spierdijk J. *Anaesthesia* 1990, **45**, 3; Gravenstein P. *Manual of Complications during Anesthesia* Philadelphia: Lippincott, 1991.
2. Hall M. *Lancet* 1856, **1**, 393.
3. Heiberg J. *Med. Times Gaz.* 1874, Jan. 10th.
4. Nunn J. F. *J. Roy. Soc. Med.* 1985, **78**, 983.
5. Guedel A. E. *JAMA* 1933, **100**, 1862.
6. Nandi P. R. et al. *Br. J. Anaesth.* 1991, **66**, 157.
7. Drummond G. B. *Br. J. Anaesth.* 1991, **66**, 153.
8. Brewer N. et al. *Curr. Res. Anesth. Analg.* 1934, **13**, 257.
9. Jacobs H. B. *JAMA* 1972, **222**, 1231; Pottecher T. et al. *Ann. Francaise d'Anaes. Reani.* 1984, **3**, 54.

10. Fisher J. A. *Can. Anaesth. Soc. J. 1979,* **26**, 225.
11. Nosworthy M. D. *Anaesthesia* 1948, **3**, 86.
12. Severinghaus J. W. and Mitchell R. A. *Clin. Res.* 1962, **10**, 122
13. Vella L. M. et al. *Anaesthesia* 1984, **39**, 108.
14. Ravindran R. S. *Anesth. Analg. (Cleve.)* 1981, **60**, 121.
15. Gawley P. H. and Dundee J. W. *Br. J. Anaesth.* 1981, **53**, 10073.
16. Ali J. and Ali-Khan T. *Surg. Gynecol. Obstet.* 1979, **148**, 863.
17 Mendelson C. L. *Am. J. Obstet Gynec.* 1946, **52**, 191.
18 Woolsey W. *C. N. Y. St. J. Med.* 1912, **12**, 171.
19 Hamman L. *Trans. Assoc. Am. Physicians.* 1937, **52**, 311.
20 Trendelenburg F. *Arch. klin. C'hir.* 1908, **86**, 686.
21 Pollard B. J. et al. *Anesthesiology* 1983, **58**, 373; Lee J. Alfred *Region. Anesth.* 1985, **10**, 99.
22 McKenzie P. J. *Br. J. Anaesth.* 1991, **66**, 4.
23 Johnson R. et al. *Clin. Orthop.* 1977, **127**, 123.
24 Gruber U. F. et al. *Br. Med. J.* 1980, **280**, 69.
25 McLean J. *Am. J. Physiol.* 1916, **41**, 250.
26 Kakkar V. V. *Proc. R. Soc. Med.* 1975, **68**, 263.
27 Negus D. et al. *Lancet* 1980, **1**, 891.
28 Kakkar V. V. et al. *Br. Med. J.* 1982, **284**, 375.
29 Eriksson B. I. et al. *J. Bone Joint Surg.* 1991, **73A**, 484–493.
30. Levine S. *JAMA* 1920, **75**, 795.
31. Magendie F. *J. Physiol. Exp. (Paris)* 1821.
32. Barlow J. *J. Med. Chir. Trans.* 1830, **16**, 19.
33. Thomas D. and van der Wetden C. *Anaesthesia* 1983, **38**, 1005.
34. Marshall W. K. and Bedford R. F. *Anesthesiology* 1980, **52**, 131.
35. Edmonds-Seal J. et al. *Proc. R. Soc. Med.* 1970, **63**, 831; Maroon J. C. and Albin M. S. *Anesth. Analg. (Cleve.)* 1974, **53**, 399.
36. Durrant T. M. et al. *Am. Heart. J.* 1947, **33**, 269.
37. Healy T. E. J. and Wilkins R. C. *Ann. R. Coll. Surg.* 1984, **66**, 56.
38. Lee J. Alfred *Reg. Anesth.* 1985, **10**, 99.
39. Scott D. B. et al. *Br. J. Anaesth.* 1966, **38**, 174; Scott D. B. and Slawson K. B. *Br. J. Anaesth.* 1968, **40**, 103.
40. Lincoln J. P. and Sawyer N. P. *Anesthesiology* 1966, **22**, 800.
41. O'Donevan N. et al. *Br. J. Anaesth.* 1986, **58**, 280.
42. Brock-Utne J. G. *Anesth. Analg. (Cleve.)* 1980, **59**, 921.
43. Roussak J. B. et al. *Br. Med. J.* 1984, **289**, 1579.
44. Morton H. J. V. and Wylie W. D. *Anaesthesia* 1951, **6**, 190.
45. Edwards G. et al. *Anaesthesia* 1965, **11**, 194.
46. Andrews A. D. et al. *Anaesthesia* 1982, **37**, 22.
47. Maliniak K. and Vakil A. B. *Anesth. Analg. (Cleve.)* 1979, **58**, 309; Dobb G. et al. *Br. J. Anaesth.* 1979, **51**, 967.
48. Gallagher E. G. et al. *Anaesthesia* 1988, **43**, 1011; Escolano F. et al. *Anaesthesia* 1989, **44**, 212; Dubin S. A. *Anesth. Analg.* 1989, **69**, 680.
49. Jenkin J. G. *Anesthesiology* 1984, **61**, 346.
50. Sellick B. A. *Lancet* 1961, **2**, 404.
51. Sellick B. A. *Anaesthesia* 1982, **37**, 213.
52. Howells T. H. et al. *Anaesthesia* 1983, **38**, 457.
53. Coriat P. et al. *Anaesthesia* 1984, **39**, 703.
54. Vella L. et al. *Br. Med. J.* 1985, **290**, 1173.
55. Dundee J. W. *J. Roy. Soc. Med.* 1980, **73**, 231.
56. Dundee J. W. et al. *Br. Med. J.* 1986, **293**, 583; Barsoum G., Perry E. P. and Fraser I. A. *J. Roy. Soc. Med.* 1990, **83**, 86; Dundee J. W., Yang J. and Ghaly R. G. *Lancet* 1990, **i**, 541.
57. Jones D. F. *Anaesthesia* 1980, **35**, 50.
58. Shearer E. S. *Anaesthesia* 1990, **45**, 255.
59. Fraser A. I. C. and Goat V. A. *Anaesthesia* 1983, **38**, 128.

60. Britt B. A. and Gordon R. A. *Can. Anaesth. Soc. J.* 1964, **11**, 514.
61. Budinger K. *Arch. klin. Chir.* 1894, **47**, 121.
62. Mullick S. *Surg. Gynecol. Obstet.* 1978, **146**, 821; Gilliatt R. W. *Mayo Clin. Proc.* 1981, **56**, 36l; Durkin M. A. P. and Crabtree S. D. *J. R. Soc. Med.* 1982, **75**, 658.
63. Cushing H. *Med. News* 1904, **84**, 577.
64. Klenerman L. *J. Bone Joint. Surg. (U.K.)* 1983, **65**, 374.
65. Hewer C. L. *Anaesthesia* 1953, **8**, 198.
66. Medicine and Law, *Lancet* 1984, **1**, 1306.
67. Esmarch J. F. A. *Chirurgie* 1873, **19**, 373.
68. Nightingale P. J. and Longreen A. *Anaesthesia* 1982, **37**, 322.
69. Norman J. E. *Anaesthesia* 1955, **10**, 88.
70. Sinclair R. N. *Anaesthesia* 1954, **9**, 286.
71. Lett Z. *Br. J. Anaesth.* 1964, **36**, 266.
72. Rosen M. and Lunn J. N. (ed.) *Awareness and Pain in General Anaesthesia* London: Butterworths, 1987.
73. Jones J. G. and Konieczko K. *Br. Med. J.* 1986, **292**, 1291.
74. Liu W. H. D. et al. *Anaesthesia*, 1991, **46**, 435.
75. Winterbottom E. H. *Br. Med. J.* 1950, **1**, 247; Hutchinson R. *Br. J. Anaesth.* 1961, **33**, 463; Waters D. J. *Br. J. Anaesth.* 1968, **40**, 259; Utting J. E. *Anaesth. Intensive Care* 1975, **3**, 334; Mainzer J. *Can. Anaesth. Soc. J.* 1979, **26**, 381; Blacker R. S. *JAMA* 1975, **234**, 67; Blacher B. S. *Anesthesiology* 1984, **61**, 1.
76. Flatt J. R. et al. *Anaesth. Intensive Care* 1984, **12**, 315.
77. Artusio J. F. *JAMA* 1955, **157**, 33.
78. Hargrove R. L. *J. Med. Defence Union* 1987, **3**, 9.
79. Russell I. F. *Br. J. Anaesth.* 1986, **58**, 965; Schultetus R. R. et al. *Anesth. Analg.* 1986, **65**, 723.
80. Millar K. and Watkinson M. *Ergonomics*, 1983, **26**, 585.
81. Levinson B. W. *Brit. J. Anaesth.* 1965, **37**, 544.
82. Bennett H. L., Davies H. S. and Giannini J. A. *Br. J. Anaesth.* 1985, **57**, 174; Bonke B. and Schmitz P. I. M. *Brit. J. Anaesth.* 1986, **58**, 957; Goldmann L. and Shah M. V. *Anaesthesia* 1987, **42**, 596.
83. Bonke B. et al. *Br. J. Anaesth.* 1986, **58**, 957.
84. Dixon N. F. *Preconscious Processing.* Chichester: John Wiley and Sons, 1981.
85. Bentin S., Collins G. I. and Adam N. *Br. J. Anaesth.* 1978, **50**, 1179.
86. Morris R. G. M. et al. *Nature*, 1986, **319**, 774.
87. Sokoloff L. *J. Cereb. Blood Flow Metab.* 1981, **1**, 7.
88. Hawkins R. A. and Biebuyck J. F. In: *Molecular Mechanisms in Anaesthesia (Progress in Anaesthesiology)*, vol. 2. (B. R. Fink ed.) New York: Raven, 1980.
89. Davis D. W. et al. *Anaesthesiology* 1986, **64**, 751.
90. Samra S. K. et al. *Anesthesiology* 1984, **61**, 261.
91. Smith D. S. and Chance B. *Anesthesiology* 1987, **67**, 157.
92. Phelps M. E., Mazziotta J. C. and Huang S. C. *J. Cereb. Blood Flow Metab.* 1982, **2**, 113.
93. Clark D. I. and Rosner B. S. *Anesthesiology* 1973, 38, 564.
94. Herregods L. and Rolly G. In: *Awareness and Pain in General Anaesthesia* (Rosen M. and Lunn J. N. ed.) London: Butterworths, 1987.
95. Homer D. and Stanski D. R. *Anesthesiology* 1985, **62**, 714.
96. Arden J. R., Holley H. O. and Stanski D. R. *Anesthesiology* 1986, **65**, 19.
97. Rampil I. J. and Matteo R. S. *Anesthesiology* 1987, **67**, 139.
98. Williams D. J. M. et al. *Anaesthesia* 1984, **39**, 422.
99. Chiappa H. K. and Ropper A. H. *N. Engl. J. Med.* 1982, **306**, 1140 and 1205.
100. Kriss A. In: *Evoked Potentials in Clinical Testing* (Halliday A. M. ed.) London: Churchill Livingstone, 1982, 44.
101. Thornton C. and Heneghan C. P. H. et al. *Br. J. Anaesth.* 1985, **57** 554.
102. Thornton C. et al. *Beitrage Zur Anaesthesiologie und Intensivmedizin* 1968, **2**, 201.

103. Velasco M. et al. *Neuropharmacology*, 1984, **23**, 359.
104. Herregods L. et al. In: *Awareness and Pain in General Anaesthesia*. (Rosen M. and Lunn J. N. ed.) London: Butterworths, 1987.
105. Isaac P. A. and Rosen M. *Br. J. Anaesth*. 1988, **60**, 338P.
106. Millar K. and Watkinson M. *Ergonomics*, 1983, **26**, 585; Eich E., Reeves J. L. and Katz R. L. *Anesth. Analg*. 1985, **64**, 1143.
107. Russel I. F. *Br. J. Anaesth*. 1986, **58**, 965; Schultetus R. R. et al. *Anesth. Analg*. 1986, **65**, 723.
108. Dixon N. F. *Preconscious Processing* Chichester: John Wiley and Sons, 1981.
109. Tunstall M. E. *Br. Med. J*. 1977, **1b**, 1321.
110. Schultetus R. R. et al. *Anesth. Analg*. 1986, **65**, 723.
111. Jones D. M. et al. *Br. J. Clin. Pharmacol*. 1978, **7**, 479.
112. Frith C. D. et al. *Q. J. Exp. Psych*. 1984, **36A**, 133.
113. File S. E. and Lister R. G. *Br. J. Clin. Pharmacol*. 1982, **14**, 545.
114. Bateman D. N. et al. *Br. Med. J*. 1985, **291**, 930.
115. Denborough M. H. et al. *Br. J. Anaesth*. 1962, **34**, 395.
116. Neubauer K. R. and Kaufman R. D. *Anesth. Analg. (Cleve.)* 1985, **64**, 837.
117. McGuire N. and Easy W. R. *Anaesthesia* 1990, **45**, 124.
118. Ording H. *Anesth. Analg. (Cleve.)* 1985, **64**, 700.
119. Cheah K. S. et al. *Acta Anaesth. Scand*. 1990, **34**, 114.
120. Harrison G. G. *Br. J. Anaesth*. 1977, **49**, 315; Freisen C. M. et al. *Can. Anaesth. Soc. J*. 1979, **26**, 319.
121. Rosenberg H. and Heiman-Patterson T. *Anesthesiology* 1983, **59**, 362.
122. Matthieu A. et al. *Anesthesiology* 1979, **51**, 454.
123. Michel P. A. and Fronefield H. P. *Anesthesiology* 1985, **62**, 213.
124. Willatts S. M. *Anaesthesia* 1979, **34**, 41.
125. Lee C. et al. *Anesthesiology* 1981, **54**, 61.
126. Stone H. H. et al. *Surg. Gynecol. Obstet* 1956, **103**, 313.
127. Rosenthal T. B. *J. Biol. Chem*. 1948, **173**, 25.
128. Treasure T. *Ann. R. Coll. Surg*. 1984, **66**, 235.
129. Easterbrook P. J. and Davis H. F. *Br. Med. J*. 1985, **291**, 23.
130. Johnson R. C. and Moss P. J. *Anaesthesia* 1981, **36**, 954.
131. White P. F. *Anesthesiology* 1983, **59**, 369.
132. Riding J. E. *Br. J. Anaesth*. 1975, **47**, 91.
133. Watkins J. *Anaesthesia* 1985, **40**, 797.
134. Laxenaire M. C. *Moneret-Vautin D. A. and Watkins J. Anaesthesia* 1983, **38**, 147.
135. Watkins J. *Br. J. Anaesth*. 1987, **59**, 104.
136. Watkins J. *Anaesthesia* 1985, **40**, 797; *ibid*, 1989, **44**, 157.
137. Cohen E. N. *Anesthetic Exposure in the Workplace*. New York: MTP Press, 1980.
138. Amess J. A. L. *Lancet* 1978, **2**, 339; Layzer R. B. *Lancet* 1978, **2**, 1227.
139. Layzer R. B. et al. *Neurology* 1978, **28**, 504; Brodsky J. B. et al. *Anesth. Analg. (Cleve.)* 1981, **60**, 297.
140. Mehta S. and Burton P. *Anaesthesia* 1977, **32**, 924; Vessey M. P. *Anaesthesia* 1978, **33**, 430; Vessey M. P. and Nunn J. F. *Br. Med. J*. 1980, **2**, 696.
141. Cohen E. N. et al. *Anesthesiology* 1974, **41**, 321; Knill-Jones R. P. et al. *Lancet* 1975, **2**, 807; Salo M. and Vapaavuori M. *Br. J. Anaesth*. 1976, **48**, 877.
142. Baden J. M. *Br. J. Anaesth*. 1979, **51**, 417.
143. Spence A. A. *Br. J. Anaesth*. 1987, **59**, 96.
144. Bruce D. L. et al. *Anesthesiology* 1974, **41**, 71.
145. Smith W. D. A. In: *Recent Advances in Anaesthesia and Analgesia – 12* (Hewer C. L. and Atkinson R. S. ed.) Edinburgh: Churchill Livingstone, 1976.
146. Hillman K. M. et al. *Anaesthesia* 1981, **36**, 1257.
147. Parbrook G. D. and Monk I. B. *Br. J. Anaesth*. 1975, **47**, 1185.
148. Smith G. and Shirley A. W. *Br. J. Anaesth*. 1977, **49**, 65; Ferstandig L. L. *Anesth. Analg*. 1978, **57**, 328; Smith G. and Shirley A. W. *Br. J. Anaesth*. 1978, **50**, 7001.

149. Blumberg B. S. et al. *JAMA* 1965, **191**, 541; Blumberg B. S. et al. *Ann. Intern. Med.* 1967, **66**, 924.
150. Tedder R. S. *Br. J. Hosp. Med.* 1980, **23**, 266.
151. Editorial, *Lancet*, 1990, **336**, 1103; Brattebo G. and Wisborg T., *Lancet*, 1990, **336**, 1456; Guidelines for Prevention of Transmission of Human Immunodeficiency Virus, *MMWR*, 1989, **38** (Suppl. 56).
152. Harrison C. A., Rogers D. W. and Rosen M. *Anaesthesia*, 1990, **45**, 831.
153. Helliwell P. J. *Anaesthesia* 1983, **38**, 1097.

Chapter 15

Drugs used in association with anaesthesia

ANALEPTICS AND ANTAGONISTS

The chief action of these drugs is to stimulate respiration, reverse narcotic activity of sedative drugs, restore blood pressure and reflex activity and elevate mood. When given in large doses they are mostly convulsants. Their stimulating action on respiration is greatest in non-anaesthetized or lightly anaesthetized patients. In conditions of respiratory arrest their use comes far behind that of oxygen and IPPV.

Ethamivan

This is a central and reflex (carotid body) respiratory stimulant. Well absorbed from mucosa of mouth and tongue in neonates in a dose of 0.5 ml. For neonates the dose is 0.2 ml of 5% solution intramuscularly. Adult dose 100 mg repeated.

Doxapram hydrochloride *(Dopram; Stimulexin)*

First described in 1962. A non-specific respiratory stimulant acting on peripheral chemoreceptors. Clinical doses do not reduce the analgesic effects of morphine and pethidine,[1] but reverse the depressant respiratory effects.[2] Can be given i.m., dose 1.0–1.5 mg/kg, or as an infusion at the rate of 100 ml/h, 2 mg/ml in 5% dextrose (about 3 mg/min).[3] May be useful in treatment of barbiturate overdosage.[4] The hyperpnoea produced may aid blind nasal intubation[5] and may speed recovery from general anaesthesia due to a volatile agent[6] and perhaps due to a barbiturate.[7] May reduce postoperative respiratory complications.[8] It should be used with great care in patients with hypertension, status asthmaticus, coronary heart disease and thyrotoxicosis.

In a double-blind trial doxapram was found to be the most efficient respiratory stimulant of five tested (nikethamide, prethcamide, amiphenazole and ethamivan). Ethamivan came second.[9] Issued in 5 ml ampoules and 500 ml containers for intravenous infusion. Continuous infusion is recommended.

PRESSOR AGENTS

Pressor drugs may act: (1) by liberating catecholamines; (2) peripherally, on vessels; and (3) centrally, on the heart. Drugs of this nature should not be used routinely, but only when a severe fall of blood pressure is anticipated or actually occurs.

The pressor drugs related to adrenaline may be used after intradural or extradural block and during general anaesthesia. These sympathomimetic amines may be grouped in several ways, none of them completely satisfactory.

Classification

A. Naturally occurring catecholamines that stimulate α- and β-receptors directly: adrenaline, noradrenaline and dopamine.

B. Sympathetic amines that act directly, as well as indirectly by releasing catecholamines and stimulate both α- and β-receptors, e.g. ephedrine, metaraminol and mephentermine.

C. Sympathomimetic amines that act directly on α-receptors, e.g. phenylephrine and methoxamine.

D. Sympathomimetic amines that act directly on β-receptors, e.g. isoprenaline.

The three naturally occurring catecholamines are adrenaline, noradrenaline and dopamine; they all contain the group 3:4 dihydroxybenzene (catechol).

Adrenaline, BP (*Epinephrine, USP*)

History

The adrenal glands were described by Bartholomaeus in 1563 and modern knowledge of adrenal physiology started with the description by Thomas Addison (1793–1860), of London, in 1855 of the disease which bears his name. Adrenaline was isolated by George Oliver (1841–1915), a practitioner

Table 15.1. Adrenergic receptors

Organ	Receptor type	Effect of stimulation
Heart	β₁	Increased rate, force of contraction and acceleration of conduction
Bronchi	β₂	Dilatation
Arterioles	β₂	Dilatation
	α	Contraction
Gut	α	Reduction of motility
Liver	β₁	Glycogenolysis
Muscle	β₁	Glycogenolysis

in Harrogate, and J. J. Abel of the Johns Hopkins Hospital and Sir Edward Schäfer (1850–1935) in 1894[10] from the adrenal medulla, who showed that it contained a pressor agent. Produced in crystalline form by Takamine (1854–1922)[11] (who determined its constitution and patented it under the name of 'adrenaline'),[12] and Aldrich,[13] independently, in 1901; the first hormone to be synthesized, by Friedrich Stolz (1860–1936) in 1904. [14] (The word 'hormone' (Greek = I excite) was introduced by E. H. Starling (1866–1927) of London in 1905.[15]) Adrenaline is derived from noradrenaline which is synthesized in the body from tyrosine, dopa and dopamine being intermediate stages.

Pharmacodynamics

Stimulates both α- and β-receptors. It is formed in the adrenal medulla where it is stored in intracellular granules (and at adrenergic nerve endings) and is liberated by acetylcholine (humoral transmitter) by impulses from the sympathetic preganglionic fibres supplying the medullary cells. Ampoules of adrenaline can be autoclaved once or twice without loss of potency.

Cardiovascular system. Increases the stroke volume, rate and cardiac output. It increases the incidence of dysrhythmias, by making the automatic conducting system more irritable. The systolic blood pressure rises, but the diastolic falls. Vessels in different situations react to adrenaline in different ways. While the vessels of the skin, mucosae, subcutaneous tissues, splanchnic area and kidneys are constricted (α-effects), those in muscles are relaxed after physiological doses (β-effects), constricted after large doses. While the cerebral and pulmonary arteries are constricted, blood pressure in the coronaries is likely to rise. Angina pectoris may be precipitated in patients with coronary disease, because of the augmentation of cardiac work on top of narrowed vessels. The peripheral venous pressure is increased. It is the most potent drug known to stimulate an arrested heart, but its transient and rather violent effect and the danger of ventricular dysrhythmias limit routine use as a pressor agent. Increases platelet stickiness and reduces clotting time, leading to shorter bleeding time. The cardiovascular effects of adrenaline are reduced by acidosis.[16]

The renal blood flow. This is decreased. Secretion of urine is reduced.

The respiratory system. Bronchial tone decreased, following both topical (1–100 solution in atomizer) and systemic administration. Depth of respiration slightly increased, and irregular breathing sometimes seen.

The alimentary canal. While the muscle of the gut is relaxed, the pyloric and ileocolic sphincters are contracted (both α- and β-effects) leading to ileus. The spleen contracts and empties its cells into the circulation. The secretion of the intestinal glands is inhibited.

Sweating and pilomotor activity not much stimulated in man. Dilates the pupil when carried to the eye in the bloodstream. Glycogen is mobilized from the liver, giving rise to an increase in the blood-sugar level; anti-insulin effect. Rise in metabolic rate, lipolysis, and muscle catabolism. Large doses stimulate, small clinical doses inhibit uterine tone in labour. It elevates the pain threshold.

Following injection, untoward reactions may include anxiety, restlessness from mild cerebral stimulation, throbbing headache, vertigo, pallor and palpitations; hyperthyroid and hypertensive patients are specially liable to these effects.

It must be used with the greatest care when the patient is inhaling halothane or cyclopropane or receiving mono-amine oxidase inhibitors or tricyclic antidepressants, because of the risk of the production of ventricular fibrillation. In the presence of thyrotoxicosis and hypertension, it must be given with great caution.

Should not be used with local analgesics in ring block of the digits, penis or of the external ear.

Pharmacokinetics

It is mostly degraded by conjugation with glucuronic and sulphuric acids and excreted in the urine. A smaller part is oxidized by amine oxidase and inactivated by o-methyl-transferase.

Clinical uses

(1) To produce vasoconstriction in local analgesia thereby reducing toxicity and prolonging analgesic effect; (2) to provide ischaemia in the skin and subcutaneous tissues before incisions, e.g. in thyroidectomy (1–200 000 to 1–500 000); (3) in the treatment of cardiac arrest. Given i.v., adrenaline may cause severe myocardial ischaemia.[17] Total dose should not exceed 0.5 mg (i.e. 0.5 ml 1–1000 solution); (4) in the treatment of anaphylactic shock an i.v. bolus dose of 0.1 mg should not be exceeded, but may be repeated; and (5) as a bronchodilator.

Noradrenaline acid tartrate, BP (*l-Arterenol; Norepinephrine; Levophed*)

(nor = nitrogen ohne radikol – German)

Clinically it is used for its vasopressor effects only (α-adrenergic receptor stimulant). It is the neurohumoral transmitter for sympathetic nerve endings.

History

Humoral transmission of nerve impulses described by Elliott in 1905 and proved by Otto Loewi (1873–1961) of Berlin, in 1921.[18] Properties of racemic noradrenaline described by George Barger (1878–1939) and Henry Hallett Dale (1875–1968) in 1910.[19]

Pharmacodynamics

A powerful α-receptor stimulator. Probably the major pressor amine found at postganglionic adrenergic nerve-endings responsible for reflex vascular effects, adrenaline being mainly responsible for metabolic activities.

Indications

It is of value to counteract vasodilating drugs; immediately after removal of a phaeochromocytoma[20]; in patients in whom the peripheral resistance is very low because of tissue acidosis; in the patient who has been poisoned by adrenergic blockade; in intra-aortic balloon pumping to raise the diastolic blood pressure.[21] An i.v. infusion of 5–20 μg/min can be given until the effects are obtained. Its addition to solutions of local analgesics is not recommended because it may cause hypertension.

Ephedrine, BP

A direct α- and β-adrenergic stimulator and a releaser of catecholamines from receptor sites. Introduced into Western medicine in 1924 by Schmidt and Chen.[22] The active principle (isolated in 1885 by Yamanash and named by N. Nagai (1844–1929) in 1887)[23] of ma huang, a Chinese plant. Chemically allied to adrenaline. Manufactured synthetically. Its adrenaline-like properties were described by Japanese pharmacologists in 1917.[24]

Pharmacodynamics

The laevo-rotatory form is more active. It delays the destruction of adrenaline and noradrenaline and so maintains a high blood catecholamine level. Releases stored noradrenaline from nerve endings in the vessel walls. [25] (1) A potent sympathetic stimulant. The rate and force of cardiac contraction are increased and blood pressure raised. Arterioles are constricted. The duration of effect is some 30–40 min but repeated doses are not so effective (tachyphylaxis); (2) relaxation of smooth muscle of bronchi; (3) dilates pupil; (4) stimulation of cerebral cortex and medulla with subjective feeling of apprehension, trembling and discomfort; (5) probably dilates coronary arteries; (6) increases bladder-neck tone; and (7) a local analgesic effect.

Uses

First used to control hypotension during spinal analgesia in 1927.[26] The drug has the advantage that cardiac output and venous return are increased. Has been used in states of hypotension, bronchospasm, heart block, carotid sinus syndrome, urticaria, narcolepsy, enuresis and myasthenia.

Available in ampoules of 30 mg. Dose: 3–6 mg i.v. boluses or 15–30 mg i.m.; up to 50 mg by mouth.

Metaraminol bitartrate (*Aramine*)

An α-stimulator with slight β-stimulating effects. Pharmacologically similar to ephedrine. Introduced in 1951,[27] and first used in spinal analgesia 3 years later.[28] Unlike noradrenaline and ephedrine it is not readily destroyed by tissue enzymes. It stimulates the myocardium without producing dysrhythmia. It raises both the systolic and diastolic blood pressures. Its action is partly direct on the vessel walls and partly due to the liberation of noradrenaline from stores in nerve endings or chromaffin cells. No influence on mental state. May cause reflex bradycardia, which can be abolished by atropine. After intramuscular injection, 10 min elapse before its action is seen; after intravenous injection, 2 min. Duration of effect 20–60 min.

Dosage: intramuscularly 2–10 mg; intravenously 0.5–5 mg; by infusion, 15–100 mg in 250–500 ml as a substitute for the noradrenaline drip.

Supplied in 1 ml ampoules of 1% solution.

Methoxamine hydrochloride, BPC (*Vasoxine*)

This is a synthetic vasopressor. It was synthesized in 1942.[29] It can be autoclaved, is non-irritating and is a potent agent with a rather prolonged effect, which comes on 2 min after intravenous injection and may last up to 1 h. First used to maintain blood pressure in spinal analgesia in 1950.

It has no effect on cardiac output, and causes increased peripheral resistance, and a rise in the right atrial and ventricular pressure and in peripheral venous mean pressure. Its action is peripheral on the arteries and veins (α-stimulator). Pulse rate slowed, an effect blocked by atropine.

Gives rise to no cardiac dysrhythmias and seems to be safe in the presence of halothane. Does not stimulate the higher centres. Pilomotor effect marked and causes desire to empty bladder. It reduces the urinary volume by depressing the glomerular filtration rate and constricting the renal artery. Must be used carefully in cases of hypertension, cardiac disease and hyperthyroidism. Large doses can act as a partial β-stimulator and induce ectopic beats.

Dosage: 5–20 mg intramuscularly; 2 mg intravenously.

Phenylephrine hydrochloride, BP (*Neosynephrine; Neophryn*)

An α-stimulator and in large doses β-stimulator. First described in 1910 by Barger and Dale[30] and in 1931 by Kuschinsky and Oberdisse.[31] First used as a pressor agent in spinal analgesia in 1938.[32] Chief effect is to cause vasoconstriction by direct action on vessel walls, and so can be used in place of adrenaline, together with local analgesics for infiltration or intradural block. Effect lasts 10–15 min. Has no effect on conducting tissue of heart, but may cause bradycardia from vagal stimulation, so that bradycardia, together with heart block, are contra-indications to its use. Dilates the pupil; relieves nasal congestion. Sensitizes the heart to catecholamines so that if cyclopropane or halogenated volatile anaesthetics are being used, initial dose should not exceed 2–5 mg intravenously.

Felypressin (*Octopressin*)

This is 2-phenylalanine-8-lysine vasopressin, a synthetic derivative of the octopeptide hormone vasopressin from the posterior pituitary. Causes contraction of all smooth muscle, including coronaries, but has little oxytocic or antidiuretic effect. On injection causes local vasoconstriction without secondary vasodilatation as adrenaline does. Little effect on cardiac rhythm and may be relatively safe in patients receiving tricyclic antidepressants, mono-amine oxidase inhibitors, halogenated volatile anaesthetics or cyclo-propane. Dose: up to 5 pressor units. Available in combination with prilocaine to prolong the effects and increase the efficiency of dental analgesia.

If pressor agents are required in patients inhaling halogenated vapours or cyclopropane, methoxamine or ephedrine would appear to be reasonably safe.

ADRENERGIC BETA STIMULANTS

Dopamine (*Intropin*)

A physiological precursor of noradrenaline occurring naturally and having the following actions: (1) improves cardiac contractility without increasing its rate and hence myocardial oxygen consumption, a β-adrenergic effect. Effects blocked by β-antagonists, e.g. propranolol. In high dosage has α-adrenergic stimulating effects, which can be abolished by vasodilators, e.g. phenoxyben-zamine; and (2) increases renal blood flow by vasodilatation and stimulation of 'dopamine receptors' in the renal artery; this results in diuresis and saluresis.

Effects blocked by dopamine antagonists, e.g. haloperidol.[33] Clinical effects are thus increase in cardiac output, renal blood flow and rise in arterial pressure. Can be used to treat exacerbations of chronic cardiac failure and acute reduction of cardiac output, as after cardiac surgery; it may be useful in septicaemia. Urine flow, blood pressure and cardiac output should be monitored. It is inactivated by alkalis and patients *should be normovolaemic* before its use.

It is postulated that there are two types of dopamine receptors, D1 which is mainly inhibitory, and D2, mainly stimulant. Side-effects are dose-dependent and include nausea and vomiting, dyspnoea, headache, angina, hypertension and dysrhythmia. It is given intravenously in an infusion of normal saline, Ringer-lactate or 5% dextrose, the dose being 2 µg/kg/min to increase renal blood flow; 5 µg/kg/min to stimulate cardiac β-receptors; higher dosage, e.g. 15–25 µg/kg/min stimulates α-receptors, causing decreased blood flow in all organs. Has been used in the management of kidney donors.[34] Each 5 ml ampoule contains 40 mg/ml.

Dobutamine (*Dobutrex*)

A derivative of dopamine with α- and β-stimulating effects, a synthetic catecholamine, has no specific effect on the kidney vasculature. May be useful when dysrhythmias are a problem. Dose: 2.5–10 µg/kg/min.

Dobexamine

A renal and mesenteric vasodilator, giving an increase of gut wall and muscosal blood flow improving oxygenation and function. Dose: 1–5 µg/kg/min by infusion.

Isoprenaline hydrochloride, BP (*Saventrine, Isoproterenol, USP*)

A powerful β-adrenergic stimulant drug, a synthetic catecholamine. Has inotropic and chronotropic effects on the heart and causes peripheral vasodilatation. The drug is used in cardiogenic shock to increase cardiac output and improve tissue perfusion. It may be given by intravenous drip, 1–5 mg in 500 ml 5% glucose at a rate of 0.5–10 μg/min. It also causes bronchodilatation and in the treatment of asthma may be administered orally 30 mg, three times a day (with a maximum of 840 mg daily) or by inhalation of 1% spray (isoprenaline sulphate). Heart block is sometimes treated by 30 mg sustained-action tablets 4-hourly. May increase myocardial oxygen demand and cause subendocardial ischaemia.

Salbutamol (*Ventolin*)

A selective β-stimulant with little or no β$_1$ (cardiac) stimulant action. Administered by metered aerosol inhaler, 100 μg per time, or intravenously. In high doses, however, it does stimulate the heart and is a vasodilator. Has been used during cardiac surgery, 1–15 mg in 500 ml of 5% dextrose, i.v. Maximal bronchodilatation occurs within 5 min and the duration of effect is about 4 hours. Can be given by mouth 2–4 mg 6–8-hourly. Used to treat asthma, bronchospasm and premature labour.

Terbutaline (*Bricanyl*)

Also a selective β-stimulant used in the treatment of bronchospasm. Peak action occurs 30 min after subcutaneous injection or 2–3 h after oral administration. Oral dose is 2–4 mg 8-hourly.

Gross hypertension may follow the use of ergot preparations given intravenously if the patient has already received a sympathomimetic amine, because ergometrine (ergonovine), ergotamine and ergotoxin may cause contraction of the muscular wall of blood vessels.

Following intra- or extradural sympathetic blockade, hypotension is best treated by posture, oxygen, intravenous fluid and either ephedrine or methylamphetamine.

INFLUENCE OF OTHER DRUGS ON PATIENTS GIVEN PRESSOR AMINES

1. Monoamine oxidase inhibitors

These may potentiate the hypertensive effects of sympathomimetic amines, leading to hypertensive crises and dysrhythmias.

2. Tricyclic and quadricyclic antidepressants

These may increase the cardiovascular effects of catecholamines, leading to dysrhythmias and hypertension.

3. Anaesthesia with halogenated vapours and cyclopropane

These may sensitize the heart to the dysrhythmic effects of catecholamines.

4. Chlorpromazine and promethazine

These cause the pressor activity of injected adrenaline to be reversed. They do not greatly affect the pressor activity of noradrenaline. They reduce the pressor activity of methoxamine and phenylephrine.

ADRENERGIC BLOCKING AGENTS

α-Blockers

These can be separated into the following groups:

1. The imidazolines

(a) Tolazoline, BP (*Priscol*) antagonizes the vasoconstrictive effects of the catecholamines and in addition has a direct vasodilating effect on blood vessels. Can be injected into an artery to relieve spasm (25–30 mg). (b) Phentolamine methane-sulphonate and hydrochloride, BP (*Regitine; Rogitine*). This drug has an atropine-like effect on the heart and is a direct stimulant of cardiac muscle. Short duration of action, so best given as continuous intravenous drip 1–2 mg/min. Acts as a competitive inhibitor at the receptor site and can be promptly reversed by use of α-stimulants. Dose for adrenaline overdose: 5–10 mg intravenously.

2. The chloro-ethymines

Phenoxybenzamine hydrochloride BP (Dibenyline; Dibenzyline). The blocking effects of this agent take about 30 min to develop with a duration of action of several hours until the drug is excreted. Used in phaeochromocytoma surgery and to antagonize the vasoconstriction associated with shock (together with fluid replacement). Can be given either by mouth or by drip intravenously, 1 mg/kg in 500 ml 5% glucose.

3. The Ergot alkaloids

Ergotamine and certain dehydrogenated derivatives have a feeble anti-adrenaline action but may potentiate the effects of other pressor agents especially in hypertensive patients, e.g. during labour. Their vasoconstrictor effects are due to α-adrenergic stimulation.[36]

4. The phenothiazines

Chlorpromazine and certain other related compounds have an α-blocking effect.

5. The butyrophenone derivatives

Droperidol and haloperidol.

6. Thymoxamine

Dose 0.1 mg/kg by bolus intravenous injection 2–4 hourly. Complications: severe hypotension, hypoglycaemia.

7. Doxazosin

(α_1 blocker). Dose: 1 mg up to 16 mg; peak effect 2 h after oral dose; duration 22 h.

Use of α-blockers in the shocked patient is dangerous unless adequate volume replacement has been achieved by rapid intravenous infusion and there is monitoring of central venous and arterial pressures. With these safeguards, α-blockers often produce a rise in arterial and venous PaO_2.

β-Blockers

β-Blockers competitively block the positive inotropic effect of isoprenaline but are without effect on the similar actions of calcium and digitalis glycosides. β_1-effects: cardiac, renin release; β_2-effects: bronchial, vascular, insulin release, uterine receptors.

Propranolol[37]

Propranolol is a crystalline solid soluble in water and alcohol. The L-isomer has the following effects:

Cardiovascular system

1. Slows the heart by direct action on cardiac sympathetic-β-receptors. Abolishes the tachycardia caused by isoprenaline injection. Does not depress the vagus.

2. Decreases contractile force and blocks positive inotropic effects of isoprenaline, but not those of digitalis or calcium.

3. Peripheral vascular resistance first temporarily decreased, then increased for a prolonged period.[38]

4. Reduction of blood pressure.

5. Causes slight prolongation of A-V conduction but has no effect on intraventricular conduction.

6. Propranolol is liable to precipitate and intensify heart failure.

Nervous system. The D-isomer is a powerful local analgesic. This is the 'membrane-depressant effect' or 'quinidine effect'. Sympathetic system – no stimulation. Propranolol reduces the sensation and physical effects of fear and anxiety.

Myoneural junction. Augments action of depolarizing and reduces action of non-depolarizing agents.

Respiration. Blocks sympathetic bronchial dilatation and may cause severe bronchospasm, especially in asthmatic and bronchitic patients – an effect reversed by isoprenaline and atropine. May delay time of effective fetal respiration by effect on fetal chemoreceptors.

Metabolism. Blocks lipolysis, muscle glycogenolysis, insulin release and, when combined with an α-blocker, the raised metabolic rate due to adrenaline (β_2-effect). Inhibits plasma renin activity (β_1-effect).

CLINICAL USES IN ANAESTHESIA

Protects the heart from adrenergic stimulation associated with anxiety, atropine, surgical stimulation, injected adrenaline, thyrotoxicosis, postoperative thyroid crises, phaeochromocytoma and hypercapnia, and so reduces dysrhythmias, but also cardiac output. To potentiate hypotension caused by ganglion blocking agents: it prevents tachycardia in patients with chronic myocardial ischaemia. Dose in adults: 0.5–10.0 mg i.v.

Uses of β-blockers

1. To lower arterial pressure and control angina pectoris.

2. To control sinus tachycardia and prevent dysrhythmias caused by injected adrenaline or phaeochromocytoma removal (with α-blockers).

3. To control thyrotoxicosis before surgery.

4. In obstructive cardiomyopathy.

Dangers of β-blockers

1. Bronchospasm in asthmatics (with non-selective blockers.) Atenolol, practolol and metoprolol are relatively free from this defect.

2. The non-selective blockers may cause hypoglycaemia in diabetics and mask its effects.

3. May precipitate cardiac failure in patients with decompensation.

4. Prolonged administration of practolol may cause corneal damage, psoriatic hyperkeratotic skin reactions, deafness, sclerosing peritonitis and systemic lupus erythematosus.

5. Intermittent claudication and Raynaud's phenomena may be aggravated.

Table 15.2. Some current β-blocking drugs

Cardioselective		Non-cardioselective	
No intrinsic sympathomimetic activity	With intrinsic sympathomimetic activity	No intrinsic sympathomimetic activity	With intrinsic sympathomimetic activity
Metoprolol	Practolol	Propranolol	Aprenolol
Atenolol	Acebutolol	Sotalol	Oxprenolol
Timolol	Pindolol	Labetalol	Nadolol

6. Diminished reflex response to haemorrhage.
7. Atrioventricular conduction defects may occur.
8. Fatigue, dizziness, depression, hallucinations, vivid dreams, somnolence, insomnia, myasthenic syndrome, dyspepsia, low birth-weight of offspring, delayed spontaneous respiration of offspring born by Caesarean section.
9. Reduced cardiac output in patients receiving cyclopropane anaesthesia.
10. Effects prolonged and potentiated by liver disease.
(*See also* Which beta-blocker? Breckenridge A. *Br. Med. J.* 1984, **286**, 1085.)

CALCIUM CHANNEL BLOCKERS[40]

These drugs cause blockade of the slow calcium ion influx into the contractile and conducting myocardial cells, resulting in slow conduction, prolonged refractory period and depression of contractility.[41] The different drugs in this group vary in their electrophysiological effects on the fast and slow inward currents, which accounts for the differences in their pharmacological effect.

Verapamil (*Isoptin*)

A synthetic papaverine derivative. May be given orally or intravenously, but larger doses are needed by mouth because of considerable first pass elimination in the liver. Doses: orally 80–160 mg 8-hourly; onset in 2 h, peak effect in 5 h, or intravenously, 75–150 μg/kg, onset in 2 min, duration of action 10–15 min. There is preferential uptake and binding in the AV node so that action there is longer lasting than elsewhere. Ninety per cent is bound to plasma proteins.

Its main use is the termination and prevention of paroxysmal supraventricular tachycardia. Great caution should be used if given in association with β-blockers since negative chronotropic and inotropic effects may be augmented. Contra-indications include pre-existing hypotension, sinus node dysfunction, A-V block and marked left ventricular dysfunction. May be of use in refractory ventricular fibrillation during cardio-respiratory resuscitation.[42]

Nifedipine (*Adalat*)

A dihydropyridine. Oral or sublingual dose 10–20 mg 4–8-hourly. Onset after oral ingestion 15–20 min but only 2 min when given intranasally as a spray. Little first pass liver extraction. Main clinical use as coronary and peripheral vasodilator. Antagonizes intracellular calcium, which is the necessary trigger for excitation-contraction coupling in vascular smooth muscle. Less effect on A-V node than verapamil. Dilates coronary arteries in dosage that does not depress myocardial contractility. Valuable in variable (Prinzmetal) angina due to myocardial spasm as well as classic angina. Can be used in association with β-blockers, nitrates, frusemide, anticoagulants and antihypertensives.

Diltiazem (*Tildiem*)

A benzothiazepine. Intermediate pharmacological position between verapamil and nifedipine. Oral administration 60–90 mg 8-hourly, with extensive first pass hepatic extraction; onset in 15 min with peak effect in 30 min. Intravenous dose 75–150 µg/kg.

Isradipine (*Prescal*)

Dose 3.6–13.5 mg/day; peak effect 2 h; duration 12–21 h.[43]

Amlodipine (*Istin*)

Dose 5–10 mg once daily (longer acting). Does not depress the myocardium.

Nimodipine (*Nimotop*)

Has preferential activity on cerebral vessels, used for prevention of ischaemic neurological deficits following subarachnoid haemorrhage. Dose 60 mg 4-hrly.

Nicarpidine (*Cardine*)

Vasodilator used for angina and hypertension. Dose 30 mg three times per day.

Use with volatile anaesthetic agents

General anaesthetic agents have a non-specific calcium antagonist action, which is the cause of myocardial depression and vascular dilatation. Calcium antagonists may cause a hypotensive response during general anaesthesia with volatile agents. This may occur with halothane[44] and other volatile supplements.[45] In animals, MAC values may be decreased.[46] Cessation of nifedipine therapy prior to cardiac surgery may result in post bypass hypertension.[47]

Other effects

(1) Use with muscle relaxants. The effects of non-depolarizing drugs may be potentiated.[48] A monitor should be used to regulate relaxant dosage; and (2) Cerebral blood flow. This may increase as a result of vascular dilatation.[49]

(*See also* Jones R. M. in: *Recent Advances in Anaesthesia and Analgesia – 15* (Atkinson R. S. and Adams A. P. ed.) Edinburgh: Churchill Livingstone, 1985.) For history of their development, *see* Fleckenstein A. *Circ. Res.* 1983, **52** (Suppl. 1).

ANTACIDS AND OTHER AGENTS

Magnesium trisilicate and sodium citrate

See Chapter 22 obstetrics and gynaecology.

Magnesium hydroxide (8.3%; Milk of Magnesia)

Used in obstetrics and intensive care. Dose: 10–20 ml oral.

Dimethicone with aluminium hydroxide (*Asilone*)

Reduces foaming in the stomach during gastroscopy. Dose: 5–10 ml oral.

Cimetidine (*Tagamet*)

Does not affect acid already in the stomach, but raises the pH above 2.5 in about half an hour. This histamine H_2-receptor antagonist has also been used in anaphylactic reactions. Dose: 200 mg by mouth or i.m.

Ranitidine (*Zantac*)

An H_2 receptor blocker that reduces the production of gastric acid. Like cimetidine it is used to reduce the acidity of gastric contents before induction of anaesthesia. Dose: 150 mg by mouth, by intramuscular or slow intravenous injection (50 mg, every 6–8 h), or by infusion (25 mg/h for 2 h).

Famotidine (*Pepsid*)

Used in treatment of peptic ulceration. Dose 40 mg at night.

Nizatidine (*Axid*)

Dose 300 mg at night.

Hyoscine N-butyl bromide (*Buscopan*)

Used in gastroscopy to reduce gastric motility. Dose: 10–20 mg i.v.

Metoclopramide (*Primperan; Maxolon*)

Speeds gastric emptying; anti-emetic; sometimes effective against hiccup; increases tone of cardiac sphincter, an effect counteracted by atropine. Dose averages 10 mg. Overdosage, seldom seen by anaesthetists, may cause extra-pyramidal effects.[50] A dopamine receptor antagonist.

Domperidone (*Motilium*)

It inhibits the chemoreceptor trigger zone (like metoclopramide), has a relaxing effect on the lower oesophageal sphincter and the gut, including the pylorus. When given i.v. inhibits postoperative vomiting and also that due to cytotoxic drugs.[51]

ANTICOAGULANTS

Used for the prophylaxis of venous thrombosis and for anticoagulation during arterial and cardiac surgery.

Heparin

Rapidly effective. Prepared from the liver and lungs of animals; it carries a strong electronegative charge. Part destroyed by heparinase, and partly excreted in the urine. Dose: 1000–5000 units subcutaneously 6–12 hourly for 3 days perioperatively to prevent thrombophlebitis; 100 units/kg in arterial surgery; 100–300 units/kg in extracorporeal circuits. Best given (for prolonged effect) by continuous i.v. infusion; otherwise at intervals of not more than 6 h, i.v. Dose controlled by the activated partial thromboplastin time. May be reversed by protamine sulphate, 1 mg for every 100 units of heparin remaining in the circulation, i.v. The half-life of heparin is about 1 h, but this may be prolonged for 4–8 h during surgery or after trauma.

Coumarins

Warfarin is the agent in most common use. Loading dose 0.5 mg/kg, maintenance dose varies between 2 and 30 mg daily. Preoperative dosage adjustment to an acceptable INR or prothrombin time (e.g. 2–3 times normal) is essential. There may be a reduced anticoagulant effect associated with barbiturates, due to increased metabolism, and increased bleeding with aspirin. Reversal of the coumarins by vitamin K analogues, in an emergency, may be monitored by the anaesthetist by placing serial blood samples in glass containers and timing the clotting process. Normal is 3–5 min. Duration of coumarins in common use is 6–48 h.

Antifibrinolysins

Unwelcome fibrinolysis after cardiopulmonary bypass and in the prostatic bed after prostatectomy is antagonized by tranexamic acid (0.5–1.0 g i.v. or aprotonin 50 000 units initially.

DIURETICS

Mannitol (*Osmitrol*)

This acts within minutes and last for 1–4 hours. Circulatory overload may be a problem. Mannitol is filtered by the glomeruli but none is reabsorbed by the tubules. Used for forced diuresis as after mismatched transfusions, and to reduce cerebral oedema. It remains extracellular and is inert in the body. Used as 10 or 20% solution, 0.5–1 g/kg by infusion. Extravasation causes inflammation and thrombophlebitis.

AMINOPHYLLINE

A bronchodilator. May cause gastric irritation and headache. Can be given as a suppository. Has been used for nocturnal cardiac asthma and left ventricular failure. Dose: by mouth 100–300 mg; i.v. 5 mg/kg, slowly (in patients not taking xanthine drugs). Has been used to reverse the respiratory depressant effects of morphine[52]

References

1. Dundee J. W. et al. *Br. J. Pharmacol.* 1973, **48**, 326P.
2. Gairola R. L. et al. *Anaesthesia* 1980, **35**, 17.
3. Gupta P. K. and Dundee J. W. *Anaesthesia* 1974, **29**, 40.
4. Dundee J. W. et al. *Anaesthesia* 1974, **29**, 710.
5. Davies J. A. H. *Br. J. Anaesth.* 1968, **40**, 361.
6. Robertson G. S. et al. *Br. J. Anaesth.* 1977, **49**, 133.
7. Riddell P. L. et al. *Br. J. Anaesth.* 1978, **50**, 921.
8. Gawley T. H. et al. *Br. Med. J.* 1976, **2**, 122.
9. Edwards G. and Leszcynski S. O. *Lancet* 1967, **2**, 226.
10. Oliver G. and Schäfer E. A. *J. Physiol.* 1895, **18**, 230.

11. Takamine J. *Therapeutic. Gaz.* 1901, **27**, 221.
12. Takamine J. *Am. J. Pharmacol.* 1901, **73**, 523.
13. Aldrich T. B. *Am. J. Physiol.* 1901, **5**, 457.
14. Stolz F. *Berl. Chem. Ges.* 1904, **37**, 4149.
15. Starling E. H. *Lancet* 1905, **2**, 339.
16. Stutzman J. W. and Allen C. R. *Proc. Soc. Exp. Med. Biol.* 1941, **47**, 218.
17. Horak A. et al. *Br. Med. J.* 1983, **286**, 519.
18. Loewi O. *Pflugers Arch.* 1921, **189**, 239.
19. Barger G. and Dale H. H. *J. Physiol.* 1910, **41**, 19.
20. Pratilas V. and Pratila M. G. *Can. Anaesth. Soc. J.* 1979, **26**, 253.
21. Gilston A. In: *Recent Advances in Anaesthesia and Analgesi – 13* (Hewer C. L. and Atkinson R. S. ed.). Edinburgh: Churchill Livingstone, 1979, Chap. 3.
22. Chen K. K. and Schmidt C. F. *J. Pharmacol. Exp. Ther.* 1924. **24.** 339.
23. Nagai N. *Pharm. Zeit.* 1887, **32**, 7000.
24. Amatsu H. and Kubota S. *Kyoto Igâai Zasski* 1917, **14**, 77.
25. Burn J. H. and Rand M. J. *Lancet* 1958, **1**, 673.
26. Ockerblad N. F. and Dillon T. G. *JAMA* 1927, **88**, 1135.
27. Beyer K. H. et al. *Fedn Proc. Fedn Am. Socs Exp. Biol.* 1951, **10**, 281.
28. Poe M. F. *Anesthesiology* 1954, **15**, 547.
29. Baltzly R. and Buck J. S. *J. Am. Chem. Soc.* 1942, **64**, 3040.
30. Barger G. and Dale H. H. *J. Physiol.* 1910, **41**, 19.
31. Kuschinsky G. and Oberdisse K. *Arch. Exp. Path. Pharmak.* 1931, **162**, 46.
32. Lorhan P. H. and Oliverio R. M. *Curr. Res.. Anesth. Analg.* 1938, **17**, 44.
33. Breckenridge A. M. et al. *Eur. J. Clin. Pharmacol.* 1971, **3**, 131.
34. Renal effects of dopamine, *see* Editorial, *Anesthesiology* 1984, **61**, 487.
35. Hannington-Kiff J. C. *Lancet* 1974, **1**, 1019; *Br. Med. J.* 1979, **2**, 367.
36. Wassef M. R. et al. *Br. J. Anaesth.* 1974, **46**, 473.
37. Black J. W. et al. *Lancet* 1964, **1**, 1080; *Br. J. Pharmacol.* 1965, **25**, 547.
38. Johnsson G. *Acta Pharmacol. Toxicol. (Copenh.)* 1975, **36**, Suppl. 59.
39. Dunlop D. and Shanks R. G. *Br. J. Pharmacol.* 1968, **32**, 201.
40. Glossmann H. *New Therapeutic Uses of Calcium Channel Blockers.* Berlin; Springer-Verlag, 1990.
41. Durant N. N. et al. *Anesthesiology* 1984, **60**, 298.
42. Kapur P. A. et al. *Anesth. Analg. (Cleve.)* 1984, **63**, 460.
43. Multicentre study group, *Am. J. Med.* 1989, **86**(suppl. 4a), 119.
44. Fahmy N. R. and Lappas D. G. *Anesthesiology* 1983, **59**, A39.
45. Skarran K. *Anaesthesiology* 1983, **59**, 362.
46. Maze M. et al. *Anesthesiology* 1983, **59**, 327.
47. Casson W. R. et al. *Anaesthesia* 1984, **39**, 1197.
48. Bikhaz G. B. et al. *Anestheiology* 1982, **57**, A268 and 1983, **59**, A269; Lawson N. W. et al. *Anesth. Analg. (Cleve.)* 1983, **62**, 50; Carpenter R. L. and Mulroy M. F. *Anesthesiology* 1983, **59,** A392.
49. Lynch C. and Bedford R. F. *Anesthesiology* 1983, **59**, A392.
50. Hughes R. L. *Anaesthesia* 1984, **39**, 720.
51. Brogden R. N. et al. *Drugs* 1982, **24**, 360; *Drug Ther. Bull.* 1983, **21**, 47.
52. Stirt J. A. *Anaesthesia* 1983, **38**, 275.

Chapter 16

Immediate postoperative care

The anaesthetist is directly responsible for anaesthetic aspects after surgery until the patient is conscious (patients unconscious prior to surgery are, of couse, exceptions), and that vital functions are stable and can be preserved without assistance.[1] After surgery, but before the patient has recovered to this extent, patients are normally supervised by nurses in a postoperative observation room. Such a room enables problems and complications, especially respiratory and circulatory, to be diagnosed and treated promptly. The patient is only discharged back to his ward when conscious, with an adequate ventilation and a stable circulation. In the UK, the primary medical responsibility for patient care after return to the general ward lies with the surgical team.

This period is one of considerable potential danger to the patient, and the nurses can be very busy. The anaesthetist must not leave his patient until satisfied that the patient will receive the care needed. Anaesthetists must draw the nurse's attention to any unusual features of the patient, surgery or anaesthesia, and leave clear instructions for the patient's care. It may be helpful to write these in the notes. Failure of postoperative care is an important contributing factor to mortality and morbidity associated with anaesthesia. It was the cause of 9.5% of 348 cases of death or brain damage reported to the Medical Defence Union between 1970 and 1977.[2]

History

Facilities for postoperative care were advocated by A. L. Flemming, President of the Anaesthetic Section of the Medical Institute of Birmingham in 1921.[3] The first Postoperative Observation Room (Recovery Ward) was opened in the UK in 1955.[4] Lundy at the Mayo Clinic had organized such a facility in 1942. The American Society of Anesthesiologists have issued standards for post-operative care.[5]

The postoperative observation room

Should be close to the operating theatre and part of the 'clean' area. Curtains for privacy should be available. Requirements vary with the type of surgery performed. 1.5 beds for each operating theatre served may be sufficient, although 3 beds per theatre will be needed for busy specialities. A floor space of $9.3\,m^2$ ($100\,ft^2$) per bed has been recommended,[6] with piped oxygen and suction at each bed-head. Trolleys should be easily tipped. Entonox may be valuable. An anaesthetic machine, resuscitation equipment, a bronchoscope and a ventilator should be readily available. Staffing is likely to be needed 24 hours. The CEPOD report described inadequate recovery facilities in 34 hospitals.[7]

Problems of the immediate postoperative period

These include: pain (*see* Chapter 26), respiratory obstruction, sputum retention, hypoxia, residual neuromuscular block, nausea and vomiting, hypovolaemia, hypotension, hypertension, arrhythmias, hypothermia, shivering and restlessness. Such sequelae of surgery and anaesthesia are common, occurring in perhaps 30% of patients.[8] The staff also tend to intravenous infusions, surgical problems, drains, urinary catheters, etc.

In the restless patient, look for and correct any hypoxaemia, pain, haemorrhage or a full bladder before considering a small dose of benzodiazepine, which then is often helpful.

Position of patient

The lateral position (perhaps with slight head-down tilt) is safest for the airway, with one or other knee drawn up to prevent rolling. After some orthopaedic and other procedures, it may be impossible to place the patient on the side, and there is greater risk of airway obstruction or aspiration. Head-down tilt is of little value in a patient lying on the back, owing to the angle the trachea makes with the horizontal.

Monitoring

Hypoxaemic episodes are especially common, both in the postoperative room[9] and during transfer to it from the operating theatre.[10] They are often not recognized by simple clinical observation, and not certain to be prevented by the routine administration of oxygen (although this is recommended).[11] Monitoring of the circulation and respiration should continue for as long as needed. Pulse oximetry is especially useful.

Some classic signs of haemorrhage, i.e. tachycardia and restlessness, are often absent in the postoperative ward. Measurement of the actual loss (or the CVP) assumes greater importance. Increasing girth is of little help in the diagnosis of intra-abdominal haemorrhage.

Progressive postoperative care and high dependency units[12]

The trend towards more major surgery on older and sicker patients, and the need to make best use of scarce resources, has led to the development of High Dependency Units (HDU). The nursing staff here are more numerous than on a general ward, and are trained in specialized monitoring techniques. The patients in such a unit are chosen by their need for a particular level of care, rather than by their medical or surgical speciality, as tradition has previously dictated. Support of organ failure (and in particular, IPPV) is not normally given in HDU. Patients at particular risk of postoperative complications are likely to benefit from such observation, and intravenous and extradural opiates may be given more safely. When the period of higher risk is judged to have passed, the patient may be returned (or 'progress') back to his normal ward. The more expensive facilities of an Intensive Care Unit are used only for patients whose clinical condition warrants them.

See also Eltringham R. J. et al. *Postanaesthetic Recovery*. Berlin & Heidelberg: Springer-Verlag, 1984; 'Patient flow patterns in a recovery room and implications for staffing' Bell M. et al. *J. R. Soc. Med.* 1985, **78**, 35; Mini-Symposium: The Post-operative Period. *Curr. Anaesth. Crit. Care* 1991, **2**, 3; For postoperative scoring system, *see* Thomas D. and Davis A. C. *Anaesth. Intensive Care* 1984, **12**, 125.

References

1. Green R. A. *Anaesthesia* 1986, **41**, 129.
2. Utting J. E. et al. *Can. Anaesth. Soc. J.* 1979, **26**, 472.
3. Flemming A. L. *Lancet* 1923, **2**, 227.
4. Jolly C. and Lee J. A. *Anaesthesia* 1957, **12**, 49; Discussion, *Proc. R. Soc. Med.* 1958, **51**, 151.
5. *Standards for Postanesthesia Care*. American Society of Anesthesiologists, 1988.
6. Department of Health and Social Security. *Operating Department*. Health Building Note 26. London: HMSO, 1975.
7. Buck N. et al. *Report of the Confidential Enquiry into Perioperative Deaths*. London: Nuffield Provincial Hospitals Trust and the Kings Fund for Hospitals, 1987.
8. Zelcer J. and Wells D. G. *Anaesth. Intensive Care* 1987, **15**, 168.
9. Blair I. et al. *Anaesth. Intensive Care* 1987, **15**, 147; Jones J. G. et al. *Anaesthesia* 1990, **45**, 563.
10. Pullerits J. et al. *Can. J. Anaesth.* 1987, **34**, 470.
11. Moller J. T. et al. *Anesthesiology* 1990, **73**, 890.
12. Crosby D. L. and Rees G. A. D. *Ann. R. Coll. Surg. Engl.* 1983, **65**, 391; Crosby D. L. et al. *Ann. R. Coll. Surg. Engl.* 1990, **72**, 309; *The High Dependency Unit*. London: Association of Anaesthetists, 1991.

Chapter 17

Intravascular techniques, infusions and blood transfusion

For the history of fluid administration during anaesthesia and surgery, *see* Jenkins M. T. P. In: *Anaesthesia; Essays on its History*. (Rupreht J. et al. ed.) Berlin: Springer-Verlag, 1985, 102.

INTRAVENOUS INJECTION

For technique *see* Chapter 9.

INTRAVENOUS INFUSION

May be indicated during surgery to help provide a stable circulation, or if anticipated blood loss exceeds 5% of blood volume. Suitable veins are in the arm, preferably distant from a flexure; the saphenous vein anterior to the medial malleolus; on the dorsum of the hand. *In infants* the internal or external jugular or scalp veins can be used or the umbilical vein during laparotomy. Topical lignocaine-prilocaine cream (EMLA) may be useful, especially in children.[1]

To speed up the flow, slowed down in shock by venous spasm, elevate the container, or use a hand pump or a pressure infusor. Procaine (1 ml of 1%) injected into the tubing may also be useful. A three-way tap and syringe can be used in infants.

Flow rate is influenced by pressure difference from drip chamber to vein and viscosity of fluid. For blood, the latter is 2.5 times as great at 0°C as at 37°C. Blood at body temperature runs twice as fast as blood at 10°C. Fluids must be given cautiously to patients with heart failure. The fluid infused may increase venous tone, which will be improved by adding papaverine.[2] Self-adhesive skin patches of glyceryl trinitrate have decreased the rate of infusion failure three-fold, whether due to thrombosis or extravasation.[3]

For flow through venous cannulae, *see* Kestin I. G. *Anaesthesia* 1987, **42**, 67. For the various colour codes for different sizes of cannulae, *see* Tordoff S. G. and Sweeney B. P. *Anaesthesia* 1990, **45**, 399.

When a winged 'butterfly' needle is used there is always the risk that it may damage the vein, so a small cannula with a self-sealing injection site may be preferable. Any solution run continuously into a vein will eventually lead to thrombosis. Thrombophlebitis is early warning reaction of infection to come. If ignored, and the foreign body left in place, sepsis will follow. Extravasation of intravenous fluids into the subcutaneous tissues occurs in about one-fifth of those receiving infusions. Usually no harm results but occasionally there is loss of skin, muscle and tendon, with permanent disability.[4]

Needlestick injuries

The most pessimistic forecast is that an anaesthetist has a 1 in 25 chance of infection with HIV over the course of a 40-year working life.[5] The chance for hepatitis B is likely to be higher. Gloves, avoiding re-sheathing needles and the use of new cannulae designed for greater safety may lessen the risks. In some cases zidovudine prophylaxis may be indicated after an injury involving HIV-positive blood.[6]

Thrombophlebitis from intravenous drips[7]

Prevention

1. Re-site cannula every 24 h. Avoid leg veins if possible.
2. Use a larger vein, e.g. central venous catheter rather than a peripheral cannula. (A cannula is usually 7 cm in length or less; a catheter, more.) There seems little difference between modern materials,[8] although polyurethane is relatively non-thrombogenic.[9]
3. Add hydrocortisone 10 mg/l or heparin 1 unit/ml to the infused fluid 4 times daily. Some advocate heparin bonded to the catheter.
4. If glucose is infused it should be sterilized by filtration. The pH of a glucose solution must be 3.4–5 to prevent the Maillard reaction (caramelization) during autoclaving.
5. Avoid hypertonic solutions.
6. Use of a microfilter,[10] although the need for them is not proven.[11]

The pH of intravenous fluids may be a factor in causing thrombophlebitis, as may particulate matter. Some patients develop thrombophlebitis more easily than others, e.g. those with carcinoma.

Treatment

Heparinoid ointment (monopolysaccharide polysulphate – Hirudoid) may be applied daily and the part bandaged firmly.

Central venous catheters[12]

A catheter is inserted from a more peripheral vein as far as the vena cava or right atrium. The veins that have been used include: (1) *Arm veins.* By using the basilic vein to avoid obstruction at the clavi-pectoral fascia, turning the head towards the side of the arm used, and applying digital pressure on the supraclavicular fossa, correct placement of the catheter may be achieved in 90% of cases;[13] (2) *Internal jugular vein.* The right side gives the best results. Cannulation is aided by a head-down tilt and head rotated to the other side; (*a*) The skin is punctured 3 cm above the the clavicle on the lateral border of the sternomastoid, and the needle advanced under the muscle towards the suprasternal notch; (*b*) in the relaxed, anaesthetized patient it may be possible to palpate the vein through the muscle and advance from the medial side; and (*c*) another approach is from the apex of a triangle formed by the sternal and clavicular heads of the sternomastoid to enter the vein beneath the clavicular head; (3) *External jugular vein* is less reliable; (4) *Subclavian vein.* Via skin puncture above or below the middle of the clavicle (first described in 1952), but carries risk of pneumothorax; (5) *Axillary vein*;[14] and (6) *Femoral vein*, medial to the artery below the inguinal ligament.

The catheter is connected to a simple saline manometer or a pressure transducer. Respiratory fluctuations confirms that the tip lies within the thorax. Sudden increases in pressure during systole indicate that the tip has entered the right ventricle. Catheter positions should be checked by X-ray, or by using the catheter as an ECG electrode. Complications[15] include air embolus, pneumothorax, migration of the tip, heart perforation,[16] damage to thoracic lymph duct, thromboembolism, infection by bacteria migrating from the hub or skin, and septicaemia.[17] One unusual attempt to prevent this has been with an electrical current.[18]

For pulmonary artery catheterization, *see* Chapter 18; For removal of catheters from the heart and great vessels, *see* Mehta A. B. et al. *Br. Med. J.* 1983, **286**, 937.

Infusion controllers and pumps

Can control flow given i.v., i.m., subcutaneously, intra-arterially, extra-durally or by nasogastric tube. Their accuracy is useful in infants, or for infusion of drugs. *Controllers* regulate the drops falling per min by gravity in the drip chamber. *Pumps* actively promote flow; they may be finger-pumps, rollers or pistons, and have visual or auditory warning devices. They should not influence the sterility of the infusion fluid. The drip chamber was described in 1909.[19]

Problems from infusion fluid containers

1. *Sepsis.* Growth of organisms in i.v. fluids can reach 10^6 or 10^7 organisms/ml without turbidity being detected and can cause severe septicaemia. A record of the batch number of containers used may help to trace the origin of infection. Infection also occurs where the intravenous line penetrates the skin. Giving sets should be changed every 24–48 h and always after blood has been used. Infusion teams to supervise intravenous drips have been employed.

2. *Embolism.* May be of plastic, rubber, bacterial, air or dust. Drug incompatibility may also cause precipitates.

In-line filtration is available, which removes particles during infusion without seriously impeding flow. The mesh size within a filter diminishes progressively in the direction of flow from about 10 μm down to around 0.1–0.5 μm. These filters cannot be used with blood transfusion.

How to set up a drip and keep it going, *see* Clutton-Brock T. H. *Br. J. Hosp. Med.* 1984, **32**, 162; *See also Intravenous Technique and Therapy* (Gilbertson A. A.) London: Heinemann, 1984. For long-term venous access, *see* Peters J. L. et al. *Br. J. Hosp. Med.* 1984, **32**, 230.

INTRAVENOUS FLUIDS

pH of some fluids

May vary by 1–2 pH units between batches. Typical values: normal saline, 5.0; compound sodium lactate solution (Hartmann), 6.5; 5% dextrose in water and 4% dextrose in 0.18% saline, 4.0; dextran in 5% dextrose, 4.5–5.0; dextran in 0.9% saline, 5.0–6.0; Haemaccel 7.3; Gelofusine 7.4; Sodium bicarbonate 8.4%, 7.8; Hetastarch 5.5; Pentastarch 5.0.

Glucose (Dextrose)

Five per cent solution is isotonic and may be used for fluid replacement and to keep an intravenous route open for medication. The preferred saline/glucose combination is 1/5 normal saline with 4.3% glucose; this mixture is isotonic. Both solutions have a pH of 3.5–5.5 and thrombophlebitis can be minimized by adjusting the pH to 6.8 with a phosphate buffer. When stored blood is followed by glucose, rouleaux formation with clumping occurs in the drip set. Glucose of 10% or more readily produces thrombophlebitis. Dextrose 5% is distributed throughout all body fluids and is ineffective as a replacement fluid in trauma.

Normal saline

First used in the treatment of shock in 1891.[20] About one-third of its volume is retained in the circulation. An excess can easily cause oedema. Intractable hypovolaemic shock has been treated by 7.5% sodium chloride solution.[21]

Hartmann's solution[22] (compound sodium lactate solution, BP)

One-sixth molar concentration of sodium lactate in Ringer's solution. The lactate is metabolized in the liver to form bicarbonate, to counteract acidosis. Large volumes have been used in the treatment of hypovolaemia instead of colloid.[23]

Colloids

Colloids maintain or increase plasma oncotic pressure and so help draw fluid into the intravascular space. They include the dextrans, gelatins, starches and albumin (*see below*).

Dextran 70

Dextrans are produced by the action of the bacterium *Leuconostoc messenteroides* on sucrose. Dextran 70 is a polysaccharide of MW 70 000. 6% solution in saline or 5% dextrose. Used to reduce incidence of thrombosis. It has an acid pH (4.5–6.0) and may degrade acid-labile drugs. Remains in the circulation, in gradually decreasing amount, for up to a week. Some of its larger molecules are stored in the reticulo-endothelial system. Only 25% is excreted within 3 h, and only 50% can be recovered from the urine. It is hyper-oncotic; 500 ml will usually increase the circulating plasma volume by 750 ml. Has proved useful as a plasma volume expander, and in the prevention of venous thromboembolism. Reactions to colloids, mainly mild pyrexia, are probably commonest with dextrans, especially in atopic patients. Serious anaphylactic reactions occur 1 in 12 500, some series showing much higher incidences.[24] If more than 1.5 litres are infused in any 24-h period there is interference with blood grouping and cross-matching, owing to rouleaux formation (greater as the average molecular weight of the dextran molecule rises), so specimens should be taken for this purpose before dextran is infused. If this is not done, recipient cells must be washed before testing. It may interfere with plasma protein determinations. Dextran molecules greater in size than 50 000 increase the ESR, those smaller decrease it. Large volumes can cause bleeding by interfering with platelet stickiness, enhancing fibrinolysis and blood flow.

Dextran 40

MW 40 000; half-life *in vivo*, 3 h. 10% solution which is strongly hyper-oncotic. Duration of useful plasma expansion is about 1 h. Used to increase intravascular volume, reduce blood viscosity and improve flow in the micro-circulation. Said to prevent intravascular aggregation of red cells ('sludging') and reverse peripheral ischaemia. It does not interfere with cross-matching, blood grouping or with coagulation. Contra-indicated in dehydrated patients, because it may produce viscous urine and can cause renal failure.

Gelatin[25]

Produced by hydrolysis of collagens. *Haemaccel* is 3.5% urea-linked gelatin, MW 35 000, in electrolyte solution which includes calcium 6.25 mmol/l and potassium 5.1 mmol/l. pH 7.2–7.3. *Gelofusine* is 4% succinylated (modified fluid) gelatin in normal saline, MW 30 000. pH 7.4. Short biological half-life, less than 12 h; no effect on blood crossmatching, and only a dilutional effect on clotting factors; 85% excreted by the kidney. Duration of useful plasma expansion is about 2 h.

Gelatins have an incidence of adverse reactions, most of which occur after the first few millilitres infused (serious reactions 1 in 2000 to 13000; probably less frequent with Gelofusine). Long shelf-life, reasonable cost (£4 per 500 ml) and no risks of transmitted viral diseases. Haemaccel contains calcium and should not be given through the same infusion set as citrated blood. It may also gel with fresh frozen plasma.[26] About 500 ml are needed to take the place of 600 ml of blood lost. Can help promote a postoperative diuresis.

Hydroxyethyl starch (HES)

Hetastarch (Hespan) is a 6% solution in normal saline. Number average MW 70000, weight average MW 450000. pH 5.5. Degree of substitution 0.7, i.e. 70 hydroxyethyl groups for every 100 glucose units. Pentastarch (Pentaspan) is a 10% solution in normal saline. Weight average MW 250000. pH 5.0. Degree of substitution 0.45. Pentastarch results in the greater intravascular volume expansion. Both have long intravascular lives, do not release histamine and are neither antigenic nor teratogenic. Little effect on coagulation or cross-matching. Expand plasma volume for about 14 h. Serious anaphylactoid reactions are probably less common (1 in 16000 for hetastarch) than with other plasma substitutes (except albumin).

Blood substitutes

There is a strong clinical need for a non-toxic blood substitute.

Perfluorocarbons

Various perfluorochemicals have been emulsified with phospholipid or synthetic surfactants and can carry enough oxygen to completely replace blood in animals. They have also been used as respirable liquids in man.[27] *Fluosol-DA* has been used in man as a blood substitute. It is an inert emulsion of perfluorinated decalin and tripropylamine which dissolves over 3 times as much oxygen as plasma, obeying Henry's law. It provides useful oxygen transport with a high inspired O_2 concentration.[28] Newer emulsions may carry considerably more oxygen.

Haemoglobin solutions

Solutions of polymerized haemoglobin with a 2,3-DPG analogue added may provide oxygen transport.[29] Renal toxicity of the red cell stroma remnants has been a major problem.

Haemosomes

Synthetic red cells with stroma-free haemoglobin in lecithin capsules in synthetic plasma solution.[30]

OTHER METHODS OF FLUID ADMINISTRATION

Intra-arterial transfusion

Intra-arterial transfusion was advocated in 1906 by Crile and Dolley and it was again advocated by Kemp in 1933.

Intramedullary or intraosseous infusion

Possible method for transfusion of blood or fluid in the complete absence of a suitable vein, e.g. into the marrow of the manubrium sterni or long bones in children.[31]

Rectal administration

This has been used when more conventional routes are not practical.

Hypodermoclysis

Subcutaneous administration of saline can be used, when the intravenous route is not available, retromammary or into outer side of thigh.

Hyaluronidase. A mucolytic enzyme that aids absorption of fluid injected into the subcutaneous and intramuscular tissues. It hydrolyses hyaluronic acid, was described by Duran Reynals in 1929 and first isolated in 1934 by Mayer and Palmer. It is a testicular extract.

Uses. (1) In paediatrics, where veins are difficult; and (2) in infiltration anaesthesia, where it increases the area of effective analgesia. It is no substitute for precise anatomical knowledge but may be helpful in skin and subcutaneous analgesia, hernia block, splanchnic and pudendal block, and in the reduction of fractures (e.g. Colles) under local analgesia. It may increase the toxic effects of local analgesia.

ARTERIAL PUNCTURE

Performed to measure the Pao_2, $Paco_2$, Sao_2 and pH to clarify the acid-base status and oxygenation. Bleeding diatheses, e.g. low platelet count, haemophilia, anticoagulants are relative contra-indications.

Technique

Any artery that can be compressed after puncture may be used, usually the radial (preferred), brachial, or femoral.

Radial artery. First, Allen's test may be performed (*see* Chapter 18); the wrist is extended. After palpation, the line of the artery may be marked on the skin. The needle or cannula is inserted at the level of the wrist skin crease (proximal to this the artery lies much deeper), at about 45° to the surface, with or without local analgesia. This site reduces the risk of ischaemia of the fingers; the radial artery's contribution to the superficial palmar arch is given off distal to the point of puncture.[32]

Brachial artery. Palpated medial to the biceps tendon. 1 ml of lignocaine without adrenaline is injected on each side of the artery and a weal left on withdrawal. A 23G needle is then inserted into the artery through the weal and suction is applied to the piston of the attached syringe. Blood must pulsate into the syringe under its own power because its colour is not a certain sign of arterial puncture. The needle is withdrawn and a pad applied tightly for 5–10 min to minimize haematoma formation. Air bubbles are expelled from the syringe.

Femoral artery. Palpated halfway between the pubic symphysis and the anterior superior iliac spine. The needle is advanced at 90° to the skin, between the fingertips of the other hand, which straddle the artery.

Dorsalis pedis artery. The line of the artery may be marked on the skin after palpation. The vessel presents a convex curve over the navicular and metatarsal heads, which makes entry easier, and is very superficial. In a modified version of Allen's test, the foot may be squeezed during pressure occlusion of this artery. If there is no satisfactory alternative blood supply, the blanched skin remains white until the occluding finger is taken off the dorsalis pedis.

Care of specimen. Analysis of blood gases should if possible be carried out immediately. A delay of more than 5–10 min demands that the sample be stored in ice, preferably in a well-fitting glass syringe.

BLOOD TRANSFUSION

History

First described in animals in 1666 by Richard Lower (1631–1691)[33] and in man by Benis (1625–1704) of Montpellier, France, in 1667, using calf's blood.[34] First successful man-to-man transfusion reported in 1818 by J. Blundell (1790–1878) an obstetrician of St. Thomas' Hospital.[35] Vein-to-vein transfusion given by James Hobson Aveling (1828–1892)[36] and by Higginson (of syringe fame) the following year. Transfusions were first given to alter the patient's temperament. Hustin (1882–1967) of Belgium in 1914,[37] Luis Agot of Buenos Aires, and Lewisohn[38] demonstrated the usefulness of sodium citrate as an anticoagulant. Apparatus for direct transfusion was coated internally with paraffin wax, to reduce coagulation, e.g. Kimpton's tube.[39] Glucose added to blood to prolong the life of the red cells in 1916.[40] Autotransfusion, for example in ruptured ectopics, was often used before the Second World War.[41] In 1900, Landsteiner (1868–1943)[42] of Vienna, later of New York, first observed agglutination of human red cells by serum belonging to other individuals (Nobel prize, 1930), and described three ABO groups according to the two types of agglutinogens, their combination or their absence, which can cause agglutination when brought into contact with agglutinins in the serum. The fourth group (AB) was described by the Viennese physician Decastello in 1902[43] and confirmed by Jansky of Prague and by W. L. Moss of Baltimore in 1910. In a British population, 47% of people are group O; 42% group A; 8% group B; 3% group AB; 83% are Rhesus positive, 17% Rhesus negative. The Rh system was discovered in 1939–40.[44] A plasma substitute, gum acacia, was first used in 1919.[45] Heparin described in 1916.[46] Cadaver blood was used in the USSR in the 1930s.[47]

One unit of whole blood will raise the haemoglobin about 1 g/dl. If a major operation is to be performed and the haemoglobin is less than 10 g/dl, a blood transfusion is often indicated, as tissue oxygenation can be maintained only by increasing cardiac output. A lower haemoglobin may be acceptable in otherwise fit patients if little blood loss is anticipated.[48] Before the era of blood banks (the 1940s in the UK) a register of blood donors was kept by individual hospitals so that potential donors could be sent for as required. The original glass bottles and rubber tubing gave way to disposable plastic sets in the late 1950s and this reduced the incidence of thrombophlebitis and infection. The National Blood Transfusion Service was set up in 1988 and incorporates the Regional Transfusion Centres and the Blood Products Laboratory which manufactures albumin, immunoglobulins, antithrombin III and Factors VIII and IX for the whole country. In 1946 there were about 200 000 donors in the UK, today the figure is around 2 200 000, all voluntary. Blood banks were established in the 1930s in Moscow, at the Mayo Clinic in 1935,[49] and by Bernard Fantus (1874–1940) in Cook County Hospital, Chicago,[50] and in 1939 in Barcelona during the Spanish Civil War.[51] Continuous drip blood transfusion introduced in 1935.[52] Anticoagulants included di- or tri-sodium citrate and heparin. First clinical use of citrated blood in 1914.[53] Acid-citrate-dextrose, which permitted 21 days' storage, introduced in 1943.[54]

For history of blood transfusion, *see* Keynes G. *Br. J. Surg.* 1943, **31**, 38; Farr A. D. *J. R. Soc. Med.* 1981, **74**, 301; Marshall M. and Bird T. *Blood Replacement.* London: Arnold, 1983; Schneider W. H. Bull. *Hist. Med.* 1983, **57**, 545.

Within the past few years the possibility of contracting hepatitis and HIV from donor blood, together with the ability of the laboratory to cross-match blood within 30–40 min, have made many anaesthetists more cautious in their practice of blood transfusion.[55]

Blood donors

Unsuitable donors include those with a history of jaundice; protozoal, spirochaetal, bacterial or virus infection, especially HIV-infection; those who have recently had vaccines or inoculations; or those with glucose-6-phosphate dehydrogenase deficiency. Blood donors must be negative for HBsAg but may be accepted if they carry antibody, and are also screened for antibody to hepatitis C, HIV-I and Treponema pallidum. Screening may also be introduced for HIV-II, and antibody to *Plasmodium falciparum*. Screening for cytomegalovirus is only needed if the recipient is immunocompromized.

The rarer blood groups may cause problems, e.g. Duffy, Kell, Lewis. Donors over 65 are not accepted in Britain. Donors are not accepted if at high-risk of HIV-infection.

Storage

Red cells last well in refrigerated (4–6°C) stored blood, only dying at 1% per day. More than 70% survive 24 h after transfusion. Clotting factors deteriorate progressively after 24 h storage. Citrate-phosphate-dextrose blood (CPD blood) contains no functioning platelets after 48 h. Factor V has decreased to 50% after 14 days, and factor VIII to 50% after 24 h and 6% after 21 days. Factor XI is only stable for 7 days. The other clotting factors do not begin to fall before 21 days. CPD blood plus adenine preserves its ATP and 2,3-DPG levels for up to 2 weeks with a slow fall thereafter. CPD blood can be usefully stored for up to 35 days. Each unit contains 450 ml of blood and 60 ml of CPD solution. The pH may be 6.7 and the potassium content about 20 mmol/l after 3 weeks, but some of this is reabsorbed into the erythrocytes after warming and infusion. Saline adenine glucose mannitol (SAG-M) also preserves red cells for 35 days. For alteration of blood components during storage *see* Lovric V. A. *Anaesth. Intensive Care* 1984, **12**, 246.

Red cells can be washed, suspended in glycerol and stored frozen in liquid nitrogen for many years. Expensive and 2 h needed for thawing and washing to remove glycerol. They then should be used within 6 h. Main application is military.

Various products available

1. *Whole blood* (*see above*).
2. *Red cell concentrates* have most of the plasma removed (PCV up to 80%). Useful for correction of anaemia. Plasma-reduced blood (PCV 60%) has up to 180 ml of the plasma removed.
3. *Leucocyte-poor blood*. CPD blood with the 'buffy coat' (containing leucocyte and platelet debris) removed. Used for patients sensitized to HLA, white cell or platelet antigens, or for transplant patients or those immunocompromised.
4. *SAGM blood*. Allows all the plasma to be used for production of components. Lower viscosity than whole blood. Shelf life 35 days as for CPD-adenine blood. The plasma is replaced by 100 ml of NaCl 140, adenine 1.5, glucose 50 and mannitol 30 mmol/l. PCV is about 60%.
5. *Washed red cells*. Washed in saline. Used rarely for non-haemolytic transfusion reactions to plasma proteins.
6. *Plasma*. Available as fresh frozen plasma, rich in all clotting factors and oncotic activity. Ten donors are used for a batch of pooled plasma: 4 group A, 4 group O, 1 group B and 1 group AB, to neutralize the ABO antibodies.
7. *Human albumin*.[56] Available as 4.5% or 20% albumin (the former has four times as much sodium per gram of albumin), or plasma protein fraction

(PPF), prepared by cold ethanol fractionation of pooled plasma. Four blood donations produces 20 g. Sterilized by filtration and holding at 60°C for 10 h. Virus-free. Very few serious reactions (1:33 000), but expensive (about £30 per 250 ml of 4.5%). Does not contain pseudocholinesterase.

8. *Human fibrinogen*. Limited supply.

9. *Cryoprecipitate*. Rich in factors VIII, XIII and fibrinogen.

10. *Platelets* may be transfused in severe thrombocytopenia, some leukaemias and depression of haemopoeisis by infection, tumours, drugs, etc.[57] Platelet concentrates are always contaminated with donor red cells and are usually given to patients of the same ABO group but this is not essential. Anti-D immunoglobulin should be given to Rh-negative women. Ordinary (170 μm) filters on transfusion sets remove 5% of platelets, but microfilters remove over 30% and so should not be used. The concentrate from each unit of whole blood contains about 50×10^9 platelets suspended in 50 ml plasma. The pooled concentrate from 6 units is used in adults (1 unit per 10 kg in children) and raises the count by about 60 000 per μl. Platelets can be stored at room temperature for 3 days. They last 7–10 days in the circulation.

11. *Factor VIII concentrate*. Contains 2 to 3 times per unit as much factor VIII as cryoprecipitate. Recombinant factor VIII has also been made.

12. *Factor IX concentrate*.

Indications for blood transfusion in surgery

(1) Haemorrhage (actual or anticipated) with reduction in circulating volume of over 20–30%. This figure must be adjusted according to the circumstances, especially the preoperative haemoglobin level, the cardiovascular and respiratory state and the probability of continuing blood loss; (2) severe anaemia; (3) blood-clotting disturbances; (4) extracorporeal circulation; and (5) exchange transfusion.

There is rarely any indication for whole blood even in massive transfusion. Specific component therapy has revolutionized blood transfusion. Blood conservation in elective surgery can be promoted by: (1) induced hypotension; (2) infiltration with adrenaline and saline; (3) tourniquet; (4) haemodilution; and (5) autotransfusion, *see below*.

Cross-matching

High molecular weight dextrans can cause problems in cross-matching. Drugs that provoke red cell antibodies include levodopa, methyldopa, mefenamic acid (Ponstan), and penicillin in more than 20 mega-unit doses daily.

Rh-negative blood should whenever possible be given to Rh-negative patients. This is specially desirable in: (a) Rh-negative patients of either sex who have either had a previous transfusion or may require a subsequent one; (b) Rh-negative girls and women of child-bearing age; and (c) infants who have haemolytic disease and their mothers.

In a grave emergency, if blood of the correct ABO group is given with no preliminary cross-matching, incompatibility will only occur once in 300 times.[58] Uncross-matched O Rh-negative blood may be transfused with a high degree of safety.[59] O Rh positive packed red cells may be more available, and even these may be given with minimal risk,[60] but there may be difficulty with subsequent cross-matching.

Complications

Each blood transfusion carries a certain risk and, in adults, single-unit transfusions are seldom necessary. The possible hazards can be divided into immune and non-immune:

1. Acute haemolytic reaction[61]

An increased rate of destruction usually of the donor's red cells by antibodies in the recipient's plasma, chiefly anti-A, anti-B and anti-D. May be immediate or delayed. ABO incompatibility usually causes a more immediate and severe reaction than one due to Rhesus factor. General anaesthesia and sedation mask the signs. The blood pressure and pulse rate should be taken every 5 min for the first quarter-hour with each new unit of blood. If there is a red rash, hypotension, tachycardia or cyanosis for which no other cause can be found, the transfusion should be stopped. Incidence variously reported between 1 in 3000 and 15000 transfused units.

Pathophysiology. Largely mediated by histamine released from mast cells in response to the activation of C3a and C5a cleavage products of complement by the antigen-antibody reaction. In addition, the action of anti-A or anti-B or both (IgM allo-antibodies) causes erythrocyte disruption with release of a phospholipid procoagulant (e.g. erythrocytin) and disseminated intravascular coagulation (DIC). The combination of intravascular fibrin deposition and vasospasm leads to acute cortical necrosis of the kidney. Anti-Kell antibodies were responsible for the reaction in 80% of cases in one American series.

Signs of incompatible transfusion. (A) *In the conscious*: (1) headache; (2) precordial or lumbar pain; (3) urticaria or pruritus; (4) burning in limbs; (5) bronchospasm, dyspnoea, tachycardia and restlessness; (6) suffused face; (7) nausea and vomiting; (8) pyrexia and rigors; (9) circulatory collapse; and (10) later, haemoglobinaemia, haemoglobinuria and oliguria. (B) *Under anaesthesia*: (1) hypotension; (2) tachycardia; (3) general oozing from wound; (4) urticarial rash; and (5) later, jaundice and oliguria in 5–10% of these patients.

See also Binder L. S. et al. *Br. J. Anaesth.* 1959, **31**, 217 (reprinted in 'Classical File', *Surv. Anesthesiol.* 1975, **19**, 91).

The factors affecting the severity of the reaction are: (1) quality and quantity recipient's antibody; (2) dose of antigen, i.e. volume of blood given, and antigen concentration per donor red cell; and (3) the general fitness of the recipient.

Investigation of transfusion reactions. The following are needed: (1) the blood samples used for the original compatibility test; (2) the remains of the blood used for the transfusion; (3) 10 ml of the patient's blood taken 3 h after the transfusion reaction, collected into a plain sterile bottle, and 2 ml in an oxalated bottle; and (4) a sample of urine.

Differential diagnosis. (1) Anaphylactic reaction to some other substance (e.g. a drug); (2) acute septicaemia; and (3) transfusion of thermally damaged, infected or outdated blood.

Treatment of Severe Transfusion Reaction. (1) Stop the transfusion; (2) support blood pressure with intravenous colloids or crystalloids, and inotropes or vasoconstrictors if needed; (3) oxygen to overcome the effects of intrapulmonary shunting; (4) induce a diuresis with mannitol 50 g or frusemide 100 mg; (5) check acid-base balance and electrolytes; (6) exchange transfusion in the desperate case; (7) high dose of steroids may be useful; (8) antihistamines may be indicated in the early stages but may increase hypotension; and (9) where disseminated intravascular coagulation is occurring, coagulation factors and platelets need to be replaced.

2. Delayed reaction

Four to ten days after transfusion, causes anaemia, jaundice and renal failure.

3. Other immune reactions

Can occur to leucocyte, platelet and plasma protein antigens.[62] Mild urticaria or fever is common, but rarely acute anaphylaxis results.

4. Transmission of disease

(1) *Viruses*:[63] (a) Hepatitis B,[64] 2–6 months incubation period. Jaundice may not be evident; (b) hepatitis C[65] carried by up to 1% of the population; an antibody assay is now available but sero-conversion takes about six months; (c) HIV-I (or HIV-II in West Africa); donor screening started in 1985 in Britain. Risk up to 26 per million units transfused in USA, but less than 1 per million in UK;[66] (d) cytomegalovirus; and (e) Epstein-Barr virus.

(2) *Bacteria*:[67] (a) Contaminants during collection or storage. Blood left out of the refrigerator for more than 30 min should not be used; (b) syphilis; (c) brucellosis; and (d) yaws.

(3) *Parasites*:[67] (a) Malaria. In areas where malaria is not endemic serology can exclude donors who may transmit the disease. Transfer of malaria can be prevented by giving chloroquine 600 mg to the recipient before transfusion; (b) trypanosomiasis; and (c) leishmaniasis (Kala-azar).

5. Circulatory overloading

Those with heart disease or anaemia and the elderly are especially vulnerable. The jugular venous pressure should be watched, and the central venous pressure or pulmonary wedge pressure monitored if needed. Such measurements give immediate indication of the balance between blood loss and replacement, but are influenced by many other factors. To make overload less likely, frusemide 20–40 mg i.v. can be given at the start of the transfusion. Early signs of pulmonary oedema include cough, dyspnoea, tachycardia, basal crepitations and cyanosis. Blood is usually given at 1–3 ml/kg/h.

Treatment. Stop or slow transfusion. Sit the patient up and give oxygen and frusemide. Tourniquets and venesection may be required.

6. Hypothermia

Anaesthetized patients, especially children, are vulnerable to hypothermia. Oxygen consumption increases, and cardiac arrest may occur. Prevented by using a thermostatically-controlled blood warmer. The temperature should never exceed 40°C.

7. Embolism

Blood filters[11] (20–40 μm pore size) remove micro-aggregates of more than 20 μm diameter during transfusion. Three structures are in common use: (a) surface filters; (b) depth filters; and (c) combination filters. Various materials have been used in their construction, such as woven polyester screen, nylon screen, dacron wool and polyester sponge. Must be fully primed with blood before use. They may prevent lung damage caused by micro-aggregates, but a consensus has not been reached. Problems and dangers of these filters include: slowing of rate of transfusion, complete blockage after 4–10 units of blood, embolism of particles from the filter, haemolysis and massive activation of the clotting process if fresh frozen plasma is infused through a filter. The ordinary infusion set filter pore size is about 170 μm.

8. Potassium intoxication

Stored blood may contain up to 30 mmol/l of potassium by its expiry date. May cause cardiac arrest during transfusion of whole blood. Children and patients with acidosis, hypothermia or renal failure are particularly at risk.

Signs of potassium intoxication include elevation of the T wave on the ECG and widening of the QRS complex. In emergency, slow i.v. injection of 5–10 ml of calcium chloride 10% will temporarily counteract the effects on the heart. For continuous display of plasma potassium during cardiac surgery *see* Drake H. F. et al. *Anaesthesia* 1987, **42**, 23.

9. Citrate intoxication and hypocalcaemia

A warm oxygenated adult can metabolize the citrate content of 1 unit of CPD blood in 5 min. If the transfusion is faster than this, citrate intoxication may cause tremors, arrhythmias, acidosis and hypocalcaemia. Calcium gluconate 10% 10 ml (2.3 mmol Ca^{2+}) may be required. This is most likely in cold or cyanosed patients, or those with severe hepatic disease.

In open-heart surgery and in renal dialysis, heparinized blood may be preferred (5 units/ml). Any haemorrhagic tendency can be controlled by protamine sulphate. Heparinization does not interfere with calcium stores in the body and citrate intoxication does not arise, but its shelf-life is less than 2 days.

10. pH changes

The pH of stored blood varies between 6.6 and 7.2 due to an accumulation of lactic acid, pyruvic acid, citric acid and raised Pco_2. This may be important in massive transfusion, although metabolism of citrate is likely to result in metabolic alkalosis.

11. Immune suppression

Transfusion during cancer surgery has been claimed to worsen the prognosis, particularly if whole blood is used.[68]

12. Hypomagnesaemia

During massive transfusion, with particular loss from the myocardium.

13. Transfusion-related acute lung injury

Due to transfusion of the donor's leukocyte agglutinating antibodies. Rare, but causes damage to the lung microvasculature. Washed red cells only should be used from donors who cause this problem.[69]

Massive blood transfusion[70]

Defined as total blood volume replacement by stored blood in under 24 h. It can be regarded as an organ transplant. A bleeding diathesis is common, due mainly to lack of platelets and fibrinogen, and to a lesser extent factors V and VIII. Platelets and fresh frozen plasma should be given as indicated by measurements of platelet count, fibrinogen levels and clotting times.

Autologous blood transfusion (autotransfusion)

1. *A pre-deposit programme* can be used to collect 6 or more units of blood during the 5 to 6 weeks before an operation.[71] The main drawback to this approach is the logistical support needed. The marrow of a patient on iron supplements replaces the cells in a unit of blood in 3–4 weeks. Erythropoeitin therapy would speed this further.

2. *Blood salvage.* The Solcotrans system[72] collects spilt blood in a container primed with ACD and is infused directly through a filter. Useful for recovery of postoperative drainage. The more sophisticated Haemonetics Cell Saver collects from suckers, which introduce heparin at their tips, and then centrifuges, washes and packs the red cells ready for re-transfusion. Reinfusion of up to 10 litres has been performed,[73] although haemolysis limits the rate at which blood can be collected. Autotransfusion first described in 1874,[74] and first used in 1886.[75] The need for homologous blood is not always eliminated, because salvage is incomplete and there is a delay before it is ready for transfusion.

3. *Pre-operative haemodilution.* Draw off 1–2 l of blood into anti-coagulated packs and replace with an equal volume of colloid. This means that haemodiluted blood is spilt at surgery, which is replaced by the saved blood after haemostasis is secured. Although a haematocrit of 30% is widely used, there is disagreement about the degree of haemodilution that is safe, especially in patients with vascular disease.

See also: Blood Conservation. Int. Anesthesiol. Clin. 1990, **28**(4); Turner D. A. B. *Br. J. Anaesth.* 1991, **66**, 281.

References

1. Hopkins C. S. et al. *Anaesthesia* 1988, **43**, 198.
2. Lewis G. B. J. and Hecker J. F. *Anaesth. Intensive Care* 1984, **12**, 27.
3. Wright A. et al. *Lancet* 1985, **2**, 1148.
4. Burd D. et al. *Br. Med. J.* 1985, **290**, 1579.
5. Jones M. E. *Anaesth. Intensive Care* 1989, **17**, 253.
6. Henderson D. K. and Gerberding J. L. *J. Infect. Dis.* 1989, **160**, 321: Jeffries D. J. *Br. Med. J.* 1991, **302**, 1349.
7. Lewis G. B. H. and Hecker J. F. *Br. J. Anaesth.* 1985, **57**, 220.
8. Larsson N. et al. *Acta Anaesthesiol. Scand.* 1989, **33**, 223.
9. Gaukroger P. B. et al. *Anaesth. Intensive Care* 1988, **16**, 265.
10. Annotation. *N. Engl. J. Med.* 1985, **312**, 78.
11. Derrington M. C. *Anaesthesia* 1985, **40**, 334.
12. Editorial *Lancet* 1986, **2**, 669.
13. Ragasa J. et al. *Anesthesiology* 1989, **71**, 378.
14. Taylor B. L. and Yellowlees I. *Anesthesiology* 1990, **72**, 55.
15. Ridley S. A. In: *Anaesthesia Review 8.* (Kaufman L. ed.) Edinburgh: Churchill Livingstone, 1991, 255.
16. Jay A. W. L. and Kehler C. H. *Can. J. Anaesth.* 1987, **34**, 333.
17. Corona M. L. et al. *Mayo Clin. Proc.* 1990 **65**, 979.
18. Dealler S. et al. *Lancet* 1988, **i**, 703.
19. Laurie R. D. *Lancet* 1909, **1**, 248.
20. Lane W. A. *Lancet* 1891, **2**, 626; Horrocks P. *Lancet* 1893, **2**, 1569.
21. De Felippe J. et al. *Lancet* 1980, **2**, 1002.
22. Hartmann A. F. and Senn M. J. E. *J. Clin. Invest.* 1932, **11**, 327; Lee J. A. *Anaesthesia* 1981, **36**, 1115.
23. Hillman K. In: *Recent Advances in Anaesthesia and Analgesia – 16.* (Atkinson R. S. and Adams A. P. ed.) Edinburgh: Churchill Livingstone, 1989, 105.
24. Paull J. *Anaesth. Intens. Care* 1987, **15**, 163.
25. Saddler J. M. and Horsey P. J. *Anaesthesia* 1987, **42**, 998.
26. Murray F. and Hutton P. *Anaesthesia* 1989, **441**, 392.
27. Fuhrman B. P. *J. Pediatr.* 1990, **117**, 73.
28. Faithfull N. S. *Anaesthesia* 1987, **42**, 234.
29. Winslow R. M. *Transfusion* 1989, **29**, 753.
30. Hunt C. A. et al. *Science* 1985, **230**, 1165.
31. Fiser D. H. *N. Engl. J. Med.* 1990, **322**, 1579.
32. Pyles S. T. and Scher K. S. *Surg. Gynecol. Obstet.* 1983, **156**, 227.
33. Lower R. *Phil. Trans. R. Soc.* 1666, **1**, 353; 1667, **2**, 557 (reprinted in 'Classical File' *Surv. Anesthesiol.* 1976, **20**, 589).
34. Denis J. B. *Phil. Trans. R. Soc.* 1667, **2**, 489.
35. Blundell J. *Med. Chir. Trans.* 1878, **9**, 56; Boulton T. B. 'Classical File'. *Surv. Anaesthesiol.* 1986, **30**, 1000.
36. Aveling J. H. *Trans. Obstet. Soc. Lond.* 1864, **6**, 126.
37. Hustin A. *Bull. Soc. R. Sci. Méd. Brux.* 1914, **72**, 104.
38. Lewisohn R. *Med. Rec.* 1915, **87**, 141.
39. Kimpton A. R. and Brown J. H. *JAMA* 1913, **61**, 117.
40. Rous P. and Turner J. R. *J. Exp. Med.* 1916, **23**, 219.
41. Pathak U. N. and Stewart D. B. *Lancet* 1970, **1**, 961.
42. Landsteiner K. *Zbl. Bakt.* 1900, **27**, 357; *Wien. Klin. Wochenschr.* 1901, **14**, 1132.
43. Decastello A. V. and Sturli A. *Munch. Med. Wochenschr.* 1902, **49**, 1090.
44. Landsteiner K. and Wiener A. S. *Proc. Soc. Exp. Biol. N. Y.* 1940, **43**, 223; Levene P. and Stetson R. E. *JAMA* 1939, **113**, 126.
45. Bayliss W. M. *Spec. Rep. Services Med. Comm., London* 1919, No. 25.

46. McClean J. *Am. J. Physiol.* 1916, **41**, 250.
47. Yudin S. S. *JAMA* 1936, **106**, 997.
48. Carson J. L. et al. *Lancet* 1988, **1**, 727.
49. Lundy J. S. *Clinical Anesthesia.* Philadelphia: Saunders, 1941, 606.
50. Fantus B. *JAMA* 1937, **109**, 128.
51. Duran-Jorda F. *Lancet* 1939, **1**, 773.
52. Marriott H. L. and Kekwick A. *Lancet* 1935, **1**, 977.
53. Agote L. *Ann. Int. Mod. Clin. Med. (B. Aires)* 1914-15, **1**, 24.
54. Loutit J. F. and Mollison P. L. *Br. Med. J.* 1943, **2**, 744.
55. Horsey P. J. *Br. Med. J.* 1985, **291**, 234.
56. McClelland D. B. L. *Br. Med. J.* 1990, **300**, 35.
57. Editorial. *Lancet* 1987, **2**, 490.
58. Isbister J. P. *Anaesth. Intensive Care* 1984, **12**, 217.
59. Smallwood J. A. *Br. Med. J.* 1983, **286**, 868.
60. Schmidt P. J. et al. *Surg. Gynecol. Obstet.* 1988, **107**, 229.
61. Högman C. F. *Acta Anaesthesiol. Scand.* 1988, **32**(Suppl. 89), 4.
62. Bashir H. *Anaesth. Intensive Care* 1980, **8**, 132; Waters A. H. and Murphy M. F. *Hospital Update* 1986, 565.
63. Barbara J. A. J. and Contreras M. *Br. Med. J.* 1990, **300**, 450.
64. Hoofinagle J. H. *Transfusion* 1990, **30**, 384.
65. Choo Q.-L. et al. *Br. Med. Bull.* 1990, **46**, 423; Wright R. *J. Roy. Coll. Physicians* 1990, **24**, 78.
66. Jones J. A. In: *Anaesthesia Review 7* (Kaufman L. ed.) Edinburgh: Churchill Livingstone, 1990, 177.
67. Barbara J. A. J. and Contreras M. *Br. Med. J.* 1990, **300**, 386.
68. Biebuyck J. F. *Anesthesiology* 1988, **68**, 422; Wu H.-S. and Little A. G. *J. Clin. Oncol.* 1988, **6**, 1348; Mecklin J. P. et al. *Scand. J. Gastroenterol.* 1989, **24**, 33.
69. Popovsky M. A. et al. *Am. Rev. Resp. Dis.* 1983, **128**, 185.
70. Patterson A. *Int. Anesthesiol. Clin.* 1987, **25**, 61.
71. Kay L. A. *Br. Med. J.* 1987, **294**, 137; Stehling L. *Acta Anaesthesiol. Scand.* 1988, **32**(Suppl. 89), 58.
72. Clifford P. C. et al. *Br. J. Surg.* 1987, **74**, 755.
73. Solem J. O. et al. *Acta Anaesthesiol. Scand.* 1988, **32**(Suppl. 89), 71; Lee D. and Napier J. A. F. *Br. Med. J.* 1990, **300**, 737.
74. Highmore W. *Lancet* 1874, **2**, 89; Blundell J. *Med. Chir. Trans.* 1878, **9**, 56.
75. Duncan J. *Br. Med. J.* 1886, **1**, 192.

Chapter 18

Monitoring[1]

'It is a capital mistake to theorize before one has facts'
(Memoirs of Sherlock Holmes)

There has been a little progress towards an international consensus in this field.[2]

There are five phases to the monitoring process.

(1) collect the monitor readings (data);
(2) analyse the measurements;
(3) decide if action needs to be taken;
(4) decide what action needs to be taken, if any; and
(5) compare results with other anaesthetists throughout the world.[3]

Clinical monitoring

This includes

(1) colour of skin and blood (oxygenation);

(2) pulse character and rate (cardiac performance and arterial pressure, radial pulse present – systolic pressure probably above 60 mmHg, temporal pulse present – systolic pressure probably above 100 mmHg);

(3) state of peripheral circulation (circulatory status);

(4) respiratory movement (adequacy of lung ventilation);

(5) movement of anaesthetic 'bag' (adequacy of lung ventilation, and depth of anaesthesia);

(6) temperature of skin, especially peripheries and tip of nose (body temperature, circulatory status, fluid balance, acid-base status);

(7) urine flow, seen in urine bag (> 0.5 ml/kg/h);

(8) perspiration, lacrimation (depth of anaesthesia);

(9) muscle tone and movement: (*a* relaxation; and *b* depth of anaesthesia);

(10) pupils (depth of anaesthesia, or, in crisis situations, the state of cerebral circulation);

(11) state of awareness, movement of head with respiration;

(12) clotting time of blood (collected in glass test-tube and kept warm in the hand while timing clotting);

(13) degree of filling of jugular veins (circulating volume); and

(14) listening to the surgeon's comments (state of relaxation, depth of anaesthesia).

The primary equipment for clinical measurement and monitoring is the hand, eye, nose and ear of the attending doctor. The anaesthetist should also develop a sixth sense, a subconscious mental computation of observations, time, and experience, which warns of impending events and prompts action to meet the needs of the patient.

Basic instrumental monitoring of patient:

(1) circulation. Non-invasive BP, ECG, pulse oximetry;
(2) respiration. With IPPV, airway pressure, ventilatory volume, capnography, disconnection alarms, volatile agent monitoring, pulse oximetry[4];
(3) metabolic status. Capnography, blood glucose, acid-base balance; and
(4) neuromuscular transmission. Nerve stimulators when relaxants are used.

Basic instrumental monitoring of anaesthetic machine:

(1) oxygen failure warning (alarms, analysers);
(2) airway pressure monitoring; and
(3) ventilator failure alarms.

Additional instrumental monitoring:

(1) urine output and body temperature. In many major surgical operations, pulmonary arterial catheterization may be required;
(2) transthoracic impedance apnoea alarms, intra-arterial blood pressure, intermittent or continuous blood gas analysis, transcutaneous and transconjunctival carbon dioxide[5]; and
(3) special blood tests, e.g. blood glucose, electrolytes, coagulation, hormone assays.
(4) Non-invasive cardiac output, cerebral electrical and metabolic activity and oxygenation, state of awareness, etc.

Non-invasive and minimally invasive monitoring are to be preferred if they give equally accurate or useful information as the invasive methods.

The main problems in instrumental monitoring are at the *patient interface*. For this reason, repeated clinical examination is still of primary importance. Accurate detailed recording is also fundamental. Pen and paper are the most reliable tools for this, and the design of anaesthetic records for ease of use and computer readability is an art.

Automated recording is available (*see also* Chapter 19). At the charted point of monitoring errors, the anaesthetist initials the places where the automated record makes (regrettably frequent) mistakes (e.g. when an operator nudges a blood pressure cuff during a reading, producing an erroneous result). Having to initial the scrolling record can place the anaesthetist under extra stress when things are very busy. Automated records are not regarded as infallible.

When monitors go wrong, and when monitors give inaccurate readings

A high index of suspicion should be directed to monitor accuracy. This requires constant comparison with clinical observation, always being able to see and feel the patient, and facilities for checking the performance of each monitor.

Computerization in monitoring

See Chapter 4.

Limitations of monitors

The anaesthetist must know the limitations of electronic surveillance monitoring, and where clinical signs and subjective feelings are better. The routine monitors do not necessarily detect the abnormality, due to compenstion by the body, until fatigue or overwhelming physiological insult occur, and compensation is lost, e.g. in postoperative haemorrhage, where the vascular parameters may be maintained up to the final collapse, but the feel of the peripheral pulse, the colour of the patient's skin and the nature of the patient's pain give much earlier warning. Another classic example is in post-thyroidectomy and respiratory obstruction due to haemorrhage in the deep tissues of the neck. Respiratory monitoring may remain normal up to the point of collapse and cyanosis, but the patient's subjective sensation of being 'unable to breathe properly' gives much better advance warning. Facial expression has been used as guide to respiratory failure and weaning from ventilators. Even gross abnormalities may not be detected by conventional monitors.

Pulse oximetry (Spo_2)

The measurement of oxygen saturation of the arterial blood.[7] First performed in 1913.[8] The lobe of the ear, bridge of nose, or finger is placed between a two-wavelength light source and a detector. Only pulsating signals are analysed, so skin pigmentation or venous saturation is ignored.[9] Measurement of Fio_2/Spo_2 ratios is diagnostic of changes of status and of some medical conditions, e.g. pulmonary fibrosis, and is useful in the pre-operative and postoperative phases.[10] Changes of cerebral blood flow have been predicted by use of the conjunctival oxygen tension/arterial oxygen tension index.[11]

Limitations of pulse oximetry[12]

The computed haemoglobin saturation can be confused by:
   (1) The presence of methaemoglobin, sulphaemoglobin, or carboxy-haemoglobin in the blood.[13] Methaemoglobin and sulphaemoglobin makes the apparent saturation tend to 85%. Carboxyhaemoglobin is seen as

oxyhaemoglobin. (*See* Adams A. P., *Recent Advances in Anaesthesia and Analgesia – 17* (Atkinson R. S. and Adams A. P. eds), (Edinburgh: Churchill Livingstone, 1991.)

(2) Bilirubin causes under-reading.

(3) Haemoglobin F in neonates and preterm infants (Spo_2 of 92% at Pao_2 of 13 Kpa).[14]

(4) Time-lag of indicated Spo_2 on sudden desaturation due to hypoxic hypoxia.[15]

(5) Polycythaemia of cyanotic congenital cardiac disease.[16]

(6) Weak arterial pulsation and poor peripheral perfusion.[39]

(7) Non-pulsatile arterial flow.

(8) Excessive movement or diathermy.

(9) Dyes in the blood, e.g. methylene blue.

(10) Nail varnish (weak signal)

(11) Digit too large for the sensor, causing constriction.

(12) Nasal pulse oximetry reads nearly 5% higher than digital[17]

(13) Strong ambient light.[18]

(14) Electronic failures.[19]

Response time 5–20 secs. Non-invasive, reliable and expensive. They may be inadequate in severe vasoconstriction. Readings are indicated as analogue or digital displays. Their detection of hypoxic events is not instantaneous.[20] Different models use different algorithms to calibrate the saturation.[39] There are problems of calibration at the lower end of the scale.

Arterial pressure[21]

In spite of the advent of more sophisticated physiological monitoring possibilities, this continues to hold pride of place in cardiovascular monitoring for anaesthesia and intensive care. The systolic pressure is the easiest to measure, and is necessary for calculation of the mean arterial pressure (MAP). The MAP is important for estimating organ perfusion, especially renal. The diastolic pressure is useful for estimating coronary flow.

History

Stephen Hales (1677–1761) in 1733 was the first to attempt measurement of the blood pressure of animals by direct cannulation of an artery.[22] Herrison, 1834,[23] devised a crude instrument to be placed directly over an artery for clinical measurement of blood pressure. Vierordt (1818–1884) was the first to estimate the amount of counter-pressure necessary just to obliterate the arterial pulse.[24] Etienne Jules Marey (1830–1904) in 1875 and von Basch (1837–1905) pioneered clinical sphygmomanometry.[25]

(For history of BP measurements in anaesthesia, *see* Calverley R. K. Classical File; *Surv. Anesthesiol.* 1985, **29**, 78.)

Scipione Riva-Rocci (1863–1937) of Turin introduced the blood-pressure cuff in 1896,[26] although the cuff he used was only 5 cm in width. In 1901, von Recklinghausen (1833–1910) drew attention to the importance of the width of the pneumatic cuff, and E. A. Codman (1869–1940) in 1894 and Harvey Cushing (1869–1939)[27] of Boston advocated the use of blood-pressure readings regularly during anaesthesia. Korotkoff (1874–1920) (Russian physician) in 1905[28] described the sounds heard over an artery at a point just below the compression cuff.[29]

The mercury manometer was first used to measure blood pressure in 1828 by Poiseuille (1799–1869) (Paris physiologist).[30]

The compression cuff

Too narrow a cuff, low readings; too wide, high readings. The cuff should cover approximately two-thirds of the length of the upper arm or 20% greater than the diameter of the arm. The American Heart Association recommends a 12–14 cm rubber bag, long enough to encircle half the arm, centred over the brachial artery. The cloth cover should be made of non-extensible material so that pressure is exerted uniformly. Recommended cuff widths are neonate 2.5 cm, 1–4 years 6.0 cm, 4–8 years 9.0 cm, adult 12–14 cm, for the adult leg 15 cm. A conventional cuff overestimates arterial pressure on a fat or muscular arm, and underestimates it on a thin arm or on the arm of a child.

Automatic oscillotonometer

A cuff is inflated automatically at preset intervals, to above the previous systolic pressure. Oscillations of pressure, due to emerging arterial pulsations beneath (or a second 'sensing' cuff) as the cuff pressure is steadily reduced below the systolic and then diastolic, are detected by a transducer in the monitor, analysed, and presented as systolic, diastolic and a computed mean arterial pressure. The electronics include artefact rejection, e.g. of surgeons leaning on the cuff during the measurement.

The automated oscillotonometer is accurate in children and adults.[31]

Monitors using ultrasonic detectors (2–10 MHz) placed over the brachial artery to detect arterial pulsation in a similar way to the transducers above, require protection from movement artefact.

Finger Arterial Pressure monitors (Finapres)[32] indicate non-invasive beat-to-beat pressure. This compares well with intra-arterial monitoring[33]

Low alarm limits are often set at 2/3 of the baseline values to give warning for action before the pressure reaches the limit of half the baseline value. There are many situations where the limit will be set nearer to the baseline value, e.g. in cardiac and arterial disease. High limits are often set at 4/3 of the baseline values.

Direct intra-arterial methods (*see* Chapter 17)

Indications:
    (1) expected large blood or fluid loss;
    (2) expected highly unstable arterial pressure, e.g. operations on the arterial tree;
    (3) non-pulsatile arterial flow. (e.g. cardiopulmonary bypass);
    (4) severe or prolonged induced hypotension; and
    (5) arterial blood sampling.

Radial artery cannulation is a low-risk, high-benefit method of patient monitoring. The risk of ischaemic complications (though not of partial or complete occlusion of the artery) is very slight.[34]

A needle or cannula, e.g. teflon 20–23G, is inserted into an artery and connected via a column of fluid to a transducer. Radial arterial puncture can be painful.[35]

The Dorsalis Pedis Artery is also a convenient site giving similar pressures to the aorta.[36] Other arteries have been used. The transducer is usually a semi-conductor.

Arterial occlusion can be diagnosed by thermography.[37] Arterial occlusion does not often cause distal ischaemia, because of other collateral arteries, e.g. ulnar. Allen's test may be used to detect adequate ulnar artery collateral circulation. The hand is exsanguinated by the patient making a fist actively (or passively when unconscious) while the radial artery is occluded and the palmar flush of blood from the ulnar artery observed on opening the hand.[38]

A continuous flush system delivers heparinized saline (1 unit/ml) at about 3 ml/h.[40]

The heart beat can also be monitored by the use of a precordial stethoscope, a method particularly suited to use in infants. In children and adults undergoing major surgery an oesophageal stethoscope is helpful. Also useful for diagnosis of air embolus during operation. An oesophageal probe, which incorporates stethoscope, thermistor and ECG lead has been described for paediatric use,[41] but may cause bradycardia from vagal stimulation.[42]

Cardiac output[43]

Swan-Ganz catheters[44]

These are balloon-tipped, flow-directed flexible pulmonary artery catheters, originally used for measuring pulmonary capillary wedge pressure. Cardiac catheterization was performed in the horse by Chareau and Marey in 1855, in the dog, by Claude Bernard in 1879 and in man probably by Bleichroder in 1905, who passed a catheter into his own vascular system,[45] and then by Forssman.[46]

Lategola developed the balloon tip,[47] and Swan and Ganz modified it for clinical use. Special ones are used to measure $S\bar{v}o_2$ by fiberoptics.

For cardiac output, ice-cold saline is injected into the pulmonary artery proximal to the thermistor at the tip of the Swan-Ganz catheter. Its thermodilution is proportional to the pulmonary blood flow and, therefore, to the cardiac output.[48] A microprocessor calculates the actual readings and presents the data. Pulmonary artery wedge pressure (PAWP) (a close index of left atrial pressure) is also recorded directly. Right ventricular ejection fraction can also be measured.

Computer-aided analysis of parameters and trends from a Swan-Ganz catheter is being used for 'intelligent' diagnosis-making, and control of theraputic interventions.

Indications. (a) Low cardiac output; (b) pulmonary oedema; and (c) to sample mixed venous blood; (d) septic shock.

Reliability. Certain criteria are used to ensure accuracy: (a) the mean PAWP should be less than the mean PA pressure, and infusate should flow freely through the catheter, indicating that the catheter tip is free; (b) the wedge tracing should have atrial waveform; and (c) the wedge Po_2 should be greater than the non-wedge Po_2. Room temperature fluid is as accurate as iced infusate; three measurements per determination ar be better than one, and a minimum of 15% difference between successive measurements suggests a real change of cardiac output.[49]

Errors in measurements. These are worst in spontaneously breathing patients where the instantaneous readings, especially those used in automated estimations, do not reflect accurately the waveforms throughout the respiratory cycle.[50] The wedge pressure is normally measured in end-expiration. A strip recorder should be used for manual measurement.

These catheters are inserted via standard central venous approaches, including arm veins. The supraclavicular route has the lowest incidence of misdirection. Progress of the catheter tip is monitored by X-ray control or by observation of the pressures being measured at the tip. Most pass to the right lower lobe artery. Measurements should be made in zone 3 for best accuracy.

Complications[51] include dysrhythmias, damage to the lung,[52] thromboembolism,[53] balloon rupture, infection, migration,[54] obstruction of venous return during cardiopulmonary bypass,[55] and knotting of the catheter.[56]

Some of these may be prevented by deflating the balloon of the dwelling catheter while not being used for measurements. The balloon blocks 5–15% of the lung blood vessels.

Pulmonary arterial wedge pressure

Normal pressure 5–10 mmHg. After cardiac surgery and severe myocardial infarction, fluid loading up to wedge pressures of 10–30 mmHg may occasionally be required. *See* Cardiac Output, *above. (See also* Fowler M. B. et al. *Br. Med. J.* 1980, **1**, 435.)

Non-invasive Doppler ultrasound cardiac output measurement records velocity-flow and cross-sectional area of aorta for single beats, and is reasonably accurate,[57] but not always during acute blood loss[58] Aortovelography gives reasonable sequential estimates of changes in output.[59] Thoracic impedance techniques have proved difficult in children.[60]

Combined ultrasound and Doppler probes give flow in other vessels, e.g. the umbilical artery in the fetus.[61]

Transoesophageal echocardiography is now a clinically useful tool,[62] giving information on wall motion abnormalities and ventricular function, but can cause damage.[63]

Radio-imaging with a gamma-camera after intravenous injection of 99m technetium[64] gives the left ventricular ejection fraction, either on a first-pass study or gated fraction studies. The computer multiplies this by the heart rate to give the cardiac output. This technique also gives information on the size, localization and reversibility of cardiac infarcts. Radio-thallium is also used. The echocardiogram is now also available for this purpose.

The electrocardiogram (*see also* Chapter 1)[65]

The electrocardiogram is an excellent non-invasive monitor of cardiac rhythm and especially of unexpected cardiac arrest or rate changes. For routine monitoring (not the 12-lead diagnostic trace), three electrodes are placed on the chest, as near to the heart as convenient. This increases the signal-to-noise ratio. Since 75% of ischaemic ECG patterns are best detected from the V_5 position, the electrodes should be placed on the positions CM_5 if possible: (1) left clavicle; (2) manubrium; and (3) 5th intercostal space, anterior axillary line. It does not afford a measure of the efficiency of myocardial contraction or of cardiac output; in fact normal electrical activity may occur when there is no cardiac output. If the electrodes are placed on the patient's back ST depression may be seen in the normal heart.

Artefacts

The ECG is liable to artefacts, which may be caused by disconnection of an electrode, superimposition of potential from another person in contact with the patient, improper earthing of apparatus, etc. It is possible for interference to take the form of a sine-wave giving rise to the appearance of ventricular tachycardia. Bizarre complexes occur, e.g. ST depression and widening of the QRS complex may be due to battery exhaustion.[66]

Central venous pressure (CVP)

Venous tone

About half the total blood volume is accommodated in the systemic venous system, and only about 15% in the arterial system. Alterations in venous tone play a large part in the regulation of the haemodynamics of the circulatory system.

History

Venous pressures were first measured by Stephen Hales (1677–1761) in 1733 in a mare, and first measured in man by Frey in 1902[67] and used clinically in 1910.[68] In 1931 Forssmann, a urologist, pioneered (on himself) cardiac catheterization,[69] for which he was awarded the Nobel prize in 1956. The first plastic intravenous catheter (polythene) was used in 1945.[70]

The term central venous pressure refers to the pressure in the right atrium or the intrathoracic inferior or superior venae cavae. For technique of insertion *see* Intravascular techniques, Chapter 17.

Readings

The zero must be a chosen reference level, i.e. the midaxillary line or the manubriosternal angle. Normal central venous pressure may be taken as 3–10 cmH$_2$O. High values may indicate right ventricular failure, pulmonary embolism, tamponade, or misplacement of the catheter tip into the right ventricle or pulmonary artery.

Complications

These include: (1) thrombophlebitis, infection, septicaemia; (2) pneumothorax; (3) haemothorax; (4) hydrothorax; (5) brachial plexus injury; (6) air

Table 18.1 Interpretation of CVP

When the patient is:	Usual CVP is: (cmH₂O)	When the patient has:	Usual CVP is: (cmH₂O)
Supine	+3 to +10	IPPV with PEEP	+5 to +15
Head-down	+5 to +10	Congestive cardiac	
On IPPV	+5 to + 10	failure	+5 to +10
head-up	−10 to −5	Pulmonary embolism	+5 to +20
Hypovolaemic	−5 to 0	Cardiac tamponade	+5 to +20
In ARDS	+5 to +20		

embolus; (7) pericardial effusion; (8) lymph leakage; (9) catheter breakage; and (10) arrhythmias.

Central venous pressure measurements are not a good guide to daily fluid requirements and should not be used for this purpose. A patient can easily be waterlogged or dehydrated in the presence of a normal CVP.

The reliability of right atrial pressure monitoring to assess left ventricular preload in critically ill septic patients has been questioned.[71]

Measurement of blood loss

Gravimetric method

The simplest and most commonly employed method. Blood loss is estimated by measurement of the gain in weight of swabs and towels, together with measurement of the contents of suction bottles; 1 ml of blood weighs 1 g. Weighing of swabs is said to underestimate blood loss by 25%.

Colorimetric method

Swabs and towels are mixed thoroughly with a large known volume of fluid, which is then estimated colorimetrically. Errors may occur due to incomplete extraction or contamination with bile. The patient's haemoglobin must be known. One common system uses the following formula:

$$\text{Blood loss (ml)} = \frac{\text{Colorimeter reading} \times \text{volume of solution ml}}{200 \times \text{patient's Hb (g\%)}}$$

In operations involving complex exchanges of blood (e.g. extracorporeal circulation), it may be useful to weigh the whole patient before and after operation.

Analysis of Gas Mixtures[72]

1. Oxygen

Paramagnetic analysers (described by Pauling in 1946[73]) are useful. Gases are classed as paramagnetic or diamagnetic according to their behaviour in a magnetic field. The former seek the area of strongest, the latter of weakest flux. Of the gases of interest to the anaesthetist only oxygen, nitric oxide and nitrogen dioxide are paramagnetic, others are weakly diamagnetic. This principle is used in commercial apparatus for analysis of oxygen concentrations in a gas mixture.

Small oxygen analysers may be of the polarographic or the microfuel cell type.[74]

For evaluation of oxygen analysers *see*.[75]

2. Carbon dioxide (capnography or capnometry)[76]

The infra-red analyser (first employed in 1865).[77] Gases whose molecules contain two dissimilar atoms or more than two atoms absorb radiation in the infra-red region of the spectrum. *Capnography*[78] for continuous recording of carbon dioxide in anaesthetic systems and in intensive care. A continuous sample of respired gas is withdrawn from as near to the trachea as possible, and the CO_2 content displayed (as a percentage) on a continuous recorder. Sensors placed directly in the breathing system are also available. The highest CO_2 content is found at the end of expiration, and is called the 'end-tidal CO_2' (ET_{CO_2}). In spite of theoretical interference by anaesthetic agents, especially nitrous oxide, and the fact that ET_{CO_2} is not exactly the same as Pa_{CO_2}, the measurement is extremely useful. (*See also* Capnography and pulse oximetry. Adams A. P. In *Recent Advances in Anaesthesia and Analgesia*. (Atkinson R. S., Adams A. P. eds.) Edinburgh: Churchill Livingstone, 1989.) A colorimetric device is available and has been used to identify tracheal intubation.[79]

Analysis of Capnogram. There are three areas of particular interest:
 1. The end-tidal value.
(*a*) intubation of oesophagus (or trachea);
(*b*) adequacy of ventilation;
(*c*) emboli (because the embolised area does not exchange CO_2 into alveolar gas);
(*d*) sudden changes in cardiac output; and
(*e*) malignant hyperpyrexia.
 2. The shape of the expired capnogram.
(*a*) Inspiratory effort; and
(*b*) V/Q maldistribution.
 3. Inspired portion.
(*a*) rebreathing, deliberate or accidental; and
(*b*) CO_2 rotameter on.
Capnography is useful because:
 (1) careful control of carbon dioxide levels is important in most types of surgery;
 (2) it warns of airway, intubation and ventilation errors;
 (3) it monitors special dangers such as air embolism, shock, etc.;

(4) it warns of inspired CO_2 rising (e.g. rebreathing);

(5) the shape of the capnogram may show diaphragmatic inspiratory effort (early relaxant failure) as a 'dip' at the end of expiration, or V/Q maldistribution as a rising expiratory plateau; and

(6) the efficiency of the closed system can be continuously monitored.

It can be monitored during HFPPV[80]

3 Volatile anaesthetic agents

Normally carried out by infra-red absorption, as for carbon dioxide.

4. Simultaneous analysis

Simultaneous analysis of various gases can be carried out using:

(a) *The mass spectrometer.* Molecules are ionized, accelerated by an electric field and deflected by a magnetic field. The angle of deflection is related to molecular weight. Carbon dioxide and nitrous oxide have the same molecular weight, as do carbon monoxide and nitrogen, but special electronic circuits can differentiate these gases. Response time <100 ms. One instrument can serve several operating rooms. It also has applications in intensive care.[81]

(b) *Gas chromatography.* Separation of components by means of a partition column. It accepts a discrete gas sample and takes several minutes to analyse it, but is extremely sensitive, e.g. for measurement of anaesthetic pollution.

The term is a contraction for gas–liquid chromatography and is not concerned with 'colour', the word 'chromatography' being handed down from an older technique of liquid–liquid separation in which the components were identified by colour.

Respiration

Tidal volume and minute volume (see also Chapter 2)

1. Inferential meters. Volume is inferred from the number of revolutions of a vane rotated by the gas stream. Now commercially available as small and light apparatus, which may be connected directly to a face-piece or catheter mount: (a) Wright anemometer, gas passes through ten tangential slots in a cylindrical stator ring to turn a flat two-bladed rotor. A recent development displays gas volumes on a calibrated meter and is not affected by water condensation. The Wright anemometer is a simple, robust, light-weight, accurate and cheap device, ideally suited for use in the intensive care ward. Its accuracy is slightly dependent on the wave form of the gases passing through it;[82] (b) there are various similar instruments.

2. The pneumotachograph. Continuously measures gas flow by measuring pressure drop across a resistor. It is compact and forms part of modern ventilator circuits.

3. Thoracic impedance plethysmography. The electrical impedance of the chest changes during respiration and can be used to compute volume changes.

4. Infant apnoea mats.

Blood-gas measurements[83]

History

Blood-gas measurements started by Pflüger (1829–1910) in 1872. (*See also* Astrup P. and Severinghaus J. W. *History of Gases, Acids and Bases*. Copenhagen: Munksgaard, 1986.)

Arterial oxygen tension

The oxygen electrode. This consists of a platinum cathode and a silver anode in a potassium hydroxide solution. Platinum gives up electrons to oxygen and the resulting voltage change can be measured and expressed in terms of oxygen tension. Platinum receives a deposition of protein when used in biological fluids, so the electrode system must be isolated from the blood sample by a thin gas-permeable membrane. The Clark electrode[84] is the basis of the modern oxygen electrode, although modifications have been produced.[85]

Blood samples. Must be drawn from an artery into a syringe whose dead space has been filled with heparin. The oxygen consumption of whole blood is sufficient to cause a fall in Po_2 of about 0.4 kPa/min. Samples should therefore be analysed at once, or kept cool to reduce oxygen consumption. Oxygen may also diffuse into the substance of the plastic syringe. The loss is greater when Pao_2 is high. Use of glass syringes obviates this source of error. 'Normal' values may be as low as 10 kPa (70 mmHg) in the over-70 age group, compared with 13.5 kPa (100 mmHg) in younger age groups.

Venous samples show satisfactory correlation with arterial ones for pH, bicarbonate, and Pco_2 (1 kPa higher), but not for Po_2.[86]

Transcutaneous oxygen electrodes[87]

In the Clark type electrode, the oxygen diffuses through the skin and is measured by a polarographic technique. Information concerning the blood flow in a flap of skin or in the skin after reconstructive vascular surgery, can also be obtained. (*See also* Tremper K. K. *Can. Anaesth. Soc. J.* 1984, **31**, 664.)

These give accurate and continuous measurement provided that: (1) the patient is not cold or vasoconstricted; (2) the skin under the electrode is not degenerating as a result of prolonged electrode placement; and (3) drift problems have been eliminated from the system.

Transcutaneous carbon dioxide monitoring[88]

A glass electrode with special membrane is closely applied to the skin. Voltage output is logarithmically related to the Pco_2. Response time is slow. The electrode is heated to 44°C. The cutaneous Pco_2 ($tcPco_2$) reads 0.5 kPa higher than the $Paco_2$.

Venous oxygen content

This is an index of adequate cardiac output and tissue perfusion. Normal value is 14 ml/100 ml blood. Central venous oxygen content correlates well with mixed venous oxygen content.[89]

Pulse oximetry (see above)

Arterial carbon dioxide measurement

1. The electrode consists of a pH electrode surrounded by a bicarbonate solution. The whole is contained in a membrane permeable to CO_2, which diffuses in from the blood sample, altering the pH of the bicarbonate solution. Modern machines consist of Po_2, Pco_2, and pH electrodes, are fully automated in their handling of the the blood sample and calibration, and only need 0.1 ml of blood.

2. End-expired gas analysis gives a useful non-invasive indication of $Paco_2$, using the lung as a tonometer. (*See above*).

Neuromuscular monitoring

(*see also* Chapter 10 and Neuromuscular Blockade Monitoring. Pearce A. C. In *Recent Advances in Anaesthesia and Analgesia – 16* (Atkinson R. S., Adams A. P. eds). Edinburgh: Churchill Livingstone, 1989).

Neuromuscular monitors should deliver a 50 mA supramaximal stimulus. Stimulating and recording electrodes are positioned over the ulnar nerve at or above the wrist. The median nerve has been used.[91] For analysis of the response, finger movement can be assessed manually, recording electrodes positioned over the small muscles of the hand, or a force-transducer applied to the thumb.

Neuronal monitoring

Sensory-evoked potentials (SEPs) are used for testing neurone integrity during spinal, cardiac and carotid surgery, and for unplanned awareness[92]. Transcutaneous SEPs require huge amplification of the signal and interference is always a problem.[93] See also Chapter 14.

Electromyography

See Pugh A. D. et al. *Anaesthesia* 1984, **39**, 574; *see also* Chapter 10.

The electro-encephalogram (EEG)[94]

Purpose in the ICU and during operations:

1. To assess sedation and awareness.[95] Sedation (e.g. propofol, opioids), slows the frequency progressively through the range 8 Hz (light) to 0.1 Hz (deep). Awareness is indicated by fast alpha activity. Pain may produce more

beta activity. Barbiturates in moderate doses give large slow waves, then burst suppression. Low-dose isoflurane shows 10–12Hz, reduction to delta waves and finally burst suppression with increasing concentration.

2. To monitor epileptic activity, and to control antiepileptic drug infusions, especially in paralysed patients.[96]

3. To monitor changes in conscious level.

Electrical activity of the brain in animals noted by Richard Caton of Liverpool (1842–1926), in 1875. Hans Berger (1873–1941)[97] in 1931 described alpha rhythms in man. Adrian and Matthews (1934) developed the technique of the electro-encephalogram.[98]

First used in anaesthesia in 1950[99] after a suggestion by Gibbs in 1937.[100]

Types of wave

1. *Delta waves*: 0.3–3.5 Hz; amplitude 100 μV. Occur in infants and sleeping adults, and anaesthesia.

2. *Theta waves*: 4–7 Hz, 10 μV.

3. *Alpha waves*: 8–13 Hz, 20 μV in infants, 75 in children, 50 in adults.

Augmented by closing eyes or mental repose. Reduced by visual and mental activity. A sign of awareness.

4. *Beta waves*: 14–25 Hz, 20 μV. May indicate pain.

5. *Gamma waves*: 26 Hz or more. 10 μV. Rare.

Technique

The scalp electrodes should have low impedance (5 Kohms) involving shaving, cleaning and abrasion. Positioning is on the 10–20 system, with a ground electrode on the forehead or mastoid process. A bandwidth of 0.5–30 Hz, eliminating mains interference, is reasonable for theatre and ICU use, but cardiac and skeletal activity may still intrude. Artefacts may occur due to movement of the patient or to superimposition of an electrocardiogram if an electrode is placed directly over an artery.

Changes in the EEG.

1. *Hypoxia.* Causes slowing of the frequency of the waves. After about 20 s of complete anoxia the recording becomes a straight line, e.g. after cardiac arrest. Lesser degrees of hypoxia may not affect the tracing until a level of 40% arterial oxygen saturation is reached.

2. *Hypotension.* A rapid fall of blood pressure is associated with slow high-amplitude waves or temporary cessation.

3. *Circulatory arrest.* Activity ceases. The recording can be used as a measure of cerebral circulation during cardiac massage. After cardiac arrest, the presence of alpha rhythm carries a good prognosis, whereas periods of wave suppression indicate a bad prognosis.

4. *Hypothermia.* Below 35–31°C some decrease in amplitude and frequency occurs. At 20°C there may be little activity.

Cerebral function analysing monitor (CFM or CFAM)

This has the advantage that the display is meaningful to non-specialized EEG staff. It has been used to monitor depth of anaesthesia and sedation, cerebral ischaemia during cardiopulmonary bypass and coma levels in the ICU.

An amplitude value is computed from the integrated area under an assigned classical wave (α, β, θ, δ). The mean amplitude and the 10th and 90th centiles are displayed. The normal amplitude is between 5 and 15 μV. A fall below 5 μV can indicate a fall of cerebral perfusion, with corresponding fall of cerebral function. Epileptiform fits are also displayed as spikes of amplitude above 15 μV. The CFM can be used to titrate the dose of fentanyl for sedation, aiming for just above 5 μV.[101]

Nuclear magnetic resonance[102, 103]

See Chapter 22, Neurosurgery.

Temperature[104]

The founder of clinical thermometry was C. A. Wunderlich (1815–1877), professor of medicine at Leipzig, whose classic work appeared in 1868.[105] "Before his work, fever was a disease; after it, a symptom" (Garrison).

1. *The standard mercury-in-glass clinical thermometer.*

2. *Dial thermometers.* Simple instruments: (*a*) a flat bimetallic spiral spring, which winds or unwinds as temperature changes; and (*b*) the pressure gauge (Bourdon gauge) – a hollow ribbon of metal, which winds or unwinds as temperature changes produce pressure changes within the coil.

3. *Thermocouple.* A circuit of two dissimilar metals produces an e.m.f. when the two junctions are at different temperatures. The e.m.f. is measured and calibrated according to temperature. The apparatus can be made small and it has a rapid response.

4. *Platinum resistance thermometry.* The resistance of a metal varies according to temperature, and the former is measured by means of a Wheatstone bridge. A platinum coil can be mounted within the lumen of a hypodermic needle for insertion in body tissues.

5. *Thermistor* (*therm*ally sensitive res*istor*). A small bead of semi-conductor material can be sealed into hypodermic needles. Semi-conductors have negative coefficients of resistance, which can be measured using a Wheatstone bridge.

6. *Skin thermometers.* Difficulties arise due to poor contact with the skin and because skin temperature itself falls as heat passes to the thermometer: (*a*) the magnetic thermometer – temperature affects its field strength; and (*b*) the radiometer. Infra-red rays, which are emitted by all substances at temperatures above absolute zero, are focused on a thermistor device.

The temperature can be taken from the mouth, rectum, skin, oesophagus or tympanic membrane. Evaluation of body temperature *see* Ilsley A. H. et al. *Anaesth. Intensive Care* 1983, **11**, 31; Hall G. M. *Br. J. Anaesth.* 1990.

Monitoring during transfer of patients

Between hospitals and within the hospital. This must reflect the severity of the patient's condition, and is as comprehensive as necessary. Specially designed trolleys are available, and also framed units, which fit on standard beds, to display parameters and prevent damage to expensive equipment. Battery power is of course necessary. Special problems exist in helicopters due to vibration and noise, and even the most elementary measurements may be impossible. With rail and road transfers, a smooth trip is better than a fast trip. The 'scoop and run' policy has been supplanted with a 'treat and resuscitate the patient as you go' technique.

Safety in monitoring equipment

See Chapter 3

References

1. Atkinson R. S. and Adams A. P. *Recent Advances in Anaesthesia and Analgesia – 16*. Churchill Livingstone, 1989 (Casey Blitt ed.) *Monitoring in Anesthesia and Critical Care Medicine* Edinburgh: Churchill Livingstone, 1985.
2. Winter A. and Spence A. A. *Br. J. Anaesth.* 1990, **64**, 263.
3. Shoemaker, W. C., Appel P. and Kram H. A. *Crit. Care Med.* 1989, **17**, 1277.
4. Payne J. P. and Severinghaus J. W. (ed.) *Pulse Oximetry.* Berlin: Springer-Verlag, 1986; Taylor M. B. and Whitman J. G. *Anaesthesia* 1986, **41**, 943.
5. Abraham E. et al. *Crit. Care Med.* 1986, **14**, 138.
6. Tremper K. K. and Barker S. J. *Anesthesiology,* 1989, **70**, 98.
7. Adams A. P., In *Recent Advances in Anaesthesia and Analgesia – 16* (Atkinson R. S., Adams A. P., ed.) Edinburgh: Churchill Livingstone, 1989; Yelderman N. and New W. *Anesthesiology,* 1983, **59**, 349; Payne J. P. and Severinghaus J. W. (ed.) *Pulse Oximetry.* Berlin: Springer-Verlag, 1986; Taylor M. B. and Whitman J. G. *Anaesthesia* 1986, **41**, 943.
8. Cooke A. and Barcroft J. *J. Physiol. (Lond.)* 1913, **47**, 35.
9. Striebel H. W. and Kretz F. J. *Anaesthesist* 1989, **38**, 649.
10. McKenzie A. J. *Anaesth. Intensive Care* 1989, **17**, 412.
11. Rutherford W. F. and Panacek E. A. *Crit. Care Med.* 1989, **17**, 1328.
12. Kidd J. F. and Vickers M. D. *Br. J. Anaesth.* 1989, **62**, 355–7.
13. Bardoczky G. I. et al. *Acta Anaesth. Scand.* 1990, **34**, 162.
14. Southall D. P. et al. *Arch. Dis. Child.* 1987, **62**, 882; Wasunna A. and Whitelaw A. G. L. *ibid*, 957.
15. Severinghaus J. W. and Naifeh K. H. *Anesthesiology* 1987, **67**, 551.
16. Ridley S. A. *Anaesthesia* 1988, **43**, 136.
17. Rosenberg J. and Pederson M. H. *Anaesthesia* 1991, **45**, 1070.
18. Jobes D. R. and Nicolson S. C. *Anesth. Analg.* 1988, **67**, 186.
19. Duncan F. B. *Anaesthesia* 1990, **45**, 1093.
20. Verhoeff F. and Sykes M. K. *Anaesthesia* 1990, **45**, 103.
21. O'Brien E. T. and O'Malley K. *Br. Med. J.* 1979, **2**, 851, 970, 1048, 1124.
22. Willius F. A. and Keyes T. E. *Cardiac Classics.* St Louis: Mosby, 1941, Vol. 1, 131.
23. Herrison J. *Le Sphygmomètre.* Paris: Crochard, 1834; Stephen Hales *Physiologist and Botanist* (Clark-Kennedy A. E. ed.) Cambridge University Press, 1977; Booth J. *Proc. R. Soc. Med.* 1977, **70**, 793.

24. Vierordt K. *Arch. Physiol. Heilk.* 1854, **13**, 284.
25. Von Basch S. *Z. Klin. Med.* 1883, **33**, 673.
26. Riva-Rocci S. *Gaz. Med. di Torin* 1896, **47**, 981 (reprinted in English translation In: *Foundations of Anesthesiology* (Faulconer A. and Keys T. E. ed.). Springfield: Thomas, 1965, 1043.
27. Cushing H. W. *Ann. Surg.* 1092, **36**, 32l; *Boston Med. Surg. J.* 1903, **148**, 29l (reprinted in 'Classical File', *Surv. Anesthesiol.* 1960, **4**, 419).
28. Korotkoff N. S. *Izvest. imp. Vyenno-Med. Acad. St Petersburg* 1905, **11**, 365.
29. Comroe J. H. *Anesth. Analg. (Cleve.)* 1976, **55**, 900.
30. Poiseuille J. L. M. *Archs. Gén. Méd. (Paris)*, 1828, **18**, 550.
31. Friesen R. H. and Lichtor J. L. *Anesth. Analg.* 1981, **60**, 742; Kimble K. J. et al. *Anesthesiology* 1981, **54**, 423; Hutton P. et al. *Anaesthesia* 1984, **39**, 261.
32. Dorlas J. C. et al *Anesthesiology* 1985, **62**, 342–345.
33. Kermode J. L., Davis N. J. and Thompson W. R. *Anaesth. Intensive Care* 1989, **17**, 470.
34. Slogoff S. et al. *Anesthesiology* 1983, **59**, 42.
35. Clark G. S. et al. *Anaesthesia* 1982, **37**, 78.
36. Cole P., Rushman G. B. and Simpson P. *Anaesthesia* 1976, **31**, 69.
37. Evans P. J. D. et al. *Anaesth. Intensive Care* 1977, **5**, 231.
38. Allen E. V. *Am. J. Med. Sci.* 1929, **179**, 237; *see also* Brown A. E. et al. *Anaesthesia* 1969, **24**, 532; Fandi S. K. and Reynolds A. C. *Anesthesiology* 1983, **59**, 147.
39. Clayton D. G. et al. *Anaesthesia* 1991, **46**, 3.
40. Morray J. and Todd S. *Anesthesiology* 1983, **58**, 187.
41. Inkster J. S. *Anaesthesia* 1966, **21**, 111; Baker A. B. and McLeod S. *Anaesthesia* 1983, **38**, 892.
42. Cordero E. T. and Hon E. H. *J. Pediatr.* 1971, **78**, 441.
43. Crowther J. and Jenkins B. S. *Br. J. Clin. Equip.* 1980, **5**, 34.
44. Swan H. J. C. and Ganz W. et al. *N. Engl. J. Med.* 1970, **283**, 447; George R. J. D. and Banks R. A. *Br. J. Hosp. Med.* 1983, **29**, 286.
45. Bleichroder F. *Berl. Klin. Wochenschr.* 1912, **49**, 1503: Forssmann W. T. J. *Klin. Wochenschr.* 1929, **47**, 93.
46. Harvey A. M. *Science at the Bedside, 1905–1945.* Baltimore: Johns Hopkins University Press, 1981.
47. Lategola M. and Rahn H. *Proc. Soc. Exp. Biol. Med.* 1953. **84**, 667.
48. Landais A. et al. *Acta Anaes. Scand.* 1990, **34**, 158.
49. Stetz C. W. et al. *Am. Rev. Respir. Dis.* 1982, **126**, 1001.
50. Cengiz M. et al. *Crit. Care Med.* 1983, **11**, 502.
51. Sprung C. L. et al. *Chest* 1981, **79**, 413.
52. Gomez-Arnau J. et al. *Crit. Care Med.* 1982, **10**, 694.
53. Devitt J. H. et al. *Anesthesiaology* 1982, **57**, 335.
54. Moore R. A. et al. *Anesthesiology* 1983, **58**, 102.
55. Meluch A. M. and Karis J. H. *Anesth. Analg.* 1990, **70**, 121.
56. Dumesnil J. G. and Proul G. *Am. J. Cardiol.* 1984, **53**, 395.
57. Schuster A. H. and Nanda N. C. *Am. J. Cardiol.* 1984, **53**, 257-259.
58. Kamal G. D., Symreng T. and Starr J. *Anesthesiology*, 1990, **72**, 95.
59. Haites N. E. et al. *Br. Heart J.* 1985, **53**, 123–129.
60. Donovan K. D. et al. *Crit. Care Med.* 1986, **14**, 1038–1044.
61. Huntsman R. L. et al. *Circulation* 1983, **67**, 593.
62. Haggmark S. et al. *Anesthesiology* 1989, **70**, 19; Vandenberg B. F. and Kerber R. E. *Anesthesiology* 1990, **73**, 799; de Bruijn, A. and Clements J. *Intraoperative Use of Echocardiography,* Lippincott Philadelphia 1991.
63. Urbanowicz J. H. et al. *Anesthesiology* 1990, **72**, 40.
64. Clements F. M. et al. *Br. J. Anaesth* 1990, **64**, 331.
65. *See* Rollason W. N. *Electrocardiography for the Anaesthetist* 4th ed. Oxford: Blackwell, 1980.
66. Bar Z. G. *Anaesthesia* 1984, **39**, 611.

67. Frey A. *Dt. Arch. Klin. Med.* 1902, **73**, 511.
68. Moritz F. and von Tabora D. *Dtsch. Arch Klin. Med.* 1910, **98**, 475.
69. Forssmann W. *Münch. Med. Wochenschr.* 1931, **78**, 489.
70. Meyers L. *Am. J. Nurs.* 1945, **45**, 930.
71. Knobel E. et al. *Crit. Care Med* 1989, **17**, 1344.
72. Davies N. J. H. and Denison D. M., In: *Scientific Foundations of Anaesthesia* 4th edn (Scurr C. S., Feldman S. A., Soni N. ed.) Oxford: Heinemann, 1990.
73. Pauling L. *Science* 1946 **103**, 338.
74. Cole A. G. H. *Br. J. Hosp. Med.* 1983 **29**, 469.
75. Ilsley A. H. and Runciman W. B. *Anaesth. Intensive Care* 1986, **14**, 431.
76. Endler G. C. *Anesthesiology* 1990, 72, 214.
77. Tyndal J. *Trans. R. Coll. Surg. Engl.* 1865, **4**, 139.
78. Kalenda Z. *Br. J. Clin. Equip.* 1980, **6**, 180; Kalenda Z. *Acta Anaesthesiol. Belg.* 1978, **29**, 201; Hurter D. *Anaesthesia* 1979, **34**, 578; Smallhout B. and Kalenda Z. *An Atlas of Capnography,* Zeist Netherlands: Kerlebosch, 1980; Whitesell R. et al. *Anesth. Analg. (Cleve.)* 1981, **60**, 508.
79. Goldberg J. S. et al. *Anesth. Analg.* 1990, **70**, 191.
80. Bourgan J. L. et al. *Br. J. Anaesth.* 1990, **64**, 327.
81. Gothard J. W. W. et al. *Anaesthesia* 1980, **35**, 890.
82. Bushman J. A. *Br. J. Anaesth.* 1979, **51**, 895.
83. Parker D. *Br. J. Clin. Equip.* 1980, **5**, 31; Blackburn J. P. *Br. J. Anaesth.* 1978, **50**, 51.
84. Clark L. C. *Trans. Am. Soc. Artif. Intern. Organs* 1956, **2**, 41.
85. Laver M. B. and Seifen A. *Anesthesiology* 1965, **26**, 73.
86. Williamson D. C. and Munson E. S. *Anesth. Analg. (Cleve.)* 1982, **61**, 950.
87. Rozkovec A. and Rithalia S. U. S. *Br. J. Clin. Equip.* 1980, **5**, 24; Goldman M. D. et al. *Anaesthesia* 1982, **37**, 944; Simpson R. M. and Bryan M. H. *Br. J. Hosp. Med.* 1982, **28**, 250.
88. Eberhard P. and Schafer R. *Br. J. Clin. Equip.* 1980, **5**, 224.
89. Tahvanainen J. et al. *Crit. Care Med.* 1982, **10**, 758; Jamieson W. R. E. and Turnbull K. W. *Can. J. Surg.* 1982, **25**, 538.
90. Cobbe S. M. and Poole-Wilson P. A. *Lancet* 1979, **2**, 444; Stevens A. J. *Br. J. Clin. Equip.* 1980, **6**, 112.
91. Lam H. S. et al. *Br. J. Anaes.* 1981, **53**, 1351.
92. Klasing S., Keller I. and Madler C. *Anaesthesist* 1989, **38**, 664.
93. Lam H. S. *Can. J. Anaes.* 1987, **34**, S232-S36.
94. Spencer E. M. and Bolsin S. N. C. *Intensive Care World* 1990, **7**, 34; *Int. Aesthesiol. Clin.* 1990, **28**(3).
95. Klasing S., Keller I. and Madler C. *Anaesthesist* 1989, **38**, 664.
96. Veselis et al. *Crit. Care Med.* 1989, **17**, S68.
97. Berger H. *Arch. f. Psychiat.* 1931, **94**, 16.
98. Adrian E. B. and Mathews B. H. C. *Brain* 1934, **57**, 355.
99. Courtin R. F. et al. *Proc. Staff Mayo Clin.* 1950, **25**, 197 (reprinted in 'Classical File', *Surv. Anesthesiol.* 1959, 3 August).
100. Gibbs F. A. and Gibbs L. *Arch. Intern. Med.* 1937, **60**, 154.
101. See also Chapter 1; Prior P. F. and Maynard D. E., *Monitoring Cerebral Function.* Amsterdam: Elsevier, 1986
102. Nixon C. et al. *Anaesthesia* 1986, **41**, 131; Hain W. R. and Zideman D. A. *Todays Anaesthetist* 1986, **1**, No. 2, 8.
103. Bydder G. M. and Steiner R. E. *Neuroradiology* 1982, **23**, 231; Bailes D. R. et al. *Clin. Radiol.* 1982, **33**, 395; Crooks L. E. et al. *Radiology* 1982, **144**, 843.
104. Imrie M. M. and Hall G. M. *Br. J. Anaesth* 1990, **64**, 346.
105. Wunderlich C. A. *Medical Thermometry* 2nd ed. (translated by Woodman W. B.). London: New Sydenham Society, 1871. *See also Br. Med. J.* 1965, **1**, 1449.

Chapter 19

Safety in anaesthetic practice and audit

PATIENT SAFETY

Concerns about the safety of anaesthesia have been expressed since the first reported deaths under ether and chloroform in 1847 and 1848 respectively (*see* Chapter 35). In 1896 Hewitt[1] stressed the need for education as a means to achieve safe anaesthesia. Although the need was clear for anaesthesia to be included in the undergraduate medical curriculum,[2] this was not adopted by the General Medical Council until 1912. Now, an increasing public awareness and often unrealistic expectation of surgery without morbidity and mortality have led to increased litigation and a related interest in patient safety.

The International Committee on Prevention of Anesthesia Mortality and Morbidity[3] and the Anesthesia Patient Safety Foundation[4] were started in the 1980s in the USA. The Australian Patient Safety Foundation first reported in 1988.[5] In the UK, the Association of Anaesthetists has promoted the development of large-scale audit. The *Report of the Confidential Enquiry into Perioperative Deaths* (*CEPOD*) was published in 1987.[6] The professional organizations in most countries have sub-committees to consider patient safety. The large literature details the multifactorial nature of most anaesthetic accidents:

1. The anaesthetist

Even after careful selection and training, there is a need for continuing education. Surveys of mortality and morbidity often reveal poor assessment and inadequate treatment or resuscitation of the patient before surgery. Delegation to a junior colleague or assistant may be inappropriate. Regular audit, morbidity and mortality meetings contribute to safe anaesthesia. Stylized training is useful to prepare for infrequent but particularly hazardous situations, e.g. difficult or failed intubation, cardiac arrest, unexpected cyanosis, anaphylaxis, malignant hyperpyrexia. As with pilots, computer-based simulators[7] have been developed (*see also* Chapter 4), e.g. ATTENDING,[8] the use of artificial intelligence in patient management; and

CASE,[9] a sophisticated simulator complete with mannequin, anaesthetic machine and monitors. However there is little formal assessment of practical skills in anaesthesia, neither of trainees nor their trainers.

The anaesthetist works in a complex environment[10] and behaviour will be influenced by some factors that are out of the anaesthetists control, such as climate, economy and even architecture. The provision of a safe environment depends in part on hospital administrators, although advised by the professions. The anaesthetist needs to prepare for the unexpected and be alert. Commonsense says a reasonable amount of sleep and rest is necessary before taking a patient's life into his hands. This is a legal requirement in New York State.[11] Sleep deprivation causes mood changes, but functional impairment is not always apparent.[12] But the relatively easy tasks that are so important to the safety of anaesthesia require a high level of personal arousal to perform well.[13] All anaesthetists should have skilled assistance. At least 14 of the deaths of CEPOD involved an anaesthetist without such help.

All anaesthetists, however experienced and however accident-free, should be humble enough to recognize that they may make mistakes at any time.[14] These errors may be in technique, judgement or failure of vigilance. With attention to detail, it should be possible to prevent the minor error turning to a disaster.[15] No anaesthetist (particularly a trainee) should be persuaded to treat a patient beyond his capabilities.

2. Equipment and drugs

The anaesthetist must understand the working of all equipment, and be satisfied that it has been properly maintained. Both equipment and drugs must be checked before use.[16] Accidental disconnection of parts of the breathing circuit is an ever-present hazard. Ill-fitting tapers should be discarded. Even minor leaks can have serious consequences. Some safety features are incorporated in modern anaesthetic machines: inability to deliver hypoxic gas mixtures, limits on CO_2 flow, built-in monitors. In the future, features such as digital control of gas flows and vaporizers, self-checks and servo control of vapour concentration within a circle may provide additional safety. But correct usage of such equipment will always be crucial.

The safety of electrical equipment[17] is governed by BS 5724-1 (1979) and by International Electrotechnical Commission (IEC) 601-1 (2nd ed. 1988). The Department of Health (UK) publish their evaluations as *Health Equipment Information* and issue cautionary notes (*Safety Action Bulletins*) and urgent warnings (*Hazard Notices*) to relevant parties. The last two are published in *Anaesthesia*. The correspondence columns of the journals are useful vehicles for the dissemination of safety information, and electronic bulletin boards may be more widely used in the future. In the USA the Food and Drug Administration regulates the manufacture and use of medical devices. It divides them into Classes I, II and III in increasing order of patient risk. In the European Economic Community since 1992, directives attempt to integrate the laws governing medical devices. The 'CE' mark allows their sale throughout the EEC.

The anaesthetist must be satisfied that the drug to be injected into a patient is the one intended and prepared at the correct dilution. Adverse reactions should be reported to the Committee on Safety of Medicines on the special yellow card for anaesthetic drugs. New drugs require special vigilence[18] and are marked by an inverted black triangle in the *British National Formulary* and *MIMS*.

3. Monitoring

Few doubt the contribution that monitoring has made to safe anaesthesia. Many countries have introduced minimum standards of monitoring[19] (*see* Chapter 18). These usually include the continuous presence of an anaesthetist in theatre (or briefly in the anaesthetic room if the intervening door is open) and monitors of the anaesthetic machine (oxygen failure alarm; inspired oxygen concentration; ventilator disconnect alarm), and of the patient (circulation – ECG, pulse, blood pressure; respiration – bag movement, capnography; pulse oximetry; temperature; neuromuscular transmission). Failures of tracheal intubation or ventilation of paralysed patients are common problems, and the requirement for capnography and oximetry will be strengthened.[20] The Harvard group found no major preventable intraoperative injury in the 3 years after instituting minimal monitoring standards.[21] Such standards are legally enforced in certain states and have led to some reductions in malpractice insurance premiums in the USA. An analysis of closed insurance claims in the USA over 15 years concluded that additional monitors, especially capnography and pulse oximetry, would have prevented 31.5% of the accidents.[22] Critical incident studies have yielded similar conclusions.

Time and motion studies of anaesthetists in the operating theatre[23] reveal much time *not* spent observing the patient, and an implicit reliance on monitors and their alarms. The judgement of the anaesthetist is most important.[24] Anaesthetists must know the limitations of the monitors, set appropriate alarm limits, know how to check that they are working correctly and be able to interpret the data. An excessive number of monitors may lead to distractions, complacency and a blind adherence to 'standards'. Alarms frequently sound when there is in fact no danger to the patient. There is much room for improvement in the integrated display of data and alarm states from various monitors so that unimportant information is suppressed. Standards are being drawn up for auditory and visual alarms (ISO 121 and IEC 62).

The patient is exposed to nearly as much danger in the postoperative recovery room as in theatre. Hypoxaemic episodes there are common.[25] Monitoring of the circulation and respiration should continue as needed. CEPOD reported 34 hospitals with inadequate recovery facilities. There should be a safe hand-over of the patient to recovery staff.

4. The patient

The anaesthetist plays an important part in ensuring that the correct operation is performed on the correct patient. A Medic Alert bracelet warns an attending doctor of hazards such as drug allergies, sensitivity to suxamethonium or susceptibility to malignant hyperpyrexia.

See also Gravenstein J. S. and Holzer J. F. ed. *Safety and Cost Containment in Anesthesia*. Boston: Butterworths, 1988; Dinnick O. P. and Thompson P. W. *Baillière's Clinical Anaesthesiology* 1988, **2** (2); *Risk Management in Anesthesia*. *Int. Anesthesiol. Clin.* 1989, **27**, 3; Adams A. P. In: *Recent Advances in Anaesthesia and Analgesia – 17*. (Atkinson R. S. and Adams A. P. ed.) Edinburgh: Churchill Livingstone, 1992.

ANAESTHETIC RECORDS

Pioneers in anaesthetic record-keeping include Harvey Cushing in 1895[26] and Ralph Waters in 1936.[27] E. I. McKesson's (1881–1935) 'Nargraf' machine of 1930 could produce a semi-automated record of inspired oxygen, tidal volume and inspiratory gas pressure.[28] Nosworthy's cards[29] carried details of the patient, operation and anaesthesia, and had notches to allow rapid sorting with a knitting needle.

A record should be kept of all administrations of anaesthesia. Its value is:[30] (*a*) *to contribute to patient care*. Although about 11% of an anaesthetist's time may be consumed by keeping the record,[23] it probably stimulates vigilant anaesthesia. It certainly helps any future anaesthetist caring for that patient; (*b*) *as an aid for audit* of an anaesthetist's work, the demands placed on a whole department and the clinical care of patients. Poor results achieved by a particular anaesthetist may be revealed;[31] (*c*) *for teaching*; and (*d*) *for medico-legal reasons*. Much harm may be done to an anaesthetist's defence of a civil claim if his record is not full, accurate, contemporaneous and legible. Although patient care should always take precedence over record-keeping, events should be recorded as soon as possible after they happen. Any corrections should be made in a way that will not arouse suspicion that the record has been falsified. Handwriting experts can often decipher alterations and clarify who wrote what and when.

Even the simplest record should contain the patient details, date of operation, surgeons and anaesthetists involved, operation performed, a summary of the pre-operative assessment, techniques and drugs used, record of vital signs such as pulse and blood pressure, complications, instructions to staff in the recovery room. Intravenous fluids given during operation should be recorded, including the serial numbers of any units of blood. Vital signs are traditionally recorded at 5-min intervals, although this may not be appropriate for all operations. Some record systems incorporate carbon copies, which may be retained as departmental records when the originals are filed in the case notes. *In every case, the anaesthetic technique used should be written in the theatre register, followed by the anaesthetist's signature.* The patient may have access to all his health records written after November 1991, which therefore should be composed with this in mind.

Handwritten records are still effective and common. Monitors may be connected to printers or computers to collect and store data, although there is no equivalent yet of an aircraft's 'black box' flight recorder. Anaesthetists have been noted to fail to record manually the extremes of blood pressure that are captured by automatic recorders.[32] The use of computers to record both data from monitors and other aspects of anaesthetic technique would be attractive, although the interface with the anaesthetist is often unsatisfactory in practice. A keyboard, touch-responsive screen, light pen, digitizing pad and voice recognition systems have all been tried.

See also Automated Anaesthetic Records. Kenny G. N. C. *Clin. Anaesthesiol.* 1990, **4**, 1.

MEDICO-LEGAL CONSIDERATIONS

In Britain, *criminal law* concerns offences prohibited by the state, has sanctions that punish and deter the offender, and does not compensate the victim (although the Criminal Injuries Compensation Board may do so). *Civil law* involves the private concerns of individuals and awards compensation to the victim that aims to restore him to the financial position he would otherwise have occupied. Criminal matters are rare in medical practice, although anaesthetists have been convicted of manslaughter, i.e. causing death by criminal neglect, but claims for civil offences ('torts'), usually negligence, are all too common. Criminal offences have to be proven 'beyond all reasonable doubt', but torts merely 'on the balance of probabilities'.

Negligence

To prove negligence, the plaintiff has to show that the doctor had a duty of care, that he breached that duty, and that the plaintiff has suffered damage as a result.

A duty of care exists whenever an anaesthetist acts professionally for a patient. Payment is irrelevant, although contract law may be invoked by a paying patient. The standard of care is more difficult to define. The principles have been established by the Bolam case: "the test (of negligence) is the test of the ordinary skilled man exercising and professing to have that special skill. A man need not possess the highest expert skill; it is well established law that it is sufficient if he exercises the ordinary skill of an ordinary competent man exercising that particular art".[33] A doctor is not liable for bad luck or necessarily for an error of judgement.

The conduct of an anaesthetist is often judged years later, but by the standards that prevailed at the time of the incident. His conduct should be that expected from colleagues of similar experience. A trainee is not expected to be as skilful as a senior consultant, although he is expected to know when to ask for help. Tasks should only be delegated to the competent and suitably trained. Any anaesthetist is expected to be thorough and diligent. The Health Authority may be liable if it "fails to provide doctors of sufficient skill and experience . . . if its organisation is at fault".[34] A defence must be able to muster 'a body of competent professional opinion' in support, even if it is in a minority. The trial judge is helped in his decision on these matters by 'expert witnesses' called by both sides.[35] The burden of proof is usually on the plaintiff unless the doctrine *res ipsa loquitur* (the thing speaks for itself) is invoked, in which case it is obvious, even to a layman, that negligence has occurred, and the burden of proof thus shifted to the doctor. EEC Council directive (90)482 may result in the EEC doctor having to prove in every case that he was not at fault. The plaintiff however would still have to establish the causative link between the anaesthetic and the harm done. This link is often disputed.

Note that the standards expected are effectively determined by one's colleagues in the guise of expert witnesses, and *not* by the legal profession. Very often these colleagues will sense 'there but for the Grace of God . . .'.

Damages

The causative link between the anaesthetist's negligence and the harm done to the plaintiff is usually easy to establish, and the judge (in the USA, the jury) has to set the level of damages or *quantum*. A common injury caused by anaesthetists is to patients' teeth.[36] This is often indefensible, but relatively inexpensive. Occasionally, when the patient's life is at risk because of inability to maintain the airway, maintenance of respiration takes absolute priority, and teeth or crowns may require removal to facilitate this. This may well not be negligent, but of course should be fully documented. At the other end of the scale is hypoxic brain damage or death. Damages have exceeded £1m in the UK, several times this in the USA. Health Authorities have met the cost of claims against their doctors working in NHS hospitals since 1990.

Consent[37]

Consent to treatment must be freely given after an opportunity for the patient to discuss the operation and anaesthetic. Anyone of 16 years or over and of sound mind may give valid consent. A patient who has been premedicated is unlikely to be able to do so. It is not considered necessary, or even always in the patient's best interest, to discuss all possible complications, however unlikely. Each case has to assessed on its own merits. There would be a duty to inform the patient of 'substantial risk of grave adverse consequences' unless there was 'some cogent clinical reason why the patient should not be informed'.[38] If this was the case it should be recorded in the notes. Consent forms are normally used, explained if necessary, and have been of value in subsequent litigation. *See* Health Circular (90)22 *A Guide to Consent for Examination and Treatment.*

Equipment

Under some circumstances the hospital or the manufacturer may be responsible for defects in anaesthetic equipment, although an EEC directive absolves manufacturers from product liability when an apparatus has been in use for 10 years. The anaesthetist should be familiar with his equipment, check it and be alert to the possibility of faults. He should not use equipment that may present a danger. He is responsible for informing management of the standards of monitoring and safety equipment that the profession consider a minimum, and the need for budgeting for their servicing and replacement.[39]

Product liability[40]

EEC directive 85/374 was implemented in 1988. The *producer* of a drug or anaesthetic equipment is liable for any defects and patient damage that ensues. Negligence does not have to be proved. In this context, the anaesthetist may become a 'producer' by mixing drugs before administration, or by such simple modifications to equipment as the bending of a needle to facilitate injection. Simple dilution of a drug (e.g. for paediatric use) according to the manufacturer's instructions does not make the anaesthetist a 'producer'. The implications of this have yet to be explored in case-law.

In practice

The potential for litigation should never be underestimated, nor should the stressful effect it can have upon the doctor. Much trouble may be avoided by: (*a*) *better communication* with the patient and relatives; (*b*) *careful preoperative assessment;* (*c*) *informing the patient of what to expect postoperatively*, e.g. temporary muscle weakness and numbness if a major regional block is to be given as well as general anaesthesia; the possibility of imperfect epidural blockade; presence of catheters, etc.; the use of a suppository of analgesic drug; an oxygen mask over the face; (*d*) *informing the patient of any special risks*, e.g. to fragile front teeth. He may wish to insure against damage to expensive dental work; (*e*) *keeping full, legible, contemporaneous and signed records*, particularly of any unusual events; (*f*) *compliance with the law on controlled drugs; and* (*g*) *dealing compassionately with any injury that the patient suffers*. An honest and full explanation should be given, with apologies and sympathy if appropriate. The anaesthetist however is not the correct person to judge negligence and liability, and it is unwise to admit these. The matter should be discussed with the surgeon. Expert help from a protection or defence organization should be sought as soon as possible.

Jehovah's Witnesses[41] and members of some other sects may wish to restrict some aspects of treatment, e.g. blood transfusion. The consequences of this should be explained fully in the presence of a witness. The patient should sign a statement of restriction, which should be countersigned by the witness. Special consent forms are available. An entry should also be made in the notes. With a child, his own best interests normally take priority over the wishes of his parents. Special legal procedures may be undertaken for his protection.

It may be unwise to ignore recommendations from an authoritative source, even though the individual anaesthetist may disagree, e.g. the 1986 letter from the Committee on Safety of Medicines stated that unexplained jaundice or pyrexia following exposure to halothane is 'an absolute contra-indication' to its future use in that patient.

The anaesthetist must know the exact operation that is planned on each patient. It is the surgeon's duty to decide this. It is the duty of the anaesthetist to encourage the surgeon when indicated, but also to warn him of possible dangers. If further pre-operative treatment would be beneficial to the patient and yet such warnings are ignored, it may be necessary to refuse to administer an anaesthetic, or refer the case to an experienced colleague.

Patient identification requires a clearly defined system, discipline and vigilance.[42] A patient may give the wrong name and agree to the wrong operation. The very old, the very young and the mentally ill may be unable to verify these details at all. Beware: (*a*) too much haste; (*b*) too much work; (*c*) too little rest for the anaesthetist; and (*d*) changes in the operating list.

For some legal aspects of anaesthesia in the UK: *see* Palmer R. N. In: *Hazards and Complications of Anaesthesia* (Taylor T. H. and Major E. ed.) Edinburgh: Churchill Livingstone, 1987, 511; Rosen M. and Horton J. N. In: *Medical Negligence* (Powers M. J. and Harris N. H. ed.) London: Butterworths, 1990, 586. In the USA: Cheney F. W. et al. *JAMA* 1989, **261**, 1599. For the implications of 'no-fault compensation' for anaesthesia, *see* Gibbs J. M. *Br. J. Anaesth.* 1987, **59**, 865. For the legal position of a doctor who overrides a computer system, *see* deDombal F. T. *J. Med. Ethics* 1987, **13**, 179.

Deaths associated with anaesthesia[43]

In England and Wales, deaths are normally reported to HM Coroner (in Scotland to the Procurator Fiscal) if the death: (1) occurs during an operation, or before recovery from an anaesthetic; (2) was sudden or unexplained; or (3) may have been caused by neglect, violence, poisoning, abortion or industrial injury or disease.

The sick anaesthetist

Anaesthetists are particularly prone to drug, alcohol and vapour abuse. In England, after a patient died in theatre while under the care of an anaesthetist who was an addict, a procedure was adopted in the NHS to try to protect patients from ill doctors. This is the 'Three Wise Men' approach, as detailed in HC(82)13 *'Prevention of harm to patients resulting from physical or mental disability of hospital or community medical or dental staff'*. The Association of Anaesthetists in London has set up a voluntary scheme to help sick colleagues. The Royal College of Anaesthetists has set up a parallel scheme to examine the question of competence to practise. (*See* Appendix for addresses.) The General Medical Council may act if the doctor refuses to take advice.

Data Protection Act

Those who use computers and word processors to keep information on patients' health should register as such under this act. Data held only for accounting purposes is generally exempt. Patients may then have restricted access to their medical records held in computers, but not to information that is used solely for research and will be published in a form that does not identify the patient. Access is restricted if it might damage the patient's health, harm anyone else or lead to the identification of other patients. Similarly, patients may have access to any of their non-computerized health records written after November 1991, and request correction of any inaccuracies.

AUDIT

Medical audit[44] is the process by which doctors collectively review, evaluate and improve their practice in the context of prescribed targets and standards: a systematic, critical analysis of the quality of medical care. It also impinges on resource provision and financial audit. It is now an important component of all medical practice, a professional obligation, and is educational, not disciplinary. Regular audit will be a condition for hospital accreditation[45] in the UK for training in most specialities, including surgery and anaesthesia. The Audit Commission became responsible for auditing the NHS in 1990. Health Circular (91)2 outlines the arrangements for audit mandatory in UK hospitals from 1991. The Professional Standards Review Organisation in the USA was legislated in 1972.

See also Shaw C. *Medical Audit – a hospital handbook*. London: King's Fund Centre, 1989; Secker-Walker J. In: *Anaesthesia Review 8* (Kaufman L. ed.) Edinburgh: Churchill Livingstone, 1991, 211.

Historical development

Government has attempted to regulate medicine from time immemorial. Doctors have realized that it is both more effective and to their advantage to do it themselves. 'The price of clinical freedom is eternal professional vigilance.' The 1518 charter of the Royal College of Physicians states that one of the College's functions is to uphold the standards of medicine 'both for their own honour and in the name of the public benefit'. Although outcome studies of particular operations had been published in the late 19th century,[46] the first systematic attempt to link outcome with the care in hospital was associated with the establishment of the American College of Surgeons in Illinois in 1912.[47] Some early results were so shocking that they were incinerated!

Anaesthetists have a strong record. The first large-scale survey was of 599 548 anaesthetics administered over 5 years in 10 teaching hospitals in the USA, with annual feedback of results to participating hospitals.[48] It recognized that anaesthesia, surgical care and intercurrent disease were inextricably linked. Mortality related to anaesthesia was 1 in 1560. Another important large survey at that time was of 10 098 spinal anaesthetics with no long-term neurological sequelae.[49] The CEPOD report was published in 1987 (*see below*).

Methods of audit

Audit is a cyclical process: current practice is observed; standards of practice are set; the results of current practice are compared with these standards; change is implemented; practice is observed again, and so on.

Time and resources, especially computing facilities[50] are essential. The 1989 White Paper[51] has been a useful stimulus. The Department of Health has set up a Medical Audit Co-ordinator in each Unit or District assisted by a sub-committee.[52] The Royal Colleges have convened audit committees.[53] Those responsible for inspecting facilities in hospitals that train junior medical staff will require regular audit of clinical work. In North America financial motives have also driven the audit process. Remuneration and even the right to practice may depend on satisfactory outcome.

There is a wide choice of outcomes of practice that may be observed, e.g. questionnaires of patient satisfaction, administrative data (e.g. hospital stay), studies of morbidity from complications of anaesthesia, surgical mortality. Bias is common in morbidity studies; death is an easily definable end-point. Sometimes one unexpected death may trigger a comprehensive review of patient care. Audit of the anaesthetist's involvement in obstetrics, intensive therapy and the treatment of chronic pain presents particular problems. Many comparisons of general and regional techniques have been made.[54] The reporting of 'critical incidents' (events which if uncorrected would lead to harm) are popular with some as it avoids the malpractice implications raised by some morbidity or mortality studies.[55]

Results of recent audit

Although methods vary widely, some have suggested that mortality associated with anaesthesia is falling.[56] In 1982[57] the widely-quoted figure was published of 1 death (occurring up to 6 days postoperatively) solely attributable to anaesthesia in 10000 operations in the UK.

The CEPOD report of 1987

A crucial innovation in this enquiry[6] was that both surgery and anaesthesia were audited together. It examined 4034 deaths that occurred up to 30 days postoperatively in 3 English regions over 1 year. Some half a million operations were performed in this time. Although anaesthesia, together with surgery and intercurrent disease, *contributed* to death after 1 in 1300 operations, only 3 deaths, or about 1 in 185000 operations, were *solely* due to anaesthesia.

Deficiencies were revealed (mainly related to the surgery) that were important because they were correctable, e.g. inadequate supervision of trainees; inadequate communication with superiors, especially for emergency or urgent operations; and poor results of surgeons operating in specialist areas outside their sphere of expertise. Of the operations resulting in death, 10% were considered unnecessary or unjustified. In 13.9% of cases, anaesthetists said they had been dissatisfied with the preparation of the patient for surgery and yet were persuaded to go ahead.

Recommendations included (a) clinical audit, both locally and nationally, and employers should allow time and resources for this; (b) time is well-spent preparing the patient for surgery; and (c) decisions whether to operate or not (especially on the sick or elderly) need to be taken at a senior level.

CEPOD was expanded in 1989 to a national enquiry (NCEPOD).[58]

CEPOD introduced four useful categories of surgical priority, which will help standardize the nomenclature in future surveys: *emergency* = should take place within 1 hour; *urgent* = within 24 hours; *scheduled* = within 1 to 3 weeks; *elective* = anytime.

Other reports

Surveys in other countries will naturally give different figures, e.g. in *New South Wales* mortality due to anaesthesia was 1 in 5 500 in the year 1960, but less than 1 in 26 000 in 1984.[59] The clinical problems are similar: inadequate pre-operative preparation of the patient, misplaced tracheal tubes and circuit misconnections. A 10-year analysis of accidents in *Holland* identified carelessness, lack of vigilance and failure to check as important problems.[60] A prospective survey in France has shown a similar mortality to the UK,[61] and a very low mortality (1 in 40 000) in children.[62]

Audit of other disciplines is of direct interest to anaesthetists. Centralization of *trauma care* into Trauma Centers in the USA has been shown to improve outcome.[63] A large British series, where such centres of excellence hardly exist, has shown that up to 33% of trauma deaths may be preventable.[64] The *Confidential Enquiry into Maternal Deaths* is run jointly between the Department of Health and the Royal College of Obstetricians and Gynaecologists and began in 1952. Anaesthetic assessors are involved in this enquiry.

Important results have come from studies of the legal consequences of anaesthetic complications, despite the uncontrolled method of patient selection. Data from death certificates and inquests were used to examine deaths in the *dental surgery*.[65] Although general anaesthesia in this situation is now used less, the risk of death was about 4 times greater with operator anaesthesia. Analysis of 348 cases of *death and brain damage* reported to the Medical Defence Union between 1970 and 1977 showed that two-thirds were caused by human error.[66] All claims from 1974 to 1983 made against anaesthetists in the Medical Protection Society have also been summarized.[67] The *closed insurance claims study* in the USA has been of particular importance.[68] Analysis of 1175 such claims showed that nearly a third might have been prevented by monitors of O_2 saturation and respired CO_2.[22] The commonest injury was due to problems with hypoventilation and intubation.[69] Closed claims relating to 14 cardiac arrests during *spinal analgesia*[70] showed how easy it is to give too much sedation and that α-agonists and postural change are the most effective treatment of sympathetic blockade. Six of these patients died and only one of the survivors could return to independent self-care.

See also Lunn J. N. (ed.) *Epidemiology in Anaesthesia* London: Arnold, 1986; Holland R. B. and Paull J. D. *Anaesth. Intensive Care* 1988, **16**, 92. For the audit of the activities of a district-wide anaesthetic department, *see* Verma R. *Anaesthesia* 1991, **46**, 143.

References

1. Hewitt F. W. *Practitioner* 1896, **57**, 347.
2. Buxton D. W. *Br. Med. J.* 1901, **i**, 1007.
3. Cooper J. B. *Can. J. Anaesth.* 1988, **35**, 287.
4. Cooper J. B. and Pierce E. C. *Anesth. Patient Safety Foundation Newslett.* 1986, **1**, 1.
5. Runciman W. B. *Anaesth. Intensive Care* 1988, **16**, 114.
6. Buck N. et al. *Report of the Confidential Enquiry into Perioperative Deaths.* London: Nuffield Provincial Hospitals Trust and the Kings Fund for Hospitals, 1987; Lunn J. N. and Devlin H. B. *Lancet* 1987, **ii**, 1384; Morgan M. *Anaesthesia* 1988, **43**, 91.
7. Good M. L. *Anaesthesia* 1990, **45**, 525; Schwid H. A. and O'Donnell D. *Anesthesiology* 1990, **72**, 191.
8. Miller P. L. *Anesthesiology* 1983, **58**, 362.
9. Gaba D. M. and Deanda A. *Anesthesiology* 1988, **69**, 387.
10. Weinger M. B. and Englund C. E. *Anesthesiology* 1990, **73**, 995.
11. Dyer C. *Br. Med. J.* 1988, **297**, 938.
12. Parker J. B. R. *Can. J. Anaesth.* 1987, **34**, 489; Bartle E. J. et al. *Surgery* 1988, **104**, 311.
13. Yerkes R. M. and Dobson J. D. *J. Compar. Neurol. Psychol.* 1908, **18**, 459.
14. Allnutt M. F. *Br. J. Anaesth.* 1987, **59**, 856.
15. Gaba D. M. et al. *Anesthesiology* 1987, **66**, 670.
16. Charlton J. E. *Anaesthesia* 1990, **45**, 425; *Checklists for Anaesthetic Machines.* London: Association of Anaesthetists, 1990.
17. Bruner J. M. and Leonard P. F. *Electricity, Safety and the Patient.* Chicago: Year Book Medical Publishers, 1990; Moyle J. T. B. In: *Anaesthesia Review 7.* (Kaufman L. ed.) Edinburgh: Churchill Livingstone 1990, 75.
18. Hull C. J. *Br. J. Anaesth.* 1989, **62**, 587.
19. In the USA, Eichhorn J. H. et al. *JAMA* 1986, **256**, 1017; *Anesth. Patient Safety Foundation Newslett.* 1987, **2**, 3; In Australia, Cass N. M. et al. *Anaesth. Intensive Care* 1988, **16**, 110; In the UK, *Recommendation for Standards of Monitoring during Anaesthesia and Recovery.* London: Association of Anaesthetists, 1988; Winter A. and Spence A. A. *Br. J. Anaesth.* 1990, **64**, 263.
20. American Society of Anesthesiologists. *Newsletter* 1990, **54**, 17.
21. Eichhorn J. H. *Anesthesiology* 1989, **70**, 572.
22. Tinker J. H. et al. *Anesthesiology* 1989, **71**, 541.
23. McDonald J. S. et al. *Br. J. Anaesth.* 1990, **64**, 582.
24. Orkin F. K. *Anesthesiology* 1989, **70**, 567.
25. Jones J. G. et al. *Anaesthesia* 1990, **45**, 563.
26. Beecher H. K. *Surg. Gynecol. Obstet.* 1940, **71**, 689.
27. Waters R. M. *J. Indiana St. Med. Assoc.* 1936, **29**, 110.
28. Westhorpe R. *Anaesth. Intensive Care* 1989, **17**, 250.
29. Nosworthy M. *Curr. Res. Anesth. Analg.* 1945, **24**, 221; *St. Thomas' Hosp. Rep. (London)* 1937, **2**, 54; Nosworthy M. D. *Anaesthesia* 1963, **18**, 209.
30. Gravenstein J. S. *J. Clin. Monit.* 1989, **5**, 256.
31. Slogoff S. and Keats A. S. *Anesthesiology* 1985, **62**, 107.
32. Cook R. I. et al. *Anesthesiology* 1989, **71**, 385.
33. Bolam v Friern Hospital Management Committee 1957, *2 All ER* 118.
34. Wilsher v Essex Health Authority 1986, *3 All ER* 801; HL *1 All ER* 871.
35. *Medico-Legal Reports. Appearing in Court.* London: Medical Protection Society, 1989.
36. Clokie C. et al. *Can. J. Anaesth.* 1989, **36**, 675; Boswell D. E. et al. *J. Med. Defence Union* 1990, **6**, 14.
37. Palmer R. N. *Anaesthesia* 1987, **43**, 265; *Consent. Confidentiality. Disclosure of Medical Records.* London: Medical Protection Society, 1988.
38. Sidaway v Bethlem Royal Hospital Governors and others. *1 All ER* 643 HL.
39. Schofield N. McC. *Anaesthesia* 1989, **43**, 883.

40. *Product Liability*. London: Medical Defence Union, 1989.
41. Benson K. T. *Anesth. Analg.* 1989, **69**, 647.
42. *Theatre Safeguards*. Medical Defence Societies and Royal College of Nursing, 1986.
43. Bacon A. K. *Anaesthesia* 1989, **44**, 245.
44. Hopkins A. *Measuring the Quality of Medical Care*. London: Royal College of Physicians, 1990; Devlin H. B. In: *Some Aspects of Anaesthetic Safety*. (Dinnick O. P. and Thompson P. W. ed.) *Clin. Anaesthesiol.* 1988, **2**(2), 299.
45. Baldock G. J. *Anaesthesia* 1990, **45**, 617.
46. Haidenthaller J. *Arch. Klinische Chir.* 1890, **40**, 493; Bassini E. *Arch. Klinische Chir.* 1894, **47**, 1.
47. Codman E. A. *Surg. Gynecol. Obstet.* 1914, **18**, 491.
48. Beecher H. K. and Todd D. P. *Ann. Surg.* 1954, **140**, 2.
49. Dripps R. D. and Vandam L. D. *J. Am. Med. Assoc.* 1954, **156**, 1486.
50. Ellis B. W. et al. *J. Roy. Soc. Med.* 1987, **80**, 157; Dunn D. C. *Br. Med. J.* 1988, **296**, 687; Tyndall R. et al. *Computers in Medical Audit*. London: Royal Society of Medicine, 1990.
51. White Paper: *Working for Patients – Caring for the 1990's*. London: HMSO, 1989.
52. Report of the Standing Medical Advisory Committee of the Department of Health: *The Quality of Medical Care*. London: HMSO, 1990.
53. *Guidelines to Clinical Audit in Surgical Practice* London: Royal College of Surgeons, 1989; *Medical Audit* London: Royal College of Physicians, 1989.
54. Scott N. B. and Kehlet H. *Br. J. Surg.* 1988, **75**, 299.
55. Currie M. *Anaesth. Intensive Care* 1989, **17**, 403.
56. Edwards G. et al. *Anaesthesia* 1956, **11**, 194; Dinnick O. P. *Anaesthesia* 1964, **19**, 536; Derrington M. C. and Smith G. *Br. J. Anaesth.* 1987, **59**, 815.
57. Lunn J. N. and Mushin W. W. *Mortality Associated with Anaesthesia*. London: Nuffield Provincial Hospitals Trust, 1982.
58. Campling E. A. et al. *Report of the National Confidential Enquiry into Perioperative Deaths*. London: Royal College of Surgeons of England, 1989.
59. Holland R. *Br. J. Anaesth.* 1987, **59**, 834.
60. Chopra V. et al. *Anaesthesia* 1990, **45**, 3.
61. Tiret L. and Hatton F. *Can. Anaesth. Soc. J.* 1986, **33**, 336.
62. Tiret L. et al. *Br. J. Anaesth.* 1988, **61**, 263.
63. Trunkey D. D. *Arch. Emerg. Med.* 1985, **2**, 181.
64. Anderson I. D. et al. *Br. Med. J.* 1988, **296**, 1305.
65. Coplans M. P. and Curson I. *Br. Dental J.* 1982, **153**, 357.
66. Utting J. E. et al. *Can. Anaesth. Soc. J.* 1979, **26**, 472.
67. Green R. A. In: *Anaesthesia Review 4*. (Kaufman L. ed.) Edinburgh: Churchill Livingstone, 1987, 147.
68. Keats A. S. *Anesthesiology* 1990, **73**, 199.
69. Caplan R. A. et al. *Anesthesiology* 1990, **72**, 828.
70. Caplan R. A. et al. *Anesthesiology* 1988, **68**, 5.

Section 3
CHOICE OF ANAESTHETIC

Chapter 20

Medical diseases influencing anaesthesia

Anaesthesia is now a very safe procedure in the fit healthy patient. The risk is increased when systemic disease is present.[1] The Confidential Enquiry into Perioperative Deaths (CEPOD)[2] examined 4034 deaths in 1986 occurring up to 30 days after some half a million operations in three regions of England. Only 3 deaths (1 in 185 000 operations) were attributed *solely* to anaesthesia, although it was considered a *contributing factor* to about 1 death in 1300 operations.

The anaesthetist's responsibility is to recognize risk factors and to advise surgeons and others that they should be corrected before elective surgery. The anaesthetist may be asked to help in this process if he has the time and facilities. This is more important in the case of emergency surgery where time is short and speedy correction is necessary. If the patient asks about risk, the anaesthetist must give an accurate and honest answer and therefore needs current morbidity and mortality figures at his disposal.[3] It is not the anaesthetist's responsibility to push prognostic data at a patient who does not ask to know them. *Common sense is an invaluable tool in these situations.*

Any such assessment of risk may suggest the need for invasive preoperative monitoring to measure extent of dysfunction, especially in the elderly.[4]

THE GERIATRIC PATIENT

The Age Anaesthesia Association in the UK was founded in 1987.

Assessment of risk in the elderly patient

There may be a difference between chronological and biological ages, e.g. a 90-year-old may appear as healthy and resilient as many 70-year-olds. The surgical team need to assess the operative risk and whether the operation should be postponed for medical treatment to improve the patient. Even the over-90s may present a relatively small risk.[5]

The elderly patient presents two sets of problems.

1. An increased incidence of concurrent diseases.

These may be multiple, for which he may be taking many drugs. The pathology may be 'hidden', e.g. painless peritonitis, apyrexial septicaemia, silent myocardial infarction, hence the need for minimum routine tests of full blood count, urinalysis, urea and electrolytes, chest X-ray and ECG. In one series only 13.5% of patients over 65 years had normal cardiorespiratory function.[4]

2. Altered pathophysiology[6]

General. Slower mental and physical recovery from trauma or surgery. Slower wound healing, weaker tissues, tendency to bedsores. Fragile skin and veins. Many physiological capacities reduce by 1% per year over the age of 40. Muscle weakness is common with the need for lower doses of relaxants.

Poor adaptation to hospital diet. Malnutrition, e.g. relative starvation, obesity, anaemia, vitamin deficiency, hypoproteinaemia. Osteoporosis, loss of teeth and jaw substance. Osteoarthritis and Paget's disease are common.

Slower metabolic rate, making it easier to hyperventilate. Cerebral vessels still react to a lowered Pco_2 which severely decreases brain perfusion.

Nervous system. Poor memory for recent events, making history-taking difficult. (Memory assessment by the Camden Scale: what is your name? when were you born? where do you live now? who is the reigning monarch? who is the prime minister? what is the date/day of the week today?) Less ability to 'process' data. Confusion resulting from the upheaval of hospital admission.

Deafness, especially high tones, with resulting difficulty in communication. Less elasticity of lens of eye.

Neurones are lost at up to 50 000 per day, especially in some areas, e.g. neocortex, spinal motor neurones. Nerve conduction is slowed. Pain threshold is increased. Autonomic function impaired: postural hypotension, less homeostasis in temperature control, tendency to urinary retention and constipation (exacerbated by anticholinergics and opioids).

Cardiovascular. Less elastic arteries with a rise in arterial pressure, especially systolic. Less homeostasis of vascular pressures, and intolerance to hypotension. Lowered blood volume, stroke volume and cardiac index (by 1% per year over 40). Longer circulation time. Haemoglobin slightly lower. A-V conduction blocks and arrhythmias more common. Reduced vascular stability is a particular problem during spinal or epidural analgesia.

Respiratory. Vital capacity drops, residual volume rises with age. Closing volume rises and may exceed functional residual capacity. Less elastic recoil of lungs. Ventilation-perfusion mismatch results in a lowered Pao_2. Laryngeal sensitivity is reduced and silent aspiration of gastric contents can occur. Auscultation of the lungs is much less likely to reveal existing pathology than in the young, and radiology therefore more valuable.

Body fluids. Glomerular filtration rate declines 1% per year after 40 years. Slight rises in urea (up to 10 mmol/l) and creatinine (up to 160 μmol/l). Reduced body water. Water excretion and conservation less efficient. Patients with fractured neck of femur are often dehydrated.

Pre- and Postoperative Sedation

Old people may become confused. Common causes are cerebral hypoxia due to cardiorespiratory abnormality, and deafness. Sedatives will make this worse. To produce sleep, alcohol is useful for those accustomed to it, or benzodiazepines. Hyoscine is best avoided.

Anaesthesia

There is a linear reduction in anaesthetic requirements with age.[7] MAC is reduced by 20% at 70 years. Renal and hepatic excretion of drugs is slower. Protein binding and volumes of distribution often altered. Intravenous agents are well tolerated as a rule, if dosage is kept low and they are given slowly. Etomidate is useful because it tends not to lower arterial pressure. Non-depolarizing relaxants are not as well reversed in the elderly (especially if hypothermic).

Early postoperative ambulation is usually desirable to prevent venous thrombosis, while rapid recovery of the cough reflex helps prevent postoperative atelectasis. A common cause of death is pulmonary embolism.

In old people with emphysema, general anaesthesia, maintaining spontaneous respiration, has given good results and for abdominal surgery thiopentone, nitrous oxide and oxygen may be combined with small doses of relaxants and volatile agents. Good speedy operating is useful at all times and is especially valuable in the elderly. Postoperative hypoxaemia increases with age. Oxygen therapy usually corrects this, and is given routinely until the patient has a good Sao_2 on room air (hours or days if needed).

Extra- and intra-dural analgesia is often suitable for operations below the umbilicus, but vascular instability is a risk. For the use of local analgesia in the elderly *see* Kaye K. W. *Clin. Geriatr. Med.* 1990, **6**, 85.

See also Craig D. B. et al. *Can. J. Anaesth.* 1987, **34**, 156; *Anaesthesia and the Aged Patient.* (Davenport H. T. ed.) Oxford: Blackwell, 1988; *Anesthesia in the Geriatric Patient. Int. Anesthesiol. Clin.* 1988, **26(2)**; Jones R. M. *Anaesthesia* 1989, **44**, 377; Ward R. M. and Hutton P. *Br. Med. Bull.* 1990, **46**, 156.

PREGNANCY

Spontaneous abortion or premature labour may result following general anaesthesia for surgical conditions unconnected with pregnancy, but these risks diminish with gestational age. The incidence of fetal abnormalities is not increased.[8] Ideally, surgery should be postponed until 6 weeks post-partum. If this is not possible, the second trimester is satisfactory. If anaesthesia is necessary in an emergency, it should be remembered that in the last two trimesters the $Paco_2$ is normally 4 kPa (30 mmHg), and that both cardiac output and blood volume are increased.

Threatened premature labour may be controlled by selective β_2-adrenergic agonists, salbutamol or ritodrine. Their side-effects include dysrhythmias, increased secretion of insulin, and pulmonary oedema.

The lower oesophageal sphincter becomes increasingly incompetent throughout pregnancy,[9] and returns to normal 1–2 days postpartum. Even in early pregnancy opiate premedicants are best avoided, and from the second trimester onwards consideration must be given to intubation to protect against aspiration. In a pregnancy of over 16 weeks aorto-caval compression syndrome can more than halve the maternal cardiac output and cause fetal asphyxia. Whether regional block or general anaesthesia is undertaken, such patients should be anaesthetized in the lateral position or with a wedge under the right side.[10] The reduction in plasma proteins can increase the toxicity of local anaesthetics.

Anaesthetics are not teratogenic in clinical practice, even nitrous oxide, which has a known effect on nucleic acid synthesis.[11] If the latter is used in very early pregnancy it may be wise to administer folinic acid, 20 mg orally 12 hours and 1 hour pre-operatively.[12] Some drugs are known teratogens, e.g. thalidomide, anti-cancer agents. Some can harm the fetus in a variety of other ways, e.g. steroids, antithyroid drugs, warfarin in late pregnancy, tetracycline, streptomycin, sulphonamides. Others, e.g. all narcotics, sedatives and anaesthetics cross into breast milk. Diazepam and coumarin anticoagulants present the main problems in this regard. The pH of milk is lower than that of plasma, and drugs that are weak bases can reach high concentrations.

For Obstetric Anaesthesia, *see* Chapter 22.

See also Surgical anaesthesia for the pregnant patient. Finster M. *Can. J. Anaesth.* 1988, **35**, S14; Steinberg E. S. and Santos A. C. *Int. Anesthesiol. Clin.* 1990, **28**, 58.

HIATUS HERNIA

This abnormality, often unsuspected, may result in regurgitation during induction or maintenance of anaesthesia, most commonly in middle-aged obese patients or those in late pregnancy. Such patients tend to have a reduced 'barrier pressure' (pressure differential between the lower oesophageal sphincter and stomach).

Hiatus hernia is suggested by retrosternal pain, burning or reflux into the pharynx induced by gravity. The anaesthetist should treat such patients as suffering from acute intestinal obstruction to reduce the likelihood of regurgitation and aspiration. Pre-operative administration of an H_2 antagonist (ranitidine 150 mg orally, 50 mg i.m.) or antacid (0.3 M sodium citrate, 15–30 ml) may be helpful. Metoclopramide 10 mg can be given to increase lower oesophageal sphincter tone.

CARDIOVASCULAR DISEASE

Anaesthesia may affect the heart:

1. By altering the heart rate or rhythm.[13] Dysrhythmias can be alarming even in a fit athlete.[14]

2. By directly depressing myocardial function and ardiac output.
3. If vasodilatation occurs with a relatively fixed cardiac output (valvular stenosis, constrictive pericarditis) then hypotension will be profound.
4. As a result of hypoxia and hypercapnia.

Patients with organic heart disease who compensate sufficiently to carry on their daily jobs usually tolerate anaesthesia well, provided it is carefully administered and overdosage, hypoxia, hypercapnia and hypotension avoided. Attention should be paid to the heart rate. Above 100 beats/min, the shortened diastolic interval reduces coronary perfusion time.

The following cardiovascular conditions should be detected before anaesthesia as they may lead to sudden death, especially if hypoxia or sudden alteration in the blood pressure should occur: (1) recent cardiac infarction; (2) aortic stenosis; (3) aortic reflux and aortitis involving the coronary ostia; (4) heart block with Stokes-Adams attacks; and (5) untreated hypertension.

If the cardiac output is low, suxamethonium takes longer to act (up to 2 min) and should be given in larger doses (e.g. 100 mg or more) before intubation. In the digitalized patient arrhythmias may occur following suxamethonium.

Postoperative congestive heart failure may be difficult to diagnose and can present with orthopnoea, raised venous pressure, triple rhythm or atrial fibrillation.

Cardiac risk factors

In the Goldman index[15] scores are given to the following: third sound or gallop rhythm (11); any dysrhythmia (7); age over 70 years (5); myocardial infarction within last 6 months (10); 5 or more ventricular ectopic beats per min (7); emergency surgery (4); aortic stenosis (3); abdominal or thoracic operation (3); poor general condition (3). A total over 13 gives a poor prognosis (11% life-threatening complications). The opinion of a cardiologist is advisable. Above 26, perioperative mortality is over 50%. Some have found angina, hypertension and prolonged surgery to be poor prognostic signs,[16] similarly heart failure and poor ventricular function.[17]

See also Mangano D. T. Perioperative cardiac morbidity *Anesthesiology* 1990, **72**, 153.

1. Coronary artery disease

Pre-operative assessment. Up to 15% of these patients have no abnormalities on routine examination or on their resting ECG. An exercise ECG (the changes in the ST segment relative to increase in heart rate)[18] is more sensitive. Echocardiography gives useful non-invasive information on myocardial function. Nuclear imaging of the ventricles and coronary perfusion,[19] and coronary angiography are little used before most non-cardiac surgery, although the risk of such surgery has been reduced by prior coronary artery bypass in some series.[20] Overall risk of the two operations may well be higher though. Drug therapy for angina, heart failure or hypertension should not be stopped before surgery.

Management. Intensive monitoring can reduce the incidence of cardiac complications[21] but the risk of infarction persists for up to a week after operation. Transoesophageal 2-D echocardiography is very expensive but probably the best technique for detecting abnormalities of heart wall motion and thus intraoperative ischaemia.[22] Control of dysrhythmias and cardiac failure are required in addition to good analgesia. A turbulent induction should be avoided. A balance of myocardial oxygen supply and demand must be struck with a diastolic blood pressure high enough to allow adequate coronary flow and a systolic pressure below a value that unduly increases cardiac work. There must be full oxygenation and an adequate haemoglobin level.

Careful haemodynamic control and prevention of intraoperative ischaemia can reduce postoperative infarction.[23] Nifedipine and glyceryl trinitrate are useful coronary vasodilators. Nitrates, nifedipine and nitroprusside reduce afterload and control postoperative hypertension. Tachycardia and hypertension, due for example to laryngoscopy, atropine or inadequate analgesia, may decrease coronary filling by shortening diastole. The use of opiates or β-blockade may be needed. The short action of esmolol may be particularly useful. Some workers use the cardiac rate–systolic pressure product as a rough index of myocardial oxygen demand (upper acceptable limit 20 000 in normal patients, 12 000 in those with coronary disease). Halothane is well tolerated in patients with myocardial ischaemia who are not in failure and have good ventricular function.[24] Isoflurane is a coronary vasodilator.[25] In about a quarter of patients[26] with coronary disease the anatomic pattern of abnormalities may allow isoflurane to 'steal' coronary blood from the diseased areas, but other evidence suggests that it can also lessen ischaemic damage in the myocardium.[27]

Haemodynamic stability and oxygenation should be ensured in the postoperative period. Obstructive sleep apnoea may cause large drops in oxygen saturation and myocardial ischaemia.[28]

See also Reiz S. *Br. J. Anaesth.* 1988, **61**, 68; Prys-Roberts C. *Br. J. Anaesth.* 1988, **61**, 85; Mangano D. T. *Anesthesiology* 1989, **70**, 175; Griffin R. M. In: *Anaesthesia Review 6* (Kaufman L. ed.) Edinburgh: Churchill Livingstone, 1989.

2. Cardiac infarction

First pre-mortem diagnosis by Adam Hammer (1818–1878) in 1878,[29] and classic description by W. P. Obrastow in 1910[30] and J. B. Herrick (1861–1954) in 1912.[31] Operation within 3 months of cardiac infarction carries a 25–50% risk of reinfarction, most likely to occur on the third postoperative day. Operation 3–6 months after infarction carries a 10–25% risk of reinfarction, reducing to about 5% for operation 6 months or more after infarction. Upper abdominal and thoracic operations carry the highest risk. The incidence is not related to the type of general anaesthetic used. These considerable risks must be balanced against those of not undertaking the proposed operation. Some consider the degree of ventricular impairment to be a more important prognostic factor than the presence of recent infarction.[32] Occasionally a treatable cause of myocardial infarction may be found, e.g. polycythaemia.

For perioperative infarction, *see* Haagensen R. and Steen P. A. *Br. J. Anaesth.* 1988, **61**, 24; For acute myocardial infarction, *see* Chapter 29.

3. Hypertension

Some problems of anaesthesia in the hypertensive patient: greater rise in blood pressure in response to stress, sympathetic stimuli and to some drugs; atheroma and thrombosis in the coronary and cerebral vessels; associated renal failure; the left ventricle is hypertrophied, stiff and needs a high filling pressure and reasonable time for filling; sensitivity to nodal rhythm; tendency to hypotension, especially after epidural block. The blood volume is reduced in untreated hypertensives.

Pre-operative Assessment. Treatable causes of hypertension should be sought (endocrine, renal, coarctation, etc.), as should secondary effects of hypertension on the heart (ischaemia, hypertrophy, failure), brain (ischaemia), kidneys (uraemia) and the eyes. Assessment will include chest X-ray and ECG. Medication is continued up to the time of surgery. If untreated, operation is delayed if possible to allow adequate control of blood pressure. The patient who is hypertensive due to anxiety presents a similar risk to the known hypertensive.[33] Even a single dose of clonidine or a β-blocker may be helpful. A diastolic pressure over 115 mmHg constitutes a serious risk.[34]

Management. Most moderately hypertensive patients present few problems provided care is taken with the maintenance of blood pressure and flow to coronary, cerebral and renal circulations. Normal autoregulation may be diminished. Minimal doses of anaesthetic agents are indicated. An excessive fall in blood pressure after induction can be minimized by infusion of fluids. Tracheal intubation may raise the blood pressure greatly, especially the systolic value and cause myocardial ischaemia and arrhythmias. This can be reduced by prior administration of opiates or β-blockers (e.g. atenolol 25–50 mg orally the evening before the operation). Most different anaesthetic techniques have been used successfully. Ketamine can increase cardiac work dangerously. Hypertensive patients react badly to rapid changes of posture.

Postoperatively. Severe rises of blood pressure may occur in response to pain or a full bladder. Even a small haemorrhage may cause severe hypotension. *See also* Prys-Roberts C. *Br. J. Anaesth.* 1984, **56**, 711.

4. Cardiac failure

These cases present serious risks. Diagnosis of the cause and vigorous pre-operative treatment are required. Many anaesthetic agents make cardiac failure worse, whereas opioids, benzodiazepines and phenothiazine premedicants are well tolerated. Local analgesic techniques are sometimes preferred. If operation cannot be delayed and general anaesthesia is necessary, the following points should be borne in mind: (*a*) the tachycardia normally seen on induction may be absent in these cases. Transient asystole is sometimes seen after suxamethonium. Atropine reduces this possibility; (*b*) pulmonary oedema increases respiratory work, so paralysis and IPPV may be indicated.

Nitrous oxide (one of the safest agents in this condition) may then be sufficient for analgesia; (*c*) ketamine, while maintaining blood pressure, increases left ventricular work and myocardial oxygen demand; (*d*) invasive monitoring of RA and LA pressures may be needed, which should be kept as high as the pre-operative values; and (*e*) inotropes, e.g. dopamine 5–15 µg/kg/min, and the reduction of afterload with vasodilators may be needed to maintain cardiac output. *See above* for assessment of coronary artery disease.

5. Heart block

A term introduced by W. H. Gaskell (1847–1914), first described in 1691 by Gerbezius. Stokes-Adams attacks described by W. M. Stokes (1804–1878)[35] and R. Adams (1791-1875).[36]

The block may be congenital or due to ischaemia, valvular disease, previous cardiac surgery, myocarditis. *Right bundle branch block* may be of little significance, whereas *left bundle branch block* usually indicates significant cardiac disease. *Bifascicular block* of the right bundle and the anterior fascicle of the left is less hazardous than once thought, unless it is symptomatic.

First-degree block is a lengthening of the PR interval to more than 0.2 s. *Second-degree block* has missed beats with a normal PR interval (Möbitz type II) or a progressively lengthening PR interval (Wenckebach). Wenckebach is more benign and usually responds to atropine or isoprenaline. A pacemaker is not usually needed unless there are Stokes-Adams attacks or cardiac failure. Möbitz type II may progress to third-degree or complete block under anaesthesia.

In *complete block* the idioventricular rate is about 35 beats/min, and hypotension usually occurs. The cardiac output is relatively fixed. In either Möbitz type II or complete heart block, general anaesthesia is seldom indicated until a pacemaker has been inserted. It is important to maintain cardiac output and avoid excessive vasodilatation with induction agents, blood loss, sudden postural change and pacemaker damage. Safety precautions include a standby external pacemaker and readily available drugs such as lignocaine, ephedrine and isoprenaline. Halothane and neostigmine should be used with caution.

6. Sick sinus syndrome

A severe sinus bradycardia or even sinus arrest, which may be associated with episodes of paroxysmal supraventricular tachycardia. It may be more serious under anaesthesia. It can be demonstrated by carotid sinus massage.[37] Patients may need a temporary transvenous pacing wire inserted pre-operatively.

7. Presence of a pacemaker

Diathermy (*See also* Chapter 3) can damage the pacemaker circuits, cause ventricular fibrillation by currents induced in pacing leads, inhibit the pacemaker, switch it into a fixed-rate mode or re-programme it entirely.[38] If possible diathermy is best avoided, but an operation may be undertaken safely provided that the active diathermy electrode is kept at least 15 cm from the pacemaker and the indifferent diathermy plate placed as far away from the pacemaker as possible and in a direction which ensures that the diathermy dipole will be at right angles to that of the pacemaker system. Diathermy should be used in short bursts and with the lowest possible power. Bipolar systems are safest. AC and DC electric motors seldom cause problems. External magnets should not be used as these usually allow complex re-programming. Pacemakers that sense physiological variables and change their rate are becoming more common, and are best converted into fixed-rate mode.[39] Suxamethonium-induced muscle fasciculations have inhibited a demand pacemaker.[40]

8. Supra-ventricular arrhythmias

The term 'auricular (= atrial) fibrillation' first used by Sir James McKenzie (1853–1925) in 1908.[41] The ventricular rate should be controlled pre-operatively by digitalization (0.0625–0.5 mg/day). Other drugs include β-blockers, verapamil (40–120 mg t.d.s.) or amiodarone (200–400 mg/day). Cardioversion may be needed.

Paroxysmal supraventricular tachycardia may respond to vagal man-oeuvres[42] such as a Valsalva manoeuvre, carotid sinus massage or eyeball pressure. Verapamil and β-blockers are useful. Adenosine[43] (0.05–0.25 mg/kg i.v.) has been successful in the acute situation. In *Wolff-Parkinson-White syndrome* there is an accessory bundle of Kent between the atria and ventricles which may form part of a circular conduction pattern and cause tachyarrhythmias. Disopyramide (300–800 mg/day), β-blockers and amiodar-one are all useful. Digoxin may make it worse. Some patients require extensive electro-physiological study and trans-catheter or surgical ablation of the abnormal bundle.[44]

9. Ventricular ectopic beats

Present in up to 50% of normal patients if the ECG is monitored for 24 hours. Usually indicate underlying pathology if they increase in frequency on exercise. Hypokalaemia or hypoventilation should be corrected. Controlled if necessary by lignocaine, β-blockers or withdrawing halothane.

10. Cardiomyopathy

General anaesthesia is likely to be dangerous, especially in older patients. Little can be done to make this situation safer. Regional techniques are preferred. Hypertrophic obstructive cardiomyopathy is worsened by catechol-amines and responds to β-blockers.

11. Congenital and rheumatic heart disease

Patients with damaged or defective endocardium, e.g. valve disease, ventricular septal defect, mitral leaflet prolapse with a systolic murmur, are at risk of subacute bacterial endocarditis and need antibiotic cover for certain operations, especially dental extractions, obstetric and gynaecological procedures, and endoscopies of the gut or the genito-urinary or respiratory tracts. Amoxycillin 3 g orally or 1 g i.m. (plus gentamicin 120 mg i.m. for special risk patients) is recommended. Erythromycin 1.5 g orally, clindamycin 600 mg orally or vancomycin 1 g slowly i.v. may be used for those allergic to penicillins. *See* The Endocarditis Working Party of the British Society for Antimicrobial Chemotherapy, *Lancet* 1990, **335**, 88.

Mitral incompetence. Mild reductions of systemic vascular resistance are helpful.

Mitral stenosis. The patient may be on anticoagulants for arterial and venous thromboembolism, and digoxin for atrial fibrillation. The left ventricle requires a longer diastolic filling time, so tachycardia is undesirable especially in atrial fibrillation. Mild vasodilatation is beneficial (with relief of pulmonary hypertension) but if excessive, leads to severe hypotension due to the fixed cardiac output. Minimal doses of anaesthetic are desirable and inotropes may be needed. Danger of pulmonary oedema.

Aortic stenosis. Preservation of normal sinus rhythm and heart rate is very important. Lignocaine for ventricular ectopics, atropine, practolol or defibrillation to control rate and rhythm may be required.

Aortic incompetence. Improved by mild tachycardia and vasodilatation with moderate fluid loading to maintain the diastolic pressure. Spinal blockade, however, can result in serious hypotension.

Valve prostheses. The patients are often anticoagulated, especially for a mitral prosthesis. Warfarin may be stopped up to 6 days pre-operatively, heparin given perioperatively and warfarin restarted 1–3 days later, all controlled by the international normalized ratio (INR<1.5) and the activated partial thromboplastin time (70–100 s). For some patients their warfarin may be changed to aspirin and dipyramidole. Each patient must be considered individually.[45] For management of pregnancy in patients with valve protheses, *see* Oakley C. *Br. Heart J.* 1987, **58**, 303.

12. Constrictive Pericarditis[46]

Thiopentone has a bad reputation in this disease. The heart is unable to increase its output to compensate for any drop in peripheral resistance.

ANAESTHESIA FOR THE HYPOVOLAEMIC PATIENT[47]

Operation should not be undertaken, except in cases of grave emergency, until the patient is resuscitated. As hypovolaemia worsens, peripheral pulses disappear, then central pulses, then pupils dilate, then the cardiac impulse and sounds fade before cardiac arrest.

Central venous and arterial pressure monitoring should be started. Raise the legs. Full fluid replacement (with blood, colloids or crystalloid as appropriate) before use of vasodilator drugs is imperative. Once improvement has occurred, with CVP rising, and hands and feet becoming warm and pink, the operation need not be delayed. The systolic pressure should, if possible, be restored to at least 100 mmHg (when the blood volume is probably not less than 70% of normal).

Anaesthesia. Premedication with atropine if thought necessary, given i.v. just before induction. Vomiting may occur at induction as shock, fear and anxiety are important causes of delayed gastric emptying. Shocked and recently resuscitated patients require much less anaesthesia and less relaxants than normal. Light general anaesthesia with IPPV is the method of choice. High oxygen concentrations may be needed. The aim of the anaesthetic technique is to preserve blood flow to the brain, heart and kidneys. Volatile agents must be used carefully if hypotension is not to be potentiated. Inotropic support should be ready. Regional analgesia may be very satisfactory if hypotension can be avoided. Ether and cyclopropane used to be valuable in shock as blood pressure is usually well maintained in light planes.

See also Chapter 29.

SEPTICAEMIA

For problems of the septicaemic patient, *see* Chapter 33.

PULMONARY DISEASE

Coryza

Acute coryza uncomplicated by fever or lower respiratory disease is seldom a contra-indication to minor surgery in adults.[48] Blocked nostrils may require the early use of an oropharyngeal airway. It would be sensible to postpone major elective operations on the thorax or abdomen because of the risk of chest infection, although there is little firm evidence of this. In paediatric practice there is a lower threshold to postpone surgery because children with upper respiratory infections are more likely to have postoperative pulmonary complications and hypoxaemia, especially younger children and those who have been intubated.[49] The airways are more reactive in the presence of any respiratory infection.

Chronic obstructive pulmonary disease (COPD)

This term includes all patients who have irreversible airflow limitation due to a combination of chronic bronchitis and emphysema.

1. *Chronic Bronchitis* is defined clinically by a chronic or recurrent increase in the volume of mucoid bronchial secretion sufficient to cause expectoration. Chronic hypoxia leads to polycythaemia and cor pulmonale

(blue bloater). Hypoventilation causes the arterial Pco_2 to rise and the respiratory centre becomes less sensitive. When a chest infection is superimposed, the hypoventilation is worse. Sputum should be coughed up before anaesthesia, by postural drainage for 2 h, if necessary. Induction should be smooth to avoid stimulation of cough and laryngeal reflexes. Rapid induction with tracheal intubation in light anaesthesia may provoke coughing, straining and bronchospasm. Intubation will allow better tracheobronchial cleansing. Pre- and postoperative physiotherapy is required.[50]

2. *Emphysema* is characterized pathologically by abnormally large air spaces distal to the terminal bronchiole with destruction of their walls. This causes loss of lung elastic recoil, overexpansion, early closure of airways during expiration and gas trapping. Ventilation is well maintained but hard work (pink puffer). The diaphragm is horizontal and flattened and pulls the lower ribs inwards during inspiration. The scalene and sternomastoid muscles assist inspiration.

The following points merit attention in all these patients: (1) hypersensitivity of respiratory reflexes (bucking, bronchospasm, etc.) to irritant vapours, thiopentone, secretions and intubation; (2) abnormal pattern of breathing may hamper the abdominal surgeon if respiration is spontaneous; (3) dependence on hypoxia for respiratory drive, via the aortic and carotid bodies. This is nearly abolished by anaesthesia and if the patient breathes an oxygen-rich atmosphere afterwards, carbon dioxide narcosis may go unnoticed; (4) undue sensitivity to such respiratory depressants as opiates and barbiturates; (5) in chronic bronchitis IPPV may need high airway pressures with adverse effects on the circulation, and the reduced elastic recoil of emphysema makes expiration prolonged; and (6) the disturbance of gas exchange that occurs on induction of anaesthesia is much more striking than in normal people.[51] Dyspnoea at rest and hypoxaemia have been suggested as the best predictors of the need for postoperative IPPV in patients with severe COPD.[52]

Anaesthetic management of COPD

Preoperative care. Should include cessation of smoking,[53] physiotherapy, treatment of bronchospasm or infection, loss of excess weight, and drainage of any pleural effusion.

Premedication. Antihistamines and diazepam are well tolerated. Opiates, especially pethidine, can be used cautiously. Atropine sometimes makes sputum too thick for easy suction. A bronchodilator inhaler if there is a reversible component to the airways obstruction.

Anaesthesia. Regional blocks can be very useful, although the patient may find it difficult to lie flat and avoid coughing for long periods. Good reasons can be advanced for preferring either spontaneous or controlled respiration. The former is particularly suitable for minor surgery, using a volatile agent. Paralysis, intubation and IPPV allow tracheal suction and the use of the smallest doses of depressant drugs. The use of relaxants need not be followed by difficulty in restarting respiration if reversal is adequate, even if the $Paco_2$ is lower than the patient's normal level.

Postoperative care. Humidified oxygen may be needed and physiotherapy should be given. Adequate pain relief by cautious doses of opiates or by regional blocks will help deep breathing, although evidence that the latter improve morbidity is scarce.[54] Infusion of doxapram hydrochloride 1.5–4 mg/min may be a useful respiratory stimulant and reduce lung complications in high-risk patients.[55] Postoperative IPPV may be needed, especially in obese patients.

For assessment of respiratory function *see* Schwieger I. et al. *Acta Anaesthesiol. Scand.* 1989, **33**, 527; Lawrence V. A. et al. *Arch. Intern. Med.* 1989, **149**, 280.

Asthma

A disease characterized by variable wheezing, dyspnoea or cough due to widespread airway narrowing, varying in severity over short periods of time, either spontaneously or as a result of treatment. The term 'bronchospasm' was first used by T. Willis (1621–1675). Various treatments first used: subcutaneous adrenaline, 1898; inhaled adrenaline, 1912; ephedrine, 1925; corticosteroids, 1952; disodium cromoglycate, 1967; selective β_2-adrenergic stimulants, 1968. Drugs that may cause bronchoconstriction in susceptible patients include penicillins, antisera, iodine-containing contrast media, relaxants, thiopentone and NSAIDs. These effects may be the result of IgE-mediated histamine release or a non-allergic mechanism, e.g. prostaglandin $F_{2\alpha}$, used for induced abortions, non-cardioselective β-blockers, etc. Other triggers include exercise and infection.

Anaesthetic management of patients with severe bronchial asthma

Except in emergency, patients with asthma should not be operated on until their lung condition is optimal because postoperative lung complications are more common. Use bronchodilators, physiotherapy, antibiotics if there is infection, and steroids to reduce bronchial oedema and spasm. Sedative premedication, especially antihistamines, are useful. Patients on large doses (> 1.5 mg/day) of inhaled steroids can have suppressed adrenal function and need additional steroid cover.[56] Regional techniques may be preferred if possible.

Volatile anaesthetics are bronchodilators and well tolerated. Nebulized salbutamol can be given during the operation. The following may make the asthma worse: intravenous thiopentone; clumsy inhalational induction of anaesthesia; tracheal intubation, especially if relaxation is incomplete or anaesthesia too light; stimulation of the upper respiratory tract by gastric acid, blood, mucus, etc. Acute bronchospasm following intubation may be treated with i.v. aminophylline 5 mg/kg (slowly) or salbutamol 200 µg. All β-blockers must be avoided.

See also Galant S. P. In: *Anaesthesia Review 4* (Kaufman L. ed.) 1987, 19; Dueck R. *Semin. Anesth.* 1987, **VI**, 2; for medical management *see* British Thoracic Society *Br. Med. J.* 1990, **301**, 797; and of acute severe asthma, *see* Chapter 30 and Cottam S. and Eason J. In: *Anaesthesia Review 8* (Kaufman L. ed.) 1991, 71.

Restrictive disease

The lungs and/or chest wall are stiff, all lung volumes and the diffusing capacity are reduced, the work of breathing is raised. The bronchi however may be held open by fibrotic lung, giving a high FEV_1/FVC ratio. There is often hypoxaemia. Patients with some restrictive diseases, e.g. severe scoliosis, may depend on ventilators in their everyday life.

High pressures are needed for IPPV, and a simple inhalational anaesthetic technique with minimal relaxants and narcotics is often satisfactory. Some surgery (e.g. prostate, limbs) are well-managed with regional blocks, although these patients may not be comfortable lying flat and may not be able to control their coughing. It is easy to give too much sedation.

Negative pressure ventilation may be useful postoperatively, especially in the Kelleher rotating iron lung, which aids physiotherapy and postural drainage. It supports ventilation in a way that avoids intubation and sedation, and allows the patient to eat and sleep.[57]

ANAEMIA

There is a reduction in arterial oxygen content but not in Pao_2. It should, when possible, be investigated and treated medically before operation because blood for transfusion is always in short supply. If the anaemia cannot be fully investigated pre-operatively, it should not be forgotten afterwards. Many prefer not to perform elective surgery on patients with a haemoglobin concentration of less than 10 g/dl, although some evidence suggests that 8 g/dl may be a safe lower limit in otherwise fit patients provided the operation is not likely to result in a blood loss over 500 ml.[58] The cardiorespiratory state must also be taken into consideration. Anaemia may exacerbate symptoms of atherosclerosis. Pre-operative transfusion should normally be given 24 hours before surgery, to allow time for depleted 2,3-diphosphoglycerate in the stored red cells to be restored. Anaemia results in an increased 2,3-diphosphoglycerate, which shifts the oxygen dissociation curve to the right.[59] Smoking should be prohibited to reduce the carboxyhaemoglobin, which may represent 10–15% of total haemoglobin, but which cannot transport oxygen. Grave hypoxia may not be accompanied by cyanosis.

For the use of erythropoeitin *see* Varet B. et al. *Semin. Haematol.* 1990, **27**, (Suppl.3), 25.

SICKLE-CELL ANAEMIA AND SICKLE-CELL TRAIT[60]

First described by J. B. Herrick of Chicago (1861–1954)[61] (who gave the first modern description of coronary thrombosis in 1912). A hereditary, autosomal recessive, haemolytic anaemia. The abnormal gene is carried by 60 million people world-wide, mainly in Africa. All patients of tropical African or West

Indian descent must be considered at risk, especially children. May also occur in certain parts of Italy, Greece, the Middle East and eastern India. It is due to substitution of valine for glutamic acid at position 6 of the β-chain of haemoglobin A, resulting in haemoglobin S (first described by Pauling[62] in 1949). In *sickle-cell anaemia* (homozygous, SS) 90% of the haemoglobin is S; in the *trait* (heterozygous, AS) 30–40% is S, the remainder being A. Haemoglobin S is vulnerable to reduction in Po_2 (first described in 1917).[63] Should this be less than about 5.5 kPa the reduced haemoglobin forms long complex strands called 'tactoids' which distort red cells. Their increased fragility causes a haemolytic anaemia. They also tend to aggregate, block small vessels and cause infarction. In the trait, sickling occurs at a Po_2 of about 2.7 kPa. Increasing the Po_2 does not reverse the changes. Acute crises, haemolytic, thrombotic or aplastic, may interrupt the chronic state.

Normal adults have largely haemoglobin A ($\alpha_2\beta_2$), with 2.5% haemoglobin A_2 ($\alpha_2\delta_2$). The neonate has 70% foetal haemoglobin (F, $\alpha_2\gamma_2$).

A similar but milder anaemia occurs in *SC disease* in which half the haemoglobin is S and half C. In C, lysine is substituted for glutamic acid at position 6 of the β-chain. This is commonest in West Africa. This disease commonly presents with an infarctive crisis after childbirth, surgery, trauma or cannabis.

Management

Patients with sickle-cell disease may present for surgery because of: (1) abdominal pain due to vascular lesions; (2) osteomyelitis; (3) priapism; (4) leg ulcers; (5) gallstones; (6) retinopathy; (7) general surgical diseases; and (8) obstetrics. All Negroes should be tested for anaemia and sickling before any anaesthetic, even if this means a delay. About 10% of British Negroes are at risk. If the haemoglobin is less than 11 g/dl and the sickling test positive, sickle-cell anaemia is probable.

The *Sickledex test* is a commercial macroscopic test for insoluble deoxygenated HbS. False positives may occur in dysproteinaemias. The test is unreliable in patients below the age of 2 years. A positive test does not differentiate between the disease and the trait and haemoglobin electrophoresis is needed. If the haemoglobin concentration and blood film are normal it is likely that the trait is present. Noted that anaemia can be masked by dehydration, and SC disease and sickle cell β-thalassaemia may not show a significant anaemia.

The following may precipitate sickling: (1) hypoxia; (2) hypothermia; (3) tourniquets (this may rule out intravenous regional analgesia); (4) acidosis and circulatory stasis; (5) pyrexia.

Trait. Usually symptomless and presents no special anaesthetic risks[64] except in major interventions such as thoracotomy, or the use of tourniquets. However pre-oxygenation, at least 30% oxygen during operation, postoperative oxygen therapy and good hydration are usually recommended. Intra-operative infarction can occur.

Disease. These patients are at high risk. Adequate oxygenation and hydration and avoidance of cardiorespiratory depression at all times are mandatory to prevent an *infarctive crisis*.

A transfusion of red cells should be given if haemoglobin is less than $8\,g/dl$ and major surgery is contemplated. In the emergency situation, a partial exchange transfusion is needed. The aim is to reduce the level of HbS to less than 30%. Administration of alkali is controversial. Sickling is more likely to occur in the presence of acidosis but the shift of the dissociation curve to the left with alkalinization lowers the venous and tissue Po_2. For the management of open heart surgery in patients with sickle-cell disease, *see* Reithmuller R. et al. *Anaesthesia* 1982, **32**, 324.

Regional analgesia, with the exception of Bier's block, should be preferred to general anaesthesia where suitable. Sickling can occur during what seems to be a faultless operation. Anticoagulants may be required after surgery to prevent pulmonary embolism, especially if thrombosis or pain in the bones is present, i.e. in an infarctive crisis.

Blood from a patient with sickle-cell trait can be safely donated for transfusion but not that from patients with other haemoglobinopathies.

In the *séquestration crisis*, acute severe hypovolaemia occurs. In the *aplastic crisis*, anaemia may be lethal.

See also Gibson J. R. *Semin. Anesth.* 1987, **VI**, 27; Esseltine D.W. et al. *Can. J. Anaesth.* 1988, **35**, 385.

THALASSAEMIA

First described in Detroit in 1925 by T. B. Cooley. Named after 'thalassa' = the sea (i.e. Mediterranean). Commonest single-gene disorder world-wide. There is reduced production of one or more of the globin chains, most commonly the β-chain. Occurs in a band from the Mediterranean, through the Middle East and southern Asia, as far as New Guinea. Also in some West Africans. The patient with *homozygous β-thalassaemia* (Cooley's or Mediterranean anaemia, thalassaemia major) has high levels of fetal haemoglobin (30–90% of total), the rest being HbA_2. Anaemia results from both haemolysis and impaired erythropoesis. Regular blood transfusions are needed, and iron overload can lead to heart and liver damage. There is an increased risk of infection. *Heterozygous β-thalassaemia* is the symptom-free carrier state. *β-thalassaemia* can be combined with an abnormal haemoglobin, one gene being inherited from each parent, and has many variants. HbC thalassaemia is relatively mild, but HbS thalassaemia is serious and can be clinically identical to sickle-cell disease. HbE thalassaemia is common in SE Asia and is associated with severe anaemia.

POLYCYTHAEMIA[65]

Most commonly secondary to chronic hypoxia or an erythropoietin-secreting renal tumour, but may be a primary myeloproliferative disease *(polycythaemia vera)*. The latter is rare in patients under 40 and is twice as common in males. It may be suspected in patients with a ruddy cyanosis and injected conjunctivae, especially if there is splenomegaly and pruritis. Haemoglobin level and packed cell volume are increased. The patient should be treated before operation by myelosuppressive drugs or ^{32}P, and a normal blood picture should have been present for several months before the proposed surgery. Operations on patients with uncontrolled polycythaemia carry a high risk of reactionary haemorrhage, e.g. after dental extractions, due to platelet defects as well as arterial and venous thrombosis. In emergency cases, repeated and voluminous phlebotomies may be helpful. Patients with a PCV over 50%, and certainly over 55%, are at risk of thrombosis. Below 48%, there is no greater risk than usual. Between these two lies an area of uncertainty where prophylaxis is wise.

See also Anesthesia for polycythemia vera. Sosis M. B. *J. Clin. Anesth.* 1990, **2**, 31.

METHAEMOGLOBINAEMIA AND SULPHAEMOGLOBINAEMIA

Methaemoglobin is derived from normal haemoglobin when the iron in the haem group is oxidized from ferrous to ferric. If a patient appears cyanosed in the absence of heart or lung disease, the blood should be spectroscopically examined for such abnormal pigments. Cyanosis is detected with 1.5 g/dl of methaemoglobin (compared with 5 g/dl of deoxyhaemoglobin). The reading of a pulse oximeter tends towards 85% in the presence of large amounts of methaemoglobin. Symptoms rarely occur unless 20% methaemoglobin is present. Above this, fatigue, dyspnoea, headache, dizziness and even coma and death can occur. The condition can be genetic or secondary to exogenous agents, e.g. nitrites, sulphonamides, phenacetin, *prilocaine*, bizarre poisons, etc. Not only is the oxygen-carrying capacity of blood reduced but also the dissociation curve is shifted to the left. Treatment is with reducing agents, ascorbic acid (300–600 mg daily) or methylene blue (1–2 mg/kg of 1% solution i.v. over 5 min, or 60 mg orally t.d.s.) which convert methaemoglobin back to normal haemoglobin. In extreme cases exchange transfusion may be considered.

Sulphaemoglobinaemia at levels of 0.5 g/dl will produce cyanosis. It is usually caused by drugs, particularly phenacetin or sulphonamides.

HAEMOPHILIA

First described by J. C. Otto (1774–1844) in 1803[66] and in this century by Bullock and Fildes in 1911.[67] There are some 4000 haemophiliacs in Britain. It is a sex-linked recessive disorder, although about 30% of males with the disease give no history of blood abnormality in previous generations. Female carriers may have postoperative bleeding problems. Haemophiliacs should attend a Haemophilia Centre where an official Haemophilia Card is issued. There is no such thing, surgically, as a mild haemophiliac. The partial thromboplastin time is prolonged and the bleeding time normal. Necessary surgery is possible with good laboratory backup. About 85% have *haemophilia A* (factor VIII deficiency) and 15% *haemophilia B* or *Christmas disease* (factor IX deficiency). The levels may range from <2% of normal (severe) to >45% (clinically unaffected). Factor IX is stable in stored blood but factor VIII levels are halved after just one day of storage. Some patients have developed antibodies to factor VIII, which makes them unsuitable for surgery. Female carriers can now be detected *in utero*. Haemophiliac patients are at high risk of carrying HIV and hepatitis viruses.

Operation regime

Intramuscular injections are avoided if possible. Treatment requires the transfusion of materials rich in the deficient factor immediately pre-operatively until a haemostatic level is reached (> 50% of normal values), and the maintenance of this level until healing is well advanced (a week or more for major surgery). Before an operation patients should have their blood tested for factor VIII antibody. Elective surgery is only possible if its titre is low. The available materials are fresh frozen plasma, cryoprecipitate, factor VIII and factor IX concentrates. Tranexamic acid may also be useful. The biological half-lifes of factor VIII and IX are 8–12 hours and 18 hours respectively. Factor VIII (or IX) levels should be monitored daily.

In minor surgery such as dental extraction,[68] the synthetic vasopressin DDAVP may be used. Before extraction, 0.4 μg/kg i.v. plus tranexamic acid 10 mg/kg is given. The latter is continued orally t.d.s. for 5 days. Penicillin should be given to prevent infection of the sockets (*see* Rizza C. R. *Prescriber's J.* 1984, **24**, 71).

See also Rudowski W. J. *Ann. R. Coll. Surg.* 1981, **63**, 111; Rizza C. R. and Spooner R. J. D. *Br. Med. J.* 1983, **286**, 929.

ANAESTHESIA IN PATIENTS WITH IMPAIRED RENAL FUNCTION

Most operations in well-hydrated patients cause minor changes in renal blood flow and glomerular filtration. But surgical stress and secretion of ADH often promote oliguria and fluid retention. Most patients with mild kidney disease do well unless more than 50% of the nephron mass is damaged. Under anaesthesia some degree of autoregulation may be preserved but function is seriously impaired with mean arterial pressures below 60 mmHg. Total renal ischaemia of more than 30 min duration is likely to result in damage to the tubules.

The uraemic patient may complain of nausea, vomiting or diarrhoea. There may be electrolyte imbalance, raised serum potassium, metabolic acidosis, anaemia, hypertension, cardiac failure, bleeding tendency due to abnormal platelet function, halitosis from ammoniacal decomposition of the salivary urea, drowsiness, convulsions and coma. The blood urea may not rise above normal until the glomerular filtration rate has fallen to about 25% of normal. Symptoms due to uraemia are rare until the blood urea approaches 15 mmol/l. Vomiting, if severe and persistent, may result in hypokalaemia and hyponatraemia. Dialysis patients are on sodium and water restriction and should not be overloaded by the anaesthetist. Parenteral nutrition must restrict protein while providing essential amino acids. There is anaemia, but the patients are well-adapted to low haemoglobin levels. Transfusion is unpopular with nephrologists. There may be osteodystrophy and hypercalcaemia. Aluminium in dialysis water may cause toxicity and severe dementia.

Risk factors for patients with pre-existing renal impairment include: (1) hypovolaemic hypotension; (2) liver failure or obstructive jaundice; (3) major vascular surgery; (4) major trauma; (5) sepsis; (6) patients over 50 having major surgery with massive blood transfusion; and (7) toxaemia of pregnancy and amniotic fluid embolism.

Regional analgesia may be especially suitable in uraemia, but coagulation defects should be excluded and blood pressure maintained. Premedication should be minimal. If general anaesthesia is preferred there may be a decreased tolerance towards intravenous barbiturates and narcotic analgesics due to changes in plasma proteins and blood pH. Many drugs are excreted by the kidneys, including digoxin, aminoglycosides, gallamine, thiazides, chlorpropamide and ACE inhibitors. A complete list is found in the *British National Formulary*. Blood volume, pressure and renal blood flow must be maintained. If IPPV is used then hypocapnia and high airway pressures should be avoided. Mannitol, frusemide and dopamine may be useful to maintain renal function, and calcium blockers[69] show promise. These patients are sensitive to narcotics, although diazepam is well tolerated. Suxamethonium may be safe unless the serum potassium is more than 5 mmol/l. Atracurium or vecuronium are the best choice of non-depolarizing relaxants. Nephrotoxic levels of fluoride ions (peak greater than 50 µmol/l) result from more than 2–2.5 MAC hours of methoxyflurane anaesthesia, but levels after prolonged enflurane anaesthesia only reach around 33 µmol/l, although toxic levels have been seen after just 3.5 MAC hours.[70] None the less it is probably wise to avoid enflurane anaesthesia in such patients when both halothane and isoflurane are known to have no such toxicity. Isoflurane has only resulted in nephrotoxic fluoride levels after its use as a sedative in intensive care for up to 127 hours (34 MAC-hours).[71] Desflurane causes no increases in fluoride levels after 1 MAC-hour.[72]

For anaesthesia for renal transplantation *see* Chapter 22. For a fuller discussion of the role of the anaesthetist in preventing acute renal failure *see* Byrick R. J. and Rose D. K. *Can. J. Anaesth.* 1990, **37**, 457.

LIVER DISEASE

Blood supply[73]

The average adult liver weighs 2.9 kg. Its total blood flow is normally 1.5 l/min, about 30% of this is provided by the hepatic artery, which supplies

50% of the oxygen requirement. The rest comes from the portal vein. Oxygen consumption is about 55 ml/min. General anaesthesia and surgery causes a fall in hepatic blood flow, which is greater than the fall in oxygen consumption, especially if the patient is hyperventilated, but this is probably not harmful. Epidural analgesia reduces hepatic arterial blood flow as the blood pressure drops.

Liver function tests

Imprecise indicators of liver function have a place in pre- and postoperative assessment. Abnormalities are frequently seen in asymptomatic patients, as are normal results in patients with known liver disease.[74] Tests include: (1) serum bilirubin. This may be elevated as a result of hepatocellular damage, excess formation (haemolysis) or biliary obstruction. If direct (conjugated) bilirubin predominates there is likely to be obstruction; (2) transaminases. May leak from liver cells into the bloodstream when damage occurs. Other tissues such as heart and skeletal muscle also contain transaminases, so high blood levels are not specific for liver pathology; (3) serum alkaline phosphatase. Present in bile duct cells. Blood levels are raised in biliary obstruction, but also in hepatocellular disease. Also found in other tissues; and (4) serum albumin. Normal value is 3.5–5.0 g/dl. The half-life is about 3 weeks, so falls do not occur for some time following liver damage. Albumin levels less than 2.8 g/dl usually point to significant disease. The production of globulin is unaffected by liver disease.

Liver Function

When this is abnormal, problems may arise related to anaesthetic practice: (1) protein. The liver is the principal site for the synthesis of important proteins, e.g. albumin, fibrinogen, prothrombin and factors V, VII, IX, X, XI and XIII. Also synthesis of prothrombin and factors VII, IX and X are dependent on vitamin K, which cannot be absorbed in the gut without bile salts. The prothrombin time is a sensitive predictor of potential coagulation problems. (2) lipid. Impaired lipoprotein synthesis. (3) carbohydrate. Hypoglycaemia may occur in advanced liver disease; and (4) drug metabolism. The liver is the site of many metabolic processes including the synthesis, conjugation, oxidation, reduction and hydrolysis. Drug elimination may therefore be impaired in advanced liver disease. Low levels of serum albumin may lead to changes in protein binding, thus leaving greater quantities of drugs unbound to exert their pharmacological effects.

Anaesthesia in the presence of overt liver disease

(1) *Drugs.* Elimination of induction agents may be impaired, but this is only of significance with infusion techniques.[75] There is likely to be a sensitivity to opiates. Resistance is shown to some non-depolarizing muscle relaxants, but biliary obstruction can prolong the effect of the steroidal relaxants.[76] As renal

problems often co-exist, atracurium may be the relaxant of choice. (2) *Serum cholinesterase.* The level must be at least halved before any effects on suxamethonium elimination are seen. Problems are unusual in clinical practice. (3) *Abnormal clotting.* (*a*) Decreased synthesis of factors (see above); (*b*) the half-life of coagulation factors may be shortened as a result of increased utilization (e.g. disseminated intravascular coagulation, loss into reticulo-endothelial system, excessive bleeding); (*c*) abnormal fibrinogen can be produced (dysfibrinogenaemia); (*d*) thrombocytopenia; and (*e*) impaired platelet function. Vitamin K, fresh frozen plasma and platelets may all be needed. (4) *Encephalopathy.* Advanced liver disease leads to altered mental state, neuromuscular signs, drowsiness, coma and death. High blood ammonia levels may be important in its genesis. There is always significant portal to systemic shunting. Precipitating factors include: (*a*) sedatives, which should be avoided whenever possible. Diazepam, 5 mg i.v. has been suggested as the most suitable agent; (*b*) gastro-intestinal haemorrhage or other protein load; (*c*) diuretics with disturbance of electrolyte balance; (*d*) infection; and (*e*) progression of underlying liver disease. (5) *Kidneys.* There is a risk of precipitating renal failure in jaundiced patients, especially those with biliary obstruction. Urine production should exceed 30 ml/h, and mannitol administered if necessary.

For management of liver failure *see* Corall I. and Williams R. *Br. J. Anaesth.* 1986, **58**, 234.

Risk factors

Severe impairment of liver function and high operative risk is indicated by: (1) serum albumin level below 2.8 g/dl; (2) serum bilirubin over 40 µmol/l; (3) prothrombin time >6 s longer than control; (4) grade 3 or 4 encephalopathy.[77]

PORPHYRIA (from the Greek *porphyros* = purple)

First described by Schultz in 1874 and named by B. J. E. Stokvis (1834–1902), a Dutch physician, in 1889.[78] Rare in England, prevalent in South Africa and Scandinavia. A family of inborn errors of haem synthesis. The rate-limiting enzyme of haem synthesis is the first one in the pathway, δ-aminolaevulinic acid (ALA) synthase, normally inhibited by haem. When subsequent enzymes in the pathway are deficient this inhibition fails, and abnormal precursors (porphyrins) are formed in excess. The particular precursors and the clinical pattern that results depend on which of these subsequent enzymes are abnormal. All porphyrias have a high activity of ALA synthase.

There are three acute hepatic porphyrias, which can be precipitated by drugs, that increase ALA synthase activity. They are all inherited as Mendelian dominants: (1) acute intermittent porphyria (common in Sweden, and the most common in the UK); (2) variegate porphyria (common in white South Africans); and (3) hereditary coproporphyria, in which the predominant porphyrin in the urine and faeces is coproporphyrin. Non-acute porphyrias (cutaneous hepatic porphyria and erythropoeitic porphyrias), which may be acquired or hereditary, are not sensitive to barbiturates.

The drugs that may precipitate acute attacks are barbiturates, sulphonamides, anticonvulsants, alcohol and oral contraceptives. Such attacks may also arise *de novo* or may be associated with infection or pregnancy.

Clinical features. (1) *Gastrointestinal.* Acute abdominal pain and vomiting. Surgeons are sometimes tempted to operate. (2) *Neurological.* Peripheral neuropathy, which can be bad enough to lead to respiratory failure and need for IPPV, epilepsy, psychiatric symptoms, rarely coma. (3) *Cardiovascular.* Tachycardia, raised blood pressure and even left ventricular failure during the active phase. (4) *A photosensitive disease* of the skin (not seen in acute intermittent porphyria). (5) *Urine* turns red or dark brown on standing.

Diagnosis is by spectroscopic measurement of porphyrins or their precursors, e.g. porphobilinogen in the urine or faeces. Bedside urine tests are available.

Barbiturates as premedication and thiopentone and its congeners are absolutely contra-indicated because their administration may be followed by the acute syndrome described above. If intravenous induction is planned, etomidate or ketamine[79] can be given. Propofol may also be safe.[80] Aspirin, codeine, morphine, pethidine, fentanyl and buprenorphine are suitable analgesics but pentazocine, chlordiazepoxide and phenylbutazone should be avoided. Atropine is preferred to hyoscine. For sleep chloral hydrate or trichloroethyl phosphate is suitable. Nitrous oxide, oxygen, volatile agents, relaxants and their reversal agents need not be withheld. Medicolegal rather than scientific reasons make some workers avoid regional analgesia in these patients. Bupivacaine is safe,[81] whereas lignocaine may not be. Detailed drug advice may be obtained from the Porphyria Research Unit, Western Infirmary, Glasgow.

King George III and some of his descendants probably suffered from this condition (Macalpine I. and Hunter R. *Br. Med. J.* 1966, **1**, 65).

See also Moyes D. G. In: *Lectures in Anaesthesiology* (Zorab J. S. M. ed.) Oxford: Blackwell, 1986, 65; Moore M. R. et al. *Blood Rev.* 1990, **4**, 88; Drugs and Porphyria. Magnus I. A. *Br. Med. J.* 1984, **288**, 1474.

CHRONIC ALCOHOLISM

Early recognition with very careful pre-operative assessment is required. Alcohol is eliminated by oxidation in the liver to acetaldehyde by the enzyme alcohol dehydrogenase. Chronic alcoholism damages the liver but also induces drug-metabolizing enzymes, so the response to drugs is not always predictable. Alcoholic cirrhosis may be associated with hyperventilation and arterial oxygen desaturation, the latter due to shunting of blood from peri-oesophageal and mediastinal veins to pulmonary veins. There may be peripheral vasodilatation, cardiomyopathy, congestive failure.

Anaesthesia[82]

Alcohol should not be withdrawn while awaiting operation. Diazepam is useful for sedation. Regional analgesia should be considered but coagulation may be abnormal. Isoflurane is probably the volatile agent of choice.[83] In acute alcoholism, patients withstand shock and trauma badly perhaps due to vasodilatation. There is a decreased adrenocortical response to stress.

To prevent withdrawal symptoms 8–10% alcohol in saline i.v. 500 ml over several hours may be helpful. *See also* Edwards R. and Mosher J. B. *Anaesthesia* 1980, **35**, 476; Edwards R. *Br. Med. J.* 1985, **291**, 423.

DRUG ADDICTION

Narcotics. These patients may manufacture symptoms to earn surgery and post-operative morphine. They may interfere with the wound to prolong their stay in hospital. There may be thrombophlebitis and multiple abscesses from unhygienic injections, so that central veins remain the only usable channels for intravenous therapy. Frequent history of asthma, tuberculosis, hepatitis B and HIV infection. Resistant to all sedatives. Hypotension is common in the operating theatre. Symptoms of withdrawal from narcotics include cramp, vomiting and diarrhoea, and can mimic intestinal obstruction.

Others. 9-Tetrahydrocannabinol in the blood stream, from cannabis, causes tachycardia and hypertension, which is made worse by atropine or adrenaline-containing local analgesics.[84] Cocaine can cause myocardial ischaemia and cardiomyopathy.[85] Amphetamine addiction may increase the required doses of anaesthetic agents.[86] *See also* Wood P. R. and Soni N. *Anaesthesia* 1989, **44**, 672.

AIDS (ACQUIRED IMMUNE DEFICIENCY SYNDROME)

First described in 1981 when *Pneumocystis carinii* pneumonia and Kaposi's sarcoma were reported in homosexuals in the USA. The incidence has been rising rapidly since. Caused by a lymphocytotropic retrovirus (HIV, human immunodeficiency virus) and transmitted in blood and semen, although the virus has also been found in saliva, urine and tears. Endemic in parts of Africa.

There may be a transient illness resembling glandular fever 1–2 weeks after infection, a variable symptom-free period of up to several years, and then AIDS-related complex (lymphadenopathy, fever, diarrhoea, weight loss, oral candidiasis) and finally overt AIDS with atypical pneumonias, other infections and Kaposi's sarcoma. This is invariably fatal. Most infected patients are asymptomatic carriers. Anonymous testing of over 115 000 pregnant women in inner London revealed an incidence as high as 0.49 per thousand.[87] Serum testing for HIV antibody is diagnostic and allows the anaesthetist to plan an appropriate management.

Certain groups are considered at high risk: homosexual and bisexual men, haemophiliacs, drug abusers and children of affected mothers. Patients with this condition present a hazard to staff, although seroconversion has probably occurred in only a handful of the thousands of reported needlestick injuries.[88] (Hepatitis B is transmitted more readily because of the higher replication rate of this virus.) Used needles should be placed in special containers without recapping and specimen containers sealed carefully. Extreme caution in handling body fluids and excreta is advised. Indeed, many recommend the wearing of gloves in *any* patient when there is likely to be contact with blood or saliva.[89] A (hopefully) pessimistic forecast has been made that an anaesthetist has a 1 in 25 chance of infection from needlestick injury over a 40-year working life.[90] Zidovudine prophylaxis may be indicated after injury in some cases.[91]

See also AIDS and Anaesthesia, Lee K. G. and Soni N. *Anaesthesia* 1986, **41**, 1011; Surgery and human immunodeficiency virus disease. Scannell K.A. *J. Acquir. Immune Defic. Syndr.* 1989, **2**, 43; A statement by the Royal College of Surgeons of England, 1992; HIV infection: Hazards of Transmission to Patients and Health Care Workers During Invasive Procedures, the Royal College of Pathologists, 1992.

OBESITY

Caesar said "let me have men about me that are fat" (Shakespeare, W. *Julius Caesar*, I, 2). He was no anaesthetist! This condition, usually the result of overeating, is perhaps the most common abnormality present in patients who require surgery. It is a serious handicap to surgeon and anaesthetist alike. "Whatever the quantity that a man eats, it is plain that if he is too fat, he has eaten more than he should have done" (Samuel Johnson, 1709–1784). One definition is a body mass index (weight in kg divided by the square of the height in m) exceeding 30.[92] The morbidly obese are over twice their ideal weight.

The disadvantages of obesity

1. *The respiratory system.* Oxygen consumption is increased. Chest (and even lung) compliance is reduced, increasing the work of breathing. The diaphragm is displaced headwards, and functional residual capacity is reduced below closing volume. Hypoxaemia develops, made worse by anaesthesia, in the supine or Trendelenburg positions. Increased incidence of postoperative chest complications. Hypoxic pulmonary arterial constriction with right ventricular strain. A few obese patients develop the Pickwickian syndrome,[93] somnolence due to chronic hypercapnia and hypoxia.

2. *The cardiovascular system.* Total blood volume, blood pressure and cardiac output and work increased. Tendency to coronary disease, stroke and postoperative thrombosis. Varicose veins are common.

3. *Miscellaneous*. Tendency to hiatus hernia. Higher volume of resting gastric juice, which has a lower pH than normal. Increased incidence of burst abdomen. Possibility of diabetes, cholelithiasis, gout, hepatic and renal dysfunction. Increased biotransformation of halogenated anaesthetics.

4. *Technical*. Difficult to nurse, move, lift and position on the table. Less tolerance of Trendelenburg and lithotomy positions. Awkward venesection and placement of needles for regional analgesia. Intended intramuscular injections may be placed subcutaneously. Difficult to maintain patent airway. Need for tracheal intubation increased and because of short thick neck this may be troublesome; awake intubation under local anaesthesia may even be needed. Difficulty of access for the surgeon in the abdomen, chest and mouth. If the blood pressure cuff is too small for an obese arm, inaccuracies will result. Intra-arterial monitoring may be preferred. Similar problems with tourniquets. The volume of the epidural space is decreased, reducing requirements for local analgesics.

This condition is usually preventable but seldom prevented. Pre-operative dietetic guidance should be more common. Antacid and H_2-antagonist prophylaxis may be useful.

See also Obesity Symposium, *J. R. Coll. Physicians, Lond.* 1983, **17**, 5; The perioperative management of morbidly obese patients (a surgeon's perspective), Ramsey-Stewart G. *Anaesth. Intensive Care* 1985, **13**, 399; Anesthesia and the obese patient, Brown B. R. Jr. ed. Philadelphia: F. A. Davis 1982; Brodsky J. B. *Int. Anesthesiol. Clin.* 1986, **24**, 93.

DIABETES MELLITUS

Insulin was isolated and first used to treat diabetics in 1922.[94] There is either a lack of, or a tissue resistance to insulin, the major anabolic hormone. Glucose, fat and protein metabolism are affected. Problems include:

1. High blood sugar: polyuria, thirst, pruritus, etc.

2. Ketoacidosis: severe metabolic acidosis, loss of extracellular sodium and water, circulatory collapse and coma; exacerbated by anaesthesia.

3. Peripheral vascular disease: commonly brings the patient to surgery, which may include coronary artery bypass.

4. Diabetic nephropathy: may lead to nephrotic syndrome and uraemia.

5. Peripheral neuropathy: autonomic neuropathy[95] can cause cardio-respiratory arrest, postural hypotension, gastroparesis and postoperative retention of urine. Sleep apnoea in diabetic patients with autonomic neuropathy[96] may be a particular hazard if respiratory depressant drugs are given. Sudden death may occur.

6. Poor wound healing in major surgery.[97]

7. Retinopathy and cataracts.

Most anaesthetic agents cause a slight rise in blood sugar, but this is seldom significant. Ether causes a pronounced rise and is to be avoided. Surgical mortality is higher in diabetics but this may be related only to the complications of diabetes, especially vascular disease, and not to the metabolic disturbance itself.[98]

Schemes of control for operation period

There is no single scheme to cover all cases. It is usually wiser to have a slightly increased blood sugar than to risk hypoglycaemia. The aim is to keep blood glucose around 10 mmol/l and to maintain the use of glucose by the cells. Hypoglycaemia presents the greatest danger, especially to the central nervous system. But the acidosis and hyponatraemia caused by a shortage of insulin is also dangerous. Avoiding general anaesthesia solves most of the perioperative problems. However, even for local analgesia, the patient may have to be starved.

Symptoms of hypoglycaemia: shaking and trembling, sweating, pins and needles in tongue and lips, hunger, palpitations, diplopia, slurring of speech, confusion, truculence, restlessness, epileptic fits, unconsciousness.

Symptoms of ketoacidosis: dehydration, over-breathing, acetone in the breath, hypotension, glycosuria and ketonuria, high serum potassium.

1. *Diabetics controlled by diet only.* Can be upset by surgery. Hyperglycaemia persisting beyond the first postoperative day may require insulin.

2. *Patients receiving oral hypoglycaemic drugs* (maturity-onset diabetes). *Sulphonylureas* stimulate insulin production by the pancreas, and most have a duration of action not exceeding 12–16 h. Chlorpropamide, however, has a half-life of 36 h and a duration of action up to 60 h. Fasting hypoglycaemia may occur, and the drug should be stopped 1–2 days preoperatively. Others should be withheld on the day of surgery. Insulin may be needed for a short time after major surgery. *Biguanides* decrease hepatic gluconeogenesis and increase tissue glucose use. Hypoglycaemia is not a problem. Phenformin caused lactic acidosis, and has been withdrawn.

3. *The well-controlled diabetic on insulin* (type 1 or juvenile-onset diabetes). The aim is: to prevent ketoacidosis, and to avoid hypoglycaemia. An elective operation should preferably be carried out in the early morning. For major procedures the patient should be stabilized on soluble insulin, twice daily, for 2–3 days before operation. Various regimes have been recommended for the operative period:

(*a*) The Alberti regime.[99] 10 units of insulin are added to 500 ml of 10% glucose, with 1 g of potassium chloride. This is infused intravenously at 100 ml/h. Many personalized versions of this regime exist. The important features are that the insulin is given continuously and that it is balanced with the correct amount of glucose. Earlier doubts about adsorption of insulin into the plastic of the container appear to have been unfounded. Blood glucose and potassium is estimated at the start of the operation, every 2–3 h and in the postoperative room, and appropriate changes made. The Alberti regime may be continued, with blood glucose monitoring, until the patient starts to eat again.

(*b*) Other physicians prefer to give half the normal dose of soluble insulin in the morning with 500 ml 5% glucose intravenously 6-hourly. Operation is carried out in the morning and at midday the remainder of the morning insulin dose is given unless blood glucose is less than 6 mmol/l. Bolus intravenous injections of 10 g glucose can be given if necessary. The evening dose of insulin can be given as usual unless blood glucose is below the level quoted above.

(*c*) The normal insulin dosage may be administered and glucose solution infused intravenously to maintain requirements. This approach can be used when there is no time for pre-operative stabilization with soluble insulin, but if long-acting insulin has been given there is lack of flexibility.

(*d*) Brief minor surgery may be managed by giving neither insulin nor glucose immediately pre-operatively, but giving half the normal daily requirement with a meal early postoperatively.

If surgery has to be delayed until late in the day prolonged fasting may present a threat to the diabetic patient. The pre-operative regime should then include both carbohydrate and insulin.

The Alberti regime is convenient and in common use,[100] but evidence that it provides positive benefit is poor.[101]

4. *The poorly controlled diabetic.* Shown by ketosis, glycosuria and electrolyte abnormalities. This is a medical emergency requiring the assistance of an experienced physician. Non-urgent surgery must be postponed, but operations such as drainage of abscesses or treatment of infected gangrene may be necessary to achieve control. After partial correction of acidosis with sodium bicarbonate (50 mmol if pH > 7.1; 100 mmol if pH <7.0), the *Alberti regime offers* a scheme for rapid control of the situation *(see above)*, or i.v. boluses of soluble insulin may be used. Hypokalaemia is corrected with potassium chloride 10–20 mmol/h, if the urine flow is greater than 1 ml/min. There is a real danger of vomiting during induction in the diabetic with ketosis.

Diabetic (ketoacidotic) coma[102]

The following abnormalities require treatment: (*a*) lack of insulin; (*b*) dehydration; (*c*) loss of sodium and potassium; (*d*) metabolic acidosis; and (*e*) precipitating diseases, especially infections. Insulin has a short half-life (5 min) in the blood and it is advantageous to administer small doses frequently. Sodium bicarbonate should be administered in small quantities; there is a danger that overzealous dosage may cause rapid changes in potassium level with perhaps cardiac arrest, CNS acidosis and shift the oxygen dissociation curve. The following regimen may be recommended:

1. *Insulin.* May be given as 4–6 units/h by continuous infusion (mechanical pump or burette). Adsorption to walls of the container occurs but is not important. Intramuscularly, use 20 units followed by 6 units 2-hourly. Blood sugar is measured 1–2 hourly and should fall by 3–5 mmol/l/hour. When the level falls below 11–14 mmol/l insulin may be given according to a sliding scale.

2. *Fluid and electrolytes.* Average deficit: water 6 litres, sodium 500 mmol, chloride 400 mmol, potassium 350 mmol, phosphate 1 mmol/l.

Give 1 l normal (0.9%) saline in first 30 min, 2–3 l in the next 2–3 hours, and then 500 ml/h until about 5 l has been given. Change to 4% dextrose in 0.18% saline 500 ml 4-hourly when the blood sugar falls to 10–15 mmol/l. Measure electrolytes 2-hourly and change to 0.45% saline if serum sodium rises above 150 mmol/l. Add potassium 13–20 mmol in the first hour then 26 mmol hourly, depending on the rate of fall.

3. *Sodium bicarbonate.* Only if acidaemia is severe. 100 mmol if pH is less

than 7.0, 50 mmol if pH is between 7.0 and 7.1, preferably using isotonic (1.4%) solution.

In addition: (a) blood analysis for sugar, urea, electrolytes, haemoglobin and packed-cell volume, arterial blood gases; (b) urinalysis and insertion of urinary catheter; (c) administer oxygen to maintain Pao_2 above 10 kPa; (d) nasogastric tube and stomach aspiration; and (e) monitor electrocardiogram.

Other causes of coma in a diabetic

(a) Hyperosmolar, non-ketoacidotic coma:[103] In the older patient who is dehydrated with very high blood sugar but no ketonuria. Sodium bicarbonate is not needed and hypotonic fluids (0.45% saline), insulin and potassium are given.

(b) Lactic acidosis.[104] May occur in patients treated with phenformin. Blood lactic acid levels should be determined, but the condition may be suspected when the 'anion gap' (difference between sum of sodium and potassium ions and sum of chloride and bicarbonate ions) is greater than 20. Large amounts of bicarbonate may be needed.

(c) Hypoglycaemia. Rarely presents in true coma. If blood sugar is less than 2 mmol/l, give 20 ml of i.v. 50% dextrose.

(d) Causes of coma unconnected with diabetes.

Postoperative control of diabetes

There is a tendency towards hyperglycaemia, with a peak at 4 h after operation (even more marked in cardiopulmonary patients). The subsequent daily insulin requirement will probably be raised by 10% for 2 days.[105]

The Alberti regime should give good control. Those patients who received subcutaneous insulin (half usual dose) with a 5% glucose drip, may require further insulin later that day as dictated by blood or urinary glucose monitoring 4-hourly on the day of operation, less often thereafter. A return to the patient's usual regime is made when he is eating normally. The *'sliding scale'* is still useful if diabetes becomes unstable postoperatively: 2% urine glucose or blood glucose 20 mmol/l – 20 units insulin; 1% urine glucose or blood glucose 10 mmol/l – 10 units insulin. Patients receiving oral hypoglycaemic control can usually be managed without the hypoglycaemic drugs until normal eating is resumed. In the complicated surgical case, such patients may require a temporary period of control by the Alberti regime, e.g. in the intensive therapy unit, where resistance to insulin is commonly seen. Special care should be taken following Caesarean section in a diabetic patient and after amputation of a gangrenous leg because insulin requirements may fall rapidly.

Duration of action of some agents: soluble insulin 6–8 h; lente insulin 20–30 h; chlorpropamide 60 h; glibenclamide 12-16 h; phenformin 6–8 h. A constant infusion of 5% glucose guards against hypoglycaemia. Metabolism of the lactate in Hartmann's solution may contribute to hyperglycaemia in diabetics.

β-blocking agents may cause hypoglycaemia. Glucocorticoids may result in carbohydrate intolerance. Thiazides, ethacrynic acid and frusemide may inhibit insulin secretion. Diabetic patients sometimes present simulating an acute abdomen. Hyperglycaemic coma is of slow onset, whereas hypogly-caemia can develop during an operation and cause sweating, pallor, tachycardia, dilated pupils, abnormal eyeball tension, etc. and delayed awakening. Treat as for hypoglycaemic coma. Normal diet should be restored as soon as possible in the diabetic after operation.

See also Alberti K. G. M. M. (p. 209) and Hirsch I. B. et al. (p. 346) *Anesthesiology* 1991, **74**.

SURGICAL TREATMENT OF HYPERINSULINISM

When an insulinoma is to be removed a pre-operative glucose load should be given and a 25–50% solution should be infused via a central line during the procedure according to blood sugar estimations performed every 15 min.[106] Diazoxide has been used to inhibit insulin release from the pancreas.[107]

HYPERTHYROIDISM

The Greek word for shield gives the thyroid gland its name. The commonest cause of thyrotoxicosis is Graves' disease (diffuse toxic goitre), typically in women of 20–40 years, caused by IgG auto-antibodies. If there is a goitre the anaesthetist should ask for the symptoms of thyrotoxicosis and look for atrial fibrillation and heart failure. Hyperthyroidism can occur without an enlarged thyroid. Cardiac involvement may be the presenting feature, especially in older patients. Proximal muscle weakness is also common. Treatment is with antithyroid drugs. The patient should be euthyroid before operation. An acute exacerbation, or thyroid crisis, is life-threatening. For details *see* Chapter 22.

HYPOTHYROIDISM

The word 'myxoedema' was introduced by Ord in 1878.[108] May be common (> 10%) and undiagnosed in older women.[109] Metabolism of drugs, especially sedatives and narcotics, is slowed and respiratory depression easily produced. Usually due to primary failure of the thyroid gland with high TSH levels. If due to pituitary failure the adrenal cortex response to stress is also likely to be impaired. There may also be hypothermia, hypoglycaemia, muscular weakness, pericardial effusion and even coma. Such patients are poor anaesthetic risks and correction is necessary before any operation. Oral

T_4 takes 10 days to exert its effect. Oral T_3 acts quicker and can also be given i.v. (5–20 µg given slowly 4-hourly if needed, or a drip of 0.1 mg/l in 5% dextrose at 20 drops per min) with ECG control (look for flattened T-waves or ST depression), using special caution in older patients and those suffering from angina. Mild, undiagnosed hypothyroidism in patients undergoing surgery may result postoperatively in myxoedema coma and respiratory obstruction.[110] Steroids are also beneficial in myxoedema coma.

The nitrous oxide, oxygen, volatile agent, relaxant sequence with IPPV is perhaps the most suitable anaesthetic technique. For review of anaesthetic considerations in thyroid dysfunction *see* Roizen M. F. et al. *Anesth. Clin. North Am.* 1987, **5**, 277.

DISEASES OF THE ADRENAL GLANDS

Primary adrenal failure (Addison's disease)

First described by Thomas Addison (1793–1860) of Guy's Hospital.[111] May be seen following: (1) removal, i.e. adrenalectomy; (2) destruction, e.g. tuberculosis, metastases, infarction, granuloma, autoimmune disease.

The diagnosis should be considered in unexplained cases of hyponatraemia. Patients with this complaint are susceptible to infection, to loss of sodium chloride and to narcotics. They are likely to be debilitated, pigmented, hypotensive, hyponatraemic, hypoglycaemic and perhaps tuberculous. They are bad anaesthetic risks because Addisonian crisis is easily precipitated. It starts with loss of sodium chloride in the urine and so of large amounts of water. This fluid loss is aggravated by diarrhoea and vomiting. Severe dehydration and circulatory shock follow. If such a patient is operated on and Addison's disease not diagnosed, severe postoperative collapse may occur. If the disease is recognized, adequate pre-operative treatment greatly lessens the risk. Sodium chloride, glucose and hydrocortisone should be given to maintain the blood volume as near normal as possible. Postoperative hypotension is still likely, which should be treated similarly. Thiopentone may cause a serious fall in blood pressure. Normal cortisol production is 30 mg/day, equivalent to 7.5 mg of prednisone. For anaesthesia in Addisonian crisis *see* Smith M. G. and Byrne A. J. *Anaesthesia* 1981, **36**, 681.

Waterhouse-Friderichsen syndrome[112]

Adrenal infarction, which is usually fatal ('adrenal apoplexy'). Often associated with meningococcal septicaemia and first described by Voelcker (1861–1946) in 1894.[113] Hyperpyrexia and circulatory collapse are the usual modes of death. Rarely the condition comes to operation because of associated arterial embolism or peritonitis. Hydrocortisone is indicated.

Secondary adrenal failure (ACTH deficiency)

This may result from: (1) removal of the pituitary (hypophysectomy); (2) destruction of the pituitary, e.g. tumours; Simmonds' cachexia (*see below*); or (3) inhibition of the pituitary by steroid therapy. Death due to circulatory failure may occur in patients who, having been on doses of cortisone for long periods, are suddenly deprived of it before the stress of anaesthesia and operation.[114]

Cushing's syndrome[115]

Described in 1932 by the neurosurgeon Harvey Cushing (1869–1939). Caused by cortisol overproduction, usually secondary to a corticotroph pituitary adenoma. More rarely due to an adrenal adenoma or ectopic ACTH production by a tumour. A similar clinical picture is frequent in patients on steroid medication. Most of the important features are due to tissue destruction: striae, fragile skin and capillaries, bruising, muscle weakness, osteoporosis, 'orange-on-matchsticks' appearance of the body. Hypertension, hypokalaemia and diabetes mellitus are common. Hypophysectomy is often performed.

PHAEOCHROMOCYTOMA

See Chapter 22.

DISEASES OF THE PITUITARY GLAND

Hyperpituitarism

In adults acromegaly, in children and adolescents gigantism.

Acromegaly

First described by Saucerotte (1741–1812)[116] in 1801 and by Pierre Marie (1853–1940) in 1886.[117] Due to an acidophilic or chromophobe cell adenoma of the pituitary forming after the epiphyses have fused. Slow onset with bony changes in the jaws, enlarged tongue, thickening of the mucosa of the pharynx, enlarged larynx with elongation, thickening and even calcification of the cords. There may be recurrent laryngeal nerve paralysis and laryngeal stenosis,[118] and the cricoid may be narrowed, so making intubation difficult. Careful assessment is required, perhaps with a fibreoptic laryngoscope. Blind nasal intubation may be needed. The hands become 'spade-like' and there may be kyphosis, diabetes and an enlarged thyroid. May present as carpal tunnel syndrome. Increased mortality due to cardiac and cerebrovascular disease. Sleep apnoea is common and may be central, obstructive or mixed.

Treatment is usually by hypophysectomy, although yttrium-90 implants and drug therapy (bromocriptine and octreotide) are also used. Postoperatively, there may be upper airway obstruction and intubation may have to be continued. Ulnar artery circulation in one or both hands may be impaired, so cannulation of the dorsalis pedis artery may be safer than the radial.[119] For *trans-sphenoidal hypophysectomy,* steroid cover must be commenced before the operation and continued. Thyroxine replacement will also be needed. A watch must be kept for diabetes insipidus. When the operation is performed for metastatic cancer, attention must be paid to pre-operative anaemia, pleural effusions and bony secondaries making movement dangerous because of the possibility of fractures.

Hypopituitarism (Simmonds' disease)[120]

Morris Simmonds (1855–1925). Chronic hypopituitarism is most commonly due to a pituitary tumour or iatrogenic ablation. Ischaemic necrosis of the anterior lobe after haemorrhage in labour (Sheehan's syndrome)[121] is now rare. There may be diminished production of any of the anterior lobe hormones: growth hormone, corticotrophin (ACTH), thyrotrophin, gonado-trophin and prolactin. The clinical picture depends on the pattern of such deficiencies. Substitution therapy may be required. General anaesthesia is liable to precipitate coma in these patients. Permanent deficit in posterior lobe hormones (oxytocin or vasopressin) is usually a result of hypothalamic disease.

CARCINOID TUMOURS

First described by Merling in 1838 and named by Obendorfer[122] in 1907 because less malignant than carcinoma. Arise from argentaffin Kultschitzky cells of the crypts of Lieberkuhn of the gastro-intestinal tract; can occur anywhere derived from the embryological foregut (including thyroid and bronchi) but 50–90% originate in the area of the appendix. These tumours neither metastasize nor secrete. Extra-appendicular tumours however are often malignant and about 25% of malignant carcinoids produce and secrete serotonin (5-hydroxytryptamine) and other hormones including bradykinin.

Carcinoid syndrome. There are big variations in the clinical manifestations. The syndrome does not occur unless there are liver secondaries with secretion into the hepatic veins. It may be characterized by: (1) a growing intra-abdominal malignancy; (2) cutaneous flushes with tachycardia and fall in blood pressure, which may be precipitated by food, alcohol and emotional stress; (3) profuse diarrhoea, nausea, vomiting and abdominal cramps; and (4) wheezing. Bradykinin and perhaps histamine are thought to responsible for the flushing and circulatory changes, and serotonin for the remaining symptoms. Attacks may be precipitated by: (1) compressing the tumour, e.g. palpation, abdominal straining, suxamethonium; (2) food and alcohol; (3) emotional stress; and (4) hypotension.

Long-term manifestations. Valvular fibrosis of the right side of the heart, which may require surgery, weight loss, pellagra and facial telangiectasia. The disease progresses very slowly.

Diagnosis. Confirmed by urinary excretion of 5-hydroxyindole acetic acid. Normal 2–9 mg/24 h, greater than 25 mg/24 h is diagnostic. Up to 1000 mg/24 h has been described.

Medical treatment.[123] Includes antihistamines (both H_1 and H_2 blockers), α-adrenergic blockers, aprotonin, 5-HT_1 antagonists (cyproheptadine, methysergide) and 5-HT_2 antagonists (ketanserin). Cytotoxic agents are disappointing. Octreotide, a somatostatin analogue, lowers 5-HT secretion and has been very helpful in preventing the flushing and diarrhoea.[124] Surgery may be for removal of primary or secondary tumour, or for heart valve replacement.

Anaesthesia. May be uneventful, but may provoke acute flushing and severe bronchospasm. This is particularly likely if hypotension occurs and so spinal techniques are not recommended. Morphine may cause serotonin release. Smooth induction of anaesthesia is desirable. Vecuronium is recommended as the relaxant of choice.[125] Neurolept agents are controversial. Angiotensin (starting with 1.5 mg/kg) is useful for severe intra-operative hypotension. Both ketanserin[126] and octreotide[127] have been used successfully to control the effects and release of serotonin intra-operatively. Careful monitoring should continue into the postoperative period. Awakening from anaesthesia may be delayed. The blood sugar should be monitored.

RECENT STEROID THERAPY[128]

Adrenal cortical hormones. (1) Glucocorticoids: hydrocortisone (cortisol) (20 mg/day, half-life 100 min). Cause protein breakdown, increase the blood glucose and oppose the action of insulin. They are anti-inflammatory and in large doses cause muscle wasting, skin atrophy and osteoporosis. (2) Mineralocorticoids: aldosterone (150 μg/day). Secreted in response to a reduction in extracellular fluid volume, and promotes retention of sodium and excretion of potassium by the kidneys. (3) Sex hormones.

Diminished adrenocortical reserve. (1) In Addison's disease, whether treated or untreated. (2) After bilateral adrenalectomy. (3) During steroid therapy. (4) After steroid therapy. Adrenocortical reserve can be sufficient to meet the ordinary needs of life, but inadequate to meet the extra burden of anaesthesia and operation when secretion of hydrocortisone normally rises to 300–500 mg/day.

Steroid therapy. Suppresses ACTH production by the anterior pituitary. The adrenal cortex atrophies and is unable to increase its secretion in response to the stress of anaesthesia, operation or trauma. During and after anaesthesia the main sign of deficiency of hydrocortisone is hypotension and tachycardia. There is probably a decreased sensitivity to catecholamines. The first death from this cause was reported in 1952 following therapeutic doses of cortisone.[129] As short a course as 1 week may produce this depression of the cortex. Depression usually recovers by 2 months after stopping steroids, but may last over 1 year, and in some cases of prolonged therapy may never recover. There are no satisfactory simple tests for adrenocortical reserve.[130] The response to the stress of insulin-induced hypoglycaemia is no longer performed. The rise in plasma hydrocortisone can be measured in response to 250 µg of synthetic ACTH and should be 7–20 µg/dl, but this test does not reliably identify all patients in need of steroid supplements.

Therefore it is best to assume that there is some diminution of reserve whenever a course of steroids has recently been given. Collapse is unlikely to occur more than 2 months after cessation of treatment. It is generally safer to give hydrocortisone cover than to omit it in cases of doubt.

Spinal analgesia is the only form of pain relief that does not cause a rise in blood-cortisol levels during anaesthesia, although the effects of stress are evident in the postoperative period when the local analgesic effect is over. Under general anaesthesia the rise is marked during abdominal surgery, but slight during neurosurgical operations. Anaesthesia itself causes only a mild stress reaction.

Steroid cover[131] can be provided by intramuscular injection of hydrocortisone 100 mg 6 to 8-hourly, started at the time of premedication and continued for 3 days in the case of major surgery, for 24 h following minor operations such as hernia repair, and restricted to a single injection prior to endoscopy or other brief procedure. Further doses can be given if complications ensue. Intramuscular injections give more sustained plasma levels than the intravenous route. The latter is indicated in emergency situation at the same dosage.

Synthetic steroid derivatives with glucocorticoid activity include prednisone and prednisolone (4 times as potent as cortisone), triamcinolone (5 times as potent), betamethasone and dexamethasone (30 times as potent).

Corticosteroids are often contra-indicated in patients with tuberculosis, local or systemic infection unless controlled by antibiotics, active peptic ulcer, psychosis, osteoporosis, renal dysfunction, diabetes mellitus, glaucoma, hypertension, myasthenia gravis (unless being started under careful control), thrombotic disorders, congestive heart failure and those who are pregnant.

Adverse effects of steroids: (1) increased susceptibility to infection; (2) retarded healing; (3) gastro-intestinal bleeding and perforation; and (4) fluid retention and impaired electrolyte balance.

CONNECTIVE TISSUE DISORDERS

Polyarteritis nodosa was first described in 1866 by Kussmaul (1822–1902).[132] There may be renal, gastro-intestinal, skin, cardiac and pulmonary involvement. Liver dysfunction may modify the response to muscle relaxants. Patients with systemic lupus erythematosus can produce an antibody which is an anticoagulant *in vitro*, but causes thrombosis and abortion *in vivo*.[133]

RHEUMATOID ARTHRITIS

First described by Sir Alfred Garrod in 1859; a disease of modern times (since 18th century); affects 2% of men and 5% of women over 64. Still's disease is a juvenile form. Symmetrical, peripheral polyarthritis, associated with vasculitis in various organs, heart and lung involvement and peripheral neuropathy and Sjogren's syndrome (keratoconjunctivitis sicca). Potential difficulties may arise from: (1) immobility or subluxation in the cervical spine, especially atlanto-axial. The vertebral arteries may be compressed. The odontoid peg can move posteriorly on neck flexion and compress the cord. Protective reflexes are lost during anaesthesia; (2) temporomandibular joint arthritis making laryngoscopy difficult; (3) crico-arytenoid joint arthritis and neuropathy of laryngeal muscles causing stridor. Thus there may be *difficulty in intubation* together with the need for great care after operation. Pre-operative chest and cervical spine (in flexion) radiography may be required; (4) amyloidosis of kidneys; (5) pulmonary fibrosis and obstructive airways disease can cause respiratory depression and pneumonia after operation; (6) steroid therapy; (7) fragility of skin and veins; (8) pericarditis, aortic regurgitation; (9) anaemia; and (10) peripheral neuropathy.

ANKYLOSING SPONDYLITIS

First described by B. Connor in 1693. Usually affects young men. Often familial. Starts in lumbar spine (radiological 'bamboo spine') and can spread to the cervical spine and atlanto-occipital joint, where stiffness may cause difficulty during tracheal intubation, and has led to spinal fractures. Temporomandibular or crico-arytenoid joints may also be ankylosed. Blind intubation techniques, awake intubation using a fibre-optic bronchoscope, the use of a laryngeal mask airway or even tracheostomy may be needed.

Although costo-vertebral involvement and kyphosis restrict chest expansion, the diaphragm compensates and lung function is good. Cardiothoracic and abdominal surgery need not result in pulmonary complications. Take care to ensure that adequate ventilation returns after operation. Extradural block for hip surgery may be technically easier via the sacral than the lumbar approach.

Aortic regurgitation may be severe. Unexpected postoperative cardiac death has been reported.[134] Iritis and amyloidosis may occur. *See also* Sinclair J. R. and Mason R. A. *Anaesthesia* 1984, **39**, 3; Whittmann F. J. and Ring P.A. *J. R. Soc. Med.* 1986, **79**, 457.

SCOLIOSIS

Usually idiopathic but may be due to congenital vertebral anomalies or to neuromuscular disorders: polio, muscular dystrophy, etc. Malignant hyperpyrexia has been seen in these patients. May be associated with congenital heart disease. For Harrington rod surgery, it may be necessary to wake the patient to check cord integrity during the operation. Excessive hypotension may reduce cord blood supply. A narcotic, nitrous oxide, oxygen, IPPV technique is usually satisfactory. These patients have a reduced vital capacity, and cannot increase their tidal volume. Airway obstruction is seldom a feature. Fluoroscopic assessment of diaphragmatic movement will exclude paralysis. Underventilation is a danger even before anaesthesia is induced, premedication must not depress respiration. Postoperatively, they require careful observation and administration of pain relief, and if necessary IPPV. Hypoxaemia results from ventilation–perfusion inequality. Pulmonary hypertension, right heart failure and respiratory failure can result. Ventilation by external negative pressure or nasal mask[135] may be useful.

ACHONDROPLASIA

Described in 1791 by Sommering (1755–1830), Polish-German physician and by M. H. Romberg (1795–1873) in 1817. Difficulties include the fit of face-masks, tracheal intubation due to abnormalities at the base of the skull, and restrictive chest wall disease. For Caesarean section, extradural block, although technically difficult, has been safely used.[136] *See* Berkowitz I. D. et al. *Anesthesiology* 1990, **73**, 739.

PAROXYSMAL MYOGLOBINURIA (OR RHABDOMYOLYSIS)

Acute episodes of muscle pain and weakness with myoglobinuria, sometimes following exercise. May be a deficiency of carnitine palmityl transferase. Rhabdomyolysis may follow the use of suxamethonium.[137]

MYASTHENIA GRAVIS

The myasthenic state may be present as follows:
1. *Myasthenia gravis*. First described by Thomas Willis (1621–1675)[138] in 1672 and Samuel Wilks (1824–1911) in 1877[139] and named pseudoparalytica myasthenica by Friedrich Jolly (1844–1904), the German neurologist, who also described its electrodiagnosis.[140] Name changed to myasthenia gravis in 1900.[141] The treatment of myasthenia by the anticholinesterase drug physostigmine was first described by Remen of Münster in 1932[142] and M. Walker in 1934 in Greenwich.[143] The first thymectomy for myasthenia gravis

was performed by F. Sauerbruch (1845–1951) in 191 [144] and the operation was further developed by Blalock[145] in 1936. Geoffrey Keynes did the first such operation in Britain in 1942.[146]

2. *Associated with malignancy (Myasthenic Syndrome)*. Especially oat-cell carcinoma of the bronchus. *See below.*

3. *Caused by drugs*. Aminoglycoside antibiotics: neomycin, streptomycin, gentamicin, kanamycin, polymyxin, etc. can cause a mild myasthenic state of little significance, and diagnosed by edrophonium. They will worsen true myasthenia. Penicillamine has precipitated myasthenia gravis.

Myasthenia gravis is a chronic disease that tends to relapse and remit, and is twice as common in women. It can develop any time between childhood and old age, but usually in early adulthood. An autoimmune disease in which there are circulating IgG antibodies, probably dependent on the thymus, to the acetylcholine receptor. Associated with thyrotoxicosis, collagen diseases and thymoma (in 10% of patients).[147] While severe cases are easily diagnosed, mild ones can be overlooked and may cause anaesthetic difficulties. Ocular, bulbar and other head and neck muscles are commonly involved, with ptosis, dysphagia and easy fatigue of the jaw muscles. Weakness comes on after exercise and improves following rest. Tendon reflexes are brisk.

There are also: a neonatal form in babies born of mysathenic mothers, which recovers spontaneously; rare congenital non-immune forms, which show variable responses to anticholinesterases.

A cholinergic crisis is due to over-dosage with anticholinesterase drugs. There is muscle weakness and fasciculation, lacrimation, sweating and colic.

Tests for myasthenia gravis

1. *Electromyography*. Reduction in response to a single twitch in rested muscles, and to repetitive stimuli at both high and low frequencies.

2. *Edrophonium* (10 mg i.v.). In myasthenics there is a full but temporary return of muscular power. In normal patients and myasthenics who are adequately treated there may be fasciculations, colic, salivation and diarrhoea, but muscular power is unaffected.

3. *Acetylcholine receptor antibody estimation.*[148]

Treatment

Oral anticholinesterases, e.g. neostigmine and the longer-acting pyridostigmine, are used especially in ocular myasthenia. In other cases steroids and immuno-suppressives such as azathioprine or cyclosporine have been useful. Thymectomy is considered, particularly if a thymoma is present. Plasmapheresis may produce dramatic improvement in an emergency and even maintain the patient in remission.

Preoperative preparation

The serum potassium should be normal because hypokalaemia aggravates myasthenia. A chest radiograph is desirable. Dose of anticholinesterase should be slightly reduced just before operation to avoid excess. A nasogastric tube may be in place for feeding. Sedative premedication should be minimal. Opiates should be avoided. Steroid cover is required for those receiving it regularly.

Use of relaxants in myasthenia gravis

1. The affected muscles only are hypersensitive to non-depolarizing relaxants. Myasthenics successfully treated with steroids and not requiring anticholinesterases may still show this hypersensitivity.

2. Myasthenics are resistant to decamethonium and suxamethonium, but a dual (non-depolarizing) block may follow.

Anaesthetic management

The chief concern is to ensure adequate respiration both during and after the operation, while the special difficulties to be borne in mind are muscular weakness and bronchial secretion from neostigmine. Regional analgesia, which does not depress respiration, e.g. intra- or extradural block to T10, may be suitable. Rapidly eliminated anaesthetic agents, such as isoflurane are drugs of choice, even though myasthenics are more sensitive to its neuromuscular effects.[149] Relaxants can often be avoided and spontaneous respiration used, but small doses of vecuronium or atracurium with monitoring of the neuromuscular block may be used successfully.[150] They have a short onset of action. Tracheal intubation may be advisable to ensure a perfect airway and to facilitate suction. Neostigmine should be administered with care to avoid overdosage. Intensive care facilities may be needed postoperatively. Mandatory minute volume ventilation may be beneficial in the postoperative period.

For anaesthesia for trans-cervical thymectomy, *see* Girnar D. S. and Weinrich A. I. *Anesth. Analg. (Cleve.)* 1976, **55**, 13; for trans-sternal thymectomy *see* Redfern N. et al. *Ann. R. Coll. Surg.* 1987, **69**, 289. For the natural course of myasthenia gravis, *see* Fonseca V. and Havard C. W. H. *Br. Med. J.* 1990, **300**, 1409.

Management of myasthenic emergencies

Both myasthenic and cholinergic crises are medical emergencies, which may cause severe respiratory failure, and can sometimes follow anaesthesia and surgery. A clear airway and adequate respiration must be established first, using IPPV if needed. It is advisable to withhold all drugs until the nature of the crisis has been diagnosed. The patient should be nursed in an intensive care unit. The reactions of the end-plates to neostigmine may be complex and require expert evaluation. Plasma electrolytes, particularly potassium, should be restored to normal values. Plasma exchange will produce dramatic benefit.

Myasthenic syndrome

A condition of proximal muscular weakness developing in a patient with oat-cell bronchial carcinoma, usually in older males. More rarely associated with other cancers. May present with prolonged apnoea after anaesthesia. The condition was first described as a distinct entity by Eaton and Lambert in 1957 (the Eaton-Lambert Syndrome).[151] Symptoms of muscular weakness should be sought and liver function assessed if such patients are to receive relaxants. Caused by antibodies from the tumour directed against the pre-synaptic membrane and less quanta of ACh being released for each nerve impulse. Differs from myasthenia gravis as follows: (1) it involves proximal limb muscles rather than bulbar and extra-ocular muscles; (2) the presence of aching muscular pains in the limbs; (3) diminished tendon reflexes; (4) poor response to neostigmine and other anticholinesterase medication; (5) marked sensitivity to both depolarizing and non-depolarizing blockers; and (6) electromyographic characteristics: (*a*) reduced response to single or slow stimuli; and (*b*) growth of potentials with tetanic stimulation.[152] Guanidine or diaminopyridine may have therapeutic value. Patients under anaesthesia being treated with thiotepa may have prolonged impairment of neuromuscular function, refractory to neostigmine.[153] Temporary improvement of the muscle weakness may follow surgical removal of the carcinoma. *See also* Engel A. G. *Ann. Neurol.* 1984, **16**, 519; Telford R. J. and Hollway T. E. *Br. J. Anaesth.* 1990, **64**, 363; For the use of high extradural analgesia *see* Sakura S. et al. *Anaesthesia* 1991, **46**, 560.

DISEASE OF THE NERVOUS SYSTEM

Spinal analgesia and extradural block are usually inadvisable because future symptoms and signs may be blamed (unjustly) on these methods of analgesia. A history of frequent headaches may also make spinal analgesia undesirable. But *see also* Crawford J. S. et al. *Anaesthesia* 1981, **36**, 821.

Epilepsy

Patients with epilepsy should be kept on anticonvulsants before, during and after operation. In susceptible patients, epilepsy may be triggered off by cholinergic drugs, methohexitone, mono-amine oxidase inhibitors, phenothiazines, tricyclic antidepressants, enflurane, and sudden withdrawal of barbiturates, benzodiazepines and hypocapnia. Has also been reported after propofol.[154]

Status epilepticus may have to be treated with barbiturate anaesthesia[155] if diazepam and phenytoin fails to bring control. Paradoxically, propofol infusion has also been used with success.[156] *See also* O'Brien M. D. *Br. Med. J.* 1990, **301**, 918.

Paraplegia

Patients with cord transection at or above T7 may get *autonomic hyperreflexia:* severe hypertension and arrhythmias after certain visceral stimuli, e.g. distension of the bladder or rectum. Ganglionic blockade or extradural block may be required to relieve this. About 40% of such patients about to undergo operation will require anaesthesia as it is difficult to be sure that the lesion of the cord is complete.

Suxamethonium may be dangerous in the period between about 14 days and 3 months after onset of paraplegia. It releases more potassium than usual from muscles, and the extreme hyperkalaemia can cause arrhythmias.

Additional considerations: (1) chronic infection; (2) nutritional difficulties; (3) disturbed temperature regulation; (4) problems of pain; (5) problems of respiration; (6) problems of position on the operating table; and (7) psychiatric difficulties. Blood pressure is well-controlled by general anaesthesia with thiopentone, nitrous oxide, relaxant/IPPV and halothane, although isoflurane may provoke less arrhythmias.

Dystrophia myotonica

First described by Déléage in 1890 and again in 1909.[157] Inherited as an autosomal dominant. Presents in early adulthood with: (1) expressionless face; (2) wasting of masseters, sternomastoids and forearms; (3) limb weakness with inability to let go after a handshake or to relax previously contracted muscles; (4) percussion myotonia; (5) cataracts; (6) frontal baldness; (7) atrophy of gonads; (8) involvement of external muscles of the eye; and (9) dysphagia.

It is a disorder of muscular fibre membranes with an abnormality of chloride conductance. The myoneural junction is normal. There may be respiratory muscle weakness, a low vital capacity and an increased $Paco_2$. Cardiomyopathy and conduction defects are common. This disease should be sought in a young patient with cataracts (as should diabetes).

Anaesthetic management

Pre-operatively: spirometry; look for myotonia of the diaphragm by fluoroscopy; ECG.

Respiratory depressants should be avoided before, during and after operation. Thiopentone has been reported to cause apnoea,[158] so if used should be given as careful 50 mg increments. Cardiovascular depression and dysrhythmias may occur during anaesthesia[159] and be worsened by volatile agents. Intubation is often possible without relaxants. IPPV may be required during operation and immediate postoperatively.[160]

Non-depolarizing relaxants, e.g. atracurium[161] or vecuronium[162] may be used cautiously but do not abolish myotonia. Infusion of propofol and atracurium may be suitable,[163] although sensitivity to propofol has been reported.[164] Anticholinesterase drugs may increase the myotonia. Depolarizing relaxants are hazardous. They can cause increased muscle tone, which may represent an exaggerated fasciculation and prevent intubation. It gives place to ordinary depolarizing relaxation with injection of additional doses. Spinal analgesia does not relax myotonia but injection of local analgesic into the muscle may do so. Dantrolene has been used for muscle relaxation.[165] Extradural block may be satisfactory,[166] but shivering may induce myotonia while uterine atony in the obstetric patient can result in haemorrhage. Pharyngeal muscle dysfunction may lead to aspiration.

See also Aldridge L. M. *Br. J. Anaesth.* 1985, **57**, 1119; In obstetrics, Blumgart C. H. et al. *Anaesthesia* 1990, **45**, 26; In children, Anderson B. J. and Brown T. C. K. *Anaesth. Intensive Care* 1989, **17**, 320.

Huntington's (1850–1916) chorea[167]

It is suggested that inhalation agents are the most suitable. Thiopentone may cause prolonged apnoea and should be avoided[168] or used with great care.[169] Midazolam has been proposed for induction.[170] Propofol and atracurium have also been used with success.[171] Abnormal serum cholinesterase may prolong the action of suxamethonium, although some patients respond normally.[172] *See also* Lamont A. S. M. *Anaesthesia* 1983, **38**, 295.

Hypokalaemic periodic paralysis

Dominant inheritance, in which attacks of generalized weakness lasting several hours may be precipitated by exercise, heavy meals or the stress of surgery. Potassium moves into the muscle cells. Thiopentone may cause temporary peripheral paralysis. Muscle relaxants may cause residual muscle weakness, but atracurium has been used without problem.[159]

Multiple sclerosis

Disseminated sclerosis, a term used by German pathologists in 1882, was changed to multiple sclerosis in 1946. Description systematized by J. M. Charcot (1825–1893) in 1868,[173] and by Cruveilhier in 1842. It has been suggested that general anaesthesia may cause a relapse, but this is probably not true.[174] Central neural blockade is better avoided on medicolegal grounds, although the relapse rate may be no greater following intradural block than after general anaesthesia.[175] Special anaesthetic care is not usually necessary. Relapses are more common in the three months post-partum.

See also Jones R. M. and Healy T. E. J. *Anaesthesia* 1980, **35**, 879; In obstetrics, Bader A.M. et al. *J. Clin. Anesth.* 1988, **1**, 21.

Motor neurone disease (amyotrophic lateral sclerosis)

First described by Erb (1840–1921)[176] in 1884 and by Gowers (1845–1915) in 1902.[177] A progressive disease of the over-50s which causes degeneration of the anterior horn cells in the spinal cord and bulbar palsy.

These patients may be emotionally labile. Excitement and tachycardia should be avoided. They are sensitive to barbiturates and non-depolarizing relaxants. Both should be given cautiously and their effects carefully monitored. Suxamethonium is best avoided as both hyperkalaemia and contracture may occur[178]. Inhalation agents may be suitable but the concentration of halothane should be increased with care. Respiratory depressant drugs must be used sparingly. Postoperative dysphagia may lead to aspiration. Epidural analgesia has been used safely.[179]

Duchenne muscular dystrophy[180]

Sex-linked recessive. The commonest muscular dystrophy and presents in early boyhood. Heart muscle is always involved and sudden cardiac arrest may occur during anaesthesia.[181] Usually present for orthopaedic procedures. Suxamethonium and halothane should be avoided as some patients develop malignant hyperpyrexia.[182] Temperature and ECG should be monitored throughout.[183] For complications *see* Larsen U. T. et al. *Can. J. Anaesth.* 1989, **36**, 418.

References

1. Derrington M. C. and Smith G. *Br. J. Anaesth.* 1987, **59**, 815.
2. Buck N. et al. *The report of a confidential enquiry into perioperative deaths.* London: The Nuffield Provincial Hospital Trust and the King's Fund, 1987.
3. Lunn J. N. and Devlin H. B. *Lancet* 1987, **2**, 1384.
4. Del Guerico L. R. M. and Cohn J. D. *JAMA* 1980, **243**, 1350.
5. Hosking M. P. et al. *JAMA* 1989, **261**, 1909.
6. Caird F. I. In *Oxford Textbook of Medicine.* (Weatherall D. J. et al. ed.) Oxford: Oxford University Press, 1987, 27.1.
7. Munson E. S. et al. *Anesth. Analg.* 1984, **63**, 998.
8. Duncan P. J. et al. *Anesthesiology* 1986, **64**, 790.
9. Cotton B. R. and Smith G. *Br. J. Anaesth.* 1984, **56**, 37.
10. Milsom I. and Forssman L. *Am. J. Obstet. Gynecol.* 1984, **148**, 764.
11. Konieczko K. M. et al. *Br. J. Anaesth.* 1987, **59**, 449.
12. O'Sullivan H. et al. *Anesthesiology* 1981, **55**, 645; Keeling P. A. et al. *Br. J. Anaesth.* 1986, **58**, 528.
13. Wendon J. and Bihari D. In: *Recent Advances in Anaesthesia and Analgesia – 17.* (Atkinson R. S. and Adams A. P. eds.) Edinburgh: Churchill Livingstone, 1992.
14. Abdulatif M. et al. *Can. J. Anaesth.* 1987, **34**, 284.
15. Goldman L. et al. *N. Engl. J. Med.* 1977, **297**, 845; Goldman L. *J. Cardiothorac. Anesth.* 1987, **1**, 237.
16. Peter K. et al. *Anesthesiologie und Intensivmedizin.* 1980, **9**, 240.
17. Pedersen T. et al. *Acta Anaesthesiol. Scand.* 1990, **34**, 144.
18. Kligfield P. et al. *Am. Heart J.* 1986, **112**, 589.
19. Pedersen T. et al. *Acta Anaesthesiol. Scand.* 1990, **34**, 183.
20. Hertzer N. R. et al. *Ann. Surg.* 1984, **199**, 223; Foster E. D. et al. *Ann. Thorac. Surg.* 1986, **41**, 42.
21. Rao T. L. K. et al. *Anesthesiology* 1983, **59**, 499.
22. Häggmark S. et al. *Anesthesiology* 1989, **70**, 19; Vandenberg B. F. and Kerber R. E. *Anesthesiology* 1990, **73**, 799.
23. Slogoff S. and Keats A. S. *Anesthesiology* 1985, **62**, 107.
24. Hilfiker O. et al. *Br. J. Anaesth.* 1983, **55**, 927.
25. Priebe H.-J. *Anesthesiology* 1989, **71**, 960.
26. Buffington C. W. et al. *Anesthesiology* 1988, **69**, 721.
27. Tarnow J. et al. *Anesthesiology* 1986, **64**, 147.

28. Pateman J. A. and Hanning C. D. *Br. J. Anaesth.* 1989, **63**, 648; Rosenberg J. et al. *Br. J. Anaesth.* 1990, **65**, 684.
29. Hammer A. *Wien. Med. Wochenschr.* 1878, **28**, 97.
30. Obrastow W. P. and Strascheskow N. D. *Zeit. Clin. Med.* 1910, **71**, 116.
31. Herrick J. B. *JAMA* 1912, **59**, 2015.
32. Dirksen A. and Kjoller E. *Br. Med. J.* 1988, **297**, 1011.
33. Stone J. G. *Anesthesiology* 1988, **68**, 495.
34. Foster E. D. et al. *Ann. Thorac. Surg.* 1986, **41**, 42.
35. Stokes W. M. *Dubl. Q. J. Med. Sci.* 1846, **2**, 73.
36. Adams R. *Dubl. Hosp. Rep.* 1827, **4**, 353.
37. McConachie I. *Anaesthesia* 1987, **42**, 636.
38. Bloomfield P. and Bowler G. M. R. *Anaesthesia* 1989, **44**, 42.
39. Andersen C. and Madsen G. M. *Anaesthesia* 1990, **45**, 472.
40. Finfer S. R. *Br. J. Anaesth.* 1991, **66**, 509.
41. McKenzie J. *Diseases of the Heart.* London: Froude, 1908.
42. Mehta D. et al. *Lancet* 1988, **1**, 1181.
43. Clarke B. et al. *Lancet* 1987, **1**, 299.
44. Scheinman M. *JAMA* 1990, **263**, 79.
45. Travis S. et al. *Br. J. Surg.* 1989, **76**, 1107.
46. Chevers N. *Guy's Hosp. Rep.* 1842, **7**, 387.
47. Ledingham I. McA. and Ramsay G. *Br. J. Anaesth.* 1986, **58**, 169.
48. Fennelly M. E. and Hall G. M. *Br. J. Anaesth.* 1990, **64**, 535.
49. Cohen M. M. and Cameron C. B. *Anesth. Analg.* 1991, **72**, 282.
50. Roukema J. A. et al. *Arch. Surg.* 1988, **123**, 30; Selsby D. and Jones J. G. *Br. J. Anaesth.* 1990, **64**, 621.
51. Hedenstierna G. *Br. J. Anaesth.* 1990, **64**, 507.
52. Nunn J. F. et al. *Anaesthesia* 1988, **43**, 543.
53. Jones R. M. et al. *Anaesthesia* 1987, **42**, 1.
54. Scott N. B. and Kehlet H. *Br. J. Surg.* 1988, **75**, 299; Ross W. B. et al. *Surgery* 1989, **105**, 166.
55. Jansen J. E. et al. *Lancet* 1990, **335**, 936.
56. *Drug Ther. Bull.* 1990, **28**, 45.
57. Patrick J. A. et al. *Anaesthesia* 1990, **45**, 390.
58. Carson J. L. et al. *Lancet* 1988, **1**, 727.
59. Richards D. W. and Strauss M. L. *J. Clin. Invest.* 1927, **4**, 105.
60. Bunn H. F. and Forget B. G. *Human Hemoglobins.* 2nd ed. Philadelphia: W. B. Saunders, 1985; Serjeant G. R. *Sickle Cell Disease.* Oxford: Oxford University Press, 1985; Esseltine D. W. et al. *Can. J. Anaesth.* 1988, **35**, 385.
61. Herrick J. B. *Arch. Intern. Med.* 1910, **6**, 517.
62. Pauling L. et al. *Science, N. Y.* 1949, **110**, 543.
63. Emmel V. E. *Arch. Intern. Med.* 1917, **20**, 586.
64. Eichhorn J. H. *JAMA* 1988, **259**, 907.
65. Wetherley-Mein G. and Pearson T. C. In: *Blood and its Disorders.* (Hardisty R. M. and Weatherall D. J. ed.), 2nd ed. Oxford: Blackwell, 1982, 1269.
66. Otto J. C. *Med. Reposit., N. Y.* 1803, **61**, 1.
67. Bullock W. and Fildes P. *Haemophilia.* London: Dulau Co., 1911.
68. Ah Pin P. J. *Br. Dent. J.* 1987, **162**, 151.
69. Harris D. C. H. et al. *Kidney Int.* 1987, **31**, 41.
70. Loehning R. W. and Mazze R. I. *Anesthesiology* 1974, **40**, 203.
71. Spencer E. M. et al. *Br. J. Anaesth.* 1990, **65**, 574P.
72. Jones R. M. et al. *Br. J. Anaesth.* 1990, **64**, 482.
73. Gelman S. *Can. J. Physiol. Pharmacol.* 1987, **65**, 1762.
74. Hulcrantz R. et al. *Scand. J. Gastroenterol.* 1986, **21**, 109; Laker M. F. *Br. Med. J.* 1990, **301**, 250.
75. Grounds R. M. et al. *Br. Med. J.* 1987, **294**, 397.

76. Bencini A. F. et al. *Br. J. Anaesth.* 1986, **58**, 988.
77. Pugh R. N. H. et al. *Br. J. Surg.* 1973, **60**, 646.
78. Stokvis B. J. E. *Ned. Tijdschr. Geneesk.* 1889, **25**, 409.
79. Famewo C. E. *Can. Anaesth. Soc J.* 1985, **32**, 171.
80. Mitterschiffthaler G. et al. *Br. J. Anaesth.* 1988, **60**, 109; Weir P. M. and Hodkinson B. P. *Anaesthesia* 1988, **43**, 1022; Meissner P. N. et al. *Br. J. Anaesth.* 1991, **66**, 60.
81. McNeill M. J. and Bennet A. *Br. J. Anaesth.* 1990, **64**, 371.
82. Haxholdt O. St. et al. *Anaesthesia* 1984, **39**, 240.
83. Stoelting R. K. *Can. J. Anaesth.* 1987, **34**, 223.
84. Beaconsfield F. et al. *N. Eng. J. Med.* 1972, **287**, 209.
85. Lange R. A. et al. *N. Eng. J. Med.* 1989, **321**, 1557.
86. Michel R. and Adams A. P. *Anaesthesia* 1979. **34**, 1016.
87. Peckham C. S. et al. *Lancet* 1990, **335**, 516.
88. Ruthanne M. *Abstracts of 5th International Conference on AIDS.* International Development Research Centre, PO Box 8500, Ottawa, Ontario. 1989, 63; Rogers P. L. et al. *Crit. Care Med.* 1989, **17**, 113.
89. *AIDS and Hepatitis B.* London: Association of Anaesthetists, 1988; *Recommendations of the Expert Advisory Group on Aids.* London: HMSO, 1990.
90. Jones M. E. *Anaesth. Intensive Care* 1989, **17**, 253.
91. Henderson D. K. and Gerberding J. L. *J. Infect. Dis.* 1989, **160**, 321; Jefferies D. I. *Br. Med. J.* 1991, **302**, 1349.
92. Frankel H. M. *JAMA* 1986, **255**, 1292.
93. Named for Mr Wardle's fat boy in Charles Dickens's (1812-1870) *The Pickwick Papers*, 1837; *see* Burwell C. S. et al. *Am. J. Med.* 1956, **21**, 811 (reprinted in 'Classical File', *Surv. Anesthesiol.* 1977, **21**, 477).
94. Banting F. G. and Best C. H. *J. Lab. Clin. Med.* 1922, **7**, 25.
95. Burgos L. G. et al. *Anesthesiology* 1989, **70**, 591; Bilous R. W. *Br. Med. J.* 1990, **301**, 565.
96. Rees P. J. et al. *J. R. Soc. Med.* 1981, **74**, 192.
97. McMurray J. F. *Surg. Clin. N. Am.* 1984, **64**, 769.
98. Hjortrup A. et al. *Br. J. Surg.* 1985, **72**, 783; MacKenzie C. R. and Charlson M. E. *Surg. Gynecol. Obstet.* 1988, **167**, 293.
99. Alberti K. G. M. M. and Thomas D. J. B. *Br. J. Anaesth.* 1979, **51**, 693; Thomas D. J. B. et al. *Anaesthesia* 1984, **39**, 629.
100. Dunnet J. M. *Anaesthesia* 1988, **43**, 538.
101. Hall G. M. and Desborough J. P. *Anaesthesia* 1988, **43**, 531.
102. Sanson T. H. and Levine S. N. *Drugs* 1989, **38**, 289.
103. Levine S. N. and Sanson T. H. *Drugs* 1989, **38**, 462.
104. Madias N. E. *Kidney Int.* 1986, **29**, 752.
105. Thomas D. J. B. et al. *Anaesthesia* 1983, **38**, 1047.
106. Muir J. J. et al. *Anesthesiology* 1983, **59**, 371.
107. Burch P. and McLeskey C. H. *Anesthesiology* 1981, **55**, 472.
108. Ord W. M. (1834–1902), *Med. Chir. Trans.* 1878, **43**, 57.
109. Cooper D. S. *JAMA* 1987, **258**, 246.
110. Sherry K. M. and Hutchinson I. L. *Anaesthesia* 1984, **39**. 1112.
111. Addison T. *Lond. Med. Gaz.* 1849, **48**, 517.
112. Waterhouse R. *Lancet* 1911, **1**, 577; Friderichsen C. *Jb. Kinderheilk. 1918*, **87**, 109.
113. Voelker A. R. *Middx Hosp. Rep. Med. Surg. Path. Regist.* 1894, 278.
114. Fraser C. G. et al. *JAMA* 1952, **149**, 1542.
115. Orth D. N. *New Engl. J. Med.* 1984, **310**, 649.
116. Saucerotte N. *Mélang. de Chirurg. (Paris)* 1801, **1**, 407.
117. Marie P. *Med. Rev. Paris* 1886, **6**, 297.
118. Chappell W. F. *J. Laryngol.* 1896, **10**, 142.
119. Campkin V. *Anaesthesia* 1980, **35**, 1008.
120. Simmonds M. *Dtsch. Med. Wochenschr.* 1914, **40**, 322.
121. Sheehan H. L. *Am. J. Obstet. Gynecol.* 1954, **68**, 202.

122. Obendorfer S. S. *Frankf. Z. Path.* 1907, **1**, 426.
123. Coupe M. et al. *Q. J. Med.* 1989, **73**, 1021.
124. Editorial *Lancet* 1990, **336**, 909.
125. Simpson K. H. *Br. J. Anaesth.* 1985, **57**, 934.
126. Fischler M. et al. *Br. J. Anaesth.* 1983, **55**, 920; Houghton K. and Carter J. A. *Anaesthesia* 1986, **41**, 595.
127. Marsh H. M. et al. *Anesthesiology* 1987, **66**, 89; Roy R. C. *Anaesthesia* 1987, **42**, 627; Hughes E. W. and Hodkinson B. P. *Anaesth. Intensive Care* 1989, **17**, 367.
128. Napolitano L. M. and Chernow B. *Int. Anesthesiol. Clin.* 1988, **26**, 226.
129. Fraser C. G. et al. *JAMA* 1952, **149**, 1542.
130. Clayton R. N. *Br. Med. J.* 1989, **298**, 271.
131. Symreng T. et al. *Br. J. Anaesth.* 1981, **53**, 949; Udelsman R. et al. *J. Clin. Invest.* 1986, **77**, 1377; *Drug Ther. Bull.* 1990, **28**, 71.
132. Kussmaul A. and Maier R. *Dtsh. Arch. Klin. Med.* 1866, **1**, 484.
133. Malinow A.M. et al. *Anaesthesia* 1987, **42**, 1291.
134. Bromley I. M. and Hirsch N. P. *Anaesthesia* 1984, **39**, 723.
135. Elliott M. W. et al. *Br. Med. J.* 1990, **300**, 358.
136. Wardall G. J. and Frame W. T. *Br. J. Anaesth.* 1990, **64**, 367.
137. Hool G. J. et al. *Anaesth. Intensive Care* 1984, **12**, 360.
138. Willis T. *The London Practice of Physick.* London: T. Cassell, 1685.
139. Wilks S. *Guy's Hosp. Rep.* 1877, **3** (Series 27), 7.
140. Jolly F. *Neurol. Zbl.* 1895, **14**, 34.
141. Campbell H. and Bromwell E. *Brain* 1900, **23**, 277.
142. Remen L. *Dtsch. Z. Nerven Heilk.* 1932, **128**, 66.
143. Walker M. *Lancet* 1934, **1**, 120.
144. Sauerbruch E. F. *Mitt. Grenzgeb. Med. Chir.* 1912-13, **25**, 746.
145. Blalock A. et al. *Ann. Surg.* 1939, **110**, 544.
146. Keynes G. *Br. J. Surg.* 1946, **33**, 201.
147. Weigeri C. *Arch. Psychiat. Nerv. Krankh.* 1901, **34**, 1063.
148. Wojciechowski A. J. P. et al. *Anaesthesia* 1985, **40**, 882.
149. Rowbottom S. J. *Anaesth. Intensive Care* 1989, **17**, 444; Nilsson E. and Muller K. *Acta Anaesthesiol. Scand.* 1990, **34**, 126.
150. Nilsson E. and Meretoja O. A. *Anesthesiology* 1990, **73**, 28.
151. Eaton M. L. and Lambert E. H. *JAMA* 1957, **163**, 1117.
152. Wise R. P. *Anaesthesia* 1962, **17**, 488.
153. Bennet E. J. et al. *Anesthesiology* 1977, **47**, 317.
154. Shearer E. S. *Anaesthesia* 1990, **45**, 255.
155. Lowenstein D. H. et al. *Neurology* 1988, **38**, 395.
156. Mackenzie S. J. et al. *Anaesthesia* 1990, **45**, 1043.
157. Steinert H. *Dtsch. Z. Nerven Heilk.* 1909, **37**, 58; Batten F. E. and Gibbs H. P. *Brain* 1909, **32**, 187.
158. Hewer C. L. *Br. J. Anaesth.* 1957, **29**, 180.
159. Rooney R. T. et al. *Anesth. Analg.* 1988, **67**, 782.
160. Harper P. S. *Lancet* 1989, **ii**, 1269.
161. Nightingale P. et al. *Br. J. Anaesth.* 1985, **57**, 1131.
162. Castano J. and Pares N. *Br. J. Anaesth.* 1987, **59**, 1629.
163. White D. A. and Smyth D. G. *Can. J. Anaesth.* 1989, **39**, 200.
164. Speedy H. *Br. J. Anaesth.* 1990, **64**, 110.
165. Phillips D. C. et al. *Anaesthesia* 1984, **39**, 568.
166. Harris N. E. M. *Anaesthesia* 1984, **39**, 1032.
167. Huntington G. *Med. Surg. Reporter (Philadelphia)* 1872, **26**, 317.
168. Blanloeil Y. et al. *Anaesthesia* 1982, **37**, 695.
169. Browne G. M. *Anaesthesia* 1983, **38**, 65.
170. Rodrigo M. R. *Br. J. Anaesth.* 1987, **59**, 388.
171. Kaufman M. A. and Erb T. *Anaesthesia* 1990, **45**, 889.

172. Costarino A. and Gross J. R. *Anesthesiology* 1985, **63**, 570.
173. Charcot J. M. *Gaz. Hôp. civ. milit., Paris*, 1868, **41**, 554; *C. R. Soc. Biol. (Paris)* 1868, **20**, 16.
174. Bamford C. et al. *J. Can. Sci. Neurol.* 1987, **5**, 41.
175. Bouchard P. et al. *Ann. Fr. Anaesth. Reanim.* 1984, **3**, 195.
176. Erb W. H. *Dtsch. Arch. Klin. Med.* 1884, **34**, 467.
177. Gowers W. R. *Br. Med. J.* 1902, **2**, 89.
178. Azar I. *Anesthesiology* 1984, **61**, 173.
179. Kochi T. et al. *Anesth. Analg.* 1989, **68**, 410.
180. Sethna N. F. et al. *Anesthesiology* 1988, **68**, 462.
181. Sethna N. F. and Rockoff M. A. *Can. Anaesth. Soc. J.* 1986, **33**, 799.
182. Wang J. M. and Stanley T. H. *Can. Anaesth. Soc. J.* 1986, **33**, 492.
183. Smith C. L. and Bush G. H. *Br. J. Anaesth.* 1985, **57**, 1113.

Chapter 21

Dictionary of difficult diseases

An anaesthetist faced by problems, which may arise in his patient due to an unusual disease, may find the following list useful in his choice of anaesthetic.

Aaskog-Scott syndrome Difficult intubation due to cervical spine stiffness.

Achalasia of the cardia Increased regurgitation risk.

Achondroplasia Intubation difficult due to short cervical spine. (Brimacombe J. R and Caunt J. A. *Anaesthesia* 1990, **45**, 132.) Extradural anaesthesia is possible. (Wardall G. J. and Frame W. T. *Br J. Anaesth.* 1990, **64**, 367.)

Acromegaly Airway sometimes very difficult, partly due to large tongue; intubation difficult, partly due to narrow cricoid ring. Diabetes, hypertension occur. A pituitary tumour may exert local pressure effects. Post-hypophysectomy: steroids required.

Addison's disease Hypovolaemia, hyponatraemia, hypoglycaemia. Steroids required. (*See* Chapter 20.) T. A. Addison (1793–1860), London physician.

Adrenogenital syndrome May be mistaken for pyloric stenosis. Fludrocortisone steroid cover may be required for salt loss. Pre-operative electrolyte check required. (Bongiovanni A. M. and Root A. W. *N. Engl. J. Med.* 1963, **268**, 1283, 1342, 1391.)

Aglossia-adactilia syndrome Difficult intubation due to micrognathia.

Agranulocytosis Susceptible to infections.

AIDS See AIDS and anaesthesia. (Lee K. G. and Soni N. *Anaesthesia* 1986, **41** 1011 *See also* Chapter 20.)

Albers-Schonberg disease Brittle bones, risk of fractures while moving or positioning patient. Anaemia, splenomegaly, hypercalcaemia. Heinrich Ernst Albers Schonberg (1865–1921), Hamburg physician.

Albright–Butler syndrome Renal calculi with renal failure, acidosis, hypokalaemia, hypercalcaemia. Cardiac arrythmias occur. (Morris R. C. *N. Engl. J. Med.* 1969, **281**, 1405.)

Albright's osteodystrophy (pseudohypoparathyroidism) Ectopic calcification, hypocalcaemia, neuromuscular excitability, convulsions. F. Albright (1900–1969), Boston physician.

Alcoholism Resistance to anaesthetic, cirrhosis, cardiomyopathy, perioperative withdrawal crisis (delirium tremens). See Chapter 20.

Alport syndrome Conduction deafness and renal failure in adult life.

Alström syndrome   Obese, deaf and blind by 7 years of age. Diabetes and renal failure in adult life. C. H. A. Alstrom (1903), Stockholm geneticist.

Alveolar hypoventilation (Ondine's curse)   (Wiesel S. and Fox G. S. *Can. J. Anaesth.* 1990, **37**, 122.) Apnoea during sleep.

Amoebiasis   Anaemia, dehydration, liver abscess with pulmonary complications.

Amyloidosis   Unexpected cardiac or renal failure may occur. (Welch D. B. *Anaesthesia* 1982, **37**, 63.)

Amyotonia congenita   (Kugelberg-Welander disease, Werdnig-Hoffmann disease). Spinal muscular atrophy with anterior horn cell degeneration. Ventilation problems due to muscle weakness. Very sensitive to thiopentone, respiratory depressants and muscle relaxants. (Ellis F. R. *Br. J. Anaesth.* 1974, **46**, 605.)

Amyotrophic lateral sclerosis (motor neurone disease)   Very sensitive to thiopentone, curare and respiratory depressants. Suxamethonium causes dangerous hyperkalaemia. (Rosenbaum K. J. et al. *Anesthesiology* 1971, **35**, 638.) *See* Chapter 20.

Analbuminaemia   Sensitivity to protein-bound drugs, e.g. thiopentone curare, bupivacaine.

Andersen's disease (glycogen storage disease IV)   Hypoglycaemia under anaesthesia. Dorothy H. A. Andersen (1901–1963), New York pathologist.

Andersen's syndrome   Cystic fibrosis.

Anhidrotic ectodermal dysplasia (Christ–Siemens–Touraine syndrome) Difficult intubation, heat intolerance, recurrent chest infections. (Beahrs J. O. et al. *Ann. Intern. Med.* 1971, **74**, 92.)

Ankylosing spondylitis   Difficult intubation sometimes. *See* Chapter 20.

Anorexia nervosa   Hypothermia, hypotension, hypokalaemia, anaemia. Myocardial weakness in addition to muscle weakness.

Apert's syndrome (craniosynostosis)   Difficult intubation due to micrognathia; raised intracranial pressure; other congenital defects, e.g. VSD. (Andersson H. and Gomes S. P. *Acta Paediatr. Scand.* 1968, **57**, 47; *Textbook of Paediatric Anaesthetic Practice* (Sumner E. and Hatch D. J. ed.) London: Bailliére Tindall, 1989; Eugene Apert (1868–1940), Paris paediatrician.

Arnold-Chiari malformation   Herniation of cerebellum and medulla through foramen magnum with headache, hydrocephalus, cranial nerve entrapment, torsion of brainstem, raised intracranial pressure, and signs of syringomyelia in about 50%. (Banerji N. K. and Millar J. H. D. *Brain* 1974, **97**, 157.)

Arthrogryposis (congenital contractures)   Difficult veins, difficult airway, due to micrognathia and cervical spine/jaw stiffness. Scoliosis, myopathic muscles. Sensitive to thiopentone, associated congenital heart disease in 10% of patients. Possibility of malignant hyperpyrexia. (Baines D. B. et al. *Anaesth. Intensive Care* 1986, **14**, 370; Oberdi G. S. et al. *Can. J. Anaesth.* 1988, **35**, 288, 612.)

Armadillo disease   Spontaneous myokymia of arms and legs, with absent tendon reflexes, but increased tone, abolished by relaxants and phenytoin, but not by regional blockade or sleep. (Wilton A. and Graham J. G. *Hosp. Update.* 1990, **16**, 698.)

Asbestosis   Pulmonary fibrosis. May be on steroids, may have tuberculosis.

Asplenia syndrome Associated congenital heart disease with failure.

Ataxia-telangiectasia Immunoincompetence (IgA and IgE). Recurrent infections.

Atrial fibrillation (acute) Procainamide infusion has been recommended. Cardioversion may be indicated. (Fulham M. J. and Cookson W. O. C. *Anaesth. Intensive Care* 1984, **12**, 121.)

Atrial septal defect (ASD) Antibiotic cover is usual. Decreasing systemic vascular resistance decreases the shunt, as does IPPV.

Atrioventricular block (1st degree) There may be severe bradycardia during anaesthesia. (Hayward R. et al. *Anaesthesia* 1982, **37**, 1190.)

Auto-immune anaemias May be on steroids. Respiration may be difficult to restart after IPPV.

Autonomic hyper-reflexia *See* Hutchinson R. C. *Anaesthesia* 1986, **41**, 663.

Barlow's syndrome (click-murmur mitral valve prolapse) Bradycardia resistant to atropine, dysrhythmias responding to beta blockade, and thromboembolism occur. Excessive tachycardia and anxiety should be avoided. Antibiotic cover is usual.

Bartter syndrome Electrolyte abnormalities occur, especially hypokalaemia.

Behçet syndrome Steroid cover often required. Mouth ulcers can be a problem.

Beckwith (Wiedemann) syndrome (infantile gigantism) Macroglossia with airway problems, severe hypoglycaemia. (Filippi G. and McKusick V. A. *Medicine (Baltimore)* 1970, **49**, 279.)

Beri-beri Cardiomyopathy with failure, muscular weakness.

Berylliosis Pulmonary fibrosis. May be on steroids.

Blackfan – Diamond syndrome (congenital red-cell aplasia) Thrombocytopenia, anaemia, VSD. May be on steroids.

Bloom's syndrome Defect in DNA management; X-rays are more likely to damage cells, and should be restricted.

Bowen's syndrome (cerebrohepatorenal syndrome) Renal failure, hypoprothrombinaemia, sensitivity to muscle relaxants. J. T. Bowen (1857–1941), Boston dermatologist.

Bronchiolitis fibrosa obliterans Pulmonary fibrosis. May be on steroids.

Buerger's disease Bronchitis and emphysema, peripheral vascular insufficiency. Indirect arterial pressure measurements may be inaccurate (reading too high).

Bullous cystic lung disease (For suggested technique of anaesthesia *see* Normandale J. P. and Feneck R. O. *Anaesthesia* 1985, **40**, 1182.)

Burkitt's lymphoma May be difficult to intubate. Denis B. Burkitt (1911–), of Dublin, London and Uganda.

Burns Hypovolaemia, lung burns, hyperkalaemia with suxamethonium, intubation problem sometimes. *See* Chapters 20 and 32.

Carcinoid syndrome Tricuspid valve malfunction, sudden bronchospasm, especially with cyclopropane and hypotension. *See* Chapter 20; Solares G. and Blanco E. et al. *Anaesthesia* 1987, **42**, 989.

Cardiac tamponade Low cardiac output, high venous pressure, anaesthesia and IPPV may worsen the failure.

Carpenter's syndrome (cranial synostosis with small mandible, congenital heart disease; PDA & VSD)   Intubation problems. (Andersson H. and Gomes S. P. *Acta Paediatr. Scand.* 1968, **57**, 47.) George C. Carpenter (1859–1910), London paediatrician.

Central core myopathy   See Congenital myopathy.

Cerebrocostomandibular syndrome   Difficult intubation and respiration (cleft palate, micrognathia, microthorax, tracheal abnormalities, vertebral anomalies).

Chagas disease (American trypanosomiasis)   Hepatic failure, cardio-myopathy. (Barretto J. C. *Br. J. Anaesth.* 1979, **51**, 1189.) Carlos Chagas (1879–1934), Brazilian physician.

CHARGE Association   Difficult intubation due to micrognathia, cleft palate. Also choanal atresia, microphallus and cryptorchidism. Congenital heart disease in 70%.

Chediak–Higashi syndrome (immunodeficiency, with some albinism)   Re-current infections, thrombocytopenia. May be on steroids. (Blume R. S. and Wolff S. M. *Medicine (Baltimore)*, 1972, **51**, 247.)

Cherubism   Oral airway obstruction due to macroglossia, intubation may be impossible, urgent tracheostomy may be required. Corrective surgery very haemorrhagic.

Choanal atresia   Nasal obstruction. If bilateral, severe respiratory obstruction can be an emergency, solved by an oral airway, which is taped in place. Compression of the tracheal tube by Boyle-Davis gag during surgical correction can be a problem. The child is extubated wide awake with nasal splints in place.

Chotzen syndrome (craniosynostosis)   Difficult intubation due to micro-gnathia, sometimes renal failure. (Andersson H. and Gomes S. P. *Acta Paediatr. Scand.* 1968, **57**, 47.) F. C. Chotzen, Breslau psychiatrist.

Christ-Siemens-Tourane syndrome (ectodermal dysplasia)   Difficult intu-bation due to micrognathia. No hair or teeth. Defective thermoregulation due to absent sweat glands; cooling mattress should be available. Atropine, etc. are avoided.

Christmas disease   See Chapter 20.

Chronic Granuloma disease   Lung problems due to granulomas.

Cleft palate   Difficult intubation, respiratory obstruction with heavy sedative premedication. *See* Chapter 22, Paediatrics.

Cockayne's syndrome   (Cockayne E. A. *Arch. Dis. Child* 1936, **11**, 1.) An inherited autosomal recessive disorder with progressive mental and physical retardation, deafness, blindness, bony malformations etc. Intubation may be very difficult. (Cook S. *Anaesthesia* 1982, **37**, 1104.)

Congenital analgesia   Sedation or general anaesthesia may be required and abnormal responses to drugs may be present. (Layman P. R. *Anaesthesia* 1986, **41**, 395.)

Congenital myopathy (central core disease)   Ventilation problem due to muscle weakness. Sensitivity to muscle relaxants. Malignant hyperpyrexia may occur. (Shuaib A. et al. *Medicine* 1987, **66**, 389.)

Congenital trophoblastic disease   Patients have a low plasma cholinester-ase level and elevated chorionic gonadotrophin. (Davies J. M. et al. *Anaesthesia* 1984, **12**, 1074.)

Conn's syndrome   Hypertension, hypokalaemia, oedema. J. C. Conn (1907–), Ann Arbor internist. (*See also* Chapter 20.)

Conjoined twins (Siamese twins) Intubation difficulties sometimes, adrenal failure, one infant may exsanguinate the other at operation, multiple anaesthetics required. Slow gas induction due to wider distribution of the agents. *See* Chapter 22, Paediatrics; Diaz J. H. and Furman E. B. *Anesthesiology* 1987, **67**, 965–973.

Conradi Hunermann syndrome (chondrodystrophy and mental deficiency) Renal and congenital heart disease sometimes.

Core syndrome Muscle weakness disease with ventilation problems. *See* Congenital myopathy.

Cretinism Intubation difficulties due to macroglossia, sensitivity to anaesthetic drugs. Muscle weakness may give respiratory problems and cardiomyopathy occurs. Steroid cover may be required. Hypoglycaemia and electrolyte problems occur.

Creutzfeldt–Jacob disease (*see* MacMurdo S. D. et al. *Anesthesiology* 1984, **60**, 590.)

Cri-du-chat disease (microcephaly, micrognathia, macroglossia) Difficult airway, difficult intubation, associated ASD and VSD (in 25%).

Crohn's disease Anaemia, toxaemia (sometimes very severe), hypoproteinaemia. May be on steroids. B. B. Crohn (1884–1983), New York physician.

Crouzon's disease (Craniosynostosis) Difficult intubation due to micrognathia, postoperative respiratory obstruction. Corrective operations very haemorrhagic. Coarctation of aorta occurs. (Andersson H. and Gomes S. P. *Acta Paediatr. Scand.* 1968, **57**, 47.)

Cushing's syndrome Diabetes, hypertension, hypokalaemia, sodium retention, obesity, thin skin. Harvey Cushing (1869–1939), Boston neurosurgeon.

Cutis laxa (elastic degeneration) Fragile skin, blood vessels, lung infections and emphysema common. Pendulous laryngeal and pharyngeal mucosa may obstruct breathing. (Wooley M. W. et al. *J. Pediatr. Surg.* 1967, **2**, 325.)

Cystic fibrosis Atropine may inspissate secretions. (Lamberty J. M. and Rubin B. K. *Anaesthesia* 1985, **40**, 448.) Nasal polypectomy may be required and children withstand anaesthesia well. May have chronic obstructive lung disease, airway obstruction, malnutrition and bleeding tendency. There is a risk of respiratory problems but careful humidification, asepsis and antibiotics will usually avoid these.

Cystic hygroma Respiratory obstruction after induction due to the soft tissue mass, often corrected by nasal airway, difficult intubation sometimes.

Dermatomyositis Mouth opening restricted, chest infections, anaemia, hypersensitivity to non-depolarizing relaxants. Steroid cover required. (Eisele J. H. in: *Anesthesia for Uncommon Diseases* (Katz E. and Kadis M. ed.). Philadephia: Saunders, 1973.)

Diaphragmatic hernia (congenital) Often an emergency, dyspnoea, hypoxia, acidosis, cardiac failure, pneumothorax, postoperative respiratory failure. (*See* Chapter 22, Paediatrics.)

Diastrophic dwarfism Difficult intubation due to micrognathia and short neck.

DiGeorge syndrome (immune deficiency, athymia) Chest infections, stridor, aortic arch anomalies with cardiac failure, hypoparathyroidism, hypocalcaemia, tetany. Fresh donor blood is irradiated to prevent graft-versus-host reaction.

Disseminated sclerosis (multiple sclerosis) Deterioration may follow pyrexia, and spinal (and other regional) analgesia. (Alderson J. D. *Anaesthesia* 1991, **45**, 1084; Bamford C. J. *Can. Sci. Neurol.* 1987, **5**, 41.) *See* Chapter 20.

Down's syndrome (mongolism, trisomy 21) Require very large doses of sedatives and premedication. Large tongue, small mouth, neck may be stiff; intubation difficult and upper airway may obstruct. Risk of extubation stridor, especially after cardiac surgery. Associated congenital heart disease, especially septal defects (in 50%). Extubation laryngeal spasm may occur. The eye is sensitive to atropine but large doses of hyoscine may be required for hypersalivation. Hypoglycaemia occurs easily. Asymptomatic atlanto-axial instability may be a problem so that intubation should be undertaken with great care. (Gallamnaugh S. C. *Br. Med. J.* 1985, **291**, 117; Powell J. F. *Anaesthesia* 1991, **45**, 1049.) *See* Chapter 22, Paediatrics. J. Langdon Down (1826–1896), London physician.

Drug addiction Opioid addicts may have inaccessible veins, requiring 'gas' induction. They may arrive in considerable respiratory depression from the most recent 'fix'. Drug withdrawal (or simulated withdrawal) may occur postop.

Dubowitz syndrome Difficult intubation (microcephaly, micrognathia), also hypertelorism.

Duchenne muscular dystrophy The commonest muscular disorder in childhood. Developing muscular weakness, scoliosis, obesity and falling vital capacity lead to chronic respiratory failure. Ventilatory support after operation may be necessary. (Heckmatt J. Z. *Br. Med. J.* 1987, **295**, 1014.) Frequent cardiac involvement, with occasional arrest. (Chalkaidis G. A. and Branch K. G. *Anaesthesia* 1990, **45**, 22). Atropine, opiates and non-depolarizing relaxants may well be avoided. A volatile agent may give adequate relaxation. Has been associated with malignant hyperpyrexia. (Ellis F. R. *Br. J. Anaesth.* 1974, **46**, 605; Lintner S. P. K. and Thomas P. R. *Br. J. Anaesth.* 1982, **54**, 1331; Rosenberg H. et al. *Anesthesiology* 1983, **59**, 362.); G. B. D. Duchenne (1806–1895), French neurologist. *See* Chapter 20.

Dyygue-Melchior-Clausen's syndrome Difficult intubation due to cervical spine.

Dysautonomia (Riley – Day syndrome) *See* Familial dysautonomia.

Dystrophia myotonica Respiratory failure and infections, hypertonic muscles (unable to relax after handshake), cardiac involvement in a significant proportion. Prolonged muscle spasm after suxamethonium, propofol (Speedy H. *Br. J. Anaesth.* 1990, **64**, 110), neostigmine and shivering. Hypersensitivity to respiratory depressants and nondepolarizing relaxants (which in some cases may *not* relax the myotonia). Associated with malignant hyperpyrexia, so halothane generally avoided. Isoflurane probably safe. Regional and inhalation techniques are recommended, but regional block may not produce relaxation. Prolonged apnoea may follow the injection of normal doses of thiopentone. Dystrophia in babies (*see* Bray R. J. and Inkster J. S. *Anaesthesia* 1984, **39**, 1007.) Dystrophia in obstetrics (*see* Blumgaret C. H., Hughes D. G. and Redfern N. *Anaesthesia* 1990 **45**, 26).

Ebstein's abnormality (tricuspid valve disease) Supraventricular tachycardia during induction. W. E. Ebstein (1836–1912), Göttingen physician.

Edward's syndrome (trisomy 18) VSD, patent ductus, pulmonary stenosis, micrognathia, short sternum, renal failure, clenched hands, low-set ears.

Ehlers–Danlos syndrome (collagen abnormality) Hypermobility of joints, fragile skin, veins, arteries and tracheal mucosa occur. Intubation may cause severe tracheal bruising. Spontaneous rupture of cerebral and other vessels, may be associated with aneurysms, thromboses occur; spontaneous pneumothorax (even during anaesthesia). Mitral regurgitation occurs. (Wooley M. W. et al. *J. Ped. Surg.* 1967, **2**, 325; Dolan P. et al. *Anesthesiology* 1980, **52**, 266; Ehlers E. *Derm. Zeit.* 1901, **8**, 173; Danlos H. *Bull. Soc. Franc. Dermatol. Syph.* 1908, **19**, 70.)

Eisenmenger's complex (pulmonary hypertension, intracardiac shunts, hypoxia) Decreases of systemic vascular resistance are dangerous by increasing the shunt, but vasoactive agents (and hypercapnia and further hypoxia) will cause rises of pulmonary hypertension. Strong tendency to asystole during anaesthesia. Very slow equilibration with inhaled gases, which worsen the situation by depressing the heart or increasing pulmonary vascular resistance (nitrous oxide). Ketamine has advantages. (Bird T. M. and Strunin L. *Anaesthesia* 1984, **39**, 48; Lumley J. et al. *Anesth. Analg. (Cleve)* 1977, **56**, 543; and Foster J. M. G. and Jones R. M. *Ann. R. Coll. Surg.* 1984, **66**, 153; Pollack K. L. and Chestnut D. H. Wenstrom K. D. *Anesth. Analg.* 1990, **70**, 212.)

Ellis–Van-Creveld disease (chondro-ectodermal dysplasia) Respiratory failure, congenital cardiac septal lesions.

Epidermolysis bullosa Skin and mucous membranes easily blistered with scarring. The no-touch technique is required. May be on steroids; may be associated with porphyria. Sticky tape may damage skin. Ketamine has been recommended. Steroid cover often required. (Fox W. T. *Lancet* 1979, **1**, 766; Kubota Y. et al. *Anesth. Analg. Curr. Res.* 1961, **40**, 244; Reddy A. R. R. and Wong D. H. W. *Can. Anaesth. Soc. J.* 1972, **19**, 536; Frost P. M. *Anaesthesia* 1980, **35**, 918; James I. G. and Wark R. *Anesthesiology* 1982, **56**, 323; Tomlinson A. A. *Anaesthesia* 1983, **38**, 495; James I. G. *Anaesthesia* 1983, **38**, 1106.)

Epilepsy Convulsions from perioperative drug withdrawal and enflurane. Loose teeth. *See* Chapter 20.

Erythema multiforme Post-intubation laryngeal oedema. (Cucchiara R. C. and Dawson B. *Anesthesiology* 1971, **35**, 537.)

Exomphalos and gastroschisis Post-correction respiratory failure.

Fabry's syndrome (lipidosis) Myocardial ischaemia in early adult life, renal failure.

Familial Dysautonomia (Riley-Day syndrome) Described in 1949. It is an inherited disease showing abnormally active parasympathetic system with sporadic storms of sympathetic activity. It is mainly confined to Ashkenazi Jews. The child cries without tears, is highly emotional with bouts of sweating and unexplained fluctuations of blood pressure. Reduced autonomic stability, hypersalivation, regurgitation, poor temperature control, sensitive to respiratory depressants. Intrinsic pulmonary disease may give postoperative problems. Volatile anaesthetics can cause bradycardia and hypotension and thus must be used carefully. Nitrous oxide and oxygen are usually sufficient.

IPPV often required while anaesthetized, due to CO_2 insensitivity. Dopamine hydroxylase is deficient, hypersensitivity to dopamine and other adrenergic and cholinergic drugs. Reduced sensitivity to pain. (Meridy A. W. and Greighton R. E. *Can. Anaesth. Soc. J.* 1971, **18**, 563; Cox R. G. and Sumner E. *Anaesthesia* 1983, **38**, 293; Foster J. M. G. *Anaesthesia* **38**, 391; Stenquist O. and Sigurdsson J. *Anaesthesia* 1982, **37**, 929; Sweeney B. F. et al. *Anaesthesia* 1985, **40**, 783; Axelrod F. B. et al. *Anesthesiology* 1988, **68**, 631.); Conrad M. Riley (1913–) Denver paediatrician; R. L. Day (1905–), Pittsburg physician.

Familial periodic paralysis The hyperkalaemic type is associated with paralysis after general anaesthesia, especially thiopentone and relaxants. (Streeten D. J. In: *Metabolic Basis of Inherited Disease* (Stanbury J. B. ed.) New York: McGraw-Hill, 1972.) (For anaesthesia, *see* Fozard J. R. *Anaesthesia* 1983, **38**, 294.)

Fanconi syndrome (renal tubular acidosis) Acidosis, dehydration, hypo-kalaemia, renal failure. (Morris R. C. *N. Engl. J. Med.* 1969; **281**, 1405.) Guido F. Fanconi (1903–), Zurich paediatrician.

Fanconi's anaemia Defect in DNA regeneration with with sensitivity to X-rays, which should be restricted, e.g. in ITU.

Farber's disease (lipogranulomatosis) Cardiomyopathy and renal failure. Granulomas may exist in the larynx, making intubation difficult. (Gilbertson A. A. and Boulton T. B. *Anaesthesia* 1967, **22**, 607.)

Farmer's lung Pulmonary fibrosis. May be on steroids.

Fat embolism Respiratory failure. *See* Chapter 30, Adult respiratory distress syndrome.

Favism (glucose-6-phosphate-dehydrogenase deficiency) Anaemia; haemolysis may result from sulphonamides and aspirin. (Gilbertson A. A. and Boulton T. B. *Anaesthesia* 1967, **22**, 607.)

Felty's syndrome (a form of idiopathic thrombocytopenic purpura) Anaemia, neutropenia, infections. May be on steroids. Augustus R. Felty (1895–), US physician.

Femoral hypoplasia syndrome Difficult intubation (micrognathia).

Fetal surgery (For anaesthesia, *see* Spielman F. J. et al. *Anaesthesia* 1984, **39**, 756.)

Fibrocystic disease (*See* cystic fibrosis.)

Fibrodysplasia ossificans (myositis ossificans) Difficult to intubate; reduced thoracopulmonary compliance. (Newton M. C., Allen P. W. and Ryan D. C. *Br. J. Anaesth.* 1990, **64**, 246.)

Fibromatosis (including juvenile and hyaline forms) *See* Vaughn G. C. et al. *Anesthesiology* 1990, **72**, 201.)

Fibrosing alveolitis (Hamman-Rich syndrome) Cyanosis, left heart failure. May be on steroids.

Fluid retention syndrome Risk of associated obesity, diabetes, hypo- and hyperthyroidism, depression. Worsened by steroids, cabenoxolone, NSAIDs, guanethidine, hydralazine, prazosin, calcium channel antagonists. Increased capillary permeability may cause problems during operation. (Dunnigan M. G. *Hosp. Update.* 1990, **16**, 653.)

Friedreich's ataxia Myocardial degeneration with failure and dysrhyth-mias, respiratory failure, diabetes, and peripheral neuropathy. Cases may be treated like those with amyotrophic lateral sclerosis. Non-depolarizing relaxants, carefully monitored, especially atracurium can be used (Bell C. F. et al. *Anaesthesia* 1986, **41**, 296 and *see* Bird T. M. and Strunin L. *Anesthesiology* 1984, **60**, 377.) An autosomal recessive inherited disease causing progressive ataxia and usually additional myopathy. (For anaesthesia, *see also* Bell C. F. et al. *Anaesthesia* 1986, **41**, 296.) Nicolas Friedreich (1825–1882), Heidelberg physician.

Freeman-Sheldon syndrome   Difficult intubation due to micrognathia.

Gardner's syndrome (multiple polyposis)   No specific difficulties except from laryngeal polyps.

Gargoylism   Respiratory obstruction after induction, very difficult intubation, cardiomyopathy and valve lesions.

Gaucher's disease   Thrombocytopenia, neutropenia, anaemia. Pulmonary aspiration may be a problem during anaesthesia.

Gilbert's disease (Familial unconjugated hyperbilirubinaemia)   Jaundice (for which the anaesthetic may be blamed) precipitated by minor upsets, including starvation. Nicholas A. Gilbert (1858–1927), Paris physician.

Glanzmann's disease (thrombasthenia)   Abnormal haemorrhage, platelet infusion rarely effective. May be on steroids.

Glomus jugulare tumours   (For anaesthesia, *see* Mather S. P. and Webster N. R. *Anaesthesia* 1986, **41**, 856; Braude B. M. et al. *Anaesthesia* 1986, **41**, 861.)

Glucagonoma   For anaesthetic management of glucagonoma, *see* Nicoll J. M. V. and Catling S. J. *Anaesthesia* 1985, **40**, 152.

Glue-sniffing   Unstable circulation due to grossly increased catecholamines.

Glycogenoses   *Type I* (Von Gierke's disease) Perioperative acidosis and hypoglycaemia. Diazoxide has been recommended. *Type II* (Pompe's disease) Heart failure and neuromuscular weakness, macroglossia. Rarely survive infancy. (McFarlane H. J. and Soni N. *Anaesthesia* 1986, **41** 1219.). *Type III* Perioperative hypoglycaemia. *Type IV* Perioperative hypoglycaemia. *Type V* (McArdle's disease) Muscle weakness, cardiac failure. (*See* Cox J. M. *Anesthesiology* 1968, **29**, 1221.)

Goldenhar syndrome (oculoauriculovertebral syndrome, hemifacial microsomia)   Difficult intubation and airway (small mandible, micrognathia with unilateral cleft defect, unilateral maxillary hypoplasia, cervical vertebral defects). Associated congenital heart disease (Fallot and VSD). (*See* Madan R. et al. *Anaesthesia* 1990, **45**, 49.) Atropine-resistant bradycardia can be a problem (Khan F. M. *Anaesthesia* 1991, **45**, 1102).

Golz–Gorlin syndrome (focal dermal hypoplasia)   Difficult airway due to frequent dental and facial asymmetry, and stiff neck. (Gorlin R. J. and Golz R. W. *N. Engl. J. Med.* 1960, **262**, 908.) Hypertension due to prorenin/renin production has been a problem (Yoshizumi J. et al. *Anaesthesia* 1991, **45**, 1046).

Goodpasture's syndrome   Severe repeated intrapulmonary haemorrhage with fibrosis. Hypertension, anaemia, renal failure. May be on steroids. Pre-operative plasmapheresis may be required. (Urbaniak S. J. and Robinson E. A. *Br. Med. J.* 1990, **300**, 662.) E. W. Goodpasture (1886–1960), Boston pathologist.

Gorlin syndrome   *See* Golz–Gorlin syndrome.

Gout   Dehydration, uricaemia may be worsened by methoxyflurane, ethanol and lactate.

Groenblad–Strandberg disease (pseudoxanthoma elasticum)   Fragile blood vessels with frequent rupture and bruising and displacement of i.v. infusions. Thromboses occur.

Guillain–Barré disease (acute idiopathic polyneuritis, with ventilation problems due to muscle weakness)   May require IPPV in intensive care, circulation sometimes unstable due to autonomic dysfunction. Usually self-limiting in up to 6 weeks, but much moral support needed while on IPPV. Suxamethonium may cause dangerous hyperkalaemia for up to 3 months after onset. (Smith R. B. *Can. Anaesth. Soc. J.* 1971, **18**, 199; Perel A. et al. *Anaesthesia* 1977, **32**, 257.) G. C. Guillain (1876–1961), Paris neurologist. J. A. Barré (1880–), Strasbourg neurologist.

Haemochromatosis (Bronze diabetes) and haemosiderosis   Iron deposits in liver (cirrhosis); pancreas (diabetes); joints (arthritis); skin (bronzing); and heart valves (late cardiac failure). The patient may be having weekly venesections.

Haemolytic uraemic syndrome   See Johnson G. D. and Rosales J. K. *Can. J. Anaesth.* 1987, **34**, 196.

Haemorrhagic telangiectasia (Osler-Weber-Rendu syndrome)   Post-intubation laryngeal bruising and obstruction. Risk of epistaxis.

Haemophilia   Pre-operative plasmapheresis may be required (Urbaniak S. J. and Robinson E. A. *Brit. Med. J.* 1990, **300**, 662), with factor VIII replacement. *See* Chapter 20.

Hallermann–Streiff syndrome   Difficult intubation, due to micrognathia, brittle teeth, hypoplastic nares.

Hallervorden–Spatz disease (Elejalde B. R. and de Elejalde M. M. *J. Clin. Genet.* 1979, **16**, 1.) A rare progressive disorder of the basal ganglia which occurs in late childhood and leads to death. The patients are demented and show various types of myotonia and muscular rigidity, with trismus, which would make intubation difficult. Halothane induction and maintenance relieve the dystonic posturing, which returns after operation, as with other basal ganglion disorders. (Roy R. C. et al. *Anesthesiology* 1983, **58**, 382.)

Hamman–Rich syndrome   Acute diffuse interstitial lung fibrosis.

Hand–Schuller–Christian disease (histiocytic granulomata)   Diabetes insipidus with electrolyte problems, hepatic failure, pancytopenia, respiratory failure, laryngeal involvement. May be on steroids. Intubation difficulties due to small larynx. (Lieberman P. H. et al. *Medicine (Baltimore)* 1969 **48**, 375.)

Hare lip   *See* Cleft palate. *See* Paediatrics, Chapter 22.

Hay–Wells syndrome   Difficult intubation (maxillary hypoplasia).

Henoch–Schönlein purpura   Bruising tendency.

Hepatolenticular degeneration (Kinnier–Wilson disease)   Defect in copper metabolism, hepatic failure, epilepsy, trismus, weakness.

Hermansky syndrome (thrombasthenia, albinism)   Bruising, platelet infusion may be required.

Holt–Oram syndrome (hand-heart syndrome)   Congenital heart septal defects. (Lewis M. et al. *JAMA* 1965, **193**, 1080.)

Homocystinuria   A recessive inborn error of metabolism due to deficiency of cystothionine synthetase. Thromboses, pulmonary embolism (requiring heparinization), lens dislocation, osteoporosis, mental handicap, hypoglycaemia and renal failure occur. (Carson N. A. J. *Br. J. Hosp. Med.* 1969, **2**, 439.)

Hunter syndrome (mucopolysaccharidosis II)   Thoracic skeletal abnormalities with respiratory failure, cardiomyopathy, stiff joints, laryngeal and pharyngeal involvement with obstruction, macroglossia and increased secretions, all making intubation difficult. (Gilbertson A. A. and Boulton T. B. *Anaesthesia* 1967, **22**, 607.) C. H. Hunter (1872–1965), English paediatrician.

Huntington's chorea   See Chapter 20. G. H. Huntington (1850–1916), New York neurologist.

Hurler syndrome (gargoylism, mucopolysaccharidosis I)   Death before puberty from cardiac involvement, with aortic and mitral incompetence. Difficult intubation due to macroglossia and increased secretions; chest infections, heart failure. (Wilder R. T. and Belani K. G. *Anesthesiology* 1990, **72**, 205.)

Hydatid disease   Pulmonary, hepatic, cardiac, renal and cerebral cysts may cause local problems.

Hydrocephalus   If there is a ventriculo-atrial valve in place antibiotic cover is often advised before dental treatment. The large occiput may make intubation difficult so that the body should be raised on a pillow or mattress.

Hyperkalaemic periodic paralysis   See Ashwood E. M. et al. *Anaesthesia* 1992, **47**, 579.

Hyperparathyroidism   May be associated with hypercalcaemia with danger of cardiac arrest. Risk temporarily diminished by potassium infusion. (For anaesthesia *see* The experts opine. *Surv. Anesthesiol.* 1985, **29**, 72.)

Hyperpituitarism   See Chapter 20.

Hyperviscosity syndrome   (Waldenstom's macroglobulinaemia, multiple myeloma) Thrombosis risk. Pre-operative plasmapheresis may be required. (Urbaniak S. J. and Robinson E. A. *Br. Med. J.* 1990, **300**, 662.)

Hyperthermia syndrome   See also Malignant hyperpyrexia.

Hypokalaemic familial periodic paralysis   See Chapter 20.

Hypoparathyroidism (*see also* Albright's osteodystrophy)   Hypersensitivity to sedatives and anaesthetics; hypocalcaemia with muscular weakness and tetany.

I cell disease (mucopolysaccharidosis VII)   Hernias; pulmonary problems due to thick secretions, with airway obstruction, and chest wall deformities. Difficult to intubate because of stiff neck. Cardiac valvular lesions coexist.

Ichthyosis   A congenital condition in which there may be difficulty in fixing an extradural catheter to the skin, if adhesives are used. (Smart G. and Bradshaw E. G. *Anaesthesia* 1984, **39**, 161.)

Idiopathic myoglobinuria   See Chapter 20.

Idiopathic thrombocytopenic purpura   Bruising, haemorrhage. Heparin and aspirin are avoided. May be on steroids. Platelet infusions for surgery, rebound thromboses after splenectomy.

Infective mononucleosis   Airway obstruction due to enlarged tonsils may prove fatal. (Catling S. J. et al. *Anaesthesia* 1984, **39**, 699; Carrington P. and Hall J. I. *Br. Med. J.* 1986, **292**, 195.)

Insulinoma   (For removal of, *see* Muir J. J. et al. *Anesthesiology* 1983, **59**, 371.) *See* Chapter 20.

Ivemask syndrome   Asplenia, situs inversus, dextrocardia, cyanotic heart disease.

Jaw, congenital fusion of in a neonate (Seraj M. A. et al. *Anaesthesia* 1984, **39**, 695).

Jervell–Lange–Nielsen syndrome Deafness with cardiac dysrhythmias, long QT interval and enlarged T wave. Risk of cardiac arrest. Pacemaker insertion may help. (Jervell A. et al. *Am. Heart J.* 1957, **54**, 59.) For anaesthesia, *see* Medak R. and Benumof J. L. *Br. J. Anaesth.* 1983, **55**, 361; Freshwater J. V. *Br. J. Anaesth.* 1984, **56**, 655; Ryan H, Can. J. Anaesth. 1988, **35**, 422.

Jehovah's Witnesses Blood transfusion refused. These patients sign a special consent absolving the doctors from problems arising from failure to transfuse blood or blood products. (For anaesthesia, *see* Clarke J. F. M. *Br. J. Hosp. Med.* 1982, **27**, 487; Wickham N. W. R. and Hardy R. N. *Hosp. Update* 1982, **8**, 1433; Harris T. J. B. et al. *Anaesthesia* 1983, **38**, 989 and in heart surgery, Henderson A. M. et al. *Anaesthesia* 1986, **41**, 748; Wong D. H. W. and Jenkins L. C. *Can. J. Anaesth.* 1989, **36**, 578.)

Jeune's syndrome Lung problems due to chest wall deformity.

Kaposi's sarcoma Pigmented sarcoma of the skin. May be associated with AIDS. M. K. Kaposi (1837–1902), Austrian dermatologist.

Kartagener's syndrome Dextrocardia, sinusitis, bronchiectasis (due to defective ciliary function), immunoincompetence. (Miller R. D. et al. *Chest* 1972, **62**, 130.)

Kasabach–Merritt syndrome Rarely survive more than a few weeks from birth, enlarging haemangioma with haemorrhage and thrombocytopenia. May be on steroids.

Kearns–Sayer syndrome The reaction to muscle relaxants is normal, but complete and sudden heart block may develop during anaesthesia. (D'Ambra M. N. et al. *Anesthesiology* 1979, **51**, 343.)

Kelly–Paterson syndrome (Plummer-Vinson syndrome, sideropenic dysphagia) In the very advanced case, regurgitation on induction.

King Denborough disease Malignant hyperpyrexia association.

Klinefelter syndrome Crush fractures of osteoporotic vertebrae. May be very large in adult life. H. K. Klinefelter (1912–), Baltimore physician.

Klippel–Feil syndrome (congenital fusion of cervical vertebrae) Difficult intubation; cleft palate; neurological defects, scoliosis and VSD may coexist (Katz J. and Kaddis E. B. *Anesthesia and Uncommon Diseases*. Philadelphia: Saunders, 1973.) (Klippel M. and Feil A. *Soc. Anat. Paris Bull. et Memb.* 1912, **14**, 185.) For anaesthesia *see* Naguib M. et al. *Can. Anaesth. Soc. J.* 1986, **33**, 60.

Klippel–Trenaunay syndrome (angio-osteohypertrophy) High output failure, thrombocytopenia, cleft palate, short wide neck and inability to extend neck.

Kneist's syndrome Difficult intubation due to stiff neck.

Kugelberg Welander muscular atrophy Respiratory problem due to muscle weakness.

Kwashiorkor Difficult to intubate due to pterygoid fibrosis. Low serum electrolytes and serum cholinesterase.

Larsen's syndrome (multiple joint dislocations) Difficult intubation due to unstable neck, pulmonary infections. (Wooley M. W. et al. *J. Ped. Surg.* 1967, **2**, 325.)

Laryngotracheoesophageal cleft   *See* Armitage E. N. *Anaesthesia* 1984, **39**, 706.

Laryngomalacia   Upper airway obstruction, especially in the paediatric patient.

Laurence–Moon–Biedl syndrome   Obesity, polydactyly, mental retardation; associated congenital heart disease, renal failure with diabetes insipidus.

Leber's disease   Congenital optic atrophy. There may be idiopathic hypoventilation with sensitivity to diazepam and mild analgesics. *See* Hunter A. R. *Anaesthesia* 1984, **39**, 781.

Leopard syndrome   Multiple leopard skin spots, hypertelorism, severe pulmonary stenosis. (*Scott. Med. J.* 1983, **28**, 300; Rodrigo M. R. C. et al. *Anaesthesia* 1990, **45**, 30.)

Leprechaunism   Abnormal endocrine state, mentally defective; hyperinsulinism, hypoglycaemia, renal failure.

Leprosy   Leprosy patients are often on steroids. Some parts of the body may be analgesic.

Lesch–Nyhan syndrome (hyperuricaemia)   Renal failure before puberty.

Letterer–Siwe disease (histiocytosis)   As for leukaemia; gingivitis with very loose teeth, intrinsic lung disease.

Leukaemia   Anaemia, thrombocytopenia, veins may be difficult. May be on steroids.

Lingual vein thrombosis   Severe upper airways obstruction, mouth breathing impossible, nose breathing difficult, laying down may be impossible. Helium/oxygen mixture useful until fibreoptic intubation achieved (approaching the patient in the sitting position from the front, the fibreoptic 'picture' is reversed).

Lipodystrophy   Liver failure, renal failure, diabetes, with anaemia. Halothane is to be avoided.

Lowe syndrome (oculocerebrorenal syndrome)   Renal failure, hypocalcaemia, acidosis.

Ludwig's angina   Difficult intubation due to infection swelling of floor of mouth, with trismus.

Lyme disease   Spirochaetal disease named after the town of origin. Intense pain requiring opioids, myocarditis occurs 6 weeks after initial attack, with A-V block. Treated by penicillin, tetracycline, ceftriaxone. Anaesthesia is postponed until remission. *See* Bateman D. E. *Hosp Update*, 1990, **16**, 677.

McArdle's disease (glycogenosis V)   A hereditary myopathy causing glycogen to accumulate in muscle, with weakness and respiratory problems, and cardiomyopathy. Atracurium appears to be a safe agent for the production of muscle relaxation in short procedures. Suxamethonium is to be avoided. *see* Rajah A. and Bell C. F. *Anaesthesia* 1986, **41**, 93.

Macroglossia, acute   Intubation and airway problem. *See* Holmes W. and Ball I. M. *Today's Anaesthetist* 1986, **No. 2**, 26.

Mafucci syndrome (enchondromas and haemangiomas)   Anaemia, sensitivity to vasodilator drugs, fragile bones, labile blood pressure.

Malignant disease   *See Anaesthesia and Malignant Disease* (Filshie J. and Robbie D. S. ed.) Edward Arnold, London, 1989.

Mandibulofacial dysostosis (Treacher–Collins syndrome)   Micrognathia, difficult intubation. Coexistent congenital heart disease sometimes. Tracheal ventilation via a 16 G needle has proved useful. (Smith R. B. et al. *Br. J.*

Anaesth. 1974, **46**, 313; Collins E. and Treacher J. *Trans. Ophthal. Soc. UK. 1900,* **20**, 190.)

Maple syrup urine disease (branched chain ketonuria with neuropathy)   A metabolic disease of children involving an accumulation of keto-acids and amino-acids in the blood and urine, with abnormalities of blood sugar and electrolytes. *See* Delaney A. and Gal T. J. *Anesthesiology* 1976, **44**, 83.

Marchiafava–Michaeli syndrome (auto-immune haemolytic anaemia with paroxysmal nocturnal dyspnoea)   Venous thromboembolism. May be on steroids.

Marfan's syndrome (arachnodactyly, congenital connective tissue disorder)   Emphysema, cataracts, high arched palate, pneumothorax, coronary thrombosis, dissecting aneurysms, easily dislocated joints, aortic and mitral regurgitation, kyphoscoliosis. (Wooley M. W. et al. *J. Ped. Surg.* 1967, **2**, 325.) Young patients with this syndrome are a high anaesthetic risk group (Verghese C. *Anaesthesia* 1984, **39**, 917). *See also* Annotation, *Br. Med. J. 1982,* **285**, 464. B. J. A. Marfan (1858–1943), Paris paediatrician (1896).

Maroteaux–Lamy syndrome (mucopolysaccharidosis IV)   Cardiomyopathy, respiratory failure, (partly due to chest wall deformity), anaemia, thrombocytopenia. (Gilbertson A. A. and Boulton T. B. *Anaesthesia* 1967, **22**, 607.)

ME (myalgia encephalitis) (postviral weakness)   Caution with dosage of anaesthesia and non-depolarizing relaxants due to debility and reduction of muscle mass. In the extreme case, reduction of myocardial muscle is a risk.

Meckel's syndrome (Mekel–Gruber syndrome)   Microcephaly, micrognathia, congenital cardiac disease, and polycystic kidney; difficult intubation, renal failure. Encephalocoele and cleft palate may be present. J. F. Meckel (1781–1833), anatomist from Halle.

Median cleft face   Difficult intubation due to micrognathia.

Meig's syndrome (ovarian cyst with embarrassing pleural effusion)   The effusion may be tapped before anaesthesia. J. V. Meig (1892–1963), Boston gynaecologist.

Methaemoglobinaemia   Made worse by prilocaine. *See* Chapter 20.

Mikulicz's syndrome (salivary and lachrimal gland enlargement)   Difficult airway and intubation sometimes, due to glandular enlargement. It has been suggested that atropine and hyoscine are best avoided. J. von Mikulicz Radecki (1850–1905), Breslau surgeon.

Moebius' syndrome   A rare congenital abnormality of the cranial nerves. Difficult intubation due to micrognathia. *See* Krajcirik W. J. et al. *Anesth. Analg. (Cleve.)* 1985, **64**, 371.

Mongolism   See Down's syndrome.

Morquio's syndrome (mucopolysaccharidosis)   Kyphoscoliotic dwarfs with atlanto-axial instability, making intubation difficult. Respiratory and cardiac failure by early adult life. Aortic incompetence. (Gilbertson A. A. and Boulton T. B. *Anaesthesia* 1967, **22**, 607; Birkinshaw K. J. *Anaesthesia* 1975, **30**, 46.)

Moschkowitz disease (a form of thrombocytopenic purpura)   Renal damage. May be on steroids.

Motor neurone disease   Hypersensitivity to all muscle relaxants. Laryngeal incompetence. Lung cancer may be present. *See also* Amyotrophic lateral sclerosis.

Moya-moya disease A rare abnormality of the cerebral circulation with narrowing or occlusion of the anterior and middle cerebral arteries, first described in Japan in 1961. For anaesthesia *see* Bingham R. M. and Wilkinson D. J. *Anaesthesia* 1985, **40**, 1198; Brown S. C. and Lam A. M. *Can. J. Anaesth.* 1987, **34**, 71.

Mucopolysaccharidosis A hereditary connective-tissue disorder with deposition of abnormal amounts of mucopolysaccharides in body tissues. May be difficulties with airways and intubation because of secretions. Pre-operative tracheostomy may occasionally be required. Other problems, very slow recovery, with breath holding, bronchospasm and frequent cyanosis, postoperative dehydration and chest infection. A light premedication with oral diazepam and glycopyrronium, and antibiotics for those with valvular lesions has been described. (Baines D. and Keneally J. P. *Anaesth. Intensive Care* 1983, **11**, 198; Kempthorne P. M. and Brown T. C. K. *Anaesth. Intensive Care* 1983, **11**, 203; King D. H. et al. *Anaesthesia* 1984, **39**, 126; Brown T. C. K. *Anaesth. Intensive Care* 1984, **12**, 178; Herrick I. A. and Rhine E. J. *Can. J. Anaesth.* 1988, **35**, 67.)

Multiple myelomatosis Pathological fractures, especially of vertebrae, care needed in positioning. Hypercalcaemia, anaemia, hyperviscosity, renal failure, coagulopathies.

Multiple mucosal neuroma syndrome May make intubation difficult.

Multiple endocrine adenomatosis type IIb Includes phaeochromocytoma.

Multiple sclerosis *See* Disseminated sclerosis.

Muscular dystrophy Weak flaccid skeletal and eventually cardiac muscles. Sensitivity to atropine, opiates and non-depolarizing relaxants, may not reverse after anticholinesterase drugs. May be confined to ocular muscles (Robertson, J. A. *Anaesthesia* 1984, **39**, 251). May be associated with malignant hyperpyrexia. (Ellis F. R. *Br. J. Anaesth.* 1974, **46**, 605.)

Myasthenia gravis and myasthenia congenita *See* Chapter 20. (Dalal F. Y. *Anaesthesia* 1972, **27**, 61.) Preoperative plasmapheresis may be required. (Urbaniak S. J. and Robinson E. A. *Br. Med. J.* 1990, **300**, 662.) Isoflurane is useful (Nilsson E. and Muller K. *Acta Anaesth. Scand.* 1990, **34**, 126).

Myasthenic syndrome Often due to carcinomatous myopathy, more commonly seen in older men. For anaesthesia during treatment with 3,4 diaminopyridine, *see* Telford R. J. and Hollway T. E. *Br. J. Anaesth.* 1990, **64**, 363.

Myositis ossificans Difficult intubation sometimes due to stiff neck. In severe cases, reduction of thoracic compliance with respiratory failure. May be on steroids.

Myotonia congenita (Thomsen's disease) *See* Dystrophia myotonica. (Ravin M. et al. *Anaesth. Analg.* 1975, **54**, 216.) A. J. T. Thomsen (1815–1896), Danish physician.

Nemaline myopathy Inadequate ventilation due to muscle weakness. Sensitivity to non-depolarizing relaxants. Malignant hyperpyrexia association.

Neurofibromatosis Fibromas may occur in larynx or heart, excessive response to relaxants, rarely associated with phaeochromocytomas. (*See* von Recklinghausen's disease.) F. D. von Recklinghausen (1833–1910), German pathologist.

Neuromuscular syndromes (associated with malignant disease)   (Croft P. *Br. J. Hosp. Med.* 1977, **17**, 356.)

Niemann–Pick disease (sphingomyelin infiltration, xanthomatosis)   Anaemia, thrombocytopenia, respiratory failure.

Noack's syndrome (craniosynostosis)   Sometimes difficult to intubate due to micrognathia. (Andersson H. and Gomes S. P. *Acta Paediatr. Scand.* 1968, **57**, 47.)

Noonan syndrome   Micrognathia, short, webbed neck, pectus excavatus, heart disease, pulmonary stenosis, VSD, renal failure.

Ollier disease   Great care required with joints.

Opitz Frias syndrome   The hypospadias dysphagia syndrome; the G syndrome. Rare congenital condition with genital and craniofacial abnormalities. (Opitz J. M. et al. *Birth Defects* 1969, **5**, 95.) For anaesthesia *see* Bolsin S. N. and Gillbe C. *Anaesthesia* 1985, **30**, 1189.

Orofacial-digital syndrome   Cleft palate may coexist. Renal failure occurs.

Osler–Weber–Rendu syndrome   See Haemorrhagic telangiectasia. W. Osler (1849–1919), physician, Baltimore and Oxford; F. Parkes Weber (1863–1962), London physician; H. J. Rendu (1844–1902), French physician.

Osteogenesis imperfecta (fragilitas ossium)   Fragile bones, teeth easily damaged, excessive haemorrhage during surgery. Occasional respiratory problem due to chest wall deformity. Malignant hyperpyrexia association. (Robinson C. and Wright D. J. *Today's Anaesthetist* 1986, **1**, No. 2, 22; Cunningham A. J. et al. *Anesthesiology* 1984, **61**, 91.)

Osteopetrosis   Similar to osteogenesis imperfecta.

Pancreatitis   Severe toxaemia and shock, hypocalcaemia, relaxant reversal difficulties.

Paramyotonia congenita   Weakness and myotonia induced by exposure to cold. Sensitivity to relaxants, electrolyte abnormalities. Halothane and suxamethonium better avoided.

Paraplegia   Autonomic instability, liability to bed-sores. Hyperkalaemia may follow suxamethonium. For neuromuscular monitoring in tetraparesis *see* Fiacchine F., Bricchi M. and Lasio G. *Anaesthesia* 1990, **45** 128.

Parkinson's disease   Restriction of movement of chest wall may give postoperative chest problems. (Severn A. *Br. J. Anaesth.* 1988, **61**, 761; *ibid 1989,* **62**, 580; Marsden C. D. *Lancet* 1990, **335**, 948.)

Patau syndrome (trisomy 13)   Micrognathia, difficult to intubate due to micrognathia and cleft palate. VSD and dextroversion; microcephaly with skin defects.

Pellagra   Neuropathy and difficult intubation.

Pemphigus vulgaris   For anaesthesia in an acutely traumatized patient, *see* Vatashshy E. and Aronson H. B. *Anaesthesia* 1982, **37**, 1193

Pendred's disease   Goitre may be found.

Pfeiffer's syndrome   Craniostenosis (may be very haemorrhagic operation, with difficult airway afterwards), syndactyly.

Pharyngeal pouch   Regurgitation of contents, not controlled by cricoid pressure, rapid sequence intubation, intubation under local analgesia, etc. The pouch should be emptied manually by the patient before anaesthesia, or by carefully directed large bore nasogastric tube.

Phenylketonuria   Sensitivity to opioids and barbiturates, so inhalation induction is recommended. Epileptic fits, hypoglycaemia.

Pierre Robin syndrome Micrognathia, posterior displacement of the tongue, a hypoplastic mandible with glossoptosis, small epiglottis, high arched or cleft palate. Respiratory obstruction occurs, which tends to disappear after the age of 2 years. It may be necessary to suture the tongue to the alveolar ridge of the mandible to relieve respiratory obstruction. Such cases may be very difficult to intubate. The child should be nursed in the prone position both before and after operation.

Plummer–Vinson syndrome *See* Kelly–Paterson syndrome. H. S. Plummer (1874–1936), Mayo Clinic physician; P. P. Vinson (1890–1959), US surgeon.

Pneumatosis cystoides intestinalis Nitrous oxide is contra-indicated. *See* Sutton D. N. and Ooskitt K. R. *Anaesthesia* 1984, **39**, 776.

Pneumoconiosis Pulmonary fibrosis and emphysema, excessive sputum, reduced compliance, cyanosis. May be on steroids.

Polyarteritis nodosa See Chapter 20.

Polycystic kidneys Renal failure, pulmonary cysts may coexist with danger of pneumothorax; 1 in 7 have cerebral aneurysms. Polycystic liver may coexist.

Polycythaemia *See* Chapter 20.

Polymyositis *See* Dermatomyositis.

Polysplenia Associated congenital heart disease.

Pompe's disease *See* Glycogenoses; difficult to intubate because of macroglossia. Respiratory problems due to muscle weakness, and cardiomyopathy.

Porphyrias Paralytic crises precipitated by barbiturates, hydroxydione, diazepoxide, anticonvulsants, nikethamide and other non-anaesthetic drugs. *See* Chapter 20. Regional anaesthesia is possible. McNiell M. J. and Bennet A. *Br. J. Anaesth.* 1990, **64**, 371.)

Potter's syndrome (Potter E. L. *Am. J. Obstet. Gynecol.* 1946, **51**, 855 and 559; Potter E. L. *Obstet. Gynecol.* 1965, **25**, 3.) Oligohydramnios in the mother and renal agenesis, typical facies and pulmonary hypoplasia in the baby. In spite of intubation, ventilation may be impossible (Van der Weyden, *Anaesth. Intensive Care* 1982, **10**, 90).

Prader–Willi syndrome Patients have (after the neonatal phase) extreme obesity, polyphagia, dental caries, congenital muscle hypotonia (with respiratory problems), mental retardation, hypogonadism and sometimes cardiovascular abnormalities. Blood glucose should be maintained during fasting. May be very large in adult life. (Mayhew J. F. and Taylor B. *Can. Anaesth. Soc. J.* 1983, **30**, 565; Yamashita M. et al. *Canad. Anaesth. Soc. J. 1983*, **30**, 179.) A. P. Prader, H. Willi (1900–71), Zurich paediatricians. (Prader A. et al. *Schweiz. Med.* Wochenschr. 1956, **86**, 1260.)

Prematurity See Chapter 22, Paediatrics.

Progeria (premature ageing) Myocardial ischaemia, hypertension, cardiomegaly.

Progressive external ophthalmoplegia (PEO) All induction agents used intravenously should be given slowly and in small dosage (James R. H. *Anaesthesia* 1986, **41, 216**).

Progressive muscular dystrophy See Chapter 20.

Prolonged Q-T syndrome An inherited condition causing attacks of dysrhythmia leading to syncope. Should be treated with β-blockers. *See* O'Callaghan A. C. et al. *Anaesth. Intensive Care* 1982, **10**, 50.

Prune belly syndrome (pseudoxanthoma elasticum), (congenital absence of abdominal muscles)   Inability to cough due to muscle weakness, causes postoperative respiratory problems. Renal failure may coexist. (Hannington Kiff J. G. *Br. J. Anaesth.* 1970, **42**, 649; Henderson A. M. et al. *Anaesthesia* 1987, **42**, 54.)

Pulmonary cysts   Increase in size with possible rupture during anaesthesia.

Pulmonary hypertension (primary)   For extradural analgesia in, *see* Davies M. J. and Beavis R. *Anaesth. Intensive Care* 1984, **12**, 165.)

Reiger's syndrome   As for Dystrophia myotonica. The teeth are abnormal.

Rett syndrome   Females with dementia, autism, movement disorders and abnormal respiratory control. (Maquire D. and Bachman C. *Can. J. Anaesth.* 1989, **36**, 478.)

Rheumatoid arthritis and Still's disease   Difficult intubation, difficult veins, poor spontaneous respiration. May be on steroids. *See* Chapter 20.

Rickets   Kyphoscoliotic respiratory limitation, difficult spinal analgesia, hypocalcaemia.

Riley–Day syndrome   *See* Dysautonomia and Familial dysautonomia.

Ritter disease   Fragile skin, difficult veins.

Romano–Ward syndrome   (Romano C. et al. *Clin. Pediatr.* 1963, **45**, 656 and Ward O. C. *J. Irish Med. Assoc.* 1964, **54**, 103.) Congenital delay of depolarization and prolonged QT interval. May cause sudden death at any age during induction of anaesthesia; transvenous pacing and stellate ganglion block have been used to prevent this *see* Callaghan M. L. et al. *Anesthesiology* 1977, **47**, 67; Ponte J. and Lund J. *Br. J. Anaesth.* 1981, **53**, 1347.

Rubinstein syndrome (microcephaly, chronic lung disease)   Associated congenital heart disease.

Russel–Silver syndrome   (Francis G. A. *Today's Anaesthetist* 1990, **5**, 81.) Short stature, facial asymmetry, micrognathia, macroglossia, *café-au-lait* spots, sweating, fasting hypoglycaemia and mental deficiency. Difficult airway and intubation, blood glucose monitoring required.

Saethre–Chotzen syndrome   *See* Chotzen.

San Filippo syndrome (mucopolysaccharidosis III)   No specific problems. (Gilbertson A. A. and Boulton T. B. *Anaesthesia* 1967, **22**, 607.)

Sarcoidosis   Pulmonary and laryngeal fibrosis, cardiac failure, dysrhythmias, hypercalcaemia. May be on steroids.

Scleroderma   Diffuse thickening of skin, fibrosis leading to muscle degeneration in the diaphragm, which may contribute to respiratory problems. Blood pressure is difficult to measure, poor lung compliance. Difficult intubation due to restricted mouth opening, difficult veins, regurgitation, respiratory failure, hypovolaemia, hypotension, renal failure, prolonged action of local analgesics in the peripheries. May be on steroids. (Birkhan J. et al. *Anaesthesia* 1972, **27**, 89; Sweeney B. *Anaesthesia* 1984, **39**, 1145; Iliffe G. D. and Pettigrew N. M. *Br. Med. J.* 1985, **286**, 337.)

Scurvy   Anaemia, bruising, loose teeth.

Sebaceous naevus disease   Congenital cardiac disease may coexist.

Sheie disease (mucopolysaccharidosis V)   Hernias, joint stiffness, aortic incompetence in adult life.

Shprintzen syndrome   Difficult to intubate (micrognathia). Deafness and congenital cardiac abnormalities occur.

Shy–Drager syndrome   (Shy G. M. and Drager G. A. *Arch. Neurol.* 1960, **2**, 511; King D. H. et al. *Br. J. Anaesth.* 1984, **39**, 126.) (central nervous and autonomic degeneration)   Highly labile blood pressure, ephedrine suitable for hypotensive crises. Cardiac dysrhythmias occur. For anaesthesia, *see* Hutchinson R. C. and Sugden J. C. *Anaesthesia* 1984, **39**, 1229.)

Siamese twins   *See* Conjoined twins.

Sick sinus syndrome   Uncoordinated atrial activity; Dissociation of atrial from ventricular rhythm, with tendency to ventricular fibrillation. Usually in elderly men. (Reid D. S. *Br. J. Hosp. Med.* 1984, **31**, 341). *See also* Chapter 20.

Simmonds' syndrome and Sheehan's syndrome (post-partum pituitary necrosis)   As for Addison's disease. M. S. Simmonds (1855–1925), Hamburg pathologist; Sheehan H. L. (1900–), British pathologist.

Sickle-cell disease   *See* Chapter 20.

Silver syndrome (dwarfism, micrognathia)   Difficult intubation sometimes. (*see* Russel–Silver syndrome.)

Sipple syndrome (multiple endocrine adenomatosis)   As for phaeochromocytoma (*see* Chapter 20).

Sjogren's syndrome (keratoconjunctivitis sicca)   Worsened by atropine and hyoscine, improved by humidification. H. S. Sjogren (1899–), Stockholm ophthalmologist.

Smith–Lemli–Opitz syndrome (micrognathia, mentally defective, hypoplasia of thymus)   Difficult intubation, infection problems and intrinsic lung disease.

Spinal muscular atrophy   (Seddon S. J. *Anaesthesia* 1985, **40**, 821.)

Sponylometaphyseal dysplasia   Difficult to intubate due to neck.

Sprengel's syndrome   Difficult intubation due to neck.

Stevens–Johnson syndrome   *See* Erythema multiforme. Fragile skin, difficult veins. Cardiomyopathy occurs. A. M. Stevens (1844–1945), US paediatrician; F. C. Johnson (1897–1934), US paediatrician.

Stickler's syndrome (progressive arthro-ophthalmopathy)   Progressive myopia, retinal detachment, secondary glaucoma, pain and stiffness of joints with hypotonia, kyphoscoliosis, maxillary hypoplasia, occasionally cleft palate, deafness, possible intubation problems. (*See* Stickler G. B. et al. *Proc. Mayo Clin.* 1965, **40**, 433; Stickler G. B. and Pugh D. G. *Proc. Mayo. Clin.* 1967, **42**, 495.)

Still's disease (juvenile chronic polyarthritis)   Airway maintenance may be difficult because of limited movement of the jaws and of the cervical spine. Atlanto-axial subluxation due to erosion of the odontoid process may be present. Blind nasal intubation, or the use of the fibreoptic laryngoscope may be necessary. Ketamine is a useful drug here. (Smith B. L. *Abstr. 8th World Congress, Manila*, 1984, **2**, A 114 and D'Arcy J. et al. 1976, *Anaesthesia* **31**, 624.) G. F. Still (1868–1941), London paediatrician.

Sturge–Weber syndrome (cavernous angioma of face with intracranial involvement)   Epilepsy and hemiparesis may occur. W. A. Sturge (1850–1919), F. Parkes Weber (1863–1962), English physicians.

Syringomyelia   Occasional respiratory failure.

Systemic lupus erythematosus   Anaemia, bruising, renal and respiratory failure, nasal skin involvement. May be on steroids.

Takayasu's disease (ITA)   See Thorburn J. R. and James M. F. M. *Anaesthesia* 1986, **41**, 734. Inflammatory occlusion of aorta and major bronchus. Extension of neck may occlude carotid arteries. May be on steroids and anticoagulants.

Tangier disease (analphalipoproteinaemia)   Sensitivity to muscle relaxants, ischaemic heart disease, anaemia, thrombocytopenia.

TAR syndrome (thrombocytopenia, absent radius)   Fallots tetralogy occurs.

Thalassaemia   Haemolytic anaemia, intubation difficulties have been described. Homozygous form fetal Hb, heterozygous forms HbC, HbE, HbS with sickling problems. *See* Chapter 20.

Total body irradiation   In children, with high dosage, *see* Lo J. N. and Buckley J. J. *Anesthesiology* 1984, **61**, 101.

Thrombocytopenic purpura   Bruising, haemmorhage. Pre-operative plasmapheresis may be required (Urbaniak S. J. and Robinson E. A. *Br. Med. J.* 1990, **300**, 662).

Tourette syndrome   For anaesthetic implications *see* Morrison J. E. and Lockhart C. H. *Anesth. Analg. (Cleve.)* 1986, **65**, 200.

Tracheo-oesophageal-fistula   Milk aspiration into lungs, stomach full of air, causing respiratory embarrassment. IPPV difficult with low fistula. For anaesthesia in adults, *see* Chan C. S. *Anaesthesia,* 1984, **39**, 158, *See* Paediatrics, Chapter 22.

Treacher–Collins syndrome   See Mandibulofacial dysostosis.

Tricuspid incompetence   Antibiotic cover is usual. Afterload reduction and preload increases have proved helpful. (Stone J. G. et al. *Anesth. Analg. (Cleve.)* 1980, **59**, 737.)

Trisomy 13   See Patau syndrome.

Trisomy 18   See Edwards' syndrome.

Trisomy 21   See Down's syndrome.

Trisomy 22   Severe hypoglycaemia during perioperative starvation.

Tuberous sclerosis   Renal failure, cardiac rhabdomyomas with dysrhythmias, lung cysts, which may rupture. Ash leaf and *café-au-lait* spots.

Turner's syndrome   (XO chromosome with micrognathia, short webbed neck, aortic coarctation and stenosis, and renal anomalies) Difficult intubation, prolonged effects from renally excreted drugs. (Strader E. A. et al. *J. Pediatr.* 1971, **79**, 473.)

Urbach–Wiethe disease (mucocutaneous hyalinosis)   Difficult intubation due to small laryngeal opening.

Urine drinking   In psychiatric patients. produces moderate to severe hyponatraemia.

VATER syndrome   VSD and intrinsic pulmonary disease. Renal failure occurs.

Ventricular septal defect (VSD)   'The louder the murmur, the smaller the defect'. Antibiotic cover is usual. Mild reduction of systemic vascular resistance is desirable. Hypovolaemia is to be avoided.

von Gierke's disease (glycogen storage problems with hepatic and renal failure)   Perioperative starvation gives severe hypoglycaemia and acidosis. (Cox J. M. *Anesthesiology* 1968, **29**, 1221.)

von Hippel–Lindau syndrome (haemangioblastomas)   Associated with phaeochromocytoma; hepatic and renal failure. (Steiner A. C. et al. *Medicine* 1968, **47**, 371.)

von Recklinghausen's disease (neurofibromatosis) May have fibromas of pharynx, larynx (making intubation difficult) and heart; may have phaeochromocytoma, kyphoscoliosis, multiple lung cysts and renal failure. There is an excessive response, sometimes, to non-depolarizing relaxants and suxamethonium. (Manser J. *Br. J. Anaesth.* 1970, **42**, 183; Brasfield R. D. and Das Gupta T. R. *Ann. Surg.* 1972, **175**, 86; Baraka A. *Br. J. Anaesth.* 1974, **46**, 701; Fisher M. M. *Anaesthesia* 1975, **30**, 648; Van Aken H. et al. *Anaesthesia* 1982, **37**, 827.)

von Willebrand's disease (pseudohaemophilia) Defective platelet adhesiveness with Factor VIII deficiency. Controlled by tranexamic acid, 1 g, and desmopressin (DDAVP), 24 µg, given slowly, i.v., 1 h before operation, 4 h after operation, and 24 h after operation. Tranexamic acid is then continued, 1 g orally, 8-hourly, for a week. Cryoprecipitate is considered if this treatment fails to correct coagulopathy. Salicylates are avoided. E. A. von Willebrand (1870–1949), physician, Finland.

Weaver's syndrome Rare developmental condition with unusual craniofacial appearance and micrognathia with airway and intubation problems. May be very large in adult life. (Weaver D. D. et al. *J. Pediatr.* 1974, **84**, 547.) *See* Turner D. R. and Downing J. W. *Br. J. Anaesth.* 1985, **57**, 1260.

Weber–Christian disease (global fat necrosis) Adrenal failure, occasional constrictive pericarditis. Subcutaneous fat is carefully protected at operation. (Spirak J. L. et al. *Johns Hopkins Med. J.* 1970, **126**, 344.)

Wegener's granuloma (ulceration of midline structures of face) Possible airway involvement causes difficulties, also renal failure. May be on steroids. F. Wegener (1907–), Berlin pathologist.

Welander's muscular atrophy (peripheral muscular atrophy) Very sensitive to thiopentone, relaxants and opiates. (Ellis F. R. *Br. J. Anaesth.* 1974, **46**, 605.)

Werdnig–Hoffman disease (infantile muscular atrophy) Respiratory failure, worsened by relaxants and opioids. (Ellis F. R. *Br. J. Anaesth.* 1974, **46**, 605.) G. W. Werdnig, Graz neurologist; J. Hoffman (1857–1919), Heidelberg neurologist.

Werner syndrome (type I endocrine adenomatosis) Renal failure, severe hypoglycaemia, bronchial carcinoid tumours, hypercalcaemia. (Werner P *Am. J. Med.* 1963, **35**, 205)

Werner syndrome (premature ageing) (cf. Hutchinson Gilford syndrome; progeria) Myocardial ischaemia, diabetes, hypercalcaemia. (McKusick V. A. *Heritable Disorders of Connective Tissue*, 4th ed. St. Louis: C. V. Mosby Co., 1972.)

William's syndrome Congenital stenosis of aortic and pulmonary valves may coexist. Hypercalcaemia occurs in infancy (20%). Stellate blue eyes.

Wilm's tumour Anaemia (7 g/dl is the limit), IVC obstruction may occur.

Wilson's disease (hepatolenticular degeneration from copper deposits) Hepatic and renal failure, with ventilatory problems and difficulty reversing relaxants. (Gilbertson A. A. and Boulton T. B. *Anaesthesia* 1967, **22**, 607.) S. A. Kinnear Wilson (1877–1937), London neurologist.

Wiskott Aldrich disease Anaemia and clotting problems.

Wolf–Hirschorn syndrome A rare chromosomal abnormality. Patients have poor intrauterine growth, severe psychomotor retardation, characteristic facies, and various midline fusion abnormalities. (Lazuk G. I. et al. *Clin.*

Genet. 1980, **18**, 6.) Malignant hyperpyrexia may occur. Anaesthetic management, *see* Ginsburg R. and Purcell-Jones G. *Anaesthesia* 1988, **43**, 386.

Wolff–Parkinson–White syndrome   ECG shows prolonged QRS and short PR interval due to various cardiac disorders; worsened by neostigmine. Tachycardia produces ST depression, so hyoscine preferred to atropine for premedication. Paroxysmal supraventricular tachycardia may accompany induction of anaesthesia, and progress to ventricular fibrillation. Prevention by transvenous pacing. Termination of paroxysmal supraventricular tachycardia with phenylephrine (Jacobson L. et al. *Anaesthesia* 1985, **40**, 657), propranolol 0.01 mg/kg i.v. or verapamil 0.1 mg/kg slowly, i.v. DC cardioversion should be immediately available. Gallamine should be avoided. (Starre P. J. A. *Anesthesiology* 1978, **48**, 369.) L. W. Wolff; J. P. Parkinson; Paul Dudley White, US cardiologists.

Wolman's disease   Anaemia and clotting problems.

(*See also* Morton L. T. *A Medical Bibliography*, 3rd ed. London: Deutsch, 1970; Magalini S. 1. *Dictionary of Medical Sydromes*. Philadelphia: Lippincott, 1971; Jones A. E. P. and Pelton D. A. *Can. Anaesth. Soc. J.* 1976, **23**, 207; Stoetling P. *Anesthesia and Coexisting Disease*. Philadelphia: Saunders, 1982.)

Chapter 22

Surgical operations and choice of anaesthetic

INTRODUCTION

The conduct of simple anaesthetic techniques

Intravenous cannulation is performed[1] and appropriate monitoring instituted.

1. The intravenous induction agent is given until loss of the eyelash reflex. Nitrous oxide and oxygen is given and a volatile agent is increased steadily at about 1% after each 5–10 breaths (pausing or giving more intravenous agent if breath-holding occurs). Anaesthesia is deepened until respiration is quiet and regular. An airway can be inserted if necessary, provided that there is no tongue movement on opening the mouth or foot movement on depressing the chin (Ballantine's sign)[2]. Surgery may then begin.

2. Where intubation and relaxation are required, e.g. for abdominal surgery, the intravenous induction agent is followed by a relaxant and the patient intubated after an appropriate interval. IPPV is maintained with nitrous oxide, oxygen and volatile (or other) agent at about MAC_{50} as long as the relaxant (or any subsequent relaxant) is acting.

There are of course multitudes of variations on these themes, but the aim is to find a balance between the four principles of an anaesthetic: absence of awareness, analgesia, relaxation and attenuation of the stress response (the 'quadrant of anaesthesia'). The emphasis on any one of these will depend on the operation being performed and the needs of the patient.

The concept of balanced anaesthesia started in 1911 when George Washington Crile (1864–1943) of Cleveland, Ohio, taught that 'psychic' stimuli must be obliterated by light general anaesthesia, while the noxious impulses due to surgery must be blocked by local analgesia, the so-called theory of anoci-association.[3]

In 1926 John S. Lundy (1894–1972) of the Mayo Clinic introduced the term 'balanced anaesthesia' for a combination of agents such as premedication, regional analgesia and general anaesthesia with one or more agents, so that pain relief was obtained by a nice balance of agents and techniques.[4]

Rees and Gray[5] of Liverpool divided anaesthesia into three basic components: (1) narcosis; (2) analgesia; (3) relaxation. It was later renamed[6] the 'triad': (1) narcosis; (2) reflex suppression; (3) relaxation.

Anaesthesia (or analgesia) may be regarded as a process of modification of the normal physiological reflex response to the stimuli provided by surgery and anaesthesia: (1) inhibition of the afferent part of the reflex system; (2) depression of the central synaptic mechanisms of co-ordination; and (3) block of the efferent part of the reflex arc.

Attenuation of the stress response to surgery

This is a hormone-mediated response to the noxious effects of surgery, a reaction designed to preserve life in trauma. However, in the anaesthetic situation, although these responses are often helpful, they may have disadvantages, e.g. the accelerated clotting cascade may lead to venous thrombosis. The stress response includes the 'fear, fight and flight' activity of adrenaline, resistance to the effects of insulin and the secretion of endogenous steroids and growth hormone.

Attenuation of the stress response is achieved with short-acting opioids in doses in excess of those required for simple analgesia, and also by the use of regional blockade during and after surgery. The disadvantages of attenuation of the stress response is that protective reflexes, e.g. vascular reflexes during epidural analgesia, are also attenuated.

References

1. Nitescu P. et al. *Acta Anaesth. Scand.* 1990, **34**, 120; Gunawardene R. D. and Davenport H. T. *Anaesthesia* 1990, **45**, 52.
2. Ballantine R. I. W. *Anaesthesia* 1982, **37**, 214.
3. Crile G. W. *Lancet* 1913, **2**, 7; *Surg. Gynecol. Obstet.* 1911, **13**, 170; *Ann. Surg.* 1908, **47**, 866; *Boston Med. Surg. J.* 1910, **163**, 893 (reprinted in 'Classical File', *Surv. Anesthesiol.* 1966, **10**, 291).
4. Lundy J. S. *Minnesota Med.* 1926, **9**, 399 (Reprinted in 'Classical File', *Surv. Anesthesiol.* 1981, **25**, 272.)
5. Rees G. J. and Gray T. C. *Br. J. Anaesth.* 1950, **22**, 83
6. Gray T. C. *Ir. J. Med. Sci.* 1960, **419**, 499.

Abdominal and general surgery

History

The abdomen was seldom opened before the 1880s; McBurney did an appendicectomy in New York in 1898, Billroth performed a partial gastrectomy in Vienna in 1881; Dean sutured a perforated duodenal ulcer in 1894 at the London Hospital, Lawson Tait did a cholecystectomy in Birmingham in 1879, Conrad Ramstedt did a pyloromyotomy in Münster in 1911 and Dragstedt performed a vagotomy in 1943 in Chicago. Reginald Fitz (1843–1913) described the surgical treatment of acute appendicitis in Boston in 1886.

Requirements for general anaesthesia

1. Unconsciousness (unless regional analgesia is employed), with complete absence of awareness.
2. Prevention of gastric contents entering the glottis.
3. Suppression of reflex responses to surgical stimuli.
4. Good relaxation of the anterior abdominal wall.
5. Reasonably rapid return of consciousness and of the upper respiratory tract reflexes.
(For Vomiting and Regurgitation; Prevention and Treatment, *see* Chapter 14. For Management of the Acid Aspiration Syndrome, *see* Chapter 14.)

Effect of anaesthetic drugs on the gut

Halothane increases the blood supply of the gut, and hypocapnia due to hyperventilation reduces it. Morphine increases the tone of the bowel especially in diverticular disease. Diazepam inhibits the tone of the gut and may even cause ileus. β-blockers may decrease the lumen of the bowel. Metoclopramide increases the tone of the small bowel, an action opposed by atropine. Pretreatment with glycopyrronium may enable neostigmine to be given without causing too much bowel constriction,[1] but this has been contradicted.[2] The use of opioid drugs does not appear to interfere with the radiological interpretation of operative cholangiography, nor to increase spasm of the sphincter of Oddi.[3]

Central neural blockade increases blood flow in the colon.

A technique of general anaesthesia for abdominal surgery

1. Intravenous induction, using 2.5% thiopentone or alternative agent.
2. Injection of a non-depolarizing relaxant in a dose sufficient to allow easy intubation, giving time for maximal neuromuscular block to occur (up to 3 min), during which the lungs are gently inflated with a nitrous oxide–oxygen mixture (if there is a risk of vomiting or regurgitation and consequent aspiration of stomach contents, suxamethonium may be preferred, to allow more rapid intubation).
3. Tracheal intubation after optional spraying of the larynx with no more than 3 ml of 4% lignocaine solution, followed by careful inflation of the tracheal cuff.
4. Maintenance with a nitrous oxide–oxygen mixture and IPPV, supplemented with either a narcotic analgesic drug, or minimal concentrations of a volatile agent, to ensure complete unconsciousness. Additional doses of the non-depolarizing relaxant may be given as required, such doses being monitored by clinical response or a nerve stimulator.
5. At the termination of the operation, an anticholinesterase is injected to overcome neuromuscular block, preceded by atropine or glycopyrronium to counteract its muscarine-like effects. The nerve stimulator may be used to gauge the adequacy of reversal.

6. When spontaneous respiration is established, tracheobronchial suction and oesophageal toilet, deflation of the cuff and removal of the tracheal tube can be effected. The patient is then transferred to his bed to receive oxygen by catheter or mask. He will normally be turned on to his side to facilitate nursing.

7. Monitoring throughout the perioperative period may include arterial blood pressure, ECG, capnography, temperature, oximetry, etc.

Alternative techniques

These include:

1. Use of volatile agent as the main drug to provide anaesthesia and relaxation of the abdominal wall, e.g. halothane, enflurane, isoflurane, with small doses of a relaxant in a subsidiary role.

2. Regional block with or without general anaesthesia to provide unconsciousness, e.g. extra- or intradural, abdominal field block.

3. Muscle relaxant drugs may be given by infusion.

Hiccup is a troublesome reflex, too often associated with present-day methods of light anaesthesia. Its exact cause is not understood, but it is likely to be associated with a high nervous tone, and light anaesthesia. The best method of prevention and treatment is the use of *adequate* amounts of a relaxant drug. It may also yield to: (1) increase in analgesia, e.g. by injection of a narcotic analgesic drug; (2) inhalation of concentrated ether vapour for a few breaths; (3) increased depth of general anaesthesia; (4) block of vagus nerves near cardia. This also has prophylactic value; (5) intravenous injection of methylphenidate (Ritalin), 20 mg, or metoclopramide;[4] (6) intravenous ephedrine, 5 mg perhaps repeated once;[5] (7) instillation into the nose of 5 ml of ice-cold water.[6]

Preparation for emergency operations

Fluid and electrolyte balance must be corrected when possible.

The problem of regurgitation and vomiting is not confined to obstetrical and emergency abdominal operations, and if there is suspicion that the stomach is not empty a nasogastric tube (6–12 gauge, 4–7 mm diameter) should be passed through the nose[7] or an oesophageal tube (gauge 12) passed through either the nose or mouth. The stomach should then be aspirated with the patient supine and on each side in turn. When there is retroperistalsis, e.g. in acute intestinal obstruction, the stomach may refill from the duodenum between the time of emptying and the introduction of the tracheal tube with the risk of the inhalation of intestinal contents.

The hydrodynamics of regurgitation

See Chapter 14.

Rapid sequence induction and intubation

The technique to induce anaesthesia followed almost immediately by tracheal intubation (so-called 'crash induction') is designed to forestall the dangers of vomiting, regurgitation and aspiration of stomach contents. Following pre-oxygenation, the induction dose of thiopentone is immediately followed by an intubating dose of suxamethonium. Pre-curarization is probably unwise. An assistant who must be properly trained, applies cricoid pressure as the patient loses consciousness, while the anaesthetist proceeds to tracheal intubation and inflation of the cuff. Cricoid pressure is released and the tube tested for correct positioning. When suxamethonium is contra-indicated, an alternative technique is to inject vecuronium or alcuronium immediately before the thiopentone; this gives reasonable intubating conditions earlier than when any other non-depolarizing agent is used.

Perforated peptic ulcer

The operation, first performed in the UK by Dean,[8] is usually short and the patient may be shocked; he is very liable to postoperative chest complications. His stomach is likely to contain vomitable material. Precautions must be taken to prevent aspiration of gastric contents during induction of anaesthesia. Most workers prefer the pre-oxygenation, thiopentone, relaxant, nitrous oxide, oxygen hyperventilation technique described above with a volatile supplement if necessary.

Operations for peptic ulcer

First gastrectomy by Theodore Billroth (1825–1897) in 1881 in Vienna;[9] first gastrojejunostomy in 1884 by Anton Wolfler (1850–1907);[10] first vagotomy in 1943.[11] Before operation, many surgeons like the patient to swallow a nasogastric tube, so that the stomach can be aspirated and kept empty. This is a most unpleasant experience for the patient. Other workers favour the passage of an oesophageal or nasogastric tube after anaesthesia has been induced.

Acute intestinal obstruction

Factors to be considered are:
1. The degree of circulatory collapse.
2. The presence or absence of regurgitation or vomiting. The former is a passive process requiring no muscular force; the latter is a muscular reflex act. The former is aided by a head-down tilt and rendered less likely if the head is tilted upwards 45°.
3. The degree of distension.
4. The degree of electrolyte and fluid imbalance. This must be controlled with infusion of Hartmann's or other appropriate solution. The moderately dehydrated patient has lost 6% of total body fluids. The severely dehydrated patient has lost 10% of total body fluids, and shows loss of skin elasticity, sunken eyes, dry tongue and oliguria.

5. In all bowel operations, except those of the shortest duration, nitrous oxide inhaled into the lungs may be partially excreted into the gut, causing distension.[12] In both normal people and those with intestinal obstruction, much fluid is excreted by the proximal small intestine, only to be reabsorbed lower down. In high obstruction, this subsequent reabsorption is prevented. Low obstruction gives rise to distension. Vomiting causes loss of chlorides and alkalosis, and consequently great fluid loss and dehydration. Distension causes interference with circulation of the bowel wall, and pressure on the great veins results in reduced venous return to the heart, hypotension and interference with cardiac action due to increased intra-abdominal pressure. If this cannot be relieved, PEEP may be beneficial.[13]

Biochemical changes in intestinal obstruction include: (1) haemoconcentration; (2) metabolic alkalosis; (3) diminution of serum chlorides; (4) increased blood urea and non-protein nitrogen; (5) metabolic acidosis in low back obstruction; and (6) abnormalities of potassium metabolism.

The stomach should be emptied by either a nasogastric or a wider bore oesophageal tube, preferably the latter. Grave illness does not make this any less necessary. The tube should be taken out before induction of anaesthesia but may be reintroduced after induction and retained until the return of the reflexes. A patient with increasing cyanosis, tightly clenched jaws and faeculent material issuing from the nose is a truly terrifying sight, and one which carries a bad prognosis. That which cannot be easily treated had better be prevented.

General anaesthesia is safer in ill subjects. The actual agents and techniques used to produce general anaesthesia vary with different workers.

Intra- and extradural analgesia (with or without a light general anaesthetic) produce good relaxation, contract the bowel and do not interfere with the cough reflex (when used alone). They produce hypotension and are questionable in shocked and debilitated patients, e.g. where systolic blood pressure is below 100 mmHg.

Burst abdomen

This may be caused by poor surgical technique, indifferent anaesthesia, the nature of the patient's disease and his nutritional state. It is a serious complication and carries a high mortality from acute peritonitis, atelectasis, intestinal obstruction, renal or cardiac failure. Prolapse of a small piece of bowel or omentum into the wound is usually only the tip of the iceberg so that only too frequently the whole incision must be examined and completely resutured. This can only be done successfully with full relaxation. Care must be taken to protect the lungs from stomach contents during induction and from atelectasis after operation.

Operations on the colon and rectum[14]

Maximal relaxation is necessary and contracted intestines an advantage. Extra- or intradural analgesia with light general anaesthesia, or light general anaesthesia with a muscle relaxant are suitable. Adequate intraoperative fluid replacement must be maintained during colon resection and anastomosis, which is a prerequisite for successful healing.[15]

The authors prefer either a combination of thiopentone, volatile agent, relaxant and nitrous oxide–oxygen given through a large orotracheal tube with controlled respiration, or a continuous or single injection extradural block combined with light general anaesthesia and spontaneous (or occasionally assisted) respiration. This avoids the use of neostigmine.[16] There is evidence that patients operated on for colorectal cancer survive longer if they are not given blood transfusions during their operations.[17] Both halothane and central neural blockade increase colon blood flow whereas the hypocapnia, which may be associated with hyperventilation, decreases it.

Neostigmine may contribute to a breakdown of an intestinal anastomosis by the production of early and intense peristalsis. Neither atropine nor glycopyrronium effectively abolish the increase in intraluminal pressure of total colon activity after neostigmine given to reverse a non-depolarizing relaxant.[2] Halothane given towards the end of the operation may prevent this. For pre-operative preparation *see* Chapter 5.

Biliary tract surgery

First successful cholecystectomy by Lawson Tait (1845–1899) in Birmingham in 1879[18] and Carl Johan August Langenbuch (1876–1901) of Berlin in 1882.[19] First cholecystogram by Evarts Ambrose Graham (1883–1957) of St Louis in 1924.[20] First exploration of common duct for stone by Thornton in 1891.[21] Vitamin K analogue may be necessary before operation. Anaesthetic technique is similar to that used for gastric operations. High elevation off a gallbladder bridge may cause hypotension by interfering with venous return by obstructing the vena cava. The dynamics of the biliary ducts must be considered in connection with pre- and postoperative pain relief in patients with biliary disease. Normally the increase in intrabiliary pressure required to overcome the tone of the sphincter of Oddi does not cause pain. Analgesics (e.g. morphine and pethidine) may, by stimulating this sphincter to contract, increase the intrabiliary pressure up to $20\,cmH_2O$ and thus produce pain. Fentanyl raises intrabiliary pressure but the effect wanes within 25 min. Cholinergic drugs have a similar effect. The use of opioid drugs does not appear to interfere with the radiological interpretation of operative cholangiography, nor to increase the low incidence of spasm of the sphincter of Oddi.[3] To relieve biliary colic, therefore, the dose of analgesic must be great enough to cause cerebral depression. The following drugs lower intrabiliary pressure by relaxing the sphincter: (1) amyl nitrate; (2) glyceryl trinitrate 1 mg; and (3) papaverine 30 mg. Atropine, even up to 2 mg, is disappointing in this respect. With biliary obstruction gallamine is often suitable.[22] If a choledochogram is required, apnoea for up to 30 s may be necessary. To relax spasm of the sphincter of Oddi during cholecystography, glucagon 10 ml may be helpful (in the absence of insulinoma or phaeochromocytoma).[23] The usual techniques for pain relief in operations in the upper abdomen are employed postoperatively.

Cases of *acute haemorrhagic pancreatitis* are bad anaesthetic risks no matter what agent and method are used; thus obscure abdominal emergencies should have serum amylase tests done so that operation can be avoided. Hypocalcaemia may complicate pancreatitis and may result in difficult reversal of non-depolarizing relaxants.[24] Intravenous aprotinin (Trasylol), an inhibitor of kallikrein, has been recommended.

(For history of choledochoscopy *see* Ashby B. S. *Ann. R. Coll. Surg. Engl.* 1985, **67**, 279.)

Portal hypertension

Endoscopic injection of oesophageal varices.

Problems: severe haemorrhage; anaemia; coma; extreme sensitivity to most anaesthetic drugs; cardiovascular instability; respiratory failure; alcoholic history; blood flooding the airway; full stomach; ammonia intoxication; cross-infection risk for personnel; etc. General anaesthesia is to be avoided if possible, and conducted with great caution if necessary.

Liver transplantation

First successful orthotopic liver transplant by Thomas Earl Starzl of Denver in 1963[25]. This presents complex problems. The anaesthetic technique recommended consists of nitrous oxide, oxygen, relaxant and IPPV with occasional analgesic supplements. Atracurium is the relaxant of choice. Large blood transfusions are required and metabolic acidosis is likely to occur. Rises in serum potassium are common during operation but hypokalaemia may be a feature later on. Transplantation of an ice-cold liver produces a fall in body temperature. Aprotinin has been used successfully to reduce blood loss during transplantation.[26]

Haemorrhoidectomy

Surgical assault on the anal region results in severe pain, reflex response, e.g. movement of body muscles, reflex laryngeal spasm (Brewer-Luckhardt reflex).

To overcome these, pain requires surgical anaesthesia; muscle movement requires deep anaesthesia or a relaxant, laryngeal spasm requires a tracheal tube, deep anaesthesia, or a relaxant. All can be controlled by regional analgesia. Light general anaesthesia alone has no place here. Some surgeons require maximal relaxation of the anal sphincter whereas others prefer a certain amount of tone to be retained. The choice is between:

1. *Deep general anaesthesia.* Thiopentone (0.25–1 g), nitrous oxide and oxygen, in addition to the use of a volatile inhalation agent.

2. *Extradural sacral block.* 15–20 ml of 1.5% lignocaine or 10–15 ml of 0.5% bupivacaine with adrenaline (*see* Chapter 25). Extradural injection into the sacral canal (0.5% bupivacaine) at the conclusion of the operation greatly reduces postoperative discomfort. It can be given by the anaesthetist or surgeon.

3. *Low intradural block* (S4–5), e.g. lignocaine 5% 50–75 mg or 0.5% bupivacaine plain, or heavy solution, 2 ml between L4 and L5 with patient sitting.

4. *Local infiltration* with lignocaine or bupivacaine. From a point 2.5 cm (1 in) posterior to the anus, with the index finger of the left hand in the rectum, 1.5% lignocaine–adrenaline solution is injected: total amount, 25 ml. Only one site of injection used, and anus and anal canal are ensheathed by a cylinder of solution.[27]

All regional techniques can be combined with light general anaesthesia.

Hernia

A pioneer surgeon was Edoado Bassini (1844–1924) of Italy.[28] General anaesthesia is usually employed, e.g. thiopentone, nitrous oxide–oxygen, analgesic and relaxant. Other workers use a volatile inhalation agent. Ilioinguinal nerve block, with infiltration of the neck of the sac, as an adjunct to general anaesthesia allows lighter planes of anaesthesia and also provides postoperative pain relief. It can also be used without general anaesthesia. Intra- and extradural block are suitable in fit patients and must be carried to T10; if the cord is to be under tension, to T7 and if the peritoneum is to be under tension, to T5. For extradural block, 25–30 ml of 1.5% lignocaine or 12–15 ml of 0.5% bupivacaine. For intradural block, 1.4–1.6 ml of 5% lignocaine hyperbaric solution or 3–4 ml of hyperbaric bupivacaine 0.5%. For regional field block, *see* Chapter 24. Bupivacaine, 0.25% solution, infiltrated 30–45 min before the incision, gives efficient and prolonged postoperative analgesia.[29] Very suitable for day-stay surgery.[30]

Postoperative chest complications frequently follow these operations, especially in fit young men who smoke cigarettes, no matter what anaesthetic agent is used. They should, consequently, be advised to avoid smoking for the month preceding operation, and be taught how to breathe deeply and how to cough effectively. In addition, they will require vigorous 'shake-up' physiotherapy after operation.

Operations for incisional hernia require profound relaxation.

The chief danger in operation for *strangulated hernia* is from aspiration of stomach contents into the chest during induction of anaesthesia.

Ventral hernia

General anaesthesia, together with a muscle relaxant, is suitable. Bucking and coughing on the tracheal tube during extubation, with consequent strain on suture lines, should be prevented.

For fit adult patients, extra- or intradural analgesia can be used, to facilitate wound closure by contracting the bowels. Giant ventral hernia repair may embarrass postoperative respiration. This is managed either by elective postoperative mechanical ventilation or by performing a two-stage operation.

Mastectomy

First radical mastectomy performed by William Stewart Halsted (1852–1922) of Baltimore in 1891.[31] A faultless airway coupled with adequate ventilation minimizes oozing as does a table tilted upwards (although the risk of air embolism is increased in this position). Only light general anaesthesia is required and many anaesthetists avoid intubation for local removal of breast tumours.

Anaesthesia in varicose vein surgery

Ligation was proposed by Friederich Trendelenburg (1844–1927) in 1890.[32] Charles Mayo (1865–1939) of Rochester, Minn. described the removal of the long saphenous vein in 1906.[33] The malleable wire stripper first used in 1954.[34]

A head-down tilt reduces blood loss. The anaesthetic technique should enable the patient to move his legs as soon after operation as possible. Ligation of the short saphenous venous system can often be carried out with the patient in the lateral position. Maintenance of a free airway in a patient in the prone position may require tracheal intubation.

References

1. Kaufman L. *J. R. Soc. Med.* 1983, **76**, 693.
2. Child C. S. *Anaesthesia* 1984, **39**, 1083.
3. Chisholm R. J. et al. *Anaesthesia* 1983, **38**, 689.
4. Vasiloff N. *Can. Anaesth. Soc. J.* 1965, **12**, 306.
5. Sohn Y. Z. et al. *Can. Anaesth. Soc. J.* 1978, **25**, 431.
6. Milo E. M. et al. *Abst. 8th World Congress. Manila* 1984, **2**, A412.
7. Tucker A. and Lewis J. *Br. Med. J.* 1980, **2**, 1128.
8. Dean H. P. *Lancet* 1894, **1**, 1191.
9. Billroth T. (1829–1894) *Wien. Med. Wochenschr.* 1881, **31**, 162.
10. Wolfler A. (1850–1917), *see* Dagensheim G. A. *Surg. Clin. North Am.* 1978, **58**, 927.
11. Dragstedt L. and Owen F. M. *Proc. Soc. Exp. Biol. Med.* 1943, **53**, 152.
12. Eger E. I. and Saidman L. J. *Anesthesiology* 1965, **26**, 61; Lewis G. B. H. *Br. J. Anaesth.* 1984, **56**, 1370 (correspondence).
13. Burchard K. W. and Ciombor D. M. *Surg. Gynecol. Obstet.* 1985, **161**, 313.
14. Kraske P. (1851–1930) *Dtsch. Ges. Chir.* 1885, **14**, 445; Miles E. *Lancet* 1908, **2**, 1812.
15. Foster M. E. et al. *Br. J. Surg.* 1985, **72**, 831.
16. McLaren A. D. *Br. Med. J.* 1981, **2**, 675.
17. Blumberg L. et al. *Br. Med. J.* 1985, **290**, 1037; Fielding L. P. *Br. Med. J.* 1985, **291**, 842.
18. Lawson Tait R. *Med. Times Gaz.* 1879, **2**, 594.
19. Langenbuch L. K. (1864–1901) *Berl. Klin. Wochenschr.* 1882, **19**, 725.
20. Graham E. and Cole W. *JAMA* 1924, **82**, 613.
21. Thornton J. *Lancet* 1891, **1**, 525.
22. Ramzan I. M. et al. *Anesth. Analg. (Cleve.)* 1981, **60**, 289.
23. Bordley J. K. and Olson J. E. *Surg. Gynecol Obstet.* 1979, **149**, 583.
24. McKie B. D. *Br. J. Anaesth.* 1969, **41**, 1091.
25. Starzl T. E. et al. *Surg. Gynecol. Obstet.* 1963, **117**, 659.
26. Mallet S. V. et al. *Lancet* 1990, **336**, 886.

27. Feeley M. et al. *J. Irish Coll. Phys. Surg.* 1974, **3**, 83.
28. Bassini B. E. (1846–1924) *Arch. Klin. Chir.* 1890, **40**, 429; Halsted W. S. (1852–1922) *Johns Hopkins Hosp. Bull.* 1893, **4**, 17; Tanner N. C. *Br. J. Surg.* 1942, **29**, 285.
29. Kingsnorth A. N. et al. *Ann. R. Coll. Surg. Engl.* 1979, **61**, 451.
30. Flanagan L. and Bascom J. U. *Surg. Gyneol. Obstet* 1981, **153**, 557.
31. Halsted W. S. *Johns Hopkins Hosp. Rep.* 1891, **2**, 255; *Ann. Surg.* 1894, **20**, 497; 1907, **46**, 1.
32. Trendelenburg, Friedrich (1844–1924) *Beitr. klin. chir.* 1890, **7**, 195; Lee J. Alfred *Regional Anesthesia* 1985, **10**, 99.
33. Mayo C. H. *Surg. Gynecol. Obstet.* 1906, **2**, 385.
34. Myers T. T. and Cooley J. C. *Surg. Gynecol. Obstet.* 1954, **99**, 733.

Cardio-thoracic anaesthesia

THORACIC ANAESTHESIA

Any underlying lung disease is usually obvious clinically and assessed by lung function tests (*see* Chapter 1). Added problems are posed by smoking and the cardiac disease that often coexists. It is not always easy to advise on the extent of any proposed lung resection, and predict outcome, especially if postoperative lung collapse or infection occurs.

History and development

The following landmarks stand out in overcoming the problems of open pneumothorax, pulmonary collapse and secretions:

The Fell–O'Dwyer apparatus for artificial respiration using a bellows and tracheal tube[1] was used in a thoracotomy by Rudolph Matas (1860–1957) of New Orleans,[2] and by Theodore Tuffier (1857–1929) and Hallion of Paris.[3]

Ferdinand Sauerbruch (1875–1951) the pioneer thoracic surgeon of Breslau, assistant to Von Mickulicz (1853–1905), suggested operating in an airtight chamber with pressure reduced by 7 mmHg, while the anaesthetist and the head of the patient were outside (negative pressure breathing).[4] Leopold Brauer (1865–1951) did the reverse by enclosing the head of his patient in a positive pressure chamber.[5] M. Tiegel developed a positive pressure apparatus used later by Sauerbruch.[6]

Apnoea was produced by deep ether anaesthesia by Brat and Schmieden.[7] An apparatus for mechanical artificial respiration was devised by Janeway and Green.[8]

Franz Volhard (1872–1950) showed that the positive pressure technique caused hypercapnia. This led to the introduction of insufflation techniques by C. A. Elsberg (1871–1948),[9] who adapted the animal work of S. J. Meltzer (1851–1920) and Leopold Auer (1875–1948).[10] Elsberg also advocated direct vision intubation,[11] instead of blind oral intubation as practised by Franz Kuhn (1866–1929),[12] while he also showed the need for periodic lung inflation during operation. The double-lumen tube designed for differential broncho-spirometry[13] was soon employed in thoracic operations.

The first use of endobronchial (one lung) anaesthesia was described in 1932 by Gale and Waters,[14] while a bronchus blocker was described by Archibald, at the suggestion of Harold R. Griffith, in 1935.[15] Clarence Crafoord (1899-1984) of Stockholm reported his method of artificial respiration by means of Frenckner's mechanical spiro-pulsator,[16] developed at the suggestion of the Swedish surgeon K. H. Giertz, former assistant to Sauerbruch, in 1938.[17] This was developed and simplified by Guedel[18] and Nosworthy[19] who advocated controlled breathing by intermittent pressure on the reservoir bag of a closed system, using cyclopropane. This had been introduced by Guedel and Treweek, using ether.[20] Cyclopropane had great popularity during the decade following 1935. Muscle relaxants have now made controlled respiration straightforward. Early ventilators were by Pinson,[21] Trier Morch (then of Denmark)[22] and Blease.[23]

Ferdinand Sauerbruch is credited with the first paravertebral thoracoplasty for pulmonary tuberculosis. The operation was first suggested by the German physician, L. Brauer (1865-1951). Morriston Davies performed the first such operation in the UK in 1912, and Tudor Edwards and Roberts the first pneumonectomy in the UK in 1935 at the Brompton Hospital.

See also Mushin W. W. and Rendell-Baker L. *The Principles of Thoracic Anaesthesia, Past and Present.* Oxford: Blackwell, 1953; McLellan I. In: *Anaesthesia: Essays on its History* (Rupreht J. et al. ed.) Berlin: Springer-Verlag, 1985, 126; for history of endobronchial anaesthesia, see White G. M. J. *Br. J. Anaesth.* 1960, **32**, 235; for history of the various tubes used in thoracic anaesthesia, *see* Pappin J. C. *Anaesthesia* 1979, **34**, 57.

Open pneumothorax and lung collapse

The lungs normally are kept inflated by the difference between atmospheric pressure in the alveoli and the negative pressure (about $-5\,cm\ H_2O$) in the potential space between the two layers of pleura. This balances the elastic recoil of the lung, and the tendency of the chest wall to spring outwards.

When the chest is opened, the negative pressure is lost and the elastic recoil causes collapse of the lung on that side. The mediastinum, unless fixed by adhesions, shifts to the other side, compresses the healthy lung and may interfere with cardiac function. If the lung is adherent to the chest wall, these effects may not be marked. The lung collapse causes shunting, hypoxia and a high pulmonary vascular resistance. If breathing spontaneously, the healthy lung breathes in and out partly from the trachea and partly from the other lung. This transfer of gas from one lung to the other is 'pendelluft', effectively increases dead space and can be lethal. These problems are overcome with IPPV, perhaps with the addition of PEEP.

Other advantages of IPPV are: (*a*) the extent of lung movement in the operating field can be adjusted to suit the surgery; (*b*) deep anaesthesia is not needed; (*c*) it allows control of secretions (*see below*); and (*d*) it provides respiratory support for a patient with lung disease. The major disadvantage of IPPV is air leak from the lung if there is a bronchopleural fistula, or the creation of an air leak by rupture of emphysematous bullae.

Pulmonary secretions

The patient with excessive secretions is uncommon, but it occurs in lung abscess, bronchiectasis, bronchopleural fistula and tumours, when infected secretions lie distal to an obstructed bronchus. Improvement may be obtained by pre-operative postural drainage and antibiotics.

Methods for preventing the spread of secretions into healthy parts of the lungs during surgery include: (*a*) *regional analgesia* and preserving the cough reflex, e.g. for drainage of empyema; (*b*) *tracheal suction*, every 10 min and especially after the position is changed or the lungs manipulated; (*c*) *surgical clamping of a bronchus*, as soon as the chest is open; (*d*) *posture*. In the lateral position, tilted 35° head-down for a left thoracotomy and 55° for a right thoracotomy, secretions from the diseased upper lung will flow into the trachea for suction and not contaminate the healthy lung. In the prone position the same is true when tilted 10° head-down (Overholt[24] – requires a special table; Parry Brown).[25] Useful in children undergoing lobectomy who are too small for bronchial blockers, and in upper lobectomies in adults. Alternatively, secretions can be retained in the diseased lobe by posture, e.g. sitting for lower lobectomy in bronchiectasis. An empyema is often drained with the patient sitting, especially if there is any chance of bronchopleural fistula with its risk of the patient drowning in his own secretions; and (*e*) *endobronchial intubation* and blocking with inflatable cuffs.

Endobronchial instrumentation[26]

Isolation of one lung or major lobe has the following advantages: (*a*) secretions and blood are confined to the diseased area; (*b*) any bronchopleural fistula is isolated; and (*c*) the lung to be operated upon is collapsed and still. Methods include the use of a double-lumen (commonest) or single-lumen endobronchial tube. The former are not designed for use in children, but single-lumen bronchial tubes may be used. Bronchial blockers are now used very rarely.

1. Double-lumen endobronchial tubes

One lumen ends just above the carina, the other extends into one main bronchus. The *Robertshaw*[27] red rubber tube in three sizes (small, medium, large) was much used. There are versions to intubate left and right main bronchi, the right-sided tube having a slotted bronchial cuff to allow inflation of the right upper lobe. The two tubes separate proximally for connection to two catheter mounts. The longer bronchial tube has a cuff that seals it in the main bronchus; a second cuff seals the whole tube in the trachea. Both cuffs have pilot balloons, blue for bronchial and red for tracheal cuff. *Disposable PVC double-lumen tubes* with specific introducers are more commonly used now. They are easier to pass, and may cause less damage and be more economical.[28] Coaxial double-lumen tubes have been used.[29]

The tube is passed into the trachea using an ordinary laryngoscope, and then advanced blindly until the fork, where the tubes separate, is opposite the lips. The tracheal and bronchial cuffs are then inflated in turn, and checks made for leaks and correct positioning by inflating down each tube and auscultating the lung. Either lung can be ventilated, isolated or collapsed at will. Accurate placement may be difficult owing to alterations in anatomy or as a result of pathology, and may be checked further by fibreoptic bronchoscopy, and eventually by the surgeon palpating the tube.

The *Carlens* double-lumen tube was the first and was originally used for differential bronchospirometry.[30] It has a left-sided endobronchial tube, and a carinal hook to aid positioning, although this does not always make intubation easier and may cause trauma.

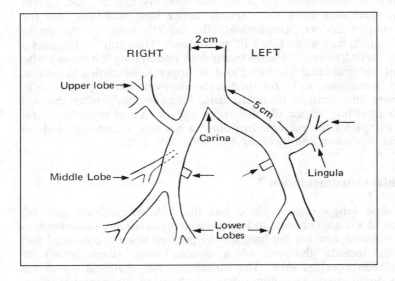

Figure 22.1 Diagram of tracheobronchial tree

2. Single-lumen endobronchial tubes

Normally left-sided, but if right-sided, the bronchial cuff is slotted to allow ventilation of the upper lobe. A tracheal cuff allows ventilation of both lungs and helps anchor the tube. *Macintosh and Leatherdale*[31] described two tubes for right-lung surgery: (*a*) a left-sided endobronchial tube with bronchial and tracheal cuffs and a small right-sided channel used to aspirate secretions or distend the right lung; (*b*) an endotracheal tube combined with a left endobronchial cuffed suction blocker. The *Green–Gordon* tube[32] is right-sided, has a tracheal cuff and carinal hook, and is used for surgery on the left lung. *Magill* endobronchial tubes are very long Magill tracheal tubes.[33] The *Machray* modification has a short cuff.[34] The *Pallister* left endobronchial tube has a tracheal cuff and two bronchial cuffs, in case one is ruptured, as may happen during sleeve resection of the right upper lobe bronchus.[35] These last three are best inserted over a rigid[33, 36] or fibreoptic[37] bronchoscope. An intubating bronchoscope is the same diameter for its entire length, and has no lip at its tip, unlike a diagnostic bronchoscope. The *Univent* is an endotracheal tube incorporating a movable bronchial blocker with a lumen for suction, giving oxygen or high-frequency ventilation.[38]

Endobronchial intubation in infants

An uncuffed tube, 1 cm longer than the distance from mouth to carina measured on the lateral chest radiograph, will tend to enter the bronchus on the opposite side to the bevel. The bevel is cut for the desired side, the tube passed into the bronchus and rotated through 180° so that the upper lobe orifice is not obstructed. The bevel needs an extension on the right side to allow for the more proximal position of the right upper lobe orifice.[39]

Endobronchial blockers

Passed through a rigid bronchoscope. Described by *Vernon Thompson*[40] and *Magill*[41] but now seldom needed. Fogarty or Swan-Ganz catheters have been used in children.[42]

Problems of endobronchial tubes

(a) *Difficulty with insertion*, especially if anatomy is abnormal or distorted; (b) *dislodgement*, during positioning the patient, and movement of the head and neck. The margin of safety in the positioning of left-sided tubes is double that of right-sided tubes, and the former should be used if possible;[43] (c) *trauma*, to larynx and airways; (d) *kinking*, of thin-walled single-lumen endobronchial tubes; (e) *arterial hypoxaemia* during one-lung anaesthesia.[44] Collapse of the upper lung and hypoxic pulmonary vasoconstriction increase its vascular resistance. None the less, blood does flow through this collapsed lung and the shunt causes hypoxaemia that is little improved by ventilation with 100% oxygen. The lower lung will be at a disadvantage too, as its FRC will be reduced with some atelectasis. These problems can be helped by: (1) using a tidal volume large enough (about 12 ml/kg) to reduce lower lung atelectasis, but not so large as to divert blood flow to the upper lung; (2) PEEP often worsens hypoxaemia in this situation by diverting blood to the upper lung and by reducing cardiac output. However the hypoxaemia is severe, cautious application of PEEP may improve oxygenation;[45] (3) insufflating, intermittently inflating, applying CPAP or using high-frequency jet ventilation in the collapsed lung with 100% oxygen. Careful monitoring of arterial saturation is needed; and (4) clamping the pulmonary artery when a pneumonectomy is performed; (f) *hypercapnia*, which is seldom a problem in practice.

Anaesthetic technique for thoracotomy[46]

While median sternotomy is used for open heart operations and access to the thymus, retrosternal goitres and anterior mediastinum, lateral thoracotomy is used for all other thoracic operations, including closed heart operations. For the problems posed by mediastinal masses, *see* Pullerits J. and Holzman R. *Can. J. Anaesth.* 1989, **36**, 681. Oat-cell bronchial carcinoma may be associated with *myasthenic syndrome* where there is marked sensitivity to all relaxants, *see* Chapter 20. Bleomycin therapy can cause pulmonary fibrosis, aggravated by a high FIo_2.

Standard premedication, including a vagolytic drug, is used. Atrial fibrillation may occur during or after thoracotomy, especially for pneumonectomy, and the patient is often digitalized pre-operatively.[47] Many anaesthetic sequences have been used with success. Thiopentone, relaxant, nitrous oxide, with some narcotic and some volatile agent is popular. Smaller doses of relaxant are needed for thoracotomy than for upper abdominal surgery.

IPPV is essential once the chest is open (*see above* under 'Open Pneumothorax and Lung Collapse'). Most prefer endobronchial techniques, but they are not essential for successful thoracic surgery. *The majority of lung resections can be carried out with ordinary tracheal tubes, IPPV and intermittent suction.* The decision to use an endobronchial instrument will depend on the operative procedure, the pathology, the equipment available, and the anaesthetist's experience. High-frequency jet ventilation[48] during routine thoracotomy probably offers no advantage over conventional one or two-lung IPPV.[49]

Analgesia is particularly important after this painful operation to allow adequate respiration and coughing, and can be instituted pre-operatively. The following may be used:[50] (*a*) i.m. or i.v. opiates; (*b*) rectal non-steroidal anti-inflammatory drugs (diclofenac or indomethacin 100 mg 12-hourly); (*c*) cryoprobe of the intercostal nerves from inside the chest gives good analgesia, which lasts for weeks, but may cause persistent scar symptoms; (*d*) paravertebral block of the intercostal nerves provides good unilateral analgesia over several segments; (*e*) thoracic extradural block, probably no better than (*d*); (*f*) lumbar extradural opiates;[51] and (*g*) transcutaneous nerve stimulation. If sputum retention is troublesome postoperatively, minitracheostomy may be needed.[52]

Technical Points

1. *Severe blood loss may occur.* At least one large-bore cannula is essential. A central venous catheter is very useful.

2. *Positioning.* Care must be taken to avoid injuries due to pressure or to the brachial plexus by traction on the upper arm.

3. *Bronchial suturing* is usually performed with the bronchus clamped and presents no problem. Some surgeons feel that the clamp may increase the risk of bronchopleural fistula. Use of a double-lumen tube gives control of the opposite lung, and helps the anaesthetist test the bronchial stump for leaks.

4. *Closure of the chest.* The lungs should be fully expanded before closure. It is wise to interrupt ventilation as the suture needle is inserted into the chest wall. Residual air in the pleural cavity can be removed by an intrapleural drain connected to an underwater seal or a Heimlich disposable flutter valve.[53]

5. *Accidental pneumothorax.* May occur on the contralateral side during thoracotomy with mediastinal dissection. Also during any operation near the pleura (e.g. cervical sympathectomy, nephrectomy, thyroidectomy) and

during local blocks (brachial plexus block, intercostal nerves). Suspected if the pattern of spontaneous respiration is altered and breath sounds are absent. Diagnosed by radiography. The hole in the pleura should be closed if possible and the lung fully inflated. Puncture of the lung itself will usually close spontaneously but chest drains may be required as a safety precaution.

Some particular operations

Pneumonectomy

A right pneumonectomy removes 55% of the patient's lung tissue, and if the function of the remaining lung is compromised the patient is in a precarious position postoperatively. The major problems are pulmonary hypertension worsened by hypoxia, and oedema of the remaining lung from mechanical damage, reduced lymph drainage and left ventricular failure. Atrial fibrillation is common and pre-operative digitalization may help.[47]

Either the lateral or prone position may be used. Can be performed under ordinary endotracheal anaesthesia, but pus can collect behind an obstructing carcinoma, and a double-lumen tube is preferable. A left-sided tube may be used even for a left pneumonectomy, by withdrawing it for the bronchial suture.

Low pressure suction (less then $5\,cmH_2O$) applied postoperatively to the pleural drain will help prevent mediastinal shift, but care must be taken if the pericardium has been incised as this may cause the heart to herniate through the opening.

Lobectomy

Upper lobectomy is sometimes carried out for carcinoma along with a segment of the main bronchus (sleeve resection). There will be a large air leak and difficulty with ventilation unless one-lung anaesthesia is used. *Lower lobectomy* is usually for tumour, but may be for bronchiectasis in children, and the volume of sputum may be large. In older children a Magill blocker may be useful. In young children with copious sputum the sitting position should be considered.

Otherwise an ordinary tracheal tube is satisfactory for lobectomy or segmental lung resection. There may be considerable alveolar air leak afterwards, which decreases when IPPV is stopped. Occasionally negative pressure must be applied to the drain to keep the lungs expanded.

Tracheal stenosis

Pre-operative dilatation may allow passage of a tracheal tube with inflation of the cuff beyond the operation site. Difficulties are more likely in children. Insertion of tracheal stents has been managed with high-frequency jet ventilation (HFJV), or venturi ventilation and partial cardiopulmonary bypass.[54] A bronchoscope can be used to place catheters for HFJV beyond an obstruction, although a free outflow for the gas must be provided to prevent lung distension.[55] Resection of central airway tumours with the Nd-YAG laser may need HFJV with air to avoid the risk of fires, together with total intravenous anaesthesia.[56]

Lung cysts and bullae

Large cysts compress surrounding lung tissue, and may have a valvular communication with a bronchus allowing gas to pass in more easily than out. IPPV and coughing may therefore cause further distension or even a tension pneumothorax. Careful induction is needed, keeping respiration spontaneous until the cyst has been isolated with a double-lumen tube or bronchial clamp. If the cysts are bilateral, HFJV should be considered in order to minimize barotrauma.[57] Avoid nitrous oxide, which may distend lung cysts within minutes because of its much greater solubility than nitrogen. A tension pneumothorax should be aspirated through a large needle or drain through the second intercostal space anteriorly.

Pulmonary hydatid cysts are common in the Middle East. They can be bilateral and multiple, and need excision if they become large. They may erode the bronchial wall and become infected. Accidental rupture of the cyst into the bronchi during surgery risks dissemination of the disease. Endobronchial instrumentation is often indicated.

Lung abscess

May be caused by aspiration, obstruction by tumour or spread from elsewhere. Pre-operative postural drainage, physiotherapy and antibiotics are the mainstays of treatment, but lung resection may be needed. Endobronchial instrumentation protects against contamination of the bronchial tree.

Bronchopleural fistula

Most commonly presents after pneumonectomy, especially if right-sided. This produces two complications: (1) a gas leak from the lung, which may make ventilation impossible, but usually is small; and (2) a collection of fluid in the pleural cavity or post-pneumonectomy space may flood the bronchial tree. A bronchial blocker in the bronchial stump may easily be pushed through the weakened suture line, converting a small fistula into a large one. Ideally a double-lumen tube is used to isolate the opposite lung, maintaining spontaneous respiration until this is achieved. This has been done using only a propofol infusion.[58] The experienced anaesthetist, however, may simply use suxamethonium to perform a bronchoscopy and then pass an endobronchial tube. HFJV may be valuable in diminishing any gas leak. For the radiological characteristics of bronchopleural fistula following pneumonectomy, see Lauckner M. E. et al. Anaesthesia 1983, **38**, 452.

Drainage of empyema

Because general anaesthesia may be dangerous with an unsuspected bronchopleural fistula, an empyema is usually drained under local analgesia in the sitting position. General anaesthesia is, however, necessary for rib resection and operations more extensive than simple drainage, and in children. The presence of a possible bronchopleural fistula will normally require a double-lumen tube. Awake intubation under local analgesia in the sitting position may be best with a large fistula or empyema.

Oesophagectomy

The patient's general condition is often poor due to lack of nutrition. Assessment and treatment to correct nutritional and electrolyte deficiencies are therefore important. A short period of enteral nutrition (or parenteral if needed) pre-operatively may be of great benefit (*see* Chapter 34). The operation may be long and bloody, and may involve opening the abdomen as well as the thorax.

Thymectomy

Pioneers in the operation of thymectomy for myasthenia gravis have been Sauerbruch (in 1912–13), Blalock,[59] and Keynes.[60] The connection between thymus enlargement and myasthenia was noticed by Carl Weigert in 1845. The approach is transcervical, or by splitting the sternum when one or both pleural cavities may be opened. For pre-operative and anaesthetic management, *see* Chapter 20.

Lung transplantation[61]

In single lung transplants in patients with emphysema, the remaining diseased lung is very compliant and tends to be ventilated at the expense of the transplanted lung. Double lung transplants have been successful.[62] Best results are in patients with fibrotic lung disease,[63] although the sepsis associated with cystic fibrosis may be a problem when immunosuppressed. Conventional one-lung anaesthesia may be used for single lung transplants. Problems include haemorrhage as adhesions are separated, pulmonary hypertension when the pulmonary artery is clamped and postoperative accumulation of lung water (due to ischaemia before implantation, denervation and section of lymphatic drainage in new lung). All efforts are made to avoid cardiopulmonary bypass, although respiratory support with extracorporeal gas exchange may be needed as a bridge to transplantation.

Bronchoscopy

History

A cylindrical metal tube, illuminated by candle-light to examine body cavities, was invented in 1807 by Bozzini (1773–1809).[64] In 1895 Gustav Killian (1860–1921) of Freiburg used a laryngoscope to peer below the cords.[65] Modern bronchoscopy was developed by Chevalier Jackson (1865–1958) in the USA and by Victor Negus (1887–1974) in the UK in the early years of this century. Diffusion respiration first described (in dogs) by Draper and Whitehead in 1944[66] and apnoeic oxygenation in man in 1947 by Draper[67] and later by Holmdahl.[68] The fibreoptic bronchoscope was introduced in 1968 by Ikeda.[69]

Rigid bronchoscopy

1. Topical analgesia. See section in Chapter 24. Not popular, but safer than general anaesthesia if the patient has respiratory obstruction, is particularly dyspnoeic or is expectorating large amounts of blood or pus. Vocal cord movements may also be assessed, which cannot accurately be done under anaesthesia.

2. *General anaesthesia.* Patient is premedicated according to general condition. Benzodiazepines are useful, remembering that awareness may occur with a totally i.v. technique. The haemodynamic effects of rigid bronchoscopy are similar to those of laryngoscopy (*see* Chapter 11), but greater and of longer duration.[70] Topical analgesia of the larynx and trachea will help prevent laryngospasm and undue straining during and after light i.v. anaesthesia. Small doses of intermittent suxamethonium prevents coughing and relaxes the larynx for insertion of the bronchoscope. Respiration is maintained by:

(*a*) The Sanders injector.[71] Intermittent flow of oxygen via a small tube in the mouth of the bronchoscope entrains air by the Venturi effect to inflate the lungs despite the open proximal end. The injector can be permanently fixed to the bronchoscope, and pipeline oxygen used (410 kPa) with three different injector sizes (SWG 16 for adults and small adult, 18 for adolescent and 19 for child, infant and suckling). This technique is the most satisfactory, and can also be used for laryngeal microsurgery. Modifications include: (i) transtracheal ventilation through a 14 G cannula; (ii) use of the oxygen side-arm of the bronchoscope to increase FIo_2; (iii) use of Entonox as the driving gas to prevent awareness, but the air entrainment will make this of little use; and (iv) high-frequency jet ventilation. Very little air entrainment occurs at rates over 1 Hz. May reduce coughing.

(*b*) The ventilating bronchoscope allows IPPV at the same time as the operator visualizes the bronchial tree through a window.

(*c*) Intermittent ventilation, using a tracheal tube pushed into the mouth of the bronchoscope. Useful in the occasional case when the Venturi injector is inadequate.

(*d*) Deep inhalational anaesthesia, performing bronchoscopy as anaesthesia lightens. Gives a limited time, but ether in air is effective in children, as is halothane and nitrous oxide in oxygen.

If massive haemorrhage occurs after biopsy, a bronchus blocker or an endobronchial tube should be passed at once. These instruments should always be available during bronchoscopy. After the procedure, reflexes must return rapidly, and the patient placed in the lateral position to allow drainage of blood, etc. on the left side after left bronchus biopsy and vice versa, to prevent blood soiling normal lung.

Removal of an inhaled foreign body[72]

Most common in children and in the right lung, and is removed via a rigid bronchoscope under inhalation anaesthesia. Respiratory obstruction may be present and can act as a valve so that a segment of lung becomes hyperinflated. These cases can be dangerous and need experience.

Fibreoptic bronchoscopy

This instrument allows most extensive visualization of the larynx and bronchial tree, and is much more comfortable under local analgesia than the rigid instrument. Anaesthetic techniques include:

1. *Topical analgesia.* The patient may be sitting or supine. The instrument is passed through a nasopharyngeal airway, directly through a naris or through the mouth, after topical analgesia to the nose, pharynx, larynx, trachea and bronchial tree. Further analgesia may be applied through the suction channel of the bronchoscope as needed, bearing in mind the rapid absorption of local analgesic drugs through the bronchial mucosa. The segmental divisions can be inspected. Sedation and analgesia, with, e.g. midazolam and fentanyl, may be helpful. Transbronchial lung biopsy is usually performed under topical analgesia.

2. *General anaesthesia.* Passed down a rigid bronchoscope (when the Sanders injector functions normally) or a standard tracheal tube. IPPV is also possible using a rubber diaphragm to provide an airtight seal, although the fibreoptic instrument (diameter up to 6.5 mm) will partially obstruct the lumen. For lengthy examinations, a high-frequency jet ventilator may be used, perhaps with a Mallinckrodt 'Hi–Lo' tracheal tube, which also allows the PEEP generated by the expiratory obstruction to be monitored.

Oesophagoscopy

Pioneered by Kussmaul (1822–1902) in 1869 and by Von Mikulicz (1829–1905) in 1881.[73]

Relaxation of the postcricoid sphincter is needed for rigid oesophagoscopy, and may be achieved using muscle relaxants or deep anaesthesia. In obstructive lesions, regurgitation may occur from a dilated oesophagus above the lesion. A tracheal tube should be passed and suction should always be available. The technique should allow rapid return of reflexes. At the end of the procedure the pharynx must be sucked clear of blood, etc. and the patient turned on the side. Oesophagoscopy may cause trauma, perforation and bleeding after biopsy or with oesophageal varices. Intermittent thiopentone and suxamethonium, using IPPV with oxygen and nitrous oxide, or spontaneous respiration using a volatile agent are both satisfactory techniques.

The flexible fibreoptic instrument usually requires no more than i.v. diazepam sedation.

Mediastinoscopy

These patients may have obstruction of the superior vena cava and the trachea. An armoured endotracheal tube may be advisable, and the anaesthetist should be prepared for haemorrhage.

CARDIAC ANAESTHESIA[74]

History of Cardiac Surgery[75]

First drainage of pericardium for suppurative pericarditis by Hilsman in 1875.[76] First successful suture of heart wound by Rehn (1849–1930) in 1896.[77]

First operation for relief of valvular disease by Tuffier (1857–1929) in 1914.[78] First pericardectomy for pericarditis by Delorme (1847–1929) in 1898,[79] and Hallopeau (1876–1924) in 1921. Valvulotomy for valvular disease by Elliott Cutler (1888–1947) and Levine in 1923.[80] Digital dilatation of mitral valve through atrium by Souttar (1875–1964) in 1925.[81] Cardiac catheterization by Bleichroder in 1912 (on himself),[82] Forssmann (1904–1979) in 1929[83] and Cournand in 1941.[84] Angiocardiography by Robb and Steinberg in 1938.[85] Ligation of patent ductus by Gross and Hubbard in 1939,[86] Surgical treatment of tetralogy of Fallot by Blalock (1899–1964) and Taussig.[87] Removal of foreign body from heart by Harken in 1946. Surgical treatment of coarctation of the aorta by Clarence Crafoord and Nylin[88] in Stockholm. Pulmonary valvulotomy for the relief of pulmonary stenosis by Brock.[89] Valvuloplasty for mitral stenosis by Harken and colleagues.[90] Pump oxygenator used in man by Gibbon.[91] Selective coronary angiography by Sones in 1958.[92] Resection of aortic aneurysm by De Bakey in 1958.[93] Deep hypothermia, to 20°C or below, by Drew.[94] Starr replaced the aortic valve in 1963.[95] Saphenous vein bypass grafting by Garrett in 1964.[96] The internal mammary artery was not used until 1970. Pioneering work on suture of small blood vessels by Carrel (1873–1944) in 1907.[97] First cardiac transplant carried out in man by Barnard in 1967[98] and Shumway in 1968.[99]

Anaesthetic Problems in Cardiac Surgery

1. *Effects of the disease process*, e.g. poor ventricular function, which may be further depressed by anaesthetic drugs and hypoxia, pulmonary oedema, valvular stenosis restricting cardiac output that cannot increase to compensate for a fall in vascular resistance. Anaesthetic agents must therefore be given with particular care. The function of other organs, especially lungs, liver and kidney may be impaired.

2. *Open pneumothorax. See above* under 'Thoracic Anaesthesia'.

3. *Blood loss and replacement.* Haemorrhage can be sudden and rapid. It is easy to overload the circulation in the presence of a failing left ventricle.

4. *Surgical manipulations of the heart* may cause ectopic beats, asystole, other dysrhythmias or hypotension, especially in the presence of acid-base or electrolyte disturbances.

5. *The problems of cardiopulmonary bypass* (and perhaps hypothermia), which allows surgery on a heart that is isolated from the circulation without damage to vital organs. *See below.*

Closed heart surgery without bypass

Premedication with morphine is well tolerated. Hyoscine is often added. Most anaesthetists will wish to avoid the tachycardia produced by atropine. An intravenous infusion is started before induction, and some patients merit arterial cannulation under local analgesia so that changes in arterial pressure during induction and tracheal intubation may be monitored continuously. The ECG and saturation are monitored as usual. After pre-oxygenation, minimal intravenous anaesthetic provides a smooth induction without undue depression. A slow circulation time delays the response. A small dose of benzodiazepine before giving thiopentone or methohexitone allows lower doses and less disturbance of the circulation. Intubation is performed using either suxamethonium or a non-depolarizing muscle relaxant, and IPPV continued with nitrous oxide, oxygen, and opiate or volatile supplements if needed.

Blood must be immediately available. Additional monitoring may include central venous pressure, body temperature and urine output. During manipulation of the heart, a close watch should be kept of the heart's rhythm and function. Direct observation of the heart can be most informative. If manipulation causes bradycardia with hypotension, a short period of rest may be required. The lungs must be fully expanded before the chest is closed. Oxygen therapy is important in the immediate postoperative period.

Closed mitral valvotomy[100]

Performed with success in some cases of pure mitral stenosis with an uncalcified valve. Other closed valvotomies are very unusual.

Patent ductus arteriosus

The ductus is a wide channel between the distal part of the aortic arch and the pulmonary artery in fetal life. If closure does not occur after birth, blood flows from the aorta to the pulmonary artery, the reverse of flow in intrauterine life. The left side of the heart dilates to cope with the increased flow through it. Less blood flows down the aorta and the diastolic blood pressure is low. Cyanosis only occurs if pulmonary vascular disease has developed, or if other congenital abnormalities exist. There is a continuous murmur, and there may also be pulmonary regurgitation. Endocarditis is a hazard. The ductus is easily torn when it is ligated, especially in an adult, with major bleeding.

Coarctation of aorta

Surgery is more risky in an adult because of associated hypertension, coronary artery disease and cerebral aneurysms. Enlarged collaterals in the chest wall prevent a severe rise in pressure when the aorta is clamped. Induced hypotension has a place to reduce blood loss from these collaterals and make the actual suturing of the aorta easier. The blood pressure should be rising again when the clamps are removed. If the collaterals are poorly developed (as in children) and the pressure distal to the coarctation is therefore low, the blood supply to the spinal cord may be at risk. Hypothermia or an assisted circulation[101] in the descending aorta has been used.

Pericardectomy

Constrictive pericarditis limits diastolic expansion of the heart. The rise in atrial pressure leads to venous congestion, ascites, peripheral oedema and sometimes atrial fibrillation. The blood pressure may almost vanish on inspiration (pulsus paradoxus). These patients present considerable risks. Cardiac output may not be able to increase if there is a sudden fall in peripheral resistance, and intravenous induction needs great care. An inhalational induction can also be used. The surgical procedure is lengthy and involves considerable manipulation of the heart. Blood loss should be replaced precisely, because the circulation is easily overloaded.

Cardiac tamponade

The patient depends on a tachycardia and vasoconstriction to maintain the blood pressure. Treatment of medical cases is normally by aspiration, but in the postoperative case open drainage is needed. Pulsus paradoxus is not a useful sign in these latter patients. IPPV may cause severe hypotension before the pericardium is opened, and adrenaline 10–20 μg may be useful, repeated if necessary.

Open heart surgery with cardiopulmonary bypass

Used when the surgery needs a circulatory arrest longer than the 7 min, which is normally considered safe under conventional hypothermia, e.g. surgery of the coronary arteries[102] (the commonest operation), heart valves, septal defects and other more complex congenital abnormalities. Extracorporeal circulation (bypass) is made possible by anticoagulation with heparin and its reversal with protamine.

Assessment

Ventricular function is assessed from the history, examination and data at cardiac catheterization. A high LVEDP (left ventricular end-diastolic pressure) of over 15 mmHg, a low ejection fraction of under 50% and abnormalities of ventricular wall motion indicate poor function. Left main stem coronary stenosis presents a high risk. Any pressure gradients across valves and calculated valve areas should be noted. Pulmonary arterial pressure and vascular resistance is important in patients with mitral stenosis or congenital disorders. Dental assessment should have been carried out. Cardiac drugs are usually continued until surgery. Relatively heavy premedication with opiates and/or benzodiazepines is usually well-tolerated, unless the patient is needing inotropic support.

Anaesthesia

Similar considerations apply as for surgery without cardiopulmonary bypass. Before bypass is instituted the anaesthetist must be prepared to control arterial pressure, dysrhythmias and any LV dysfunction. If the latter is severe, inotropic support (adrenaline 5–20 μg/min) and rapid progression to bypass is needed. Tracheal intubation, skin incision and sternal splitting are the most stimulating events. IPPV with nitrous oxide and oxygen is used perhaps with opiate or volatile supplements. Halothane and enflurane are myocardial depressants. Isoflurane is a systemic and coronary vasodilator, and so may cause coronary steal. Most feel that this is unlikely to be significant at the low concentrations used and without severe hypotension, and there is even evidence that isoflurane may protect the myocardium against ischaemia.[103]

A different approach, used more in the USA, is to employ IPPV and relaxation, but with large doses of opiates given slowly as the sole anaesthetic agent, e.g. morphine (1–5 mg/kg), fentanyl (up to 50 or even 100 µg/kg) or equivalent doses of alfentanil or sufentanil. Such doses usually give good cardiovascular stability and suppress the endocrine response to stress. Disadvantages include the need for longer postoperative respiratory support, possible awareness and chest wall rigidity.

Monitoring (*See also* Chapter 18.)

1. Myocardial ischaemia. The ECG warns of ischaemia (CM5 lead best) and dysrhythmias. An endocardial pacemaker wire may be inserted pre-operatively, and an epicardial wire used intra- and postoperatively. Transoesophageal echocardiography will detect abnormalities of wall motion usually due to ischaemia.

2. Pulse oximetry.

3. Arterial pressure. Usually by cannulation of the non-dominant radial artery. Flow is non-pulsatile during bypass. Rapid changes may occur.

4. Central venous pressure. Indicates right ventricular filling pressure. During bypass, a rise in CVP suggests obstruction or malposition of the venous lines. At the end of operation high pressure may be caused by over-transfusion or myocardial insufficiency; low pressure by inadequate transfusion. Two or more catheters, or a multi-lumen catheter, may be inserted into the internal jugular vein. One is then used for pressure measurement and another for drug administration.

5. Left atrial pressure. Can be measured directly via a catheter inserted by the surgeon, but risks embolization. Otherwise a Swan-Ganz[104] pulmonary arterial catheter may be used to measure wedge pressure.

6. Cardiac output. Special Swan–Ganz catheters may be used for thermal dilution measurements, and for mixed venous oxygen saturation.

7. Capnography. Hyperventilation may be harmful if the cerebral perfusion is compromised.

8. Cerebral perfusion. An EEG may indicate the adequacy of cerebral perfusion. Pupil sizes will warn of gross differences between the hemispheres.

9. Temperature. In the nasopharynx for core (or brain) temperature. Toe or bladder temperature may be used for peripheral temperature and gives an index of peripheral vasodilatation.

10. Urine flow. A simple index of adequate renal perfusion and thus cardiac output. Urine output should be recorded every half-hour, and should normally exceed 0.5 ml/kg/hour. Initially during bypass, output is very small, but becomes high as rewarming occurs and the priming solution is excreted.

11. Biochemistry. Especially serum potassium and glucose. The latter is of particular interest because there is evidence that cerebral ischaemia causes more damage if there is hyperglycaemia. Some avoid giving dextrose solutions.[105]

12. Arterial blood gases. See below.

Cardiopulmonary bypass[106]

The extracorporeal circulation incorporates a pump(s), a heat exchanger and an efficient oxygenator for gaseous exchange. Damage to blood must be minimal at the flows chosen, and the apparatus must be capable of sterilization or be disposable.

Blood flow. Perfusion flows used in adults vary from 1.0 to 2.4 l/min/m^2 body surface area. Venous blood is taken from the right atrium or both venae cavae separately, and returned via an arterial cannula inserted into the aorta or femoral artery. Lower flows help keep the heart cold if cardioplegic arrest is used, and may cause less damage to the blood. Flow is almost non-pulsatile and generates a mean arterial pressure of about 30–50 mmHg. This pressure can be adjusted with small doses of vasoconstrictor or vasodilator drugs. It must be remembered that while rewarming and suturing of the proximal anastomoses during coronary artery grafting, the myocardium is still dependent on the diseased coronaries for its supply.

Acid-base balance. Most operations are performed under moderate hypothermia at 25–28°C. CO_2 is more soluble at low temperatures and so the Pco_2 drops and the pH rises, if the values measured in the blood-gas machine at 37°C are corrected to body temperature. CO_2 may be added to the oxygenator gas mixture to avoid this apparent respiratory alkalosis. This is the '*pH-stat*' approach.[107] Hibernating mammals adopt this strategy.

More recently, it has been pointed out that poikilotherms maintain their ventilation and allow their Pco_2 to fall (and pH to rise) as their body temperature falls. This maintains electrochemical neutrality or the ratio of H^+ to OH^- constant. This means that the fraction of the histidine imidazoles in proteins which are unprotonated is constant. This is the '*alpha-stat*' approach, as this fraction is called alpha. It keeps the major buffer systems, and perhaps enzyme function, at their most effective.[108] In practice it means that Pco_2 and pH should not be corrected for temperature when considering acid-base status, and that the apparent respiratory alkalosis should be accepted despite the possibility of cerebral vasoconstriction. Some evidence suggests that alpha-stat is the better policy, but the case is far from proven.[109]

Anticoagulation.[110] A control activated clotting time (ACT)[111] is measured before giving heparin, 2–3 mg/kg or 90 mg/m^2 body surface area, before arterial cannulation. A long control value may indicate rare antithrombin III deficiency, which requires greatly increased heparin dosage. The ACT should exceed 300 s before starting bypass. ACT is measured by adding 2 ml of blood to 12 mg of celite, which reduces the clotting time to 90–130 s. Additional heparin during bypass is given according to the ACT, but is not always needed.

Heparin is reversed with protamine 3–4 mg/kg after bypass, given over several minutes. If given too fast, hypotension may occur as a result of systemic vasodilatation, or sometimes intense pulmonary arterial constriction perhaps after the release of thromboxane A_2 in the lung.[112] Patients who are allergic to fish, have been on isophane insulin, or who have had a vasectomy may be allergic to protamine.

For cardiopulmonary bypass in patients with cold agglutinins, *see* Park J. V. and Weiss C. I. *Anesth. Analg.* 1988, **67**, 75.

Haemodilution. The pump is primed with crystalloid, colloid (which may include blood) or a mixture of both so that the calculated haematocrit will drop to about 20–25% on bypass. Heparin and usually mannitol are added. This haemodilution economizes on bank blood, may cause less lung damage and improve tissue capillary perfusion. Before bypass 500–1000 ml of blood may be taken from the patient into anticoagulated bags and the patient given colloid to replace it. This blood is then reinfused after bypass to restore the haematocrit to over 30%.

Oxygenators. Bubble oxygenators are satisfactory for most cases, although they do damage all three types of blood cell. The polypropylene or silcone used in membrane oxygenators is less damaging to blood, but more expensive and takes rather longer to set up.

Blood loss. Although there is no venous return to the heart during bypass, blood reaches the heart from: (*a*) the coronary circulation; (*b*) bronchial arteries via pulmonary veins (may be considerable in conditions such as Fallot's tetralogy); and (*c*) incompetent aortic valve. This heparinized blood is returned via suckers to the bypass reservoir.

Suction causes blood cell damage, and may be reduced by: (*a*) arrest of coronary circulation by a clamp across the aortic root. The heart is arrested and the myocardium protected against ischaemic damage by an ice-cold potassium-containing cardioplegic solution injected into the coronary circulation. For short periods ventricular fibrillation may be induced; and (*b*) hypothermia to 15–20°C, *see below*.

Blood replacement. Via a cannula in an arm vein used solely for this purpose. It may also be added to the pump during bypass, when the proportion of blood in the patient and in the pump varies somewhat with vascular tone. After bypass, blood is given according to the clinical state, the CVP, the appearance of the atria and the apparent blood loss. It may be given from the pump reservoir as long as the arterial cannula is still in place.

Hypothermia. Ventricular fibrillation occurs when body temperature falls below about 28°C, and asystole at even lower temperatures. Under deep hypothermia (15°C) cell metabolism is so low that total circulatory and ventilatory arrest is safe. The period for which this is true was taken to be 1 hour, but may be shorter.[113] The operating field is still and dry, and this is used for repair of the aortic arch and of some congenital defects. On rewarming, the heart can be defibrillated above 30–32°C.

Postoperative care

Patients are nursed in an intensive care area with full monitoring continued as needed. Artificial ventilation is often maintained until cardiovascular stability and rewarming is complete, although patients who have had uneventful coronary artery surgery are extubated immediately in some centres. Postoperative pain from a median sternotomy is not severe and is treated by conventional analgesics.

Cardiovascular support. Inotropic drugs and/or vasodilators are often needed after discontinuing bypass and are usually continued for a while. *See* Chapter 29 for details. Phosphodiesterase inhibitors have been useful in patients awaiting heart transplantation.[114] If drug therapy fails to maintain cardiac output, the intra-aortic balloon pump[115] should be considered. This is inserted percutaneously into the femoral artery and advanced to the descending aorta. The balloon is inflated in diastole (to help coronary perfusion) and deflated in systole (to reduce afterload). It can increase the output of a failing heart by 10–20%, is relatively simple and provides useful but limited assistance.

If the patient's condition is not improved (such a situation is also seen after massive infarction or particularly in those awaiting transplantation), various other mechanical devices have been used to assist the failing ventricles.[116] They include[117] the haemopump, a spinning turbine placed in the left ventricle after surgery; extracorporeal centrifugal pumps; either implanted or external ventricular assist devices and a totally artificial heart.

Complications of cardiopulmonary bypass

1. Excessive Bleeding. Occurs especially with repeat surgery. The problems arise after bypass and may be due to: (1) pre-operative bleeding diathesis, especially treatment with anticoagulant, antiplatelet or thrombolytic drugs; (2) inadequate neutralization of heparin; (3) fibrinolysis and fibrinogen depletion (less than 1 g/l); (4) platelet sequestration and dysfunction; (5) failure of surgical haemostasis.

Bleeding usually responds to careful surgical technique, more protamine if indicated by the ACT and fresh frozen plasma. Platelets are not usually needed. Antifibrinolytic therapy (tranexamic acid 1 g) reduces loss.[118] Reduction in Von Willebrand factor may occur (and so a failure of platelet adhesion) and is treated with cryoprecipitate or desmopressin 0.3 µg/kg over 15 min.[119] The plasmin and kallikrein inhibitor, aprotonin, has been used with success,[120] although it probably acts on platelets.

2. Gas embolism. From an empty venous reservoir, faulty oxygenator, leaks and faults in the bypass circuit, or ejected from the heart before air has been completely removed. Retrograde cerebral perfusion can minimize brain damage after massive gas embolism. Bubble detectors and filters in the arterial line are used. Even with meticulous technique small bubbles can be introduced, so nitrous oxide should be avoided for up to 20 min after bypass to prevent their expansion.

3. Brain damage.[121] May be global or focal, and caused by ischaemia, embolism of gas bubbles, blood clot, calcific fragments from a stenosed aortic valve or fat droplets. More subtle neuropsychiatric sequelae and personality changes also occur. Dysfunction may be worsened by hypocapnia before bypass,[122] low perfusion pressure and hyperglycaemia.[123] Cerebral autoregulation may be better preserved with the alpha-stat approach to acid-base balance.[124] The contribution that drugs can make to the lessening of brain damage is slight. However, doses of thiopentone large enough to make the EEG flat (about 40 mg/kg) have been shown to reduce cerebral complications after surgery involving an open left ventricle, although this study was at normothermia.[125] Also the calcium channel blocker nimodipine 0.5 µg/kg/min during surgery has resulted in a minor improvement in some neuropsychological tests after CPB.[126]

4. Awareness. The need to avoid both myocardial depressant drugs just before discontinuing bypass, and nitrous oxide because of possible bubble emboli, can leave the patient with very little anaesthetic. The risk of awareness is inherent in the technique of bypass. Sweating at this stage can be striking, but probably because warm blood is perfusing the hypothalamus.

5. *Lung changes*. Due to: (1) poor LV function, high pulmonary venous pressure and pulmonary oedema; (2) post-perfusion lung syndrome. Activation of the complement and kallikrein cascades causes neutrophils to aggregate in the pulmonary circulation. These affect vascular tone and capillary permeability. Gas and particulate emboli also contribute to the development of an inflammatory response, which can progress to full-blown adult respiratory distress syndrome: perivascular oedema and haemorrhage, congestion and thickening of inter-alveolar walls, patchy collapse, intra-alveolar haemorrhage, disturbance of ventilation-perfusion relationships; (3) fentanyl is sequestered in the lungs during bypass and released again afterwards; and (4) phrenic nerve damage due to cold solutions applied to the heart.[127]

6. *Cardiac tamponade*. Clots may block drainage of the pericardium and tamponade results.

7. *Hypertension* after coronary artery surgery is controlled by vasodilators, e.g. sodium nitroprusside, but this may increase pulmonary shunting.[128]

8. *Postoperative hypothermia*. Rewarming on bypass may leave some vascular beds still cold. As these are gradually re-opened postoperatively, body temperature falls. Vasodilatation during bypass and monitoring of peripheral temperature helps avoid this problem.

9. *Kidney and liver dysfunction*. Although haemolysis and haemoglobinuria occurs during bypass, it usually clears spontaneously. Development of renal failure is more related to the cardiovascular state before and after the operation. The same is true of jaundice and liver dysfunction.

Surgery for dysrhythmias

Accessory conducting pathways that are causing intractable dysrhythmias may be ablated by an electric shock delivered down a special cardiac catheter. Alternatively subendocardial resection is carried out at cardiopulmonary bypass.[129] Either method requires extensive electrophysiological mapping of the conducting tissues. Apart from the dysrhythmias themselves, these patients do not present any unusual anaesthetic problems.

Anaesthesia for cardiac transplants

The main indications for the operation are coronary artery disease and cardiomyopathy. Anaesthetic problems do not differ from those of any open heart operation in a seriously ill patient. Active infection or malignant disease are contra-indications. The specific immunosuppressive action of cyclosporin has greatly improved results.

Heart-lung transplants are technically easier than heart-only transplants and are performed for primary pulmonary hypertension, primary lung disease and cardiomyopathies. The tracheal anastomosis heals better than a bronchial anastomosis. If the recipient's heart is normal it may be used for transplantation into a third patient. Obliterative bronchiolitis has been a late complication. Long-term results are improving.[130]

Cardiac catheterization

Usually performed under local analgesia and sedation, except in small children.

Insertion of indwelling pacemakers

The sternal pacemaker was used in 1954,[131] the first transvenous endocardial pacing in 1958,[132] and the first totally implanted system a few years later.[133] Patients should seldom present for anaesthesia without adequate pacing. The apparatus itself is now usually implanted in the chest wall under local analgesia. For patients with pacemakers who require other surgery, *see* Chapter 20.

Cardioversion[134]

First described in 1962.[135] Anaesthesia is necessary because the shock is painful, more so at higher strengths. Although barbiturates may be used, some have noted fewer dysrhythmias using benzodiazepines, e.g. diazepam 2.5 mg increments up to 0.3 mg/kg, or midazolam increments up to 0.2 mg/kg.

References

1. Fell G. *Buffalo Med. J.* 1887, Nov.; O'Dwyer J. P. *NY Med. J.* 1885, **42**, 145.
2. Matas R. *Ann. Surg.* 1899, **29**, 951.
3. Tuffier T. and Hallion J. *C. R. Biol. (Paris)* 1896, **48**, 951.
4. Sauerbruch F. *Zbl. Chir.* 1904, **31**, 146; *Mitt. Grenzgeb. Med. Chir.* 1904, **13**, 399.
5. Brauer L. *Mitt. Grenzgeb. Med. Chir.* 1904, **13**, 483.
6. Tiegel M. *Zentbl. Chir.* 1908, **22**, 369; *Beitr. Klin. Chir.* 1909, **64**, 358.
7. Brat H. and Schmieden V. *Münch. Med. Wochenschr.* 1908, **55**, 2421.
8. Janeway H. H. and Green N. W. *JAMA* 1909, **53**, 1975; *Ann. Surg.* 1910, **52**, 58.
9. Elsberg C. A. *Ann. Surg.* 1910, **52**, 23.
10. Meltzer S. J. and Auer L. *J. Exp. Med.* 1909, **11**, 622.
11. Killian G. *Münch. Med. Wochenschr.* 1898, **45**, 844.
12. Kuhn F. *Dt. Z. Chir.* 1905, **76**, 148.
13. Bjork V. C. and Carlens E. *J. Thorac. Surg.* 1950, **20**, 151.
14. Gale G. W. and Waters R. M. *J. Thorac. Surg.* 1932, **1**, 432.
15. Archibald E. *J. Thorac. Surg.* 1935, **4**, 335.
16. Frenckner P. *Acta Otolaryngol.* 1934, Suppl. 20, 100.
17. Crafoord C. *Acta Chir. Scand.* 1938, Suppl. 54.
18. Guedel A. E. *Anesthesiology* 1940, **1**, 13.
19. Nosworthy M. D. *Proc. R. Soc. Med.* 1941, **34**, 479.
20. Guedel A. E. and Treweek D. N. *Curr. Res. Anesth. Analg.* 1934, **13**, 263.
21. Pinson K. B. and Bryce A. G. *Br. J. Anaesth.* 1944, **19**, 53.
22. Morch T. *Proc. R. Soc. Med.* 1947, **40**, 603.
23. Musgrove A. H. *Anaesthesia* 1952, **7**, 77.
24. Overholt R. H. et al. *J. Thorac. Surg.* 1946, **15**, 384.
25. Parry Brown A. I. *Thorax* 1948, **3**, 161; *Proc. R. Soc. Med.* 1973, **66**, 339.

26. Dunne N. M. and Gillbe C. E. In: *Thoracic Anaesthesia* Gothard J. W. W. (ed.) *Clin. Anaesthesiol.* 1987, **1**(1), 79.

27. Robertshaw F. L. *Br. J. Anaesth.* 1962, **34**, 576; Black A. M. S. and Harrison G. A. *Anaesth. Intensive Care* 1975, **3**, 299.

28. Linter S. P. K. *Anaesthesia* 1985, **40**, 191.

29. Conacher I. D. *Anaesthesia* 1991, **46**, 400.

30. Carlens E. *J. Thorac. Surg.* 1949, **18**, 742; Bjork V. O. and Carlens E. *J. Thorac. Surg.* 1950, **20**, 151; Bjork V. O. et al. *Anesthesiology* 1953, **14**, 60.

31. Macintosh R. R. and Leatherdale R. A. L. *Br. J. Anaesth.* 1955, **27**, 556.

32. Green R. and Gordon W. *Anaesthesia* 1957, **12**, 86.

33. Magill I. W. *Proc. R. Soc. Med.* 1936, **29**, 643.

34. Machray R. *Tuberc. Index* 1958, **13**, 172.

35. Pallister W. K. *Thorax* 1959, **14**, 55.

36. Mansfield R. E. *Anaesthesia* 1957, **12**, 477.

37. Aps C. and Towey R. M. *Anaesthesia* 1981, **36**, 415; Watson C. B. In: *Thoracic Anaesthesia* Gothard J. W. W. (ed.) *Clin. Anaesthesiol.* 1987, **1**(1), 33.

38. Hultgren B. L. et al. *Anesthesiology* 1986, **65**, A.481.

39. Cullum A. R. et al. *Anaesthesia* 1973, **28**, 66.

40. Rusby N. L. and Thompson V. C. *Postgrad. Med. J.* 1943, **19**, 44.

41. Magill I. W. *Newcastle Med. J.* 1934, **14**, 67.

42. Cay D. L. et al. *Anaesth. Intensive Care* 1975, **3**, 127.

43. Benumof J. L. *Anesthesiology* 1987, **67**, 729.

44. Kerr J. H. In: *Thoracic Anaesthesia* Gothard J. W. W. (ed.) *Clin. Anaesthesiol.* 1987, **1**(1), 61.

45. Klingstedt C. et al. *Acta Anaesthesiol. Scand.* 1990, **34**, 421.

46. Benumof J. L. *Anesthesia for Thoracic Surgery* Philadelphia: W. B. Saunders, 1987.

47. Ritchie A. J. et al. *Ann. Thorac. Surg.* 1990, **50**, 86.

48. Lunkenheimer P. P., Whimster W. F. and Sykes M. K. (ed.) *Acta Anaesthesiol. Scand.* 1989, **33**, (Suppl.90).

49. Jenkins J. et al. *Anaesthesia* 1987, **42**, 938; Howland W. S. et al. *Anesthesiology* 1987, **67**, 1009.

50. Conacher I. D. *Br. J. Anaesth.* 1990, **65**, 806.

51. Patrick J. A. et al. *Anaesthesia* 1991, **46**, 85.

52. Wain J. C. et al. *Ann. Thorac. Surg.* 1990, **49**, 881.

53. Heimlich H. J. *Hosp. Topics* 1965, **43**, 122; Harriss D. R. and Graham T. R. *Br. J. Hosp. Med.* 1991, **45**, 383.

54. Sherry K. M. et al. *Anaesthesia* 1987, **42**, 61.

55. Larsson S. and Nordberg G. *Anesth. Analg.* 1987, **66**, 471.

56. Blomquist S. et al. *Acta Anaesthesiol. Scand.* 1990, **34**, 506.

57. McCarthy G. et al. *Anaesthesia* 1987, **42**, 411.

58. Donnelly J. A. and Webster R. E. *Anaesthesia* 1991, **46**, 383.

59. Blalock A. et al. *JAMA* 1945, **128**, 189.

60. Keynes G. *Lancet* 1954, **1**, 1197; *Ann. R. Coll. Surg.* 1953, **12**, 88.

61. Conacher I. D. *Br. J. Anaesth.* 1988, **61**, 468; Smyth R. L. et al. *Respir. Med.* 1989, **83**, 459; Dark J. and Corris P. *Thorax* 1989, **44**, 689.

62. Cooper J. D. et al. *Am. Rev. Respir. Dis.* 1989, **139**, 303.

63. Conacher I. D. et al. *Anaesthesia* 1990, **45**, 971.

64. Bozzini P. *Der Lichleiter*. Weimar, 1807.

65. Killian G. *Münch. Med. Wochenschr.* 1898, **45**, 844.

66. Draper W. B. and Whitehead R. W. *Anesthesiology* 1944, **5**, 262, 524.

67. Draper W. B. et al. *Anesthesiology* 1947, **8**, 524.

68. Holmdahl M.-H. *Acta Chir. Scand.* 1956, Suppl. 212, 1.

69. Ikeda S. et al. *Keio Med. J.* 1968, **17**, 1.

70. Hill A. J. et al. *Anaesthesia* 1991, **46**, 266.

71. Sanders R. D. *Delaware St. Med. J.* 1967, **39**, 170; Spoerel W. E. *Can. Anaesth. Soc. J.* 1969, **16**, 61.

72. Moussalli H. *Br. J. Hosp. Med.* 1981, **25**, 300.
73. Kussmaul A. *Dtsch. Arch. Klin. Med.* 1869, **6**, 456; von Mikulicz-Radecki J. *Wien. Med. Presse* 1881, **22**, 1405.
74. Kaplan J. A. (ed.) *Cardiac Anesthesia* Philadelphia: W. B. Saunders, 1987; Hensley F. A. and Martin D. E. *The Practice of Cardiac Anesthesia* Boston: Little Brown, 1990.
75. McKeown K. K. *Can. Anaesth. Soc. J.* 1982, **29**, 325.
76. Hilsman F. A. *Schrift. Univ. Kiel* 1875, **2**, 20.
77. Rehn L. *Zentbl. Chir.* 1896, **23**, 1048.
78. Tuffier T. *Bull. Acad. Méd. Paris* 3rd series, 1914, **71**, 293.
79. Delorme E. *Gaz. d'Hopit.* 1898, p.1150; Hallopeau P. *Bull. Mém. Soc. Chir. Paris.* 1921, **47**, 1120.
80. Cutler E. and Levine S. A. *Boston Med. Surg. J.* 1923, **188**, 1023.
81. Souttar H. S. *Br. Med. J.* 1925, **2**, 903; Ellis R. H. *Anaesthesia* 1975, **30**, 374.
82. Bleichröder F. *Berlin. Klin. Wochenschr.* 1912, **49**, 1503.
83. Forssmann W. *Klin. Wochenschr.* 1929, **8**, 2085.
84. Cournand A. and Ranges H. A. *Proc. Soc. Exp. Med. Biol.* 1941, **46**, 462.
85. Robb G. and Steinberg I. J. *J. Clin. Invest.* 1938, **17**, 507.
86. Gross R. E. and Hubbard J. P. *JAMA* 1939, **112**, 729.
87. Blalock A. and Taussig H. B. *JAMA* 1945, **128**, 189.
88. Crafoord C. and Nylin K. G. *J. Thorac. Surg.* 1945, **14**, 347.
89. Brock R. C. *Br. Med. J.* 1948, **1**, 1121.
90. Harken D. E. et al. *N. Engl. Med. J.* 1948, **238**, 804.
91. Miller B. J. et al. *Med. Clin. North Am.* 1953, **37**, 1609; Gibbon J. H. *Minn. Med.* 1954, **37**, 171; Kirklin J. W. et al. *Ann. Surg.* 1956, **144**, 2.
92. Sones F. M. and Shirley E. K. *Mod. Concepts Cardiovasc. Dis.* 1962, **31**, 735.
93. De Bakey M. E. et al. *J. Thorac. Cardiovasc. Dis.* 1958, **36**, 369.
94. Drew C. E. et al. *Lancet* 1959, **1**, 745.
95. Starr A. et al. *Circulation* 1963, **27**, 779.
96. Garrett H. E. et al. *Cardiovasc. Cent. Bull.* 1964, **3**, 15.
97. Carrel A. *Johns Hopkins Hosp. Bull.* 1907, **18**, 18.
98. Barnard C. N. *S. Afr. Med. J.* 1967, **41**, 1271.
99. Shumway N. and Lower R. R. *Ann. N. Y. Acad. Sci.* 1964, **120**, 773 (*see also* Cooley D. *Surg. Clin. North Am.* 1978, **58**, 895).
100. Bailey C. P. *Dis. Chest* 1949, **15**, 377.
101. Buckels N. J. et al. *Thorax* 1988, **43**, 1003.
102. Streisand J. B. and Wong K. C. *Br. J. Anaesth.* 1988, **61**, 97.
103. Priebe H.-J. *Anesthesiology* 1989, **71**, 960.
104. Swan H. J. C. et al. *N. Engl. J. Med.* 1970, **283**, 447.
105. Lanier W. L. *Anesth. Analg.* 1991, **72**, 423.
106. Tinker J. H. (ed.) *Cardiopulmonary Bypass: Current Concepts and Controversies.* Philadelphia: W. B. Saunders, 1989.
107. Tinker J. H. and Campos J. H. *J. Cardiothorac. Anesth.* 1988, **2**, 701.
108. Murkin J. M. *J. Cardiothorac. Anesth.* 1988, **2**, 705.
109. Bashein G. et al. *Anesthesiology* 1989, **71**, 7.
110. Stow P. J. and Burrows F. A. *Can. J. Anaesth.* 1987, **34**, 632.
111. Gravlee G. P. et al. *Anesth. Analg.* 1988, **67**, 469.
112. Lowenstein E. and Zapol W. M. *Anesthesiology* 1990, **73**, 373.
113. Treasure T. *Ann. R. Coll. Surg. Engl.* 1984, **66**, 235.
114. Watson D. M. et al. *Anaesthesia* 1991, **46**, 285.
115. For development, *see* Kantrowitz A. *Surgery* 1953, **34**, 678; Dunkman W. B. et al. *Circulation* 1972, **46**, 465; Curtis J. J. et al. *Mayo Clin. Proc.* 1977, **52**, 723.
116. Hill J. D. *Ann. Thorac. Surg.* 1989, **47**, 167.
117. Glenville B. *Hosp. Update* 1991, **17**, 89.
118. Horrow J. C. et al. *J. Thorac. Cardiovasc. Surg.* 1990, **99**, 70.
119. Editorial. *Lancet* 1988, **i**, 155.

120. Royston D. et al. *Lancet* 1987, **ii**, 1289; Van Oevren W. et al. *J. Thorac. Cardiovasc. Surg.* 1990, **99**, 788.
121. Hilberman M. (ed.) *Brain Injury and Protection during Heart Surgery* Boston: Martinus Nijhoff, 1988; Shaw P. J. et al. *Q. J. Med.* 1989, **267**, 633.
122. Nevin M. et al. *Lancet* 1987, **ii**, 1493.
123. Fitch W. In: *Anaesthesia Review 5.* (Kaufman L. ed.) Edinburgh: Churchill Livingstone, 1988, 119; Nakakimura K. et al. *Anesthesiology* 1990, **72**, 1005.
124. Murkin J. M. et al. *Anesth. Analg.* 1987, **66**, 825.
125. Nussmeier N. A. et al. *Anesthesiology* 1986, **64**, 165.
126. Forsman M. et al. *Br. J. Anaesth.* 1990, **65**, 514.
127. Editorial. *Lancet* 1990, **335**, 1373.
128. Möllhoff T. et al. *Br. J. Anaesth.* 1990, **64**, 493.
129. Irish C. L. et al. *Can. J. Anaesth.* 1988, **35**, 634.
130. Glanville A. R. et al. *J. Roy. Soc. Med.* 1990, **83**, 208.
131. Zoll P. M. *N. Engl. J. Med.* 1954, **247**, 768; Weinrich W. L. et al. *Surg. Forum* 1957, **8**, 360.
132. Forman S. and Schwedel J. B. *N. Engl. J. Med.* 1959, **261**, 943.
133. Chardick W. M. et al. *J. Thorac. Cardiovasc. Surg.* 1961, **42**, 816.
134. De Silva R. A. et al. *Am. Heart J.* 1980, **100**, 881.
135. Lown R. et al. *JAMA* 1962, **182**, 548.

Day-stay (day-case) surgery

History

Extensively practised in Belfast and in Glasgow during the first decade of this century.[1] Also in the US.[2]

Indications

For patients whose operation normally lasts up to 30 min, is not likely to be associated with severe postoperative pain, the use of drains or catheters, or complicated by postoperative haemorrhage. Patients should be generally fit and the social and domestic arrangements suitable. Particular indications include surgery in children.[3] Another advantage is the reduced incidence of hospital-acquired infections.[4]

Patients must be accompanied home and not travel by public transport. They should be supported for 24 hours. The mental attitude towards illness and pain must be healthy.

Postponement should occur if medical disease is found on the day of admission.[5] Provision should be made for admission overnight if postoperative sequelae or unexpected complications occur.

Selection of patients

Often done by surgeons, who may need guidelines from the anaesthetist. ASA grades 1 or 2 and age under 70 years are acceptable. In practice this means no interference with lifestyle by medical conditions. Obesity is a problem. Under 0.5 kg/cm or 35 lb/ft of height is quite acceptable. Particular care is necessary before accepting patients for day-case general anaesthesia with the following conditions: ischaemic heart disease, insulin-dependent diabetes, those on steroid medication, those living more than 1 hour's journey from the hospital, those living alone, and those with acute respiratory infection or chronic respiratory failure.

A pre-operative history and general examination in the surgical clinic, anaesthetic clinic or at domiciliary visit is performed. Co-operation with the family doctor is important. Pre-operative standardized check-lists,[6] which the patient or his relatives fill in, are useful.

Questions appearing on a typical check-list

It would be very helpful if you would answer the questions below in your own time. You may be asked for more details when you see the doctor. What do you weigh? Can you do normal activities? Is your general health good? Have you ever had an operation? If so, what? Have you ever had an anaesthetic? If so, did you have any problem with it? Have your relatives had any problems with anaesthetics? Have you had any Medical illnesses? If so, which ones? Are you taking any sort of medicine, pill or tablet? If so, which ones? Are you allergic or sensitive to any medicine? Or anything else? Do you smoke? How much? How many stairs can you climb quickly before you get short of breath? Do you have a cough or wheeze? Do you get pain in the chest or palpitations? Have you had heart surgery or a 'stroke'? Do you know if you are anaemic? Do you have someone to take you home and stay with you for the night after the operation?

The day of operation

Pre-operative and postoperative instructions (e.g. fasting or inability to drive) should be in writing and easy to understand. Regional analgesia may be considered.

Oral temazepam[7], triazolam, or antacids[8] suitable for premedication if required.

Technique

Ideally the day-stay theatre should be adjacent to the day-stay ward and the postoperative observation room. Operations should be performed early in the day. Premedication should be minimal or avoided completely. Infants should be put first on the list to prevent hypoglycaemia from starvation. The anaesthetic is only started when the surgeon and operating team are ready and the anaesthetic should be the lightest compatible with safety. Only agents that are rapidly eliminated are used, e.g. propofol for induction of anaesthesia,[9] alfentanil, nitrous oxide, isoflurane, enflurane, or desflurane.[10] Suxamethonium may cause muscle pains the following day unless precautions are taken. Tracheal intubation is not contra-indicated. Diazepam and fentanyl have a rebound effect 4–8 hours after administration which although not greater than the initial effect, may be dangerous. [11] Midazolam may be the benzodiazepine of choice when full general anaesthesia is not required. Local analgesia on its own or combined with light general anaesthesia has the advantage of excellent postoperative pain relief. In suitable patients both intra- and extradural block may be employed. [12] Cryo-analgesia has also been described. [13]

Recovery from anaesthesia[14]

Assessment of recovery and fitness to go home is usually undertaken by an experienced nurse. It is more important for the patient to be escorted home and public transport avoided than for any particular test to be carried out. Someone should stay with the patient until the next day.

Factors to be taken into account in assessing recovery include: (1) awakening; ability to answer questions and obey commands;[15] (2) stable arterial pressure and pulse; (3) can swallow and cough; (4) fitness to go to the bathroom without feeling faint; Romberg's test and stabilometry;[16] (5) has eaten and drunk without nausea and passed urine; (6) fitness to return home; have their unwritten postoperative instructions and medications, if any. Reaction time tests may be performed; (7) fitness to go out alone, usually allowed the day after anaesthesia. Research tools to assess this include the EEG, the track tracer, psychomotor tests, choice reaction tests;[17] (8) fitness to go to work; usually the following day (depending on the surgery).

Assessment of fitness to drive

Views differ. The drugs used, their amounts and timing are important in assessment. An interval of 48 hours has been suggested[18] whereas others think a shorter time is safe.[19] Perhaps a median time is 24 hours. Following the injection of local analgesics, one hour after the return of normal function.[20]

See also T Commission on the provision of surgical services; guidelines for day-stay surgery. *R. Coll. Surg. Engl.* 1985; Bradshaw E. G. and Davenport H. T. (eds) *Day Case Surgery, Anaesthesia and Management.* London: Arnold, 1989; White P. F. (ed). *Outpatient Anesthesia* Edinburgh: Churchill Livingstone, 1990; *Drug Ther. Bull.*, 1991, **29**, 23.

References

1. Calwell H. G. *Br. Med. J.* 1980, **1**, 115; Nicholl J. H. *Br. Med. J.* 1909, **2**, 753.
2. Waters R. M. *Am. J. Surg. (Anesth. Suppl.)*, 1919, **33**, 71.
3. Kay B. *Acta Anaesth. Scand.* 1966, suppl 25, 421; Davenport H. T. et al. *Can. Anaesth. Soc. J.* 1971, **105**, 498; Atwell J. D. et al. *Lancet* 1973, **2**, 895; Armitage E. N. *Lancet*, 1975, **2**, 21.
4. Natof H. E. In *Anesthesia for ambulatory surgery* (Wechler B. V. ed.), Lippincott Philadelphia, 1986.
5. Gabbay J., Francis L. *Brit. Med. J.* 1988, **297**, 1249.
6. Ogg T. W. *Br. Med. J.* 1976, **1**, 82; Knight R. F. In: *Clinics in Anaesthsiology preparation for Anaesthesia* 1986, **4**, 509. (Stevens A. J. ed.), Kent, Pitman 1980; Rollasoon W. N. and Hems G. *Ann. R. Coll. Surg. Engl.* 1981, **63**, 45.
7. Beechey A. P. C. et al. *Anaesthesia* 1981, **36**, 10.
8. *See* Brown B. R. ed. *Outpatient Anaesthesia* Davis, Philadelphia, 1978.

9. *Drug Ther. Bull.* 1990, **28**, 19–20
10. Padfield A. and Mullins S. R. C. *Anaesthesia* 1980, **35**, 508.
11. Adams A. P. and Pybus D. A. *Br. Med. J.* 1978, **1**, 278.
12. Atkinson R. S. and Lee J. A. *Anaesthesia* 1985, **40**, 1059.
13. Wood G. J. et al. *Lancet* 1979, **2**, 479; Wood G. J. et al. *Anaesthesia* 1981, **36**, 603.
14. *See also*, Korttila K. *Anaesthesia* 1976, **31**, 724; Fahy A. and Marshall M. *Br. J. Anaesth.* 1969, **41**, 433; Ogg T. W. *Br. Med. J.* 1972, **4**, 573; Ogg T. W. *Proc. R. Soc. Med.* 1975, **68**, 414; Brindle G. F. and Soliman M. G. *Can. Anaesth. Soc. J.* 1975, **22**, 613; Smith B. L. and Young P. W. *Anaesthesia* 1976, **31**, 181.
15. Steward D. G. *Can. Anaesth. Soc. J.* 1975, **22**, 111.
16. Steward D. G. *Can. Anaesth. Soc. J.* 1978, **25**, 4.
17. Doenicke A. et al. *Can. Anaesth. Soc. J.* 1967, **14**, 567.
18. Havard J. *Br. Med. J.* 1978, **1**, 1595; Routh G. S. *Br. Med. J.* 1979, **1**, 673.
19. Baskett P. J. F. and Vickers M. D. *Lancet* 1979, **1**, 490.
20. Seppala J. et al. *Drugs* 1979, **17**, 389; Ashton H. *Adverse Drug Reactions* 1983. Feb. 98.

Dental anaesthesia

History

For the early uses of nitrous oxide in dentistry, *see* Chapter 7. After the introduction of ether and chloroform, nitrous oxide fell into disfavour, until interest was revived in its use for dental extractions over 100 years ago by G. Q. Colton and T. W. Evans. The latter demonstrated his method in London on 31 March 1868.[1] Other pioneers of nitrous oxide anaesthesia include Edmund Andrews (1824–1904) who used it with oxygen, Sir F. Hewitt, who advocated sound teaching and practice in the use of anaesthetics in dental surgery and designed an apparatus,[2] and E. I. McKesson (1881–1935) whose demand-flow machine is still in use.[3] Nasal administration became commonly used in dentistry around the turn of the century[4] although Clover and Alfred Coleman had used it in 1868.[5] The addition of oxygen to nitrous oxide in dental anaesthesia was popularized by Frederick Hewitt. In the first 50 years of the century if pure nitrous oxide was administered, the patient would pass through the stages of analgesia and excitement until the stage of surgical anaesthesia was reached. Oxygen was then added to prevent hypoxia, but the amount was carefully regulated because the margin between too light anaesthesia and dangerous hypoxia is small. Some degree of hypoxia was accepted.

The dangers of fainting when the patient is held in the sitting position were pointed out by Bourne.[6] The Society for the Advancement of Anaesthesia in Dentistry has been active since 1958.[7] Diazepam first used in dental surgery in 1966.[8] The first local dental block was given by R. J. Hall,[9] Halsted's assistant in New York's Roosevelt Hospital in 1884; in the UK by W. A. Hunt of Yeovil.[10]

Apparatus for dental surgery anaesthesia

Anaesthetic machine with spare gas supply and volatile agents. Full intubation set. Full resuscitation set. Intravenous infusions with crystalloids colloids and range of cannulae. Atropine and suxamethonium. Emergency drugs. Monitors – ECG, arterial pressure, pulse oximetry, nerve stimulator.

Uptake and elimination of nitrous oxide[11]

During dental anaesthesia peak inspiratory flow-rates may be between 30 and 200 l/min, tidal volumes between 300 and 3000 ml, and respiratory minute volume between 1 and 50 l/min. The arterial blood concentration of nitrous oxide reaches an initial plateau within 10 min. In this time, depending upon factors such as inhaled concentration, alveolar ventilation and cardiac output, the arterial tension will be over 90% of the inhaled tension. On discontinuing, blood levels fall rapidly over 10 min.

Four 'zones' of nitrous oxide anaesthesia have been described:

1. Moderate analgesia (6–25% N_2O inhaled); 25% N_2O is more potent than 10 mg morphine.
2. Dissociation analgesia (26–45%); 30% gives rise to psychological symptoms and lack of ability to concentrate. This is more severe at 45%.
3. Analgesic anaesthesia (46–65%). Near complete amnesia. Patient may respond to commands.
4. Light anaesthesia (66–80%). Complete analgesia and amnesia. Not possible to communicate with patient.

Posture during dental chair anaesthesia

The supine position for dental anaesthesia is favoured because of the dangers of hypotension and inadequate cerebral perfusion (fainting). A faint is vasovagal syncope.[12] Some workers feel that the sitting position discourages regurgitation of stomach contents and helps to prevent soiling of the pharynx with blood and debris. The dependent position of the legs is always to be avoided because blood may pool in them.

Selection of patients for general anaesthesia in the dental surgery

Whenever possible, local techniques are to be preferred but general anaesthesia may be required: (*a*) in small children, especially when removal of teeth in different quadrants of the mouth is planned; (*b*) in adults when multiple extractions are to be performed on a single occasion; (*c*) in the presence of acute sepsis; (*d*) following failed local analgesia, for any reason; and (*e*) when the patient is too apprehensive to co-operate with local methods.

Some difficult types of ambulant dental surgery patient

1. Patients who are frightened and have a poor command of themselves. These are difficult to control and may need premedication. Intravenous induction is usually indicated.

2. Patients who resist all anaesthetics, e.g. alcoholics; vigorous young men. In addition to larger doses of induction agents, short-acting opioids and even muscle relaxants may be needed.

3. Children under 4 years. Premedication is helpful. A sympathetic but firm approach should be used. The authors favour nitrous oxide–oxygen and halothane, using a face mask for induction. Above the age of 12, most children can be treated as adults. At the age of about 7, intravenous induction is easier.

4. Obesity. Difficult veins; difficult airway.

5. Patients who have missed periods and may be pregnant. Elective general anaesthesia is undesirable during pregnancy.

6. Patients who are anaemic.

7. Patients with decompensated heart disease. These are best managed in hospital.

8. Patients with hypertension. The risk is sudden, severe hypotension. Volume loading with a plasma expander is a good prophylactic.

9. Diabetics. *See* Chapter 20.

10. Patients on steroid therapy. 100 mg hydrocortisone may be given intravenously just prior to anaesthesia.

11. Patients on mono-amine oxidase inhibitors (MAOIs). These drugs are contra-indications to the use of pethidine and related compounds. Additionally, pressor drugs should not be used in patients taking these antidepressants. Pressor drugs may be needed at any time during dental anaesthesia.

12. The physically or mentally handicapped require careful management. Even for conservation, it may be necessary to administer general anaesthesia with tracheal intubation. Premedication is important and combinations such as temazepam 20 mg and droperidol 2–5 mg (in adults) orally 2 h before induction have been recommended. Sedation by diazepam before local analgesia or general anaesthesia is also useful. Initial dose in children up to the age of 10 years is 1 mg/year, i.v. In older patients 15–20 mg.

A suggested pre-operative questionnaire:

A. Are you reasonably physically fit?

B. What drugs or medicines do you take?

C. Have you ever received a general anaesthetic before? If so, how did it affect you?

D. How old are you?

E. What do you weigh?

F. Are you pregnant?

G. Have you ever had a heart attack, 'stroke', or angina?

H. What diseases do you suffer from (if any)?

I. Have you any allergies? If so, to what are you allergic?

J. Do you faint easily?

Relative contra-indications to general anaesthesia in the dental surgery

1. Patients whose stomachs may not be empty.
2. Patients with acute infections or tumours in the region of the upper airways, which cause or may cause obstruction.
3. Sickle-cell disease.
4. Severe coronary disease.
5. Cerebral vascular disease.
6. Extreme obesity.
7. Severe chronic bronchitis and obstructive airways disease.
8. Spastic states.
9. Haemophilia.
10. Patients on medication with certain drugs, e.g. MAOIs, anticoagulants.

It is unwise to allow patients who have received intravenous anaesthetics to return home alone, to drive a car or to cook or go shopping on the day of the anaesthetic.

Anaesthesia administration in the dental surgery

The stomach and bladder should be empty, the nose should be blown and dentures removed. The anaesthetist must be sure that the patient is fit for the proposed operation and tight garments must be loosened. Premedication may or may not be given, but the patient should be treated sympathetically and the procedure explained. Any suggestion that pain and discomfort will ensue is to be avoided. Dental forceps and other instruments should be prepared unobtrusively and an atmosphere of calm confidence adopted.

The patient should lie in the horizontal position, with the head rest adjusted to allow surgical access. The hands may be placed in the trouser pockets or arms comfortably folded. A restraining seat belt may be valuable in the robust individual. Saliva must be swallowed before consciousness is lost to prevent it irritating the larynx and causing cough.

After insertion of a mouth prop and i.v. cannula, anaesthesia is induced by intravenous injection or, for 'gas induction', the patient is instructed to breathe through the nose while the inhalation mixture (usually nitrous oxide–oxygen and volatile agent) is administered by nasal mask; 30% oxygen is recommended in the mixture. Some anaesthetists prefer to induce anaesthesia with a face-mask, substituting a nasal inhaler when the patient has lost consciousness. Surgical anaesthesia is marked by loss of eyelash reflex, eyeball movements and then fixation, relaxation of the jaw. The hiss of the expiratory valve is good evidence of free nasal respiration. The patient may be intubated if necessary.[13]

The anaesthetist has several duties to perform simultaneously during the dental operation. These include: (1) maintenance of a clear airway. This may be difficult if the patient is not intubated, and during operations on the lower jaw when there is a tendency to flex the head and obstruct respiration; (2) provide counter-pressure, if required by the dental surgeon, and hold the head and jaw securely; (3) see that a dental pack is used to prevent inhalation of blood and debris and to discourage mouth breathing; (4) observe the vital signs, pulse and respiration, and take early action should untoward reactions (e.g. fainting) occur. Pulse monitors may not function well during the conditions of dental chair anaesthesia, but a finger can usually palpate the superficial temporal artery; (5) the anaesthetist must sometimes assist in the insertion of mouth gags, particularly when extractions on both sides of the mouth are necessary; and (6) observation of the dials and gauges of the anaesthetic apparatus at all times to make sure that connections are maintained and that cylinders do not run empty unnoticed. *Unobstructed breathing through the nose is essential.*

As soon as the operation is complete, pure oxygen may be given with advantage for a few minutes before removal of the mask. The patient must be carefully observed at this stage, to ensure that blood clot or debris is expelled from the mouth and not inhaled, and to control any signs of excitement during the recovery. Fainting can also occur *after* the operation is completed, and the anaesthetist must be prepared to elevate the legs and apply other appropriate treatment.

Sedation in the dental surgery

(*See also* Sedation techniques for dental inpatients below).

1. Diazepam first used for this purpose in 1966 and 1968.[14] The cardiac output and stroke volume are decreased. The patient should be prepared as for general anaesthesia and should be supine. The drug is given at a rate of about 2.5 mg each half minute until drowsiness, slurred speech and drooping eyelids are evident: usual dose between 12 and 20 mg. At this point either light general anaesthesia or local analgesia is administered. Atropine premedication reduces troublesome salivation, while amnesia is usually present. Local burning or even thrombosis at the injection site may be seen. Complete recovery may take several hours, although long before this the patient may sit up in the dentist's waiting room. Flumazenil 0.1–0.5 mg has proved useful for reversal of benzodiazepines.

The combination of diazepam with methohexitone may cause severe cardiovascular depression.

2. Narcotic analgesics, e.g. alfentanil, fentanil, sufentanil, pethidine or pentazocine, can be given intravenously before nitrous oxide anaesthesia or to supplement diazepam. Grave respiratory depression must be avoided. Naloxone (0.1–0.4 mg i.v.) should be available for reversal of these opioids.

4. 'Ultra-light' methohexitone. *See below.*

Monitoring in the dental surgery

'Finger on the pulse'. (1) ECG. Adhesive electrodes may be placed on arms and leg. Ventricular ectopic beats are common during extractions; (2) arterial pressure. An automated monitor with good artefact rejection is best. The cuff may also be placed on leg (ankle); (3) pulse oximetry. Very highly recommended; (4) capnography. Technically extremely difficult to get a reliable sample.

Complications of dental surgery anaesthesia[15]

1. Hypoxia. Even when 30% oxygen is given during dental anaesthesia arterial hypoxia is likely to occur unless a perfect airway is maintained. This can be difficult when the surgeon exerts pressure during extractions in the lower jaw. Obstruction can occur as a result of malposition of packs and it is possible for the nasal mask to obstruct the nasal openings. It can be caused by the tongue, enlarged tonsils and adenoids, and laryngeal spasm. The latter may be due to irritation by foreign material such as blood, saliva or dental debris, as well as by anaesthetic vapours. Nasopharyngeal airways may be helpful.[16] There is evidence that some deaths in the dental surgery may result from hypoxia. *Airway obstruction is just as likely during 'total intravenous anaesthesia'.*

2. Excitement. A quiet calm commentary by the anaesthetist helps to allay fears during a 'gas induction' and allows the patient to know that the anaesthetist is aware that the patient is still awake. Struggling during the excitement stage is less common when potent supplements such as halothane are used. In sturdy and frightened patients intravenous induction is indicated and extra doses may be given.

3. Mouth-breathing. This dilutes the mixture delivered by nasal masks from the anaesthetic apparatus. In frightened or difficult patients and in small children the full face-mask should be used for induction. Mouth-breathing may occur due to the premature insertion of mouth gags or faulty positioning of a mouth pack. The oropharyngeal barrier, formed by apposition of the dorsum of the tongue and the palate, may be opened by mouth gags, operator's fingers, packs or anything that depresses the tongue.

4. Contamination of the trachea. Regurgitation, vomiting and inhalation of blood or tooth fragments. Lung abscess may result.[17] Tracheal soiling may also occur in conscious patients sedated with diazepam. A powerful sucker should always be available.

5. Respiratory arrest. This may be due to: (*a*) respiratory obstruction and is treated accordingly; (*b*) breath-holding in light anaesthesia. Treatment careful deepening of anaesthesia; (*c*) apnoea due to severe hypoxia Treatment is by inflation of lungs with oxygen; (*d*) grave cardiovascular depression – and full resuscitation required; (*e*) apnoea due to deep anaesthesia. Treatment is by inflation of the lungs with oxygen. In practice it may be difficult to make the diagnosis between over-light and over-deep anaesthesia.

6. Cardiac dysrhythmias. There is evidence of increased sympathetic activity during dental anaesthesia,[18] shown by tachycardia and an increase in circulating catecholamines. Parasympathetic responses can also occur. Ventricular dysrhythmias have been reported during dental anaesthesia in the ambulant patient.[19] The incidence may be up to 38% when halothane is given, but does not occur with intravenous methods.[20] Atropine increases the incidence of dysrhythmias during nitrous oxide–oxygen and halothane anaesthesia in children.[21] Beta-blocker premedication produces a significant reduction[22] as does local analgesia. Patients who have abnormalities of rhythm are likely to have delayed recovery. Pulse monitors are not reliable detectors of ectopic beats in the dental chair, due to movements of the patient. Dysrhythmias have been reported in patients receiving tricyclic antidepressants.[23] Gingival retraction cord, used to produce ischaemia, is impregnated with 8% racemic adrenaline and so may cause severe dysrhythmias in patients under halothane; a death has been reported from this cause.[24] Cord impregnated with either zinc chloride or aluminium sulphate can be used instead to reduce bleeding. Enflurane is associated with a lesser incidence of dysrhythmias in dental patients than halothane[25] but is less convenient to use. For the ECG in dental anaesthesia, *see* Rollason W. N. *SAAD Digest* 1983, **5**, 112. For management of ventricular fibrillation, *see* Chapter 31.

7. Fainting and hypotension. Bourne has drawn attention to the possibility of fainting during the administration of nitrous oxide in the dental chair.[6] The pulse should be continuously monitored, and should the patient even become pale, he must be immediately tilted into the head-down position to prevent cerebral ischaemia. If this is neglected, delayed recovery from anaesthesia, permanent cerebral damage from hypoxia or even death may result.

It is an arguable proposition that all dental operations should be performed with the patient in the horizontal position.[26] (Collapse and death has also followed local analgesia.[27])

Causes of hypotension during dental anaesthesia may include: (*a*) emotional factors, operative before or during early stages of anaesthesia; (*b*) hypoxia. Some subjects faint when given hypoxic mixtures (10% oxygen), even in the absence of anaesthesia; (*c*) pressure on the carotid sinus area when supporting the jaw; (*d*) bradycardia and hypotension due to surgical stimulation of vagal reflexes; and (*e*) cessation of anaesthesia. Anaesthesia may protect against syncopal reactions, which become manifest at the end of the procedure.

8. Nausea and vomiting. This can be reduced if hypoxia is scrupulously avoided, or if droperidol 0.25 mg i.v. is given. This does not delay recovery.[28] Other antiemetics may be used.

9. Deaths. It is often difficult to determine the true cause of death, but hypoxia and pulmonary oedema feature in a number of reports. Cardiomyopathy presents a special risk and diabetic autonomic neuropathy is important (*see* Chapter 20).

10. Minor morbidity. Following extraction under local or general anaesthesia there is a high incidence of sore lips, inability to open mouth and eat normally, drowsiness, nausea, vomiting, giddiness and headache.[29]

11. Pain. Oral analgesics, one hour prior to induction, or short-acting opioids during the procedure, may be used.

12. Hazards to dental and nursing staff. Occupational exposure to nitrous oxide may cause depression of vitamin B_{12} activity resulting in measurable changes in bone marrow secondary to impaired synthesis of deoxyribonucleic acid (DNA).[30]

Mouth packs

These perform vital functions: (1) to soak up blood and saliva; (2) to discourage mouth-breathing; and (3) to prevent soiling of the lower respiratory tract. They may be: (*a*) moist cellulose flange packs[31] (one for each side of mouth). Placed by the operator; or (*b*) gauze, 12-fold, 8 cm by

120 cm (at least 14 cm outside the mouth at all times) or a strip of gamgee tissue.

Packs need to be inserted carefully into the retromolar space between the underside of the tongue and the teeth on the side to be operated on, with its free end on the opposite side.[32] The tongue should be displaced upwards and medially, to touch the soft palate, not the posterior pharyngeal wall. This discourages mouth-breathing.

See also Deaths and dental anaesthetics. Lewis B. *Br. Med. J.* 1984, **286**, 3; Deaths associated with dentistry. Coplans M. P. and Curson I. *Br. Dent. J.* 1982, **153**, 357.

Regional analgesia

See Chapter 24.

Sedation techniques for dental inpatients

While general anaesthesia is a controlled state of unconsciousness accompanied by partial or complete loss of protective reflexes, 'deep sedation' is a depressed level of consciousness with some blunting of protective reflexes, although it remains possible to arouse the patient. 'Conscious sedation' is a light level of sedation with full activity of protective reflexes and ability to respond to verbal command. Such sedation is combined with potent analgesia, either local analgesia, or parenteral analgesics.

Sedative techniques

1. Intravenous benzodiazepine, e.g. diazepam 10–20 mg slowly over 2 min until a degree of ptosis is observed.[33] Diazepam may be painful on injection and can cause venous thrombosis. The competence of the laryngeal closure reflex may be impaired for 5–10 min following intravenous diazepam. Combination with pentazocine has been recommended; dose 30 mg.[34] Midazolam has advantages over diazepam, with faster onset of sedation, quicker recovery and fewer sore arms. Average dose, 2–3 mg, given slowly, so minimizing hiccups and respiratory depression.[35]

2. 'Ultra-light' anaesthesia with intermittent methohexitone. Scrupulous attention must be paid to the airway and the insertion of a pack to prevent inhalation of water or tooth powder. This technique has been criticized on the grounds that clinical studies have shown respiratory obstruction, arterial hypoxaemia, tachycardia, fall in peripheral resistance, and unsatisfactory operative conditions and patient tranquillity in an unacceptable proportion of patients.[36]

3. Total Intravenous Anaesthesia, using, for example propofol. *See* Chapter 9.

4. The Jorgensen technique[37] (The Loma Linda Dental School, Univ. of California). The aim is to provide good sedation while work is carried out under local analgesia.

5. Relative analgesia.[38] the Quantiflex apparatus has been used to provide inhalation of sub-anaesthetic concentrations of nitrous oxide during conservation under local analgesia. Nitrous oxide 25% with oxygen 75% gives inhalation analgesia.[39] (*see above*.)

Parenteral analgesics in common use include alfentanil, fentanyl and ketamine. Dihydrocodeine, although effective in the relief of pain in labour, after operation, and of skeletal origin, is reported to act as an anti-analgesic when given after dental extraction.[40]

See also Matthews R. A. *Dental Local Analgesia*. Bristol: Wright, 1982.

Anaesthesia for dental inpatients

Dental patients are admitted to hospital and treated as inpatients when either the dental procedure or anaesthetic facilities exceeds the scope of the outpatient department, or when the general condition of the patient contra-indicates outpatient anaesthesia.

Pre-operative assessment and premedication are usual. The anaesthetic technique usually involves nasotracheal intubation and a throat pack to prevent aspiration of blood and debris. Complications and hazards include:

1. Epistaxis and nasal trauma due to passage of a nasal tube. Can be minimized by prior spraying of the nasal mucosa with a vasoconstrictor (e.g. cocaine 4%).

2. Sore throat. Due to the insertion of a throat pack, when bruising and abrasion of the mucus membrane of the palate and fauces can readily occur.

3. Muscle pains due to suxamethonium.

4. Ventricular dysrhythmias have been reported as a result of surgical stimuli during dental extractions.[41] (*See above*.) Premedication with a β-blocker reduces the incidence. Less common if halothane avoided.

The types of patient who present for inpatient operation because of their general physical condition include:

1. Mental defectives and spastics, who are difficult to manage in the dental surgery under local analgesia.[42]

2. Cardiac patients, who require especially careful anaesthetic management. It is a good plan to precede anaesthesia by the inhalation of 100% oxygen for 10 min. In the presence of valvular lesions, antibiotic cover should be given to prevent subsequent development of subacute bacterial endocarditis. Antibiotics are also necessary in patients with hip prostheses.

3. Cases of chronic respiratory disease, particularly where there is gross derangement of ventilation/perfusion relationships. (see Chapter 20.)

4. Those with a haemorrhage disorder, e.g. haemophilia, Christmas disease, thrombocytopenia, or where there is a history of severe post-extraction haemorrhage. Pre-operative clotting screen is performed, and if necessary appropriate treatment arranged.

The haemophilic patient

For details of management *see* Chapter 20. Extreme gentleness is required during anaesthesia to avoid trauma. An oral tube is preferred to a nasal, and throat packs are not used. Surgery should include meticulous haemostasis.

Faciomaxillary operations

For history of faciomaxillary surgery and anaesthesia, *see* Ward T. *Ann. R. Coll. Surg. Engl.* 1975, **57**, 67.

Fractured jaw

This may be part of a grave emergency complicated by intraoral haemorrhage, obstructed airway and associated injuries (including head injury and loss of consciousness). In these very severe cases the protective laryngeal reflexes may be obtunded with danger of aspiration of blood, teeth and other debris. Securing a clear airway is the first priority. However, most mandibular fractures are unilateral and do not require urgent treatment. In others trismus may be a feature. The operative treatment of jaw injury can usually be carried out as an elective procedure. Fractures of the maxillae can be classified according to the Le Fort scheme.[43] There may be associated periorbital oedema and epistaxis, and cerebrospinal rhinorrhoea is not infrequent. Diplopia may occur with orbital fracture. Respiratory problems occasionally arise if the mobile maxilla approximates to the posterior pharyngeal wall or the dorsum of the tongue.

The anaesthetist who is asked to deal with a fractured mandible and/or maxilla should look out for: (1) associated injuries, especially: (*a*) head injuries – loss of consciousness, depressed fractures, raised intracranial tension; (*b*) chest injuries – pneumothorax or haemothorax; (*c*) abdominal injuries – ruptured viscera and (*d*) major bone fractures. The presence of associated injuries results in increased haemorrhage and shock; (2) presence of blood and debris in the pharynx, larynx and trachea. There may be respiratory obstruction and the laryngeal reflexes may be obtunded. Occasionally it is necessary to bronchoscope the patient for tracheobronchial cleansing; (3) possibility of swallowed blood, which may be regurgitated as anaesthesia is induced. It is seldom practical to ask the patient to swallow an oesophageal tube; and (4) the possibility of food in the stomach.

First-aid treatment may include: (1) in the unconscious patient, it may be wise to pass a tracheal tube, usually via the nose. Rarely a tracheostomy may be required; (2) temporary fixation with dental wire of large displaced fragments of bone; (3) pharyngeal (or tracheobronchial) cleansing; and (4) treatment of shock, if present, by blood transfusion, etc.

Anaesthetic technique for the faciomaxillary case

Premedication. In the emergency case it is wise to restrict premedication to atropine or hyoscine. Respiratory depressants are to be avoided. An anti-emetic drug is used to prevent postoperative vomiting (when the jaws have been wired together).

Induction. The following should be available: two or more good laryngoscopes; experienced dedicated, and adequate help; an operating table or trolley that can be instantly tipped; suction, instantly available and switched on; and equipment for emergency cricothyroid puncture. Rarely bronchoscopy may be indicated. The usual precautions to prevent regurgitation of stomach contents should be taken.

Rapid sequence induction is usually carried out. Visualization of the larynx may be rendered difficult if blood and debris are present – but the shattered tissues do not resist introduction of the laryngoscope and intubation can usually be performed without difficulty. The anaesthetist should be as gentle as possible in order to avoid further mobilization of the fracture.

A nasotracheal tube is usually preferred. This may be cuffed.[44] A pharyngeal pack can also be inserted, which should be removed and pharyngeal toilet performed immediately before the jaws are wired together.

Maintenance By inhalation anaesthesia. Smooth anaesthetic technique is desirable, with rapid return of reflexes at the end of operation and absence of vomiting, coughing and straining. Anti-emetic drugs may be used with advantage in premedication or postoperatively.

If the jaws have been wired together the patient should leave theatre with a nasopharyngeal airway in situ. A pair of wire cutters should remain near the patient, so that they can be used in an emergency to free the jaws, and the mouth and pharynx can be sucked out. The nursing attendants should know how to use the instrument and which wires to cut. In fact on occasion it may be life-saving, e.g. in the presence of severe respiratory obstruction.

References

1. Evans T. W. *Br. J. Dent. Sci.* 1868, **11**, 196, 318.
2. Hewitt F. W. *Anaesthetics and their Administration.* London: Griffin, 1893; Hewitt F. W. *The Administration of Nitrous Oxide and Oxygen for Dental Operations.* London: Ash, 1897.
3. McKesson E. I. *Br. Med. J.* 1926, **2**, 1113.
4. Coleman F. *Dent. Rec.* 1942, **62**, 143, 167.
5. Clover J. T. *Br. Med. J.* 1868, **2**, 491; Coleman A. *Br. J. Dent. Sci.* 1868, **11**, 128.
6. Bourne J. G. *Lancet* 1957, **2**, 499.
7. *Drummond-Jackson's Dental sedation and Anaesthesia.* London: SAAD, 1979.
8. Davidau A. *Rev. Stomatol.* 1966, **67**, 589.
9. Hall R. J. *N. Y. Med. J.* 1884, **40**, 643.
10. Hunt W. A. *Br. Dent. J.* 1886, Jan.
11. *See also* Green R. A. and Coplans M. P. *Anaesthesia and Analgesia in Dentistry.* London: Lewis, 1973.
12. Lewis T. *Br. Med. J. 1932*, **1**, 873.
13. Sale J. P., et al. Anaesthesia, 1985, **40**, 3.
14. Davidau A. *Rev. stomatol.* 1966, **67**, 589; Brown P. R. H., Main D. M. G. and Lawson J. I. M. *Br. Dent. J. 1968*, **125**(2), 498.
15. *See also* Love S. H. S. In: *General Anaesthesia for Dental Surgery* (Hunter A. R. and Bush G. H. ed.) Altrincham: Sherratt, 1971, p. 104; Love S. H. S. *Br. J. Anaesth.* 1968, **40**, 188.
16. Doctor N. H. *Anaesthesia* 1977, **32**, 273.
17. Brock R. C. *Guy's Hosp. Rep.* 1947, **96**, 141.
18. Edmondson M. D. et al. *Br. Med. J.* 1972, **2**, 47; Taggart P. et al. *Br. Med. J. 1976*, **2**, 787; Al-Khishali T. et al. *Anaesthesia* 1978, **33**, 184.
19. Kaufman L. *Proc. R. Soc. Med.* 1966, **59**, 731; Ryder W. *Anaesthesia* 1970, **25**, 46.
20. Ryder W. *Proc. R. Soc. Med.* 1971, **64**, 82; Ryder W. and Townsend D. *Br. J. Anaesth.* 1974, **46**, 760; Bradshaw E. G. *Anaesthesia* 1976, **31**, 13.
21. Thurlow A. C. *Anaesthesia* 1972, **27**, 429; Whalley D. G. et al. *Br. J. Anaesth.* 1976, **48**, 120.
22. Ryder W. et al. *Anaesthesia* 1971, **26**, 508.
23. Plowman P. E. and Thomas W. J. W. *Anaesthesia* 1974, **29**, 576.

24. Hilley M. D. et al. *Anesthesiology* 1984, **60**, 587.
25. Wright C. J. *Anaesthesia* 1980, **36**, 775; Ryder W. and Wright P. A., *Anaesthesia* 1981, **36**, 532; Barker G. I. and Briscoe C. E. *Brit. J. Anaesth.* 1981, **53**, 1079.
26. Bourne J. G. *Studies in Anaesthetics.* London: Lloyd-Luke, 1967, p. 131.
27. Tomlin P. J. *Anaesthesia* 1974, **29**, 551; Coplans M. P. and Curson I. *Br. Dent. J.* 1976, **141**, 255.
28. O'Donovan N. and Shaw J. *Anaesthesia* 1984, **39**, 1172.
29. Muir V. M. J. *Anaesthesia* 1976, **31**, 171.
30. Sweeney B. et al. *Br. Med. J.* 1985, **291**, 567.
31. Drummond-Jackson S. L. *Br. Dent. J.* 1964, **116**, 15.
32. Coplans M. P. and Barton P. R. *Br. Dent. J.* 1964, **116**, 209.
33. Verrill P. *Br. Dent. J.* 1969, **127**, 85.
34. Sykes P. *Br. Med. J.* 1977, **2**, 832; Corrall I. M. et al. *Anaesthesia* 1979, **34**, 850.
35. Rosenbaum N. L. *Br. Dent. J.* 1985, **158**, 139.
36. Wise C. C. et al. *Br. Med. J.* 1969, **2**, 540; Mann P. E. et al. *Anaesthesia* 1971, **26**, 3; Thornton J. A. *Proc. R. Soc. Med.* 1971, **64**, 83. *Drummond-Jackson's Dental Sedation and Anaesthesia* (Sykes P. ed.). London: SAAD, 1979.
37. Jorgensen N. B. and Leffingwell F. *Dent. Clin. North Am.* 1961 (July), 299; Jorgensen N. B. et al. *J. Soc. Cal. Dent. Clins.* 1963, **31**, 7; *see also* Bourne J. G. *Studies in Anaesthetics.* London: Lloyd-Luke, 1967, 116; Jorgensen N. B. and Hayden J. *Sedation: local and general anesthesia in dentistry.* 3rd ed. Philadelphia: Lea & Febiger, 1980.
38. Langa H. *Relative Analgesia in Dental Patients.* Philadelphia: Saunders, 1976; Young T. M. et al. *Br. Dent. J. 1976,* **141**, 34.
39. Edmunds D. H. and Rosen M. *Anaesthesia* 1984, **39**, 138.
40. Seymour R. A. et al. *Lancet* 1982, **1**, 1425.
41. Kaufman L. *Proc. R. Soc. Med.* 1966, **59**, 731.
42. Diamond D. W. and Cochrane D. F. *Anaesthesia* 1976, **31**, 190.
43. McGregor I. A. *Fundamental Techniques of Plastic Surgery.* Edinburgh: Churchill Livingstone, 1972.
44. Davies J. A. H. *Anaesthesia* 1967, **22**, 153.

Endocrine glands

1. THYROID GLAND

The great pioneer of surgery of the thyroid was Theodore Kocher (1841–1917) of Bern. He received the Nobel Prize in 1909, the first, and for many years the only, surgeon to be so honoured. Antithyroid drugs (thiourea) were first used in 1943.[1]

Thyroid function

Clinical assessment can be supplemented by: (1) measurement of total serum thyroxine (T_4) which is 99.96% bound to thyroid binding globulin (TBG), albumin and a pre-albumin; (2) TBG levels, tri-iodothyronine (T_3) uptake tests, which measure unoccupied T_4 binding sites, and free T_4 levels directly;

(3) serum T_3; (4) serum thyroid-stimulating hormone (TSH) and thyrotropin-releasing hormone (TRH); (5) thyroid scan; (6) serum cholesterol (high in myxoedema).

Preoperative preparation

When surgery is advised the patient should first be rendered euthyroid. Antithyroid drugs[2] or radioactive iodine (^{131}I) take some months to be fully effective. β-blockade controls the hyperdynamic circulation within hours.[3] Iodine was used to treat goitre in 1821 by J. F. Coindet (1774–1834), Swiss physician, and is used today in the immediate pre-operative period. Lugol's iodine (iodine 5%, potassium iodide 10%) 0.1–0.3 ml t.d.s. (Jean G. A. Lugol, 1786–1851, of Paris) or potassium iodide tablets 60 mg t.d.s. Carbimazole increases vascularity of the thyroid and the change to potassium iodide is usually made 7–10 days pre-operatively. Propranolol (e.g. 40 mg q.d.s.), which acts peripherally and does not affect the gland, may be combined with potassium iodide before and perhaps immediately following operation. It is important to check the possibility of respiratory obstruction from retrosternal goitre, compression of the trachea or its deviation by radiography.

Anaesthesia for thyroid surgery

Respiration may be spontaneous (using a laryngeal mask or an endotracheal tube) or controlled. Coughing must be prevented by a volatile agent, topical analgesia or by muscular paralysis. In very large goitres, difficulties are more likely to be surgical rather than anaesthetic.[4] An endotracheal tube is essential if: (1) the trachea is deviated or compressed; (2) goitre is retrosternal; (3) malignancy is suspected; or (4) the vocal cords move abnormally when viewed through a laryngeal mirror in husky, stridulous patients.

Stimulation of the recurrent laryngeal nerve causes spasm of the corresponding cord, with a high-pitched crowing sound, when patient is not intubated. If nerve is divided, the cord first becomes abducted and flaccid; later it assumes the cadaveric position between abduction and adduction. Later still, some voluntary control is gained.

Hyperextension of the neck is unnecessary and should be avoided. A head-up tilt reduces venous oozing. Infiltration of the skin and subcutaneous tissues with 1 in 200 000 to 1 in 500 000 adrenaline reduces oozing from skin flaps. The addition of bupivacaine to the adrenaline does not relieve postoperative pain.[5] Dysrhythmias can be greatly reduced by normal blood gases or by β-blockers. The eyes should be protected from the risk of drying and ulceration of the exposed cornea. Special care is necessary if there is exophthalmos.

The trachea and pharynx should be aspirated at the end of the operation, but coughing is to be avoided because it may contribute to reactionary haemorrhage. The cords can be examined as the effects of any muscle relaxant wear off to check that they move normally. Postoperatively aspirin is useful for muscular neck pain.

Respiratory obstruction after thyroidectomy

The causes may be:

1. Reactionary haemorrhage. This may cause pressure on the trachea and requires immediate restoration of the airway and evacuation of the haematoma. The glottis can be completely hidden by submucosal blood and emergency cricothyrotomy may be needed.

2. Oedema of the larynx. Usually on the second or third day after operation. Diagnosis is by indirect laryngoscopy and if stridor becomes troublesome a tracheal tube or tracheostomy will be required. Oedema of the pharynx may also be a cause of obstruction.[6]

3. Recurrent laryngeal nerve injury.[7] This may be transient or permanent. The former is not uncommon, and even if bilateral need not cause obstruction unless there is also oedema. Permanent injury to one nerve is not serious, unless the patient earns his living with his voice, because the opposite cord compensates for the immobile cord. Routine examination of the larynx before and after thyroidectomy has shown that one-third of cases of unilateral paralysis resulting from trauma to the recurrent nerve are symptomless even if the paralysis is permanent. Treatment is unnecessary.

Permanent injury to both cords is very serious because both voice and airway are impaired owing to the narrow glottis. Either a permanent tracheostomy or an operation to widen the glottis is required, certainly if the obstruction is severe enough to cause insomnia.

4. Collapse of trachea. Can occur due to erosion of the cartilages by a large goitre, but is rare unless the actual tracheal cartilage is removed in malignant cases. The unsupported walls of the trachea may collapse and cause partial or even total obstruction when the tube is removed. It should be replaced immediately. Tracheostomy may be necessary.

5. Injury to the superior laryngeal nerve. This is rare but can be suspected if there is: (*a*) a change in the voice; or (*b*) difficulty in swallowing. The former is due to cricothyroid paralysis (external branch), the latter to sensory loss (internal branch). The condition soon improves. In a series of over 300 thyroidectomy operations, the operation carried a hazard to the voice in 5% of patients, with permanent damage, measured by sophisticated methods, in 3%. There is as great a need for surgical care of the superior laryngeal nerve as for the recurrent branches.[8]

6. Mucus or blood in the airway.

Other complications

1. Thyroid crisis. Now rarely seen. There may be abdominal pain, fever, diarrhoea, gross nervousness and restlessness with tachycardia and dysrhythmias. An acute abdomen may be suspected. A sudden crisis in an unsuspected thyrotoxic patient after operation requires careful administration of β-blockers, and possibly α-blockers, together with potassium iodide and hydrocortisone. Mild tachycardia or pyrexia during the first few postoperative days may indicate a lesser degree of thyroid overactivity and may be prevented by oral potassium iodide.

2. *Postoperative hypoparathyroidism.* A low serum calcium (normal 2.2–2.6 mmol/l) requiring calcium gluconate 10%, up to 20 ml slowly i.v. There may be tetany, and Chvostek's and Trousseau's signs may be present. *See also* Roizen M. F. et al. *Anesth. Clin. North Am.* 1987, **5**, 277.

2. PARATHYROIDS

The parathyroids help maintain a normal serum calcium (2.2–2.6 mmol/l), together with diet, kidney function and vitamin D. Primary hyperparathyroidism is due to excessive secretion of parathormone, usually by a single adenoma (80% of cases). Rarely there is diffuse hypertrophy of the glands, multiple adenomata or carcinoma. 10–15% are familial, part of multiple endocrine neoplasia types I or II. It may be associated with renal stones, bone pain progressing to osteitis fibrosa cystica, loss of appetite, nausea, thirst, and mental changes. There is a short Q-T interval on the ECG. In advanced cases polyuria causes water and sodium depletion, and renal failure may ensue. Large quantities of i.v. fluids and frusemide to promote calcium excretion are required. Rarely, surgery may proceed into the chest. After parathyroidectomy the serum calcium falls and there may be tetany, requiring calcium gluconate 10% (up to 20 ml slowly i.v.), or 1-α-hydroxycholecalciferol (2–4 µg daily).

3. ADRENAL CORTEX

Conn's syndrome described in 1955.[9] Excessive production of aldosterone. In 60% of cases it is from an adrenal cortical adenoma, which requires excision. Clinical features include hypertension, hypokalaemic alkalosis and hypokalaemic nephropathy.[10] Pre-operative management includes correction of metabolic disturbances and potassium depletion (spironolactone or amiloride, and potassium supplements). Anaesthetic management is likely to be complicated by large swings of blood pressure and control may be difficult. Temporary hypoaldosteronism can occur after operation and may require fludrocortisone 50–300 µg daily.

See Shipton E. A. & Hugo J. M. *Anaesthesia* 1982, **37**, 933; Hanowell S. T. et al. *Anesth. Rev.* 1982, **9**, 36.

4. ADRENAL MEDULLA

Phaeochromocytoma was first reported by Frankel in 1886[11] and named by Ludwig Pick (1868–1935), of Berlin.[12] A tumour of chromaffin cells of neuro-ectodermal origin. May be familial, part of multiple endocrine neoplasia types II and III. Usually in the adrenal medulla but 10% occur in chromaffin tissue elsewhere, e.g. the paravertebral space, near the aortic bifurcation in the organ of Zuckerkandl, the coeliac plexus or even in the bladder. Of the adrenal tumours, 10% are bilateral and 10% are malignant. Even when benign, the excessive secretion of adrenaline and noradrenaline is dangerous. The patient exhibits headaches, sweating and hypertension, either paroxysmal or continuous, but postural hypotension is common. Accounts for less than 0.1% of hypertensives. Catecholamines can cause a cardiomyopathy and the tumour can present with heart failure.[13] Diagnosis is by estimation of urinary catecholamines and their metabolites and the failure of pentolinium or clonidine to suppress tumour catecholamines. The tumour is localized by MRI or CT,[131]I meta-iodobenzylguanidine imaging or by selective venous catheterization.[14] It can be as large as 3 kg. In one series 85% of patients with these tumours were diagnosed only at autopsy.[15]

Pre-operative care

Adequate pre-operative α-adrenergic blockade is essential to allow blood volume to be restored to normal and to prevent dangerous rises of blood pressure during surgery, e.g. phenoxybenzamine 10 mg t.d.s., increased by 10 mg increments until the recumbent diastolic pressure is 90–100 mmHg without postural hypotension. Prazosin may be added, which causes less tachycardia. Therapy should continue for at least 1 week pre-operatively. The presence of a stuffy nose is a good guide to adequate blockade. β-adrenergic blockade is indicated for tachycardia or dysrhythmia, e.g. propranolol 40 mg orally, 8-hourly. It should not be started before α-blockade, otherwise a paradoxical rise in blood pressure will result. The ECG must be free of ST/T changes for over 1 week.

Anaesthetic technique

Premedication should be anxiolytic. Droperidol has caused a hypertensive crisis.[16] Direct intra-arterial blood pressure recording is started before induction. General anaesthesia with relaxation is usually employed, but agents that cause sympathetic stimulation or histamine release are to be avoided. Excessive hypertension caused by catecholamine release when the tumour is handled may be controlled by the use of sodium nitroprusside. Some patients become suddenly hypotensive after tumour excision (although catecholamine levels may take over a week to return to normal). An adrenaline or noradrenaline infusion should be ready for this situation. Angiotensin may be needed if this is inadequate. Hypoglycaemia should be sought, especially in the presence of β-blockade.[17] Recovery from anaesthesia can be slow.

If phaeochromocytoma presents in early pregnancy it is normally excised in mid-trimester. If later, excision is combined with operative delivery of the infant.[18] The sympathetic supply to the adrenals is from T8 to L1.

See also Hull C. J. *Br. J. Anaesth.* 1986, **58**, 1453; Roizen M. F. et al. *Anesth. Clin. North Am.* 1987, **5**, 269; Pullerits J. et al. *Can. J. Anaesth.* 1988, **35**, 526.

References

1. Askwood E. B. *JAMA* 1943, **122**, 78.
2. Cooper D. S. *New Engl. J. Med.* 1984, **311**, 1353.
3. Klein I. and Levey G. S. *Am. J. Med.* 1984, **76**, 167.
4. Swadia V. N. et al. *Br. J. Anaesth.* 1981, **53**, 963.
5. Park G. R. et al. *J. R. Coll. Surg. Edin.* 1983, **28**, 295.
6. Bexton M. D. R. and Radford R. *Anaesthesia* 1982, **37**, 596.
7. *See also* Mountain J. C. et al. *Surg. Gynecol. Obstet.* 1971, **133**, 1; Stewart G. R. et al. *Br. J. Surg.* 1972, **59**, 379.
8. Kark A. E. et al. *Br. Med. J.* 1984, **289**, 1412.
9. Conn J. W. *J. Lab. Clin. Med.* 1955, **45**, 6.
10. Vaughan N. J. A. *Lancet* 1981, **i**, 120.
11. Frankel F. *Virchow Arch. Path. Anat.* 1886, **103**, 244.
12. Pick L. *Berl. Klin. Wochenschr.* 1912, **19**, 16.
13. Sardesai S. H. et al. *Br. Med. J.* 1990, **63**, 234.
14. Bravo E. L. and Gifford R. W. *N. Engl. J. Med.* 1984, **311**, 1298.
15. St John Sutton M. G. et al. *Mayo Clin. Proc.* 1981, **56**, 354.
16. Brinquin L. et al. *Ann. Fr. Anesth. Reanim.* 1987, **6**, 204.
17. Levin H. and Heifetz M. *Can. J. Anaesth.* 1990, **37**, 477.
18. Mitchell S. Z. et al. *Anesth. Analg.* 1987, **66**, 478; Harper M. A. et al. *Br. J. Obst. Gynaecol.* 1989, **96**, 594.

Neurosurgical anaesthesia[1]

History

First successful diagnosis and surgical removal of a cerebral tumour took place in 1885.[2] Sir Victor Horsley (1857–1917) of London removed an extradural spinal cord tumour for the first time in 1884. He began to develop neurosurgery as a separate specialty, having been appointed surgeon to the National Hospital for Nervous Diseases, Queen Square in 1886. This influenced Harvey Cushing (1869–1939) of the Massachusetts General Hospital in Boston (who introduced the silver clip to arrest haemorrhage in 1911 and pioneered the use of diathermy in 1928[3] and whose anaesthetist was Walter M. Boothby), and Walter Dandy (1886–1946) of Philadelphia (who described ventriculography in 1918[4] and air encephalography in 1919).[5] Egas Moniz of Lisbon used cerebral angiography in 1927.[6] The first planned operation for cerebral aneurysm was reported in 1932,[7] and the first localization of a cerebral tumour by EEG in 1936[8] and by radio-isotopes in 1948.[9]

Horsley preferred chloroform anaesthesia whereas Cushing favoured ether. A death under anaesthesia in 1893 stimulated Cushing to introduce the ether chart, a record of pulse, BP and respiration during major surgery.[10] Early pioneers of neurosurgical anaesthesia in the UK, many of them part-time general practitioners, included Zebulon Mennell (1876–1959, appointed to the National Hospital in 1911),[11] Maxwell Brown and John

Gillies in Edinburgh, Noel Gillespie and John Challis at the London Hospital, Oliver Jones in Oxford, and Harry Brennan and Andrew Hunter in Manchester. Local analgesia was also used before the availability of muscle relaxants. Even the introduction of tracheal intubation in the 1930s and 1940s could not avoid hypercapnia and raised venous pressure, due to expiratory resistance, resulting in a swollen brain. Paralysis and IPPV is now usual, except for minor operations such as burr-hole biopsy or for some stereotactic procedures.

See also Dott N. *Proc. R. Soc. Med.* 1971, **64**, 1051; Hunter A. R. In: *Anaesthesia: Essays on its History* (Rupreht J. et al. ed.) Berlin: Springer-Verlag, 1985, 148.

SPECIAL PROBLEMS IN NEUROSURGERY

(1) Control of intracranial pressure (ICP) and cerebral blood flow. Control of ventilation and $Paco_2$ is particularly important; (2) maintenance of the airway. The tracheal tube and connections are often inaccessible; (3) Control of venous pressure by absence of straining or coughing at any stage of the operation. Even a short period of straining may cause cerebral oedema persisting for hours; (4) length of surgery; (5) positioning in the sitting, lateral or prone positions requires special care; (6) air embolism in head-up positions; (7) induced hypotension may be needed; (8) brain retraction or surgical trauma may affect vital structures; (9) postoperative care of airway and respiration; and (10) fits.

The operating microscope, ultrasonic devices that remove abnormal tissue without unnecessary destruction of normal brain and new ways of reaching previously inaccessible lesions at the base of the skull, have all contributed to an improved surgical prognosis.

CEREBRAL HAEMODYNAMICS

Intracranial contents are: brain 80% (which is one-seventh ECF, and three-quarters water), cerebral blood volume 12% and cerebrospinal fluid 8%. All are incompressible and restricted within the rigid skull, although some venous blood and CSF may be squeezed out into the jugular veins and the spinal canal respectively. The brain weighs about 1.5 kg (but only 50 g when suspended in CSF) and its total blood flow is 750 ml/min (15% of cardiac output). Grey matter has a higher blood flow than white matter (70 and 20 ml/min per 100 g respectively). Over two-thirds comes from the carotid arteries, the rest from the vertebrals. Its oxygen consumption is about 50 ml/min (20% of that for the whole body). Different regions of the brain have differing functions and patterns of blood flow. The status of important areas may not be reflected in global measurements. Blood flow and metabolism are normally tightly coupled.

Cerebral blood flow below about 20 ml/min per 100 g cause EEG changes. Values below 10 ml/min per 100 g cause impaired ionic homeostasis and histological changes of ischaemia.

Factors affecting cerebral blood flow (CBF)

Regional blood flow is closely related to local brain metabolism. Global CBF is affected by:

1. *Arterial P_{CO_2}*. Linear response between a P_{CO_2} of 2.7 kPa (20 mmHg) when CBF is halved, and 10.7 kPa (80 mmHg) when CBF is doubled. Little change outside these values. Mediated through the associated changes in H^+ concentration. CBF returns to normal over about 24 hours if the change in P_{CO_2} is maintained, as CSF bicarbonate is adjusted. This limits the period that hyperventilation is of value in reducing ICP. Reactivity to CO_2 indicates healthy cerebral (and spinal) vessels, is increased by volatile agents and may not be seen in abnormal areas of brain.

2. *Arterial P_{O_2}*. Inhalation of 100% oxygen only reduces CBF by 10%. The P_{O_2} must be reduced below 6.7 kPa (50 mmHg) before CBF starts to rise.

3. *Cerebral perfusion pressure*. This is mean arterial blood pressure minus ICP (or cerebral venous pressure, whichever is the higher). *Autoregulation* maintains a steady CBF as perfusion pressure varies between 50 and 150 mmHg. Both these pressure limits are higher with sympathetic stimulation and in hypertensives. Vasodilators or cervical sympathectomy allows a lower blood pressure to be tolerated than when sympathetic tone is high (e.g. in haemorrhage). As with CO_2 reactivity, autoregulation is a sign of healthy brain. Impaired by volatile agents.

4. *Venous and intracranial pressures*. A rise in venous pressure will raise the ICP, which tends to lower CBF because: (*a*) cerebral perfusion pressure is lowered; and (*b*) a high ICP compresses the cerebral vessels. The normal brain compensates to some extent. Abrupt rises in venous pressure during straining or coughing may cause serious falls in CBF, especially if arterial pressure also falls (e.g. during induction).

5. *Autonomic system*. Extensive sympathetic supply, mainly from the superior cervical ganglion, but relatively little effect. α_2 stimulation causes vasoconstriction, β_1 stimulation causes dilatation. A vasodilator parasympathetic supply derives from the facial nerve.

6. *Temperature*. CBF falls by 20–50% if body temperature is dropped 10°C. Hyperthermia increases CBF.

7. *Blood viscosity*. CBF rises as viscosity falls and *vice versa*.

8. *Age*. Falls by about 0.5% per year in later life, and this fall is confined to the grey matter.

9. *Drugs*. All inhalation agents are cerebral vasodilators but this effect can be modified by hyperventilation. Any resultant rise in ICP is greater in patients with a space-occupying lesion, and 'shift' may occur at the level of the tentorium or foramen magnum. Ketamine is also a cerebral vasodilator and increases CBF. Other intravenous anaesthetics (e.g. barbiturates, propofol, etomidate, benzodiazepines) reduce CBF together with a drop in cerebral metabolism. *See below.*

Cerebral steal and inverse steal

Brain pathology may produce maximal local vasodilatation or a loss of normal regulation. In these circumstances, a rise of $Paco_2$ may dilate vessels in surrounding normal brain and 'steal' blood from the abnormal area. The converse may happen if $Paco_2$ falls, and blood be diverted to the abnormal part ('inverse steal' or Robin Hood effect). The clinical importance of these possibilities is uncertain.

Intracranial pressure (ICP)

Normal ICP is 10–15 mmHg, and varies slightly with both the heartbeat and respiration. The zero level is taken to be the base of the skull or the external auditory meatus. Measured by an intra-ventricular catheter, a subdural or extradural transducer. All can be inserted via a burr-hole. An approximate value of ICP can be obtained from a CT scan.

Raised ICP[12] occurs with coughing, sneezing, straining, etc. Raised pathologically with: (*a*) pressure from outside, e.g. bony tumour or craniostenosis; (*b*) space-occupying lesions, e.g. neoplasm, abscess or haematoma; (*c*) hydrocephalus; (*d*) venous obstruction and PEEP; (*e*) arterial dilatation, e.g. high $Paco_2$; (*f*) cerebral oedema; and (*g*) head-down position.

Raised ICP causes headache, vomiting, papilloedema, drowsiness, bradycardia and hypertension (Cushing reflex). Neurogenic pulmonary oedema may occur. If ICP equals arterial blood pressure, cerebral blood flow cannot occur.

Decreased ICP occurs after: (*a*) dehydration or blood loss; and (*b*) removal of a space-occupying lesion. It is of little significance.

As a space-occupying lesion grows, ICP rises little at first because (by the Monroe-Kellie hypothesis) there is a corresponding decrease in volume of cerebral venous blood and CSF. The pressure-volume curve is still flat. Later, however, this compensatory mechanism fails, and then a small rise in intracranial volume (e.g. hypercapnia or volatile agents causing arterial dilatation; coughing or turning the neck causing venous distension) causes a big rise in ICP. Measurement of intracranial compliance may indicate how nearly this danger point has been reached.

Cerebrospinal fluid

See Chapter 1.

Techniques of anaesthesia for neurosurgery

CT and MRI scanning now means that the anaesthetist first sees the patient before major surgery, rather than before a diagnostic procedure. Many patients are generally fit, but those having surgery for cerebrovascular or cervical spine disorders or for secondary tumours may have important associated disease.

Local analgesia

May be considered where facilities for skilled administration of general anaesthesia are not available. Any coughing, straining or respiratory obstruction under general anaesthesia will be hazardous if ICP is raised. Since most of the brain is insensitive to surgical stimuli, local analgesia is useful in e.g. decompression of a haematoma when ICP may be rising rapidly, burr-hole biopsy or cortical mapping. Sometimes the patient's co-operation is required during the operation, e.g. localization of subjective phenomena.

The skin and scalp may be infiltrated with 0.5% lignocaine with adrenaline 1 in 200 000 to cut down oozing. The bone is only slightly sensitive and drilling, though uncomfortable, is usually tolerable. The only sensitive parts of the brain are the dura mater at the base of the skull, the dural sheath around arteries, especially in the region of the middle meningeal artery, and the dura on cranial nerves in the posterior fossa and at the base of the brain, especially the trigeminal ganglion.

Unsuitable for children and unco-operative adults, and for long operations. Alterations in level of consciousness, fits or vomiting may occur, sometimes needing respiratory support. The patient may need restraint. Oxygen blown under the towels near the mouth prevents a feeling of suffocation. Full monitoring is used.

General anaesthesia

The brain should be soft, the veins uncongested, ICP low and CBF adequate for the cerebral metabolic rate.

Premedication

Sedative drugs, particularly narcotic analgesics, should be avoided with: (*a*) raised ICP; (*b*) head injury; and (*c*) the prone, sitting or steep head-up position with spontaneous respiration. A modest dose of temazepam will calm an anxious patient without leading to confusing postoperative drowsiness. Glycopyrrolium is a useful anti-sialogogue.

Induction

Coughing and straining can raise the venous pressure for up to half an hour, and must be avoided. Thiopentone and a short-acting opioid (fentanyl 0.2–0.3 mg) are commonly used.

The airway

Any rise in ICP on intubation may be obtunded by the opioid and perhaps an extra dose of thiopentone and/or lignocaine 1-1.5 mg/kg i.v. If the latter is used it is best given 4 min before laryngoscopy.[13] Topical analgesic spray is commonly used. It does little to prevent the rise in ICP, but helps avoid coughing and straining on the tube. A generous dose of relaxant is better in this regard and gives best conditions for laryngoscopy. Jugular venous obstruction can be caused by laryngoscopy.

Care should be taken to prevent disconnections and kinking. Reinforced tubes may be used. The tube is *securely* fixed with strapping rather than tapes, which can cause venous obstruction. IPPV is almost universal for neurosurgery, but spontaneous respiration may be used for some infra-tentorial operations if it is felt that the pattern of breathing may indicate the proximity of the surgeon to vital structures. In either case there should be no obstruction, especially to expiration. Adequate muscle relaxation means that airway pressures are kept to a minimum.

Choice of anaesthetic agents[14]

Intravenous Barbiturates. Cerebral metabolism and blood flow are reduced by similar amounts. This may amount to 30% in light (burst suppression on the EEG) and 50% in deep thiopentone anaesthesia (isoelectric EEG). The latter requires repeated administrations. There is no added advantage in giving doses higher than those needed to cause an isoelectric EEG, as metabolic activity to maintain neuronal integrity persists. Evoked potentials are unaffected. ICP is reduced. But in head injuries other agents (e.g. mannitol) are probably as good, and outcome is not improved. Thiopentone may protect the brain from incomplete ischaemia (e.g. as may occur during cerebral vascular surgery) if given in burst suppression dosage (3–7 mg/kg) before the ischaemia occurs, or by infusion shortly afterwards to equilibrate throughout the brain. Inverse steal may contribute to this protection. Haemodynamic and respiratory support are likely to be needed.[15] Barbiturates are of no value after cardiac arrest because the EEG will be flat anyway.

Other induction agents. Ketamine raises cerebral blood flow with little change in metabolic rate. It retains a place for children undergoing diagnostic radiological procedures. Midazolam suppresses cerebral metabolism to only a limited extent. Etomidate and propofol have similar effects to thiopentone, but myoclonus after etomidate may increase ICP.

Narcotic analgesics. Little effect on cerebral blood flow (CBF), and CO_2 reactivity is preserved.

Muscle relaxants. Do not penetrate the blood-brain barrier and have no direct effects on the brain. Suxamethonium increases muscle afferent discharge, which can raise CBF and ICP unless the patient is adequately anaesthetized or has been pretreated with a non-depolarizing agent. Atracurium may release histamine, and its metabolite laudanosine is a cerebral stimulant. Curare may drop the blood pressure, and pancuronium raise it. Vecuronium has no effect on the brain, and is preferred, although phenytoin therapy may increase requirements.

Nitrous oxide. 15% N_2O was used by Kety and Schmidt as the diffusible indicator in their classic measurement of CBF.[16] Little effect on cerebral metabolism, probably increases blood flow and so may increase ICP in susceptible patients. These effects are of little significance because they are readily modified by barbiturates, opiates and hyperventilation. Nitrous oxide diffuses into air-filled spaces, e.g. air embolism and perhaps the subarachnoid space after dural closure. The latter is not a problem clinically. Should be turned off if air embolism occurs. Commonly used in neurosurgery.

Isoflurane.[17] Only a mild cerebral vasodilator with little impairment of autoregulation. No increase in CBF below 1–1.5 MAC (1.15–1.7%). May increase ICP in susceptible patients, but this can be controlled by hyperventilation. No evidence that it is harmful to introduce isoflurane before lowering the $Paco_2$. Reactivity of the cerebral circulation to CO_2 is preserved or enhanced by all volatile agents.

All the volatile agents tend to decrease the amplitude and increase the latency of evoked potentials. Isoflurane decreases cerebral metabolism and the EEG becomes isoelectric at the relatively low concentration of about 2 MAC. This is similar to thiopentone, and isoflurane offers some protection against incomplete global or regional ischaemia, although some steal may occur in the latter case. Useful for carotid artery surgery, and for all intracranial surgery.

Halothane. Most potent cerebral vasodilator of the volatile agents, but decreases metabolism to a moderate degree. CBF is tripled and autoregulation abolished at 1 MAC (0.75%). The associated rise in ICP is prevented by prior reduction of $Paco_2$ to about 3.3 kPa (25 mmHg) by hyperventilation, even in patients with tumours. May worsen regional ischaemia by cerebral steal.

Enflurane. Cerebral vasodilator (less than halothane, more than isoflurane). CBF doubled at 1 MAC (1.68%). May increase ICP in susceptible patients, but this causes little problem in normal doses and with prior hyperventilation. Tends to cause EEG discharges and sometimes convulsions over about 1.5 MAC (2.5%), especially if the $Paco_2$ is low. This can be used to identify the focus in surgery for epilepsy. Little used otherwise in neurosurgery.

Thiopentone or propofol, fentanyl, vecuronium and 70% nitrous oxide plus isoflurane is a widely-used combination.

Hyperventilation

The $Paco_2$ should be lowered before introducing a volatile agent, although this is not essential with isoflurane. Many workers aim for a $Paco_2$ of about 3.5 kPa (26 mmHg). This gives near-maximal cerebral vasoconstriction, lowered ICP and an excellent surgical field. Some prefer less hyperventilation if possible. Below 2.7 kPa (20 mmHg) there is no improvement in ICP and EEG and metabolic signs of cerebral ischaemia occur, mainly because of the left-shifted dissociation curve.

High frequency ventilation may also be used, although it may be difficult to achieve such a low $Paco_2$. The brain may show less respiratory movement, and a lower mean airway pressure should cause less venous congestion.

Monitoring

In addition to the normal monitoring, invasive intra-arterial pressure measurement is used for intracranial and high spinal cord surgery. Changes in ICP and surgical manipulation, particularly in the posterior fossa, can cause profound changes in pulse and blood pressure, and so these should be reported to the surgeon. Any difference in height between the arterial pressure transducer and the brain must be considered for the calculation of cerebral perfusion pressure. It is helpful to measure body temperature and degree of neuromuscular blockade. Blood gas analysis complements oximetry and capnography. If excessive bleeding is expected, e.g. cerebral vascular surgery, or if air embolism is a possibility, a central venous line is useful.

Electrophysiological monitoring[18]

1. *Electroencephalogram.* Usually a 16-channel record on huge amounts of paper, but computer processing of the signals enables them to be presented in form useful for monitoring purposes,[19] e.g. the cerebral function analyzing monitor. Normal rhythms are: alpha (8–12 Hz, the dominant rhythm), beta (18–30 Hz), theta (4–7 Hz) delta (less than 4 Hz). As CBF drops the fast rhythms disappear, slow rhythms predominate and the voltage drops. The EEG can detect cerebral ischaemia during carotid artery surgery. *See also* Chapter 18.

2. *Sensory evoked potentials.*[20] Unlike EEGs these test specific neural pathways and are less influenced by anaesthetics, but the voltages measured are smaller and so computer averaging techniques are needed. They are difficult to record in the electrically hostile environment of an operating theatre, and are influenced by other factors such as body temperature and $Paco_2$. Agreed criteria for their interpretation do not exist.

Somatosensory (SSEP) and brainstem auditory (BAEP) evoked potentials are the most useful intra-operatively. (Visual evoked potentials show too much variation.) Used to detect: (*a*) awareness or depth of anaesthesia; and (*b*) damage to the nervous system during surgery. Characteristic positive (P) and negative (N) voltage peaks occur, e.g. N20, a negative peak in SSEPs occurring 20 ms after the stimulus (i.e. with a *latency* of 20 ms). Ischaemia, injury and inhalational anaesthetics tend to decrease SSEP amplitude and increase latency. Intravenous agents have less effect. BAEPs test brainstem pathways, e.g. during surgery for acoustic neuroma, and are short latency. SSEPs are used (especially with extradural sensors) to help check spinal cord integrity during, for example, operations to stabilize the spine. This is more reliable than the 'wake-up' test. Descending pathways also may be assessed by cortical stimulation.[21]

Control of intracranial pressure (ICP)

A raised ICP produces a tight dura and brain, and makes retraction more hazardous. Methods of reducing ICP:

1. *Hyperventilation.* Is of value for at least 24 h, until the CSF pH returns towards normal (*see* above).

2. *Diuretics.* Hyperosmotic agents: mannitol ($C_6H_{12}O_6$). A hexahydric alcohol related to the hexose sugars. An isomer of sorbitol. Solutions (e.g. 20%) can be sterilized by autoclaving. Dose 0.5–1.5 g/kg i.v. over 10–20 min, which starts to lower ICP in 5 min, is maximal at 45 min, and lasts up to 4–6 h. The larger doses are no more effective, but last longer. Shrinks brain ECF, but may also produce cerebral vasoconstriction and reduce CSF production. Lowers blood viscosity, which augments cerebral blood flow for a given perfusion pressure. Some do not give it before a bone flap is raised, to avoid tearing of bridging veins. Disadvantages: initial transient rise in blood

volume, and ICP, if given too fast; excessive fluid depletion; small rebound rise in ICP later; may increase ICP if blood–brain barrier is disrupted; and may precipitate heart failure. Often combined with a loop diuretic, e.g. frusemide 0.5–1 mg/kg. A urinary catheter is needed. Other agents, e.g. urea, have been used but damage veins and cause more rebound increase in ICP. Oral glycerol has also been used.

3. *Removal of CSF.* (Up to 150 ml.) Via a needle or catheter in the lateral ventricle. Catheters are less likely to block if drained against a pressure of about 15 mmHg. Spinal drainage is useful for aneurysm surgery, but can cause tonsillar herniation if there is a space-occupying lesion.

4. *Control of arterial and venous pressures.* Hypotensive agents and head-up tilt.

5. *Steroids.* Dexamethasone 4 mg 6-hourly gives a rapid, if temporary, clinical improvement in patients with oedema around tumours, but the reduction of ICP is often delayed. Of no value in head injuries.[22]

6. *Intravenous anaesthetics and lignocaine.* Cause cerebral vasoconstriction. The latter (1–1.5 mg/kg) is used to prevent coughing and ICP rises at intubation and extubation.

7. *Hypothermia.* Reduces ICP and provides some protection against brain ischaemia, as the ischaemic time is doubled to about 8 min at 30°C. This is achieved by surface cooling, but is rarely used now. Profound hypothermia (15°C) with cardiopulmonary bypass is still occasionally used for surgery on giant aneurysms.[23]

Postoperative care

IPPV may be necessary. Neurological deterioration may result from haematoma or oedema formation. Localizing signs are eagerly sought. Relatively few workers use routine ICP monitoring postoperatively, preferring to rely on clinical assessment and CT scanning when indicated. The need for analgesia after intracranial surgery is small. Codeine phosphate is effective and causes little sedation. Antiemetics are often needed. Phenytoin is often given after supratentorial surgery to reduce incidence of fits, although its efficacy is uncertain.[24] Hyponatraemia due to inappropriate secretion of antidiuretic hormone may follow trauma or some tumours.

PARTICULAR OPERATIONS AND PROCEDURES

Intracranial aneurysms

Operation is performed to prevent re-bleeding, which is most likely early after the first bleed. The desire for early surgery is tempered by the danger of vasospasm in the first few days, and by the poor prognosis of patients with significant neurological deficit. The sympathetic outflow after subarachnoid haemorrhage can cause asymptomatic widespread ST and T-wave changes on the ECG, which do not necessarily mean coronary artery disease and need not contra-indicate surgery. Although the CT scan may indicate the site of the aneurysm, angiography is needed to define it more precisely. Its exact site will determine the surgical approach and be important in assessing risk. Surgery is normally performed on relatively fit patients. The microscope is used. The aim is to clip the aneurysm neck. If this is not possible then wrapping with a reinforcement material or perhaps embolization or ligation of a feeding artery is performed. Hypotension is often used (*see below*). Giant aneurysms can need cardiopulmonary bypass and profound hypothermia (15°C).[23] Rupture of the aneurysm as the dissection proceeds is not uncommon, when severe blood loss will occur. Postoperative recovery can be complicated by cerebral vasospasm, hydrocephalus and hyponatraemia. Spasm can be treated by keeping the blood pressure high with fluid loading and inotropes, or with nimodipine 1–2 mg/h i.v. or 60 mg 4-hourly orally.[25] Prostaglandins and polypeptides from platelets may be factors causing vasospasm.

Controlled hypotension

Useful during the removal of vascular tumours (e.g. meningioma) as well as in aneurysm surgery. It also reduces ICP. An aneurysm becomes easier to dissect and to clip, and may be less likely to burst. The mean arterial pressure may be reduced to 50 mmHg for the placement of the clip. Nitroprusside is easily controllable, but is a cerebral vasodilator and may increase ICP slightly. Some therefore use trimetaphan before the dura is opened, because it is not a cerebral vasodilator, but this gives fixed and dilated pupils for some hours after operation. Autoregulation is impaired after induced hypotension, especially if volatile agents have been used too, and postoperative IPPV may be needed. Isoflurane and adenosine[26] are also effective hypotensive agents. For the techniques of controlled hypotension *see* Chapter 13.

Posterior fossa craniotomy

Performed in the prone, semi-prone (park-bench) or sitting position, and needs careful attention to positioning. Cerebral venous pressure is harder to keep low in the prone position or if the head is flexed. Particular hazards: (*a*) *air embolism* in the sitting position (*see below*); (*b*) *hypotension* in the sitting position. Prevented by bandaging and elevating the legs, fluids and pressor drugs; (*c*) *surgical damage to vital brainstem structures*. The pattern of spontaneous respiration has been used to indicate brainstem integrity, but the improved surgical field obtained by IPPV is striking. In the paralysed patient, proximity to these vital structures is indicated by dramatic changes in pulse, cardiac rhythm and blood pressure; (*d*) *hydrocephalus,* due to CSF obstruction in the 4th ventricle; (*e*) *cranial nerve damage.* Stimulation of the trigeminal nerve during excision of an acoustic neuroma may cause hypertension. Vagal stimulation may also occur, with bradycardia and hypotension. Damage may cause postoperative laryngeal obstruction. Glossopharyngeal damage will predispose to postoperative aspiration; and (*f*) *massive swelling of the face and tongue* may occur up to 36 hours postoperatively and obstruct the airway.[27]

Air embolism in neurosurgery

Venous air embolism is common if the patient is in the sitting position, which is also sometimes used for surgery of the cervical spine. Many veins in the occipital muscles and other tissues of the back of the neck do not collapse readily after they have been divided, but are held open, allowing air to be sucked in. The mastoid emissary vein is a particularly common site for air entry, as are the major dural sinuses. Portals of entry within the dura are relatively uncommon. For signs, diagnosis and treatment, *see* Chapter 14.

An oesophageal or precordial stethoscope may pick up the typical murmur of air in the heart, end-tidal CO_2 falls rapidly, and a Doppler ultrasonic probe over the precordium or in the oesophagus will detect small amounts of air. Diathermy interferes with the latter, so in practice it is of least value when it is most needed. Although significant amounts of air may be aspirated through a correctly-placed right atrial catheter, serious air embolism is best prevented by good surgical technique and prompt flooding of the surgical site with saline if air is suspected. N_2O should be discontinued. The cerebral venous pressure is quickly raised by compressing the jugular veins, either manually or by a special cuff around the neck.[28] PEEP is unlikely to raise the venous pressure enough. An aviation type of anti-gravity suit worn around the lower limbs and inflated to 8 kPa can raise the CVP by about 1 kPa (7.5 mmHg) for the duration of surgery, which approaches the pressure difference between the wound and the right atrium (12.5 cm of blood).[29] It is rather cumbersome to use.

A patent foramen ovale is a common (25–35%) incidental finding at post mortem,[30] but can be readily detected preoperatively by contrast Doppler echocardiography.[31] Paradoxical air embolism can occur through a PFO, because the atrial pressure gradient can reverse transiently at certain phases of the cardiac cycle, even if the mean LA pressure exceeds mean RA pressure. PEEP and infusion of colloid make little difference to the likelihood of paradoxical embolism.[32] A small bubble of air entering the left side of the heart in the sitting position is likely to enter a cerebral or coronary artery.

The only certain way of avoiding the problem of air embolism is to abandon the sitting position in neurosurgery. Although the sitting position results in less blood loss and cranial nerves may be less damaged, and the excellent conditions obtained are beloved by some surgeons, there is little evidence that ultimate clinical outcome is improved.[33]

Craniofacial surgery

The main problems are airway difficulties and heavy blood loss.

See Goat V. A. In: *Recent Advances in Anaesthesia and Analgesia–16* (Atkinson R. S. and Adams A. P. ed.) Edinburgh: Churchill Livingstone, 1989, 139.

Trans-sphenoidal surgery

Usually for pituitary tumours. Not suitable for supra-sellar extensions. Fluoroscopy and the operating microscope are used. Although operating through an unsterile part of the body, meningitis is surprisingly rare. The operation is well-tolerated, with minimal trauma and blood loss. Diabetes insipidus is uncommon. Vasoconstrictors should be applied to the nasal mucosa. The patient should be warned that the nose will be packed when he awakes. Full steroid cover is needed.

Operation for intractable epilepsy

Electrophysiological mapping of the cortex during craniotomy may be done in specialized centres under i.v. sedation and local analgesia.[34]

Carotid artery surgery[35]

The problems are: (1) elderly patients with arterial disease, associated coronary heart disease and perhaps hypertension. The patients are often taking aspirin; (2) prevention and recognition of ischaemia of the brain; and (3) reflex bradycardia from manipulations near the carotid sinus (prevented by infiltration of local analgesic, or i.v. atropine). The angiograms and transcranial Doppler studies help assess the adequacy of collateral circulation.

Regional block (cervical plexus) has been advocated because it allows continuous neurological assessment,[36] but will not prevent embolic damage. General anaesthesia is usual, and allows control of blood gases and the blood pressure. Older methods of assessing brain oxygenation include jugular venous Po_2 and 'stump' pressure (in the occluded carotid artery), and are not always satisfactory. Regional CBF, blood velocity in the middle cerebral artery and the EEG[37] can all be studied intra-operatively in some centres. Some surgeons use carotid shunts to minimize the interruption in blood supply to the brain. The blood pressure should be kept near-normal, using inotropic agents if necessary. Isoflurane may provide a measure of cerebral protection. $Paco_2$ is best kept at normal values. The neurological outcome after a period of cerebral ischaemia is probably worse if the blood sugar is high, so dextrose solutions are best avoided.[38] The place of specific measures (e.g. barbiturates) to protect the brain in this setting is uncertain. N-methyl-D-aspartate antagonists may be of value in the future.

Postoperative hypertension can be controlled by vasodilators, e.g. hydralazine 5–20 mg i.v. Lower cranial nerve palsies (IX, X and XI) may occur postoperatively.

Operations on the vertebral column

Usually performed for degenerative and disc disease, or for tumours[39] or extradural haematoma. The first operative cure of prolapsed disc was in 1934.[40] Tumours of the spinal cord may interfere with intercostal or even the phrenic nerve roots. Operations may be carried out in the lateral, prone or 'Muslim praying' position; the sitting position being used for cervical and upper thoracic operations, and supine for anterior cervical fusion.

Bleeding from extradural veins is the chief problem. Any increase in abdominal pressure, from coughing, straining or incorrect positioning, forces blood through the vertebral veins and distends them. For lumbar surgery, if the patient is supported prone with the weight on the upper chest and the pelvis so that the abdomen is free, and the lumbar spine flexed, then the extradural veins collapse. This also prevents hypotension due to vena caval obstruction. Special padded frames with an adjustable angle of flexion are available. Full relaxation helps. The arms may be placed above the head, giving excellent venous access.

IPPV is usual. Induced hypotension should not be necessary, especially if extradural block is combined with general anaesthesia. Damage to the bowel, IVC and aorta has occurred if the surgeon pierces the anterior longitudinal ligament.[41] During high spinal surgery, cardiac dysrhythmias may occur. Cervical cord surgery may be followed by sleep apnoea (Ondine's Curse).[42] The surgeon may stimulate the carotid sinus during an anterior approach to the cervical spine. Lumbar microdiscectomy has even been done as a day-case.[43]

Excision of the odontoid peg and spinal fusion may be needed in patients with rheumatoid arthritis. It is approached through the mouth. Atlanto-axial instability is also common in Down's syndrome, often asymptomatic and so a hazard for the unwary anaesthetist.[44] Lateral radiographs of the cervical spine should be performed in neck flexion and extension.

For the implications of cervical spine pathology in airway management *see* Crosby E. T. and Lui A. *Can. J. Anaesth.* 1990, **37**, 77.

Anaesthesia for diagnostic procedures

The same considerations for monitoring and control of ICP and CBF are needed as for major neurosurgery. Conditions for the anaesthetist are never easy in a radiology department.

Ketamine (2 mg/kg i.v. or 10 mg/kg i.m.) may be used for diagnostic procedures in children, e.g. CT scanning, myelography or lumbar puncture. The airway should be maintained without the need for tracheal intubation.

Cerebral angiography

Popularized by Egon Moniz[6] of Portugal of leucotomy fame in 1927. Both carotids and both vertebrals may be studied with a catheter inserted percutaneously via the femoral artery under local analgesia, perhaps with i.m. or i.v. sedation. The flushing and retrobulbar pain associated with the injection of contrast is much less with the small volumes needed for digital subtraction angiography. This also gives better pictures without the need to control the $P\text{co}_2$. Some use general anaesthesia and IPPV, believing the hypocapnia and cerebral vasoconstriction to improve the quality of the angiograms. Direct carotid puncture is performed much less commonly.

Angiographic techniques are also used in the treatment of arteriovenous malformations (embolization) or cerebral aneurysms (balloon occlusion).[45]

Myelography

First performed with Lipiodol in 1922.[46] In children this is often performed under general anaesthesia with tracheal intubation and IPPV. Changes of posture may be sudden and extreme, to encourage movement of contrast to the site of interest. The examination room may be darkened and careful monitoring is required. In adults local analgesia is used.

Computerized tomography

1. CT Scanning. First described in 1973.[47] The head must be completely still for the several seconds taken for imaging each slice. General anaesthesia may be required in unco-operative adults and young children. Ketamine is useful, or tracheal intubation and the use of a very long Bain system, allowing machine and monitors to be outside the room, with the patient in sight through a window or camera. Contrast is often given i.v. to improve scan quality.

2. MRI Scanning.[48] Nuclear magnetic resonance discovered in 1946,[49] but not used for imaging until 1973.[50] MRI exploits similar computing techniques to CT. Immobility is vital for good images. The patient is placed in a strong magnetic field (about 0.5 Tesla) and exposed to radiofrequency pulses. Protons in certain atoms, especially hydrogen, realign themselves with the magnetic field, emitting an RF signal that induces microvoltages in the detector coils. The decay of this RF signal is described by two time constants T_1 and T_2, directed with and transverse to the magnetic field respectively. Imaging is achieved by varying the field strength across the body.

X-rays are avoided, but the magnetic field can: (1) attract ferromagnetic materials inside or outside the body, e.g. older vascular clips, laryngoscope batteries, gas cylinders and anaesthetic equipment.[51] Also such materials distort the image; (2) cause malfunction of pacemaker circuits, analogue and digital watches and magnetic storage media; (3) cause T-wave changes on the ECG of no clinical significance and (4) induce tiny currents inside the body, which seem to be harmless. The scanners are claustrophobic and noisy.

The anaesthetic machine and ventilator are best placed remotely, and a long circuit used with a suitably low expiratory resistance. A coaxial circuit may need modifying to achieve this. Monitoring is difficult as even non-ferromagnetic wire connections to the patient may degrade the image, but methods include: apnoea mattress; capnography sampling through a long capillary; non-invasive blood pressure using long connectors; pulse oximetry is often possible. Equipment placed in high magnetic fields needs special design.[52] The patient has to be removed from the body of the scanner in an emergency.

3. Positron emission tomography (PET). Not in widespread clinical use.

Thermocoagulation of the roots of the trigeminal nerve

Hypertension and dysrhythmias may occur.

Electroconvulsive therapy (ECT)[53]

Convulsions were first used in psychiatry in 1934 by Meduna of Budapest, who employed a relative overdose of cardiazol.[54] Cerletti and Bini induced them electrically in 1938;[55] Bennett used curare in 1940[56] before its use in anaesthesia, to modify cardiazol-induced convulsions; Holmberg and Thesleff used suxamethonium in 1951.[57] For ECT machines, *see* Mikhail W. I. et al. *Br. J. Hosp. Med.* 1984, **31**, 369.

Relative contra-indications

(1) Myocardial infarct or major cerebrovascular accident within 3 months; (2) congestive cardiac failure; (3) severe osteoporosis or a major fracture; and (4) raised intracranial pressure. Pulse rate, blood pressure, cardiac output and catecholamine levels rise during the fit[58] and ventricular arrhythmias may be seen, although severe bradycardia or even asystole can occur just after the passage of the electric current. These circulatory changes are no worse than those following defaecation or coughing, and are usually well tolerated, even in hypertensives and other patients with mild heart disease. Esmolol 100 mg has been used to obtund them.[59] In mid-pregnancy, ECT does not appear to harm the fetus.[60] Well tolerated in old age. Postictal confusion may occur. For ECT in patients with a pacemaker, *see* Jauhar P. et al. *Br. Med. J.* 1979, **1**, 90.

Technique

Atropine premedication (0.3–0.4 mg i.v.) may be given to prevent the initial bradycardia. Then thiopentone (2 mg/kg) or methohexitone (1 mg/kg) is given i.v., followed by suxamethonium 25–40 mg. The use of propofol (1.5 mg/kg) is controversial. Although reported to have convulsant properties,[61] it has also been used to control status epilepticus[62] and shortens the duration of the fit of ECT.[63] It is not clear whether this reduces the efficacy of treatment. When muscle fasciculation ceases, the lungs are inflated with oxygen and the electric current is applied. In the absence of limb movements, a modified convulsion is likely if: (1) there is a pilomotor reaction (seen in half the patients); and (2) the pupil fails to contract when inspected or hippus is seen. Ventilation by face-mask is continued until muscle power has returned. Monitoring is difficult during the fit.

Any damage to teeth and lips is likely to occur during the passage of the current rather than during the convulsion, because the stimulus produces maximal direct stimulation of the muscles of mastication, unmodified by neuromuscular blockade. Teeth should be separated by a suitable rubber bite block. Pain after suxamethonium is rare. Prolapsed disc and long bone fracture can occur. A ruptured urinary bladder has been reported following ECT.[64]

BRAIN PROTECTION

Various measures have been put forward to 'protect' the brain from ischaemic insults.[65] Hypothermia is the only established intervention that does so.

Cerebral oxygen consumption falls progressively with temperature, and the EEG becomes isoelectric below about 21°C. Enough barbiturate will produce a flat EEG, but cerebral oxygen consumption can only be reduced by about 50%. Isoflurane behaves similarly. Both barbiturates and isoflurane may offer some protection against incomplete ischaemia.

None of these agents have been useful given *after* an ischaemic insult. Calcium channel blockers (nimodipine), free radical scavengers and NMDA (*N*-methyl-D-aspartate) receptor antagonists are all under investigation. ICP and blood glucose should be carefully controlled.

See also Rogers M. C. and Kirsch J. R. *JAMA* 1989, **261**, 3143; Murdoch J. and Hall R. I. *Can. J. Anaesth.* 1990, **37**, 663 and 762.

MANAGEMENT OF ACUTE HEAD INJURIES[66]

The brain may be damaged by contusion, haemorrhage, oedema and microscopic diffuse axonal injury. The latter is important for long-term prognosis.

Initial treatment

First aid – airway management (lateral position because vomiting is likely), control of haemorrhage, speedy hospitalization. The first few minutes after the injury are crucial in determining the ultimate outcome. Subsequent treatment is then directed towards prevention of further brain injury.

1. Ventilation and adequacy of the airway are assessed. Oxygenation of the brain must be maintained. If tracheal intubation is needed it should be performed as a rapid sequence induction, after pre-oxygenation, thiopentone and suxamethonium, and with cricoid pressure. The provision of the best conditions for intubation is less important than any transient rise in ICP after suxamethonium. Nasal tubes should be avoided if CSF drainage from the mouth, nose or ears suggests a base of skull fracture, because they can be passed into the cranial cavity by mistake. Precautions should be taken in case of instability of the cervical spine (radiography if there is time; immobilization of the neck if there is not). The chest should be examined for injury; a chest drain may be indicated to prevent a tension pneumothorax. If sedation is needed for a ventilated patient, a propofol infusion 3 mg/kg/h is satisfactory, with a relaxant if needed.[67]

2. Blood gases. Hypoxia, hypercapnia and acidosis must be avoided. IPPV should be used early to correct any deterioration in blood gases. Neurogenic pulmonary oedema (NPO) is a rare complication of head injury, and is treated by IPPV, control of ICP and vasodilators to counteract the intense sympathetic outflow, which causes NPO.

3. Circulation. Arrest any serious haemorrhage and maintain an adequate blood pressure. Blood loss from scalp wounds may require transfusion. It may not be wise to insert a CVP line from the neck if this is also injured. Disturbances of body temperature, fluid balance and fat embolism may occur.

4. *Neurology.* Assess level of consciousness by the Glasgow Coma Scale,[68] which uses the best verbal and motor responses on scales of 1 to 5, and eye opening on a scale of 1 to 4. The total score can thus range from 3 to 14. Look for lateralizing signs (limb movements, pupil sizes and reflexes). CT or MRI scans[69] if available. IPPV may be needed to control decerebrate spasms. Hypothermia, barbiturates[70] and steroids[22] have no place in head injuries.

5. *Associated injuries.* Should be sought, especially to the neck. The patient may have taken drugs or alcohol. Uncomplicated head injury should not prevent the urgent treatment of abdominal injuries, compound limb fractures or haemothorax, although treatment of faciomaxillary fractures can usually be delayed.

6. *Control of ICP.* Many centres insert an ICP monitor (*see above*) if the Glasgow Coma Scale Score is 8 or less. It also allows assessment of ICP waveform,[71] cranial compliance and the importance of a small haematoma. It cannot reflect regional variations in ICP, however, and there is little evidence that measurement of ICP improves outcome.[72] IPPV to a $Paco_2$ of 4–4.5 kPa (30–34 mmHg) is recommended. One has to weigh the possible reduction in ICP against ischaemia caused by the cerebral vasoconstriction. Lower values of $Paco_2$ have no benefit. Mannitol 0.5–1.0 g/kg is effective, but for a limited time.

7. *Fits.* May be overt, or seen on the EEG of a paralysed patient. Voltage on the cerebral function monitor should be 5–15 µV. (Less may indicate ischaemia.) Fits markedly increase the brain's need for oxygen and must be controlled with barbiturates, phenytoin or benzodiazepines. IPPV may well be needed if large doses are used.

8. *Blood sugar.* The dangers of hypoglycaemia are well-known, but hyperglycaemia may increase the brain damage after ischaemic episodes.[38]

Anaesthesia for acute head injury surgery

Anaesthesia may be required for diagnostic procedures, evacuation of haematoma, elevation of a depressed fracture or for other associated injuries. There may be considerable blood loss. Pain relief may also be required after non-cranial surgery in the presence of a head injury.

Each case needs individual assessment. Special care will be needed over the ICP, airway (there may be bleeding into the airway with a fractured base of skull), ventilation, full stomach, aspiration, hypovolaemia and associated injuries. An antacid regime is used if the patient is conscious. A rapid sequence induction and tracheal intubation is usually indicated. Fractures through the base of the skull or the sinuses may allow pneumoencephalus if face-mask ventilation is used, which may worsen with nitrous oxide.[73]

Intracranial haematoma

May be extradural, often from the middle meningeal artery, subdural or intracerebral. Urgent operation is especially needed for the first. The results can be dramatic. Physical signs are a progressive: (1) increase in coma score; (2) dilatation of a pupil; (3) bradycardia and hypertension; and (4) hemiparesis opposite to the side of the injury. Confirmed by CT scan. If the clinical picture progresses to apnoea, the prognosis is grave, even when instantly remedied by IPPV. Burr-holes under local analgesia may be performed with success, but formal craniotomy is often needed immediately after CT scanning.

Transportation of patients with head injuries[74]

The airway must be secure. Tracheal intubation is preferable if in any doubt, because this will be much more difficult if it has to be performed during the journey. Facilities must be carried for intubation and IPPV with oxygen in all cases (tubes can fall out). Suction equipment must be available. Propofol infusions are useful for control of the patient during transport.

An intravenous cannula is sited before leaving, with a pressure infusor because head-room is limited in an ambulance. ECG, pulse and blood pressure should be monitored, although the latter may be difficult. Normal drugs for resuscitation should be available, as well as thiopentone, suxamethonium, steroids and diuretics. The doctor and nurse may be advised to take travel sickness pills!

Prognosis

The long-term effects of head injury can seldom be assessed at the time of admission to the intensive therapy unit. In general, younger patients have a better prognosis. Of those patients in coma for 6 h or more, mortality is around 50%. Permanent disability may result. Even if physical recovery is good, social and personality problems may arise.

Brainstem death[75]

First described clinically in 1959,[76] and more recently challenged.[77] For this diagnosis *all* the following signs must be present, in addition to a clear diagnosis of the underlying condition,[78] for at least 12 h: pupils have no response to light. Caloric and oculovestibular reflex absent. (There should be no wax in the ear.) The 'doll's-eye reflex' does not mean that there is brainstem death. Absent corneal, gag and carinal reflexes. No response to pain inflicted on head. No spontaneous respiration for 4 min in the absence of hypothermia and hypoxia, with a $Paco_2$ of 6.7 kPa (50 mmHg) or more, provided that no drugs that affect these reflexes persist in the body. If blood gas analysis is not available, ventilate with 100% oxygen for 10 min and then 5% CO_2 in oxygen for 5 min before disconnection.

In the UK the diagnosis is made by two senior doctors independently, the interval between such examinations depending on the clinical situation. The time of death is at completion of the last test. Other countries differ, e.g. in France the two examinations must be performed at least 24 hours apart. Spinal reflexes may persist after brainstem death. EEG or cerebral angiography can confirm brainstem death. This is not necessary in the UK, but is more often used in the USA.

***Brainstem death and organ donation.*[79]**

Problems in the management of the brain dead for organ donation are hypotension, arrhythmias, oliguria, diabetes insipidus and coagulopathy. The 'rule of 100's' is useful:[80] keep systolic blood pressure over 100 mmHg using volume loading and, if needed, dopamine up to 5–10 µg/kg/min; keep urine output over 100 ml/h by maintaining the cardiac output, dopamine infusion and frusemide 20–40 mg; keep Pao_2 over 13.3 kPa (100 mmHg), and haemoglobin over 100 g/l. Some details vary with the organ(s) to be retrieved. For the lung, any tracheal suction should be performed in a sterile manner, oxygen toxicity avoided and 5 cmH$_2$O PEEP used to prevent atelectasis. For the kidney, give mannitol 0.5 g/kg before excision to ensure good urine flow. For the heart or heart/lungs, the donor may be put on total bypass and hypothermia, or *in situ* or bench perfusion used.[81]

ANAESTHESIA AND SPINAL CORD INJURY

If the patient's lowest functional root is C5 he is totally dependent on others; if it is C7 he has enough use of his arms to be more independent. Vital capacity is an important measure of respiratory reserve. If below 1 l, postoperative respiratory support is likely to be needed. Hypotension may need pressor drugs. Neurogenic pulmonary oedema may be seen after high cord injuries. Non-particulate antacids and H$_2$ antagonists are normally given as prophylaxis against gastro-intestinal bleeding.

After the stage of spinal shock (which can last up to several weeks) *autonomic hyperreflexia*[82] may result from painful stimuli, transurethral surgery, bladder distension, etc. There is vasodilatation above the injury, and constriction below. Hypertension, bradycardia, arrhythmias and even myocardial ischaemia can occur. General anaesthesia can also precipitate this response, and spinal blockade may be preferable, although its height can be difficult to predict. From about 1 week after the injury until several months later, *suxamethonium* may cause dangerous hyperkalaemia.[83]

See also Alderson J. D. and Frost E. A. M. *Spinal Cord Injuries: Anaesthetic and Associated Care.* Oxford: Butterworth-Heinemann, 1990.

References

1. Campkin T. V. and Turner J. M. *Neurosurgical Anaesthesia and Intensive Care*, 2nd ed. London: Butterworth, 1986; Michenfelder J. D. *Anesthesia and the Brain.* New York: Churchill Livingstone, 1988; *Clinical Neuroanesthesia* (Cucchiara R. F. and Michenfelder J. D. eds.) New York: Churchill Livingstone, 1990.
2. Bennett A. H. and Godlee R. J. *Med. Chirurg. Trans.* 1885, **68**, 243.
3. Cushing H. *Surg. Gynecol. Obstet.* 1928, **47**, 751.
4. Dandy W. *Ann. Surg.* 1918, **68**, 5.
5. Dandy W. *Ann. Surg.* 1919, **70**, 397.
6. Moniz E. *Rev. Neurol.* 1927, **2**, 72.
7. Dott N. M. (1897–1974) *Trans. Med.-chir. Soc. Edinb.* 1932, n.s. **47**, 219.

8. Walter W. G. *Lancet* 1936, **2**, 305.
9. Moore G. E. *J. Neurosurg.* 1948, **5**, 392.
10. Cushing. H. *Boston Med. Surg. J.* 1903, **148**, 250; Beecher H. K. *Surg. Gynecol. Obstet.* 1940, **71**, 689.
11. Hunter A. R. *Anaesthesia* 1983, **38**, 1214.
12. North B. and Reilly P. *Raised Intracranial Pressure.* Oxford: Butterworth-Heinemann, 1990.
13. Wilson I. G. et al. *Anaesthesia* 1991, **46**, 177.
14. Michenfelder J. D. *Anesthesia and the Brain.* New York: Churchill Livingstone, 1988.
15. Nussmeier N. A. et al. *Anesthesiology* 1986, **64**, 165.
16. Kety S. S. and Schmidt C. F. *J. Clin. Invest.* 1948, **27**, 476.
17. Moss E. *Br. J. Anaesth.* 1988, **63**, 4.
18. Electrophysiology and Anesthetic Practice. *Int. Anesthesiol. Clin.* 1990, **28**(3).
19. Thomsen C. E. et al. *Br. J. Anaesth.* 1988, **63**, 36.
20. Lam A. M. *Can. J. Anaesth.* 1987, **34**, S32.
21. Loughnan B. A. and Hall G. M. *Br. J. Anaesth.* 1989, **63**, 587.
22. Braakman R. et al. *J. Neurosurg.* 1983, **58**, 326; Dearden N. M. et al. *J. Neurosurg.* 1986, **64**, 81.
23. Spetzler R. F. et al. *J. Neurosurg.* 1988, **68**, 868; Thomas A. N. et al. *Anaesthesia* 1990, **45**, 383.
24. Shaw M. D. M. and Foy P. M. *J. Roy. Soc. Med.* 1991, **84**, 221.
25. Pickard J. D. et al. *Br. Med. J.* 1989, **298**, 636.
26. Lagerkranser M. et al. *Acta Anaesthesiol. Scand.* 1989, **33**, 15.
27. Howard R. et al. *Anaesthesia* 1990, **45**, 222.
28. Sale J. P. *Anaesthesia* 1984, **39**, 795; Pfitzner J. and McLean A. G. *Anaesthesia* 1985, **40**, 624.
29. Brodrick P. M. and Ingram G. S. *Anaesthesia* 1988, **43**, 762.
30. Thompson T. and Evans D. C. *Q. J. Med.* 1930, **23**, 135.
31. Konstadt S. N. et al. *Anesthesiology* 1991, **74**, 212.
32. Black S. et al. *Anesthesiology* 1989, **71**, 235.
33. Black S. et al. *Anesthesiology* 1988, **69**, 49.
34. Archer D. P. et al. *Can. J. Anaesth.* 1988, **35**, 338.
35. Cebul R. D. and Whisnant J. P. *Ann. Intern. Med.* 1989, **111**, 660.
36. Luosto R. et al. *Scand. J. Thorac. Cardiovasc. Surg.* 1984, **18**, 133.
37. McFarland H. R. et al. *J. Cardiovasc. Surg.* 1988, **29**, 12.
38. Fitch W. In: *Anaesthesia Review 5* (Kaufman L. ed.) Edinburgh: Churchill Livingstone, 1988, 119; Nakakimura K. et al. *Anesthesiology* 1990, **72**, 1005.
39. Tindall S. *Anesth. Analg.* 1987, **66**, 894.
40. Mixer W. J. and Barr J. S. *N. Engl. J. Med.* 1934, **211**, 210.
41. Ewah B. and Calder I. *Br. J. Anaesth.* 1991, **66**, 721.
42. Vella L. M. et al. *Anaesthesia* 1984, **39**, 108.
43. Editorial. *Lancet* 1988, **1**, 394.
44. Editorial. *Lancet* 1989, **i**, 24; Powell J. F. et al. *Anaesthesia* 1990, **45**, 1049.
45. Molyneux A. J. *Hosp. Update* 1990, **16**, 683.
46. Sicard J. A. and Forestier J. *J. Neurosurg.* 1922, **20**, 721.
47. Hounsfield G. N. *Br. J. Radiol.* 1973, **46**, 1016 and Ambrose J. p.1023; New P. F. J. et al. *Radiology* 1974, **110**, 109.
48. Menon D. K. et al. *Anaesthesia* 1992, **47**, 240; Peden C. J. et al. *Anaesthesia* 1992, **47**, 508.
49. Purcell E. M. et al. and Bloch F. et al. *Phys. Rev.* 1946, **69**, 37 and 127.
50. Lauterbur P. *Nature* 1973, **242**, 190.
51. New P. F. J. et al. *Radiology* 1983, **147**, 139.
52. Ramsay J. G. et al. *Br. J. Anaesth.* 1986, **58**, 1181.
53. Selvin B. L. *Anesthesiology* 1987, **67**, 367.
54. Major R. H. *History of Medicine.* Springfield, Ill.: Thomas, 1954, **2**.
55. Cerletti U. and Bini L. *Boll. Atti Acad. Med.* 1938, **64**, 136.
56. Bennett A. E. *JAMA* 1940, **114**, 322.
57. Holmberg A. G. and Thesleff S. *Nord. Med.* 1951, **46**, 1567.

58. Wells D. G. and Davies G. G. *Anesth. Analg.* 1987, **66**, 1193.
59. Kovac A. L. et al. *Can. J. Anaesth.* 1991, **38**, 204.
60. Views, *Br. Med. J.* 1984, **288**, 1239; Repke J. T. and Berger N.G. *Obstet. Gynecol.* 1984, **63**, 39S.
61. Shearer E. S. *Anaesthesia* 1990, **45**, 255.
62. Mackenzie S. J. et al. *Anaesthesia* 1990, **45**, 1043.
63. Dwyer R. et al. *Anaesthesia* 1988, **43**, 459; Rampton A. J. et al. *Anesthesiology* 1989, **70**, 412; Boey W. K. and Lai F. O. *Anaesthesia* 1990, **45**, 623.
64. Irving A. D. and Drayson A. M. *Br. Med. J.* 1984, **288**, 194.
65. Michenfelder J. D. *Anesthesia and the Brain.* New York: Churchill Livingstone, 1988, 181.
66. Coonan T. J. *Can. J. Anaesth.* 1989, **36**, S26.
67. Farling P. A. et al. *Anaesthesia* 1989, **44**, 222.
68. Teasdale G. and Jennett W. B. *Lancet* 1974, **2**, 81.
69. Jenkins A. et al. *Lancet* 1986, **2**, 445.
70. Ward J. D. et al. *J. Neurosurg.* 1985, **62**, 383.
71. Lin E. S. et al. *Br. J. Anaesth.* 1991, **66**, 476.
72. Gelpke G. J. et al. *J. Neurosurg.* 1983, **59**, 745.
73. Finch M. D. and Morgan G. A. R. *Anaesthesia* 1991, **46**, 385.
74. Andrews P. J. D. et al. *Lancet* 1990, **335**, 327; Gentleman D. and Jennett B. *Lancet* 1990, **335**, 330.
75. Conference of the Royal Colleges and Faculties, *Br. Med. J.* 1976, **2**, 1187; *Lancet* 1979, **i**, 261; Report of Ad hoc Committee of the Harvard Medical School. *JAMA* 1977, **237**, 982; Searle J. and Collins C. *Lancet* 1980, **i**, 641; Jennett B. *Br. J. Anaesth.* 1981, **53**, 1111.
76. Mollaret P. and Goulon M. *Rev. Neurol.* 1959, **101**, 3.
77. Hill D. J. In: *Intensive Care: Developments and Controversies* Dobb G. J. (ed.) *Clin. Anaesthesiol.* 1990, **4**(2), 601.
78. e.g. Coad N. R. and Byrne A. J. *Anaesthesia* 1990, **45**, 456.
79. Bodenham A. et al. *Br. Med. J.* 1989, **299**, 1009.
80. Gelb A. W. and Robertson K. M. *Can. J. Anaesth.* 1990, **37**, 806.
81. Ghosh S. et al. *Anaesthesia* 1990, **45**, 672.
82. Schonwald G. et al. *Anesthesiology* 1981, **55**, 550.
83. Fraser A. and Edmonds-Seal J. *Anaesthesia* 1982, **37**, 1084.

Obstetrics and gynaecology

OBSTETRIC ANAESTHESIA AND ANALGESIA

History

Non-pharmacological methods. Hypnosis has been used periodically since Anton Mesmer first wrote about it in 1777, and childbirth without pain, employing *relaxation* and a *naturalistic* approach, is an old and frequently revived technique (Grantley Dick-Read, 1890–1959).[1]

The *decompression suit* was proposed in 1959.

Sedatives and analgesics. During the last century, *chloral hydrate* (Liebreich 1869), *tincture of opium* and *bromide* formed a popular analgesic mixture, designed to encourage sleep, rather than to relieve pain. This gave place to *barbiturates* in the years following the introduction of barbitone by Emil Fischer and von Mering in 1903. Phenobarbitone appeared in 1912,[2] Pernocton[3] and pentobarbitone[3] came later[4], and Somnifaine in 1924.[5]

Morphine has been used with success in labour[6] since its isolation by Serturner in 1806; fetal respiratory depression is its chief disadvantage. It was hoped, in vain, that papaveretum would be without this stigma.[7] It was first used in obstetrics by Jaeger in 1910.[8]

Morphine and hyoscine were used in the technique of Dammerschlaf (twilight sleep) by von Steinbuchel of Graz[9] and by Carl Joseph Gauss of Freiburg, later of Würzburg,[10] following the use of the mixture as a true anaesthetic.[11] *Hyoscine* alone was used in large doses in 1928,[12] but it produced far too much restlessness (the central anticholinergic syndrome[13]). *Pethidine* was used by Benthin in Germany in 1940. Naloxone, a major advance in the treatment of respiratory depression in mothers and infants, was first used by Clark in 1971.[14]

Ketamine was first used in obstetrics by Akamatsu in 1974.[15]

Agents introduced into the rectum to relieve the pains of labour started in 1847[16] when ether was employed. *Ether and oil* had a vogue;[17] *bromethol* was first used in 1927 and was closely followed by paraldehyde.[18] Various drugs of the *phenothiazine* group have been used, and promazine was for a time popular. Synergistic prescriptions of drugs, such as rectal oil ether, morphine and magnesium sulphate, were at one time warmly recommended.[19] *Diazepam* was investigated by Bepko.

See also Gaton D. *Anesthesiology* 1977, **46**, 132.

Regional techniques. Soon after Bier gave the first intradural spinal block in 1898, it was used in labour.[20] The so-called controlled 'spinal' was used in 1928.[21] Saddle block was described in 1946.[22] Sacral extradural block was described for use in labour by Stoeckel,[23] *paracervical block* by Gellert[24] and *paravertebral block* of T11 and T12 by Cleland.[25] Eugen Bogdan (1899–1975) of Bucharest worked out the afferent pathways of labour pains[26] and gave continuous extradural sacral cinchocaine in 1931.[27] This work was independent of that of Cleland. Lumbar extradural analgesia was described in 1928.[28] and *continuous caudal* (sacral extradural) block in 1938.[29] This was ably popularized by R. A. Hingson.[30] *Continuous lumbar extradural* block was reported some time later.[31]

Pudendal block was first described by Muller in 1908.

Inhalation methods. Ether was the first and was given by J. Y. Simpson on 19 January 1847.[32] The following year, Walter Channing, Professor of Obstetrics at Harvard, published his book *A Treatise on Etherisation in Childbirth*, illustrated by 581 cases.

Chloroform was proposed as a substitute for ether, also by Simpson[33] and he gave it for the first time on 8 November 1847. When Scottish Calvinists objected on moral[34] and scriptural grounds to the relief of pain in labour (Genesis, 3, 17: "In sorrow shall thou bring forth children"), Simpson quoted to them, knowing his Bible, Genesis, 2, 21: "And the Lord God caused a deep sleep to fall on Adam, and he slept, and He took one of his ribs and closed up the side instead, thereof". Simpson thus yielded up the pride of place as the first obstetric anaesthetist to God. Pain relief in labour only became really respectable when John Snow gave chloroform to Queen Victoria during the birth of her eighth child, Prince Leopold, in 1853 (*narcose à la reine*), a technique described in his book *On Chloroform and Other Anaesthetics* (*see also* the 7th edition of this Synopsis). The most common way of administration was the open drop method or by blowing air over chloroform vapour.[35, 36] The drug was first used in the USA by A. K. Gardner in 1848. *Divinyl ether* was used by Wesley Bourne in 1935.[37] *Cyclopropane* had a short popularity in obstetrics just as it had in general surgery, especially in Montreal and Madison.[38] *Trichloroethylene* was found to be a useful analgesic in labour soon after its first use in surgery and early reports came from Barnet[39] and from London[40] *Nitrous oxide* has had a long reign and is still a valuable analgesic today. First used in 1880[41] it was revived in 1915.[42] A method of self-administration was described by that pioneer of anaesthesia, Guedel.[43] Yet another advance was the introduction of the gas air machine by R. J. Minnitt (1890–1974) of Liverpool[44] and its modifications. This method of self-administration held the field in the UK for some years but was given up because it could well cause fetal hypoxia. *Nitrous oxide with oxygen* was used in 1949[45] and the pre-mix of nitrous oxide and oxygen in equal volumes (Entonox) was advocated by Tunstall in 1961[46] and is extensively used today. *Methoxyflurane* has been found to be safe when given in a low concentration for short periods.[47] The Leboyer technique calls for calm, and soft music at delivery.[48] Underwater delivery also had some popularity.

First Caesarean section, with a surviving mother, in England took place in Lancashire by James Barlow, in 1793.

Important concepts in the history of obstetric analgesia include the description of the *supine hypotensive syndrome*,[49] the description of the *acid aspiration syndrome*[50] and one easy way of reducing the effects of this by routine administration of an antacid mixture before anaesthesia.[51]

Safe and pain-free childbirth is a dream for the future rather than a reality today. This long catalogue of worthy effort, extending back for more than a hundred and forty years, will surely be added to in the days to come.

Fetoscopy was first performed by Scrimgeour in 1973.[52] Amniocentesis was done as early as 1930.[53]

See also Poppers P. J. The history and development of obstetric anaesthesia. In: *Anaesthesia, Essays on its History* (Rupreht J. et al. ed.) Berlin: Springer-Verlag, 1985.

Pregnancy

Pregnancy and labour produce remarkable physiological and psychological changes in the mother.

1. Circulatory system. The enlarged uterus pushes the diaphragm upwards. This results in a change in position of the heart, which is lifted upwards, shifted to the left and anteriorly, and rotated towards a transverse position. The electrocardiogram may show a large Q-wave and inverted T-waves in Lead III. Heart rate increases during pregnancy, reaching a peak between 28 and 36 weeks to about 10–12 beats above normal. There is a significant increase in cardiac output, which reaches a peak 30–50% above normal at term.[54] Whereas the healthy heart compensates well for these changes, the diseased heart may be severely taxed. Peripheral resistance is reduced in pregnancy, and mean blood pressure reaches its lowest point at the time of maximal cardiac output. Venous pressure is normal, except where the gravid uterus may compress the inferior vena cava. Blood volume is increased, plasma volume more than red cell volume, so that haematocrit falls, and uterine blood flow is markedly increased.

2. *Respiratory system.* Upward displacement of the diaphragm results in decrease of vertical diameter of the thorax and increase in transverse diameter. X-rays show increased lung markings probably due to an increase of blood volume in the pulmonary vessels. Minute ventilation rises to levels of 50% above normal. Both the diaphragmatic and the thoracic excursion is increased, at least in the upright position. Functional residual capacity is decreased from the 20th week. Closing volume is greater than functional residual capacity in about half of women in late pregnancy.[55] $Paco_2$ falls by the 12th week of pregnancy to about 4 kPa (30 mmHg) and stays low until term. Pao_2 is sometimes reduced at term and may be higher in the sitting than in the supine position.[56] Oxygen consumption rises during the last trimester due to the metabolic needs of the uterus, placenta and fetus. Basal metabolic rate is increased by about 15%. Smoking during pregnancy is associated with smaller babies and higher perinatal mortality.[57] Carboxyhaemoglobin may be a factor.

3. *Fluids and electrolytes.* Water and salt retention occur. Probably related to the secretion of steroids by the placenta.

4. *Endocrine glands.* There is hyperplasia of the anterior pituitary, thyroid and adrenal cortex.

5. *Psychology.* The impact of pregnancy and parturition may have a considerable emotional effect.

For discussion of the altered pharmacokinetics and adverse reactions to drugs used in pregnancy, *see Br. J. Hosp. Med.* 1982, **28**, 559.

There is no evidence that nitrous oxide should not be given in early pregnancy.[58]

Supine hypotensive syndrome of late pregnancy[59]

This is a condition of circulatory depression due to diminished venous return caused by the gravid uterus pressing on the inferior vena cava and perhaps the aorta. Most patients compensate by blood flowing through the azygos system via the paravertebral veins (not possible if an adrenaline containing local analgesic solution has constricted them). It is relieved by a pillow under one side or the adoption of the lateral position.

Analgesia in vaginal delivery

The ideal procedure should: (1) produce efficient relief from pain, with consciousness between pains and good co-operation from the patient; (2) not depress the respiration of the fetus; (3) not depress the uterus, causing prolonged labour; (4) be non-toxic; and (5) be safe for mother and child.

No agent at present in use fulfils all these conditions. Analgesia is not necessary in every case of labour and sympathetic explanation may be all that is required.

I. Non-pharmacological methods

Since drugs administered may cross the placenta to depress the fetus, any method that avoids or restricts their use deserves attention.

1. *'Natural childbirth'*. A naturalistic approach with emphasis on the attainment of relaxation of muscles. Patients are taught the art of relaxation and given exercises in a course of lectures and demonstrations.[60] Psychoprophylaxis in labour (Lamaze preparation).[61]

2. *Transcutaneous nerve stimulation (TENS)*. Beneficial in an important group of patients[62] with moderate to severe contraction pains in an otherwise reasonably normal labour. This technique is rapidly gaining ground in Europe because it is easy to apply, totally non-toxic, and frequently effective. Commonly, four electrodes are placed, one either side of the spine in the lower thoracic region (T10) and one either side of the spine at the sacral area. The patient may control up to three levels of intensity of stimulus, and can switch off if she wishes. Some patients find mental concentration difficult while TENS is operating.

3. *Decompression suit*.[63]

4. *Hypnosis*.

II. Sedatives and analgesics

1. *Simple oral sedatives*. Chloral hydrate, a soporific and mild analgesic, is excreted by the kidneys. A safe dose is 2 g. Can be given in tablet form as dichloralphenazone (Welldorm) or as trichlorethyl phosphate (Triclofos).

2. *Opioids*. The English National Board for Midwifery allow pethidine to be used by midwives acting alone if certain rules are observed. It depresses fetal respiration, increases uterine activity and relaxes spasm of the cervix. It is very useful in cases with a rigid, slowly dilating os. Fetal depression due to pethidine can be reversed by intramuscular injection of naloxone 200 μg.[64] Morphine is also used. In small doses, it increases the intervals between pains; in larger doses it may depress contractions.

3. *Diazepam*.[65] Rapidly crosses the placenta. Produces amnesia and reduces maternal apprehension without causing untoward effect on the fetus in reasonable dosage. Dose: 0.1–0.3 mg/kg i.m., not normally exceeding 30 mg.[66] Dose: 5–10 mg i.v. It is not an analgesic drug.

PLACENTAL TRANSFER OF DRUGS

All drugs found in maternal blood cross the placenta to some extent unless they are altered or destroyed in passage, especially those with a high lipid solubility and low degree of ionization.[67] Placental vascular activity and metabolism also play a part.

III. Regional analgesia[68]

AUTONOMIC NERVE SUPPLY OF UTERUS

1. Sympathetic (motor to upper uterine segment). The middle thoracic segments from T6 downwards, perhaps as low as L2, via splanchnic nerves and coeliac, aortic, renal and hypogastric plexuses, and thence with blood vessels to the great cervical ganglion of Frankenhauser. In addition, some of the motor supply of the body of the uterus may come from below the sensory supply, i.e. T11–L2.

2. Visceral afferent (sensory from uterus).[25, 69] Block of these eases pain of the first stage of labour, with the exception of those near the end of this stage. Eleventh and 12th thoracic (and possibly 1st lumbar). Fibres go from uterus (ganglion of Frankenhauser) via sympathetic nerves to pelvic, hypogastric and aortic plexuses, enter the sympathetic chain at the level of L5 and ascend in the chain, entering the cord via the white rami of T11 and T12, and the 11th–12th posterior thoracic roots and thence up posterior columns of cord. Block of the sympathetic chain between L5 and T12 gives the same freedom from first-stage labour pains as block of the 11th–12th thoracic ganglia.

3. Visceral afferent and efferent parasympathetic (inhibitory to uterus; sensory and motor to cervix). Second, 3rd and 4th sacral nerves, directly to great cervical ganglion of Frankenhauser.

SOMATIC AFFERENT NERVES OF LOWER BIRTH CANAL

The inferior rectal, perineal and dorsal nerve of the clitoris – from the pudendal nerve (S2, 3, 4). The ilio-inguinal (L1) and the genitofemoral (L1, 2). There are twenty nerves transmitting labour pains, namely: (1) the visceral afferents of the 11th and 12th thoracic – pain of uterine contraction; (2) the posterior roots of the 2nd, 3rd and 4th sacral nerves, carrying pelvic afferents (Henry Head, 1861–1940) – pain of cervical dilatation; (3) The rectal, perineal and pudendal branches of the sacral plexus – pain of perineal stretching; and (4) the ilio-inguinal and genitofemoral branches of the lumbar plexus.

With all forms of regional block, blood pressure fall must be avoided because of the risk of fetal hypoxia, and to prevent this, the patient should be nursed in the lateral position or a wedge used to prevent caval compression. If it occurs the legs should be elevated, plasma-volume expander infused and oxygen administered. Pressure should not be allowed to fall below 90 mmHg. The initial and most useful treatment of hypotension is the rapid infusion of a plasma-volume expander. Pressor drugs do not necessarily improve the blood flow to the uterus. It is best to avoid the α-stimulating pressor drugs. Recommended are ephedrine 12–25 mg i.v. or metaraminol as an intravenous drip. Intravenous injection of ergometrine soon after a patient has received a vasopressor may cause dangerous hypertension.

The postpartum uterus contracts well. Obstetric paralysis due to pressure of the fetal head or the forceps on the lumbosacral trunk may occur even with intradural or extradural analgesia Neuropathy if due to the block itself is likely to be bilateral and to have a segmental (radicular) rather than a peripheral distribution.

1. Subarachnoid block (intradural, 'spinal')[70] (*see also* Chapter 25).

Can be used for mid or low forceps extraction, for Caesarean section or for normal delivery. For normal delivery or for outlet forceps with episiotomy, block should extend to S1 (saddle block, to denote a zone of analgesia of the perineum and perianal region, without involvement of the legs). Uterine muscle can function without neural control and may have its own intrinsic pacemakers. Successful uterine activity leading to delivery can occur in the presence of a total spinal block.[71]

Hyperbaric 5% lignocaine or hyperbaric amethocaine (dose: 1 ml) is injected between L4 and L5 in either the sitting position or in the lateral position with the vertebral canal inclined caudally. After an interval of a minute or so the patient is turned to the supine position with lateral tilt. The onset of analgesia takes less than 5 min.

Isobaric 0.5% bupivacaine in a dose of 3 ml is also satisfactory[72] with the patient in the lateral position for the injection, and immediately placed in the supine position with a wedge under the loin. It has been suggested that 0.5% bupivacaine with fentanyl 10 µg added is the best solution for Caesarian Section.[73] The use of 32G spinal catheters may have a place in labour, when only small doses of local analgesic drug are required.[74] This may also prove to be a useful route for the administration of spinal narcotics during labour.[75]

For high forceps or intrauterine manipulation, block should reach T10 to abolish the traction pain associated with a high forceps delivery, which will result if the sacral nerves alone are blocked. Spinal analgesia does not influence the course of established labour provided the level of block is not above T10 and blood pressure is maintained.

Perineal analgesia removes the bearing-down reflex but saddle block does not greatly delay normal labour if, when the cervix is fully dilated, the patient is encouraged to bear down during the pains.

In both subarachnoid and extradural (epidural) block, a given dose of local analgesic solution may ascend higher in pregnant than in non-pregnant patients, so doses should be given with care.[76] One hypothesis is that as the patient is turned from the lateral position some degree of aortocaval compression occurs, distending extradural veins, and forcing the analgesic solution cephalad.[77] This may have implications for giving test doses during extradural block[78]

Advantages of intradural block: (1) no fetal respiratory depression; (2) excellent relaxation of pelvic floor muscles; (3) absence of aspiration of stomach contents and risk of asphyxia, Mendelson's syndrome, pneumonia, etc.; (4) delivery of patient while she is conscious; and (5) can be quickly performed and has a rapid onset.

If used in congestive heart failure, for forceps delivery, to help spare the mother the exertion of pushing out the baby, subarachnoid injection should be made immediately the cervix is fully dilated, and forceps applied.

Postoperative headaches have always been a problem for a nursing mother, but the incidence is considerably minimized if fine needles, e.g. 26G,[79] 29G[80] or pencil-point needles with no bevel, e.g. 24G Sprotte[81] or 22G Whitacre. It has been suggested that the target should be an incidence of less than 1% severe headache (a patient willing to undergo a blood patch) and less than 4% failure.[82]

2. Extradural (epidural) lumbar block[83] (see also Chapter 25).

Indications. The aim is to reduce pain, prevent exhaustion and preserve morale. Indications are: (1) pre-eclamptic toxaemia; (2) slow, unbearably painful labour; (3) cardiac and respiratory distress; (4) premature or high-risk fetus; (5) multiple pregnancy; (6) breech delivery; (7) diabetes; (8) incoordinate action of uterus; (9) total failure of conventional analgesia; and (10) operative delivery, if the patient must be conscious.

Contra-indications. Near-absolute contra-indications are: (1) patient unwilling (note: some mothers who were initially willing, are retrospectively resentful of having received an epidural block); (2) haemorrhagic disease or anticoagulant therapy; (3) local sepsis; (4) lack of experience of anaesthetist and inadequate supervision; (5) inadequate facilities (apparatus or personnel) for immediate resuscitation should untoward events occur; (6) shock, hypotension, hypovolaemia; (7) neurological disease; (8) back deformities, previous back trouble, previous spinal surgery, or difficult anatomy (perhaps including obesity); (9) previous Caesarean section, because it is feared that analgesia may prevent recognition of a rupture of the uterus, although some workers disagree; (10) severe heart disease and hydramnios; and (11) existing supine hypotension.

Technique. Catheter design may be important. One with a closed tip and three lateral holes may be preferable to one with a single end hole.[84] The catheter may be introduced in the L2–3 or L3–4 interspace. It should not be advanced more than a short distance into the extradural space as it may take an undesired direction. The markings on the needle and catheter are useful here.[85] Head-down tilt may aid spread to T10. Warming of the solution has been recommended.[86] Combined extradural and spinal block has also been advocated[87] Drugs used include:

1. Bupivacaine 0.125%–0.5%. There is evidence that risks to the fetus, if they exist, are less than with lignocaine.[88] There is no advantage to be gained by adding adrenaline, which does not prolong duration of the block and does not protect against maternal toxicity unless the dosage is large.[89] Block may be patchy. Onset time: up to 0.5 h. Duration: 3 h. Infusion rate of bupivacaine (following an initial dose of 7–10 ml of 0.25%) is 10 ml/h[90] using a syringe pump.

2. Lignocaine 1.5%. The block is of very rapid onset and satisfyingly complete. Duration: 1–2 h. Maternal plasma concentration at delivery is directly related to total dose of lignocaine. Carbonated lignocaine solutions have given better results in clinical practice.[91]

3. Mepivacaine 1.5%. More likely to give rise to side-effects in the mother.

4. Prilocaine. This may cause methaemoglobinaemia and a blue baby.

5. Chloroprocaine has a rapid onset of action but is of short duration. It may be used for the initial injection to obtain analgesia quickly. Its analgesic effects may wear off suddenly. *See* Chapter 25.

6. Etidocaine, 1% solution, is a good agent for Caesarean section,[92] but is not favoured for normal delivery because it causes a high degree of motor block.

7. Opioids, diluted in 5–10 ml of saline. Morphine 2 mg; diamorphine 1 mg; buprenorphine 0.15 mg (may last 24 hrs); fentanyl 0.1 mg (a single bolus with the first dose of local analgesic intensifies analgesia, speeds its onset, overcomes any 'patchiness', and lasts up to 6 h); and methadone 10 mg (lasts about 12 h). Solutions without preservatives should be used. Cardiovascular effects are minimal. Maternal respiratory depression and nausea may occur if the above doses are exceeded. The method is especially valuable after delivery in Caesarean section.[93] An alternative is to infuse opioid and local analgesic into the epidural space using a syringe pump, throughout labour[94] Patient Controlled Analgesia (PCA) has been used by this route.[95]

Difficulties. All reported series indicate failure to achieve complete pain relief in a proportion of cases. This may take the form of unblocked segments. This should be openly explained to the patient beforehand. Extradural block may increase the need for instrumental delivery.[96]

MATERNAL COMPLICATIONS

Occur in 1 in 400 cases of epidural analgesia for labour.[97]

1. Life-threatening (1 in 30000 cases): (a) intravenous injection of local analgesic, with convulsions and cardiovascular collapse; and (b) intrathecal injection, with respiratory failure and cardiovascular collapse.

2. Serious (1 in 13500 cases): (a) introduction of foreign material into the extradural space; (b) extradural haematoma; and (c) extradural infection.

3. Moderate (1 in 2000 cases): (a) hypotensive crisis; (b) hypertensive crisis; (c) hyperalgesia; and (d) spinal headache if the dura has been punctured.

4. Prolonged (1 in 2000 cases): (a) backache at site of injection; (b) leg pain; (c) numbness and weakness; (d) pressure sores; and (e) burns from skin preparation material.

5. Mildly disturbing (1 in 1600 cases): (a) 6th cranial nerve palsy; (b) Horner's syndrome[98]; (c) catheter broken off in epidural space; and (d) injection of local analgesic into wrong catheter (intrauterine).

6. Pseudocomplications: Many unconnected symptoms are blamed on the epidural, e.g. headache, backache, leg ache, arm pain and numbness. Careful neurological examination usually enables an accurate diagnosis to be made.

3. Extradural sacral block – continuous caudal block[99]

Whatever the merits or demerits of continuous caudal block throughout labour, there is no doubt about the excellence of a single injection given for forceps delivery. Continuous caudal block is relatively safe for mother and child, gives superlative relaxation and good analgesia of the lower birth canal. Lignocaine 1–1.5% solution 16–20 ml or bupivacaine 0.5% 10–15 ml are the recommended agents and doses. Should continuation of the analgesia be required, topping-up doses of 10 ml can be given when necessary. The method should only be used when every means of resuscitation is to hand. High spread can occur following sacral injection as evidenced by reports of meiosis and ptosis.[100] It is not without its disadvantages and is accompanied by a high forceps rate and increased frequency of anomalies of rotation, e.g. persistent occipitoposterior position and mid-transverse arrest of the head. The third stage is short and post partum blood loss minimal. The method is useful in uterine inertia and in cervical dystocia. The pain following episiotomy can be relieved by sacral extradural morphine, 4 mg dissolved in 20 ml of saline, relief lasting up to 12 h.[101]

The dangers are: (1) accidental subarachnoid block; (2) infection; (3) broken needle; and (4) intrafetal injection.

For relief of first-stage pain, block must reach T11 and T12: for painless delivery, block of the sacral nerves is necessary.

Technique. See Chapter 25. A Tuohy needle and catheter are used.

Solutions used:

1. Bupivacaine (0.125%-0.5%). For first-stage pains, 16–20 ml injected

with the patient horizontal; for second-stage, 5–10 ml with patient sitting for 10 min, to block sacral nerves. Bupivacaine can produce a 'patchy' result, (improved by concurrent fentanyl), and may take a long time to work (up to 0.5 h).

2. Lignocaine (1–1.5% 20 ml). This gives a block up to T11. In most cases, patients in labour show a higher level of analgesia than in normal women using the same dose. Repeated injections have decreasing effect. The block is swift and complete.

4. Trancutaneous electrical nerve stimulation (TENS)

The electrodes are applied over the mid-lumbar region, 3–10 cm from the midline. Analgesia is frequently surprisingly good, and may safely be used in combination with other forms of pain relief.

5. Pudendal nerve block and local infiltration

This may be used for: (*a*) normal delivery – the sensory nerve supply of the vulva comes from the ilio-inguinal nerve anteriorly and from the perineal branch of the posterior cutaneous nerve of the thigh posteriorly; (*b*) episiotomy; (*c*) outlet forceps; and (*d*) repair of lacerations.

Indications may include fetal distress, delayed second stage, assisted breech delivery and multiple pregnancy. It can be used for forceps delivery because it is associated with less danger, both for the mother and for the baby, than general anaesthesia. This block is usually carried out by the obstetrician.

6. Paracervical nerve block

Seldom performed today, and then usually by the obstetrician.

Administration of analgesia by midwives

The English National Board for Midwifery lays down rules relating to analgesia in labour administered by midwives working alone. A practising midwife must not, on her own responsibility, administer an inhalation analgesic unless:

1. She has received special instruction in the essentials of obstetric analgesia at an institution approved by the Board, and has satisfied the institution or Board that she is thoroughly proficient in the use of the apparatus.

2. The patient has at some time during the pregnancy been examined by a registered medical practitioner who has signed a certificate that he finds no contra-indication to the administration of analgesia by a midwife. Should the patient subsequently contract an illness requiring medical attention, the onus is on the midwife to obtain confirmation that the certificate remains valid. In Scotland, the patient must be examined by a registered medical practitioner within 1 month of confinement and a certificate signed that the patient is fit for the administration of analgesic agents.

3. One other person, acceptable to the patient, who in the opinion of the midwife is suitable for the purpose, is present at the time of the administration, in addition to the midwife.

The following apparatus are approved by the Board for the use of midwives: The Entonox Apparatus (approved in 1965) for administration of premixed nitrous oxide – oxygen (50% of each).

Since 1970 a midwife has been allowed to top-up extradural catheters, always provided that: (*a*) she has been trained in the technique; (*b*) the first dose has been given by the anaesthetist; and (*c*) analgesia obtained is satisfactory and no obstetric complications have arisen. Even so, competent help should be readily available should maternal collapse occur. This will often be the anaesthetist.

Pethidine can be administered by the midwife in doses of 100 mg; not more than 200 mg may be given to any one patient.

The midwife can also administer the following drugs: chloral hydrate, syrup of chloral, pentazocine, ergotamine maleate, naloxone, oxytocin, and promazine.

IV. Inhalation analgesia

NITROUS OXIDE

Nitrous oxide does not interfere with uterine contractions, nor has it any effect on the fetus.

Premixed nitrous oxide – oxygen.[102] The mixture is very acceptable to the patient. It is important to check that the machine is working well, cylinders contain gas and dentures are removed. Inhalation must begin some seconds before the onset of pain. If the patient holds her own mask, it will fall from her hand, should unconsciousness supervene: this is a safety factor. Nitrous oxide 50% and oxygen 50% (Entonox) is used. Self-administration in labour has been shown to increase maternal Pao_2 at the time when placental flow is greatest.[103]

Late second-stage pains are fairly regular, and it is often possible to commence inhalation a minute before the pain is expected and to continue until the pain is maximal, followed by bearing down. In this way, the blood is saturated with nitrous oxide during the most agonizing phase of the contraction.

General anaesthesia[104]

There is a definite maternal death rate which includes anaesthetic complications.[105] Commonest causes of death are hypertensive states including eclampsia; and pulmonary embolism. Other deaths are associated with: (1) aspiration of stomach contents; (2) hypoxia associated with difficulty in tracheal intubation; (3) hypotension from any cause, including accidental subarachnoid injection during an intended epidural; (4) inadequate blood transfusion, too little, and too late; and (5) amniotic fluid embolus and existing maternal diseases, e.g. cardiac disease, sickle cell anaemia.

Equipment

Apparatus for the administration of general anaesthesia should be accompanied by: (1) laryngoscopes and tracheal tubes; (2) efficient suction; (3) a table that can be rapidly placed in the head-down position; (4) the means to produce a lateral tilt; (5) resuscitation equipment including provision for the administration of oxygen and appropriate drugs; (6) intravenous cannulae and infusion sets, with appropriate fluids; and (7) full monitoring equipment.

Prevention of vomiting during anaesthesia in labour

(*See also* Chapter 14.) Vomiting is always a real danger during labour as the patient may not be suitably prepared, while the gastric emptying time is delayed. There may, too, be associated hiatus hernia. (Promethazine, because of its antanalgesic effect, should not be given as an anti-emetic in labour).[106]

Diet. A satisfactory regimen must be instituted to lessen the likelihood of acid stomach contents being present should general anaesthesia be required. It has been suggested[107] that patients be classified as 'normal' or 'high-risk' cases:

1. 'Normal' cases. Unlikely to require general anaesthesia. The aim is to provide a light, easily digestible diet and to avoid large pieces of meat or vegetables with a high-fibre content. Fried food should be avoided and the ingestion of milk curtailed. Sieved foods are allowed. Drinks should not contain more than 5% glucose because stronger solutions delay gastric emptying. Small meals 3-hourly are preferable to large meals. Normal labour does not retard gastric emptying time,[108] but food and drink should be of the low residue, low fat type.

2. 'High-risk' cases. In these cases the obstetric history suggests that operative delivery may be required. Patients can be placed in the 'high-risk' category even if it is planned to use regional analgesia. Aspiration of vomitus can occur during spinal analgesia for Caesarean section. In these patients, once active labour is established, they should be given nothing by mouth except antacids. They should receive intravenous fluids, 500 ml 5% dextrose, 4-hourly. Both pethidine and diamorphine delay gastric emptying time,[109] and so does maternal fatigue and exhaustion.

3. The Use of Antacids. Antacids, such as sodium citrate (20 ml of 0.3 M) should be given 2-hourly to reduce gastric acidity and immediately before induction of anaesthesia. There is evidence that the antacid may 'layer' in the stomach unless the patient is rolled from side to side to ensure mixing. Oral H_2 blockers, cimetidine, 300 mg or ranitidine 150–300 mg.[110] one hour before anaesthesia, may contribute to safety.[111]

Before induction of anaesthesia, a No. 10 oesophageal tube may be passed to empty the stomach if the anaesthetist cannot guarantee safety from aspiration of gastric contents without it. Airway problems may arise from: (1) *Gross obstruction* by solid or liquid material. (2) *Mendelson's or the acid pulmonary aspiration syndrome.*[50] This serious condition was thought by Mendelson to be due to acid irritation of material at a pH of 2.5 or below, but has been shown to occur with fluid of a neutral pH as well.[112] Aspiration of alkali may also be harmful. The normal pregnant fasting gastric secretion has a pH of 1.5. The signs and symptoms are cyanosis, dyspnoea, tachycardia, bronchospasm and in fulminant cases either acute oedema of the lungs or acute respiratory failure. The chest X-ray shows a regular 'butterfly-shaped' hilar mottling, initially without evidence of atelectasis. An interval of some hours may separate the initial aspiration from the development of symptoms. Most commonly seen in obstetric patients. For treatment *see below*.   (3) *Bronchopneumonia and its later complications*, e.g. lung abscess or bronchiectasis.

PREVENTION OF MENDELSON'S SYNDROME

Aspiration of stomach contents during general anaesthesia can be made less likely by:

1. Giving only fluid and semi-solid food during labour.
2. The insertion of a No. 10 oesophageal tube before induction of anaesthesia.
3. Use of cricoid pressure (*see* Chapter 14).
4. Use of metoclopramide, 10 mg i.v., increases the lower oesophageal sphincter tone and so may reduce the incidence of regurgitation. Development of Mendelson's syndrome after regurgitation is made less likely by antacids, e.g. 0.3 sodium citrate, and H_2 blockers (*see above*). Cimetidine, 200 mg i.v. 60–90 min before induction results in a gastric juice of pH 5 on induction. Cimetidine crosses the placental barrier.[113] Ranitidine is also widely employed;[114] famotidine, 40 mg nizatidine, 150 mg may be considered.[115] The acid pulmonary aspiration syndrome can occur without definite vomiting or obvious regurgitation. Patients for sterilization by tubal section and ligation in the immediate post-partum days may also be at risk.

TREATMENT OF MENDELSON'S SYNDROME

1. Milder cases may be treated by: (*a*) the Trendelenburg position; and (*b*) pharyngeal suction.
2. Severe cases may require, in addition to careful tracheobronchial cleansing, aspiration and lavage with solution of 1% sodium bicarbonate, oxygen therapy and postoperative IPPV. Hydrocortisone in large doses reduces the inflammatory reaction and aids bronchodilatation. The same precautions are necessary to prevent aspiration during the puerperium (e.g. for sterilization) as during labour.

Drugs used by anaesthetists in obstetrics

Intravenous agents

A dose of 100–250 mg of thiopentone for induction is unlikely to seriously depress fetal respiration, but larger amounts are probably undesirable. Propofol is also useful, but limited by rapid offset and hypotension. Other induction agents are also suitable. Opioids are reserved for after the baby is delivered, with the possible exception of alfentanil.

Muscle relaxants

Clinical doses of relaxants are usually without harmful effects on the fetus, although some may cross the placenta, especially gallamine. Suxamethonium is normally used in the rapid sequence (crash) induction. Small doses of non-depolarizing relaxants are then used. 'Normal' doses are not necessary, and may be difficult to reverse at the end.

Nitrous oxide

The only complication of nitrous oxide is awareness during operation, especially when less than 70% of the inspired gas is nitrous oxide.[116] (Full oxygenation at this level is monitored by pulse oximetry.) Awareness may be prevented by the addition of a small amount of volatile agent, e.g. isoflurane 1% (there is a decrease of 30% in MAC values at term, due to high circulating progesterone levels), and by an opioid after delivery.

Inhalation agents

Low concentrations used as an adjuvant to nitrous oxide to prevent awareness are unlikely to affect the fetus if given for a short period and do not depress uterine retraction.

Ketamine

Ketamine increases uterine tone in the first and second, but not in the third trimester of pregnancy.[117] Has been used as the sole agent for forceps delivery, manual removal of the placenta and similar procedures, and as an induction agent prior to Caesarean section. Should be avoided in eclampsia or hypertension. In large doses, it may cause fetal respiratory depression.

Ergometrine

Ergometrine, is a powerful oxytocic and an α-adrenergic agonist. If given to a patient under the influence of another α-stimulator, e.g. a pressor drug, can produce widespread vasoconstriction with hypertension, bronchoconstriction and even acute pulmonary oedema. Should be used carefully in patients with Raynaud's disease, since collapse due to intense vasoconstriction has been reported.[118] Although it is usually a myocardial depressant, it may cause ventricular ectopic beats. It causes vomiting in almost half of patients.[119] It is suggested that it may contribute to the occurrence of Mendelson's syndrome.[120]

Synthetic oxytocin (*Syntocinon*, 10 units i.v.)

This drug may result in transient dilatation of vessels containing both α- and β-receptors and so may result in hypotension, unless the legs are in the lithotomy position or the patient in a head-down tilt. Oxytocin is preferred if a myometrial stimulant is required in a patient who has recently been given a pressor agent.[121] Not emetic.

Anticoagulants

Patients on long-term anticoagulant therapy should be managed by a change to heparin at 36 weeks, because it does not cross the placenta. It should be reversed before any extradural block is considered and not restarted until at least 24 h after removal of the catheter.

Hyperventilation in obstetric anaesthesia

A fall of maternal $Paco_2$ below 2.85 kPa causes fetal acidosis as a result of reduction in placental blood flow.[122] It is desirable to keep $Paco_2$ at or above 4 kPa which is normal for the pregnant mother at term.

Operative obstetric procedures

Anaesthesia for caesarean section

The ideal anaesthetic or analgesic provides: (1) absolute safety, especially from aspiration of stomach contents. This includes proper airway management during general anaesthesia with readiness to deal with the problem of failed intubation should it arise; (2) absence of respiratory depression of the fetus; (3) absence of psychic trauma to mother and awareness during operation; and (4) absence of toxicity in mother and infant. The fetal mortality following elective section is greater than that following normal delivery. Abdominal relaxation is achieved with relatively small doses of non-depolarizing relaxants.

PREMEDICATION

1. Atropine or hyoscine to prevent salivation and bradycardia.
2. If sedation is essential, diazepam, 5 mg orally, is the preferred drug.[123]
3. Sodium citrate, 15 ml, 0.3 M is given p.o. and/or H_2 blockers e.g. ranitidine, to antagonize gastric acidity.
4. Metoclopramide 10 mg, to hasten gastric emptying, increase oesophageal sphincter tone and combat nausea.
5. Analgesics are not indicated until the delivery of the baby, but pethidine may have been given during earlier labour.

GENERAL ANAESTHESIA

Proper measures to prevent aspiration of stomach contents must be taken (*see* Chapter 14). The apparatus should be checked. A standard induction technique is: preoxygenation for 3 min, thiopentone 4 mg/kg, suxamethonium 100 mg, cricoid pressure, tracheal intubation, nitrous oxide–oxygen, non-depolarizing relaxant. The risk of awareness can be reduced if a trace of volatile agent, e.g. 1% isoflurane, is added. Atracurium, mivacurium and vecuronium are useful relaxants in Caesarean section because of their short duration of action, rapid clearance and minimal placental transfer. Oxygen concentrations up to 66% used to be advocated. The disadvantage is that the mother may become aware of events during the operation.[124] Lateral tilt is employed to present caval compression. Half doses of relaxant are all that is necessary in Caesarean section. The abdominal muscles are stretched during pregnancy and muscle tone is seldom a problem.

Morphine, pethidine or methadone are given to the mother as soon as the baby is delivered, to deepen anaesthesia.

Hyperventilation has been used as an aid to the production of unconsciousness. Respiratory alkalosis in the mother may, however, produce hazard to the fetus, by reducing placental blood flow and oxygen transfer.[125]

EXTRADURAL LUMBAR BLOCK

Extradural block for Caesarean section does not decrease the amount of placental blood flow to the fetus.[126] Previous Caesarean section is not necessarily a contra-indication to extradural block in a subsequent labour, provided that careful monitoring for a ruptured scar is well maintained. (Scar pain and 'peritoneal pain' are uncommon signs of rupture. Sudden reduction or cessation of contractions are more usual signs of rupture.)

MANAGEMENT OF EPIDURAL ANALGESIA FOR CAESAREAN SECTION

One suggested technique:

1. Explanation of having to lie still for at least an hour; being draped; breathing oxygen; the premedication antacids; and the risks.

2. Consent.

3. Premedication H_2 blockers the night before and one hour before; 15 ml 0.3 M sodium citrate, orally, 10 min before starting the block.

4. A drip is set up, and baseline arterial pressure, pulse, oxygen saturation and other parameters are noted.

5. A lumbar epidural catheter is inserted. 4–5 ml of plain 0.5% bupivacaine or 1.5% lignocaine test dose is injected up the catheter. Added adrenaline is usually avoided[127] The patient is sat up for 5 min; testing for hypotension and paralysis. If there is none, a further 5 ml analgesic solution, perhaps with added fentanyl 100 μg is injected up the catheter to achieve block of the sacral roots. The patient is laid flat again and a further 5 ml analgesic solution injected up the catheter.[128] If the block has not extended to T6, after 10 min a further 5 ml analgesic solution is injected. When the block has reached T6, a left lateral tilt is put on, and the surgeon may proceed. Monitoring continues as before. Local analgesic may be infused by syringe pump, especially if this has been going on in earlier labour.

6. At delivery, synthetic oxytocin is given i.v., and diamorphine 5 mg in 10 ml saline given epidurally (Diamorphine is one of the quicker-acting opioids).

7. Epidural opioid analgesia may be continued in the postoperative phase, with antiemetics if necessary. Itching may be noticed.

8. The systolic pressure should be maintained at 90 mmHg or above by infusion of fluids intravenously, and if necessary by i.v. ephedrine. Hartmann's solution, 2 l given rapidly while the block is taking effect, goes some way to preventing hypotension.[129] Vomiting is not uncommon. Oxygen may be given to the mother. One of the advantages of extradural lumbar block for Caesarean section is that the mother may remain awake with active cough reflexes. Even very nervous patients can be managed in this way if they are treated sympathetically and the surgeon is gentle. However, the anaesthetist must be prepared to proceed to full general anaesthesia at any time.

Lignocaine, 2% solution given extradurally for Caesarean section (elective) caused no neurobehavioural problems in the newborn.[130]

It would seem that extradural analgesia reduces uterine activity; it increases the forceps delivery rate.[131] Slow controlled induction of extradural analgesia greatly reduces the risk of local analgesic toxicity.[132]

EXTRADURAL SACRAL (CAUDAL) BLOCK

After a test dose of 10 ml, 20 ml bupivacaine 0.5% or lignocaine 1.5% are injected, followed by 5–10 ml every 10 min until analgesia reaches the eighth thoracic dermatome. Severe hypotension is a major risk of this technique, so prophylactic 'volume loading' and perhaps ephedrine are needed.

INTRADURAL BLOCK (SUBARACHNOID BLOCK)

Block should reach at least to the costal margin and can be obtained with bupivacaine 0.5% plain, 3 ml injected with the patient in the right lateral position and afterwards turned on to her back on a table with a slight head-down tilt with a wedge under the right hip and shoulder to remove pressure, especially at the pelvic brim, on the vena cava from the gravid uterus.

Lateral tilt is used to avoid pressure of the gravid uterus on the vena cava. The enlarged uterus, by interfering with the movements of the diaphragm, tends to produce hypoxia of the mother so oxygen may be given to the mother from the outset. The systolic blood pressure should not be allowed to fall below 90 mmHg. (*See also* above.)

COMPLICATIONS OF REGIONAL BLOCK FOR CAESAREAN SECTION

See Maternal complications for epidural analgesia for labour (above). Visceral pain may occur during the operation.[133] Following intra- or extradural block, the pressor agents to be avoided are methoxamine and phenylephrine, which may reduce the blood supply to the placenta. Ephedrine does not possess these disadvantages.[134]

Great care is required, especially in control of arterial pressure and in adequate oxygenation of the mother and hence of the child. Hypotension can be treated by a lateral tilt, elevation of the legs, infusion of plasma-volume expander, ephedrine and oxygen administration.

LOCAL INFILTRATION

This is without serious effect on the mother or child, but is unsuitable for frightened or uncontrolled patients. The surgeon's co-operation is essential for success: he performs the injections himself.[135]

Intradermal and subcutaneous infiltration is carried out in the line of the incision and solution should be deposited for about 2.5 cm on each side of the midline. Extra solution is injected into the pyramidales and into the retropubic space of Retzius. Solution injected into the rectus sheath will improve relaxation. The parietal peritoneum is infiltrated, likewise the tissue overlying the lower segment if the classic operation is not to be employed.

Complications of anaesthesia for caesarean section

ACID ASPIRATION SYNDROME

(*See above*).

AWARENESS[136]

This is a problem when light anaesthesia, nitrous oxide–oxygen with relaxants, is employed. The use of adjuvants is essential, e.g. isoflurane 0.8%, halothane 0.5% or enflurane 1.0%. Even so, an incidence of 2.5% has been quoted as an irreducible minimum. The use of a tourniquet on one arm to prevent entry of muscle relaxant and allow the patient to use her hand on command has been advocated.[137] Following reversal of muscle relaxant at the end of operation, a patient's response to command within 15 s of nitrous oxide cessation suggests that there has been a risk of awareness.

Pseudo-awareness is when the patient thinks that what happens as she awakes postoperatively, is happening during the operation.

CAVAL COMPRESSION SYNDROME

In the supine position the inferior vena cava is compressed by the gravid uterus at term. In 6% of patients this results in bradycardia, fall of cardiac output and hypotension of significant degree. Caval compression syndrome may be *latent* or *overt*. In either case placental blood flow is reduced. This may result in fall of Pao_2 and metabolic acidosis in the fetus. These ill effects are less when the fetus descends during labour and when the patient is put in the lateral position or when a tilt to the left is used on the operating table. Tilt to the left is preferred, but if this is not effective tilt to the right can be tried.

FAILED INTUBATION

Failure to intubate the patient has resulted in maternal death as a result of hypoxia. The following procedure has been recommended should tracheal intubation fail:[138] (1) maintain cricoid pressure; (2) patient put on left side, head down; (3) give oxygen by IPPV; (4) if ventilation easy, ventilate with nitrous oxide–oxygen and volatile supplement (isoflurane) and continue by face-mask when spontaneous respiration is restored; (5) pass wide-bore stomach tube via mouth, aspirate and instil 30 ml sodium citrate before withdrawal; (6) continue anaesthesia for operation with lateral tilt; and (7) if oxygenation proves difficult (3, *above*), allow patient to resume consciousness, and consider regional technique or general anaesthesia by face-mask with spontaneous respiration. Caval compression combined with hypoxia can precipitate cardiac arrest, so it is important to keep the patient in the lateral position until oxygenation is assured. The laryngeal mask airway may have a place.[139] This is best inserted when the patient is breathing spontaneously,[140] although this has been questioned.[141]

Other obstetric operations

ANAESTHESIA FOR EXTERNAL VERSION

Thiopentone and a muscle relaxant will relax the abdominal wall, although not the uterus. Where uterine tone prevents version, deep anaesthesia with a volatile agent is required.

ANAESTHESIA FOR INTERNAL VERSION

If the obstetrician requires a well-relaxed uterus, high into which his hand and arm must be introduced, deep anaesthesia is required, e.g. with isoflurane. The technique used should avoid the risk of aspiration of stomach contents and provide relaxation of the muscles of the pelvic floor and perineum.

ANAESTHESIA FOR FORCEPS DELIVERY

(1) Thiopentone, suxamethonium and nitrous oxide–oxygen, given through a cuffed tracheal tube. (2) Extradural block. (3) Low spinal analgesia has much to be said in its favour because it removes the risk of aspiration of gastric contents. Extradural sacral block is excellent, if time is available. The disadvantage of these regional techniques is the time they take to perform (in what is a semi-urgent situation). (4) Pudendal block is fast and efficient.

ANAESTHESIA FOR BREECH DELIVERY

1. In assisted breech delivery, good oxygenation and a smooth induction at the right time are necessary. In the first and early second stages, pethidine 100–150 mg and nitrous oxide–oxygen if necessary. When the presenting part appears, an episiotomy can be done under infiltration analgesia and pudendal block, and this gives adequate pain relief. For delivery of the aftercoming head by forceps, anaesthesia is not induced until the scapulae are delivered. If it is then necessary, it must be induced rapidly by rapid-sequence induction (*see below*). Regional analgesia (intra- or extradural block) not contra-indicated.[142]

ANAESTHESIA FOR RETAINED PLACENTA

Frequently the demand for manual removal of the placenta comes for a patient who merely has a slow third stage of labour. There is no shock or any hurry. Occasionally, however, the patient may be shocked and a retraction ring may form an obstruction. Standard techniques are satisfactory. Deeper anaesthesia may be necessary. In the absence of facilities for general anaesthesia, nitrous oxide, analgesia or intravenous opioids (e.g. sub-apnoeic doses of fentanyl or alfentanil) make the manoeuvre of manual removal tolerable. In an emergency and to save life in severe postpartum haemorrhage it may be justified to remove the placenta from a collapsed patient without any analgesia.

ANAESTHESIA FOR THE OBSTETRIC FLYING SQUAD[143]

The idea of the obstetrical flying squad was suggested by Professor Farquhar Murray of Newcastle on Tyne in 1929, and organized in Glasgow in 1933 and in Newcastle two years later. This raises problems of the unusual location. In the absence of properly trained anaesthetists or where distances are short, it is best to transfer the patient to hospital. Equipment may include: (1) a portable anaesthetic machine; (2) suction apparatus; (3) case for drugs and accessories; (4) plasma expanders for intravenous infusion and group O Rh-negative blood, and giving sets; and (5) self-inflating bag.

See also Chapter 31. Less popular than in former years.

ANAESTHESIA FOR VAGINAL TERMINATION

Thiopentone and nitrous oxide–oxygen, with or without a narcotic analgesic or volatile agent. Halothane is better avoided. Ketamine affords good operative conditions with reduced blood loss.

Management of some obstetric emergencies

This is the task of obstetricians. However, in practice, anaesthetists are often called in to advise, and to help with resuscitation.

ECLAMPSIA AND PRE-ECLAMPTIC TOXAEMIA (PET)

This occurs after the 20th and more often after the 24th week of pregnancy.

Mild pre-eclampsia is defined as a diastolic pressure above 90 mmHg with proteinuria less than 25 g/l.

Severe pre-eclampsia is said to exist when one or more of the following are present: (*a*) systolic pressure above 160 or diastolic above 110 mmHg on repeated estimation; (*b*) rapidly increasing proteinuria; (*c*) oliguria (less than 400 ml urine in 24 hours); (*d*) cerebral or visual disturbance; and (*e*) pulmonary oedema or cyanosis.

Eclampsia is manifest if convulsions occur at any time. There may be hypertension, reduced blood volume, increased fluid in extravascular compartment, increased risk of premature placental separation and convulsions.

Death can occur from: (*a*) heart failure; (*b*) inhalation of saliva or vomit; (*c*) cerebral haemorrhage; (*d*) hepatorenal failure. The so-called HELLP syndrome may occur (Haemolysis, Elevated Liver enzymes, Low Platelets). Management guidelines have been suggested;[144] (*e*) disseminated intravascular coagulopathy (DIC). Thrombocytopenia is said to occur in one third of patients, but prolonged bleeding time is unlikely with counts above 100 000.[145] Platelet screening is advised.[146] Hepatic rupture has been reported.[147] Renal failure may be associated with haemoglobinuria and can require dialysis; and (*f*) laryngeal oedema has been reported[148] and can cause intubation problems.

Management. The anaesthetist should be informed at an early stage. Treatment is supportive until the fetus is delivered, which usually brings the condition to an end, although convulsions can occur in the immediate post-delivery period. Early delivery is advantageous. Control of convulsions may be by: (*a*) established anticonvulsant drugs, e.g. diazepam in 5–10 mg increments or 10 mg/h by infusion (may cause fetal depression), chlormethiazole 0.8% in 5% dextrose at 20 ml/min (may cause undue sedation or water overloading), phenytoin 10 mg/kg in 100 ml saline at 50 mg/min followed 2 h later by half this dose with a maintenance dose 12 h later of 200 mg 8 hourly orally or i.v.; (b) magnesium sulphate is popular in some countries, loading dose 40–80 mg/kg followed by infusion at 2 gm/hr. Side-effects include neuromuscular blockade directly related to serum magnesium levels,[149] reduction of perepheral resistance, increase of cardiac output and anti-adrenergic effects in animals.[150] Magnesium is not currently popular in Britain, but a case can be made for[151] and against.[152] See also, Maheshwari R. et al. J. Postgrad. Med. 1989, 35, 66; Crowther C. Br. J. Obstet. Gynaecol. 1990, 97, 110; Domisse J. Br. J. Obstet. Gynaecol. 1990, 97, 104; James M. F. M. In: Recent Advances in Anaesthesia and Analgesia–17. Atkinson R. S. and Adams A. P. Edinburgh: Churchill Livingstone, 1991.

AMNIOTIC FLUID EMBOLISM[153]

A rare and dangerous complication of delivery first recognized in 1926.[155] but clinical features described in 1941.[154] Its signs and symptoms may wrongly be attributed to anaesthesia. A sudden infusion of amniotic fluid into the maternal circulation, after rupture of the membranes, gives rise to an acute shock-like state characterized by: (1) respiratory distress; (2) cyanosis; (3) chest pain; (4) peripheral vascular collapse; (5) coma; (6) disseminated intravascular coagulopathy with hypofibrinogenaemia and excessive bleeding, which may occur without collapse and be the first sign of the condition; effect on blood-clotting mechanism described in 1950;[156] and (7) convulsions, which must be differentiated from those of eclampsia or toxicity of local analgesics.

The mortality is high. Chest X-ray reveals bilateral peri-hilar mottling. ECG shows right heart strain. Pulmonary artery and central venous pressures are raised. The pulmonary bed may be blocked by fibrin deposits.

Diagnosis is definite when elements of amniotic fluid are found in maternal tissues, especially blood, urine, lungs and sputum.

Treatment may include: (1) blood transfusion; (2) administration of fresh frozen plasma or fibrinogen to combat defibrination; (3) vasopressors (ephedrine is preferred as it does not cause pulmonary vasoconstriction); (4) artificial ventilation with oxygen; (5) bronchodilators; (6) steroids; (7) possibly digitalis; and (8) heparin (very low dose, 100–500 units) has been recommended to prevent continued fibrinogen-fibrin conversion.[157]

DISSEMINATED INTRAVASCULAR COAGULOPATHY (DIC)[158]

May follow haemorrhage, abortion, hydatidiform mole, intrauterine fetal death, amniotic fluid embolism. (1) continued bleeding; (2) destruction of fibrin and fibrinogen by plasma fibrinolysins; and (3) conversion of prothrombin to thrombin may be inactivated by release of heparin-like substance in amniotic fluid. Normal fibrinogen is 150–700 mg/dl. Less than 150 mg/dl is dangerous.

Diagnosis. Clotting screen shows widespread abnormalities, often with Fibrin Degradation Products (FDPs)

Treatment. (1) Fresh frozen plasma (FFP); (2) if there is a circulatory fibrinolysin give aminocaproic acid, 4–5 g, initial dose i.v. over 1 h, then 1 g 8-hourly; (3) when heparin-like factor diagnosed, give 20–50 mg protamine sulphate i.v. slowly. Clotting screen analysis is repeated frequently to assess effects of therapy. 500 ml blood contains less than 1 g of fibrinogen, 1000 ml plasma provides 3 g; and (4) blood transfusion is usually required. The prognosis is not good. Intensive care is often needed.

SHOCK

Causes of shock in the obstetric patient include: (1) haemorrhage, e.g. antepartum or postpartum haemorrhage, lacerations of birth canal, retained placenta, uterine atony; (2) traumatic: acute inversion of the uterus; surgical trauma; (3) septic shock; (4) supine hypotensive syndrome (*see below*); (5) amniotic fluid embolism; and (6) anaphylaxis.[159]

SICKLE-CELL DISEASE AND PREGNANCY[160]

MYASTHENIA GRAVIS IN PREGNANCY[161]

ACUTE INVERSION OF THE UTERUS

Shock is out of proportion to blood loss. Immediate replacement of blood or fluid is necessary with general anaesthesia.

Resuscitation of the newborn

One of the earliest papers on treatment was 'The Asphyxia of the Stillborn Infant and its Treatment', by Marshall Hall in 1856.[162] Intrauterine respiration of the fetus, the rhythmical amniotic tide into and out of the air passages, was first demonstrated by J. F. Ahfelt (1843–1929), Leipzig obstetrician, in 1888 and then by the Italian, Ferroni, in 1899.[163]

The fetal blood haemoglobin is 15–20 g/100 ml and when fully saturated carries 22 vol% of oxygen. But because of the low oxygen partial pressure at which maternal blood gives up its oxygen, fetal haemoglobin is only 50% saturated. Brown fat is important in heat regulation of the newborn.

In the newborn the amount of carbonic anhydrase is half that found in adult blood so that release of carbon dioxide in lungs is handicapped.

During the process of birth, anaerobic glycolysis may aid the survival of the infant, should respiratory embarrassment occur, energy being released from glycogen.

Fluctuation in maternal carbon-dioxide tension may contribute to respiratory difficulties in the newborn, especially in premature infants. Maternal $Paco_2$ may fall as a result of hyperventilation towards the end of the first stage of labour, reducing placental blood flow, but may rise during the second stage as a result of breath-holding.

Intrapartum fetal monitoring

The signs of intrauterine hypoxia are irregularity of the fetal heart rate going on to tachycardia or bradycardia. In a cephalic presentation, the presence of meconium indicates hypoxic relaxation of the fetal anal sphincter.

Estimation of the pH of fetal blood as an index of fetal hypoxia has proved most useful. A pH of 7.15 indicates critical hypoxia.

Causes of hypoxia in fetus and newborn

1. Maternal hypoxia. Pao_2 may be reduced at term (*see above*). Factors such as altitude, reduced FIo_2 or the presence of haemoglobinopathy may cause further problems. Oxygen consumption is increased in late pregnancy. Maternal hypotension, maternal cardiac failure.

2. The trauma of labour.

3. Placental infarction or premature separation; prolapse or knotting of cord.

4. Fetal respiratory failure: The diagnosis of fetal asphyxia during labour is confirmed by measuring the pH of fetal blood. (*a*) *Central*. Due to: (*i*) immaturity of respiratory centre, perhaps associated with gross fetal abnormality; (*ii*) damage to respiratory centre from trauma or from cerebral oedema due to diabetes or hydrops fetalis; (*iii*) oxygen lack perhaps associated with intrapartum fetal asphyxia; and (*iv*) narcotics and sedatives given to mother. The threshold of maternal respiratory centre differs from that of the fetal centre, as a level of narcosis harmless to the mother may be depressing to the fetus. All anaesthetics, except nitrous oxide and oxygen, and all analgesic agents, other than chloral in reasonable dosage, depress the fetal respiratory mechanism, an effect made worse by any hypoxia of the mother during labour. The placenta acts as no barrier to these agents. There is definite evidence that hypoxia of the fetus during labour, and of the baby at birth or shortly afterwards, may be followed by impaired cerebral function in later life. The danger is increased with premature infants. (*b*) *Peripheral*. Due to: (*i*) immaturity of lungs; (*ii*) respiratory obstruction; (*iii*) muscular weakness; (*iv*) fetal lungs full of liquor amnii or meconium; and (*v*) intranatal pneumonia.

The baby recovering from asphyxia first takes a series of gasps, which give place to a series of single prolonged inspirations. Finally, rhythmic inspiration and expiration set in. Periodic breathing is not of bad prognostic significance in newborn babies and is common in premature infants.

Management of asphyxia of the newborn

The fetal circulation can withstand 10–15 min of hypoxia but deficient cerebral blood flow may cause permanent damage. The fetus *in utero* is cyanosed. The normally delivered child should breathe rhythmically from the beginning, air replacing liquor amnii. Alveoli are opened up by the negative pressure exerted by normal respiratory movements ($-50\,cmH_2O$) as in crying. In respiratory depression, respiration begins differently, in gasps – the most primitive respiratory movement, involving many more muscles.

Monitoring neonatal status

Virginia Apgar[164] (1909–1975) of New York City described a system whereby the condition of a neonate can be assessed, one (or more) minutes after birth. A score of 0, 1 or 2 is given in each of five variables: heart rate, respiratory effort, muscle tone, colour and reflex irritability. The maximum score is 10. A single clinical assessment at 1 min does not distinguish between primary apnoea (which will usually recover without treatment) and terminal apnoea (when active resuscitation is required). Important factors are: (*a*) changes in heart rate before resuscitation; (*b*) whether gasping precedes an improvement in colour or vice versa; and (*c*) whether or not apnoea supervenes in a baby who has initially gasped or cried. Some anaesthetists prefer to omit colour and use the A − C (Apgar minus colour) score. Subtle effects on the neonate's nervous system may be caused by drugs, local and general, used in obstetric pain relief.[165]

Table 22.1 Apgar Scoring System

		Respiratory	Muscle tone	Colour	Reflex Irritability
	Heart rate	Effort	Muscle tone	Colour	Irritability
0	Absent	Absent	Flaccid	Blue or white	No response
1	Slow, less than 100	Weak cry, hypoventilation of limbs or feet	Some flexion	Blue hands	Some movement
2	100 or over	Crying lusty	Well flexed	Healthy pink	Active movement

Indications for oxygen and IPPV by mask in the newborn

(1) Central cyanosis; (2) bradycardia; and (3) failure to cry on stimulation. Face-mask resuscitaton may be successful if Head's reflex[166] stimulates spontaneous respiration; if it does not, intubation will be required. It requires skill and may cause damage.

Indications for intubation of the newborn and short-term IPPV

The following guidelines may be considered when the baby's condition deteriorates in the minutes following birth: (1) central cyanosis for more than 3 min; (2) bradycardia less than 100 bpm for more than 3 min; (3) apnoea for more than 3 min; (4) 'white asphyxia', i.e. skin vasoconstriction; (5) cardiac arrest or depression; and (6) Apgar score of 0–2.

The cyanosis will fail to respond to oxygen therapy in the presence of cyanotic heart disease, severe tracheo-oesophageal fistula, large diaphragmatic hernia and severe respiratory distress syndrome.

The upper air passages are cleared by suction, using a catheter (No. 6 FG). Skin stimulation, passive limb movements, slapping, etc. are also very valuable, while oxygen is given via a nasal catheter or face-mask and neonatal inflating bag 30–40 puffs per min. In feeble babies, a small stomach tube should be passed to evacuate the stomach of liquor amnii and prevent its aspiration into the lungs.

If no improvement takes place within 3–4 min the trachea is intubated and the lungs inflated with oxygen. Any baby born apnoeic, flaccid or with a slow heart beat should be intubated. The laryngoscope should have a straight blade.

The tracheal tube used should have an internal diameter of 2.5–3.5 mm. Various designs are available.

The infant is ventilated by: (1) a Jackson Rees modification of Ayre's T-piece, with manual compression of the reservoir bag; or (2) pressure from an oxygen supply. A small hole in the tubing is occluded by the finger to build up controlled pressure so that frequent half-second puffs of oxygen can be given. The pressure needed to expand the newborn lung is usually about 4 kPa (30 cmH$_2$O), but may be double this for a few inflations. Pressures greater than this may cause rupture of the lung. Excessive pressures are avoided by use of a blow-off device, set for 30 cmH$_2$O. Should pneumothorax occur, its presence may be confirmed by X-ray and relief obtained by insertion of an i.v. cannula in the mid-axillary line, which is then connected to a source of suction.

To intubate a neonate the patient should be on a flat table with no pillow. The head should not be over-extended. The straight blade of the infant laryngoscope should be inserted posterior to the epiglottis from the right side of the mouth and then lifted vertically, but gentleness is required. Rhythmic inflation of oxygen often has beneficial results (probably because of changes in intrabronchial pressure rather than because of expansion of collapsed alveoli). There is evidence that a positive pressure of 30–50 cmH$_2$O applied through a tracheal tube for repeated short periods will cause a collapsed lung to expand. Estimation of blood gases and electrolytes is desirable.

Closed chest massage, if required, can be carried out by pressure of two fingers over the midsternum 60 times/min. In a baby who is hypotonic and is not responding, continued resuscitation beyond 30 min is unlikely to result in a favourable outcome.

Premature babies must not be given pure oxygen for any length of time. If they are cyanosed they may receive 40% oxygen for short periods only, thus reducing the danger of retrolental fibroplasia.[167]

Steps should be taken to prevent fall in temperature during resuscitation. Procedures should be carried out under a heat lamp, the infant should be wrapped up as soon as possible, and the rectal temperature taken using a low-reading thermometer.

Drugs. Injection into the umbilical vein of naloxone, 0.01 mg/kg repeated, i.v. or i.m., will counteract any respiratory depression following injection of pethidine or morphine into the mother.

Respiratory distress syndrome

The idiopathic respiratory distress syndrome of the newborn is the commonest cause of death in liveborn premature infants. The incidence is related to the degree of prematurity and is rare in infants born at term. One baby out of every 200 born alive dies of respiratory failure in the first few days of life. An equal number have respiratory distress but recover normal function. The distress may show itself from birth or may come on several hours later, and is characterized by severe retraction of the chest wall during inspiration, cyanosis, a respiratory rate above 60/min and an expiratory grunt. Recovery is usual in those babies who survive beyond the third day. The lungs are grossly atelectatic, and the radiographic appearances are those of 'ground glass'. The alveoli and terminal bronchioles are lined by a hyaline membrane, first described in 1925.[168] The material interfering with ventilation is probably formed from the lung itself and not inhaled. Lack of surfactant in the alveolar spaces is causal. Surfactant is a lipoprotein containing dipalmitoyl lecithin. Its function is to confer stability on the terminal air spaces, or to act as an anti-atelectasis factor. It increases in the amniotic fluid from the 33rd week of pregnancy. The ratio between this and another surface active phospholipid, sphingomyelin, can be determined by amniocentesis and may enable those infants who are at high risk to be diagnosed. The condition is most frequently seen in premature babies, and in babies born to mothers suffering from diabetes, toxaemia or placenta praevia. Neonatal respiratory function is related to the total lipid, phospholipid and lecithin content of amniotic fluid.

If inadequate respiration causes acid-base imbalance, hyperkalaemia may occur. It has also been suggested that routine transfusion of blood from the placenta may reduce the incidence of the condition. The infant should be nursed in an incubator in a humid atmosphere and at a temperature of 35°C (95°F) to minimize oxygen consumption. Careful monitoring of blood gases and pH is mandatory, and metabolic acidosis corrected by sodium bicarbonate, which may be given orally or intravenously. The atmosphere should be oxygen enriched to maintain an arterial oxygen tension as near normal as possible. IPPV and CPAP may be required. This can be achieved with and without tracheal intubation.

GYNAECOLOGY

First successful removal of an ovarian cyst in 1817 by Ephraim McDowell (1771–1830), of Kentucky,[169] and first successful closure of a vesicovaginal fistula in 1852 by James Marion Sims (1813–1883), of New York.[170] First successful surgical treatment of ruptured ectopic pregnancy by Lawson Tait of Birmingham (1845–1899).[171]

Main problems – haemorrhage, postoperative vomiting and deep vein thrombosis.

Abdominal operations call for profound relaxation to prevent damage to muscles and the upper abdominal peritoneum from abrasion by packs. They can be performed under spinal analgesia, either intradural or extradural, or under general anaesthesia.

For Wertheim's hysterectomy[172] (Ernst Wertheim, 1864–1920, of Vienna) extradural block up T5 is recommended and light general anaesthesia is a useful adjunct as there may still be some surgical stimulation outside the field of the block.

The Trendelenburg position is unphysiological and should be maintained for as short a time as possible. It may lead to headache, regurgitation and a steep rise in CVP.[173] The less steep it is the better for the patient's respiratory and cardiovascular function. Levelling of the table should be gradual, with a watch on venous and arterial blood pressure.

Vaginal operations can be performed under extradural lumbar or sacral block (*see* Chapter 25) or general anaesthesia. Stretching of the cervix or trauma to the perineum may produce laryngeal spasm, requiring a deeper plane of anaesthesia or a small dose of a muscle relaxant. Spinal analgesia combines afferent block, muscular relaxation and moderate hypotension and ischaemia. *For dilatation and curettage*, intravenous induction, with nitrous oxide and oxygen, with or without a volatile agent is satisfactory.

Anaesthesia for laparoscopy.[174] Laparoscopy was first employed in 1910, using a cystoscope.[175] It is not a minor procedure and is accompanied by an increase in blood glucose, plasma cortisol, prolactin and growth hormone.[176] The patient is usually in a steep Trendelenburg position. A distended stomach may be injured by the operator; it must be prevented, or if present, deflated. The injected gas, usually CO_2, may cause cardiovascular disturbances due to the raised intra-abdominal pressure. These include rise or fall of arterial pressure, central venous pressure and heart rate. Hypercapnia causes increase in circulating catecholamines, peripheral vascular resistance and sometimes hypokalaemia.[177] peak levels of $Paco_2$ may not arise until after completion of the operative procedure. CO_2 embolus has been reported.[178] Studies[179] using impedance cardiography suggest that a moderate fall in stroke volume and cardiac output is related to the volume of gas used for peritoneal insufflation. The gas may accidentally be injected into the aorta, inferior vena cava, retroperitoneal tissues causing caval compression, hollow viscera or abdominal wall. The intra-abdominal pressure should probably not exceed $30\,cmH_2O$, a pressure adequate for good surgical exposure. The gas is absorbed but can be removed from the bloodstream by hyperventilation and IPPV. These changes are less frequent if N_2O is substituted for CO_2, although the risk of explosion from diathermy is introduced. The risk will be increased if gas from an injured viscus enters the peritoneal cavity.[180] Light general anaesthesia through a tracheal tube, with IPPV and relaxants, is a suitable combination and preferable to techniques of spontaneous respiration when the incidence of dysrhythmia is high, although nitrous oxide, oxygen and enflurane, with spontaneous respiration is stated to give good results.[181] Gross obesity, marked anxiety and the presence of peritoneal adhesions are relative contra-indications. The gas must be let out at the end of the operation or shoulder pain may result, lasting several days.[182]

Pneumothorax has been reported, presumably due to the passage of gas through congenital defects in the diaphragm.[183] Other complications reported include brachial plexus palsy (poor positioning) and regurgitation of gastric contents.

Termination of pregnancy. It is most important to check in these patients that the stomach is empty before induction. For the vaginal operation, thiopentone with nitrous oxide and oxygen, diazepam or neurolept agents, is usually satisfactory. Halothane relaxes the uterus, but halothane 0.5% is a

suitable agent for termination in the first trimester.[184] Light general anaesthesia with IPPV and a relaxant is suitable for the abdominal operation. Ergotamine tartrate, intravenously, raises venous as well as arterial tone and in patients with pre-existing heart disease may result in angina or acute pulmonary oedema. It may cause bronchospasm, nausea and vomiting. Oxytocin, 5 units, may be preferable.
For anaesthesia for operations during pregnancy, *see* Chapter 20.

References

1. Dick-Read G. *Childbirth without Fear*. 4th ed. London: Heineman; Brown F. J. *Antenatal and Postnatal Care*. London: Churchill Livingstone, 1976.
2. Loewe S. *Dtsch. Med. Wochenschr.* 1912, **38**, 947.
3. Vogt E. *Medsche Klin.* 1928, **24**, 24.
4. O'Sullivan J. V. and Craner W. W. *Lancet* 1932, **1**, 119: Irving F. C. et al. *Surg. Gynecol. Obstet.* 1934. **58**, 1.
5. Cleisz L. *Presse méd.* 1924, **32**, 1001
6. Kormann E. *Monat. Gerburts. Frauenkrank* 1860, **32**, 114
7. Sahli L. *Münch. Med Wochenschr.* 1909, 26.
8. Jaeger W. *Zentbl. Gynäk.* 1910, No. 46.
9. Steinbuchel R. von *Zentbl Gynäk* 1902, No. 48
10. Gauss C. J. *Arch Gynaek* 1906, **78**, 579. (*See also* Greenwood W. O. *Scopolamine-Morphine* London: Froude. 1918; the 5th edition of this Synopsis, 1964).
11. Korff B. *Münch. Med. Wochenschr.* 1901, **48**, 1169
12. van Hoosen B. *Curr. Res. Anesth. Analg.* 1928, **7**, 1963.
13. Duvoisin R. and Katz R. *JAMA* 1968, **206**, 1963
14. Clark R. B. *J. Arkansas Med. Soc.* 1971, **68**, 128
15. Akamatsu T. J. et al. *Anesth. Analg. (Cleve.)* 1974. **53**, 284; Dundee J. W. *Proc. R. Soc. Med.* 1971, **64**, 1159.
16. Pirogoff N. I. *C. R. Hebd. Séanc. Acad. Sci, Paris* 1847, **74**, 7879; Secher O. *Anaesthesia* 1986, **41**, 829.
17. Gwathmey J. T *N. Y Med. J* 1913, **98**, 1101.
18. Rosenfeld H. H. and Davidoff R. B. *Surg. Gynecol. Obstet.* 1935, **60**, 235.
19. Gwathmey J. T. *Am. J. Obstet. Gynecol. N. Y* 1965, **26**, 456
20. Kreis A. *Zentbl. Gynäk.* 1900, 747; Doleris Malartie and Dupaigne, *Report to Acad. Med. Paris* 22 January 1901.
21. Pitkin G. P. and McCormack F. C. *Surg. Gynecol. Obstet* 1928, **47**, 713.
22. Adriani J. and Roma-Vega D. *Am. J. Surg.* 1946, **71**, 12.
23. Stoeckel D. *Zentbl Gynäk.* 1909, **33**, 3; Oldham. S. P. *Kenty Med. J.* 1923, **21**, 321.
24. Gellert P. *Msehr. Geburtsh. Gynäk.* 1926, 73.
25. Cleland J. G. P. *Surg. Gynecol Obstet.* 1933, **57**, 51.
26. Bogdan E. C. *R. Soc. Biol. (Paris)* 1930, **105**, 25
27. Bogdan E. *Bull. Soc. Obstet. Gynaecol (Paris)* 1931, **20**, 35
28. Pickles W. and Jones. S. *N. Engl. J. Med.* 1928, **199**, 988.
29. Graffagnino P. and Seyler L. W. *Am.. J Obstet. Gynecol.* 1938, **35**, 597.
30. Hingson R. A and Southworth J. L. *Am. J. Surg.* 1942, **58**, 92; Edwards W. B. and Hingson R. A. *Am. J. Surg.* 1942, **57**, 459 (reprinted in 'Classical File', Surv. Anesthosiol. 1980, **24**, 275): Hingson R. A. and Edwards W. B. *Curr. Res. Anesth. Analg.* 1942, **21**, 301.
31. Flowers C. E. et al. *Curr. Res. Anesth. Analg.* 1949, **28**, 181
32. Simpson. J. Y. *Mon. J. Med. Sci.* (Lond. and Edin.), 1846–47, n.s, 1.
33. Simpson. J. Y. *Lond. Med. Gaz.* 1847, **5**, 935.
34. Farr A. D. *Anaesthesia* 1980, **35**, 896.
35. Little D. M. *Surv. Anesthesiol.* 1980, **24**, 272.

36. Junker F. E. *Med. Times, Lond.* 1869 **1**, 171.
37. Bourne W. *JAMA* 1935, **105**, 2047
38. Bourne W. *Lancet* 1934, **2**, 20; Griffith H. R. *Curr. Res. Anesth. Analg.* 1935, **14**, 253; Knight R. T. *Curr. Res. Anesth. Analg.* 1936, **15**, 63.
39. Elam J. *Lancet* 1943.
40. Freedman A. *Lancet* 1943, **2**, 696.
41. Klikowitsch H. *Arch. Gynaek.* 1881, **17**, 81; Richards W. et al. *Anaesthesia* 1976, **31**, 933.
42. Webster J. C. *JAMA* 1915, **24**, 812.
43. Guedel A. E. *Indianap. Med. J.* 1911, **14**, 476; *N. Y. Med. J.* 1912, **95**, 387.
44. Minnitt R. J. *Proc. R. Soc. Med.* 1934, **27**, 1313.
45. Seward E. H. *Proc. R. Soc. Med.* 1949, **42**, 745.
46. Tunstall M. E. *Lancet* 1961, **2**, 964.
47. Major V. et al. *Br. Med. J.* 1966, **2**, 1554.
48. Leboyer F. et al. *N. Engl. J. Med.* 1980, **302**, 655; Editorial, *N. Engl. J. Med.* 1980, **302**, 685
49. Hansen R. *Klin. Wochenschr.* 1942; Holmes F. J. *J. Obstet. Gynaecol. Br. Emp.* 1958, **64**, 229.
50. Mendelson C. L. *Am. J. Obstet. Gynecol.* 1946, **52**, 191 (reprinted in 'Classical File', *Surv. Anesthesiol.* 1966, **10**, 599).
51. Taylor G. and Pryse-Davies J. *Lancet* 1966, **1**, 288.
52. Scrimgeour J. B. in: *Antenatal Diagnosis of Genetic Diseases* (Emery A. E. H. ed.) Edinburgh: Churchill Livingstone, 1973.
53. Menees, T. O. et al *Am. J. Roetengenol.* 1930 **24**, 353.
54. Sweet M. *Br. J. Hosp. Med.* 1976, **15**, 351.
55. Bevan D. R. et al *Br. Med. J.* 1974, **1**, 13.
56. Ang C. K. et al. *Br. Med. J.* 1969, **4**, 20
57. Butler N. R. et al. *Br. Med. J.* 1972, **2**, 127; Cole P. V. et al. *J. Obstet. Gynaecol. Br. Commonw.* 1972, **79**, 782; Hardy J. B. and Mellitus E. D. *Lancet* 1972, **2**, 1332.
58. Crawford J. S. and Lewis M. *Anaesthesia* 1986, **41**, 900.
59. Hansen R. *Klin Wochenschr;* 1942, **21**, 301; Holmes F. *J. Obstet. Gynaecol. Br. Emp.* 1958, **64**, 229.
60. Dick-Read G *Childbirth without Fear*, 4th ed. London: Heineman, 1960.
61. See *N. Engl. J. Med* 1976, **294**, 1205.
62. Robson J. E. *Anaesthesia* 1979, **34**, 357; Stewart P. *Anaesthesia* 1979, **34**, 361.
63. Heyns O. S. *J. Obstet. Gynaecol. Br. Emp.* 1959, **66**, 220; Ginsburg J. *Br. J. Anaesth.* 1973, **45**, (Suppl.), 790.
64. Weiner P. C. et al. *Br. Med. J.* 1977, **2**, 228, 229.
65. Flowers C. et al. *Obstet. Gynecol. NY* 1969, **34**, 68.
66. Moir D. D. and Thorburn J. *Obstetric Anaesthesia and Analgesia*, 3rd ed. London: Baillière. Saunders, 1985.
67. Ginsberg J. *Am. Rev. Pharmacol.* 1971, **11**, 387.
68. See also Atkinson R. S. in: *Practical Regional Analgesia* (Lee J. A. and Bryce-Smith R. ed.) Amsterdam: Excerpta Medica, 1976; Moir D. D. *Obstetric Anaesthesia and Analgesia* 2nd ed. London: Baillére Tindall, 1980; Lee J. A., Atkinson R. S. and Watt M. J. *Lumbar Puncture and Spinal Analgesia*, 5th ed. Edinburgh: Churchill Livingstone, 1985.
69. Abural E. *Bull. Soc. Obstet. Gynaec. de Paris*, 1930, **19**, 165; Cleland J. G. P. *Surg. Gynecol. Obstet.* 1933, **57**, 51.
70. Kestin I. G. *Br. J. Anaesth.* 1991, **66**, 596; Russell I. F. *Curr. Opin. Anaesthesiol.*, 1991, **4**, 340.
71. Moore D. C. *Anaesthetic Techniques for Obstetrical Anaesthesia.* Springfield: Thomas, 1964.
72. Sprague D. H. and Russell I. F. *Anaesthesia* 1983, **37**, 346.
73. Randalls B. et al *Br. J. Anaesth.* 1991, **66**, 314.
74. Benedetti C. and Tiengo M. *Lancet* 1990, **ii**, 225.
75. Naulty J. S. et al *Anesthesiology* 1990, **73**, (Suppl. 3A), A964; Norris M. C. et al. *Anesthesiology* 1990, **73**, (Suppl. 3A), 983; El-Naggar M. et al. *Anesthesiology* 1990, **73**, (Suppl. 3), 970.

76. Morgan B. *Anaesthesia* 1990, **45**, 148.
77. Russell I. F. *Br. J. Anaesth.* 1983, **55**, 309.
78. Tunstall M. E. *Br. J. Anaesth.* 1991, **67**, 227.
79. Barker P. *Anaesth. Intensive Care* 1990, **18**, 553.
80. Carrie L. E. S. and Collins P. B. *Br. J. Anaesth.* 1991, **66**, 145.
81. Cesarini M. et al. *Anaesthesia* 1990, **45**, 656.
82. Lyons G. and Macdonald R. *Br. J. Anaesth.* 1991, **67**, 222.
83. van Steenberge A. *Curr. Opin. Anaesthesiol.* 1991, **4**, 345.
84. Michael S. et al. *Anaesthesia* 1989, **44**, 578.
85. Lee J. A. *Anaesthesia* 1960, **15**, 186; 1962, **17**, 249; Doughty A. *Anaesthesia* 1974, **29**, 63.
86. Howie J. E. and Dutton D. A. In: *Epidural and Spinal Analgesia in Obstetrics* (Reynolds F. ed). London: Bailliere Tindall, 1990, 162.
87. Carrie L. E. S. *Br. J. Anaesth.* 1990, **65**, 225.
88. Reynolds F. and Taylor G. *Anaesthesia* 1970, **25**, 14.
89. Reynolds F. and Taylor G. *Br. J. Anaesth.* 1971, **43**, 436.
90. Evans K. R. L. et al. *Anaesthesia* 1979, **34**, 310.
91. Nickel P. M. et al. *Regional Anaesthesia* in press; Cole C. P. et al. *Anesthesiology* 1985, **62**, 348.
92. Lund P. C. et al. *Br. J. Anaesth.* 1977, **49**, 457.
93. Vella L. M. et al. *Anaesthesia* 1985, **40**, 741; Reynolds F., *Br. J. Anaesth.* 1989, **63**, 251.
94. Enever G. R. et al. *Anaesthesia* 1991, **46**, 169.
95. Baldwin A. M. et al. *Anaesth. Intensive Care* 1991, **19**, 246.
96. Walton P. and Reynolds F. *Anaesthesia* 1984, **39**, 218.
97. Crawford J. S. *Anaesthesia* 1985, **40**, 1219.
98. Evans J. M. et al. *Anaesthesia* 1975, **30**, 774.
99. Edwards W. B. and Hingson R. A. *Am. J. Surg.* 1942, **57**, 459 (reprinted in 'Classical File' *Surv. Anesthesiol.* 1980, **24**, 275); *JAMA* 1943, **121**, 225; Hingson R. A. et al. *Anesth. Analg. Curr. Res.* 1961, **40**, 119.
100. Curran J. et al. *Anaesthesia* 1975. **30**, 765.
101. Macdonald R. and Bickford Smith P. J. *Br. J. Anaesth.* 1982, **56**, 1202.
102. Tunstall M. E. *Lancet* 1961, **2**, 964; *Br. Med. J.* 1963, **2**, 915; Gale C. W. et al. *Br. Med. J.* 1964. **1**, 732; MacGregor W. G. et al. *Anaesthesia.* 1972, **27**, 14; Dolan P. F. and Rosen M. *Lancet* 1975, **2**, 1030.
103. Davis J. M. et al. *Br. J. Anaesth.* 1975, **47**, 370.
104. Crowhurst J. A. *Curr. Opin. Anaesthesiol.* 1991, **4**, 349.
105. Morgan B. M. *Anaesthesia* 1980, **35**, 334.
106. Vella L. et al. *Br. Med. J.* 1985, **290**, 1173.
107. Crawford J. S. *Principles and Practice of Obstetric Anaethesia.* 5th ed. Oxford: Blackwell. 1986.
108. Crawford J. S. *Lancet* 1983, **1**, 271.
109. Nimmo W. S. et al. *Lancet* 1975, **1**, 890.
110. Andrews A. D. et al. *Anaesthesia* 1982, **37**, 22.
111. Johnston J. R. et al. *Anaesthesia* 1982, **37**, 33.
112. Alexander I. G. S. *Br. J. Anaesth.* 1968, **40**, 408: Bannister W. K. and Sattilaro A. J. *Anesthesiology* 1962, **23**, 251; Vandam L. D. *N. Engl. J. Med.* 1965, **273**, 1206; Heaney G. A. M. and Jones H. D. *Br. J. Anaesth.* 1970, **51**, 266; Whittington R. M. et al. *Lancet* 1979, **2**, 228; Bond Y. K. et al. *Anesthesiology* 1979, **51**, 452.
113. McCaughey W. et al. *Anaesthesia* 1981, **36**, 167.
114. McAuley D. M. et al. *Anaesthesia* 1983, **38**, 108.
115. Gallagher E. G., et al. *Anaesthesia* 1988, **43**, 1011–1014; Escolano F et al. *Anaesthesia* 1989, **44**, 212–215; Dubin S. A. *Anesth. Analg.* 1989, **69**, 680–683.
116. *See* Rorke M. J. et al. *Anaesthesia* 1965, **23**, 585; Marx G. F. and Matter C. V. *Can. Anaesth. Soc. J.* 1971, **18**, 587; Crawford J. S. et al. *Br. J. Anaesth.* 1976, **48**, 661; Palahiuk R. J. et al. *Can. Anaesth. Soc. J.* 1977, **24**, 586.
117. Galloon S. *Can Anaesth. Soc. J.* 1971, **18**, 600.

118. Valentine B. H. et al. *Br. J. Anaesth.* 1977, **49**, 81.
119. Moodie J. E. and Moir D. D. *Br. J. Anaesth.* 1976, **48**, 571; Moir D. D. and Amoa A. B. *Br. J. Anaesth.* 1979, **51**, 113.
120. Crawford J. S. *Anaesthesia* 1985, **40**, 498.
121. Johnstone M. *Br. J. Anaesth.* 1972, **44**, 826.
122. Levinson G. et al. *Anaesthesia* 1974, **40**, 340.
123. Crawford J. S. *Anesthesia* 1979. **34**. 892.
124. Hutchinson R. *Br. J. Anaesth.* 1961, **33**, 463; Waters D. J. *Br. J. Anaesth.* 1968, **40**, 259.
125. Skoldebrand A. et al. *Acta Anaes. Scand.* 1990, **34**, 79.
126. Lindblad A. and Marsal K. *Br. Med. J.* 1984, **288**, 132.
127. Skoldebrand A. et al. *Acta Anaes. Scand.* 1990, **34**, 85.
128. Thompson E. M. et al. *Anaesthesia* 1985, **40**, 427.
129. Hallworth D. et al. *Anaesthesia* 1982, **37**, 53.
130. Kileff M. E. et al. *Anesth. Analg. (Cleve.)* 1984, **63**, 413.
131. Bates R. G. and Helm C. W. *J. R. Soc. Med.* 1985, **78**, 890.
132. Thompson E. M. et al. *Anaesthesia* 1985, **40**, 427.
133. Alahuhta S. et al. *Acta Anaes. Scand.* 1990, **34**, 99.
134. Russell I. F. *Anaesthesia* 1983, **37**, 346; Brownridge P. *Anaesth. Intensive Care* 1984, **12**, 334.
135. Ranney B. and Strange W. F. *Obstet. Gynecol. NY* 1975, **45**, 163.
136. Brahms D. *Anaesthesia* 1990, **45**, 161.
137. Tunstall M. E. *Br. Med. J.* 1977, **1**, 1321; Tunstall M. E. *Anaesthesia* 1979, **34**, 316; Wilson M. E. *Br. Med. J.* 1980, **1**, 1270.
138. Tunstall M. E. in: *General Anaesthesia* (Gray T. C. et al. ed.) 4th ed. London: Butterworths, 1980.
139. McClure S., Regan M. and Moore J. *Anaesthesia* 1990, **45**, 227; Freeman R. and Baxendale B. *Anaesthesia* 1990, **45**, 1094.
140. King T. A. and Adams A. P. *Br. J. Anaesth.* 1990, **65**, 400.
141. O'Sullivan G. and Stoddart P. A. *Br. J. Anaesth.* 1991, **67**, 225.
142. Crawford J. S. *Br. J. Anaesth.* 1977, **49**, 19.
143. Dallas S. H. *Br. J. Anaesth.* 1967, **39**, 969; Whitford J. H. et al. *Br. J. Anaesth.* 1973, **55**, 1153.
144. Patterson K. W. and O'Toole D. P. *British Journal of Anaesthesia* 1991, **66**, 513
145. Schindler M. et al. *Anaesth. Intensive Care* 1990, **18**, 169.
146. Barker P. and Callendar G. C. *Anaesthesia* 1991, **46**, 64; Trotter T. N. et al. *Anaesthesia* 1991, **46**, 590.
147. Loevingen E. H. et al. *Obstet. and Gynecol* 1985, **65**, 281.
148. Tillman H. A. *Can. Anaesth. Soc. J.* 1984, **31**, 210.
149. Ramathan J. et al. *Am. J. Obstet. Gynecol.* 1988, **158**, 40.
150. James M. F. M. et al. *Magnesium* 1987, **6**, 314 *ibid*, **7**, 37.
151. Dinsdale H. B. *Arch. Neurol.* 1988, **45**, 1360.
152. Kaplan P. W. et al. *Arch of Neurol.* 1988, **45**, 1360.
153. Morgan M. *Anaesthesia* 1979, **34**, 20; Annotation, *Lancet* 1979, **2**, 398; Moore P. G. et al. *Anaesth. Intensive Care* 1982, **10**, 40.
154. *Brazil-Medico* 1926, **2**, 301.
155. Steiner P. E. and Lusbaugh C. C. *JAMA* 1941, **117**, 1245.
156. Weiner A. E. et al. *N. Engl. J. Med.* 1950, **243**, 597.
157. *See also* Scott J. S. *Br. J. Hosp. Med.* 1969, **2**, 1847.
158. Preston F. E. *Br. J. Hosp. Med.* 1982, **28**, 129.
159. Slater R. M. et al. *Anaesthesia* 1985, **40**, 655.
160. Tuck S. M. *Br. J. Hosp. Med.* 1982, **28**, 125.
161. Coaldrake I. A. and Livingstone P. *Anaesth. Intensive Care* 1983, **11**, 254.
162. Marshall Hall (1790–1857). *Lancet* 1856, **2**, 601 (reprinted in 'Classical File'. *Surv. Anesthesiol.* 1977, **21**, 398).

163. Boddy K. and Robinson J. S. *Lancet* 1971, **2**, 1231; Boddy K. and Mantell C. D. *Lancet* 1972, **2**, 1219.
164. Apgar V. *Curr. Res. Anesth. Analg.* 1953, **32**, 260 (reprinted in 'Classical File'. *Surv. Anesthesiol.* 1975, **19**, 401): Calmes S. H. In: *Anaesthesia: Essays on its History.* (Rupreht J. et al. ed.) Berlin: Springer-Verlag, 1985, p. 45.
165. Dubowitz V. *Br. J. Anaesth.* 1975, **47**, 1005; Brazelton T. B. *Clinics in Developmental Medicine.* No. 50, 1973, London: SIMR-Heinemann.
166. Head Hy, J. *Physiol. (Lond.)* 1889, 10; 1 and 279.
167. Terry T. L., *Am J. Ophthalmol.* 1942, **25**, 203.
168. Johnson W. C. and Meyer J. R. *Am. J. Obstet. Gynecol.* 1925, **9**, 151: Strang L. B. *Br. Med. Bull.* 1963, **19**, 45.
169. McDowall E. *Elect. Rep. Analyt. Rev.* 1817, **7**, 242.
170. Sims J. M. (1813–1883) *Am. J. Med. Sci.* 1852, **23**, 59.
171. Tait L. *Med. Times Gaz. 1881*, **2**, 654.
172. Wertheim E. (1864–1920). *Archs f. Gynaek.* 1900, **61**, 627.
173. Taylor J. and Weil R. H. *Surg. Gynecol. Obset.* 1967, **124**, 1005.
174. *See also* Atkinson R. S. In: *Recent Advances in Anaesthesia and Analgesia*–12 (Hewer C. L. and Atkinson R. S. ed.) Edinburgh: Churchill Livingstone, 1976; Nuefeld J. S. et al. *Surg. Gynecol. Obstet.* 1978, **147**, 705; Cuschieri A. *Br. J. Hosp. Med.* 1980, **24**, 252.
175. Jacobeus H. C. *Münch. Med. Wochenschr.* 1910, **57**, 2090.
176. Cooper G. M. et al. *Anaesthesia* 1982, **37**, 266.
177. Hassan H. and Tomlin P. J. *Anaesthesia* 1979, **34**, 897.
178. Clark C. C. et al. *Anaesth. Intensive Care* 1977, **5**, 650.
179. Lenz R. J. et al. *Anaesthesia* 1976, **31**, 4.
180. Cameron A. E. et al. *J. R. Soc. Med.* 1983, **76**, 1015.
181. Harris M. N. E. et al. *Br. J. Anaesth.* 1984, **56**, 1214.
182. Dodson M. E. *Br. J. Anaesth.* 1978, **50**, 169.
183. Calverly R. K. and Jenkins L. C. *Can. Anaesth. Soc. J.* 1973, **20**, 679.
184. West S. L. et al. *Anaesthesia* 1985, **40**, 669.

Ophthalmic surgery

In intraocular surgery, a sudden rise in intraocular tension from the normal 15–25 mmHg following coughing, vomiting, contraction of the orbicularis oculi or straining may cause displacement of iris or vitreous into the wound, and so in the past these operations have been usually performed under local analgesia. (It was, in fact, the poor quality of the general anaesthesia available in Vienna in the 1880s that stimulated Carl Koller to seek practical means of producing local analgesia of the eye, and to employ cocaine for this purposes – so initiating the whole concept of local analgesia in surgery.) Now, following modern improvement in general anaesthetic technique, cataract operations in the younger patients are usually done under careful general anaesthesia, taking great pains to avoid coughing and similar disturbances. There is now a swing towards local methods (*see below*).

Extraction of the lens nucleus for cataract was first described by Jacques Daviel, French oculist (1696–1762), in 1753. The ophthalmoscope was invented in 1851 by H. L. F. von Helmholtz (1821–1894).

Tone of pupil

Dilatation. Drops of 0.5% tropicamide with maximum effect in 40–60 min, wearing off in a few hours. Effects of atropine last many days. It is parasympatholytic and weakens the sphincter muscles of the pupil; both are potentiated by phenylephrine 10%. Effects reversed by 0.5% pilocarpine, which stimulates muscle fibres of the pupillary sphincter. Thymoxamine reverses the action of phenylephrine. The risks of causing acute closed-angle glaucoma is very small.[1]

Innervation of the eye

(1) Motor. Superior oblique muscle from 4th cranial nerve. Lateral rectus from 6th. All other extraocular muscles from the 3rd nerve. Orbicularis oculis from the 7th. (2) Sensory. Optic nerve conveys vision. Other sensation from ophthalmic division of the 5th nerve. (3) Parasympathetic. Fibres arise from the Edinger–Westphal nucleus and run with the 3rd nerve to synapse in the ciliary ganglion, then via the short ciliary nerves. Stimulation of the parasympathetic causes constriction of the pupil and of the ciliary muscle. (4) Sympathetic. Fibres from T1 synapse in the superior cervical ganglion and travel via the carotid plexus to join the long and short ciliary nerves. Stimulation produces dilatation of the pupil.

Local analgesia

Advantages. (1) Safer; (2) less postoperative nausea and vomiting; (3) early ambulation and feeding; (4) less bleeding; (5) less risk of pulmonary embolism; (6) less upset of biochemical processes; (7) less postoperative restlessness; (8) less postoperative lung pathology; and (9) less postoperative coronary or cerebral thrombosis.[2] Loss of memory function in the elderly after cataract extraction under general anaesthesia is no worse than after regional analgesia plus sedation.[3]

Disadvantage. Lack of control of the patient. Difficulty in controlling intraocular pressure.[4]

Technique of analgesia of cornea and conjunctival sac. Drops of 4% lignocaine should be instilled into the conjunctival sac every 2 min on five occasions; 2–4% cocaine may be used when prolonged intense analgesia is required. This will give analgesia and vasoconstriction of the cornea and conjunctiva, but not of the iris or ciliary body; nor will it produce analgesia in a glaucomatous eye. Cocaine has the disadvantage that it produces dilatation of the pupil (bad in glaucoma), slight cloudiness of the cornea, while it irritates and dries the corneal epithelium. Amethocaine 0.5 or 1%, which lasts longer, does not have these effects and can also be used for tonometry. If the local analgesic drug is dissolved in methylcellulose, stinging of the eye will not result when instillation into the conjunctival sac takes place. Adrenaline can be added to these local analgesics to produce ischaemia. Oxybuprocaine has been used for local analgesia.[5]

Infraorbital block (*see* Chapter 24) from the infraorbital canal below the eye produces analgesia of the central part of the lower lid; lacrimal block, its lateral part; supra- and infratrochlear block, its medial part. These can all be reached as they emerge from the skull.

The lacrimal, supraorbital, supra- and infratrochlear nerves together supply the upper lid, the upper part of the lacrimal fossa, and the upper canaliculus.

Akinesia or facial nerve block is necessary before all intraocular operations under local analgesia, to prevent blepharospasm.

1. Van Lint's technique.[6] The first method for producing akinesia in operations for cataract extraction. From a point 1 cm behind the lateral margin of the orbit at the level of the inferior margin, solution is injected first upwards and then horizontally between the muscles and the bone.

2. O'Brien's technique.[7] From a weal just in front of the tragus, below the zygomatic process, a needle injects solution over the condyloid process of the mandible.

Retro-bulbar (retro-ocular) block.

This must be done before operation under local analgesia on the globe of the eye. After topical analgesia of the cornea and conjunctival sac, the long and short posterior ciliary nerves and ciliary ganglion are blocked within the muscle cone. These supply the uveal tract and cornea and reduce the tone of the extraocular muscles. Retro-ocular block dilates the pupil, causes exophthalmos, reduces intraocular pressure and makes prolapse of the vitreous less likely. Hyaluronidase (6–10 turbidity-reducing (TR) units to each ml of solution) aids spread. Facial nerve block is used to paralyse the extraocular muscles. Two per cent lignocaine or prilocaine is a suitable solution, 2 ml (4 ml for enucleation).

1. Superior,[8] through the superior rectus, with the patient looking downwards, from a weal just above the middle of the tarsal plate. A 5 cm needle is used and is inserted 3–4 cm backwards, slightly inwards and downwards. During movement of the needle, injection is continuous as a safeguard against injuring veins.

2. Inferolateral, from a weal at the inferolateral margin of the orbit. A 5-cm needle is inserted backwards along the floor of the orbit, until its tip is posterior to the eye at the apex of the orbit: 1–2 ml of solution are injected. A transconjunctival approach may also be employed. Deposition of a little solution is also necessary in superior rectus.

Retrobulbar haemorrhage. This is likely to follow puncture of a vessel by the needle used for retrobulbar block. It results in a rise in intraorbital pressure with proptosis and requires postponement of the operation.

Retro-bulbar block using bupivacaine has been reported as resulting in brainstem anaesthesia with apnoea, needing IPPV and intubation.[9]

Periocular block[10]

The block is advocated as simple to perform with a low incidence of complications.

Solution used. Equal mixture of 2% lignocaine and 0.5% bupivacaine to which 500 units hyaluronidase are added. Total volume used 12–15 ml, occasionally 20 ml (especially in the elderly when fluid is likely to leak out from the space).

Technique. (1) Lower Block. Skin weal in lower lid, just superior to inferior orbital rim, 1.5 cm medial to lateral canthus. Needle advanced through weal with bevel towards orbit (blunt 1.25 inches Atkinson needle recommended). 'Pop' felt as needle passes through lower orbital septum. Needle point is advanced towards equator of eye, angled supero–medially, and 4 ml injected at a depth of about 2.5 cm. Tension within orbital tissues monitored by testing eyeball movement using lid palpation. Often there is a temporary proptosis and conjunctival oedema. On needle withdrawal, 1 ml is delivered to the orbicularis oculi muscle. (2) Upper Block. Skin weal to upper lid 1–2 mm medial and inferior to the supra–orbital notch. Needle is advanced through the weal aimed at the roof of the orbit, parallel to nose. The needle is advanced posteriorly over eyeball to a depth of about 2 cm. Then it is directed medially and advanced 0.5–1.0 cm and 2–3 ml injected and eyeball tension checked. 1 ml injected into substance of orbicularis oculi on withdrawal. A pressure cuff is applied to the eye for 10–20 min. Degree of blockade is checked 5 min after application. If there is mobility still present a further 3–4 ml is injected (lower injection for infero-lateral and upper injection for supero-medial movement).

Mechanism. Thought to be by diffusion of solution to branches of cranial nerves 3, 4, 5, 6 and 7 and to ciliary ganglion.

Advantages. (1) Technique is easy to learn and perform; (2) reduced incidence of serious complications (retro-bulbar haematoma, optic nerve damage, intradural injection); and (3) no need for the often painful facial nerve block.

Disadvantages. (1) Time consuming to undertake; (2) minor complications include peri-orbital ecchymosis and subcutaneous spread of solution to opposite eye; (3) global perforation possible in large myopic eyes; and (4) larger volumes of solution required than for retrobulbar block, with need for close monitoring.

General anaesthesia

Intraocular pressure.[11] Ideally the eye should be soft before the anterior chamber is opened, because a sudden decompression may produce stresses, which can in turn result in haemorrhage. General anaesthesia should not cause a rise in intraocular pressure. Anaesthesia should aim at reduction of choroidal vascular congestion, which in turn causes reduction in intraocular tension. Choroidal blood flow is affected by $Paco_2$ (similar in effect to the cerebral circulation).

Intraocular pressure may be lowered by: (1) mechanical methods, pre-operative use of a pressure pad, or manual milking of fluid from the anterior chamber immediately prior to start of the operation; (2) hypocapnia (IPPV); (3) hypotension; (4) reduction of central venous pressure; (5) acetazolamide; and (6) intravenous anaesthetics, narcotic analgesics and volatile anaesthetic agents (provided $Paco_2$ is not allowed to rise).

Intraocular pressure is raised by: (1) hypercapnia; (2) coughing, sneezing, straining and other causes of raised central venous pressure; (3) suxamethonium; (4) locally administered atropine (in narrow-angle glaucoma); and (5) local steroids.

When the blood pressure rises, the intraocular pressure does not greatly alter but when it is less than 85 mmHg the intraocular pressure falls.[12] Drainage of the anterior chamber is increased by contraction of the ciliary muscle, e.g. eserine; decreased by relaxation, e.g. atropine. (*See* Review on anaesthesia and intraocular pressure. Murphy D. F. *Anesth. Analg. (Cleve.)* 1985, **54**, 520.)

Advantages. (1) Co-operation of patient ceases to become a problem; (2) no risk of retrobulbar haematoma from injection of local analgesic drug; (3) less of an ordeal for the patient; and (4) quiet atmosphere in theatre facilitates delicate surgery.

Anaesthetic drugs in ophthalmic surgery

Premedication. Drugs used must not contribute to postoperative vomiting. Narcotic analgesics are better avoided for this reason. Phenothiazine or benzodiazapine drugs are often employed, e.g. lorazepam, 5 mg in healthy young adults, reducing to 1 mg in older patients, by mouth.

Atropine. This with other mydriatics raises the intraocular pressure only in the presence of glaucoma with a narrow angle between the cornea and iris, a genetically determined state not usually detected prior to the onset of glaucoma. Atropine may precipitate an acute attack of glaucoma in these patients, but dilatation of the pupil is without risk in the majority of patients with glaucoma.[13] Sensitivity to atropine drops into the conjunctival sac does not contra-indicate intramuscular or intravenous atropine. Pilocarpine drops, 1%, overcome this danger by constricting the pupil.

Adrenaline. Does not dilate the pupil if instilled into the conjunctival sac. Adrenaline is rapidly absorbed from the conjunctival sac and may cause systemic effects. One drop of 1 in 100 solution contains 1.4 mg.

Morphine. Contracts the pupil from stimulation of the 3rd cranial nerve nucleus.

Suxamethonium. This increases intraocular tension but the rise is probably confined to the period of apnoea and so is no reason for banning this useful aid to intubation. The average rise is 7–8 mmHg.[14] It comes on in 30 s, is maximal at 2 min and has disappeared in 6 min after injection.[15] It should not be used during an operation when the eye is already open, for fear of precipitating vitreous prolapse, e.g. in penetrating injury.[16]

The mechanism of the rise in intraocular pressure is not fully understood. It may be that contraction of the extraocular muscles is important, but there is evidence that pressure rises even when these muscles have been detached from their insertions.[17]

These effects can be minimized by the injection, 3–5 min beforehand, of a small dose of a non-depolarizing relaxant (but this view has been disputed).

The intravenous injection of *acetazolamide*, 500 mg immediately before induction of anaesthesia, largely prevents rise in intraocular pressure due to suxamethonium. It is a carbonic anhydrase inhibitor and interferes with the secretion of aqueous. Its other effects include diuresis, depression of the central nervous system, potassium loss, metabolic acidosis and alteration of the response of the respiratory centre to carbon dioxide. It has no effect on either the pupil size or the drainage from the eye.

Non-depolarizing relaxants. Reduce the tone of extraocular muscles and produce apnoea. Gallamine blocks the oculocardiac vagal reflexes. IPPV has the advantage that rise in the $Paco_2$ with associated rise in intraocular pressure can be prevented. It allows light planes of anaesthesia to be maintained with rapid recovery on completion of surgery.

Intravenous and intramuscular agents. Thiopentone is popular for the induction of anaesthesia. It reduces the tension in normal and glaucomatous eyes. Anti-emetic agents may be used to reduce the incidence of vomiting.

Inhalation agents. Halothane, isoflurane and enflurane given to supplement nitrous oxide and oxygen, or with oxygen alone, in a non-rebreathing, partially rebreathing or closed system, offer good conditions, with quiet respiration and minimal postoperative nausea and vomiting. Intraocular pressure falls, even when arterial pressure is maintained, but is more certain when hypotension occurs. The $Paco_2$ can be prevented from rising if muscle relaxants and IPPV are used to maintain it at normal levels.[18] Intraocular pressure falls if $Paco_2$ remains normal.[19]

Ecothiopate iodide (phospholine iodide, an organophosphate derivative of choline). Low levels of serum cholinesterase amounting to a twofold reduction in one-third of patients can occur within a few days of commencing the use of drops of this agent in the treatment of glaucoma.[20] Although a 50% reduction in enzyme activity should not prolong apnoea with suxamethonium for more than 10–15 min a non-depolarising agent may be preferred. The effects of these drops on the enzyme level lasts 2–4 weeks after the cessation of treatment.

Some suitable general anaesthetic techniques

1. Squint. Intravenous thiopentone, suxamethonium, tracheal tube, and nitrous oxide–oxygen–halothane with spontaneous respiration or muscle relaxant and IPPV. The oculocardiac reflex is discussed below.

2. Intraocular operations. Intracapsular extraction, removal of the lens with its capsule, is the operation now usually done for cataract. The binocular microscope for operating was first used as a colposcope in 1953 and first used in ophthalmology at Tübingen, its employment having been stimulated by Julius Lempert in otology in 1938.[21] Lysis of the zonule supporting the lens was described by Joaquin Barraquer of Barcelona in 1958. Extraction of the lens by first touching it with a cryoprobe (temperature −30°C) was described by T. Krawitz of Poland in 1961.

Some suitable techniques are: (1) thiopentone, muscle relaxant, nitrous oxide and oxygen, supplementation with a volatile or intravenous agent and IPPV; and (2) spontaneous respiration can be allowed, particularly if the surgeon is quick. Volatile agents must be given in sufficient concentration to ensure that coughing does not occur. Coughing on the tube is to be avoided, and if the eye is open this complication may be disastrous because vitreous can be extruded and eyesight may be lost. An alternative to the use of a tracheal tube is the laryngeal mask. In cases of difficult or impossible intubation a Charles airway adaptor[22] can be useful, although the jaw still needs support.

Corneal grafts. The first corneal graft[23] was carried out in 1906 in Austria. Tudor Thomas of Cardiff was a pioneer in the 1920s in the UK. Operations to restore eyesight after damage to the front of the eye require anaesthesia as for intraocular operations.

Insertion of implants following cataract surgery. Harold Ridley used the first intraocular lens implant in 1948,[24] a technique developed by D. P. Choyce.[25] The principles of anaesthesia are the same as for other intraocular procedures.

Vitriectomy. Diseased and fibrosed vitreous is removed and replaced by a balanced salt solution. General anaesthesia is required with complete immobility of the patient for several hours. A microscope and a small fibreoptic light source are used, in a darkened theatre. Sulpha-hexafluoride is employed to fill the vitrectomized eye to prevent retinal detachment. Nitrous oxide can diffuse into the eye with considerable increase in its volume and must be discontinued at this stage and alternative drugs employed to maintain anaesthesia. Repeated operations at short intervals may be required. Non-depolarizing relaxants, IPPV and full monitoring techniques are recommended.[26]

Retinal Detachment. Meticulous anaesthesia is required and a smooth, quiet emergence and postoperative period are wanted in order to reduce the likelihood of further detachment.

Glaucoma. Patients have often received medical treatment with drugs such as cholinergics and anticholinesterases (e.g. ecothiopate). Acetazolamide can cause dehydration and metabolic acidosis. Systemic atropine is not contra-indicated in normal dosage. The anaesthesist should avoid agents and techniques that cause a rise in intraocular pressure.

Perforating eye injuries. Smooth anaesthesia is the order of the day. Induction of anaesthesia must avoid coughing and straining because these are associated with an acute rise in intraocular pressure with the danger of loss of vitreous fluid and even the danger of loss of sight when the eye is open as a result of trauma. Surgery is rarely urgent and the optimal time of operation must be discussed with the surgeon. Each case must be judged on its merits, attention being paid to: (1) urgency of surgery; (2) likelihood of the presence of stomach contents; and (3) possible difficulty of tracheal intubation. Few anaesthetists have personal experience of a large series of cases. A suitable technique for many cases includes preoxygenation, thiopentone induction, generous dose of non-depolarizing relaxant, intubation as soon as conditions are considered right, use of cricoid pressure and maintenance along the usual lines. There are workers of experience who have used suxamethonium for intubation without vitreous loss, especially when there is judged to be a risk of aspiration of stomach contents.[27] In a few patients other injuries may have to be considered.

3. Examination of the eyes in small children. Spontaneous breathing without a tracheal tube using a small mask for halothane with nitrous oxide and oxygen is satisfactory. Ketamine has been suggested (e.g. 2 mg/kg i.v. or 10 mg/kg i.m.)

4. Tonometry in infants. This is required when buphthalmos is suspected. Nitrous oxide–oxygen–halothane is satisfactory.

5. Laser treatment. When applied to the retina, this can be carried out without general anaesthesia; a few drops of local analgesic solution in the conjunctival sac allows treatment without major discomfort.

Special points

(1) All disturbances causing movement, cough or contraction of the orbicularis oculi must be avoided because they may increase the intraocular tension with resulting iris prolapse or vitreous prolapse; (2) postoperative vomiting and coughing should be minimized for the same reason; (3) postoperative restlessness may be due to a full bladder; (4) congenital cataract may be associated with dystrophia myotonica or with diabetes; and (5) *Oculocardiac reflex* (Aschner's reflex), first described in 1908.[28] A variety of stimuli arising in or near the eye may cause abnormalities of the rate or rhythm of the heart. Anaesthesia appears to make the heart vulnerable to increased vagal tone, especially in the young. It is suggested that patients with blue or grey eyes are less likely to develop an oculocardiac reflex dysrhythmia than similar patients with brown or hazel eyes.[29] Cardiac standstill is the danger, preceded by bradycardia, especially following traction on the medial rectus, or pressure on the eyeball, so that adequate cardiac monitoring should accompany these interventions. Gallamine and atropine intravenously are useful preventatives. Glycopyrronium has a similar effect but causes less tachycardia.[30] Hyoscine butylbromide, 10–20 mg i.v. (Buscopan) has been recommended.[31] Retro-bulbar injection of local analgesic solutions is not as efficient. The oculocardiac reflex may also be seen during operations for the correction of facial fractures[32] in patients with the Marcus Gunn syndrome[33] and in operations on the empty orbit.[34]

See also Elliott J. and Morrison J. D. In: *Anaesthesia for Eye, Ear, Nose and Throat Surgery*. 2nd ed. (Morrison J. D., Mirakhur R. K. and Craig H. J. L. ed.) Edinburgh: Churchill Livingstone, 1985.

References

1. Phillips C. I. *Br. Med. J.* 1984, **288**, 1779.
2. Backer C. L. et al. *Anesthesiology* 1979, **51**, Suppl. 61; Backer C. L. et al. *Anesth. Analg. (Cleve.)* 1980, **59**, 257.
3. Karkunen U. and John G. *Acta Anaesth. Scand.* 1982, **26**, 294.
4. Bricker S. R. W., McGalliard J. N. and Mostafa S. M. *Anaesthesia* 1990, **45**, 36.
5. Christensen C. *Acta Anaesthesiol. Scand.* 1990, **34**, 165.
6. Van Lint A. *Ann. Oculist.* 1914, **151**, 420.
7. O'Brien C. S. *Arch. Ophthalmol.* 1929, **1**, 447.
8. Macintosh R. R. and Ostlere M. *Local Analgesia. Head and Neck.* 2nd ed. Edinburgh: Livingstone, 1967, 121.
9. Editorial, *J. Neuro-ophthalmol.* 1981, **1**, 172; Smith J. L. *Ann. Ophthmol.* 1982, **14**, 1005; Chang J. L. et al. *Anesthesiology* 1984, **63**, 789.
10. Fry R. A. and Henderson J. *Anaesthesia* 1990, **45**, 14.
11. *See also* Jay J. L. *Br. J. Anaesth.* 1980, **52**, 649; Le May M. *Br. J. Anaesth.* 1980, **52**, 655; Holloway K. B. *Br. J. Anaesth.* 1980, **52**, 671; Rose N. M. and Adams A. P. *Anaesthesia* 1980, **35**, 569.
12. Schreuder M. and Linssen G. A. *Anaesthesia* 1972, **27**, 165.
13. Foulds W. S. *Br. J. Anaesth.* 1980, **52**, 643.
14. Katz R. L. *Anesthesiology* 1968, **29**, 70.
15. Pandey K. et al. *Br. J. Anaesth.* 1972, **44**, 191.
16. Feneck R. O. and Cook J. H. *Anaesthesia* 1983, **38**, 120.

17. Craythorne N. W. B. et al. *Anesthesiology* 1960, **18**, 44.
18. Adams A. P. et al. *Br. J. Ophthalmol.* 1979, **63**, 204.
19. Adams A. P. et al. *Anaesthesia* 1979, **34**, 526.
20. McGavi D. D. M. *Lancet* 1965, **2**, 272.
21. Lempert J. *Arch. Otolaryngol.* 1938, **28**, 42.
22. Charles H. *Br. Med. J.* 1937, **1**, 449.
23. Zirn E. A. *von Graefes' Arch. Ophth.* 1906, **64**, 580.
24. Ridley H. *Lancet* 1952, **1**, 118.
25. Choyce D. P. *Intraocular Lenses and Implants.* London: Lewis, 1964.
26. Mirakhur R. K. *Ann. R. Coll. Surg. Engl.* 1985, **67**, 34.
27. Libonati M. M. et al. *Anesthesiology* 1985, **62**, 637; Bourke D. L. *Anesthesiology* 1985, **63**, 727.
28. Aschner S. *Wien. Klin. Wochenschr.* 1908, **21**, 1529; Dagnini G. *Bol. della Sc. Med.* 1908, **8**, 380.
29. Fry E. N. S. and Hall-Parker B. J. P. *Br. Med. J.* 1974, **4**, 659.
30. Myers E. F. *Anesthesiology* 1979, **51**, 350.
31. Fry E. N. S. *Anaesthesia* 1975, **30**, 549; Fry E. N. S. and Hall-Parker B. J. P. *Br. J. Ophthalmol.* 1975, **59**, 529.
32. Robideaux V. *Anesthesiology* 1978, **49**, 433.
33. Gunn M. *Trans. Ophthalmol. Soc. UK* 1883, **3**, 283; Kwik R. S. H. *Anaesthesia* 1980, **33**, 46.
34. Kerr W. J. and Vance J. P. *Anaesthesia* 1983, **38**, 883.

Orthopaedic Operations

Orthopaedics, a term introduced in 1741 by Nicolas Andre, professor of medicine in Paris in a book entitled *Orthopaedia, or the Art of Correcting Deformities in Children*. First performance of: open plating of fractures by Sir Wm Arbuthnot Lane in 1903; the intermedullary nail (Gerhard Kuntscher of Hamburg, 1967); the Smith-Petersen nail, 1939; and the Charnley arthroplasty, 1970.

Plaster of Paris bandages first used by Anthonius Mathijsen (1805–1878), a Flemish surgeon, in 1852.

Manipulations, requiring good relaxation for a short time, are conveniently done under thiopentone or methohexitone, a relatively large dose being given just before the surgeon is ready to produce his trauma. A relaxant can be added if required. Preoxygenation is beneficial.

The application of a tourniquet or Esmarch bandage.[1] (Johan Friedrich August von Esmarch, 1823–1908, of Kiel) to the lower limb causes a rise in central venous pressure and arterial pressure, which may be serious in handicapped patients, with actual or potential congestive cardiac failure. The pressure in a pneumatic tourniquet should be the systolic pressure plus 30–50 mmHg in the arm and plus 50–70 mmHg in the leg; duration of inflation in the arm should not exceed 1 hour and in the leg, 1.5 h, and should be used with the greatest care in patients with ischaemic vascular disease and if sickle-cell trait is present. Application of an Esmarch bandage may cause the release of a blood clot causing pulmonary embolism.[2] The acidosis resulting from ischaemia in the limb may precipitate a crisis in a patient with sickle-cell disease (*see* Chapter 20). A tourniquet may also be associated with postoperative deep vein thrombosis,[3] and with changes of blood levels of drugs.[4]

The pressure gauges of tourniquets used for surgery and anaesthesia, especially if IVRA is used (*see* Chapter 24), should be tested at least monthly to ensure that their measurements are reasonably accurate.[5]

The Esmarch bandage should not be used as a tourniquet.

Leg amputations may be done under unilateral intradural spinal analgesia, a method well tolerated in old people undergoing amputation for gangrene; care must be taken, hopefully to keep the block unilateral, by maintaining the lateral position for 20–30 min after subarachnoid injection with the diseased side down. Because of the possibility of phantom limb pain, in amputees this may not be the first choice.[6]

Otherwise thiopentone, nitrous oxide–oxygen with or without a relaxant, a narcotic analgesic, a tracheal tube, or volatile agent. Refrigeration analgesia can be used. Meticulous pre-operative preparation and postoperative care together with low-dose heparin can improve the prognosis of this potentially dangerous operation.[7]

For operations on the limbs, more use should be made of various techniques of regional analgesia including intravenous regional analgesia, and sciatic nerve and lumbar plexus compartment block,[8] and wrist and finger block, etc., particularly for prolonged postoperative pain relief.[9]

Internal fixation of hip fractures

A pioneer of the surgery of fracture of the neck of the femur was the Norwegian, Marius Nygaard Smith-Petersen (1886–1953), working in Boston.[10]

Main problems. The patient is usually elderly and often handicapped by cardiovascular and respiratory conditions, diabetes, anaemia, dehydration, mental deterioration and sometimes hypothermia. Many will be suffering from hypoxaemia, perhaps due to fat embolism, and this will be made worse by operation. Abnormalities should be detected and if possible treated before surgery; postponement of the fixation for a few days after injury will not increase morbidity or mortality. A femoral nerve block will ease the pain during movement of the patient.[11]

Extradural methadone may have a place.[12]

Anaesthesia. Any reasonable method of anaesthesia, if carefully applied and if dosage is kept low, is usually safe on the operating table, but postoperative morbidity and mortality may be influenced by the technique employed.[13]

There are arguments for and against most of the commonly employed procedures, including spontaneous respiration with minimal volatile agent, narcotic analgesic and IPPV with barbiturate, nitrous oxide, oxygen and a relaxant; hypocapnia, with attendant cerebral vasoconstriction is undesirable. Patients in poor condition may be managed by a combination of femoral nerve block, i.v. ketamine and diazepam.[14] Intermittent ketamine, with or without diazepam, is reported to give better results than IPPV with relaxant.[15] Extradural and intradural blocks give good results and reduce postoperative hypoxaemia.[16] Postoperative analgesia may be satisfactorily obtained by lateral cutaneous nerve block.[17]

Sequelae and complications. Mortality is often more than 20% in patients over 80 years,[18] is chiefly due to chest infections and to pulmonary embolism. Oxygen therapy and plasma volume expanders may be necessary in the postoperative period.

Arthroplasty of the hip joint (total hip replacement)

Problems. The age and size of some patients; bleeding during and after operation; and possible lateral position of the patient. The use of polymethyl methacrylate cement to fix the prostheses to the bone, first used in 1953,[19] has been followed by hypotension and even by cardiac standstill, probably due to vasodilatation caused by the systemic absorption of the monomer. The prior infusion of 500 ml of a suitable plasma volume expander will go a long way to counteract this, and a head-down tilt of the table may be helpful. When this cement is used for arthroplasty of the knee joint, the tourniquet prevents absorption of the monomer and consequent blood pressure fall. The surgical contortions may cause injury to leg veins leading to thrombophlebitis. Cardiovascular collapse during this operation may also be due to air embolism. An attempt to prevent this by flushing the marrow cavity of the femoral shaft with CO_2 has been made.[20]

Anaesthesia. Many agents and techniques are described, including spontaneous respiration with a volatile agent, and IPPV with relaxant and nitrous oxide and oxygen and narcotic analgesic, which may inhibit the hormonal response to surgery. Tracheal intubation is usual and an intravenous drip mandatory. Bleeding is always a problem and is not lessened by neurolept anaesthesia. Some workers advocate hypotensive anaesthesia and if this technique is used, sodium nitroprusside may be preferable to trimetaphan.[21] Central neural blockade by lowering the blood pressure reduces bleeding and may reduce the incidence of thrombophlebitis. Maintenance of blood pressure by ephedrine, under spinal analgesia does not necessarily increase bleeding.

Complications and sequelae. Thrombophlebitis occurs in about 20% of patients after operation[22] and every method of prevention deserves attention (*see* Chapter 14). With extradural block there is improved fibrinolysis and so less tendency for clot formation than if a general anaesthetic is given.[23] Fat embolism is not infrequent and may account for some cases of postoperative hypoxaemia. Air embolism may occur.[24] Infusion of plasma volume expander 0.5–1 l before use of cement, normally prevents a hypotensive response. Blood transfusion is likely to be required, bearing in mind postoperative oozing.

Arthroplasty of the knee joint

The problems are somewhat similar to total hip replacement, but the monomer effects and blood loss occur when the tourniquet is removed at the end. Epidural block is a satisfactory answer to the considerable problem of postoperative pain.

Spinal fusion

Hypotensive anaesthesia has been recommended to reduce bleeding. The anterior approach in the neck may result in vocal cord paralysis.

Operations on unstable cervical spines

The patient should be intubated and placed on the operating table with the cervical collar and traction still in place so that the position is not altered. This may be difficult, but the patient usually adopts the position providing the clearest airway. Intubation may be difficult and may require great care.[25] Fixation interferes with the anaesthetist's manoeuvres. Severe flexion deformity of the cervical spine may cause difficulty with intubation. This may be accomplished by fibreoptic intubation, under topical analgesia.[26] *See also* Chapter 11. Transoral excisions of odontoid processes, and fixations, present, in addition, problems of the shared airway.

Manipulation and Plaster-of-Paris in children

Ketamine has a place in the management of small children who require repeated manipulation and application of Plaster-of-Paris.

Arthroscopy

General anaesthesia is usually necessary because of pain and avoids damage to the instrument from movement. Postoperative pain relief may be achieved by injection of 0.5% bupivacaine, 10 ml, into the joint after operation. Air embolism has been reported. Arthroscope designed in 1960.[27] For history, *see* McGinty J. B. *J. Irish Coll. Phys. Surg.* 1981, **11**, 63.

Operations for kyphoscoliosis[28]

The main problems are prolonged surgery, heat loss, blood loss, poor access to the patient who will be on a Toronto frame, pre- and postoperative respiratory failure, metabolic acidosis before and after operation, postoperative ileus and severe postoperative pain. In addition, some surgeons may request a 'wake-up test' in which the patient is woken up in the middle of the operation and asked to move his toes, to exclude possible cord compression.[29] The alternative is spinal cord monitoring.[30] At the end of the operation, during which a narcotic, relaxant, nitrous oxide and oxygen technique, with IPPV is usually satisfactory, the muscle relaxant is reversed after the patient is placed supine, to prevent coughing while being moved. A rapid wake-up allows early assessment of toe movement. For severe postoperative pain, a morphine infusion has proved useful, PCA or extradural opioid block.

Laminectomy

First classic description of a prolapsed disc in 1934.[31] Surgery of the thoraco-lumbar spine demands scrupulous anaesthetic technique and careful positioning to avoid an increase in pressure in the extradural veins; the main problem is to produce an ischaemic field. Some workers infiltrate the skin incision and interspinal region with adrenaline saline solution to aid haemostasis. Extradural lumbar block has also been used with success and this we recommend in suitable patients.

Anaesthesia for *bone-marrow harvest*, for transplantation, *see* Filshie J. and Pollock A. N. *Anaesthesia* 1984, **39**, 480.

Pain after *Keller's operation* for hallux valgus can be relieved by infiltration of the pseudarthrosis with bupivacaine.[32]

For more detailed information, *see* Loach A. *Anaesthesia for Orthopaedic Patients*. London: Arnold, 1983.

References

1. Esmarch J. F. A. von (1823–1908), *Der erste Verband auf dem Schlaftfelde*. Kiel, 1869; Lee J. Alfred *Regional Anesthesia* 1985, **10**, 99.
2. Mihic D. N. *Anesthesiology* 1984, **60**, 526; Pollard P. J. et al. *Anesthesiology* 1983, **58**, 373.
3. Zahavi J. et al. *Lancet* 1980, **2**, 663. ; Klenerman L. *J. R. Soc. Med.* 1982, **75**, 31.
4. Schmitt H. et al. *Acta Anaesthesiol. Scand.* 1990, **34**, 104.
5. Klenerman L. *J. Bone Joint Surg.* 1962, **44B**, 937; Klenerman L. *J. R. Soc. Med.* 1982, **75**.
6. Murphy J. P. and Anandaciva S. *Anaesthesia* 1984, **39**, 188.
7. Mann R. A. M. and Bissett W. I. K. *Anaesthesia* 1983, **38**, 1185.
8. Edmonds-Seal J. et al. *J. R. Soc. Med.* 1980, **73**, 111.
9. Brands E. and Callanan V. I. *Anaesth. Intensive Care* 1978, **6**, 256.
10. Smith-Petersen M. N. et al. *Ann. Surg.* 1931, **23**, 715; *Surg. Gynecol. Obstet.* 1937, **64**, 287.
11. Berry F. R. *Anaesthesia* 1977, **32**, 576; Brands E. and Callanan V. I. *Anaesth. Intensive Care* 1978, **6**, 256.
12. Nyska M. et al. *Br. Med. J.* 1986, **283**, 1347.
13. McLaren A. D. et al. *Anaesthesia* 1978, **33**, 10; McKenzie P. J. et al. *Br. J. Anaesth.* 1980, **52**, 49; Sikorski J. M. et al. *Br. Med. J.* 1985, **290**, 439; Spreadbury T. H. *Anaesthesia* 1980, **35**, 208.
14. Howard C. B. et al. *Anaesthesia* 1983, **38**, 993.
15. Sikorski J. M. et al. *Br. Med. J.* 1985, **290**, 439.
16. McKenzie P. I. et al. *Br. J. Anaesth.* 1980, **52**, 49.
17. Jones S. F. and White A. *Anaesthesia* 1985, **40**, 682.
18. *B. J. Anaesth.* 1990, **64**, 403.
19. Kiaer S. *C. R. du 5ième Cong. Internat. de Chir. Orthop.* 1953, 534; Haboush J. J. *Bull. Hosp. Joint Dis., N. Y.* 1953, **14**, 242.
20. Harvey P. B. and Smith J. A. *Anaesthesia* 1982, **37**, 714.
21. Vazeery A. K. et al. *Br. J. Anaesth.* 1983, **55**, 783.
22. Harris W. H. et al. *J. Bone Joint Surg.* 1974, **56A**, 1552.
23. Modig J. et al. *Br. J. Anaesth.* 1983, **55**, 625.
24. Michel R. *Anaesthesia* 1980, **35**, 858.
25. Doolan L. A. and O'Brien J. F. *Anaesth. Intensive Care* 1985, **13**, 319.
26. Ovassapian A. et al. *Anesthesiology* 1983, **58**, 370.
27. Bedford A. et al. *J. R. Soc. Med.* 1979, **72**, 6.
28. Harrington H. *J. Bone Joint Surg.* 1962, **44A**, 591; Kafer E. R. *Anesthesiology* 1980, **52**, 339.
29. Abbott T. R. and Bentley G. *Anaesthesia* 1980, **35**, 298.
30. Shimogi K. et al. *Spinal cord Monitoring and Electrodiagnosis* Berlin: Springer-Verlag.
31. Mixter W. J. and Barr J. S. *N. Engl. J. Med.* 1934, **211**, 210.
32. Porter K. M. and Davies J. *Ann. Roy. Coll. Surg. Eng.* 1985, **67**, 292.

Otorhinolaryngology

In throat and nose surgery, the problems of anaesthesia are related to the fact that the operations are carried out on the upper respiratory tract. The anaesthetist must preserve a clear airway, while allowing the surgeon adequate access, and must take steps to prevent soiling of the trachea and bronchial tree with blood and debris. The problems are most evident during operations on the larynx itself.

The following factors should be considered when surgery is to be carried out on the upper respiratory tract:

1. Premedication must be adequate, but not heavy enough to cause a sluggish cough reflex after operation.

2. Smooth induction will reduce the incidence and degree of haemorrhage.

3. No topical analgesic should be applied to the larynx or trachea (except in ear surgery), because the cough reflex must be brisk after operation.

4. Entrance of blood and debris into the lungs must be prevented by the use of an inflatable cuff on a tracheal tube and/or efficient pharyngeal packing.

5. The use of a slight reversed Trendelenburg position minimizes venous oozing.

Induction with thiopentone, intubation using a relaxant, and maintenance with nitrous oxide, oxygen and a volatile agent, with or without narcotic analgesic, can usually be relied on to provide a safe and smooth technique.

Intranasal operations

If topical or regional analgesia is not used, general anaesthesia should be maintained through an orotracheal tube sealed off with a cuff or a pharyngeal or nasopharyngeal pack. These packs should not be removed until the return of the patient's cough reflex. Forgetfulness to remove a pharyngeal pack on the other hand, is one of the easiest mistakes for an anaesthetist to make and can readily prove fatal. Connections to the tube can conveniently be led down over the patient's chest. In this position, particularly if the surgeon asks for flexion of the neck, there is a liability for the tube to kink; using non-kinking tube, such as a nylon-reinforced or Oxford tube, is advantageous. Muscle relaxants will aid intubation, but care must be taken to see that the cough reflex is active at the end of the operation. General anaesthesia may be combined with topical application of vasoconstrictors to the nose (e.g. cocaine 1–10%) to reduce bleeding, or injection into the nasal septum of octopressin and prilocaine[1] (*see* Chapter 24) and block of the sphenopalatine ganglion, which carries the vasodilator fibres to the nasal blood vessels.

Anaesthesia for manipulation of fractured nasal bones

The safe technique involves tracheal intubation with cuff and/or pack to prevent aspiration of blood should haemorrhage occur. The anaesthetic agents should permit rapid return of protective reflexes. If Plaster-of-Paris is applied, the closed eyes may be protected with adhesive tape.

Tonsillectomy in children

Premedication

Provision of the right psychological atmosphere is of the greatest value in obtaining smooth induction of anaesthesia without tears. Both pre-operative crying and tachycardia are reported to increase bleeding in these operations. Sedative premedication must be given carefully because of possible depressant effect on the cough reflex. When the facilities of a postoperative observation room are available and the nursing supervision before and after operation is skilled and alert, heavy basal narcosis can be prescribed so that the child arrives in the anaesthetic room asleep. Oral trimeprazine 3 mg/kg body weight or temazepam syrup 0.2 mg/kg, given 2 h pre-operatively, or narcotic analgesics on a weight basis. Atropine or hyoscine can be given orally or by injection. The oral dose may be twice that given intramuscularly. Where skilled nursing facilities do not exist it is safer to avoid all sedative premedication and use atropine or hyoscine alone for premedication. This is especially true before guillotine tonsillectomy when rapid return of reflexes is essential.

Dissection tonsillectomy

A secure airway demands a tracheal tube, which may be nasal or oral (if adenoids are to be curetted). An oral tube may be kept clear of the operative field if a Doughty blade on the Boyle–Davis gag is used.[2] The use of a tube allows the plane of anaesthesia to be more easily maintained, reduces oozing and obviates respiratory obstruction. IPPV can be combined with it or the patient allowed to breath a volatile agent spontaneously. The alternative is endopharyngeal insufflation using the BD gag, in which case the patient should be taken well down into Plane 3 before the mouth is opened (seldom employed today).

Nitrous oxide, oxygen and a volatile agent, or thiopentone and relaxant are satisfactory techniques. The aim should be to have the patient coughing within a minute or two of the completion of the operation. A nasal tube is very satisfactory for adult tonsillectomy

Adenoids can be curetted either with the tracheal tube *in situ* or after its withdrawal when the cough reflex has been reestablished.

The patient should be returned to the ward in the tonsil position (semi-prone, prevented from rolling on to his face by a pillow beneath the chest, and prevented from rolling supine by bringing the lower arm behind the body) and remain in this position until full consciousness is regained. Aspirin, because it interferes with blood clotting, should not be used for one week before operation, or for the relief of postoperative pain.

Guillotine tonsillectomy

A technique popularized in 1910 in the USA and in the UK[3] and now seldom used. For details of management, *see* earlier editions of this Synopsis.

Anaesthesia for post-tonsillectomy haemorrhage

This can be a grave responsibility. It is wise that experienced anaesthetists should be in charge of such difficult cases. The patient is likely to have a stomach full of blood clot and to be shocked. Visible blood loss is only a fraction of total haemorrhage. Blood loss is replaced by transfusion, before reinduction of anaesthesia. After atropine premedication anaesthesia may be induced by the thiopentone, suxamethonium rapid intubation ('crash') technique (*see above*). Some workers prefer induction with an inhalation agent with the patient in the lateral position, initially. Orotracheal intubation is usually employed, but cuffed tubes are not usually recommended in small children. Perioperative suction is likely to be necessary and vomiting of blood after operation must be expected with care taken to prevent its aspiration into the trachea. Aspiration via a gastric tube passed before leaving theatre is advisable. It gets rid of some of the blood.

Anaesthesia in upper respiratory tract obstruction

This may occur: (1) at the lips; (2) in the mouth; (3) in the nose; (4) in the pharynx; (5) in the larynx; and (6) in the trachea.

Signs. Stridor; dilating alae nasi; rib and intercostal retraction; use of accessory muscles, e.g. scalenes and sternomastoids; indrawing over clavicles; and perhaps cyanosis.

Symptoms. Dyspnoea; anxiety; restlessness and inability to sleep.

Diagnosis. Inspiratory stridor suggests obstruction at or above cords; expiratory stridor suggests obstruction in bronchial tree; and inspiratory with expiratory stridor suggests tracheal obstruction. Soft tissue X-rays of the neck may be useful.

These cases present difficulties because of:

1. Trismus, e.g. in Ludwig's angina, which may not relax with suxamethonium.

2. Voluntary use of accessory muscles of respiration to overcome respiratory obstruction associated with the lesion; if this is present, fatal hypoxia may follow loss of consciousness. Thus tracheostomy under local analgesia may be necessary before the induction of general anaesthesia. Blind nasal intubation in the conscious patient after spraying the nares and larynx with local analgesic solution (cocaine 4% in the nares) may be the method chosen by experienced workers in some cases. General anaesthesia should only be contemplated when the anaesthetist is experienced and confident that he can control the airway and ventilate the lungs. Premedication must not depress respiration. Halothane in oxygen allows smooth induction, and rapid recovery should problems arise, with high inspired oxygen.

A peritonsillar abscess can be opened under lignocaine or cocaine topical analgesia with the head low. Light general anaesthesia in the same position, with a mouth gag and sucker to hand, is permissible in patients without severe respiratory obstruction.

In severe upper respiratory obstruction, tracheostomy may be necessary before induction of general anaesthesia, or even during induction in an emergency.

When inducing general anaesthesia in a patient with an acute infection of the neck or chronic laryngeal obstruction, who is hypoxic, apnoea must not be produced until it is certain that the lungs can be inflated. Oxygen, 100%, should be given for 10 min, followed by a smooth oxygen–halothane induction. Early passage of a nasopharyngeal tube will remove any respiratory obstruction due to trismus, or the presence of a bulky or oedematous tongue or pharynx. Blind nasal intubation can then be carried out. A rather small tube, e.g. size 6.5 or 7, is easier to insert than a larger one, and is permissible for short operations.

Laryngectomy

First performed by Theodor Billroth (1829–1924) in Vienna in 1874.[4] The available methods are:
1. With no pre-existing tracheostomy. A cuffed tracheal tube is passed, and a tracheostomy performed towards the end of the operation.
2. Tracheostomy performed immediately before the operation under general or local analgesia with the insertion of a cuffed tube through the opening.
3. Anaesthesia through a pre-existing tracheostomy opening.

Anaesthetic management

It is important to assess the likelihood of narrowing of the laryngeal aperture by growth clinically (stridor, indirect laryngoscopy), by peak flow meter and from soft-tissue X-rays of the neck. When there is obvious respiratory difficulty, it is wise to intubate or to perform a preliminary tracheostomy under local analgesia. If there is any doubt, it is better to omit respiratory depressant drugs and give atropine or hyoscine alone for premedication.

During induction of anaesthesia care must be taken that control of the airway is maintained. In some cases where there is respiratory obstruction it is difficult to inflate the lung using a bag and mask. Distortion of the normal anatomy by tumour or oedema may render intubation difficult. In these circumstances it may be justifiable to give a sleep dose of thiopentone through an indwelling needle. Nitrous oxide and oxygen are given, and ability to inflate the lungs tested by manual compression of the reservoir bag. If this is readily achieved suxamethonium follows, the larynx sprayed with 4% lignocaine, and a large-sized cuffed tracheal tube passed. (Occasionally it is only possible to pass a small tube, and a range of tubes should be available.) Anaesthesia is continued with standard methods. The use of muscle relaxants and IPPV ensures good gas exchange during light anaesthesia, but the anaesthetist must be vigilant when the tracheal tube is changed to the tracheostomy tube and be on the watch at all times for accidental disconnection. Ventilation should not be interrupted for more than a brief moment. Spontaneous respiration can also be allowed, using nitrous oxide, oxygen and a volatile agent. The aim is to secure quiet respiration with laryngeal reflexes obtunded. Obstructed inspiration may lead to a negative pressure in neck veins with the danger of air embolism. Construction of a tracheostomy early in the operation simplifies airway management. When the larynx is severed from the trachea, the tracheal tube is removed. The surgeon inserts a sterile tube via the tracheostome.

An intravenous drip should be set up. Blood transfusion may be required, particularly if block dissection of the neck is undertaken. After laryngectomy, parenteral nutrition may be undertaken until the suture lines are healed.

For *laryngofissure*, a cuffed tube is inserted from the mouth before the early dissection is done. After a planned tracheostomy a tube is placed in the trachea by the surgeon and connected to the anaesthetic machine.

Carotid sinus syndrome shown by either or both bradycardia and hypotension may follow dissection round the carotid bulb. Should these signs not disappear following the cessation of surgical stimulus, atropine may be required. This may also be associated with other operations in the neck, e.g. thyroidectomy.

Pharyngolaryngectomy

One-stage operations using colon or stomach as replacement are lengthy and pose additional problems:

1. Space around the patient is restricted, and it is important that the anaesthetist has adequate access.

2. Hypotension and cardiac dysrhythmias can occur during mobilization of the oesophagus and transference of stomach or colon to the neck.

3. Rupture of the trachea has occurred.[5] Should this happen, it becomes impossible to ventilate the lungs until an endobronchial tube is passed below the site of rupture.

4. Total thyroidectomy is also performed. Thyroxine will be required as replacement therapy. Calcium metabolism may be disturbed due to removal of the parathyroids.

5. Postoperative intravenous feeding will be necessary.

Laryngoscopy

Problems include: (1) need for relaxation of the jaw and cords; (2) facility to observe cord movement in some cases; (3) rise of blood pressure and dysrhythmias associated with manipulation of the larynx; (4) quick recovery of laryngeal reflexes with absence of spasm; and (5) the possible presence of lesions that cause obstruction to the airway.

Local analgesia. Topical lignocaine 4%.

General anaesthesia. Using nitrous oxide, oxygen and a volatile agent. A long plastic 5- or 6-mm cuffed tracheal tube is inserted through the nose so that the tube lies between the arytenoids. Suxamethonium, either in repeated doses or by continuous drip, and IPPV allow early return of reflexes. Awareness must be avoided. A ventilating laryngoscope, employing Sanders insufflation technique for bronchoscopy, can be used.[6] A fibreoptic instrument may be helpful to visualize the larynx and to act as an introducer to facilitate tracheal intubation in difficult cases.

Microsurgery of the larynx

First use of operating microscope for microsurgery of larynx by Scalco in 1960.[7] This demands meticulous anaesthetic management to provide a relaxed patient who is absolutely immobile with full return of the protective reflexes at the end of the procedure. The following techniques have been recommended:

1. Thiopentone, nitrous oxide, oxygen and non-depolarizing relaxant or volatile agent. Topical analgesia helps to ensure smooth quiet resumption of respiration. An oral or nasal tracheal cuffed tube of 5–6 mm internal diameter is used.[8] Its use allows adequate pulmonary ventilation using IPPV without encroaching on the surgical field. The cuff prevents blood from trickling down the trachea. The patient is placed in the lateral position before extubation.

2. Deep halothane anaesthesia followed by nasopharyngeal insufflation of halothane has been recommended in children. Spontaneous respiration is maintained, and the tube does not reach the larynx. Topical lignocaine spray is helpful.

3. The Sanders oxygen injector, as used to maintain pulmonary ventilation during bronchoscopy, can be modified for attachment to the laryngoscope used for microsurgery. If the injector is placed below the cords there is little risk of blowing a blood clot down the tracheobronchial tree. This can be achieved by puncture of the cricothyroid membrane and passage of an intravenous catheter, which replaces the jet.[9] Alternatively, the thin catheter can be passed via the mouth.[10] An injector device can also be made for insertion into the trachea through the cords.[11] There is a risk of hyperinflation of the lung and surgical emphysema if upper airway obstruction prevents free exhalation.[12] The problem is that during expiration, blood and mucus may shoot up all over the surgeon.

Laser surgery to the larynx

The surgeon, using the operating microscope, guides the laser beam to excise lesions of the larynx. It is necessary that the target should remain quiescent, but when regular movements occur (as with the use of the Sanders injector), the surgeon can time his manipulations to coincide with the rhythm produced by the anaesthetist. When a tracheal tube is used, there is a danger of ignition of the tube by the laser in the presence of a nitrous oxide–oxygen mixture, with results likely to be fatal. Techniques to maintain ventilation, using a full relaxant technique include:

1. Use of a metal tube that will not ignite.[13]
2. Protection of the tube by wrapping it in aluminium tape.
3. Avoidance of a tube, ventilation being maintained by a Sanders injector attached to the surgeon's laryngoscope.
4. Patients with a pre-existing tracheostomy are best managed by retaining the silver tracheostomy tube in position.

The medical laser

The laser is a light beam (*L*ight *A*mplification by *S*timulated *E*mission of *R*adiation) of radiation that can be focused on to a very small spot. The CO_2

surgical laser vaporizes tissue on this spot but surrounding tissue is hardly affected by the temperature rise; coagulation damage is therefore closely confined. It is sufficient for the control of bleeding, with minimal oedema formation and good healing. These are attractive features in surgery of the larynx. Lasers can also be focused into an optical fibre for endoscopy work.

All surgical lasers present potential hazard to both patients and staff. The eyes and skin of patients must be protected. Lasers can also ignite combustible materials.

Injuries to larynx and trachea (including cut throat)

These may occur as a result of accident or attempted suicide. The wound may be open and clear or there may be considerable tissue destruction. Closed injuries may cause haematoma or surgical emphysema. First-aid treatment includes haemostasis by digital pressure or surgical clip. Intravenous fluids may be required. A clear airway must be established and pneumothorax excluded or if necessary treated. Spinal cord lesions can occur. The patient should be nursed in head-down position to prevent air being sucked into an open vein.

Anaesthesia may be hazardous due to blood and debris in the airway and a full stomach. Gastric tubes or cricothyroid pressure may be contra-indicated if there is a risk of increasing tissue damage. The first priority is maintenance of the airway and, if necessary, a tracheal tube must be passed in the awake patient. The method of anaesthesia will depend upon assessment of the individual case. Local analgesia is sometimes indicated. Muscle relaxants must not be used unless the anaesthetist is confident of maintaining ventilation. Tracheostomy is occasionally necessary. The fibreoptic laryngo-scope has proved useful when obstruction is due to a damaged epiglottis.[14] *See also* Flood I. M. and Astley B. *Br. J. Anaesth.* 1982, **54**, 1339.

Tracheostomy

P. F. Bretonneau (1778–1862) of Tours performed a tracheostomy (for diphtheria) in 1825.

General anaesthesia

Patients in the intensive therapy unit may already have a tracheal tube in place. If not, an orotracheal tube is inserted after induction of light general anaesthesia with muscle relaxants if necessary. The cuff of the tracheal tube should not be deflated before the trachea is opened and the tube should not be withdrawn through the cords until the tracheostomy tube is satisfactorily in place. This allows ready replacement of the original tube should difficulties arise. Care should be taken when patients are already on mechanical ventilation or when muscle relaxants are used so that there is a rapid and smooth transfer of anaesthetic connections from one tube to the other.

Local analgesia

Emergency tracheostomy under local analgesia is rarely justified today as tracheal intubation to ensure a clear airway throughout the procedure offers a positive advantage. It should be undertaken only when respiratory obstruction prevents introduction of a tracheal tube. Extension of the neck to facilitate surgical access may actually increase the degree of obstruction in some cases.

Anaesthesia for tracheal resection

Anaesthesia for resection of tracheal stenosis can be performed using high-frequency jet ventilation.[15] *See also* Harrison M. J. *Anaesthesia* 1985, **40**, 708; and Chapter 22, Thoracic.

Anaesthesia for excision of pharyngeal pouch

Pharyngeal pouch first described by Ludlow of Bristol in 1764.[16] The anaesthetist may be asked to pack the pouch with gauze, after induction, to help with its identification. Contents of the pouch may spill into the pharynx during induction.

Excision of pharyngeal pouch

The patient may have undergone recurrent chest infections due to aspiration of pouch contents. The anaesthetist should be aware of this possibility associated with induction of anaesthesia. Cricoid pressure does not prevent regurgitation from the pouch. Endoscopy may be carried out to identify the pouch and pack it with gauze prior to neck exploration. This can be removed by the anaesthetist when it is no longer required. Sometimes operative treatment may be carried out endoscopically when the 'carina' between pouch and oesophagus is removed by diathermy.

Operations on the middle and inner ear

A. F. von Troeltsch (1829–1890) invented the otoscope in 1860 and performed the first mastoid operation for suppurative otitis media in 1861. Julius Lempert, New York otologist pioneered fenestration in 1938.

Myringotomy

For all patients other than young children, an aerosol spray of 10% lignocaine can be directed towards the upper wall of the auditory canal, so that the solution runs downwards on to the drum and so avoids pain and coldness on the drum head. Otherwise general anaesthesia is required. When the operating microscope is used, a tracheal tube helps to avoid airway obstruction and provides a still field. Vagal cardiac arrest may occur if the 'vagal' area of the tympanic membrane (supplied by the auricular branch) is incised. Atropine will prevent this.

Mastoid operations

Some surgeons like to be able to observe facial twitching should the facial nerve be stimulated by manipulations in the vicinity. Immediate steps can then be taken for decompression should injury be demonstrated. For this reason some surgeons and anaesthetists avoid the use of muscle relaxants. The operations of *myringoplasty, tympanoplasty* and *stapedectomy* are greatly facilitated by the provision of an ischaemic field.[17] This may be provided by the use of standard techniques (*see* Chapter 13).

In all ear operations there are theoretical considerations that may arise due to diffusion of nitrous oxide into the middle ear if it is used for anaesthesia.[18] Nitrous oxide will cause increased pressure within the middle ear with bulging of the intact drum. When the patient is breathing a nitrous oxide mixture spontaneously, middle ear pressure can increase by $39 \, mmH_2O$ per minute; with IPPV it may increase by $63 \, mmH_2O$ per minute, and these pressures can be reached within 5 min.[19] This may be important during operations such as myringoplasty. The problem is avoided if nitrous oxide is discontinued 30 min before anticipated placement of the graft. Anaesthesia may be maintained with intravenous agents or combinations such as oxygen and halothane until surgery is completed. Air may be used for IPPV.[20]

References

1. Taylor S. et al. *Anaesthesia* 1984, **39**, 520.
2. Doughty A. G. *Lancet* 1957, **1**, 1074.
3. Whillis S. S. and Pybus F. C. *Lancet* 1910, **2**, 875; Sluder G. *JAMA* 1911, **56**, 867.
4. Gussenbauer C. *Arch. f. Klin. Chir.* 1874, **17**, 343.
5. Loach A. B. *Anaesthesia* 1974, **29**, 448.
6. Sanders R. D. *Del. State Med. J.* 1967, **39**, 170; Albert S. N. *Br. J. Anaesth.* 1971, **43**, 1098; Lee S. T. *Br. J. Anaesth.* 1972, **44**, 874.
7. Scalco A. N. et al. *Ann. Otol. Laryngol.* 1960, **69**, 1134.
8. Koo M. K. T. *Anaesth. Intensive Care*, 1980, **8**, 469; Atkinson R. S. In: *Recent Advances in Anaesthesia and Analgesia – 12.* (Hewer C. L. and Atkinson R. S. ed.) Edinburgh: Churchill Livingstone, 1976; Coplans M. P. *Anaesthesia* 1976, **31**, 430.
9. Spoerel W. E. et al. *Br. J. Anaesth.* 1971, **43**, 932; Smith R. B. *Anesth. Analg. (Cleve.)* 1974, **53**, 225.
10. Carden E. and Ferguson G. B. *Laryngoscope* 1973, **83**, 691; Smith R. B. et al. *Br. J. Anaesth.* 1974, **46**, 313.
11. Norton M. L. et al. *Am. J. Otol. Rhinolaryngol.* 1976, **85**, 656; Rontal M. et al. *Laryngoscope* 1980, **90**, 1162.
12. Chakrabarti K. et al. *Br. J. Anaesth.* 1973, **45**, 733; Spoerel W. E. and Greenway R. E. *Can. Anaesth. Soc. J.* 1973, **20**, 369.
13. Hunton J. and Oswal V. H. *Anaesthesia* 1985, **40**, 1210.
14. Davies J. R. *Br. Med. J.* 1979, **2**, 610.
15. Rogers R. C. et al. *Anaesthesia* 1985, **40**, 32; Selby D. G. et al. *Anaesth. Intensive Care* 1982, **11**, 166.
16. Ludlow A. quoted by Hunter W. *Med. Observations and Enquiries* 1767, **3**, 85.
17. Condon H. A. *Clin. Otolaryngol.* 1979, **4**, 241; Eltringham R. J. et al. *Anaesthesia* 1982, **37**, 1028; Rollason W. N. et al. *Anaesthesia* 1983, **38**, 590.
18. Davis I. et al. *Anaesthesia* 1979, **34**, 147.
19. Casey W. F. and Drake-Lee A. B. *Anaesthesia* 1982, **37**, 896.
20. Perreault L. et al. *Canad. Anaesth. Soc. J.* 1981, **28**, 136.

Paediatric anaesthesia

Safety in paediatric anaesthesia, *see* NCEPOD.[1] For morbidity and mortality in the perioperative period, *see* Cohen M. M., Cameron C. B. and Duncan P. G. *Anesth. Analg.* 1990, **70**, 160.

It is almost impossible to generalize about 'paediatric anaesthesia' because this age group comprises three or four distinct age subgroups, with differing physiology and pharmacology. They will therefore be considered somewhat separately.

The special considerations fall into the following groups:

1. Differences as a result of anatomical size, e.g. body weight, narrowness of cricoid ring.

2. Differences as a result of physiology, e.g. temperature homeostasis.

3. Differences as a result of pharmacology, e.g. relatively larger volume of distribution of many drugs.

4. Differences as a result of psychology, e.g. intense dependence on parents.

THE NEONATE

Defined as an infant during the first 28 days of life. The mature 3 kg infant is normally one-third the length, has one-ninth the body surface and one-twentieth the weight of the average adult. The head is large compared with the body, and the neck muscles are inadequately developed to maintain the head in position without support. The physiology of the neonate differs from that of the adult in many ways.

Respiration

In comparison with adults, neonates have a larger proportion of dead space in their lungs. Their ribs are nearly horizontal in the position of deep inspiration, and the diaphragm is pushed up by the large liver, hence respiration is rapid (30 breaths/min), diaphragmatic, and may easily become deficient. The lungs are much less efficient ventilating organs than they eventually become, with a respiratory surface per unit weight one-third that of adults. To compensate for this, the respiratory rate is increased in infants. Bucking does not occur in the first 3 months of life, although the laryngeal reflexes are very active because the child is living on fluids. In infants, the tongue is often pushed against the palate, causing respiratory obstruction under anaesthesia.

The respiratory pattern of the neonate may be one of three types. (1) *Regular:* inspiration and expiration taking equal time in the cycle with no expiratory pause. (2) *Cogwheel:* a definite and extended inspiratory pause following a lengthened expiratory phase; (3) *Periodic:* bouts of regular pattern, interrupted by apnoeic intervals or groups of shallow respirations. Periodic respiration may be seen in premature infants, or as a result of birth injury or hypoxia of the respiratory centre.

Because of the variations seen in respiratory patterns it is difficult to measure a 'normal' rate in the neonate, although average figures of 30–40 min have been found. Average tidal volumes for the neonate $V_T = 7$ ml/kg or 20 ml. The trachea bifurcates at the level of T2. The airway is narrow and this causes a high airway resistance with low compliance.

In infants, a negative pressure is sometimes created in the stomach during inspiration and gas may be sucked in. To relieve this a catheter should be used as a stomach tube if the abdomen is distended or if breathing is laboured.

Alveolar ventilation is 100–150 ml/kg/min (cf. 60 ml/kg/min in adults) and the MV/FRC ratio is 5:1 (cf. 1.5:1 in adults).

Intubation may be difficult because of the relatively large head, unless the anaesthetist is constantly doing this type of work. A small amount of mucus secretion may cause considerable obstruction to respiration. The Bullard laryngoscope may help.[2]

The cardiovascular system

In the fetus the left ventricle drives blood through the aorta to the body tissues and to the placenta in the proportion of one-third to two-thirds. Oxygenated blood from the placenta mixes with venous blood in its return to the heart. About half of this mixed blood passes through the foramen ovale to the left heart. The other half flows to the right heart for the pulmonary circulation, although a variable part of this passes through the ductus arteriosus to the aorta.

At birth, when the umbilical cord is tied, systemic arterial resistance rises because blood passing formerly to the placenta now has to pass through the arterial system to the body tissues. At the same time, as regular respiration is established, there is a profound reflex fall in pulmonary vascular resistance, and an increase in blood flow to the lungs. Pressure in the pulmonary artery falls and a reversal of flow occurs in the ductus arteriosus. The lumen of this vessel decreases in size over the next 7–10 days and is usually finally obliterated. The foramen ovale also closes. At birth the BP averages 80/50 mmHg. Falls of systemic vascular resistance in neonates can cause serious right-to-left shunts.

The blood volume of the neonate is about 70–90 ml/kg, and haemoglobin is 17–21 g/dl. Cyanosis appears at high Sp_{O_2} because of this haemoglobin concentration. Normal pulse rate 120–140 min. Only 30% of the myocardium is contractile mass (cf. 60% in adults), and the neonate is less able to increase its stroke volume. Cardiac sympathetic innervation is incomplete, vagal tone is higher, and thus bradycardia occurs much more easily.

Body water is 75% of body weight (cf. 50% in adult), and of this, 45% is extracellular fluid (cf. 16% in adult).

Metabolism

Brown fat is an important source of energy in the newborn whose metabolic rate is nearly twice that of the adult. It contains β-adrenergic receptors.

Asphyxia at birth can result in exhaustion of carbohydrate reserves in muscles, liver and myocardium, leading to hypoglycaemia and acidosis. The normal neonate has a mild metabolic acidosis and respiratory alkalosis. Exposure to cold can also give rise to the same changes. Administration of glucose is indicated, particularly if infants are starved prior to surgery. Hypoglycaemia may be present if the patient is starved for undue periods pre-operatively, especially below the age of 4 years and below a weight of 15.5 kg. Hyperventilation during anaesthesia will compensate for metabolic acidosis but the calculated dose of bicarbonate should be given at the end of operation when spontaneous respiration is resumed. Blood-sugar estimations should be done in these circumstances. Figures below 1.5 mmol/l may be found. It may be necessary to infuse strong glucose solutions, 20% or 25%, into central veins. To prevent hypoglycaemia, children should, if possible, be operated on early in the day.

Oxygen consumption is 6–8 ml/kg/min. (cf. 3 ml/kg/min in adults) Heat loss is of the order of 50% by radiation to cold walls of rooms or incubators, in addition to conduction, convection and evaporation. It has recently been appreciated that it may be unwise to nurse babies naked in an air temperature of 35°C, and it is more logical to use 'double-glazing' of the incubator or use a radiant heat shield. Draughts are to be avoided. Space blankets retain heat at first but are ineffective later when wet. Neonates have reduced renal function, especially urea concentrating capacity. Full function reached by 2 years. Fetal albumin has a lower affinity for drugs than adult.

Stress response

Under light non-narcotic anaesthesia, the stress response is even greater than the adult.[3] Administration of opioids requires intensive monitoring and 1:1 nurse:patient ratio.

The complicated neonate

Has all the problems of the neonate plus the added dangers of its particular condition. The neonate may suffer from respiratory distress syndrome, haemorrhagic disease of the newborn with jaundice, birth trauma, hypoglycaemia, or infection. Congenital disease may be present. Venepuncture is difficult. There is sensitivity to non-depolarizing relaxants but resistance to suxamethonium. Hypothermia must be avoided.

Dehydration is recognized clinically by thirst, sunken eyes and fontanelle, oliguria, loss of skin turgor, empty veins, dry mouth and acute weight loss. Moderate dehydration represents a water deficit of about 75 ml/kg body weight. Biochemical estimation of electrolytes and glucose is required for calculated exact replacement of deficits. Special infant ventilators have been designed.[4] The usual problems of infection exist.[5]

The premature child

These children are more complex than usual up to 6 months of age (longer if there are residual organ disorders). Their problems include relative sensitivity to volatile anaesthetics at birth (compared with full term babies) possibly due to: (*a*) high progesterone levels; (*b*) high β-endorphins;[6] and (*c*) immature central nervous system. They have a lower than usual body lipid content.

Immature cardiovascular system. Nitrous oxide, associated with a small increase in cardiac output, is useful. Volatile agents cause dose-dependent depression of baroreceptor activity leading to hypotension (and failure of heart-rate response to it)[7] and chemoreceptor activity, leaving the pre-term child vulnerable to hypoxia without protective reflexes. For this reason, most pre-term babies are intubated, and remain so after anaesthetic until awake. They are monitored postoperatively as if they were still anaesthetized.

Immature respiratory system. With smaller tidal volumes, greater respiratory rates (30–60/min), and high alveolar ventilation (100–150 ml/kg/min). High metabolic rate and oxygen consumption (6–8 ml/kg/min).

Immature hepatic metabolic processes. (E.g. paracetamol is metabolized as sulphate in neonates and glucuronide in adults.) The average rate of drug metabolism is 20% of the adult value up to 2 months of age. (At 3 years it is 5 times the adult rate.)[8] Glucose, electrolytes and calcium are frequently out of balance.

Fragile intracerebral blood vessels. Greater risk of spontaneous intracerebral haemorrhage.

Enflurane in particular depresses muscle power, and is useful for abdominal relaxation, but may also depress respiration. Nitrous oxide has minimal effect on muscle power. MAC halothane of preterm infants of 1–6 months is 1.2%, and isoflurane 1.8–1.9%.[9]

Anaesthesia in the neonate[10]

The choice lies between: (1) a 'volatile' technique; (2) balanced anaesthesia with relaxant and IPPV; and (3) ketamine[11] has a longer elimination half-life than in older children.[12]

With inhalation induction, anaesthesia comes on more rapidly and awakening is more rapid than in adults. A reliable intravenous infusion is an important prerequisite in neonatal anaesthesia.

In premature infants, perioperative apnoea is a danger so that operative IPPV with normocapnia may be indicated, and for the first postoperative 18–24 h, respiratory monitoring, with facilities for IPPV should be considered. IPPV, presents the problem of severe overventilation, due to difficulty in setting low enough flows on many rotameters. One solution to this is to ventilate with 4% carbon dioxide in the fresh gas mixture, keeping the end tidal tension at about 4 kPa.

It has been advised that, where possible, operation before the 44th week of conceptual age, should be postponed.[13] Vitamin K treatment for clotting problems may well be required. Causes of postoperative apnoea in the neonate are: (1) immaturity; (2) hypothermia, 34°C or below; (3) overdosage of relaxant; (4) overdosage with inhalation agent; (5) potentiation of non-depolarizing relaxant with volatile agents; (6) concurrent aminoglycoside antibiotics; (7) overdosage of narcotic analgesics; and (8) a combination of the above.

Tracheal intubation in small babies

This is almost routine during anaesthesia. Many workers use a straight blade, the tip of which is placed posterior to the epiglottis. A tube with internal diameter of 2.5–3 mm is suitable for neonates. An assistant, skilled in holding the baby, prevents side-to-side movement by a hand either side of the head, both for awake and anaesthetized intubation.

When intubated, there must be a leak of air between tube and trachea, to prevent pressure on the mucosa, with subsequent development of subglottic stenosis.

The risk of misplacement of the tube in the oesophagus is always present and detecting it requires vigilance.

See also Hatch D. J. and Sumner E. *Current Topics in Anaesthesia Series – 5, Neonatal Anaesthesia.* London: Arnold, 1986; Sumner E. and Hatch D. J. *Textbook of Paediatric Anaesthetic Practice* 1989, London: Bailliére Tindall, 1989.

Monitoring (*See also* Chapter 18)

As always, careful clinical observation of the condition of the patient throughout the operation is vital.

Circulation. A precordial stethoscope acts as a useful monitor of heart sounds, rate and rhythm. An oesophageal stethoscope can be used where a precordial stethoscope is impracticable. Pulse monitors and electrocardiogram are routine. Lead 3 or CM_3 may give the best signal. The ECG monitor should show heart rate, since bradycardias are more frequent. Average normal heart rates (bpm) are: birth 135; 1 month 160; 6 months 140; 1 year 120; 3 years 100. For blood pressure measurements, it is important that cuffs are of the correct size (*see* Chapter 18). Too narrow a cuff gives a reading which is too high and vice-versa; the bag should almost encircle the upper arm. The automated oscillotonometer is accurate.[14] Monitors using ultrasonic detectors require protection from movement artefact. Finger arterial pressure monitors[15] indicate non-invasive beat-to-beat pressure. For pulse oximetry *see* Metabolic status, below.

Respiration. A stethoscope attached to the side-arm of a T-piece provides audible monitoring of respiration. Apnoea alarms may be needed in the ward. An ingenious oesophageal probe has been described, which combines a stethoscope, thermistor and ECG lead.[16] Use of disposable oesophageal probes is now routine.

Metabolic status. Pulse oximetry (Spo_2) and percutaneous oxygen tension (TC Pao_2) monitoring makes continuous observation of the Pao_2 a realistic proposition. Pulse oximetry has some inaccuracies due to haemoglobin F, bilirubin and lag time (*see* Chapter 18), but is very useful in the sudden-cyanosis situations of paediatric anaesthesia. Capnography is possible, but technically more difficult to obtain a proper alveolar sample in small babies, e.g. under 8 kg,[17, 18] overcome by automatic fresh gas flow interruption during expiration and a capnograph with a rapid response time. Temperature is important. Urine flow is useful in major operations.

Blood loss and replacement

The blood volume of an neonate is small, 85 ml/kg (about 250 ml in the newborn), and so blood replacement must be accurate. This can be done with the help of calibrated small suction bottles, swab weighing or colorimetric methods to estimate blood loss. Blood transfusion can be undertaken from small reservoirs, or a three-way tap and 20-ml syringe can be used to transfuse an accurate volume in replacement. Replacement should be commenced when 10% of the estimated blood volume has been lost. Blood should be warmed to prevent hypothermia. For autotransfusion *see* Church J. J. and Davidson A. M. *Anaesth. Intensive Care* 1979, **7**, 178.

Fluid balance

It is rare for pre-operative fluid and electrolyte balance to require correction during the first 12 h of life but 0.25% normal saline with 5% dextrose is suitable in small babies. Haemoglobin, haematocrit, electrolytes and blood sugar should be available before major surgery. In infants over 12 h of age correction of fluid and electrolyte abnormalities is of major importance. During operation Ringer lactate 2 ml/kg/h is recommended,[19] using a burette or infusion pump. In the perioperative period, glucose-containing fluids are suitable until normal oral ingestion can be resumed.

Nutrition

The neonate requires energy in excess of 0.45 MJ/kg/day in order to grow. For enteral and parenteral nutrition, *see* Chapter 34. Aseptic technique must be scrupulous.

Temperature

The patient loses 580 cal for every 1 gram of water evaporated. This amount alone is enough to reduce the temperature of 580 grams of the patient's body water by 1°C.

The newborn rapidly loses heat if placed in a cold environment. The heat-regulating mechanisms are immature in the premature infant and in the mature newborn baby for some weeks. The newborn maintains its body heat through the metabolic activity of brown fat, which is to be found mainly around the kidneys and back. This fat has a rich blood and β-adrenergic nerve supply and the cells are profusely equipped with mitochondria. It may be deficient in small or premature babies. Care must be taken that undue heat loss does not occur on the operating table.

Routes of heat loss. Conduction (e.g. to operating table); convection (e.g. due to draughts); radiation (worsened due to a baby's large surface area, especially the head, which should be covered); and evaporation (of perspiration, exhaled vapour and water from exposed viscera). Drapes provide an efficient insulation of the exposed surface of the infant. Cold blood transfusion may also produce hypothermia. It should be warmed. Cold stress and hypoxia both lead to hypoglycaemia. For operations on babies below 10 kg, a warming mattress is very important.[20] Temperature is, of monitored at rectum, oesophagus, axilla or nasopharynx. The response to cold may be shivering, which increases oxygen consumption. (A 10°C fall of room temperature increases oxygen consumption by 50%). Neonatal environmental thermal neutrality is 33°C and 35°C for the premature. Hypothermia moves the oxyhaemoglobin dissociation curve to the left, reducing oxygen delivery to the tissues.

Relaxants in neonates

In babies, muscular relaxation requires neither deep anaesthesia nor large doses of relaxants. Protrusion of the intestines from the belly is due to diaphragmatic breathing and distension due to gas in the bowel, not to the muscular tone of the abdominal wall.

The neonate is more sensitive to non-depolarizing relaxants than the adult, although this sensitivity gradually decreases over the first 2 months of life.[21] Less acetylcholine is released in infants. Postoperative difficulties may be experienced if anticholinesterase drugs are not used, if hypothermia is allowed to occur, or when there is potentiation by volatile agent, hypokalaemia or antibiotics are administered.

Suxamethonium is probably the preferred relaxant in neonates for short operations and they require at least twice the dose (dose for weight) to produce comparable results as in adults. A dose of 5 mg can be given and repeated many times if necessary. It sometimes causes bradycardia in infants.

Opioids and postoperative analgesia in neonates

Neonates are very sensitive to opioids, with reduced clearances and prolonged duration of action. They also have smaller respiratory reserves. Administration of opioids requires intensive monitoring and 1:1 nurse:patient ratio.

Intraoperative bolus doses: morphine 25 µg/kg (for inhibition of stress response, 60 µg/kg); fentanyl 1–3 µg/kg (spontaneously breathing), 5–10 µg/kg (IPPV);[22] alfentanil for analgesia, 10–20 µg/kg bolus, then infusion 1 µg/kg/min, for stress response inhibition, 50–120 µg/kg; sufentanil 1–3 µg/kg, for stress response inhibition, 5–20 µg/kg[23]; pethidine 0.5 mg/kg. If other opioids have been given for premedication, these doses are reduced. Postoperative analgesia is under scrutiny. On one hand, it is seen as desirable, but on the other, NCEPOD revealed deaths from postoperative analgesics[1]. Regional blockade is appropriate in neonates and infants.[24]

Anaesthesia for some neonatal operations

Abdominal surgery

In neonates, muscular relaxation does not require deep anaesthesia or relaxants, except in special cases such as when a large volume of viscera has to be returned to the peritoneal cavity. The Jackson–Rees modification of Ayres T-piece is very convenient for both spontaneous breathing and IPPV.

PYLORIC STENOSIS

The commonest disease requiring surgery in the first 6 months of life. Commoner in males and after the age of 2 weeks. The operation of pyloromyotomy was performed by Dufour[25] in 1908 and by Conrad Ramstedt (1868–1963) in 1911.[26] *This operation is not an emergency procedure.*

Preoperative preparation (in collaboration with paediatricians).[27]

1. Fluid and electrolyte replacement is the major consideration.

2. Loss of gastric acid results in metabolic alkalosis and low serum chloride.

3. There is marked loss of sodium and potassium in the urine in an effort to conserve hydrogen ions.

4. Classic signs of dehydration occur: (*a*) weight loss (0.5–1 kg); (*b*) oliguria; (*c*) dry mouth; (*d*) sunken eyes; (*e*) depressed fontanelles; and (*f*) loss of skin elasticity.

5. The result is an ill, dehydrated, alkalotic, hypochloraemic, hyponatraemic, hypokalaemic infant.

6. Treatment is by intravenous infusion, initially normal saline with potassium chloride 20–40 mmol/l, until urine flow restarts, then 0.45% saline in 2.5% glucose with potassium chloride 20–40 mmol/l until urine flow is normal, then 0.18% saline in 4.3% glucose. A suitable drip flow-rate is 2–3 ml/kg/h. The glucose is important to prevent hypoglycaemia. Surgery should not be undertaken until the chloride is at least 90 mmol/l and the bicarbonate 24–30 mmol/l. Occasionally, intravenous feeding is required.

7. Via a gastric tube, hourly gastric washouts continue until the washout fluid is returned clear and odourless. The serum standard bicarbonate should be below 30 mmol/l before anaesthesia.

Premedication. Atropine or hyoscine: 0.1 mg i.m.

General anaesthetic technique.

1. Perioperative body warming, precordial or oesophageal stethoscope and other routine monitoring.

2. Suction on the gastric tube.

3. Inhalation or intravenous induction and cricoid pressure. Intubation with 3 mm (or smaller) tracheal tube, perhaps facilitated by suxamethonium 1–2 mg/kg i.v., or 5 mg/kg i.m. (which will last up to 20 min).

4. Maintenance with inhalational agents, supplemented if desired by relaxants and IPPV.

5. Extubation with the child awake, preferably lying on the side.

6. Postoperative 0.18% saline in 4.3% glucose until the child is back on partial or full feeds, usually the same day.

Local analgesic technique. The maximum dose is 8 mg/kg of 0.25% lignocaine with adrenaline 1–400 000. A useful technique in the absence of a competent anaesthetist but results are no better than after general anaesthesia.[28] Ketamine as sole anaesthetic is not recommended.[29]

DIAPHRAGMATIC HERNIA

Diagnosis. Shortly after birth, the child may have cyanosis resistant to oxygen; dullness of the chest, absent breath sounds, and later bowel sounds on the affected side of the chest (usually left). Chest X-ray confirms the diagnosis. There are areas of pulmonary hypoplasia on the affected side, mediastinal shift and compression of the opposite lung.

Initial management. (1) Intubation of the trachea and gentle IPPV. The chest should not be inflated with a face-mask, as this merely fills the stomach and intestines and worsens the degree of compression; (2) insertion of a gastric tube to prevent aeration of the gut; (3) measurement and correction of acidosis; and (4) prevention of hypothermia, dehydration and hypoglycaemia.

Perioperative Management. The physiological problem is that some of these neonates revert to transitional circulation, with decreased pulmonary vascular bed, high pulmonary vascular resistance, and reopening of the ductus arteriosus and foramen ovale. Tolazoline, 2 mg/kg bolus, followed by the same dose infused over each hour, has been used to control these problems. Profound muscular relaxation may be required for short periods. Rapid infusion of colloids, e.g. plasma, may be required to counteract cardiovascular collapse during surgery. Postoperative elective IPPV with nasotracheal tube in severely ill cases. To cope with possible pneumothorax, a chest drain may be inserted into each side.

See also Marshall A. and Sumner E. *J. R. Soc. Med.* 1982, **75**, 607.

OMPHALOCELE

This requires emergency operation because rupture of the thin sac covering the intestines will result in peritonitis. May be associated with the Beckwith–Wiedemann syndrome. Anaesthetic management is similar to that for diaphragmatic hernia. Prolonged ileus is a common complication and problems of fluid and electrolyte balance and parenteral nutrition may have to be solved. Peritonitis is a common cause of death and intestinal obstruction due to adhesions may occur. The overall mortality is high.

Tracheo-oesophageal fistula with oesophageal atresia

Aspiration of food and secretions usually results in pneumonia within a few days of birth. Operation is a hazardous procedure and successful operations were not carried out before 1939 when Leven and Ladd (independently) in the USA performed multistage operations. Primary oesophageal anastomosis was introduced by Haight in 1941.

There are various anatomical variations. Much the commonest finding is the blind upper oesophageal pouch, with a fistula between the posterior trachea and lower oesophagus.

Anaesthetic management may be difficult. Pre-operative care includes safe transfer to a special unit with avoidance of hypothermia. A tube should be passed into the blind upper end of the oesophagus for suction. Controlled respiration via a tracheal tube is generally advocated. It is imperative that the anaesthetist be able to use effective suction in the airway at all times and a suitable fine catheter must be available. IPPV can result in gastric distension. Fortunately this is only a serious problem in a minority of cases, when gastrostomy may be necessary for its relief. Good relaxation enables ventilation to be carried out at minimal pressures. Accurate replacement of blood is essential.

Recommended techniques. Premedication: atropine or hyoscine 0.05 mg/kg. An intravenous infusion is set up. Awake intubation may be performed (but asleep intubation in the premature child because of the risk of intracerebral haemorrhage) then nitrous oxide–oxygen, volatile agent and muscle relaxants, if necessary. The upper oesophageal pouch should be intubated to remove secretions. Care must be taken to avoid intubation of the fistula and inflation of the stomach.

Postoperative care

Neonates require special postoperative care after major surgery. Attention must be paid to: (1) environmental temperature; (2) feeding. A weight loss of 44 g/day/kg birth-weight may occur in the first 2 days of life. It is possible for the blood sugar (normal level 3 mmol% at birth) to fall to very low levels if early feeding is not commenced – oral feeding is preferable if possible; (3) acidaemia. If present must be corrected; (4) oxygen therapy with pulse oximeter monitoring. Respiratory failure is a not an uncommon complication and especially if opioids are administered. Assisted respiration may be necessary – rates of 60–80/min may be required using air enriched with oxygen; Po_2 estimation can be obtained using umbilical artery catheters; (5) cross-infection is a particular hazard; and (6) jaundice. This may occur in any sick newborn baby. After surgery, haematomas provide an additional source of bile pigments.

Postoperative analgesia. Opioid infusions are used, especially where IPPV is employed, e.g. morphine 0.1 mg/kg/h. Aspirin is avoided because of risk of Reye's syndrome.

LARGER CHILDREN

Children up to 10 years of age. The tidal volume (7 ml/kg), FRC (30 ml/kg) and deadspace (2 ml/kg) are similar to adults. Resting respiratory rate decreases throughout childhood towards the adult rate. Body lipid content rises up to 9 months of age, falls up to 6 years, and then rises again towards puberty.

Preanaesthetic assessment. Is congenital or general medical disease present? Has the child had an exanthem or upper respiratory tract infection (URTI) recently? If the child has a runny nose, is it due to allergy, teething or URTI? Elective anaesthesia should probably be postponed in the presence of a URTI. Has the child had an anaesthetic before, and if so, was it happy? How does the child feel about injections?

Preanaesthetic preparation. Fasting – no solid food for 6 h, a drink of 5% glucose 4 h pre-operatively, is an average guide. Infants may have the last drink 2 h before anaesthesia, other considerations permitting.[30] Laboratory testing, as appropriate.[31]

Premedication. Morphine and papaveretum are very widely used, but care is needed in infants (*see* Opioids in neonates above). Some anaesthetists aim to give heavy premedication so that children arrive in the theatre suite asleep; they can then be anaesthetized by gravity nitrous oxide and halothane without the patient regaining consciousness. Other anaesthetists prefer to establish rapport with the child and to provide an environment without fear; light premedication is given and the child 'talked' to sleep, anaesthesia being induced by inhalation or intravenous routes. Sedative premedication may not be necessary when the weight is less than 10 kg. Trauma, anxiety and pain may all delay emptying of the stomach. Metoclopramide 0.1 mg/kg i.m. may help here.

Routes of sedative premedication[32]

1. *Oral.* Some anaesthetists do not like this method because of the danger of vomiting and because absorption of drugs from the alimentary tract is uneven. Others find it a satisfactory method, acceptable to the child.

Benzodiazepines. Temazepam syrup (2 mg/ml): 0.3 mg/kg (short acting, 2–4 h).

Trimeprazine tartrate. This is a phenothiazine derivative and has a central sedative, antihistaminic, anti-emetic and spasmolytic action. It has none of chlorpromazine's anti-adrenaline properties. Its side-effects may include dryness of the mouth, vertigo, depression and fainting. Available in a palatable syrup as Vallergan Forte (6 mg/ml), dose 3–4 mg/kg 1.5 h before anaesthesia. Also given in a dose of 2 mg/kg 2 h pre-operatively followed by intramuscular opioid 1 h later. The 'Liverpool regime' is trimeprazine, 1.5 mg/kg orally 3 h pre-operatively, then morphine 0.25 mg/kg 1 h pre-operatively.

Analgesics. E.g. paracetamol 5–10 mg/kg.

Chloral and related agents. Chloral elixir, 35 mg/kg; dichloralphenazone (contra-indicated in porphyria), 35 mg/kg; and triclofos, 70–100 mg/kg. All 1–2 h before anaesthesia. May also be given before an intramuscular opioid premedication.

2. *Rectal.* E.g. methohexitone, 20 mg/kg; thiopentone, 40 mg/kg; diazepam 0.2 mg/kg with or without opioid. Nursing care must be good.

3. *Intramuscular.* Papaveretum 0.3–0.4 mg/kg and hyoscine, 0.01 mg/kg premixed. Pethidine, 1 mg/kg up to 5 years, 2 mg/kg over 5 years (maximum 75 mg). Pethidine/promethazine mixture is available. Morphine, 0.1 mg/kg up to 5 years, 0.2 mg/kg over 5 years (maximum 10 mg). Pentazocine is avoided because of severe hallucinations.

Atropine 15 µg/kg and hyoscine 10 µg/kg are well tolerated by children and are useful as salivation is often profuse. The drugs may also be given by mouth. Hyoscine may be preferred because of its anti-emetic action and sedative effect. Glycopyrronium 5 µg/kg (max. 200 µg) is satisfactory.

Anaesthesia

Should parents be allowed in the anaesthetic room? Some parents exert a helpful and calming influence on the patient, especially mentally deficient ones. Other parents generate tension and fear by body language and ill-chosen words (e.g. 'pain', 'hurt', 'afraid'). Sometimes those parents who demand to be present are the least helpful ones. If a parent wishes to be present, it should be requested at the pre-operative visit, and not at the last minute.

The classic method of anaesthesia, in infants and children with spontaneous respiration, of various mixtures of anaesthetic gases and vapours is widely used. Inhibition of the stress response with analgesics is important.[35] Nitrous oxide and opioids are suitable but opioids carry the risk of respiratory depression, and require great care.

Intravenous induction of anaesthesia

For a nomogram to estimate drug dosage in children, *see* Wilson M. E. and McCleod K. R. *Anaesthesia* 1982, **37**, 951.

A 27 SWG needle is helpful. Topical analgesia of the skin, e.g. using EMLA (Eutectic Mixture of Local Analgesics) cream,[34] applied an hour before, helps. EMLA does have complications.[35] More than two attempts at venepuncture should not be allowed in the conscious child, unless the skin analgesia has worked perfectly. (*See also* Whitelaw A. and Valman B. *Br. Med. J.* 1980, **2**, 602.) To facilitate intravenous puncture, a light shining from the side, casting a shadow is helpful. Suitable veins include those on the back of the hand, the dorsum of the foot, the internal saphenous vein (in front of the medial malleolus, and scalp veins in babies. Intravenous induction of anaesthesia with a sleep dose of thiopentone, is common, followed by a relaxant, intubation and IPPV with a nitrous oxide–oxygen mixture, with or without volatile agent or opioid. There should be a small leak of air between tube and trachea.

INTRAVENOUS AGENTS

1. Thiopentone 2.5 mg/kg in infants; 5 mg/kg in children. Laryngeal reflexes remain active.[36] The effects are similar to those seen in the adult. There is a progressive fall in the dose of thiopentone required for anaesthesia throughout later childhood.

2. Methohexitone 1.5 mg/kg of 1% solution, has triexponential decay, shorter $T_{1/2\alpha}$ (2.4 min) and $T_{1/2\beta}$ (23 min), than adults, with higher clearance (18.9 ml/kg/min), giving faster postoperative psychomotor recovery than thiopentone.

3. Propofol 2–2.5 mg/kg.[37] Hypotension (−24%) and apnoeas (> 30 sec in 13%) are similar to adults.

4. Etomidate 0.2 mg/kg with opioid premedication, 0.4 mg/kg without.[38] *See also* Chapter 9.

5. Ketamine 2 mg/kg i.v. or 6 mg/kg i.m. Elimination half-life 100 min in children.[39] Recommended for diagnostic procedures and minor operations in small children and infants and to control restlessness before induction of general anaesthesia. Particular examples are orthopaedic manipulations, burns dressing, radiology, e.g. radioisotope scanning and radiotherapy, examinations under anaesthesia of eye, rectum, etc. Recommended when scarring of the neck as a result of burns produces an airway problem during induction of anaesthesia for plastic surgery. The agent may produce

hallucinations even in children but this can be reduced if recovery is allowed to be quiet and if diazepam is given before and after. Infusion dose 40 µg/kg/min.

'Gas' induction of anaesthesia

Suxamethonium, syringes needles and tracheal tubes should be immediately available in the anaesthetic room. Gas induction is indicated if there is difficulty finding a vein, where the child has needle-phobia, EMLA cream has been unsuccessful or forgotten, and the anaesthetist feels it is the best approach. Intravenous access is gained at the earliest possible opportunity.

A suitable method is to allow nitrous oxide, halothane 1% and oxygen to flow from a mask or tube held closely above the patient's face. Telling the child an interesting story helps enormously. A flow of about 10 l/min may be required for this. When consciousness is lost, after about 2 min, the mask is applied to the face and the gas flow reduced, and the percentage of halothane increased steadily. The child equilibrates with halothane 30% faster than the adult.[40] Halothane is well tolerated by children in whom the risk of halothane-associated hepatitis on repeated administration is very small.[41]

Enflurane, being more pungent, is not as easy to use, and should be avoided in children with a history of epilepsy. Isoflurane is also more difficult than halothane – about 10 breaths are allowed between each 1% rise of concentration. Reduced incidence of breath-holding, coughing and laryngo-spasm make halothane safer than enflurane and isoflurane. Desflurane can be used in a similar way, expensively, or in a ready-charged closed system (with difficulties due to leaks and deadspace). Cyclopropane 50% gives a rapid induction (35 s) but laryngeal spasm and excessively deep anaesthesia can occur with alarming speed. (The safe distance for monitor electrics while using cyclopropane is 2 m, and it should not be used in investigation rooms.) For management of laryngeal spasm, *see* Chapter 7.

It is quite acceptable to change the volatile agent to isoflurane or enflurane after induction as above. This may be indicated by the appearance of arrythmias. Isoflurane 1–2 MAC does not depress cardiac output[42] The volatile agents greatly potentiate non-depolarizing muscle relaxants in children.

MAC VALUES AND PHYSIOLOGICAL EFFECTS

MAC is highest at 1 year of postconceptual age (e.g. 2 months after full-term birth), being about 1.5 times the young adult value. At 32 weeks gestation (e.g. an 8-week preterm baby) it equals the adult figure. MAC falls steadily through childhood and adolescence to reach adult levels by the mid 20s.

Nitrous oxide 70% or 2.5 mg/kg morphine reduces the MAC of halothane by 61–63%. High dose sufentanil reduces it by 90%. However, opioids have a ceiling effect, and may not prevent awareness.

Hypotension (about 25% reduction at 1 MAC, about 50% reduction at 2 MAC of halothane, enflurane and isoflurane) is largely heart rate-dependent and responds to atropine. Systemic vascular resistance is slighly increased with nitrous oxide, unchanged with halothane, slightly reduced with enflurane, and halved at 2 MAC isoflurane.

Cerebral blood-flow (at constant MAP and $Paco_2$), is unaltered at 0.5 MAC of the volatiles, but thereafter increased most by halothane (doubled at 1 MAC, quadrupled at 1.5 MAC), and least by isoflurane (unaltered at 1.2 MAC).

Nitrous oxide is particularly useful because of the 'second gas effect' during induction, absence of cardiovascular and respiratory depression, rapid onset and offset, dilution of over-high oxygen tensions, reduction of volatile requirement, near-absence of metabolism and powerful analgesic effect.

Care must be taken that dead space is not too high when small children and infants are anaesthetized by these methods, but previous fears about mask deadspace have proved ungrounded because of 'streaming' of gas within them.

The closed system should not be used unless specially designed apparatus is available to minimize deadspace, such as the absorber of Cope.

Monitoring in paediatric anaesthesia

See Neonatal monitoring, above and Chapter 18.

Children require the same clinical and basic instrumental monitoring, of which pulse oximetry is a great aid.[43] Temperature monitoring is routine if a child is on a warm mattress (in case of hyperpyrexia). Routine capnography is revealing as far as further specialized instrumental monitoring is concerned, indwelling arterial cannulas are likely to be required in cardiac, intracranial, and craniofacial operations, phaeochromocytomas, neuroblastomas, transplantations and complex spinal operations.

Central venous pressure monitoring has similar indications to the adult (*see* Chapter 18), also in neuroblastoma surgery and in children with unstable circulation due to congenital heart disease. The antecubital fossa approach is very difficult in small children. The subclavian approach has the problem that passage of a cannula from the right subclavian vein to the SVC is difficult unless aided by a guide-wire. Swan-Ganz catheters are likewise difficult to insert and maintain in infants, partly due to the reactivity of the pulmonary vasculature. In neonates, alternative information about transitional circulation may also be obtained indirectly from pre- and postductal Pao_2. Cardiac output measurements via Swan-Ganz catheters require great technical care if errors are to be avoided. Non-invasive Doppler ultrasound cardiac output measurement records velocity-flow and cross-sectional area of aorta for single beats, and is reasonably accurate.[44] Aortovelography gives reasonable sequential estimates of changes in output.[45] Thoracic impedance techniques have proved difficult in children.[46]

Left atrial pressure monitoring lines for cardiac surgery can be inserted at operation via the right upper pulmonary vein. Coagulation monitoring (baseline and after each 50% of blood-volume loss) includes: (*a*) platelet count (platelets needed if below 50000/mm³); (*b*) prothrombin time and partial thromboplastin time (fresh frozen plasma needed if 25% prolonged); (*c*) clotting time (can be performed at any time in the theatre itself); and (*d*) fibrinolysins.

Neuromuscular monitors should deliver a 50 mA supramaximal stimulus. Positioning of stimulating and recording electrodes on the infant wrist is a problem. The median nerve has been used.[47] Sensory-evoked potentials (SEPs) are used for testing neurone integrity during spinal, cardiac and carotid surgery, and for unplanned awareness. Transcutaneous SEPs require huge amplification of the signal and interference is always a problem.[48]

Blood glucose and calcium levels should be monitored. Bilirubin/kernicterus (unconjugated bilirubin, 300 μmol/l) is especially dangerous in sick children with congenital intestinal malformations.

Malignant hyperpyrexia is uncommon in children but its occasional occurrence still calls for vigilance.[49]

Anaesthetic equipment for children

One or more 'Paediatric trolleys' are organized containing all the special equipment required.

Deadspace and resistance to respiration must be minimal; weight and size of the equipment, with its tubing, must be suitable for small children; valves must not cause undue obstruction; inhaled gases should be humidified; the reservoir bag should be smaller than in adults so that its movements with respiration can be seen easily; for spontaneous respiration, a 'one-way' valve may be satisfactory; the face-mask must fit well to the contours of the face (e.g. the Rendall Baker mask); the Magill attachment (Mapleson-A) or Bain coaxial circuit is suitable in older children, if the fresh gas flow exceeds the alveolar ventilation, during spontaneous respiration.

Ayre's T-piece[50] and Jackson Rees[51] modification

This has a minimal resistance to respiration. *See* Chapter 6. Jackson Rees[51] modified the system by fitting a 500-ml bag with an open tail to the expiratory limb. This makes controlled ventilation and easy monitoring of respiration possible. During spontaneous respiration the fresh gas flow should be 150 ml/kg to eliminate rebreathing. During controlled ventilation the input need only be 100 ml/kg body weight with a minimum flow of 3 l/min. This is likely to produce a $Paco_2$ of about 4 kPa. A flow of 3 l/min is recommended during neonatal anaesthesia. (For detailed analysis of the T-piece, *see* Froese A. B. and Rose D. K. In: *Some Aspects of Paediatric Anaesthesia* (Steward D. J. ed.) Amsterdam: Elsevier, 1982.)

Intubating a child

Indications: (1) difficult or obstructed airway; (2) many patients under 6 months or under 5 kg; (3) full stomach; (4) hypoventilation requiring IPPV; (5) use of relaxants requiring IPPV; (6) operations limiting access to the airway; and (7) operations over 1 h.

It may be performed under deep anaesthesia or relaxant. Awake intubation causes rises of intracranial pressure.[52] It is similar to the adult, except that the larynx appears to be more anterior, and the epiglottis is doubly curved and more floppy. A straight-bladed laryngoscope is often helpful, especially in the smaller child, and this is inserted posteriorly to actively lift the epiglottis out of the way.

The smallest part of the trachea is the cricoid ring and the tracheal tube should be *a loose fit in this indistensible ring* evidenced by a small gas leak on IPPV, to avoid mucosal damage. The shoulder of the Cole tube was very prone to cause this damage. Preshaped RAE tubes with Murphy eyes are very convenient. Uncuffed tubes are used below the age of 10 years. Longer-term intubation is usually done with a PVC nasal tube. There is always the risk of misplacement of the tube in the oesophagus, and this must be checked for at every intubation.

$$\text{Internal tube diameter (mm)} = \frac{16 + \text{age in years}}{4}$$

$$\text{Tube length to teeth (cm)} = \text{internal diameter (mm)} \times 3$$

Difficult intubations in children

The Bullard laryngoscope has been developed for these situations. It has a long thin rigid blade (over which the tube is passed), and fibreoptics.[53] For those situations where intubation is sometimes difficult, *see* Chapter 21. Flexible fibreoptic intubation may be used.

Subglottic stenosis is a special case. It may be easy to intubate the larynx, only to find that the tube will not pass down the trachea. It should not be forced, but replaced with a smaller one.

It is still necessary to have a small leak between tube and trachea.

Complications of intubation in children: (1) disconnections; (2) displacements (down, bronchial and up, oesophageal; (3) obstruction by kinking and secretions; and (4) after extubation, sore throat (50%), hoarse voice, subglottic oedema. Highest incidence between 1 and 3 years, especially in Down's syndrome[54] (3–10% of intubations in the past), epithelial damage (due to ischaemic pressure or chemical irritation).

IPPV

Controlled respiration has the advantage that it relieves the respiratory muscles of work and ensures adequate gas exchange. The Jackson-Rees system or a paediatric ventilator[55] is suitable. Anaesthesia can be maintained at light levels with nitrous oxide–oxygen and a muscle relaxant, and recovery is rapid. The risk to be avoided is severe hypocarbia (< 21 mmHg or 3 kPa). Small babies have a reduced FRC and airways closure may cause problems during spontaneous respiration.

Extubating a child and recovery from anaesthesia

Extubating a child in stage 2 anaesthesia is likely to cause coughing, straining and laryngospasm. Most infants can be extubated awake (i.e. stage 1 or lighter), except after intraocular surgery, where a cough on the tracheal tube as they pass through stage 2 should be avoided. In this case, and in older children, extubation may be done in stage 3 plane 1, and the child left (with extra oxygen) to awaken very quietly under close supervision in the postoperative recovery room. The tracheal tube, laryngoscope and T-piece can be left close by in case reintubation is needed. Postoperative recovery staff monitor (and initiate correction of) breathing, colour, Sp_{O_2}, airway patency and peripheral pulse.

Intraoperative opioids in children

Fentanyl 1–10 µg/kg (may cause significant muscle stiffness). Sufentanil 0.1–10 µg/kg, has a place in cardiac anaesthesia because of its cardiostability, especially if bradycardia is prevented. *See* Chapter 9.

Muscle relaxation in children

The volatile agents (especially isoflurane and enflurane) greatly potentiate (by 4–5 times)[56] non-depolarizing muscle relaxants in children. The usual relaxants and reversing drugs are satisfactory; infants require only half the dose of neostigmine.[57] *See* Table 22.2.

Table 22.2 Some suggested doses

	Neonate		Child	
Drug	Initial dose (mg/kg)	Repeat dose (mg/kg)	Initial dose (mg/kg)	Repeat dose (mg/kg)
Atracurium	0.5	0.25	0.5	0.25
Vecuronium	0.1	0.05	0.1	0.05
Doxacurium	0.03	0.01	0.03	0.01
Mivacurium	0.1	0.1	0.2	0.1
Tubocurarine	0.25–0.8	0.1	0.25–0.8	0.1
Pancuronium	0.06	0.01	0.1	0.02
Alcuronium	0.2	0.05	0.25	0.1
Gallamine	1.0	0.25	2.0	0.5
Suxamethonium	2–3	1.0	1.0	1.0
Pethidine i.m.	0.5	0.5	1.0	1.0
Morphine i.m.	0.1	0.1	0.15	0.15
Fentanyl i.v.	0.01			0.01
Alfentanyl i.v.	0.1			0.1
Methohexitone i.v.	–	–	2–4	1–2
Thiopentone i.v.	–	–	4–8	2–4
Propofol i.v.	1–3			
Atropine	0.01		0.02	–
Hyoscine	–	–	0.01	–
Trimeprazine	–	–	3 (oral)	–
Rectal thiopentone	–	–	40	
Ketamine i.m.	–	–	5–10	5–10
Ketamine i.v.	–	–	1–2	1–2

Suxamethonium. Infants are resistant to it (in spite of low cholinesterase levels) due to their greater ECV (40% of body weight cf. 18% in adults), and require twice the dose. Intramuscular dose 5 mg/kg for infants, 4 mg/kg for children. Phase 2 block may occur over 4 mg/kg. Suxamethonium in children (even in single doses) causes more bradyarrhythmias than in adults.

Side effects. Muscular fasciculation is not seen in infancy and there is no rise in intragastric pressure under 4 years of age; the rise in older children is less than in adults.[58] Cricoid pressure is effective in preventing regurgitation. Suxamethonium should be preceded by atropine, 0.05 mg/kg to reduce the greater muscarinic effects seen in children. Hyperkalaemia is insignificant except after burns, paraplegia and tetanus. Post-suxamethonium/halothane myoglobinaemia is prevented by previous low-dose nondepolarizing relaxants. Successful use of suxamethonium in open-eye injuries in children has been reported.[59] Suxamethonium is best avoided in children with Duchenne progressive muscular dystrophy because of cardiac effects and risk of malignant hyperpyrexia (MH).[60] In children known to have MH, a nitrous oxide–oxygen–opioid non-depolarizing relaxant technique is recommended.[61] Suxamethonium exacerbates congenital dystrophia myotonica with body rigidity preventing respiration and intubation. Such myotonia has also rarely followed the use of neostigmine in this condition.

Intermediate-acting relaxants

Neonates and infants are slightly more sensitive to vecuronium and atracurium than older children.[62] Compared with adults, vecuronium is slightly longer acting in infants,[63] and slightly shorter in children. Infusion doses: atracurium, 5–10 µg/kg/min (depending on concomitant 'volatiles');[64] vecuronium, 1.4–2 µg/kg/min (depending on concomitant 'volatiles').[65] Onset: 2 min. Bradycardia during intubation is unusual. Histamine release from atracurium is less marked in children, but occasionally significant.[66]

Mivacurium is short-acting, hydrolysed by plasma cholinesterase. Dose: 0.1–0.2 mg/kg. Onset: 1.8 min. Duration: 10–20 min. There is some histamine release.[67]

Longer-acting relaxants

The vagolytic action of pancuronium is useful because infant cardiac output is very rate-dependent, but the hypertension it generates may be undesirable in neonates and hypertensive heart disease. Most neonates and infants are slightly more sensitive to pancuronium and tubocurarine, but a few are markedly resistant.

Doxacurium is almost devoid of cardiovascular side-effects. Dose: 30 µg/kg; Onset: 1 min; Duration: 45–60 mins.[68] Children with Duchenne progressive muscular dystrophy (*see* Chapter 21) or myasthenia gravis (*see* Chapter 20) require reduced doses of non-depolarizing relaxants, or none at all.

The acute abdomen in children (e.g. acute appendicitis)

Vomiting and acid regurgitation risk. In children, cimetidine 10 mg/kg by mouth, 2–3 h before induction of anaesthesia reduces the volume of gastric juice and increases the pH above 2.5.[69] Rapid sequence induction is indicated. It is exceptionally rare for the small leak between tube and trachea to allow soiling of the trachea by gastric contents.

Sedation techniques

The Toronto mixture is in common use for infants (pethidine 25 mg; promethazine 6.25 mg; chlorpromazine 6.25 mg; in 1 ml: the dose is 0.06–0.08 ml/kg up to 14 kg.[32]

Rectal pentobarbitone 2–4 mg/kg or diazepam (in propylene glycol for rapid and predictable absorption) 0.5 mg/kg. Ketamine remains useful.

Regional analgesia

This is receiving more attention now that it has been shown that lignocaine 4 mg/kg or bupivacaine 2–3 mg/kg introduced into the body are safe doses. Extradural sacral, penile, ilio-inguinal and sciatic nerve block[70] (in fact the whole panoply of regional techniques), for pain relief in the perioperative period give good results.

TIVA in children

See Chapter 9 for general principles. Children require rather larger doses of propofol, e.g. induction 2–2.5 mg/kg, and MIR 15–20 mg/kg/h. Analgesics are required, especially alfentanil 10–20 µg/kg bolus and 1 µg/kg/min, stopped 10 mins before the end of surgery. Relaxants are infused as appropriate.

'Complicated' children

The congenital or medical condition needs to be defined (the casenotes will be large) and optimized before anaesthesia. They may have had many hospital visits and be highly cautious about anaesthetics.

Perioperative hyperpyrexia

This is likely to occur: (1) when the child is pyrexial; (2) in hot climatic conditions; (3) when there are too many coverings over the child, particularly if these include macintosh sheets; and (4) inhibition of sweating following atropine premedication may interfere with heat loss. Hyperpyrexia is an aetiological factor in ether convulsions. A mattress with circulating water coils placed under the patient may be useful for cooling.

Intravenous infusions in children

Infusion sets should include a burette, so that small and measured volumes of fluid can be given. Infusion pumps and heaters may be required.

Anaesthesia for some paediatric operations

Cleft Palate and Hare-lip in Infants

Many surgeons prefer to operate when the child is about 10–16 weeks old for hare-lip and about 1 year old for the palate. The child should be fit and healthy.

Atropine alone is suitable as premedication. Anaesthesia can be induced by any suitable method. An orotracheal tube is essential and may be used in conjunction with a Dott mouth gag. An Oxford or other non-kinking tube is recommended. Introduction may be hindered by an anteriorly displaced premaxilla obstructing the field of vision. To prevent the blade of the laryngoscope from sinking deeply into the wide cleft, gauze packing or adhesive tape can be used or the gap can be bridged by a spatula. Following removal of the tube and a careful oropharyngeal toilet, a patent airway can be ensured by a suture through the tongue. May be associated with the Pierre-Robin syndrome (*see* Chapter 21) and/or congenital heart disease.

Tumours about the face and neck

Cystic hygromas and other tumours may occur in these regions and may make tracheal intubation difficult.

The following method of guided blind tracheal intubation for cases of cancrum oris has been described:[71]

A Tuohy needle is introduced through the cricothyroid membrane and sterile vinyl plastic tubing threaded through the cords from below to coil up in the pharynx. A length of polythene tubing with a blunt hook is pushed through the nose to engage the vinyl catheter, which is brought out through the nose. A Magill cuffed tracheal tube is then passed round the catheter and afterwards withdrawn. The Bullard laryngoscope may be helpful.[72] Ketamine may have a place. Fibreoptic intubation facilities should be available.

Anaesthesia in asthma

Common sense dictates that anaesthesia during an attack is undesirable. For patients on long-standing steroid therapy, pre-operative injection of hydrocortisone will be required. Bronchospasm during the operation may be due to problems with a tracheal tube, e.g. irritation of the carina.

Anaesthesia for removal of inhaled foreign body

Should never be undertaken unless the services of an experienced bronchoscopist and anaesthetist are available. IPPV can force the foreign body further down. (*See* Baraka A. *Br. J. Anaesth.* 1974, **46**, 124; Moussali H. *Br. J. Hosp. Med.* 1981, **25**, 300; Bush G. H. and Vivori E. *Br. J. Hosp. Med.* 1981, **26**, 102.)

Anaesthetic management of major spinal surgery in children

The surgical approach to the spine is via vascular tissues and blood loss can be large. Good intravenous lines and monitoring are essential.

Scoliosis[73] which is progressive, is likely to result in long-term cardiorespiratory deterioration. Total lung capacity and vital capacity are both reduced. FEV may be diminished as a result of mechanical inefficiency of the respiratory muscles. Airways closure encroaches on the FRC earlier than in normal subjects. Abnormal ventilation/perfusion ratios may result in relative arterial hypoxaemia. During operation, full cardiovascular and respiratory monitoring is usual. General anaesthesia with muscle relaxation and IPPV is the rule. Some surgeons require the patient to wake up so that the integrity of the cord, after distraction of the spine, can be tested;[74] others use evoked potentials.[75] The wake-up technique must be explained to the patient beforehand and the timing of supplementary doses of muscle relaxant and fentanyl must be carefully gauged. Blood loss at operation may be considerable and deliberate hypotension is often used. Elective IPPV may be employed postoperatively.

Neurosurgical operations

These require light general anaesthesia via an orotracheal tube. Isoflurane and halothane are useful agents in children, since respiration is usually quiet, but hypoventilation is to be avoided. Ketamine is useful for diagnostic procedures.

Operation for hydrocephalus. Intubation may be difficult due to the large forehead, which makes visualization of the larynx awkward.

Meningocele. Careful anaesthetic technique is required. The operation is performed in the face-down position. Tracheal intubation is mandatory. Controlled ventilation is likely to be required as spontaneous respiration, mainly diaphragmatic, is embarrassed in this position.

Posterior fossa exploration. In infants IPPV is recommended with close attention to replacement of blood loss, avoidance of heat loss, with wrapping of abdomen and legs in bandages and elevation of the legs. Central venous pressure measurement is helpful.

Circumcision

Standard techniques of general anaesthesia are suitable. Tracheal intubation is seldom necessary but laryngeal spasm may occur; this requires temporary cessation of the surgical stimulus, then deepening of anaesthesia. Caudal block (0.25% plain bupivacaine, 0.25 ml/kg, or 1 ml/year, performed while the child is anaesthetized, gives good postoperative analgesia as does penile block and dressings incorporating lignocaine ointment or EMLA cream. *See* Chapter 24.

Conjoined twins[76]

These babies may require several anaesthetics, depending on how they are joined. *Radiological investigations* require quiet babies. Each twin must be anaesthetized separately. Two anaesthetists should therefore be available.

Narcosis of the first twin may be difficult. If there is a significant common circulation the anaesthetic agent will be drained away to the other twin so that the speed of induction is slowed. Conversely, the second twin is anaesthetized more readily because it has already received some anaesthesia from the first. Depending on the site of union, intubation may be technically difficult. Ketamine has a place in the management of these sometimes difficult cases.

Operations for separation of conjoined twins are likely to be long and to be associated with blood loss. (*See also* Harrison V. L. et al. *Anaesth. Intensive Care* 1985, **13**, 82; and Roy M. *Anaesthesia* 1984, **39**, 1225.)

Burns dressings

Problems arise when small children require frequent anaesthesia for burns dressings. Excessive starvation is to be avoided. Multiple halothane administrations are undesirable. Possible techniques include neurolept analgesia, ketamine and inhalation analgesia (e.g. nitrous oxide).

Diabetic patients (See also Chapter 20)

The juvenile type of diabetes is very labile and demands particular care at the time of surgery. In the severely ill, frequent estimations of electrolytes and acid-base balance are required. The anaesthetist should aim for a rapid return of consciousness at the end of the operation without vomiting. It is usually wise to seek the advice of a paediatrician regarding the insulin regimen.

Postoperative pain[77]

Regional analgesia can be used when appropriate (*see* Chapters 24, 25). Great care is needed when giving opioids to infants, not only because of respiratory depression, but also because cardiac output is also very rate-dependent, with serious results from opioid bradycardia. (*See* Opioids in neonates, above). For infants over 5 kg in weight, codeine phosphate, 1 mg/kg is satisfactory but should not be given i.v. because it causes a severe fall in cardiac output. For children on ventilators pethidine 1 mg/kg or morphine 0.2 mg/kg is satisfactory. Older children may be given narcotic analgesics on a weight basis. Morphine has been used as a continuous infusion by syringe pump in a dose of 1 mg/kg in 50 ml of saline at 1 ml/h following major surgery. Aspirin is avoided because of risk of Reyes Syndrome.

Vomiting in children after operations

Below the age of 3 there is a low incidence. Vomiting is common after operations for hernia, tonsils and adenoids, squint and after cardiac catheterization.

Airway and respiratory emergencies in paediatrics

1. Asphyxia of the newborn.
2. Choanal atresia.[78] Nearly always posterior. If bilateral, the infant will breathe through the mouth. The airway must be kept patent by opening the mouth, keeping the child crying, or insertion and taping down of an oropharyngeal airway until surgical correction can be performed.
3. The Pierre Robin syndrome.[79] *See* Chapter 21.
4. Laryngomalacia.[80] The commonest congenital cause of stridor. This is caused by incomplete development of the laryngeal cartilages. Inspiratory obstruction to respiration occurs as the flaccid structures are drawn in. Usually improves after the age of 18 months.

Common causes of stridor in children are (in order): laryngotracheitis, laryngotracheobronchitis, congenital stridor, acute epiglottitis and spasmodic laryngitis.

Resuscitation in paediatrics

The basic life support system applies. The majority of paediatric cardiac arrests are respiratory in origin. The airway is more difficult and more variable than in adults. A pharyngeal foreign body or two is more common. External cardiac massage is easier than in adults and can achieve 50% of normal cardiac output, and can be done with two fingers in infants, with great care to avoid compressing the upper abdomen. Note that absent pulses may be due to surgery, and scars should be looked for. Tracheal intubation is the best way of ensuring efficient ventilation, but in inexperienced hands oesophageal misplacement is a risk. Venous access is more difficult than in adults, with the external jugular the simplest, and then the femoral. The subclavian and internal jugular veins are possible.

There is a real risk of giving over-large doses of resuscitation drugs and fluids. Some doses include:

Atropine 0.02 mg/kg
Adrenaline 10 μg/kg[81]
Sodium bicarbonate 1 mmol/kg
Calcium chloride 10 mg/kg
Glucose 1 g/kg
Lignocaine 1 mg/kg
Frusemide 1 mg/kg
Dopamine 5–10 μg/kg
Isoprenaline 0.1 μg/kg/min
DC defibrillation 2 J/kg

See also Hatch D. J. In: *Recent Advances in Anaesthesia and Analgesia – 15* (Atkinson R. S. and Adams A. P. ed.) Edinburgh: Churchill Livingstone, 1985; Steward D. J. *Management of Paediatric Anaesthesia* 2nd ed. London: Churchill Livingstone, 1985; Hatch D. J. and Sumner E. *Neonatal Anaesthesia* 2nd ed. London: Arnold, 1986; Sumner E. and Hatch D. J. (ed.) *Clinics in Anaesthesiology, Pediatric Anaesthesia*. London: Saunders, 1985;

Sumner E. and Hatch D. J. (ed.) *A textbook of Paediatric Anaesthetic Practice*, Edinburgh: Churchill Livingstone, 1990.

Children in the ITU

These present the usual problems, compounded by different anatomy, physiology, pharmacology and psychology (*see above*). For outcome after assisted ventilation in children with acquired immunodeficiency syndrome, *see* Notterman D. A. et al. *Crit Care Med.* 1990, **18**, 18.

References

1. NCEPOD 1989 (Campling E. A., Devlin H. B. and Lunn J. N. ed.), 1990.
2. Borland L. M. and Casselbrant M. *Anesth. Analg.* 1990, **70**, 105.
3. Anand K. J. S. and Hichey P. R. *Anesthesiology* 1987, **67**, A502.
4. Chakrabarti M. K. et al. *Br. J. Anaesth.* 1990, **64**, 374.
5. Diaz-Blanco J. et al. *Crit. Care Med.* 1989, **17**, 1335.
6. Moss I. R. et al. *J. Pediatr.* 1982, **101**, 443.
7. Gregory *Can. Anaesth. Soc. J.* 1982, **29**, 105.
8. Morselli P. L. et al. *Handbook of Clinical Pharmacokinetics* (Gimaldi M. and Prescott L. ed.) New York: Adis Health Science Press, 1983.
9. LeDez K. M. and Lerman J. *Anesthesiology* 1987, **67**, 301–307.
10. Waugh R. and Johnson G. G. *Can. Anaesth. Soc. J.* 1984, **31**, 700.
11. Friesen R. H. and Henry D. B. *Anesthesiology* 1986, **64**, 238.
12. Cook D. R. *Can. Anaesth. Soc. J.* 1986, **33**, (Suppl), 38.
13. Liu L. M. P. et al. *Anesthesiology* 1983, **59**, 506.
14. Friesen R. H. and Lichtor J. L. *Anesth. Analg.* 1981, **60**, 742; Kimble K. J. et al. *Anesthesiology* 1981, **54**, 423.
15. Dorlas J. C. et al. *Anesthesiology* 1985, **62**, 342.
16. Inkster J. S. *Anaesthesia* 1966, **21**, 111.
17. Sasse F. J. *J. Clin. Monit.* 1985, **1**, 147–148.
18. Badgewell J. M. et al. *Anesthesiology* 1987, **66**, 405.
19. Bush G. H. In: *General Anaesthesia* (Gray T. C. and Nunn J. F. ed.) 3rd ed. London: Butterworths, 1971, Vol. 2. Chapter 31.
20. Goudsouzian N. G. et al. *Anesthesiology* 1973, **39**, 351.
21. Goudsouzian N. G. *Br. J. Anaesth.* 1980, **52**, 205.
22. Koehntop D. E. et al. *Anesth. Analg.* 1986, **65**, 227.
23. Moore R. A. et al. *Anesthethesiology* 1985, **62**, 725.
24. Lloyd-Thomas A. R. *Br. J. Anaesth.* 1990, **64**, 85.
25. Dufour H. and Fredet P. *Revue Chir.* 1908, **37**, 208.
26. Ramstedt W. C. *Med. Klin.* 1912, **8**, 1702.
27. Connor M. E. and Drasner K. *Anesth Analg.* 1990, **70**, 176.
28. Gray D. W. et al. *Ann. R. Coll. Surg. Engl.* 1984, **66**, 280.
29. *See* Bush G. H. *Anaesth.* 1984, **39**, 381; Battersby E. F. et al. *Anaesth.* 1984, **39**, 381.
30. Splinter W. M., Stewart J. A. and Muir J. G. *Can. J. Anaesth.* 1990, **37**, 36.
31. Connor M. E. and Drasner K. *Anesth. Analg.* 1990, **70**, 176.
32. Laub M. et al. *Anaesth.* 1990, **45**, 110.
33. Raftery S. and Warde D. *Br. J. Anaesth.* 1990, **64**, 167.
34. Wahlstedt C. et al. *Lancet* 1984, **2**, 106; Hopkins C. S. et al. *Anaesth.* 1988, **43**, 198; Gunawardene R. D. and Davenport H. T. *Anaesth.* 1990, **45**, 52; Bjerring P. and Arendt-Nielsen L. *Br. J. Anaesth.* 1990, **64**, 173.

35. *Br. J. Anaesth.* 1990, **64**, 403.
36. Jonmarker C. et al. *Anesthesiology* 1987, **67**, 104.
37. Purcell-Jones G. et al. *Br. J. Anaesth.* 1987, **59**, 1431–1436.
38. Kay B. *Br. J. Anaesth.* 1976, **48**, 207.
39. Grant I. S. et al. *Br. J. Anaesth.* 1983, **55**, 1107.
40. Brandom B. W. et al. *Anesth. Analg.* 1983, **62**, 404.
41. Wark H. J. *Anaesth.* 1983, **38**, 237.
42. Neal M. B. et al. *Anesthesiology* 1984, **61**, A437.
43. Cohen D. E. et al. *Anesthesiology* 1988, **68**, 181.
44. Schuster A. H. and Nanda N. C. *Am. J. Cardiol.* 1984, **53**, 257.
45. Haites N. E. et al. *Br. Heart J.* 1985, **53**, 123.
46. Donovan K. D. et al. *Crit. Care Med.* 1986, **14**, 1038.
47. Lam H. S. et al. *Br. J. Anaesth.* 1981, **53**, 1351.
48. Lam H. S. *Can. J. Anaesth.* 1987, **34**, S232.
49. Allen G. and Rosenberg H. *Anesth. Analg.* 1990, **70**, 115.
50. Ayre T. P. *Lancet* 1937, **1**, 561; Inkster J. S. *Br. J. Anaesth.* 1956, **28**, 512; Ayre T. P. *Br. J. Surg.* 1937, **25**, 131 (reprinted in 'Classical File,' *Surv. Anaesthesiol.* 1967, **11**, 400).
51. Rees G. J. *Br. Med. J.* 1950, **2**, 1419; *Br. J. Anaesth.* 1960, **32**, 132.
52. Friesen R. H. et al. *Anesth. Analg.* 1987, **66**, 874.
53. Borland L. M. and Casselbrant M. *Anesth. Analg.* 1990, **70**, 105.
54. Sherry K. M. *Br. J. Anaesth.* 1983, **55**, 53.
55. Hatch D. J. et al. *Br. J. Anaesth.* 1990, **65**, 262.
56. Ali H. H. and Savarese J. J. *Anesthesiology* 1976, **45**, 216.
57. Fisher D. M. and Miller R. D. *Anesthesiology* 1983, **58**, 519.
58. Salem M. R. et al. *Br. J. Anaesth.* 1972, **44**, 401.
59. Libonati M. M. et al. *Anesthesiology* 1985, **62**, 637.
60. Rosemberg H. and Heiman-Patterson T. *Anesthesiology* 1983, **59**, 362.
61. Michel P. A. and Fronefield H. P. *Anesthesiology* 1985, **62**, 213.
62. Nightingale D. A. *Br. J. Anaesth.* 1986, **58**, 32S.
63. Motsch J. et al. *Anaesthesist* 1985, **34**, 382.
64. Ridley S. A. and Hatch D. J. *Br. J. Anaesth.* 1988, **60**, 31.
65. Mirakhur R. K. et al. *Anesthesiology* 1984, **61**, A293.
66. Goudsouzian N. G. et al. *Br. J. Anaes.* 1986, **58**, 1229
67. Miler V. et al. *Anesth. Analg.* 1988, **67**, S149.
68. Goudsouzian N. G. et al. *Anesth. Analg.* 1988, **67**, S80; Sarner J. B. et al. *Anesthesiology* 1987, **67**, A365.
69. Yildiz F. et al. *Anaesthesia.* 1984, **39**, 314.
70. Dalens B., Tanguy A. and Vanneuville G. *Anesth. Analg.* 1990, **70**, 131; McNichol L. R. *Anaesthesia* 1985, **40**, 410; Arthur D. S. and McNicol *Br. J. Anaesth.* 1986, **58**, 760.
71. Waters D. J. *Anaesthesia.* 1963, **18**, 158.
72. Borland L. M. and Casselbrant M. *Anesth. Analg.* 1990, **70**, 105.
73. Loach A. *Current Topics in Anaesthesia. Anaesthesia in Orthopaedics.* London: Arnold, 1983.
74. Vauxelle J. et al. *Clin. Orthop.* 1973, **93**, 173; Abbott T. R. and Bentley G. *Anaesth.* 1980, **35**, 298.
75. Brown R. H. and Nash C. L. *Spine* 1979, **4**, 466.
76. Ballantine R. I. W. and Jackson I. *Br. Med. J.* 1964, **1**, 1339; Furman E. B. *Anesthesiology* 1971, **34**, 95; Tovey R. M. et al. *Anaesthesia.* 1979, **34**, 178; Chi-Ching Cho et al. *Can. Anaesth. Soc. J.* 1980, **27**, 565.
77. Lloyd-Thomas A. R. *Br. J. Anaesth.* 1990, **64**, 85.
78. Hall B. D. *J. Pediatr.* 1979, **95**, 395.
79. Robin P. *J. Med. Paris* 1923, **43**, 235; Freeman M. K. and Manners J. N. *Anaesth.* 1980, **35**, 282; Heaf D. P. et al. *J. Pediatr.* 1982, **100**, 698.
80. Holinger P. H. and Brown W. T. *Ann. Otol. Rhinol. Laryngol.* 1967, **76**, 744.
81. Goetting M. G. et al. *Crit. Care Med.* 1989, **17**, 1258.

Plastic surgery and burns

PLASTIC SURGERY

History[1]

First described in Europe by Tagliacozzi (1546–1599) in 1586.[2] Thiersch graft described in 1874;[3] Wolfe's full-thickness graft in 1875;[4] and the split-skin graft in 1929.[5] Magill and Rowbotham developed insufflation and then endotracheal anaesthesia[6] in order to aid the development of plastic surgery by Sir Harold Gillies[7] at the Queen's Hospital, Sidcup.

Anaesthesia

Skin grafts can often be removed painlessly from the thigh after block of the lateral femoral cutaneous and, if necessary, femoral nerves, or by intradermal and subcutaneous infiltration of skin. The main problems in anaesthesia for plastic surgery are: (1) access to the airway may be restricted because of facial injuries, scars, cleft palate, or because of bizarre positions requested by plastic surgeons; and (2) provision of ischaemic skin to facilitate the work of the surgeon – this may conflict with the absolute priority for cerebral perfusion, e.g. during mammoplasty with the patient in the sitting position.

For anaesthetic management of patients undergoing operations for free flap transfer it is important to ensure adequate skin blood flow with: sodium nitroprusside; light general anaesthesia; maintenance of arterial blood pressure above 100 mmHg; maintenance of normal blood gases, circulating volume, cardiac output and body temperature; and good postoperative analgesia. Central neural blockade does not prevent arterial muscle spasm.[8]

Microvascular surgery has become increasingly ambitious, and these operations can take extreme lengths of time, even into a second day.[9] The patient must be kept immobile under the operating microscope, protected from bedsores and warm. A nasogastric tube may be needed to keep the stomach empty, while anaesthetic agents chosen should not be cumulative or toxic (e.g. nitrous oxide) if used for such long periods. Isoflurane is an ideal agent. General anaesthesia is usual, although adequate pain relief may be a problem. Postoperative shivering can destroy many hours of the plastic surgeon's work. Pethidine and chlorpromazine may be useful. Regional block may be used, even as the sole technique, for operations exceeding 20 hours.[10]

The anaesthetist in the plastic unit needs to have a strong feeling for the theatrical and a good sense of humour!

BURNS[11]

The anaesthetist is more concerned with the extent and location of the burn, which determine fluid and airway management, rather than the thickness, which dictates the surgical care. Percentage of body surface burned is assessed by 'rule of nines': front and back of trunk 18% each, each leg 18%, each arm 9%, head and neck 9%, and genitalia 1%. For children the 'rule of tens' is used: front and back of trunk 20% each, each limb 10%, and head and neck 20%. The size of the patient's hand and fingers is 1% of surface area. Adults with burns exceeding 20% (or children over 10%) will need fluid resuscitation and those over 30% need the care of a burns unit. If the burn is over 60%, or if the patient's age added to the percentage burn exceeds 100, he is unlikely to survive. Many patients may be burned in the same accident, e.g. the Bradford Football Club fire.[12]

Pain. Cooling with water gives immediate pain relief, but only influences burn thickness if applied within 30 sec. Subsequent analgesia may be Entonox, increments of i.v. opiate, volatile agent, e.g. methoxyflurane, or ketamine, which has been given orally.[13]

Respiratory injury. Dry heat or sometimes inhaled irritants may damage the lining of the upper airway. If this has occurred, evidenced by oral burns, singed nasal hairs, carbon-stained sputum or any sign of upper airways obstruction, then early intubation should be performed, preferably awake using a fibreoptic laryngoscope. A naso-tracheal tube is preferred if the mouth is burnt. Complete obstruction can supervene rapidly; delay may make the identification of landmarks and intubation impossible. Tracheostomy in burned patients is associated with a high incidence of infections and of subsequent tracheal stenosis.[14]

Direct thermal damage is rare below the trachea, but pulmonary damage results from inhalation of irritants, e.g. aldehydes from wood smoke, oxides of nitrogen and sulphur and hydrochlorides, or from chemical burns, e.g. phosgene. Copious sputum, wheezing, pulmonary oedema, infection and an ARDS-like picture develop some 4–10 days after the burn. Carbon monoxide and cyanides are also inhaled. COHb over 15% is significant. COHb over 50–60% or a plasma cyanide over 130 µmol/l is likely to be fatal. Some pulse oximeters can measure COHb. Blood gases and chest radiography should be performed, and humidified oxygen given by mask if Pao_2 is below 10 kPa, or to shorten the half-life of COHb. Ventilatory support may be needed. Regular steroids increase mortality, but a single large dose given early may benefit,[15] and methylprednisolone was used in the Falklands.[16]

Escharotomies may be needed to allow adequate respiration in the presence of circumferential burns of the trunk.

Fluid therapy. Capillaries in the burnt tissue become leaky and large amounts of fluid and plasma proteins are lost into the extracellular space, mostly in the first 2–3 hours.[17] Intravenous infusion will probably be needed and perhaps central venous or even pulmonary wedge pressure monitors. The patient should be weighed, and a urinary catheter may be needed with careful asepsis. Haemoglobin, PCV, plasma and urine electrolytes should be measured.

There are many different formulae for calculating fluid requirements. A common one in the UK is that of Muir and Barclay:[18]

Fluid requirement (ml) = 0.5 × body weight (kg) × area of burn (%)

This volume is given (in addition to normal water and electrolyte needs) as colloid (human albumin), 4-hourly for the first 12 h, 6-hourly for the next 24 h, and then as needed to keep the PCV normal.

In parts of the U.S. up to 4 ml/kg/% area of burn are given as lactated Ringer's solution in the first 24 h. Another regimen is hypertonic saline (Na 250 mmol/l) to keep the urine output greater than 1 ml/kg/h for the first 24 h, and 0.5 ml/kg/h after that.[19] This may be difficult because of the high secretion of vasopressin. In the Falklands conflict a mixture of Hartmann's solution and gelatin solution was used.[16] Blood may be needed to replace red cells damaged by deep burns, to keep PCV up to 35%.

Metabolic and immune effects. The hypercatabolism and rise in metabolic rate following burns is greater than after other forms of trauma. This compensates for the loss of heat by evaporation and impairment of vasoconstriction. The hypothalamic thermostat is reset at a higher temperature. There is a rise in plasma catecholamines, cortisol, glucagon, and particularly in vasopressin.[20] Hyperglycaemia is common. Energy requirement is 20 kcal/kg + 50 kcal/% burn, and may exceed 17 MJ/24 h (4000 kcal). Protein needed is 1 g/kg + 2 g per % burn. Palatable food is best but will often need to be supplemented by enteral tube feeding and sometimes parenteral nutrition. During anaesthesia, the increased metabolism requires a high alveolar ventilation. All aspects of the immune response are suppressed. Infections are a particular danger, and are treated energetically as they arise. Aminoglycosides, ticarcillin, azlocillin are commonly used.

Problems for the anaesthetist after the initial resuscitation

1. *The need for repeated procedures*, e.g. dressings. This may be done with neurolept analgesia, e.g. droperidol 0.1–0.2 mg/kg and phenoperidine 0.03–0.05 mg/kg supplemented by Entonox if needed. Ketamine, 2 mg/kg i.v. or 10 mg/kg i.m., is useful in children or where scarring of the neck makes airway maintenance difficult, but it does not always prevent aspiration.

2. *Further major operations*, such as tangential excision of burnt tissue under general anaesthesia is associated with considerable haemorrhage. IPPV with large tidal volumes is needed. Propofol and alfentanil infusions have been successful.[21] Controlled hypotension[22] or the use of tourniquets if possible has been advocated to reduce blood loss.

3. *Practical difficulties*, of venous access, applying a face-mask, difficult airway if the neck is scarred, and siting the blood pressure cuff, ECG electrodes or oximeter probe. An oesophageal stethoscope is useful. The patient may need to be placed in an unusual position on the operating table.

4. *Associated trauma to other organs.*

5. *Deep venous thrombosis.*

6. *Suxamethonium* may cause a dangerous rise in serum potassium and cardiac arrest, especially if given between 3 and 8 weeks after the burns, due to increased number of extra-junctional receptors. Others recommend the avoidance of this drug at any time between 5 days and 4 months after.

7. *Resistance to the action of non-depolarizing relaxants.*[23] ED_{95} doubled (peak effect 2 weeks after burn) possibly for the same reason.

8. *Renal failure*, associated with either haemoglobinuria or myoglobinuria. Urine output should be watched closely. Alkalinization of the urine may be protective.

9. *Loss of drugs*, into oedema fluid and because of decreased binding proteins. Aminoglycosides and cimetidine may need higher doses.

See also Brown J. M. In: *Recent Advances in Anaesthesia and Analgesia – 15* (Atkinson R. S. and Adams A. P. ed.) Edinburgh: Churchill Livingstone, 1985, 155; Martyn J. A. J. *Acute Management of the Burned Patient* W. B. Saunders, 1990; Robertson C. and Fenton O. *Br. Med. J.* 1990, **301**, 282.

References

1. Bodenham D.C. *Ann. R. Coll. Surg. Eng.* 1981, **63**, 233; Bennett J. P. *J. R. Soc. Med.* 1983, **76**, 152.
2. Mercuriali G. *De decoratione* 2nd ed. Frankfurt, 1586.
3. Thiersch C. *Arch. Klin. Chir.* 1874, **17**, 318.
4. Wolfe J. R. *Br. Med. J.* 1875, **2**, 360.
5. Blair V. P. and Brown J. B. *Surg. Gynecol. Obstet.* 1929, **49**, 82.
6. Bodley P. *Proc. R. Soc. Med.* 1978, **71**, 839.
7. Gillies H. D. *Plastic Surgery of the Face.* Oxford: Oxford Medical Publications, 1920.
8. Aps C. et al. *Ann. R. Coll. Surg. Engl.* 1985, **67**, 177.
9. Caplan R. A. and Long M. C. *Anesth. Analg.* 1984, **63**, 353.
10. Shanahan P. T. *Anesth. Analg.* 1984, **63**, 785.
11. For history of the treatment of burns: Wallace A. F. *Hosp. Update* 1980, **6**, 375; McGinty J. B. *J. Irish Coll. Phys. Surg.* 1981, **11**, 63.
12. Griffiths R. W. *Br. Med. J.* 1985, **291**, 917.
13. Morgan A. J. and Dutkiewicz T. W. S. *Anaesthesia* 1983, **38**, 293.
14. Lund T. et al. *Ann. Surg.* 1985, **201**, 374.
15. Head J. M. *Am. J. Surg.* 1980, **139**, 508.
16. Williams J. G. et al. *Br. Med. J.* 1983, **286**, 775.
17. Arturson G. *Acta Anaesthesiol. Scand.* 1985, Suppl. 82, 55.
18. Muir I. *Intensive Care Med.* 1981, **7**, 49.
19. Monafo W. W. et al. *Surgery* 1984, **95**, 129.
20. Crum R. L. *Arch. Surg.* 1990, **125**, 1065.
21. Reyneke C. J. et al. *Br. J. Anaesth.* 1989, **63**, 418.
22. Szyfelbein S. K. *J. R. Soc. Med.* 1982, **75**, Suppl. 1, 26.
23. Martyn J. A. J. et al. *Anesth. Analg.* 1982, **61**, 614.

Radiology

(*See also* Neurosurgery, above.)

General considerations

An increasing number of diagnostic and therapeutic procedures taking place in X-ray departments do not require general anaesthesia. Interventional radiology has applications in biopsy procedures, decompression and drainage of abnormal collections of fluid, extraction of stones and vascular procedures. Coronary angioplasty allows treatment of some cases of coronary artery occlusion, although facilities must be available for cardiopulmonary bypass procedures if required. Those working in the radiology department must be competent to treat cardiopulmonary collapse.

Patients are frequently managed under sedation rather than general anaesthesia. The principles of sedation are the same as those needed in other situations,[1] but there is also the need to work with dim lighting sometimes, to protect the staff from exposure to radiation (which may mean observation of the patient from a distance) and to work in situations remote from the main theatre block. It is important, therefore, that good assistance and monitoring facilities are available. Children are a special problem in that co-operation may be difficult and general anaesthesia is more likely to be required. *See also* Paediatrics, above.

There should be regular cardiopulmonary resuscitation drills for the Radiology staff together with the availability of respiratory care equipment, oxygen, plasma volume expander, suction, atropine, diphenhydramine, steroid and adrenaline. Reactions to intravenous contrast media are more likely to occur in patients with strong allergic, asthmatic, atopic or cardiac histories. *See also* Chapter 14 for principles of management.

All varieties of arteriography, including aortography, cerebral, femoral and brachial are rendered virtually painless by the use of the newer low osmolar contrast media iohexol, iopamidol, iogalate and, to a less extent, metrizamide. They are much more expensive however.[2]

References

1. Willats S. M. In: *Recent Advances in Anaesthesia and Analgesia – 16* (Atkinson R. S. and Adams A. P. ed.) Edinburgh: Churchill Livingstone, 1991.
2. Grainger R. G. *Br. Med. J.* 1984, **289**, 144.

Urology

Max Nitze of Berlin (1848–1906) developed the first electrically illuminated cystoscope in 1879.[1] Sir Peter Freyer (1852–1921) developed suprapubic prostatectomy in London in 1901. Terence Millin's retropubic operation first performed in 1945. Although Hugh Young had used an endourethral knife in 1908 to remove a small prostatic adenoma blindly, wire loop resection only became practical in 1926 when Maximilian Stern used both diathermy and special optics. By 1945 transurethral resection was the standard operation for benign prostatectomy in the US, but not for another 15 years in the UK.[2]

For anaesthesia in patients with impaired renal function, *see* Chapter 20.

Cystoscopy

If *general anaesthesia* is used, there must be: (1) complete loss of sensation; (2) relaxation of bladder sphincters and abdominal wall; and (3) no straining, coughing or respiratory obstruction. These can be difficult to accomplish smoothly, especially in old men with chronic obstructive lung disease. It should never be undertaken lightly and may require tracheal intubation. Spontaneous respiration using oxygen, nitrous oxide and volatile agent with a small dose of i.v. narcotic is a common technique. Cystoscopy is often repeated at intervals.

Topical analgesia, e.g. lignocaine 1 or 2% gel may be satisfactory, especially in women, or if a flexible fibreoptic cystoscope is used in men, but should not be used after recent instrumentation or in the presence of urethral bleeding. Severe cystitis makes local analgesia unsuitable because distension of the bladder with irrigating fluid causes painful spasm. *Extradural sacral block* or *intradural spinal analgesia* is very satisfactory. Sympathetic supply to the bladder is from T11 to L2.

Transurethral resection of the prostate (TURP)[3]

General anaesthesia, either with spontaneous respiration or IPPV, may be supplemented by caudal extradural block to reduce bleeding and for postoperative pain. Intradural spinal block is also very satisfactory, e.g. 2–4 ml heavy or plain bupivacaine 0.5%. The block must reach at least T10. Transurethral and perineal local analgesia has also been employed.[4]

Glycine 1.5%, at a pressure of less than 70 cmH$_2$O, is widely used for irrigation. Although slightly hypotonic (2.1% is isotonic) it is non-electrolytic and prevents dissipation of diathermy current during resection. Glycine[5] has a half-life of 85 min. Metabolic products include oxalate, which may precipitate in the renal tubules if urine flow is low during the first 10 postoperative days, and ammonia, which is a cerebral depressant. Glycine is an inhibitory neurotransmitter and may cause transient blindness. The amount that may be absorbed via the prostatic veins is typically around 700 ml or 20 ml/min, but can reach several litres, depending on the surgical skill, pressure of irrigant and duration of operation.

It can result in *TURP syndrome*:[6] water intoxication, cerebral oedema, pulmonary oedema, hypoxia, nausea, vomiting, headache, fibrinolysis, bradycardia, hypertension, cardiac arrest, convulsions and coma. Burning sensations of the hands and face are early symptoms. The dilutional hyponatraemia may prolong the action of non-depolarizing relaxants, and cause QRS widening and T-wave inversion. Bacteraemia may confuse the clinical picture. Ideally the syndrome should be prevented by close observation of the patient and by monitoring the serum sodium. General anaesthesia will obscure the early symptoms. End-tidal ethanol levels after marking the irrigant with 1% ethanol have also been used as a measure of amount absorbed.[7] Intravascular sodium electrodes have been used. A sodium level below 120 mmol/l should be treated. The fully established syndrome is more difficult to manage. Treatment includes loop diuretics, e.g. frusemide 20–80 mg, water restriction, hypertonic saline (500 ml of 1.8%, 100 ml of 5%, 20 ml of 30%) with CVP monitoring, inotropic agents or even dialysis. Various sugars including sorbitol 5% have also been used as irrigants.[8] Cold irrigating solutions may cause hypothermia.[9]

Blood loss during this operation is difficult to measure, but is usually about 7–20 ml/g prostate resected. It will be increased by raising venous pressure (straining, overtransfusion, excessive absorption of irrigant), prolonged operation time and release of plasminogen activators from the prostate. Tranexamic acid 0.5–1 g may be useful. Blood loss is usually less with regional neural blockade than with general anaesthesia.

Transurethral resection of bladder tumour

Significant glycine absorption is much less likely in this operation. Irrigation with normal saline is used postoperatively to prevent clot retention. Bladder perforation may occur. Stimulation of the obturator nerve may cause adduction of the patient's legs. Muscle relaxants or obturator nerve block will prevent this.

Abdominal prostatectomy[10]

Better if the prostate is especially large. Relaxation is required and considerable haemorrhage may occur. General anaesthesia with IPPV is often used. Caudal or lumbar extradural analgesia (7–15 ml of plain bupivacaine 0.5% for the latter) is a useful supplement. Spinal intradural block to T10 with 2–4 ml heavy or plain bupivacaine 0.5%, is satisfactory. It provides relaxation and reduces bleeding. (*See also* Chapter 25.) During transvesical prostatectomy there is considerable heat loss.

Circumcision

Babies and children may be given a normal intravenous or inhalational induction and spontaneous respiration maintained using oxygen, nitrous oxide and volatile agent. Laryngeal spasm may easily develop if anaesthesia is too light, and may need the surgery to be interrupted, the application of CPAP or even suxamethonium and intubation. Some prefer intubation and IPPV, using a volatile agent and a narcotic. *In adults* spontaneous respiration is generally used.

Extradural sacral block with bupivacaine 0.25%, 0.25–0.5 ml/kg, is an extremely useful adjunct, especially in children.[11] Penile block is a good alternative, blocking the dorsal nerves with 0.25% bupivacaine, 0.25 ml/kg in children, or 10 ml in adults. Postoperative sedation or β-blocker for 3 days may help prevent painful erections after operation.

Priapism

Erection may occur under anaesthesia when the penis is handled and can be difficult to treat. It may even preclude the insertion of a cystoscope. Deepening anaesthesia, topical local analgesics, dorsal nerve block,[12] glyceryl trinitrate,[13] or intracorporeal metaraminol 1 mg[14] may help. Benzodiazepines[15] or terbutaline 0.25–0.5 mg i.v.[16] have been used with success, as has ketamine in children.[17]

Vasectomy

Innervation of the scrotum and its contents is derived from T10–L2 (splanchnic) and S2–3 (somatic). This operation is often done under local infiltration analgesia, but some surgeons prefer general anaesthesia because there is less likelihood of haematoma formation. This may be partly due to the postoperative sedation and the short bed-rest required. Traction on the cord may result in bradycardia or even asystole. Atropine or glycopyrronium should be available and some give it pre-operatively.

Nephrectomy

First performed by Gustav Simon (1824–1913) of Heidelberg, in 1870.

Nerve supply to kidney and ureter arises from T10–L2. The pain of ureteric colic may be relieved by atropine, probanthine, hyoscine-butyl bromide (Buscopan), non-steroidal anti-inflammatory drugs and narcotic analgesics. The bladder, lower ends of the ureters and the prostate are supplied by filaments of the inferior hypogastric plexus. This is formed from the sympathetic T11 to L2, and parasympathetic S2–4.

IPPV in the lateral position impairs respiratory efficiency, for although the lower lung has the higher blood flow, it receives less ventilation. A reduction of minute volume of 9% occurs in the lateral position with spontaneous breathing. Use of the kidney bridge further impairs lung function and predisposes to dependent atelectasis. When the patient is turned on his back at the end of the operation the lower lung should be fully inflated. Use of the kidney bridge in the lateral position may also cause inferior vena caval obstruction, leading to sudden severe hypotension. The patient may also be placed supine with a sandbag under the loin.

Renal tumours are extremely vascular. The anaesthetist should be prepared for torrential bleeding, and set up a wide-bore i.v. cannula. General anaesthesia with relaxant, IPPV, nitrous oxide, volatile agent plus narcotic is usual, although spontaneous respiration may be employed. Both intradural and extradural analgesia up to T8 may be used, but is best combined with general anaesthesia because the lateral position is uncomfortable and is likely to embarrass the respiration of overweight patients. Ureteric tone is not greatly affected.

Rarely, the pleura is damaged during kidney operations; the resulting collapse of the upper lung may prove dangerous unless IPPV is employed. An underwater drain may be required. Tumour embolus causing collapse and cardiac arrest is an occasional complication of operations for carcinoma of the kidney.

Total cystectomy

Much bleeding may occur, but there is an impressive reduction when employing extradural blockade. Circulatory monitoring is likely to include intra-arterial and central venous cannulae. A diuretic (e.g. frusemide 20 mg) is often requested at the end of the procedure.

Haemodialysis

Insertion of a Scribner shunt involves the insertion of an arterial and venous cannula with connecting link, in either the arm or leg. General anaesthesia and local infiltration with lignocaine have been used but are not always satisfactory. Regional analgesia has been advocated: axillary brachial plexus block with 10–20 ml 0.5% bupivacaine for the arm; sciatic (15–20 ml) and femoral (10 ml) blocks for the leg.

Anaemia is usually present; there may be impaired excretion of some of the drugs used; intravenous infusions must not be given into the arm with the fistula; and suxamethonium should be avoided if the patient is hyperkalaemic. The further rise is likely to be less than 0.7 mmol/l with a single dose of 1 mg/kg but may be greater with repeated doses or in the presence of peripheral neuropathy.[18]

Renal transplantation

First transplantation of a kidney by Richard H. Lawler (1935–1982) in 1950.[19] Immunological basis of tissue rejection described by Medawar in 1944.[20] Over 80% of first transplants function for more than a year, and the perioperative mortality is less than 1%. Patients awaiting renal transplantation are in end-stage renal failure and have had repeated haemodialysis. Some will have already had nephrectomies. Hypertension, anaemia, pulmonary oedema, and infections are common, and multiple drug therapy is likely. Neurological problems include mental changes, tremor, convulsions, coma, peripheral and autonomic neuropathy and myopathy. Problems during the operation include the maintenance of a stable cardiovascular system, and fluid and electrolyte balance.

Pre-operative preparation

There is a limited time available for the correction of anaemia, acidosis and electrolyte imbalance. As there is an increased risk of aspiration, antacid, ranitidine or metoclopramide is given. Pre-operative transfusion seems to confer no additional immunological advantage over cyclosporin.[21] Erythropoeitin is very expensive but may be used in the most anaemic patients.

Technique[22]

Sedative premedication with an oral benzodiazepine may benefit the hypertensive, anxious patient. Some insert a multi-lumen internal jugular venous catheter before induction, which spares the arm veins and provides useful monitoring during and after the operation. Suxamethonium may be used for intubation despite the risk of hyperkalaemia if it is felt that the risk of aspiration warrants it. IPPV is continued with nitrous oxide, oxygen, a volatile agent or fentanyl. Enflurane is best avoided because it is metabolized to fluoride. Atracurium is often the preferred relaxant because its elimination does not depend on renal function, but the need for relaxation in this extra-peritoneal operation is slight. An automated oscillotonometer (on the opposite arm to any shunt) is used in preference to intra-arterial measurement to spare any trauma to the artery. There may be a rise in blood pressure on release of the vascular clamps. Regional techniques are not usually favoured. Fluid overload and potassium-containing fluids are to be avoided. Transfusions should not be used if possible as they may lead to haemosiderosis. Cryoprecipitate or desmopressin 0.3 µg/kg may counter any bleeding diathesis. Diuretics and low-dose dopamine are used to encourage urine output from the graft. Immunosuppression is usually with prednisolone, cyclosporin and azathioprine.

Lithotripsy and lithotomy

Renal stones can now be treated without open operation in many cases. Bacteraemia is likely and should be covered by antibiotics.

Percutaneous nephrolithotomy involves the passage of a telescope into the renal pelvis under radiological control, irrigation with saline, and electrohydraulic fragmentation until the stone can be extracted. Large volumes of saline may be absorbed if the pressure is allowed to rise above 75 cmH$_2$O in the pelvis.[23] The patient is semi-prone, and IPPV is often used, although neural blockade up to T8 may be satisfactory.

Extracorporeal shock-wave lithotripsy (ESWL) fragments the stone by acoustic shockwaves. It is non-invasive but painful. The patient is placed in a water bath to allow the shock to be focused on the stone. Arrhythmias are minimized by the shockwave being triggered 20 ms after the R wave. As many as 2500 shocks may be given at one treatment. Other problems include: variable length of procedure (up to 1–2 hours); awkward positioning of the patient with poor access in an emergency; transfer of blood from the periphery into the thorax when immersed in water and back again at the end, with accompanying swings in blood pressure; use of image intensifier; and noise of the shockwaves. Lumbar extradural analgesia up to T4 using a catheter has been widely used.[24] Methadone has been a useful addition to bupivacaine.[25] Intradural analgesia is too inflexible, general anaesthesia technically difficult. Local infiltration plus intercostal and intrapleural block is not adequate for the older machines,[26] although just local infiltration (or even no analgesia at all) seems satisfactory for the newest generation.[27] Air used to identify the epidural space may be hazardous to the surrounding structures when the shockwave passes through.[28] Postoperative backache, nausea and vomiting are common. ESWL is contra-indicated in pregnancy or with an uncorrectable bleeding disorder. Care must be taken if the spine is deformed, if the arteries in the abdomen are calcified or if the patient has a cardiac pacemaker.

For sedation, *see* Chapter 9.

References

1. Nitze M. *Wien. Med. Wochenschr.* 1879, **29**, 779, 806.
2. Blandy J. P. In: *Trans-urethral Resection* (Blandy J. P. ed.) 2nd ed. London: Pitman, 1975, Chapter 1.
3. Hatch P. D. *Anaesth. Intensive Care* 1987, **15**, 203.
4. Sinha B. et al. *J. Urol.* 1986, **135**, 719.
5. Hahn R. G. *Acta Anaesthesiol. Scand.* 1988, **32**, 53; Wang J. M-L. et al. *Anesthesiology* 1989, **70**, 36.
6. Browne B. *Curr. Opin. Anaesthesiol.* 1989, **2**, 735; Jensen V. *Can. J. Anaesth.* 1991, **38**, 90.
7. Hahn R. G. *Anaesthesia* 1990, **45**, 577; Hultén J. et al. *Anaesthesia* 1991, **46**, 349.
8. Norlen H. et al. *Scand. J. Urol. Neprhrol.* 1986, **20**, 9.
9. Harioka T. et al. *Anaesth. Intensive Care* 1988, **16**, 324.
10. Freyer P. *Lancet* 1900, **1**, 774.
11. Armitage E. N. *Clins. Anaesth.* 1985, **3**(3), 535.
12. Papworth D. P. *Can. J. Anaesth.* 1987, **34**, 428.
13. Snyder A. R. and Ilko R. *Anesth. Analg.* 1987, **66**, 1022.
14. Block T. et al. *Urologe* 1988, **27**, 225.
15. Baraka A. and Sibai A. N. *Anesth. Analg.* 1988, **67**, 596.
16. Shantha T. R. *Anesthesiology* 1989, **70**, 707.
17. Benson T. H. et al. *Anesth. Analg.* 1983, **62**, 457.
18. Walton J. D. and Farman J. V. *Anaesthesia* 1973, **28**, 626.
19. Starzl T. E. *Surg. Clin. North Am.* 1978, **58**, 552.
20. Medawar P. B. *J. Anat.* 1944, **78**, 879.
21. Opelz G. *Transplant. Proc.* 1987, **19**, 149.
22. Cottam S. and Eason J. In: *Anaesthesia Review 8* (Kaufman L. ed.) Edinburgh: Churchill Livingstone, 1991, 159.
23. Sugai K. et al. *Br. J. Anaesth.* 1988, **61**, 516.
24. Silbert B. S. et al. *Anaesth. Intensive Care* 1988, **16**, 310.
25. Drenger B. et al. *Br. J. Anaesth.* 1989, **62**, 82.
26. Stromskag K. E. and Steen P. A. *Anesth. Analg.* 1988 **67**, 1181.
27. Wilbert D. M. et al. *J. Urol.* 1987, **138**, 563.
28. Bromage P. R. and Bonsu A. K. *Anesth. Analg.* 1988, **67**, 484.

Vascular surgery

Anaesthesia for peripheral vascular surgery

Pre-operative assessment: Are there other manifestations of arterial disease? What is the cardiac status, and does the patient need coronary artery surgery first? Is the patient a smoker or ex-smoker and has lung function been affected? Has the arterial disease affected renal function? Have there been signs of cerebral arterial insufficiency?

Main problems

Poor cardiovascular reserve, with tendency to vascular accidents, massive transfusion, clotting problems, high blood viscosity. The haemoglobin level and red cell count are often high, and abnormal fibrinogens also contribute to this viscosity. Haemodilution with dextran 70 or other colloid is often beneficial. Severe and widespread peripheral vascular disease; non-invasive physiological measurements will be needed before, during and after the operation.[1]

Techniques

The blood pressure and carbon dioxide levels should be well maintained. An IPPV technique is commonly used because of the poor general condition of these patients. These operations are often prolonged, with risks of cooling, atelectasis, and rapid blood loss. Massive transfusions or cell-saving techniques are employed. There is still a great need for synthetic oxygen carriers. Extradural or other regional blockade is helpful, especially in the postoperative period.

Anaesthesia for carotid artery surgery

See Neurosurgery, above.

Elective aortic aneurysm

Cardiovascular instability.[2] Monitoring often includes intra-arterial, central venous and pulmonary arterial pressure measurements, as well as the usual minimal monitoring (*see* Chapter 18). Clotting mechanism control calls for intraoperative pathology tests of coagulation and electrolyte status. Epidural catheters are inserted before anticoagulation and are cared for in the ITU after operation. Antibiotic cover is common. After major vascular cases, the peripheral circulation may remain 'shut down' for 3–5 h. During this time some crystalloid infusions go into 'the third space'. Then, over a matter of half-an-hour, the peripheral circulation 'opens up' with falls of peripheral resistance, and venous and arterial pressure. Lactate is washed into the circulation from the peripheral tissues, causing further cardiac failure. Intravenous colloid infusion and cardiac support may be needed. Ileus, bowel ischaemia, and temporary renal failure occur. Second and subsequent operations are common. Small doses of dopamine and dopexamine are beneficial.

Anaesthesia for leaking aortic aneurysm

First resection of an aortic aneurysm performed in 1951.[3] This condition carries a high mortality. Patients are usually in poor general condition and suffering from shock, ileus due to retroperitoneal haematoma, or haematemesis from leakage into the duodenum from the aneurysm. The patient may already have suffered irreversible brain and cardiac damage. Large volumes of blood will be required with the usual risks that may follow massive transfusion, such as a failure of clotting mechanism, accidental hypothermia, and calcium and potassium imbalance requiring intravenous calcium. Blood filters and warmers are used. Autotransfusion is useful. Several large-bore drips are needed for high-speed massive transfusion until the clamps are on, and bleeding is controlled. Monitoring as above. Metabolic acidosis occurs.

If the ruptured aneurysm extends above the renal arteries the outlook is especially grave because this causes renal and spinal cord ischaemia with irreversible damage.

The technique of general anaesthesia should provide tracheal intubation free from the risk of aspiration of stomach contents with induction preferably in the head-down position because of the associated shock. Reduction of intra-abdominal pressure by anaesthesia may lead to renewed bleeding; induction should take place in the operating room, so that an aortic clamp can be applied rapidly. Maintenance should be light general anaesthesia with non-depolarizing relaxants. The patient is in a critical shocked condition. It may be necessary to proceed with operation without waiting for resuscitative measures. Blood transfusion is started as quickly as possible. Coughing and straining are to be avoided because the aneurysm may rupture. It may therefore be wise to avoid pre-operative passage of an oesophageal tube. The blood supply to the spinal cord may be compromised during aortic surgery. Infrarenal cross clamping affects spinal haemodynamics.[4] Monitoring as for elective aneurysms, above.

Postoperatively, it is convenient to nurse the patient in an intensive care unit for cardiorespiratory and renal support and analgesia.

Anaesthesia for ruptured thoracic aorta

This may be required for surgical repair following trauma in road traffic accidents. Cardiopulmonary bypass may be necessary. *See* Cardiothoracic surgery, above.

See also Cunningham A. J. In: *Recent Advances in Anaesthesia and Analgesia – 17*, (Atkinson R. S. and Adams A. P. ed.) Edinburgh: Churchill Livingstone, 1992.

References

1. Clifford P. C. *Br. J. Hosp. Med.* 1984, **32**, 82.
2. Quinton L. et al. *Acta Anaesthesiol. Scand.* 1990, **34**, 132.
3. Dubost C. et al. *Arch. Surg.* 1952, **64**, 405.
4. Gamulin Z. et al. *Anesthesiology* 1984, **66**, 394.

Chapter 23

Anaesthesia in abnormal environments

ABNORMAL AMBIENT PRESSURE

Low pressures – high altitude

Still measured in feet by pilots, but in metres by mountaineers. Barometric pressure decreases exponentially with altitude, halving every 18 000 ft (5.5 km). Temperature decreases linearly at 2°C per 1000 ft up to 40 000 ft, where it is −60°C. In a pressurized jet plane flying at 40 000 ft (12.2 km), or in Concorde up to 60 000 ft (18.3 km), passengers are in effect at about 5000 to 8000 ft (1.5 to 2.4 km). Unpressurized aircraft do not fly much above 10 000 ft (3 km).

Problems of anaesthesia at altitude[1]

Well over 10 million people live at altitudes over 3000 m, and some hospitals in the Andes are above 5000 m. It is necessary to remember that gas partial pressure, rather than concentration, determines its potency.

1. Hypoxia. Inspired and arterial Po_2 are low. High concentrations of oxygen (at least 40%) should be given both during and after anaesthesia. *Venturi oxygen masks* deliver the correct concentration at altitude, as the increased flow through the oxygen flow-meter (*see* 4 below) offsets the error that would otherwise occur. The Po_2 will of course be less.

2. Nitrous oxide is therefore limited to 60%, and the partial pressure of even this concentration decreases as P_B decreases. Since its MAC is over 100% at sea-level it is of little use as an anaesthetic at 1500 m and of no value whatsoever at 3000 m.

3. Cylinder pressure gauges are reliable because the pressures involved are so high compared with ambient.

4. Flow-meters read low at altitude because of the low gas density, especially at higher flows. The error is about 20% at 3000 m. It should affect all gases to the same extent, but this may not be true at lower flows, and analysis of Fio_2 is essential.

5. Vaporizers. Since SVP of a vapour does not change with barometric pressure (but only with temperature), the amount of anaesthetic delivered at a given dial setting, and hence its partial pressure, is the same whatever the altitude. However, its concentration will increase as P_B decreases. Any changes in the splitting ratio are slight. So the clinical effect that can be expected from a given dial setting is the same at all ambient pressures.

6. *Gas and vapour analyzers.* These all measure partial pressure, but often present the result as percent concentration, assuming P_B is that of sea-level. Thus the true concentration will be underestimated at altitude.

7. *Low temperatures* are associated with altitude.

8. *Pathophysiology* of both the unacclimatized and acclimatized resident at high altitude. Changes include hyperventilation, respiratory alkalosis, which gradually becomes compensated, polycythaemia, pulmonary hypertension, fluid retention, and pulmonary or cerebral oedema. Acute pulmonary oedema requires descent to lower levels and IPPV if possible. Acetazolamide 250 mg 2 or 3 times a day is useful prophylaxis.[2]

9. *Anaesthesia.* The hypoxic respiratory drive is important. Sensitivity to opiates may occur. There is a high incidence of spinal headache. Other regional techniques are satisfactory.

Anaesthesia in space

This has not yet proved necessary. Possible problems[3] would include weightlessness, the increase in central blood volume and CVP, the resulting diuresis and naturiesis, motion sickness, negative nitrogen balance, osteoporosis and reduction in red cell mass.

Table 23.1. Barometric pressure P_B and moist inspired oxygen pressure P_{IO_2} (mmHg), and the inspired oxygen concentration needed to make P_{IO_2} its sea-level value of 150 mmHg, for various altitudes and depths. Note that alveolar water vapour tension is always 47 mmHg. In practice, P_B on Everest's summit is slightly higher, and has been measured at 253 mmHg.[4]
HPNS = high-pressure nervous syndrome

Altitude (ft)	(km)	P_B mmHg	P_{IO_2} mmHg	F_{IO_2} needed for P_{IO_2} to be 150 mmHg	Notes
63 000	19.2	47	0	–	Blood boils
40 000	12.2	141	20	–	
29 028	8.848	236	40	79%	Summit of Mt. Everest
20 000	6.1	349	63	50%	May lose consciousness without added O_2
18 000	5.5	380	70	45%	
10 000	3.0	523	100	32%	
6 000	1.8	609	118	27%	
0	0	760	150	21%	
Depth (m)					
10		1 520	309	10%	
50		4 560	945	3.3%	Lower limit of diving breathing air
200		15 960	–	0.9%	
500		38 760	–	0.4%	HPNS precludes diving lower than this

High pressures – diving

Pressure increases linearly with depth, 1 atmosphere for each 10 m of sea-water. Divers may fall ill or be injured when saturation diving, i.e. working for several days under pressures as high as 20–30 atmospheres absolute (ATA), which are those on the continental shelf 200–300 m deep. Doctors require training to work under these conditions. Surgery would take place in a large compression chamber back at base, with the medical team also at high pressure.

Problems of anaesthesia at depth[5]

Many factors should be considered, including: (1) air-breathing over 50 m deep may cause nitrogen narcosis: 15% loss of cognitive skills and 5% loss of manual dexterity at 6 ATA. Overcome by the use of oxygen-helium mixtures; (2) acute cerebral oxygen toxicity (convulsions, death) results from a P_{IO_2} that exceeds 2 ATA; chronic pulmonary oxygen toxicity may occur in saturation diving when the P_{IO_2} should not exceed 0.5 ATA. This limits the F_{IO_2} to less than 2% at 25 ATA; (3) high-pressure nervous syndrome (tremor, loss of fine movement control, disorientation) occurs at about 500 m, but may be less especially if compression is rapid (over 1 m/min). Caused by direct effects on enzymes; (4) rapid gas compression raises temperature; helium's high thermal capacity has a big effect on body heat balance; (5) blood samples are decompressed before analysis outside the chamber. Blood gas analysis is impossible; (6) pressure reversal of the effects of all general anaesthetics, around 30% loss of potency at 31 ATA; (7) cuffs on tracheal tubes and Foley catheters should be filled with water, not air; (8) voice communication with helium-containing mixtures is difficult; (9) glass containers, e.g. of drugs, may implode on compression; opening them beforehand may render them unsterile; (10) bubbles of gas appearing in any local analgesic solution injected into the body; and (11) the skin of divers shows an increase in Gram-negative organisms, such as *Proteus* and *Pseudomonas*.

Possible techniques: (1) ketamine, the anaesthetic agent least affected by pressure reversal, or propofol infusion; (2) intravenous regional analgesia for limb injuries; and (3) for major procedures, morphine 2–3 mg/kg with muscle relaxants and IPPV with air. Inhalational agents are precluded because the chamber atmosphere is recycled. A small ventilator powered by gas, e.g. Penlon, is suitable.

ABNORMAL AMBIENT TEMPERATURE

Low temperatures

These may be encountered at altitude, at sea or in polar regions, particularly under field conditions. Mean skin temperature below 33°C causes discomfort and shivering. The patient must be kept warm, and techniques of local analgesia are often unsatisfactory. Some liquid nitrous oxide may form in Entonox cylinders below −7°C.

Tropical conditions

Many drugs deteriorate if stored at too high temperatures, e.g. atracurium, suxamethonium. The filling ratio of nitrous oxide and carbon dioxide cylinders is 0.75 in temperate climates, but 0.67 in the tropics, to prevent excessive pressure if ambient temperature rises. Tropical conditions do not prevent the use of open ether. Rubber articles are liable to perish. Dehydration is common.

SITUATIONS OF UNUSUAL DIFFICULTY

Anaesthesia may have to be administered without the facilities of the modern general hospital: (1) following major disasters (earthquake, nuclear explosions, mining and other industrial accidents, transport accidents); (2) on board ships at sea; (3) during exploration of remote regions; (4) in underdeveloped countries; and (5) in military surgery.

Major accident procedures

Most hospitals have major accident procedures which are rehearsed regularly. Emergency boxes are kept containing resuscitation equipment, lights, distinctive protective clothing, etc. Anaesthetic equipment may include a self-inflating bag (e.g. Ambu), face-masks, tracheal tubes, laryngoscopes, drugs, etc. Infusion fluids in plastic containers, cannulae, giving sets and a manual pressure pump are also included. Boxes should be lightweight, able to be carried by one person and have clear labelling and an inventory. Communications between the accident site and the hospital can be unreliable.[6]

See also Report of the Working Party on the Management of Patients with Major Injuries London: Royal College of Surgeons, 1988; *Medicine for Disasters* (Baskett P. and Weller R. ed.) London: Butterworths, 1988; Coad N. R. et al. *Anaesthesia* 1989, **44**, 851.

Apparatus for field use

Apparatus for intravenous anaesthesia is easily carried. Medical gases are likely to be in short supply. Volatile agents may be vaporized in air, or perhaps oxygen-enriched air. Draw-over apparatus[7] is useful, and should be light and portable. Tracheal tubes may make anaesthesia safer. Where laryngoscopes are not available, simple equipment can be improvised[8] or various blind techniques used (*see* Chapter 11). A Venturi system for oxygen enrichment is economical. A portable container, weighing just 4.3 kg when full, is available containing 1.2 l of liquid oxygen (equivalent to 1000 l of gas), and can deliver up to 15 l/min or power gas-driven ventilators.[9]

Inhalation apparatus

1. Open masks. In the first 80 years of general anaesthesia, many millions of patients were managed satisfactorily this way, which cannot be discarded even today. Halothane can be used for induction with ether for maintenance. Atropine should be given beforehand.

2. Epstein Macintosh Oxford vaporizer (EMO).[10] Draw-over ether vaporizer, and can be used with Oxford bellows for IPPV. Has a water jacket heat sink and is temperature and level-compensated. Holds 450 ml of ether.

3. Oxford Miniature vaporizer.[11] Delivers up to 3.5% halothane and was designed to smooth induction with ether. Has a sealed water jacket but is not temperature compensated. Holds 20 ml.

4. Penlon draw-over vaporizer.[12]

5. Flagg can.[13] Devised during the First World War. The patient breathes in and out through a can containing ether. Such a simple device may be improvised from available material e.g. coffee jar, food tins, and control over vapour strength achieved by admitting air as a diluent.[14]

6. Triservice anaesthetic apparatus (Penlon).[15] Used with success in the Falkland Islands war in 1982.[16] Consists of a Laerdal self-inflating bag, valve and mask resuscitator connected to two Oxford Miniature vaporizers (for trichloroethylene and halothane) and an oxygen supplementation attachment. The vaporizers are modified by the addition of feet and their capacity increased to 50 ml. In its box the apparatus weighs 25 kg and is rugged enough to be dropped by parachute. Has been much used by the services and for disasters. May be used with enflurane or isoflurane,[17] or low concentrations of isoflurane may be supplemented with i.v. ketamine, midazolam and alfentanil.[18] Arrangements for preoxygenation have been described.[19]

Techniques in the field

Intravenous apparatus, induction agents, muscle relaxants and self-inflating bags are easily carried and may be used in conjunction with tracheal tubes and portable apparatus as described above. Halothane is probably the most widely used inhalational agent. Techniques include:

1. Thiopentone, muscle relaxant, either ether from an EMO vaporizer or halothane from an Oxford Miniature vaporizer, intubation and IPPV with air (possibly with added oxygen) using the Oxford inflating bellows.[20]

2. Ketamine,[6,21] i.v. or i.m., may be useful in the rare accident case where access to the airway is difficult, and when the patient may be shocked. A suitable agent where evacuation to hospital is not available.

3. Entonox is valuable for treatment of trapped casualties.[6] Properly administered it produces good analgesia without reduction of blood pressure or loss of consciousness.

4. Portable mechanical ventilation have been used in the field.[22]

See also Boulton T. B. and Cole P. V. *Anaesthesia* 1966, **21**, 268, 379, 513; 1967, **22**, 101, 435; Farman J. V. *Anaesthesia and the E.M.O. System.* London: English Universities Press, 1973; Freyer M. E. and Boulton T. B. *Anaesthesia* 1977, **32**, 189; Perel A. *Battlefield Anesthesia.* In: *Internat. Anesthesiol. Clin.* 1987, **25**, 175.

Anaesthesia in developing countries

The greatest challenge to practitioners of Western anaesthesia is to see that the most relevant information is brought to all those who need it. Gifts of books and journals may be more welcome than outdated complex equipment. Great skills of improvisation are seen in the developing countries. The anaesthesia will depend largely on the facilities available. Regional techniques are widely used.

See Farman J. V. *Anaesthesia* 1981, **36**, 712; Ezi-Ashi T. I. et al. *Anaesthesia* 1983, **38**, 729 and 736; Prior F. N. *Br. Med. J.* 1984, **288**, 1750; Sankaran B. In: *Lectures in Anaesthesiology 1985/1* (Zorab J. S. M. ed.) Oxford: Blackwell, 1985, 1; Fenton P. M. *Anaesthesia* 1989, **44**, 498.

Operating theatre equipment. See Bewes P. *Br. Med. J.* 1984, **288**, 1284.

Use of oxygen concentrators. See Easy W. R. et al. *Anaesthesia* 1988, **43**, 37; Wilson I. H. et al. *Br. J. Anaesth.* 1990, **65**, 342; Pedersen J. and Nyrop M. *Br. J. Anaesth.* 1991, **66**, 264; Dobson M. B. *Anaesthesia* 1991, **46**, 217.

Anaesthesia in the dark

Diminution of room lighting, or near-total darkness, may be requested during microsurgery, endoscopy and radiological procedures. The patient is then exposed to the hazards of unrecognized cyanosis, respiratory obstruction, exhaustion of gas cylinders, etc. Monitoring is at its most valuable. When lights *have* to be extinguished, the anaesthetist should pay particular attention to the following points: (1) spot lighting must be on continuously for inspection of the patient; (2) gas cylinders, particularly oxygen, contain adequate reserves; (3) tracheal intubation may reduce the danger of airway obstruction; (4) monitoring of vital parameters by the senses of hearing and touch, and by electronic means; and (5) in some anaesthetic machines, vital parts may be fluorescent.

References

1. James M. F. M. and White J. F. *Anesth. Analg.* 1984, **63**, 1097.
2. *Drug Ther. Bull.* 1987, **25**, 45.
3. West J. B. *J. Appl. Physiol.* 1984, **57**, 1625.
4. West J. B. et al. *J. Appl. Physiol.* 1983, **54**, 1188.
5. Cox J. and Robinson D. J. *Br. J. Hosp. Med.* 1980, **23**, 144.
6. Finch P. and Nancekievill D. G. *Anaesthesia* 1975, **30**, 667.
7. Mackie A. M. *Anaesthesia* 1987, **42**, 299.
8. O'Donohoe B. P. et al. *Anaesthesia* 1988, **43**, 970.
9. Ramage C. M. H. et al. *Anaesthesia* 1991, **46**, 395.
10. Epstein H. B. and Macintosh R. R. *Anaesthesia* 1956, **11**, 83.
11. Parkhouse J. *Anaesthesia* 1966, **21**, 498.
12. Merrifield A. J. et al. *Br. J. Anaesth.* 1967, **39**, 50.
13. Flagg P. J. *The Art of Anaesthesia.* 7th ed. Philadelphia: Lippincott, 1954.
14. Boulton T. B. *Anaesthesia* 1966, **21**, 513.
15. Houghton I. T. *Anaesthesia* 1981, **36**, 1094.

16. Bull P. T. et al. *Anaesthesia* 1983, **38**, 770; Jowitt M. D. and Knight R. J. *Anaesthesia* 1983, **38**, 776.
17. Kocan M. *Anaesthesia* 1987, **42**, 1101.
18. Restall J. et al. *Anaesthesia* 1990, **45**, 965.
19. Johnson T. W. *Anaesthesia* 1988, **43**, 713; Wilson I. H. et al. *Br. J. Anaesth.* 1990, **65**, 342; Lowe D. M. and McFadzean W. *Br. J. Anaesth.* 1991, **66**, 196.
20. Boulton T. B. *Anaesthesia* 1978, **33**, 769.
21. Dobson M. B. *Anaesthesia* 1978, **33**, 868; Fiel M. S. El. *J. Irish Coll. Phys. Surg.* 1981, **11**, 69; White P. F. et al. *Anesthesiology* 1982, **56**, 119.
22. Harries M. G. *Anaesthesia* 1983, **38**, 279.

Section 4
REGIONAL TECHNIQUES

Chapter 24

Regional analgesia[1]

Enthusiasm is strong for these techniques, as the sole technique for surgery, for supplementary analgesia, and for postoperative or chronic pain management.

History

Modern local analgesia began with the introduction of cocaine into medical practice in 1884 by Koller.[2]

The ether spray was used by B. W. Richardson in 1866,[3] 'freezing', and the ethyl chloride spray in 1880 by Rothenstein and in 1890 by P. Redard.[4]

Karl Ludwig Schleich (1859–1922) in Berlin (1892)[5] and Reclus (1847–1914) in Paris (1890)[6] popularized infiltration analgesia, while nerve block, the mandibular, was employed by Halsted and Hall in New York in 1884.[7] As a result of acting as their own guinea-pigs during their researches on the new drug, they became cocaine addicts. First textbook on the subject by J. L. Corning, *Local Anaesthesia in General Medicine and Surgery*. New York: Appleton 1886. Arthur E. Barker, in 1899, with β-eucaine[8] was using infiltration analgesia at University College Hospital.[9] Braun (1856–1917) introduced adrenaline in 1903 in local analgesia,[10] which was first isolated in pure form in 1897.[11] The term 'block' first used by G. W. Crile of Cleveland.[12]

Substitutes for the toxic cocaine soon came. Giesel's tropococaine appeared in 1891; Fourneau's stovaine in 1904,[13] and Einhorn's novocaine (procaine) described in 1899,[14] in 1904, popularized by Heinrich Braun in 1905.[15] Amethocaine described in 1931.[16] Miescher and Uhlmann introduced Nupercaine in 1929.[17] Lofgren and Lundqvist synthesized lignocaine in 1943, and Gordh was the first to use it in 1948.[18] Oil of cloves (eugenol) first used as a local analgesic in dentistry in 1890.[19]

The hypodermic trocar and cannula was described by Rynd (1801–1861) of Meath Hospital and County Infirmary, Dublin in 1845,[20] and by Alexander Wood, a general practitioner, of Edinburgh who used a modified Ferguson syringe in 1855.[21] The latter also popularized hypodermic therapy for the treatment of neuralgia by injecting morphine near to the seat of the pain. Luer all-glass syringes appeared in Paris about 1896; Luer-Lok syringes in the

US in 1925. *See also* Schwidetsky O. *Anesth. Analg. Curr. Res.* 1944, **23**, 34; Jones N. H. *J. Hist. Med.* 1947, **2**, 201. Until the 1920s, regional analgesia was almost exclusively in the hands of surgeons. For early history of regional analgesia *see* Matas R. *Am. J. Surg.* 1934, **189**, 362.

'Regional anaesthesia' was a term first used by Harvey Cushing (1869–1939) in 1901 to describe pain relief by nerve block.[22]

For history of limb blocks, *see* Bryce-Smith R. In: *Practical Regional Analgesia* (Lee J. A. and Bryce-Smith R. ed.). Amsterdam: Excerpta Medica, 1973, Chapter 3.

In the UK, R. R. Macintosh, J. Alfred Lee and R. J. Massey Dawkins have been pioneers and practitioners of regional techniques. Prominent and pioneering workers in regional analgesia in the USA have included R. A. Hingson, J. S. Lundy, G. P. Pitkin, G. Labat, Lincoln Sise, R. D. Dripps, L. Vandam, J. J. Bonica, D. C. Moore, P. C. Lund, P. R. Bromage and Alon Winnie. The American Society of Regional Anesthesia was founded in 1920 by G. Labat and resuscitated in 1976 with A. P. Winnie as president. The journal *Regional Anaesthesia* first published in 1976. For the history of regional block in the USA *see* Moore D. C. In: *Anaesthesia: Essays on its History* (Rupreht J. et al. ed.) Berlin: Springer-Verlag, 1985, 128.

GENERAL CONSIDERATIONS

Advantages of regional analgesia

Effects of drug limited to part of body to be operated on; after-effects usually less than after general anaesthesia, e.g. pulmonary complications and venous thromboembolism.

Relative indications for regional analgesia

1. Avoidance of some of the dangers of general anaesthesia, e.g. known impossible intubation, severe respiratory failure and cases where relaxant problems are expected.
2. The patient specifically requests regional analgesia.
3. For high-quality postoperative pain relief.
4. General anaesthesia not available.

Relative contra-indications to regional analgesia, when used alone

(1) In children under 10; (2) in the unco-operative or restless; (3) in psychotics; (4) in those rare patients in whom local anaesthetics do not produce analgesia; and (5) in long operations when the patient may become uncomfortable and restless.

Regional analgesia is used less frequently than it might be because of: (1) time taken to induce (0.5 h with bupivacaine or ropivacaine, faster with lignocaine); (2) the fear of failure; (3) the fear of neurological complications;

(4) the unpopularity of the awake patient at operation; and (5) for postoperative analgesia, where they are supremely good, 'one-shot' blocks wear off in a few hours. (This can be overcome, almost anywhere in the body by inserting an ordinary epidural catheter at the blocksite, which can be 'topped up' with local anaesthetic as often as needed).

Local analgesic drugs are water-soluble salts of lipid-soluble alkaloids. Each molecule is composed of an aromatic portion, intermediate chain and an amide portion. Procaine, chloroprocaine and amethocaine have ester linking the aromatic end of the molecule and the intermediate chain; lignocaine, prilocaine, mepivacaine, bupivacaine, ropivacaine and etidocaine have an amide group between the aromatic part of the molecule and the intermediate chain. Ester-linked drugs are degraded by hydrolysis and amides by oxidative dealkylation in the liver. Overall clearance rate is fastest with prilocaine, then lignocaine, mepivacaine and finally bupivacaine and ropivacaine. Anaphylactoid reactions are well documented in the case of ester-linked agents, but extremely rare when amide-linked drugs are administered.

With the exception of cocaine (a vasoconstrictor) and lignocaine (no effect on vessels), local analgesic drugs are vasodilators. Vasoconstricting agents such as adrenaline may be added to local analgesics to delay absorption and also to prevent haematoma formation if a small local vein is damaged by the needle.

Adrenaline and noradrenaline do not prolong the action of local analgesic solution applied topically.

Most of the local analgesic drugs are available as hydrochlorides in modified Ringer's solution. Those containing adrenaline are often acid with a pH of 4 or 5, and contain a reducing agent sodium metabisulphite to prevent oxidation of the adrenaline. In addition, a small amount of preservative and fungicide may be added.

Regional analgesia is supremely useful and effective in postoperative pain relief. Sensory block, without motor block is indicated, and the smaller the area of the body blocked, the better, because some patients do not like having large numb or paralysed areas. Either the longer-acting analgesics, or regular top-ups using a catheter placed at the blocksite, or both, are most effective.

Theories of impulse conduction along nerve fibres

The nerve membrane consists of a bimolecular framework of phospholipid molecules associated with a globular protein mosaic. Non-specific channels, one permeant to sodium and the other to potassium, are thought to be controlled by gates, which are voltage-dependent. Myelinated nerves are protected by the myelin sheath, which acts as an insulator. The impulse propagation has been studied in the squid axon because of its great size compared with the mammalian fibre. There is a resting potential of $-70\,mV$ on the outside of the membrane, which rises to about $-55\,mV$, the firing threshold, before it jumps up to $+40\,mV$ to form an action potential, which constitutes a change of over $100\,mV$.

This is associated with movement of sodium ions inwards and potassium ions outwards, through their respective channels. The membrane becomes depolarized. During recovery, the ions reverse the direction of their movement across the cell membrane.

Impulse blockade.[23] The local analgesic solution prevents depolarization of the nerve membrane. As the concentration increases, the height of the action potential is reduced, the firing threshold is elevated, the spread of impulse conduction is slowed and the refractory period lengthened. Finally, nerve conduction is completely blocked.

It is thought that local analgesic drugs exert their effect by bonding to the internal mouth of the sodium channel.[24] It is likely that specific receptors exist to which molecules of local analgesic drug become attached. Expansion of the membrane also occurs during impulse blockade; this may be the cause of conduction block or may just be an associated phenomenon.

The weak nerve block of perineural opioids is of a conduction type (although opioid receptors have been demostrated in peripheral nerves), is short-lived, and is not reversed by naloxone. (*See* Arendt-Nielsen L. et al. *Acta Anaesthesiol. Scand.* 1991, **35**, 24; Gissen A. J. et al. *Anesth. Analg.* 1987, **66**, 1272.)

Site of action

The site of action of local analgesic drugs (and of general anaesthetics) is at the surface membrane of cells of excitable tissues. In a myelinated nerve the site of action is the node of Ranvier (1835–1909). Two or three adjacent nodes must be affected to prevent conduction; at least 6 mm and perhaps 10 mm of nerve fibre must be exposed to the local analgesic agent or else a blocked segment may be jumped.

Differential block. The minimum concentration of local drug necessary to cause block of a nerve fibre of given diameter is known as the Cm. The thicker the diameter of a nerve fibre the greater the Cm required. The A delta fibres have a Cm about half that of A alpha fibres; it is therefore possible to block pain sensation while leaving sensation to pressure or position intact. The Cm of preganglionic autonomic B fibres is similar to that of small A so that sympathetic blockade is equivalent to analgesia in spinal analgesia. In practice, the sequence of block is autonomic, sensory, and finally motor according to fibre diameter. Local analgesics affect not only nerve fibres but all types of excitable tissue, including smooth and striated muscle, e.g. in the myocardium vessels, etc., probably by interfering with the cation fluxes across the muscle-cell membranes (as in nerve tissue). In moderate doses there is inhibition of activity of ventricular ectopic foci in the heart. The membrane stabilizing effect is shared by other drugs such as phenothiazines, antihistamines, many β-blockers, barbiturates, and some antihypertensive agents, e.g. guanethidine.

Uptake

Local analgesic drugs are lipoid-soluble bases that act by penetrating lipoprotein cell membranes in the non-ionized state. In order to make a suitable solution for injection, the non-ionized base has to be converted to the ionized state.

The blocking quality of a local analgesic drug depends on its: (1) potency; (2) latency (time between injection and maximum effect), which in turn depends on nerve diameter, local pH, diffusion rate and concentration of the local drug; (3) duration of action; and (4) regression time (time between commencement and completion of pain appreciation).

Dissociation constants (pKa). The pKa is the pH at which a local analgesic drug is 50% ionized and 50% non-ionized (base). Therefore, local analgesic drugs with pKa values close to physiological pH tend to have a rapid onset of action. The degree of ionization of a molecule is important and the pKa is a measure of this. It may be calculated from the Henderson-Hasselbalch equation, pH = pKa + log base/cation. Most local analgesic agents are weak bases with pKa between 7 and 9, and are relatively insoluble in water. Examples of pKa are: lignocaine, 7.87; amethocaine, 8.50; bupivacaine, 7.74; procaine, 8.92. They are usually prepared for clinical use as the acid salt. The non-ionized form is lipid soluble and can spread through tissues and penetrate membranes; the cation is the active agent that produces the pharmacological effect. pH of local analgesic solution may be lowered by addition of adrenaline, sodium metabisulphite (antioxidant) and glucose. When the buffering effect of the tissue is low, local analgesic drugs may be less effective. This occurs in inflamed tissues. Mucous membranes also have minimal buffer reserve and this is one reason why higher concentrations of drugs are needed for topical analgesia.

Carbonated local analgesic solutions. The manufacture is difficult and expensive, and are commercially available only in Canada and West Germany. Carbonated lignocaine and prilocaine produce a shorter latent period and more intense blockade than the hydrochloride salts,[25] but trials of carbonated bupivacaine have proved disappointing.[26]

For further information about impulse conduction and impulse blockade by local analgesic drugs, *see Lumbar Puncture and Spinal Analgesia; Intradural and Extradural* 5th ed. (Lee, J. A. et al. ed.) Edinburgh: Churchill Livingstone, 1985.

Biotransformation

Ester-linked drugs are hydrolysed in the plasma by plasma cholinesterase, the rate depending on substitution in the aromatic ring of the molecule. Half-life in plasma varies from less than 1 minute (chloroprocaine) to 8 min (amethocaine) and is prolonged in the presence of atypical cholinesterase.

Amide-linked drugs undergo biotransformation in the liver, the rate of clearance being dependent on hepatic blood flow and drug extraction by the liver.[27] Hepatic blood flow may be altered in general anaesthesia and as a result of administering vasoactive drugs. Extraction by the liver may be diminished in conditions such as cirrhosis, congestive cardiac failure, hypothermia and the administration of cimetidine. Half-life is likely to vary between 1.5 and 3 hours.

Toxicity

The following factors influence toxicity: (1) quantity of solution; (2) concentration of drug; (3) presence or absence of adrenaline; (4) vascularity of site of injection; (5) rate of absorption of drug, e.g. rate is rapid from bronchial mucosa; (6) rate of destruction of drug; (7) hypersensitivity of patient; and (8) age, physical status and weight of patient. Toxic signs not always related to dosage.

A study of plasma concentration of local analgesic drugs suggests that higher levels are reached after lignocaine than after prilocaine in equal dosage. Addition of adrenaline to the local infiltration reduces the plasma concentration of lignocaine but not of prilocaine. Higher plasma levels are found after intercostal block than after extradural injection.[28] Plasma concentrations of local analgesic drugs correspond very poorly with the patient's body weight; the site of injection is far more important.[29] There is no maximum safe dose for all procedures. Skeletal injuries, including dislocation of the shoulder joint have been caused by convulsions due to the toxicity of local analgesic agents.[30]

1. Central nervous system

Central stimulation followed by depression, restlessness, hysterical behaviour, vertigo, tremor, convulsions and respiratory failure. Treatment consists of: (1) artificial ventilation with oxygen or air; and (2) intravenous or intramuscular suxamethonium or just sufficient thiopentone to control convulsions (10–150 mg). Diazepam may be useful. A rise in $Paco_2$ increases tendency to convulsions, so treatment should include hyperventilation with oxygen.

2. Cardiovascular system

Hypotension. Acute collapse – primary cardiac failure. This has followed moderate amounts, given intravenously, of etidocaine and bupivacaine.[31] Feeble pulse and cardiovascular collapse, bradycardia, pallor, sweating, and hypotension. This type of intoxication may be due to a rapid absorption of the drug. *Treatment.* Elevate legs; give oxygen by IPPV; rapid intravenous infusion; raise blood pressure; cardiac massage if necessary. Resuscitation after the longer acting drugs, bupivacaine and etidocaine, may be difficult and lengthy.[32] High-energy shock electrical defibrillation may be required.[33]

3. Respiratory depression

This may progress to apnoea from medullary depression or respiratory muscle paralysis. It may have delayed onset.

4. Allergic phenomena

Allergy, a term introduced by C. P. von Pirquet (1874–1929) in 1906. Rare: may take form of bronchospasm, urticaria or angioneurotic oedema.[34] Well documented in association with the use of ester-linked agents, including contact dermatitis in personnel handling procaine.[35] Cross-sensitivity can occur. Allergy to amide-linked agents is extremely rare but has been reported.[36] Injections of adrenaline, hydrocortisone and oxygen therapy by IPPV and i.v. colloid solutions may be necessary.

Reactions to vasoconstrictor drugs may include pallor, anxiety, palpitations, tachycardia, hypertension and tachypnoea and may respond to a β-blocker. Care should be taken in patients receiving mono-amine oxidase inhibitors or tricyclic antidepressants.

Toxicity may occur as a result of simple overdosage, by inadvertent intravenous injection, or because of susceptibility of the patient to normal dosage. Injection with a moving needle, together with frequent aspiration testing, minimizes risk of intravenous injection. No preservatives, such as phenol, chlorocresol or sodium sulphite, should be used when any large volume of local analgesic solution is to be injected. Allergic reactions may be due to methylparaben, sometimes used in commercial preparations of local analgesic solutions as a stabilizing agent.[37]

Toxic signs are often due to intravenous injection.

There is evidence that local analgesic drugs may have cytotoxic effects, although harmful clinical consequences are difficult to find.[38]

Improving duration and quality of local analgesia

1. Addition of adrenaline, e.g. 1 in 200 000 to 1 in 500 000 solution.
2. Free base is liberated quickly due to rapid buffering and liberation of CO_2, which diffuses across cell membranes. Thus the analgesic base is brought closer to nerve tissue more rapidly and in higher concentration, resulting in a more widespread and more intense block. The amount of free base available determines the rate of diffusion of the local analgesic solution. Adjusting the pH to about 7 (alkalinization) reduces the time of onset and the duration of analgesia. Substitution of the carbonated salts of local analgesic drugs for the hydrochloride, the pH of carbonated salts (6.5) is relatively higher than other acid salts so that speedy buffering occurs with liberation of free base and CO_2 which diffuses to lower the pH inside the nerve sheath (diffusion trapping).[39]

Premedication

Adequate premedication is essential for successful local analgesia in major surgery. The subject is set out in the chapter on Spinal analgesia.

Table 24.1 Some dosages of local analgesics

Drug	Minimum effective concentration	Maximum dose for 70kg adult when used 'plain'	Maximum dose for 70kg adult when used with adrenaline 1 in 200 000
Lignocaine	0.25%	200 mg (40 ml of 0.5%)	500 mg (100 ml of 0.5%)
Bupivacaine	0.175%	150 mg (30 ml of 0.5%)	150 mg (30 ml of 0.5%)
Ropivacaine	0.25%	250 mg (50 ml of 0.5%)	Not yet defined
Prilocaine	0.5%	400 mg (80 ml of 0.5%)	600 mg (120 ml of 0.5%)

In children, the above adult doses do not apply, but the dose can be calculated on a 'dose for weight' basis, eg. the maximum dose for a 7 kg child would be one tenth of the adult dose.

Methods of local analgesia

1. Simple topical application of local analgesic to the operative site, e.g. on to the ovaries at ovarian cystectomy or into the knee at meniscectomy under general anaesthetic, for effective postoperative analgesia. Intrapleural analgesia is a modification of this.

2. Infiltration analgesia[40] to abolish the pain due to surgical intervention and to ease pain associated with trauma and the injection of irritant drugs. The direct injection of drugs into the area to be incised and between bone ends in fractures.

3. Field block. The injection of a local analgesic so as to create a zone of analgesia around the operative field.

4. Nerve block (conduction anaesthesia). The injection of a solution of local analgesic drug near the nerve or nerves supplying the area to be operated on. The use of a peripheral nerve stimulator increases the accuracy of needle placement and the success of the block.[41]

5. Refrigeration analgesia.

6. Intravenous local analgesia.

7. Topical or surface analgesia.

8. Central neural blockade (*see* Chapter 25).

PHARMACODYNAMICS AND PHARMACOKINETICS OF DRUGS USED IN LOCAL ANALGESIA

A molecule of local analgesic drug possesses an aromatic or lipophilic group and a hydrophilic group with a linking chain between them, which may be an ester (COO—) or an amide (NH.CO—).

A. Ester-linked drugs

1. Cocaine (Benzoyl methylecgonine hydrochloride)[42]

A derivative of the nitrogenous base ecgonine and an ester of benzoic acid. Cocaine is extracted from the leaves of *Erythroxylon coca*, a shrub indigenous to Bolivia and Peru, which the natives have chewed for centuries for their stimulant effect; 100 g of leaves yield 200 mg of cocaine. Easily decomposed by heat sterilization. Cocaine is soluble in water and alcohol. It is an excellent surface analgesic and vasoconstrictor, 4% being a suitable strength. It is often toxic when injected.[43] A dangerous drug of addiction. Duration of effect, 20–30 min. Solutions should be protected from the light. pKa 8.7. (For history of coca plant, *see* Christensen E. M. *Anaesthesia* 1947, **2**, 4; *Time Magazine* 1981, 6th July, p. 42; Images of cocaine (Leader) *Lancet* 1983, **2**, 1231.)

History. Specimens of the leaves and bark of the plant containing cocaine were brought to Europe in the middle of the 19th century by Dr Scherzer, scientific officer in an Austro-Hungarian round-the-world voyage in the naval frigate *Novara*. Several sacks of the leaves were made available to Viennese investigators and an alkaloid was isolated in 1855 by Gaedcke. Niemann (1840–1921), a pupil of Wohler (1800–1882), purified *Erythroxylon* and described its numbing effects and named the alkaloid in 1860;[44] its local analgesic effects were noticed in 1868 by Moreno y Maiz, surgeon-in-chief to the Peruvian Army,[45] and also by von Anrep (1852–1902) of Wurzburg in 1878.[46] Was prescribed by Freud (and used by Sherlock Holmes) for its stimulating effects and as a cure for morphine addiction.[47] Carl Koller (1858–1944), introduced to cocaine by Sigmund Freud (1856–1939), proved its use in surgery (of the cornea) in 1884[48] using 2% solution in water; this was reported on 15 September 1884, at the Congress of Ophthalmology at Heidelberg.[49] The drug was originally prepared by Merck of Darmstadt. Used by W. C. Burke of South Norwalk, Connecticut, for removal of a revolver bullet from a hand (5 minims of 2% solution) in November 1884, in urology by F. N. Otis (1825–1900) in 1884 in New York, and also by R. J. Hall (1856–1897) and William Stewart Halsted (1852–1922)[50] at the Roosevelt Hospital in New York, each of whom injected it into his own arms[51] and each becoming an addict. First synthesized in 1924.[52]

PHARMACODYNAMICS

Central nervous system. This is stimulated from above downwards:

On the cortex, excitement and restlessness are caused and mental powers increased. There is euphoria, agitation, decreased sleep, anxiety, hyperexcitability, psychosis, paranoia, suicidal tendency, violence and confusion. In higher dosage convulsions (prevented by diazepam and reduced by D-1 antagonists[53]) are followed by apnoea and death associated with hyperthermia. Calcium channel blockers increase toxicity.[54]

The sympathetic nervous system is stimulated. As cocaine is a powerful vasoconstrictor, adrenaline added to it is not only unnecessary but also increases the risks of cardiac dysrhythmia and ventricular fibrillation. The two drugs should not be used together.[55]

It inhibits mono-amine oxidase. It is not destroyed by cholinesterase.

Cardiovascular system. Small doses increase the pulse rate, raise the blood pressure and potentiate the effects of adrenaline on capillaries (dilatation or constriction). Dysrhythmias may occur, but can be reversed by beta blockade. Cutaneous vasoconstriction prevents heat loss. Hypertension and vasospasm may lead to vascular accidents.

Eye. Mydriasis, perhaps due to sympathetic stimulation; there is blanching of the conjunctiva from vasoconstriction, clouding of the corneal epithelium and, rarely, ulceration, together with excellent analgesia. Used as 1% solution for analgesia. Eserine counteracts the mydriatic effect of cocaine and atropine increases it. Now seldom employed in ophthalmology.

Treatment of overdose.[56] Diazepam 5–10 mg slowly, repeated to control fits and agitation. (Other antiepileptic drugs have been used successfully.) Oxygen, active cooling and rehydration may also be needed.

PHARMACOKINETICS

Absorption. From all mucous membranes, including the urethra and bladder. There is some evidence that stronger solutions are absorbed less readily than weaker solutions, owing to the increased vasoconstriction they produce. In nose and throat surgery, used as 1% to 20% solution. Can be employed usefully as a spray to produce ischaemia of the nose, e.g. before nasal intubation.

Excretion. Cocaine is detoxicated in the liver, one metabolite being ecognine, a CNS stimulant. About 10% is excreted by the kidneys, unchanged.

A safe dose of cocaine for surface analgesia is 2 ml of 4% solution. It was for years used to overcome drowsiness due to chronic morphine addiction in the treatment of severe pain in terminal disease (e.g. in the Brompton cocktail).[57]

2. Procaine hydrochloride, BP (Novocain, Planocaine, Ethocaine, Neocaine)

p-amino-benzoyl-diethyl amino-ethanol hydrochloride. pKa 8.9. The standard local analgesic agent until the advent of lignocaine. Synthesized by Alfred Einhorn (1856–1917) of Munich in 1899.[14] Like amethocaine, it inhibits the bacteriostatic action of *p*-aminosalicylic acid and the sulphonamides. Should be stored in a cool place to retard hydrolysis.

For infiltration, the strength used is 0.25–1%; for nerve block, 1–2%. Procaine 5.05% in water is iso-osmotic, with pH of 6.4. Hydrolysed by serum cholinesterase, diethyl amino-ethanol and *p*-aminobenzoic acid being formed. Biotransformation requires absorption into the bloodstream as neural tissue and cerebrospinal fluid lack esterases.

Analgesia lasts from 45 to 90 min when adrenaline is added. Relatively non-toxic.

Procaine has been recommended as the agent of choice in patients with a history of malignant hyperpyrexia.[58] A concentration of 5% may be necessary for successful extradural block.[59]

Procaine intravenously has been recommended for the treatment of malignant hyperpyrexia, in almost toxic doses.

3. Chloroprocaine hydrochloride

An ester of para-aminobenzoic acid. Has been in use in the USA since 1952. Quick onset of effect, but analgesia may disappear suddenly. Rapid hydrolysis makes it relatively non-toxic and it is not easily transferred across the placenta. Effect lasts about 45 min. Used as a 2 or 3% solution, pKa 8.7. Initial dose for obstetrical extradural block 8–10 ml, which can be followed by bupivacaine or ropivacaine.[60] The most acid of local analgesic agents commonly used (3% solution has pH of 3.3). Paraplegia has been reported following its use, particularly after intradural injection for which it is not recommended. This may be due to sodium metabisulphite in the commercial solution.[61]

4. Amethocaine hydrochloride, BP (Pantocaine, Pontocaine, Decicain, Butethanol, Anethaine, tetracaine, USP)

Synthesized by O. Eisleb in Germany in 1928. pKa 8.2. Solutions prepared under sterile conditions remain sterile and bactericidal. Like cocaine, it may cause cardiac asystole or ventricular fibrillation. Used for topical and corneal analgesia in 0.5% solution. The solution can be boiled once or twice without deterioration, but is rendered inactive by alkalis. It should be protected from light. For infiltration the usual strength is 1 in 2000 to 1 in 4000, preferably with adrenaline. Up to 200 ml of 1 in 2000 solution with adrenaline can safely be used for infiltration analgesia. It is hydrolysed completely by serum cholinesterase but four times more slowly than procaine. None is found in bile or urine. Used for intradural block.

The maximum dose is 100 mg or 1.5 mg/kg of body weight. Large doses are unwise and maximum for surface analgesia should be 8 ml of 0.5% solution in two or three divided doses with an interval of 5 min between each dose. A lozenge containing 60 mg amethocaine is available. Absorption from the bronchial tree – when analgesia for bronchoscopy is being induced – is almost as rapid as that following intravenous injection.

Its effect lasts longer than that of procaine and lignocaine, roughly 1.5–3 h. Onset of analgesia slow. For intradural block, 0.5–1% solution may be used; for extradural block 0.25–0.5% with adrenaline. The addition of adrenaline greatly reduces its toxicity; toxic signs are similar in appearance and treatment to those of cocaine.

5. Oxybuprocaine

Bradycardia may be a problem,[85] but unlikely when used for surface analgesia for tonometry (0.4% solution less irritant to the conjunctiva than amethocaine; duration 5 min).

B. Amide-linked drugs

1. Lignocaine hydrochloride, BP (Xylocaine, Duncaine, lidocaine, USP)

The most commonly used local analgesic agent in the UK. A tertiary amide, synthesized by Nils Lofgren (1922–1953) and Lundqvist in 1943 in Sweden.[62] First used by Gordh (1907–) of the Karolinska Hospital, Stockholm in 1948.[63] Very stable, not decomposed by boiling, acids or alkalis. The pKa is 7.86. Solutions of 0.25–0.5% for infiltration, with adrenaline 1 in 250 000; 4% for topical analgesia, in surgery of throat, larynx, pharynx, etc. For nerve block 1.5–2% with adrenaline, and for extradural block 1.2–2% with adrenaline. For corneal analgesia 4%; this causes no mydriasis, vasoconstriction or cycloplegia. For urethral analgesia 1–2% in jelly and for tracheal tubes 5% as an ointment. Toxicity not great, but cardiovascular and central nervous symptoms of poisoning may occur. Can be toxic when ingested orally.

The clearance of lignocaine is reduced in the presence of propranolol, with increased risk of toxicity. As in the case of prilocaine, the metabolism of lignocaine can give rise to the formation of methaemoglobin. It is neither a vasodilator nor does it interfere with the vasoconstrictive action of adrenaline. It has a cerebral effect, causing drowsiness and amnesia. It is metabolized by oxidases and amidases from microsomes in the liver, but this is retarded in chronic liver disease.[64] It is excreted renally, hastened when the urine is acid.

Duration of effect of 1% solution, 1 h; with adrenaline, 1.5–2 h. Has rapid onset. Has been given intravenously in 40-mg doses at 5-min intervals, to potentiate the analgesia of thiopentone-gas-oxygen-relaxant combination, and also intramuscularly in 250-mg doses as 2% solution. Has been used in the treatment of status epilepticus, and due to its cell membrane-stabilizing effect on cardiac tissue for ventricular dysrhythmias, by intravenous injection. As lignocaine may facilitate the release of calcium from sarcoplasmic reticulum, it should not be used in patients susceptible to malignant hyperpyrexia.[65] Its use in the treatment of cardiac infarction is not proven. Whereas it controls the non-dangerous unifocal ectopics, it is far less successful in cases of multifocal ectopics. Suggested maximum safe dose of lignocaine for a 70-kg man, with adrenaline, 500 mg, i.e. 7 mg/kg; without adrenaline, 200 mg, i.e. 3 mg/kg body weight.

The carbonate of lignocaine (and prilocaine) has been investigated[66] and found to give greater speed of onset and intensity of both sensory and motor block, in comparison with the hydrochloride salt, especially in the L5 and S1 segments. On injection the CO_2 diffuses out of the drug, so lowering the tissue pH and increasing the concentration of the non-ionized base.[67]

Alkalinized lignocaine may have an even faster onset. Bicarbonate bufering of the solution to pH 7.4 reduces stinging on injection, especially important around the eyes.

Toxic effects of lignocaine are twitching, convulsions, apnoea and acute cardiac failure.

2. Mepivacaine (Carbocaine, Meaverin)

This is a tertiary amine synthesized in 1956 by Ekenstam and Egner[68] and used first by Dhuner in 1956.[69] It is clinically comparable with lignocaine. It is resistant to acid and alkaline hydrolysis. The pKa is 7.8. Seventy per cent of the drug becomes protein bound (greater than in the case of lignocaine but less than bupivacaine). Most of the drug is metabolized in the liver and some has been recovered from the urine (increased by acidification). Unlike lignocaine, it is not metabolized by neonates; eliminated via the kidneys. It is claimed to be a little less toxic than lignocaine and its local analgesic effects last rather longer. The subconvulsive dose in man is 5 mg/kg.[70] When injected into the extradural space of patients in labour it passes rapidly into the fetal circulation where it may cause harm. It would appear to have few advantages over lignocaine. A dose of 400 mg should not be exceeded (about 5 mg/kg body weight). For extradural analgesia 15 ml of 2% or 20 ml of 1.5% solution; for intradural block 1–2 ml of heavy 4% solution. Has anti-dysrhythmic properties. Onset may be speeded by alkalinization (*see* Tetzlaff J. E. et al. *Reg. Anaes. 1990,* **15**, 242).

3. Bupivacaine (Marcain, Marcaine, Sensorcaine, Carbosterin)

This amide-type local analgesic drug was synthesized in Sweden by Ekenstam and his colleagues in 1957,[71] and used clinically by L. J. Telivuo (1923–1970) in 1963.[72] The base is not very soluble but the hydrochloride readily dissolves in water. The pKa is 8.2. It is very stable both to repeated autoclaving and to acids and alkalis, but solutions containing adrenaline should not be autoclaved more than twice. It is reputed to be four times as potent as both mepivacaine and lignocaine, so that a 0.5% solution is approximately equivalent to 2% lignocaine. More cardiotoxic than lignocaine and this is made worse by hypoxia, hypercapnia and by pregnancy.[73] It causes more sensory than motor block. It is not recommended for intravenous regional analgesia because leakage past the tourniquet into the bloodstream may cause toxic or even fatal complications. Duration of effect is between 5 and 16 h, one of the longest-acting local analgesics known. This may be more related to binding to nerve tissue than to its overall retention in the body. Duration of action of a local analgesic drug correlates with binding to plasma lipoproteins. The duration may be prolonged by mixing the drug with dextran 150. (*See* Tripathi M. and Krishna O. *Indian J. Med. Res.* 1990, **92**, 273.)

A small percentage of a given dose of bupivacaine is excreted unchanged in the urine. The remainder is metabolized in the liver. The N-dealkylated metabolite, pipecolyloxylidine, is found in the urine.[74] Maximal dose is 2 mg/kg body weight (25–30 ml of 0.5% solution) and the strength used is 0.125–0.75% with or without adrenaline 1 in 200 000 or 1 in 400 000; adrenaline does not greatly prolong its effect but reduces its toxicity. The carbonated form probably has few advantages over the hydrochloride salt. A plain solution of 0.5% has been much used for intradural block, either alone or made hyperbaric with dextrose, and for extradural analgesia. The pH of the 0.5% solution with adrenaline is 3.5 and its density 0.997 g/ml at 37°C.

4. Etidocaine hydrochloride (Duranest, W-19053)

This long-acting local analgesic drug is related chemically to lignocaine and was described in 1972.[75] It is a stable compound and can be autoclaved up to five times without deterioration. The onset of action is rapid and the duration of action is long (comparable to bupivacaine or ropivacaine). It is very lipid-soluble and almost completely protein-bound; metabolic pathways not yet determined. Probably retained in the body longer than other local analgesic drugs. It is probably less toxic than bupivacaine but certainly more toxic than lignocaine.[76] Gives good motor block. pKa 7.7.

The drug has been used in extradural block but in obstetric analgesia has the disadvantage that motor block is readily produced. It has been used in 0.25 and 0.5% concentration. The former may give inadequate analgesia, the latter inappropriate motor block.

Concentrations of up to 1.5% have been used with success in extradural block for surgical operations. Maximal dose: 4 mg/kg.

It is a useful topical analgesic, similar to bupivacaine or ropivacaine and stronger than lignocaine.

5. Prilocaine hydrochloride (Citanest, Xylonest, Distanest)

A close relation of lignocaine to which it is clinically comparable. A secondary amide. Described by Lofgren and Tegner,[77] tested pharmacologically by Wiedling,[78] and used clinically by Gordh in 1959.[79] A very stable compound, pharmacologically resembling lignocaine but less toxic. pKa 7.9. Whereas lignocaine is metabolized in the liver, prilocaine is metabolized also in the kidneys and lungs and more rapidly, partly by amidase. Little drug reaches the urine. This rapid metabolism may account for the methaemoglobinaemia seen after its use, especially if more than 600 mg are injected.[80] A maximal safe dose without adrenaline is 400 mg; with adrenaline 600 mg.

Methaemoglobin is continuously formed during red-cell metabolism but normally does not exceed 1% of the haemoglobin at any one time. The cause of this oxidation of haemoglobin to methaemoglobin is not prilocaine itself but one of its degradation products. The degree of cyanosis due to methaemoglobin following prilocaine varies with erythrocyte methaemoglobin reductase[81] and usually disappears spontaneously in 24 h. It is of little clinical importance unless there is severe anaemia or circulatory impairment. The presence of cyanosis indicates that 1.5 g/dl or more of the haemoglobin is circulating as methaemoglobin. There is an associated shift of the oxygen dissociation curve of the remaining haemoglobin, which hinders oxygen liberation at tissue level. Methaemoglobin crosses the placenta. A dose of 6 mg/kg or more is necessary to cause symptoms of hypoxia and is only likely to be seen after extradural block with repeated injections through a catheter. Congenital or acquired methaemoglobinaemia are probably contra-indications to the use of prilocaine. Treatment is by intravenous injection of 1% methylene blue, 1–2 mg/kg.

In extradural block the drug has been shown to give a slower onset and spread with a longer duration of effect and greater intensity than lignocaine, with less toxicity. The addition of adrenaline prolongs the duration of effect less with prilocaine than with lignocaine.

It is most useful when high dosage and strong concentration are required of a local analgesic drug as when injection is into vascular areas, e.g. pudendal block and blocks about the face and neck, and for Bier's intravenous local analgesia in 0.5% solution, for which it is most suitable,[82] and for which it can be alkalinized.[83] For topical analgesia 10 ml of 4% solution is reasonable. A rough guide to dosage is to regard 4 mg/kg as reasonably safe.

6. Cinchocaine hydrochloride (Nupercaine, dibucaine, Percain, Sovcaine, Dulzit)

Synthesized by Karl Miescher in 1925,[84] used for many years for spinal analgesia (intradural) with great satisfaction, and also for infiltration and surface analgesia. No longer commercially available in the UK.

7. Ropivacaine

Introduced as a safer alternative to bupivacaine, with a similar effect and duration.[86] (For pharmacokinetics and pharmacodynamics, *see* Katz J. A. et al. *Anesth. Analg.* 1990, **70**, 16.) Ropivacaine 0.75%, has less cardiovascular side-effects, and is useful for producing more reliable motor block, than 0.5% bupivacaine.

Has been used in many techniques with good results.[86] Peak blood levels of about 1 mg/l are found after injection of nearly 200 mg ropivacaine, unaffected by the addition of adrenaline. (*See* Hickey R. et al. *Can. J. Anaesth.* 1990, **37**, 878.)

Others

Lecithin-coated microdroplets of methoxyflurane produce long-lasting local analgesia which is stable and localized.[87]

Autoclaving of local analgesic drugs

The commonly used agents are very stable chemical compounds. Ampoules of the hydrochloride salts of lignocaine, prilocaine, mepivacaine, bupivacaine, ropivacaine, etidocaine and procaine can all be autoclaved and thereafter show no chemical change on chromatographic analysis. They are not inactivated by gamma radiation (25 Mrad).

DRUGS USED FOR VASOCONSTRICTION

For history of sympathomimetic amines, *see* Runciman W. B. et al. *Anaesth. Intensive Care* 1980, **8**, 289.

Vasoconstrictor drugs have been used in local analgesia since Braun introduced adrenaline in 1902.[88]

The adrenaline-induced contraction of the smooth muscle of vessel walls is modified to different degrees by the same molar concentrations of different local analgesic agents and by different concentrations of the same agent.[89] The vascularity of the tissues receiving the injection is also a factor to be considered in estimating the optimal concentration in a given case. Vasoconstrictors are employed: (1) to retard absorption and reduce toxicity; (2) to prolong analgesic activity; and (3) to produce ischaemia.

Adrenaline, BP (Epinephrine, USP)

The tartrate, which is synthetic, is used for injection and contains a stabilizer, potassium metabitartrite, 0.1% which increases the acidity of the solution. Many workers add their own adrenaline to local analgesic solutions, preferring this to the commercially available mixtures, in extradural block. It is used less frequently in intradural block. The hydrochloride, which is of animal origin, is for topical application. For infiltration it is probably unnecessary to use a strength greater than 1 in 200 000, although dentists employ 1 in 80 000. Discoloration indicates decomposition; it can be autoclaved once but not repeatedly. For infiltration to produce ischaemia before incision the usual amount added is 1 mg to 250–500 ml of saline, giving a 1 in 250 000 to 1 in 500 000 solution. It is probably unwise to inject more than 0.5 mg at one time. The addition of adrenaline reduces the uptake of lignocaine by the circulation more than that of the other amide-linked agents.

It is an α-adrenergic stimulant and may produce pallor, tachycardia and syncope. It should be used with the greatest care if chloroform, cyclopropane or halothane is to be given, because the combination may cause ventricular fibrillation. It has been suggested that, providing there is no hypercapnia or hypoxia, 10 ml of 1 in 100 000 adrenaline solution can be injected with safety in any 10-min period and not more than 30 ml/h.[90] Vasoconstrictors help to produce a dry operative field. Adverse reactions to adrenaline and noradrenaline are most likely to occur following intravascular injection, especially in patients with diabetes, heart disease, thyrotoxicosis, epilepsy and those receiving some halogenated anaesthetics or drug therapy involving tricyclic antidepressants or adrenergic neurone-blocking drugs.

Phenylephrine (Neosynephrine)

Used for vasoconstriction during local analgesia, 0.25–0.5 ml of 1% solution added to each 100 ml of local analgesic solution. Causes no cerebral stimulation or tachycardia.

Noradrenaline

This can be used to produce local vasoconstriction but is less effective than adrenaline because it is a weaker α-receptor stimulant. Does not stimulate the β-receptors in muscle so causes no ischaemia there. It is oxidized in the body more rapidly by amine oxidase than is adrenaline. Tricyclic antidepressants increase its pressor effects.

Felypressin (PVL-2, Octopressin)

This is 2-phenylalanine-8-lysine vasopressin and is a good local vasoconstrictor for use along with halothane, cyclopropane, etc. It is a synthetic derivative of the octapeptide hormone, vasopressin, from the posterior pituitary. It causes constriction of all smooth muscle but has little oxytocic or antidiuretic effect. May result in coronary arterial constriction, but has little influence on cardiac rhythm. Unlike adrenaline it does not alter cardiac rate or rhythm in dental surgery. Available with 3% prilocaine for dental use.

TECHNIQUES OF REGIONAL ANALGESIA

Before any large volume of local analgesic solution is injected, the following should be available: (1) an open vein; (2) a tilting table or trolley; (3) facilities for IPPV with oxygen; (4) suction equipment and catheters; (5) syringes, needles and ampoules of thiopentone, suxamethonium, diazepam and pressor drugs; and (6) fluid for infusion.

Uses of vasoconstrictors in patients on other drugs

If volatile anaesthetic agents are being given at the same time, suitable β-blocking agents should be available and of course both hypoxia and hypercapnia avoided. Some dental cartridges contain adrenaline 1 in 80 000 solution, but felypressin can be substituted. With tricyclic antidepressants, the cardiovascular effects of catecholamines may be increased. They should not be used together.

Identification of nerves

Facilitated in many nerve blocks by an electric current (6–8 V, 2 Hz) via a needle, insulated apart from its tip. Muscular contraction shows proximity to nerve.[91] Nerves can be located using voltages high enough to stimulate motor fibres without causing sensory discomfort as sensory stimulation requires a higher voltage than motor stimulation.[92]

Topical analgesia[93]
(Greek topos,'a place')
   Can be applied: (1) on gauze swabs; (2) as a liquid in a spray; (3) as a paste, cream or ointment, e.g. EMLA cream for the skin;[94] (4) as an aerosol; and (5) by direct instillation, e.g. conjunctival sac, nose and trachea.

Sites

(1) The upper air passages, e.g. 4% lignocaine, 5 ml. A 10% aerosol of lignocaine is safe;[95] (2) the nasal cavities, e.g. 4% cocaine is potentiated by sodium bicarbonate; (3) the external ear, e.g. 10% lignocaine aerosol for paracentesis; (4) the conjunctival sac, e.g. 4% lignocaine, 2–4% cocaine or 0.5% amethocaine. Stinging pain on instillation can be eased if the drug is dissolved in methylcellulose; (5) perineum and vagina in obstetrics, e.g. 10% lignocaine aerosol for spontaneous delivery or for suture of simple lacerations; (6) urethra, e.g. 1% lignocaine gel; and (7) before open wound closure.[96]

Infiltration analgesia

Popularized by C. L. Schleich (1853–1922) of Berlin in 1892. A weal is raised with a fine needle and through this weal a larger needle is used to inject the main bulk of solution. Procaine or lignocaine 0.5–1% solution, each with adrenaline, is ideal for this procedure. *For painless skin incisions, infiltration should be intradermal as well as subcutaneous.* For maximal intradermal analgesia the adrenaline should be omitted.[97] A slow, gentle technique is important, and the solution should be injected while the needle is moving to reduce the chances of intravenous injection.
   A patient taking debrisoquine (Declinax) for hypertension may develop total ischaemia in areas infiltrated with lignocaine–adrenaline solutions.[98]

As with all forms of local analgesia, the effect is not instantaneous and a proper interval must elapse between injection and incision. Patience is vital.

Transverse injection anaesthesia

A name given by Russian surgeons to a method (Vishnevsky technique) in which a transverse disc of tissue of a limb is infiltrated from skin to bone with a dilute solution of an analgesic drug, such as 0.5% procaine, in large volume. In the vernacular 'the squirt-and-cut' technique.

Field block of scalp and cranium

Anatomy

The trigeminal nerve supplies the anterior two-thirds, the posterior divisions of cervical nerves the posterior third (Fig. 24.1).

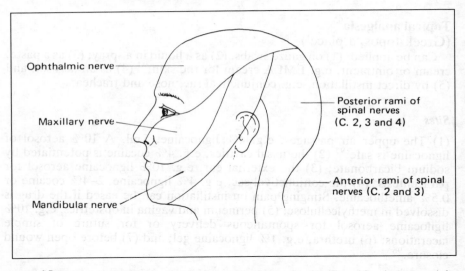

Figure 24.1 Showing the cutaneous nerve areas of the face and scalp. *(From 'Gray's Anatomy', by kind permission of the Editor.)*

There are five sensory nerves in front of the ear and four behind it. These nerves all converge towards the vertex of the scalp, so that a band of infiltration passing just above the ear through the glabella and the occiput will block them all.

Technique

Injections of 0.5% lignocaine with adrenaline solution must be made in three layers: (1) the skin, intradermal; (2) the subcutaneous tissues superficial to the epicranial aponeurosis in which the nerves and vessels lie, and also below the aponeurosis; and (3) the periosteum.

In addition, the solution should be injected into the substance of the temporalis muscle. The dura is insensitive except at the base of the skull.

For removal of sebaceous cysts or suturing of small wounds, the area is surrounded by a zone of infiltration. Periosteal injection is only necessary if bone is to be removed.

Useful in some cases of acute head injury and also to reduce haemorrhage in intracranial operations under general anaesthesia.

Nerve block for eye operations

Retrobulbar and periocular[99] blocks are used (*see* Chapter 22, Ophthalmic surgery).

Nerve block for nose operations

Anatomy

The nerve supply is from the first or ophthalmic division and from the second or maxillary division of the trigeminal nerve.

In more detail: *The skin of the nose* is supplied by the supratrochlear branch of frontal nerve of the ophthalmic; the anterior ethmoidal branch of the nasociliary (ophthalmic); and the infraorbital branch of the maxillary. *The maxillary antrum of Highmore*: its lining is supplied by the maxillary nerve via the sphenopalatine ganglion. *The frontal sinus*: frontal nerve; branch of ophthalmic. *The ethmoid region*: the anterior and posterior ethmoidal branches of the nasociliary.

The sensory supply of the nasal cavities, fifth nerve, is as follows: the anterior one-third of the septum and lateral walls by the anterior ethmoidal branch of the nasociliary nerve (division 1); and the posterior two-thirds of the septum and lateral walls by the long sphenopalatine nerves from the sphenopalatine ganglion (division 2).

Injections into the nose or orbit (ethmoid region, septum, middle turbinates, etc.) may result in total spinal block (cf. rhinorrhoea after fractured base of skull). Surgeons who do these injections must know how to treat this complication.[100]

Techniques

1. BLOCK OF MAXILLARY NERVE AND SPHENOPALATINE GANGLION

Useful for operations on antrum (e.g. Caldwell-Luc) and on upper lip, palate and upper teeth as far as the bicuspids.

Anatomy. The maxillary or second division of the fifth nerve is entirely sensory. It is given off from the middle of the Gasserian ganglion and passes forwards horizontally in the lower part of the lateral wall of the cavernous sinus until it leaves the skull through the foramen rotundum. It crosses the pterygomaxillary fissure to enter the orbit through the inferior orbital fissure and ends as the infra-orbital nerve after emerging on to the face through the infra-orbital foramen. The sphenopalatine ganglion of Meckel is situated in the pterygopalatine fossa in the upper part of the pterygomaxillary fissure, lateral to the sphenopalatine foramen. Blocking of the nerve causes analgesia in: (*a*) the lateral nasal; (*b*) inferior palpebral and superior labial nerves; (*c*) the posterior, middle and anterior superior alveolar nerves; and (*d*) the palatal nerves, which supply the skin of the upper lip, side of nose, lower eyelid and malar region, the teeth of the upper jaw and the underlying periosteum, the mucosa of the maxillary antrum and of the hard and soft palate, and the posterior part of the nasal cavity.

A weal is raised 0.5 cm below the midpoint of the zygoma, which is over the anterior border of the coronoid process, and through it a needle is introduced at right angles to the median plane of the head until it strikes the lateral plate of the pterygoid process at a depth of about 4 cm. A marker is set 1 cm from skin surface and the needle reinserted slightly anteriorly so that its point glances past the anterior margin of the external pterygoid plate and advances as far as the marker. The needle point should be in the pterygomaxillary fissure. The needle has been known to enter the pharynx or the orbit. If aspiration test is negative, 3–4 ml of 1.5% solution of lignocaine is injected and a similar amount as the needle is slowly withdrawn.

Transient paralysis of the sixth cranial nerve may result; it soon passes off.

2. BLOCK OF ANTERIOR ETHMOIDAL NERVE (MEDIAN ORBITAL BLOCK)

This is a branch of the nasociliary nerve and is blocked in the medial wall of the orbit as the nerve passes through the anterior ethmoidal foramen. A weal is raised 1 cm above the caruncle at the inner canthus of the eye. A small needle is introduced along the upper medial angle of the orbit for 3.5 cm keeping near the bone. Injection is made of 2 ml of 1.5% lignocaine.

3. BLOCK OF FRONTAL NERVE

From the same weal as in anterior ethmoid block, the needle is introduced more laterally towards the central part of the roof of the orbit where the frontal nerve lies between the periosteum and the levator palpebrae superioris. Lignocaine, 1 ml of 2% solution, is injected in close contact with the bone.

4. BLOCK OF INFRAORBITAL NERVE

The infra-orbital nerve, the terminal portion of the maxillary nerve, divides at the infra-orbital foramen into inferior palpebral, external nasal and superior labial branches. These supply the side of the nose, the lower eyelid, the upper lip and its mucosa. The infra-orbital foramen is in line with the supra-orbital notch and canine fossa – both of which are palpable – or the second upper premolar tooth; it is 1 cm below the margin of the orbit, below the pupil when the eyes look forward. The mental foramen is in the same straight line, as is also the second bicuspid tooth.

A needle is inserted through a weal 1 cm below the middle of the lower orbital margin, a finger-breadth lateral to the ala of the nose. Lignocaine, 2 ml of 2% solution, is deposited near the nerve as it issues from the foramen, not while it is in the foramen. By this injection the upper lip and tip of the nose are made insensitive.

For radical operation on the antrum, a maxillary block is indicated, together with local infiltration inside the upper lip, over the canine fossa.

For radical operation on the frontal sinus, anterior ethmoidal and frontal blocks are necessary.

For operations for dacryocystitis, anterior ethmoidal and infra-orbital blocks are required.

INTRA-ORAL NERVE BLOCK FOR EXTRA-ORAL LESIONS[101]

Useful for repair of lacerations of face and removal of skin lesions. No tissue distortion; injections less painful than through the skin.

Infra-orbital nerve. Injection in mucobuccal fold, just medial to canine tooth; 1–2 ml of solution injected, advancing needle 1 cm. The entire upper lip is anaesthetized. Can be done bilaterally.

Mental nerve. Injection between apices of premolar teeth of lower jaw of 1–2 ml of solution; lower lip anaesthetized. (*See* Smith J. S. et al. *Anaesth. Intensive Care* 1985, **13**, 407.)

Long buccal nerve. Can be blocked as it crosses the anterior border of mandible. Injection immediately in front of the ramus, in the mucobuccal fold opposite the first molar tooth. Needle is inserted just anterior to the margin of the mandible and 2–3 ml of solution injected as needle is withdrawn. Useful for blocking 'cross-over' fibres.

Topical analgesia of the nasal cavities

Sometimes managed by the surgeon. Useful in co-operative patients with reasonably patent nares.

1. Packing

The nasal cavities are first sprayed with 4–10% cocaine, all excess solution being rejected and not swallowed. With a good light and a speculum, the cavity is now packed with gauze soaked in 4–5% cocaine. Cocaine is a powerful vasoconstrictor and so adrenaline, although beloved of rhinologists, is not necessary. Trauma must be avoided.

After 10 min the packing is removed and the mucosa will be found to be avascular.

2. Sluder's method[102]

3. Use of cocaine paste[103]

Cocaine is toxic.

4. Moffett's methods[104]

The solution is a mixture of 2 ml of 8% cocaine hydrochloride, 2 ml of 1% sodium bicarbonate, 1 ml of 1 in 1000 adrenaline solution. A 2-ml syringe with bent cannula is required.

Position 1: Patient lies on left side with pillow under left shoulder and head in lateral position at angle of 45° with vertical. One-third of solution is drawn up, half being squirted into each naris along the floor of the nose.

Position 2: After 10 min, second third of solution is drawn up and is similarly divided between the two sides of the nose; patient pinches nose, turns prone, and lies on face for 10 min.

Position 3: With the remainder instilled the patient rolls on to right side as in position 1 and remains 10 min. If the septum is to be operated on, 2 ml of 1% lignocaine–adrenaline should be injected into the columella and base of septum in addition, as this area is covered by squamous epithelium, which will not absorb the topical agent.

The method gives good analgesia, free from the unpleasantness of gauze packing and its resulting mild trauma. It can also be used as cocaine 4%, omitting bicarbonate and adrenaline.

5. Curtiss' method[105]

6. Macintosh and Ostlere's method[106]

7. Bodman's method[107]

These methods of local analgesia are useful for the surgery of nasal septal defects, removal of polypi, turbinectomy, cauterization, etc.

For puncture of the antrum, cotton-wool swabs on applicators soaked in 4% cocaine solution are inserted under the middle and inferior turbinates for 10 min. The nasal cavity is then sprayed with two or three squirts of 10% lignocaine aerosol spray.

Local infiltration for dental extraction

This can be done for all teeth with the possible exception of the lower molars. Lignocaine 2% with 1 in 80 000 adrenaline solution is commonly used, and 3% prilocaine with felypressin is now also used. A 26G needle is inserted at the junction of the adherent mucoperiosteum of the gum with the free mucous membrane of the cheek and directed parallel to the long axis of the tooth; 0.5–1 ml of solution is injected superficial to the periosteum on the buccal and either the lingual or palatal side. Analgesia is tested for after 5 min by pushing the needle down the periodontal membrane on each side of the tooth to be extracted. If required more solution can be injected. Where there is infection involving teeth in the lower jaw, a 5% lignocaine solution may give better analgesia than the usual 2%. It has a shorter latency but a similar duration of activity.[108]

Mandibular (inferior dental) block

This may be required for extraction of several teeth of the lower jaw or for removal of the second or third molars. Infiltration cannot always be relied on to make these teeth insensitive. A single, well-placed injection makes one-half of the lower jaw and tongue analgesic, except for the central incisor, which gets some nerve supply from the other side, and the lateral buccal fold and molar buccal alveolar margin and gum supplied from the buccinator nerve. Both of these areas can be infiltrated with a small volume of solution to make them painless.

With the mouth open palpate the anterior border of the ramus of the mandible, the retromolar fossa and the internal oblique ridge. The needle is inserted just medial to this ridge lateral to the pterygomandibular ligament for a distance of 1.5 cm, keeping the syringe parallel to the occlusal plane of the lower teeth with its barrel over the premolar teeth of the opposite side; 2 or 3 ml of solution are now injected.

Transient amaurosis after mandibular nerve block has been reported[109] and may be due to intra-arterial injection of adrenaline with the local analgesic solution in patients whose orbital blood supply is derived from the middle meningeal artery – a rare anomaly. Unusual reactions to lignocaine in dental surgery (fixed drug eruption) may occur.[110]

Paracentesis of the eardrum

Two or three metered (10-mg) doses of lignocaine aerosol spray are applied to the superior wall of the external auditory canal and allowed to trickle down onto the eardrum. This is repeated in 2 min and the incision can be made 3 min later. Useful in co-operative children.

Lingual nerve block

The lingual nerve is the only sensory nerve supplying the floor of the mouth between the alveolar margin and the midline.

A finger in the retromolar fossa of the mandible will palpate the internal oblique line. The lingual nerve can be injected, just medial to this line, with 2 ml of 2% lignocaine. A useful method of analgesia for removing calculi from the submaxillary duct.

Facial nerve block

For hemifacial spasm.[111] The nerve is blocked as it crosses the neck of the mandible. Used also in combination with retrobulbar block for intraocular surgery.

Vagus nerve block

This was described[112] as a method of analgesia for broncho-oesophagoscopy and in the diagnosis of pain arising in the thorax, but is now seldom used.

Superior laryngeal nerve block

The internal laryngeal nerve passes forwards and downwards and pierces the thyrohyoid membrane to reach the space between the epiglottis and the pharyngeal mucosa posteriorly and the membrane in front. Its terminal twigs convey sensation from the larynx above the cords, the epiglottis, vallecula and the base of the tongue. This nerve is blocked at its point of division into the internal and external laryngeal nerve, slightly below and anterior to the greater cornu of the hyoid bone. Block of the internal branch causes analgesia of the lower pharynx, the laryngeal aspect of the epiglottis, the vallecula, the vestibule of the larynx, the aryepiglottic fold and the posterior part of the rima glottidis. There is no motor block.

1. A weal is raised over the thyroid notch in the midline, the hyoid grasped between the thumb and index finger of the left hand and displaced laterally towards the side to be injected. Through the weal, an 8-cm needle is introduced laterally and 2% procaine solution is injected as the needle is advanced to the greater cornu – but not beyond it for fear of injuring the great vessels of the neck. A further few millilitres of solution are injected as the needle is withdrawn. A similar procedure is carried out on the other side, through the same weal.[113]

2. A 22G, 4-cm needle is passed through the skin, just above the thyroid cartilage, at a point one-third of the distance between the midline and the tip of the superior cornu; it is advanced upwards and medially for 1–2 cm until a 'give' is felt as it pierces the thyrohyoid membrane, and enters the space containing the internal laryngeal nerve. With the needle moving slightly in and out, 2–3 ml of solution is injected. If the needle advances too far it may enter the pharynx and air can be aspirated.

This block causes analgesia of the posterior surface of the epiglottis and of the larynx above the cords, so that food and drink must be prohibited for an adequate period depending on the drug and strength used.

It is useful, in conjunction with topical analgesia of the nose and pharynx, to enable blind nasotracheal intubation to be performed for tracheobronchial cleansing; the coughing, which results from irritation of the larynx below the cords, soon passes off.

Topical analgesia, coupled with superior laryngeal and glossopharyngeal nerve block, gives good results for awake intubation, tonsillectomy and bronchoscopy.[114]

Transtracheal block

For technique for awake intubation, *see* Bromage P. R. *Epidural Analgesia.* Philadelphia: Saunders, 1978, 476.

Accessory nerve block

The nerve has both cranial and spinal roots. It leaves the skull through the jugular foramen, enters the deep surface of the sternomastoid, pierces it and emerges just above the midpoint of its posterior margin. It crosses the posterior triangle of the neck and enters the anterior border of the trapezius, giving motor fibres to it and to the sternomastoid.

Technique: Needle inserted 2 cm below the tip of the mastoid and 5–10 ml of solution injected into muscle.

Indications: To relax sternomastoid and trapezius muscles during physiotherapy for pain in the shoulder and neck, e.g. torticollis.[115]

Stellate ganglion block[116]

(Cervicothoracic sympathetic block)

Sympathetic block is most commonly carried out: (1) in the neck (stellate ganglion block); (2) in the abdomen (splanchnic or coeliac plexus block); and (3) in the lumbar region (L1–L4).

The stellate ganglion is formed by the fusion of the lowest of the three cervical ganglia with the first thoracic ganglion. It is irregular in size and position, being usually 1–3 cm long, and differs in the same individual on the two sides. Stellate ganglion block was first used for cerebral vascular accidents by Leriche and Fontaine in 1934[117] This should be named cervicothoracic sympathetic block, because when 10–15 ml of analgesic solution is injected into the correct plane at the base of the neck, the middle cervical, stellate and the second, third and usually the fourth thoracic ganglia and their rami are blocked. This results in interruption of all sympathetic fibres to most of the thorax, head, neck and arm (except possibly the nerve of Kuntz[118]). Certain visceral afferent fibres are also blocked, e.g. the cervical cardiac nerves.

The stellate ganglion is often blocked by spill-over following supraclavicular brachial plexus block.

Anatomy

The cervical sympathetic chain and its three ganglia lie in front of the head of the first rib and the seventh cervical and first thoracic transverse process, just behind the subclavian artery and origin of the vertebral artery. It lies posterior to the carotid sheath on the longus colli and longus cervicis muscles. It is anterior to the eighth cervical and first thoracic nerves; paraesthesia involving these nerves indicates, if stellate ganglion block is done from the front, that the needle is too deeply placed. On the right side, the apex of the lung and the dome of the pleura are anterior relations; on the left side these structures are 2.5 cm lower and so are not in such close relationship to the ganglion. Vasoconstrictor fibres pass from the stellate and the other cervical sympathetic ganglia to a plexus around the internal carotid artery. Twigs from the second and sometimes also from the third thoracic sympathetic ganglion often go directly to the upper extremity via the first thoracic nerve, thus bypassing the stellate ganglion (the nerve of Kuntz[118]). But this nerve is usually blocked by spread of the analgesic solution down to the region of the fourth thoracic ganglion.

It sends grey rami to the seventh and eighth cervical nerves, gives origin to the inferior cervical cardiac nerve, and supplies twigs to the vessels in its vicinity. It may communicate with the vagus.

Its most frequent indication is to release vascular tone, and it may need to be repeated several times.

As pointed out by Winnie[119] postganglionic sympathetic fibres are also distributed to the arm with the somatic nerves of the brachial plexus and are distributed from them to the vessels, supplying vasoconstrictor impulses to the whole limb.

Indications

There are few indications for stellate ganglion block today, although in the recent past it was widely practised. The control of the tone of intracranial vessels is now known to be more humoral than nervous. It has been used to treat quinine blindness[120] and acute deafness.[121] Its use in the treatment of blindness due to quinine poisoning is doubtful.[122] Has been used for relief of the acute pain due to herpes zoster ophthalmicus.[123]

Technique

Stellate ganglion block performed on a patient with an increased bleeding time or a decreased clotting time may result in a large haematoma in the deep planes of the neck. Long-acting drugs, e.g. 6% phenol or absolute alcohol, are used chiefly to control cardiac pain. Bilateral block should not be carried out at the same time.

1. *Paratracheal approach.*[124] The patient lies supine, chin forwards, and neck extended without a pillow. Weal raised two finger-breadths lateral to the suprasternal notch and a similar distance above the clavicle, which is on the medial border of the sternomastoid overlying the transverse process of the seventh cervical vertebra. The position can be checked by palpating the tubercle of Chassaignac and the cricoid cartilage, both of which are at the level of the sixth cervical transverse process, i.e. a little higher than the weal. A fine 5–8-cm needle is inserted directly backwards through the weal, while downward and backward pressure is exerted on the sternomastoid to draw the muscle and the carotid sheath laterally. When contact is made with bone (C7) the needle is withdrawn 0.5–1 cm so that its point lies in front of the longus colli muscle and, after careful aspiration for blood (the vertebral artery is very near) and for cerebrospinal fluid, 15–20 ml of 0.5% lignocaine or similar solution are injected. This will, if correctly placed, diffuse up and down in the fascial plane and will block the ganglia and rami from C2 to T4 inclusive. Thirty minutes may elapse before Horner's syndrome and vasodilatation of the arm appear. This technique is, in the authors' opinion, the safest and easiest.

2. *Anterior approach* (Apgar).[125]
3. *Lateral approach* (Goinard).[126]
4. *Posterior approach* (Kappis et al. 1947; Labat, 1930; White, 1940).
5. *Tissue displacement method.*[127]

Signs of successful block

(1) Horner's syndrome:[128] miosis, enophthalmos and ptosis. This does not guarantee sympathetic paralysis of the vessels of the arm; (2) flushing of the cheek, face and neck and arm. Engorged veins of arm. Increase in skin temperature; (3) flushing of the conjunctiva and sclera; (4) anhidrosis of the face and neck; (5) lacrimation; (6) stuffiness of the nostril (Guttmann's sign); (7) Mueller's syndrome: injection of tympanic membrane and warmth of face;

and (8) sympathetic block can be assessed by the cobalt blue and ninhydrin sweat tests, which are more informative than the sympatho-galvanic response.[129]

Complications and dangers of the block

(1) Pleural shock; (2) perforation of the oesophagus, with infection; (3) intrathecal injection causing a total spinal block;[130] (4) intravascular injection, e.g. sending volume of solution via the vertebral artery straight up to the medulla; (5) pneumothorax; (6) cardiac arrest – very rare, although it has resulted from surgical cervicothoracic sympathectomy (a permanent stellate block);[131] (7) alteration of voice from recurrent laryngeal nerve block; (8) phrenic nerve block; (9) brachial plexus block; (10) extradural or intradural block; (11) mediastinitis; and (12) intercostal neuralgia.[132]

Death has been reported after stellate ganglion block, so that it should not be lightly undertaken.

Field block for tonsillectomy

Anatomy

The tonsil and its immediate surroundings are supplied by the lesser palatine (from maxillary), the lingual (from mandibular) nerves, and the glosso-pharyngeal nerve, via the pharyngeal plexus, which gives off filaments that form a plexus called the circulus tonsillaris.

Technique

Half an hour before the analgesia is commenced, an amethocaine lozenge 60 mg is given, after which the mouth and pharynx should be sprayed with 4–10% cocaine solution; some operators object to this preferring to the keep the cough reflex active throughout.

Injections of 3–5 ml of 1.5% lignocaine and adrenaline are now made: (1) into the upper part of the posterior pillar; (2) into the upper part of the anterior pillar – both pillars must be made oedematous throughout their whole extent; (3) into the triangular fold, near the lower pole; and (4) into the supratonsillar fossa, after drawing the tonsil towards the middle line.

The patient should be sitting, well supported, in a chair. Adequate time must be given for the analgesic to act. Fainting is sometimes seen, and depression of the tongue by the spatula may cause discomfort.

The technique finds little favour in the UK.

Glossopharyngeal nerve block[133]

Head fully rotated to opposite side with the patient lying supine. At midpoint of a line joining the tip of the mastoid process to the angle of the jaw a needle is inserted vertical to the skin until it makes contact with the styloid process 2–4 cm deep. The needle is partially withdrawn and reinserted 0.5 cm deep to, and posterior to, the styloid process. Injection of 6 ml of solution at this point will produce analgesia of posterior one-third of tongue.

Another technique for block of the glossopharyngeal nerve is to deposit solution near the jugular foramen. A 5-cm needle is introduced through a weal just below the external auditory meatus, anterior to the mastoid process. It is advanced perpendicularly to the skin until it meets the styloid process 1.5–2 cm deep and passes it posteriorly for a further 2 cm. Analgesia involves the 9th to 12th nerves inclusive and has been maintained with a long-acting drug in cases of malignant disease in the posterior third of the tongue, and in severe cases of neuralgia. Successful block results in analgesia of the posterior one-third of the tongue, uvula, soft palate and pharynx. There is no motor block. The gag reflex is suppressed. Also used in differential diagnosis between glossopharyngeal and atypical trigeminal neuralgias. An intraoral approach has been described.[134]

Suprascapular nerve block[135] (C5–6)

The nerve is the sole pathway of somatic pain from the shoulder and acromioclavicular joints and structures surrounding them. The block does not result in any skin analgesia, but when successful, relieves pain in the shoulder-joint.

Technique

Patient should be sitting with arms to the sides and head and shoulders slightly flexed. With a skin pencil the spine of the scapula is lined in: the inferior scapular angle is located and bisected by a line which crosses the first line. A weal is raised one finger-breadth from the crossing, in the upper outer angle, and a needle inserted downwards and medially to make contact with the bone of the supraspinatus fossa, just lateral to the notch. Needle is then withdrawn and reintroduced more medially until its point lies in the notch. Paraesthesiae take the form of pain at the tip of the shoulder, and after aspiration, 10 ml of analgesic solution is injected. The block must be at the suprascapular notch as there the nerve is accessible to a needle and no afferent branches leave it before it passes through the notch. Types of shoulder pain relieved by this block include subacromial bursitis and painful abduction of the arm; calcified deposits about the capsule of the shoulder-joint. Used for pain relief, not surgery.

Cervical plexus block (C1–4)

This is paravertebral cervical analgesia. It is not commonly used but is convenient for the removal of superficial tumours and cysts from the neck.

Anatomy

Formed by the anterior primary divisions of the upper four cervical nerves, each one of which, after leaving the intervertebral foramen, passes behind the vertebral artery and comes to lie in the sulcus between the anterior and posterior tubercles of the transverse process of the appropriate cervical vertebra. Each nerve lies between the scalenus medius deeply and the levator anguli scapulae, under cover of the sternomastoid. Each of these four nerves, except the first, divides into upper and lower branches, which form three loops lateral to the transverse processes. The loops are between C1 and C2; C2 and C3; C3 and C4. The lower branch of C4 joins C5 in the formation of the brachial plexus. The upper loop is directed forwards, the lower two, backwards.

Branches are superficial (cutaneous), deep (muscular) and communicating. *Superficial branches* emerge posterior to the lateral border of the sternomastoid, near its midpoint. They are:

1. Ascending Branches. Lesser occipital (C2) and great auricular (C2 and C3). They supply skin of the occipitomastoid region, auricle, and parotid.

2. Transverse Branch. The anterior cutaneous nerve of the neck (C2 and C3) supplying skin of anterior part of neck between the lower jaw and the sternum.

3. Descending Branches. The lateral, intermediate and medial supra-clavicular nerves (C3 and C4) supplying skin of shoulder and upper pectoral region. C1 has no cutaneous branch.

Deep branches of the plexus are: (1) phrenic nerve – C3, C4 and C5; (2) anterior (deep) muscular branches; and (3) posterior muscular branches to sternomastoid, levator scapulae, trapezius and scalenus medius.

Communicating branches are: (1) sympathetic – each cervical nerve receives a grey ramus from the cervical sympathetic chain – the upper four nerves from the superior cervical ganglion; (2) to vagus; and (3) branch to hypoglossal nerve from C1 and C2, the descendens hypoglossi, which joins the descendens cervicalis (C2–C3) to form the ansa hypoglossi.

The posterior primary divisions of the cervical nerves supply skin and muscles of the back of the neck. Their cutaneous distribution spreads like a cape over the upper thorax and shoulders, and this area is made insensitive in cervical plexus block.

Nerve supply of thyroid is from middle and inferior cervical sympathetic ganglion; of the oesophagus, the vagus (and sympathetic); of the trachea, recurrent laryngeal (and sympathetic); and of the sternomastoid, the 11th cranial, and 2nd and 3rd cervical nerves.

Technique

The patient lies supine with shoulders slightly elevated and neck and head extended – as for thyroidectomy, but with his head turned away from the side to be injected. Solution used is 0.5–1% lignocaine, or one of its congeners, with adrenaline.

Deep cervical block requires the deposition of analgesic solution just lateral to the transverse processes of the 2nd, 3rd and 4th cervical vertebrae (the 6th, 7th and 8th nerves having no sensory branches in the neck, and the first is purely motor). A needle is inserted to a depth of 1.5–2 cm perpendicular to all planes of the skin so that the transverse processes are contacted.

Superficial cervical block is carried out by injecting 20 ml of analgesic solution between skin and muscle along the posterior border of the sternomastoid near its midpoint, usually just below the position where it is crossed by the external jugular vein, so as to cut off impulses from the ascending, transverse and descending superficial branches of the plexus.

Cervical plexus block gives analgesia of the front and back of the neck, the occipital region, and a cape-like area over the shoulders to below the clavicle, the skin above the third rib anteriorly and above the upper border of the scapula posteriorly. Its chief indication is in thyroidectomy.

Complications may include: (1) phrenic block; (2) intrathecal or intravascular injection; (3) vagus and/or recurrent laryngeal nerve block causing aphonia; and (4) cervical sympathetic block and Horner's syndrome.

Brachial plexus block (C5–T1)

History

Halsted (1852–1922) of New York in 1884, Matas of New Orleans[136] (1860–1957) and Crile[137] (1864–1943) of Cleveland in 1897, injected the plexus under direct vision following exposure under local infiltration (intraneural block). Hirschel injected the plexus blindly through the skin.[138] Kulenkampff, assistant to Heinrich Braun at Zwickau, after experimenting on himself, used the supraclavicular technique in 1912.[139] Patrick[140] in Sheffield published his modification of the Kulenkampff technique in 1940. Macintosh and Mushin[141] describe this method in their excellently illustrated book. The method involves blocking the plexus as it lies on the first rib, lateral to the subclavian artery. (*See* Winnie A. P. *Plexus Anesthesia*, Vol. 1. Edinburgh: Churchill Livingstone, 1983.)

Anatomy

The brachial plexus is formed from the anterior primary divisions of C5, C6, C7, C8 and T1. It forms the entire motor and almost the entire sensory nerve supply to the arm. It receives communicating branches from C4 and T2. These nerves unite to form three trunks, which lie in the neck above the clavicle. Its roots pass through the fascia-enclosed space between the scalenus anterior and the scalenus medius accompanied by the subclavian artery, invaginate the scalene fascia to form a neurovascular space; this fascia then becomes the axillary sheath or axillary perivascular space, which surrounds the plexus. This space may be entered at the supraclavicular, interscalene, axillary or infraclavicular level; a single injection into it will produce analgesia, the extent of which will depend on the volume of solution injected and the level of injection. Each trunk divides, behind the clavicle, into anterior and posterior divisions, which unite in the axilla to form cords.

The plexus is broad above and converges to the first rib. Its anterior relations are the skin, superficial fascia, platysma and supraclavicular branches of the cervical plexus, the deep fascia and external jugular vein; the clavicle is in front of its lower part, the scalenus anterior is in front of its upper part. Its posterior relations are the scalenus medius and the long thoracic nerve. Its inferior relations are the first rib, where the plexus lies between the subclavian artery anteriorly and the scalenus medius behind.

The plexus emerges from the intervertebral foramina and passes between the scalenus anterior and the scalenus medius. Close to their emergence the 5th and 6th nerves each receive a grey ramus from the middle cervical sympathetic ganglion. The 7th and 8th nerves each receive a grey ramus from the inferior cervical ganglion. The thoracic nerve receives a grey ramus from and sends a white ramus to the first thoracic sympathetic ganglion. As the plexus converges on the first rib it is enclosed in a fibrous sheath contributed by the scalenus anterior and medius muscles. It lies first above, and then to the outer side of, the subclavian vessels and just above the clavicle lies between the skin and the first rib, immediately behind the deep fascia.

The upper trunk is formed by the anterior rami of C5 and C6.

The middle trunk is formed by the anterior ramus of C7.

The lower trunk is formed by the anterior rami of C8 and T1. Behind the clavicle the trunks each divide into anterior and posterior divisions, i.e. in relationship to the axillary artery.

The posterior cord is formed by the three posterior divisions.

The medial cord is formed by the lowest anterior division.

The lateral cord is formed by the upper two anterior divisions.

Branches are given off from: (1) roots; (2) trunks; and (3) cords.

1. *Branches from roots*: The nerve to the serratus anterior (of Bell) from C5, C6 and C7. Dorsalis scapulae nerve from C5. Muscular branches to the longus cervicis (C5–C8) and the three scaleni (C5–C8), the rhomboids (C5) and a twig to the phrenic (C5).

2. *Branches from trunks*: Suprascapular nerve (C5 and C6). Nerve to subclavius (C5 and C6).

3. *Branches from cords*: From lateral cord (three): lateral pectoral (C5–C7); lateral head of the median (C5–C7); and musculocutaneous (C5, C6, C7). From the posterior cord (five): radial (C5, C6, C7, C8 and T1); axillary (C5 and C6); thoracodorsal nerve to the latissimus dorsi (C6, C7, C8); and upper and lower subscapular nerves (C5 and C6). From the medial cord (five): Medial head of the median; medial pectoral; ulnar; medial cutaneous of the forearm (all from C8 and T1); and medial cutaneous of the arm (T1).

The scalenus anterior arises from the anterior tubercles of the transverse processes of the 3rd, 4th, 5th and 6th cervical vertebrae. It is inserted into the scalene tubercle on the inner border of the first rib. The muscle lies anterior to the plexus, being separated from it below by the subclavian artery. Its lateral border, if it is palpable, is a guide to the position of the plexus.

The scalenus medius arises from the posterior tubercles of the six lowest cervical vertebrae and is inserted into the upper surface of the first rib behind the groove made by the plexus and the subclavian artery. The plexus thus lies in front of the muscle.

The first rib lies in an almost horizontal plane, being inclined slightly downwards and forwards. It passes below the clavicle at about the junction of its inner and middle thirds. Its surfaces look upwards and downwards and its borders inwards and outwards.

The head has a single articular facet, which articulates with the body of the first thoracic vertebra. The tubercle articulates with the transverse process of the same vertebra.

The upper surface has two transverse grooves: an anterior for the subclavian vein and a posterior for the subclavian artery and the lowest trunk of the brachial plexus. On the inner border, between the grooves, is the scalene tubercle. The subclavius muscle originates in front of the anterior groove and the scalenus medius is inserted behind the posterior groove. The lower surface has no costal groove; the inner border embraces the dome of the pleura; and the outer border gives origin to the first slip of the serratus anterior.

The subclavian artery extends from its origin to the outer border of the first rib. The right subclavian comes from the innominate artery, the left from the aortic arch. At its highest point, each artery is about 2 cm above the clavicle. Three parts of the artery are described: one medial, one behind and one lateral to the scalenus anterior.

The relations of the third part, i.e. the part lateral to the scalenus anterior, are: anteriorly, the skin, superficial fascia, platysma, deep fascia, descending branches of the cervical plexus, a plexus formed by the external and anterior jugular veins, and the transverse cervical and transverse scapular veins, the transverse cervical and transverse scapular arteries. Above and laterally is the brachial plexus, while below is the first rib.

The subclavian vein is separated from the plexus by the scalenus anterior. As it is well protected by the clavicle, it is unlikely to be punctured.

It has been pointed out[142, 143] that a continuous fascia-enclosed perineural and perivascular compartment exists, extending from the origins of the brachial plexus at the intervertebral foramina to the upper arm. This compartment can be entered at various levels and different volumes of local analgesic solution can be injected into it, as is the case with the extradural space, producing different effects. Thus the need for the elicitation of paraesthesiae with the needle is diminished.[143] The importance of this anatomical concept to anaesthetists should be recognized by its being known as 'Winnie's fascial compartment'. The connective tissue forming the neurovascular sheath of the plexus is denser proximally than distally. Connective tissue septa between the components of the plexus make the sheath multicompartmental and the compartments do not always inter-communicate. Thus, using any technique of block, certain nerves may remain unblocked.[144]

Supraclavicular technique

The patient should be sitting or lying supine. The head is rotated to the other side and the arm and shoulder depressed. A weal is raised 1 cm above the midpoint of the clavicle, a position: (1) midway between the sternoclavicular and acromioclavicular joints; (2) crossed by a line produced downwards from the external jugular vein, made prominent by blowing out the cheeks; (3) just lateral to the pulsating subclavian artery, often palpable; and (4) lateral to the outer border of the scalenus anterior, sometimes palpable under cover of the sternomastoid.

A needle is inserted through the weal downwards, inwards and backwards, so that it is pointing to the spine of the second to fourth thoracic vertebra, a finger meanwhile guarding the subclavian artery and drawing it slightly medially. A cough from the patient is a warning that the pleura is being irritated by the needle. If paraesthesia is felt, the needle is steadied and 30 ml of the solution is injected. The following nerves are blocked: the median, the musculocutaneous, the radial, the axillary, the ulnar, the medial cutaneous nerve of the arm and the medial cutaneous nerve of the forearm.

If paraesthesiae are not felt in the arm and hand after one or two needle thrusts, the upper surface of the first rib is contacted and the needle inserted onto it so that the pulsations of the subclavian artery are transmitted to the needle. This is at a depth of 1.2–2.5 cm. Doppler ultrasound will aid localization.[145] After a negative aspiration test, 10 ml of solution are injected between the first rib and the skin. The needle is reintroduced onto the first rib, 1 cm laterally to the first position, and 10 ml similarly injected. Third and fourth injections are made, each 1 cm lateral to the last, and at each point 10 ml is injected between skin and rib. Efficiency is improved if a nerve stimulator and an insulated needle are used. (*See* Kaiser H. et al. *Reg. Anaesth.* 1990, **13**, 143, 172.) If stimulation is felt in the second, third or fourth fingers, a successful block results in over 90% of cases. It may be incomplete if only the first and fifth fingers react to stimulation.[146]

Analgesia is rapid in onset if paraesthesiae are present; if not, an interval of 20 min may be necessary. A feeling of warmth and 'pins and needles' precedes analgesia, and motor paralysis, when it occurs, follows analgesia.

An area of skin over the point of the shoulder and another on the inner aspect of the upper arm from the axilla to its midpoint (intercostohumeral T2) are not made insensitive. A subcutaneous band of injection downwards from the acromioclavicular joint and surrounding the shoulder will render these areas analgesic. Occasionally, median nerve block at the wrist is necessary, as the palm of the hand, supplied by the middle trunk (C7) of the plexus via the median nerve, is the most resistant area to successful block.

Lignocaine 2% solution with adrenaline, or longer-acting drugs, will produce sensory and motor paralysis. Solution of 1% will give sensory loss alone for about 1 h. Nerve suturing or trimming requires the use of the stronger solutions. Toxic and ill or feeble patients should have the strength of solution and not the volume reduced.

Horner's syndrome may or may not follow injection. It is due to paralysis of the cervical sympathetic chain. For details, *see above*.

Continuous brachial plexus block.[147]

Complications

1. Paralysis of phrenic nerve often occurs.[148] At the level of the first rib, the phrenic nerve is separated from the brachial plexus by the scalenus anterior muscle. Higher in the neck it is the same fascial compartment as the upper components of the plexus. Analgesic solution injected into the tissue surrounding the plexus can therefore ascend to block the phrenic nerve. Such a block is harmless and causes no symptoms, even if bilateral, but if the patient has a respiratory difficulty, e.g. emphysema or kyphosis, or if a general anaesthetic is to be administered, the possibility of diaphragmatic paralysis must be borne in mind. There is a high hemidiaphragm on X-ray examination.

2. Puncture of vessels, including subclavian artery. Haematomata may form but cause no trouble. Intravascular injection must be avoided.

3. Pneumothorax. Due to piercing Sibsons fascia.[149] Trouble seldom occurs. The axillary approach avoids this complication. Silent pneumothorax is unlikely as air in the chest is usually accompanied by pain. Surgical emphysema may be seen, probably due to wounding of the lung by the

needle. If a radiograph shows a large area of lung collapse, air should be withdrawn from the chest. Bilateral pneumothorax may be a dangerous condition.

Pain in the chest during needling may also be due to irritation of the nerve to the serratus anterior.

4. Toxic effect of drug injected. Slow injection lessens chance of this.

5. Postoperative disability following brachial plexus block is rare, although the paralysing effects of bupivacaine or ropivacaine may last many hours.[150]

Interscalene approach (cervical approach)[151]

Described by Labat in 1927[152] but modern use is due to Alon Winnie.[153] The sheath of the plexus can be entered via the interscalene space between the anterior and middle scalene muscles at the level of C6. The patient lies supine, arms by the sides and head turned away from the side to be injected. The level of C6 may be obtained by palpation of the cricoid cartilage or of the sixth transverse process (Chassaignac's tubercle). At the edge of the sternomastoid muscle the palpating finger lies on the scalenus anterior muscle and more laterally the groove between the anterior and middle scalene muscles can be felt. A needle is inserted perpendicular to the skin and passing the external jugular vein advanced until the point is felt to enter the perivascular space by a click. After the injection of a small volume of fluid, there should be a 'flow-back' on aspiration.[154] After careful aspiration tests the desired volume of analgesic solution is injected (e.g. 25–40 ml). When this is completed the patient may be sat up and gentle massage used to aid downward spread of solution. For complete analgesia of the inner aspect of the upper arm, block of the intercostohumeral nerve (T1–2) may be required. Permanent neurological damage has been reported.[155]

Although the dangers of pneumothorax are avoided, there is risk of injection into the extradural space, into CSF or the vertebral artery, and bilateral block of the cervical and brachial plexuses.[156] The needle should not be inserted more than 3 cm.[157] Successful injection blocks both the cervical and brachial plexuses. Suitable for operations on the shoulder joint[158] and for the reduction of Colles fracture. The complications are the same as may arise from the supraclavicular approach. Bupivacaine, 30 ml of 0.375% or ropivacaine with adrenaline may be used. Complete onset of block may take 30 min. An acute exacerbation of asthma has been reported in an asthmatic patient.[159]

The subclavian (supraclavicular) perivascular technique

The recumbent patient is told to turn his head to the opposite side and to touch his knee. The tip of the anaesthetist's index finger is placed posterior to the lateral border of the relaxed sternomastoid at the level of C6 (cricoid cartilage). The tip of the finger moves medially behind the belly of the sternomastoid and enters the interscalene groove and edged inferiorly. The interscalene groove is palpated, and followed down until the subclavian artery is felt pulsating. At this point, a short-bevelled needle is inserted through the clavicular head of sternomastoid, and pushed downwards (caudally) until it enters the perivascular space, shown by paraesthesia in the arm (not the shoulder because this may be due to irritation of the suprascapular nerve) or by a click as the needle pierces the fascia. After aspiration, 20–40 ml of solution is injected slowly. The intercostobrachial and the medial brachial cutaneous nerve (C8–T1) must in addition be blocked by a few millilitres of solution injected subcutaneously over the axillary artery if a tourniquet is to be applied.

Axillary approach to brachial plexus[160]

Used by Labat in 1922,[161] by Burnham[162] a surgeon, who revived the idea of Reding,[143] concerning a fascial compartment and Eather[163] in 1958. Hirschel injected it 'blind', through the axilla, in 1911.[164] In the axilla the nerves from the brachial plexus, together with the main artery, are enclosed in a fibrous neuromuscular fascial sheath. The median and musculocutaneous nerves together with their sensory branches are anterior or anterolateral, i.e. above and beyond the artery; the ulnar nerve is inferior; the radial nerve is posterolateral or below and behind the vessel. The musculocutaneous and axillary nerves are given off high in the axilla.

Block follows if analgesic solution is injected periarterially into the fibrous neurovascular sheath.

Technique. The patient lies supine with the arm abducted at a right angle, the humerus externally rotated and the elbow flexed. The skin of the axilla is not shaved but is well cleaned and a weal is raised at the highest part of the axilla at which arterial pulsation is felt, proximal to the lower border of the pectoralis major. The pulsating vessel is identified and through the weal a 2.5–5 cm short bevelled needle is inserted until a click shows that the neurovascular sheath has been entered; a paraesthesia indicates that the point has entered the sheath. It is easy to push the needle too deeply and to thus avoid the sheath. Local analgesic solution, e.g. 20 ml of 1–2% lignocaine with adrenaline, is placed in each quadrant surrounding the vessel. Alternatively, bupivacaine or ropivacaine may be employed to a total dose of 1.5 mg/kg. The addition of potassium chloride to 0.25% solution of bupivacaine (but not to prilocaine) causes a more rapid onset of sensory block.[165] To prevent dissipation of the solution downwards in the neurovascular space, firm finger pressure is applied below the needle during and after the injection or the arm elevated. Occasionally the musculocutaneous nerve (C6), which is a continuation of the lateral cord of the plexus, is given off higher than usual and consequently escapes the effects of local analgesic solution injected in the neurovascular space. In such cases it can be dealt with by the injection of 10–15 ml of solution from a point 2.5 cm distal to the crease of the elbow joint in the cleft between the tendon of the biceps and the brachioradialis where it becomes the lateral antebrachial cutaneous nerve, or the original needle can be inserted superior to the vascular bundle and 5 ml of solution injected into the substance of the coracobrachialis muscle. Similarly, a few drops of solution may be injected just superficial to the neurovascular bundle, to block the intercostobrachial nerve, which supplies the inner and outer aspects of the upper arm. An area of skin over the point of the shoulder supplied by the intercostohumeral nerve (T1 and T2) is not blocked by this approach. Onset of analgesia takes up to 30 min. If necessary, reinforcement of the ulnar distribution will follow ulnar nerve block just proximal to the ulnar nerve sulcus above the 'funny' bone. The use of a nerve stimulator before injection increases the efficiency of brachial plexus block by the axillary route.[166]

An alternative approach is to enter the neurovascular sheath at the lowest point of the axilla just posterior to the head of biceps, where pulsation is felt. The plexus is quite superficial at this point.

Extent of block by axillary approach. Complete analgesia below the elbow joint. Good sympathetic block of arm. Shoulder joint, supplied by the suprascapular nerve (C5 and C6), not made insensitive, so reductions of dislocation of this joint cannot be performed under axillary block as they can under the supraclavicular block. A subcutaneous ring injection at the level of the initial weal may be required for the painless application of a tourniquet. Pain from ischaemia caused by an arterial tourniquet may not be completely obtunded unless a 2% solution of lignocaine, mepivacaine or prilocaine is used.

Advantages. Only one landmark, the axillary artery. No paraesthesiae so less chance of nerve damage. No possibility of pneumothorax, stellate ganglion, recurrent laryngeal nerve block or phrenic nerve block. Less pain during injection. Difficult in obesity or when the arm cannot be abducted. Continuous block, using a catheter, eases pain following trauma to the arm.[167]

Brachial plexus block is a most satisfactory method of analgesia, although less popular since the reintroduction of intravenous regional analgesia. For dislocations of the shoulder joint or elbow joint, for tendon suture, for manipulation of fractures under the X-ray screen, for suturing of lacerations, etc., the method is excellent. A tourniquet may be applied to the upper arm even in the absence of analgesia of the inner aspect of the upper arm. It is more sucessful in cases with a previously painless limb than in those with an existing painful lesion, e.g. a fracture or abscess.

Injury to the brachial plexus following brachial plexus block may be due to lack of support for the anaesthetized limb after operation.[168]

Breast surgery

Major operations on the breast are not satisfactory under regional analgesia, but biopsies can be obtained without pain using lignocaine and adrenaline.[169]

Intravenous regional analgesia

History

This was first described by Bier in 1908 who used procaine[170] but it never became popular. Its use today follows the work of Holmes in 1963, then of Oxford, who substituted the more powerful lignocaine for procaine.[171] It was also described by Riha in 1962.[172]

Intravenous injection of local analgesic agents has been used for: (1) general anaesthesia; (2) in the treatment of cardiac dysrhythmias; and (3) to produce local analgesia.

Local analgesia involves the injection of a local analgesic solution into a vein of a limb that has been made ischaemic by a tourniquet. Most useful for operations on arms but can also be used in the leg.

Technique

A cannula is inserted into a vein on the dorsum of the hand (preferably not in the forearm) and very firmly secured; another should be in a vein in the other limb in case of toxic signs. Veins in the forearm or antecubital fossa are better avoided. The limb is drained of blood by elevation for 5 min, with or without compression of the brachial artery. An Esmarch bandage,[173] the Rhys-Davies exsanguinator (an inflatable pneumatic cylinder that is easier to apply and less uncomfortable[174]) or an orthopaedic pneumatic splint[175] can also be used for this purpose. Two narrow sphygmomanometer cuffs are securely placed on the upper arm, one proximal to the other, and the upper one inflated to a pressure a little above the systolic blood pressure, before removal of the compression or pneumatic bandage (if used). Injection of the local analgesic solution now follows, and after 5–10 min, the lower cuff is inflated and the upper one released, to minimize discomfort. A tourniquet that does not occlude the brachial artery throughout the operation may result in congestion of the limb, absorption of the drug and imperfect analgesia. Close attention to detail and to the efficiency of the apparatus is most important.[176] The patient is ready for operation after an interval of 10 min. Analgesia and motor weakness continue while the tourniquet remains inflated. The block has been used successfully in children, and also on the lower extremity, in which case the cuff should be placed on the mid-calf.[181]

Note that tourniquet release can cause changes in the blood concentrations of drugs other than the local analgesic.[177] Intravenous analgesia below the knee, using prilocaine, has been used, but for perfect results requires near-toxic doses.[181]

Local analgesic solutions

Whereas 0.5% lignocaine or prilocaine[178] are effective and popular, 0.2% bupivacaine is efficient but potentially toxic and should not be used. Volumes: lignocaine or prilocaine 0.5%, 3–4 mg/kg, e.g. 30–40 ml; solutions should be free of preservative.

The information derived from angiography of the upper limb may be increased if guanethidine is used to produce sympathetic block, using the Bier technique.[179]

Cuff deflation

This is better done in stages although interosseous leak may occur. Analgesic drug is released into the circulation in a biphasic manner. There is an initial fast release of 30%, but 50% may still be present in the limb 30 min later.[180] Toxic signs may be drowsiness, twitches, jactitations or convulsions, bradycardia proceeding to asystole, hypotension and ECG abnormalities. The patient should be carefully observed during the 10 min following release of the cuff. Reinflation may be considered if signs of toxicity arise.

Contra-indications

These may include Raynaud's disease, sickle-cell anaemia and scleroderma. Reactionary oedema may follow release of the cuff, so that in plaster work a back splint should be applied and splintage completed in a few days time.

The site of action of the drug is on the peripheral nerve endings, and also on nerve trunks when stronger solutions are used.

Intravenous regional analgesia of one finger has been reported.[182]

Because of its toxicity, bupivacaine should not be used.

Intravenous sympathetic block

Guanethidine 10–20 mg with 500 units of heparin in 25 ml of saline has been used to reduce pain; a form of regional blockade.[183]

(For a full review of this subject, *see* Goold J. E. *Br. J. Hosp. Med.* 1985, **33**, 335.)

Intra-arterial local analgesia

Introduced by Goyanes, a Spaniard, in 1912.[184]

A pneumatic cuff is applied to the upper arm, and a fine, short-bevel needle, attached to a 20-ml syringe containing 0.5% lignocaine solution, is introduced into the brachial artery near the elbow. The cuff is then inflated until arterial pulsations are occluded and the solution injected intra-arterially 5 ml at a time until the desired analgesic effect is obtained. The average dose in adults is 14–15 ml, considerably less than would be required in intravenous regional analgesia. Unsuccessful attempts at intra-arterial injection may cause temporary vascular spasm, but no other complications were seen in van Niekerk and Coetzee's series of 300 cases.[185]

Distal nerve blocks

Elbow block

Intradermal and subcutaneous circles of infiltration are made just proximal to the internal epicondyle.

Median block is obtained by injecting through a weal placed midway between the outer side of the tendon of the biceps and the medial epicondyle, or from a weal 1 cm medial to the brachial artery at the bend of the elbow. The needle should be inserted in an upward direction. If paraesthesiae are felt, success is likely: 5 ml of 2% lignocaine is used. The median nerve supplies the lateral part of the palm of the hand and fingers.

Radial block together with block of the lateral cutaneous nerve of the forearm, the sensory continuation of the musculocutaneous nerve, is performed through a weal 1 cm lateral to the tendon of the biceps at the line of the bend of the elbow. The needle is directed upwards to reach the front of the outer surface of the lateral epicondyle and solution injected between the bone and the skin.

Alternatively, a weal is raised four finger-breadths proximal to the lateral epicondyle of the humerus, which overlies the point where the nerve pierces the intermuscular septum and is close to the bone. The needle is advanced perpendicularly to the skin towards the bone and 20 ml of analgesic solution is injected above and below the point of injection.

Ulnar block is performed 2 or 3 cm proximal to the point where the nerve can be palpated behind the medial epicondyle using 2–4 ml of 2% lignocaine. The ulnar nerve supplies skin on the medial side of the palmar and dorsal aspects of the hand and 5th and medial part of 4th fingers.

Wrist block

Circular lines of intradermal and subcutaneous infiltration are carried out just above the wrist-joint.

Median nerve (C5–T1). The median nerve at the wrist lies deeply between the flexor carpi radialis laterally and the palmaris longus and flexor digitorum sublimis medially. It is injected with 5 ml of 1% lignocaine immediately lateral to the tendon of the palmaris longus with the hand dorsiflexed. Attempts to elicit paraesthesiae are made, but if unsuccessful the solution is injected nevertheless. The median nerve supplies the skin of the thenar eminence and of the anterior aspects of the lateral three and a half fingers together with the skin over the dorsal aspects of their terminal phalanges. Median nerve block at the wrist or elbow may be followed by neuritis.

Ulnar nerve (C7–T1). Divides 5 cm above the wrist joint into superficial terminal or palmar mixed, and dorsal sensory branches.

The superficial terminal branch lies between the flexor carpi ulnaris tendon and the ulnar artery. It supplies the medial part of the palm of the hand and the palmar aspect of the fifth and medial side of the ring finger. The pisiform bone is immediately medial to it. Its sensory branch is blocked from a weal immediately lateral to the flexor carpi ulnaris.

The dorsal branch is anaesthetized by intradermal and subcutaneous injection along a line at the level of the ulnar styloid from the medial side of the tendon of the flexor carpi ulnaris to the middle of the back of the wrist. It supplies the ulnar border of the dorsum of the hand.

Radial or musculospiral nerve (C5–T1). The sensory nerve of the back of the lateral part of the hand. After accompanying the radial artery along the medial border of the brachioradialis, it passes 6–7 cm above the wrist joint beneath the tendon of that muscle and comes to lie beneath the skin on the extensor aspect of the lower forearm and wrist. It can be blocked by infiltrating between the skin and the bone on the posterolateral aspect of the wrist joint near the base of the thumb lateral to the radial artery.

Wrist block, with a finger tourniquet, is useful for surgery of the hand, especially if motor function is required during the operation. It does not remove the discomfort of an Esmarch bandage on the forearm.

Elbow and wrist block are often unwise in the presence of neuritis or carpal tunnel syndrome, but intravenous regional analgesia is not contra-indicated.

Nerve supply of the palm of the hand is from the ulnar and median nerves, with the radial supplying part of the thumb. (The sole of the foot is supplied by the sural and the lateral and medial branches of the tibial nerve.) The palm can be blocked at the wrist and the sole at the ankle.

Field block for operation on the digits

Two palmar and two dorsal nerves supply each digit. With a fine (25G) needle an intradermal weal is raised on the dorsum of the finger near its base. Lignocaine, 2 ml of 1 or 2% solution (or one of its congeners) is injected into the substance of the finger through this weal between the bone and the skin and repeated on the other side of the digit. The weals should be connected by 1 ml of solution between skin and bone on the dorsal aspect. Analgesia may take 15 min to become established. The palmar skin is not pierced. *Adrenaline should not be used*. Another method of blocking the finger is to inject 5–7 ml of 1% lignocaine solution in the interosseous spaces at each side of the metacarpal bone, entering from the dorsal aspect and carrying the needle almost to the palmar skin. Spread of infection due to this technique is very rare, providing that solution is not injected into infected tissue.

If a tourniquet is used, no more than 3 ml of solution should be injected; a tourniquet must not remain on the finger for more than 15 min and not used at all in patients with Raynauds's disease.[186]

A similar technique, using less solution, can be employed on the toe. Intravenous regional analgesia of one finger has been reported.[182]

Paravertebral somatic block

This method was introduced by Hugo Sellheim of Leipzig (1871–1936) in 1906[187] and developed by Läwen in 1911, who called it 'paravertebral conduction anaesthesia',[188] and by Kappis (1881–1938).[189] It involves injecting a local analgesic close to the vertebral column where the nerve trunks emerge from the intervertebral foramina.

Macintosh and Bryce-Smith, in a well-illustrated book,[190] describe the paravertebral space as a wedge-shaped compartment, bounded above and below by the heads and necks of adjoining ribs; posteriorly by the superior costotransverse ligament; medially it communicates with the extradural space through the intervertebral foramen; laterally its apex leads into the intercostal space. The base is formed by the posterolateral aspect of the body of the vertebra and the intervertebral foramen and its contents.

There is no direct communication between one paravertebral space and another, but an indirect communication exists medially through the intervertebral foramen with the extradural space. Spread from one paravertebral space to another, across the extradural space, is frequent and may involve nerves on the same or on the opposite side of the body.

When the first thoracic to second lumbar nerve roots are blocked, their rami communicantes are blocked too.

PARAVERTEBRAL CERVICAL BLOCK

Described under Cervical plexus block.

PARAVERTEBRAL THORACIC BLOCK

It is indicated for operations on the chest or abdominal wall, for relief of postoperative pain, post-herpetic pain and the pain of fractured ribs.[191]

Technique. Skin weals are raised 4 cm from the midline, opposite the lower borders of the vertebral spines. Through each weal, a needle is inserted perpendicularly to strike bone near the lateral extremity of the transverse process. It is then redirected to pass upwards and slightly medially over the upper border of the transverse process and at this point local analgesic solution is injected. Aspiration tests should be conducted to ensure that the needle point has not entered a vessel or the dura. Puncture of the pleura is also possible. (*See also* Cleland J. G. P. *Surg. Gynecol. Obstet.* 1933, **57**, 51.)

Lumbar sympathetic block

Surgical lumbar sympathectomy was described at the Mayo Clinic in 1929[192] and by Leriche (1879–1955) and Fontaine in 1934.[193] Phenol injected by Mandl in 1947.[194] A technique using phenol dissolved in a radio-opaque medium and an image intensifier has been used.[195] (*See also* Cleland J. G. P. *Surg. Gynecol. Obstet.* 1933, **57**, 51; reprinted in 'Classical File' *Surv. Anesthesiol.* 1981, **25**, 341.)

Anatomy

The sympathetic trunk in the lumbar region consists of four ganglia and their interconnecting fibres. It lies on the anterolateral aspect of the bodies of the lumbar vertebrae, immediately medial to the psoas muscle, which fills the triangular space between the vertebral bodies and the transverse processes. A tendinous arch, which gives part origin to the psoas muscle, connects the upper and lower borders of each lumbar vertebra and forms a tunnel around the side of the bone in which the lumbar vessels and the grey ramus communicans run. The lumbar arteries are posterior but the veins may be anterior. The fatty tissue occupying this tunnel is an extension of that in the extradural space and it passes through the intervertebral foramina as far forward as the sympathetic chain. The chain lies in a fascial plane bounded by the vertebral column, the psoas sheath and the parietal peritoneum. L1 is on a level with the intersection of the last rib and the outer border of the erector spinae. The L4–L5 interspace corresponds to the highest point of the iliac crests in many patients.

In the sacral region, each chain consists of four ganglia with intervening fibres lying medial to the anterior sacral foramina. Preganglionic fibres (white rami) are derived from the anterior primary rami from T4 to T12 and each ganglion gives off a grey ramus to the corresponding sacral nerve, to supply sympathetic innervation to the lower limbs. On the coccyx, the two chains unite to form the ganglion impar.

Disturbances of function of the sympathetic nervous system can produce: (1) vasospasm: (2) pain; and (3) visceral dysfunction. Sympathetic block can remedy all of these, either temporarily, for diagnosis, or permanently, by interrupting a vicious circle.

Indications

See Chapter 27.

Technique

Posterior approach.[196] The patient is placed in the prone position, with two pillows flexing the lumbar spine, or in lateral spinal position with the affected side uppermost and the spine flexed. He should be premedicated with a sedative. The procedure can be carried out in the patient's bed if necessary.

1. Skin weals are raised at points 5 cm lateral to the upper borders of the spinous processes of the 2nd, 3rd and 4th lumbar vertebrae. Successful injection at these points blocks all the vasoconstrictor impulses to the lower limb. These points lie immediately above the transverse processes of the corresponding vertebrae. A 12–16-cm needle is introduced through each weal at right angles to the skin for 4–5 cm and should encounter the transverse process; it is slightly withdrawn and directed upwards so that it passes between the transverse processes; it is also directed slightly inwards. After travelling 3–4 cm from the transverse process, the needle should make contact with the anterolateral aspect of the body of the vertebra. After careful aspiration to exclude both blood and cerebrospinal fluid, 10 ml of 1% lignocaine is injected at each site. (If force is required, needle tip is in anterior vertebral ligament or the psoas muscle and should be slightly withdrawn.) The solution spreads out in the retroperitoneal tissue. The spinal lumbar nerves run midway between the spinous processes, so if the needle point is kept in relation to the upper border of the transverse process, pain from hitting a nerve should be avoided. The lumbar arteries, branches of the aorta, with their veins must also be avoided. After 5–20 min the leg becomes less painful, its temperature increases and it becomes dry, its superficial veins dilate, and there is hyposensitivity to pin-prick.

2. A 12-cm needle is inserted at an angle of 70° through a weal three finger-breadths lateral to the superior point of the spinous process of L3. It should miss the transverse process and come into contact with the body of the vertebra in the psoas tunnel: 15–20 ml of analgesic fluid is then injected.[197]

Use of X-ray control with an image intensifier greatly adds to the accuracy of needle placement.[195] Results of chemical lumbar sympathectomy can be assessed by taking infra-red thermograms before and after the injections.[198]

For chemical sympathectomy three needles are placed against the bodies of L2, L3 and L4 and their position verified radiologically; 3 ml of either 6% phenol in water or absolute alcohol, preceded by local analgesia, are injected through each correctly placed needle.[199]

Lateral approach. See Wallace C. *Anesthesiology* 1955, **16**, 254.

For assessment and monitoring of sympathetic block, *see* Cronin K. D. and Kirsner R. L. G. *Anaesth. Intensive Care* 1979, **7**, 353.

(*See also* Klopper G. T. *Anaesth. Intensive Care* 1983, **11**, 43.)

Complications

1. Intradural injection and spinal analgesia.
2. Intravascular injection.
3. Hypotension.
4. Haemorrhage into the sheath of the psoas muscle with pain referred to the groin and upper and inner part of the thigh.
5. Neuritis of the genitofemoral nerve.

Caudal block gives the same results but is not unilateral; it produces, in addition to sympathetic paralysis, motor paresis and analgesia, which may be useful objective signs of successful sympathetic block.

(*See also* Cherr D. A. et al. *Anaesth. Intensive Care* 1978, **6**, 164; Walker P. M. et al. *Surg. Gynecol. Obstet.* 1978, **146**, 741; Goldring J. R. et al. *J. R. Coll. Surg. Edin.* 1979, **24**, 83; Cousins M. J. et al. *Anaesth. Intensive Care* 1979, **7**, 121.)

Intercostal nerve blocks

The cutaneous distribution of spinal nerves was worked out by O. Foerster (1873–1941) of Breslau and by Henry Head (1866–1940) of London.

The cutaneous nerves

Figs 24.2–24.4.

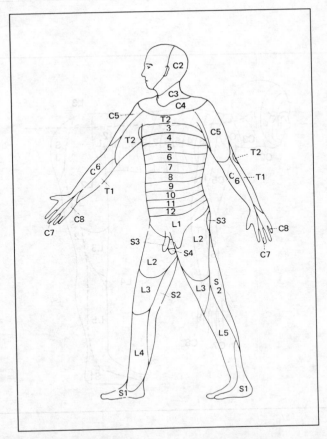

Figure 24.2–4 Distribution of cutaneous nerves (*after* Foerster O. *Brain* 1933, **56**, 1).

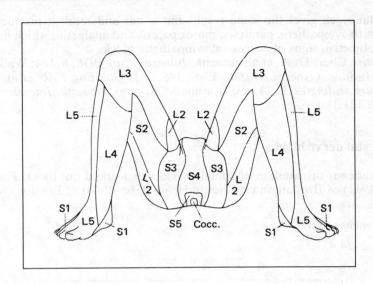

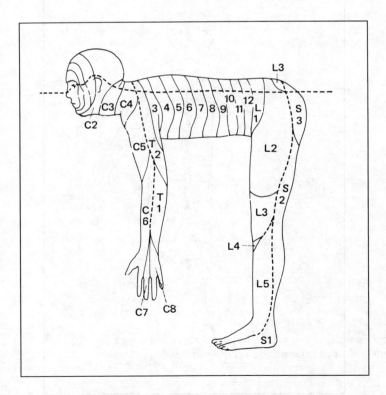

Figure 24.2–4 *Continued.*

Anteriorly.
1. The lateral, intermediate and medial supraclavicular branches of the superficial division of the cervical plexus (C3–C4) to the second interspace.
2. The anterior rami of the thoracic nerves, excluding T1.
3. The iliohypogastric and ilio-inguinal nerves (L1).
Posteriorly. The posterior rami of C2–C5; T1–T12; L1–L3; the five sacral and the coccygeal nerves.

Anatomy of spinal nerves

Typical intercostal nerves are the 3rd to 6th inclusive. Each nerve is formed by the union of the anterior (motor) and the posterior (sensory) root; the latter has a ganglion on it. The mixed spinal nerve soon divides into anterior and posterior primary divisions (rami). The thoracic or dorsal nerves then are distributed as follows:

The posterior rami are smaller than the anterior. They turn backwards and divide into medial and lateral branches (except C1, S4 and S5, coccygeal), which supply the muscles and skin of the back.

The anterior rami in the thoracic region of the 2nd to 6th nerves are each connected to the lateral sympathetic chain by a grey and a white ramus communicans. Each crosses the paravertebral space between the necks of contiguous ribs and then enters the subcostal groove where it lies below the vein and artery in a triangular space, bounded above by the rib, the posterior intercostal membrane and the internal intercostal muscle (intercostal intima)[200] until it reaches the anterior axillary line, at which point the nerves come into direct relationship with the pleura, as the innermost intercostal muscle terminates. There is a communication between each space and those contiguous to it, while analgesic solution spreads medially to surround the sympathetic chain in the paravertebral space.[200] Each intercostal nerve supplies muscular branches to the intercostal muscles and lateral and anterior cutaneous branches to supply the skin of the chest and abdomen. The 7th to 11th nerves pass below and behind the costal cartilages, between the slips of the diaphragm running between the internal oblique and transversus muscles (again between the second and third layers) to enter the posterior layer of the rectus sheath. They run deep into the rectus, pierce and supply it, and end as anterior cutaneous nerves.

The lateral cutaneous branch emerges in the midaxillary line, and divides into anterior and posterior branches, which supply the skin on the lateral wall of the chest as far forward as the nipple line.

The anterior cutaneous branch is the termination of the intercostal nerve; it supplies the skin on the front of the chest, internal to the nipple line.

Exceptions. The 1st nerve parts with most of its fibres to the brachial plexus and gives neither lateral nor anterior cutaneous branches, the skin over the first intercostal space being supplied by the descending branches of the cervical plexus (C3–C4). The lateral cutaneous branch of the second intercostal nerve crosses the axilla and becomes the intercostobrachial nerve supplying the skin on the medial aspect of the arm. The lateral cutaneous branch of the 12th thoracic nerve, which does not divide into anterior and posterior branches, crosses the iliac crest to supply the skin of the upper part of the buttock as far as the greater trochanter. The 12th thoracic and 1st lumbar nerves supply sensory branches to the anterior chest and anterior abdominal wall, the parietal pleura and the parietal peritoneum.

The 10th nerve, lateral and anterior cutaneous branches, supplies the area of the umbilicus.

The 9th, 8th and 7th nerves supply the skin between the umbilicus and the xiphisternum.

The 11th, 12th and 1st lumbar nerves supply the skin between the umbilicus and the pubis.

Technique of intercostal nerve block

1. At the angle of the ribs (Sellheim (1871–1936), 1906,[201] James, 1943[204]) At this point the nerve becomes relatively superficial, lateral to the erector spinae muscle. In this technique the rami communicantes conveying afferent impulses may be blocked by the local analgesic solution tracking medially but splanchnic analgesia will be necessary in addition for intra-abdominal surgery. The patient is arranged in the lateral spinal position with his back well arched over the edge of the table. After swabbing with antiseptic and fixing sterile towels, two lines are drawn, one on each side four finger-breadths from the middle line, the lines should extend from the spines of the scapulae to the iliac crests. At a point where the lower border of the 11th rib on the patient's upper side crosses the line, a needle is introduced (through an intradermal weal if necessary) until it makes contact with the rib. It is then partially withdrawn and advanced until it slips past the lower border of the rib for 3 mm; 2–3 ml of local analgesic solution with adrenaline is then injected, while the needle point is slightly advanced and withdrawn so as to surround the nerve with analgesic solution. The intercostal nerve is thus surrounded by a zone of solution as it lies in the subcostal groove between the intercostalis internus and the internal intercostal muscles. The needle should be mounted on a syringe, so that should the pleura be punctured no air will enter the pleural cavity.

The needle is then withdrawn until its point is just beneath the skin, so that it can act as a marker. The 10th to the 6th nerves are now injected on the upper side, followed, after turning, by the lower seven nerves on the patient's other side. The 12th nerves are deeper and require special care. Before the 6th and 7th nerves can be injected the patient's scapulae must be drawn laterally by crossing his arms over his chest. The needle pierces the trapezius, the latissimus dorsi and the two intercostal muscles. Good analgesia for up to 12 h results if the abdominal incision is subcostal. For paramedian or midline incisions, bilateral block is necessary.[200] A possible complication is pneumothorax.[201] Another is intradural injection.[203]

Posterior splanchnic block can be performed with the patient in the same position if the abdomen is to be opened.

2. In the posterior axillary line. First reported in 1915.[204] Similar injections can be carried out with the patient supine and with his arms abducted to a right angle. In this position the ribs, and so the intercostal nerves, are not so deeply placed. A block in the midaxillary line misses the lateral cutaneous nerve. Local analgesic solution injected via an extradural catheter often spreads to several spaces above and below the point of injection, external to the pleura.[187] This spread was not seen in Moore's cases.[202] Massive haematoma formation has been reported.[200, 205]

3. In the midaxillary line. It has been shown that the intercostal nerves can be blocked at the level of the midaxillary line in supine patients as effectively as at the posterior angle of the ribs.

Indications

Blocking of the lower seven intercostal nerves on each side results in analgesia of the anterior abdominal wall from just below the nipple line to a level just above the pubic bone. In addition, it produces analgesia of the parietal peritoneum and relaxation of the muscles of the anterior abdominal wall. It is especially useful when scars from previous operations disturb the relations of the abdominal wall making abdominal field block difficult. For analgesia of the viscera, splanchnic analgesia is required in addition.

To give a longer period of analgesia, 0.25 or 0.5% bupivacaine or amethocaine hydrochloride 1 in 2000 to 1 in 4000 solution may be used, 3 ml being injected at 12-hourly intervals for up to 36 hours.[205] Care must be taken to avoid a toxic dose of these and other agents and adrenaline should be added. Absorption is rapid.

Intercostal block is also useful to enable deep breathing and coughing to take place in a patient with severe postoperative abdominal pain or with fractured ribs but does not always produce good results.[206]

Blood levels of local analgesic solutions injected near the intercostal nerves rise rapidly.

A cryoprobe applied to intercostal nerves within the thorax has been used to reduce post-thoracotomy pain[207] There is evidence that more complications follow attack on the intercostal nerves from inside the thorax than when it is injected percutaneously.[208]

Intercostal block for rib resection and insertion of a drain

The surgeon is asked to mark out the position of the incision he wishes to make, and it is infiltrated intradermally and subcutaneously with 0.5–1% lignocaine solution. An intradermal and subcutaneous line of infiltration is carried out one rib above and one below the length of rib to be removed. Their lines extend 2.5 cm in front and 2.5 cm behind the proposed incision, and the extremities are joined by intradermal and subcutaneous infiltrations, so that a rectangle is marked out. The intercostal nerves within this rectangle are blocked at their posterior extremities with 2% lignocaine solution. There may be slight discomfort during the stripping of the periosteum from the rib by the surgeon.

Local block is usually the preferred method of anaesthesia in these operations. If the patient is well enough, he should sit sideways across the table, to prevent him drowning in his own pus if the abscess ruptures into a bronchus. Otherwise he is placed in the lateral position with the head and shoulders elevated. This position is also suitable for general anaesthesia.[209]

Interpleural block for intercostal nerves[210–213]

The analgesic solution is given as a single injection, or as an infusion through a cannula inserted between the ribs into the pleural space. Identifying the pleural space without causing a pneumothorax requires care. The skin may be punctured with a sharp needle just above a rib (at the angle of the rib, or in the axillary line). A semi-blunt needle, e.g. Tuohy, attached to a saline- or local analgesic-filled syringe, is inserted and loss of resistance used to identify the interpleural space. Spontaneous respiration makes puncture of the lung less likely at this point. The needle hub is occluded beween detaching the syringe and inserting the catheter, to prevent air rushing in. Various systems are available for this. Bupivacaine 20 ml of 0.5% or ropivacaine will produce a block lasting up to 4 h. Continuous infusion is less effective than intermittent injection, possibly due to regional interpleural pressure profiles. The technique is frequently used to control post cholecystectomy pain,[215] and after other abdominal operations. It has been used in chronic pain.[214]

Toxic effects are rare after boluses of 20 ml of 0.5% bupivacaine or ropivacaine with adrenaline 1 in 200 000.

Complications: Pneumothorax, damage to intercostal vessels during insertion, and toxic signs of abnormally rapid absorption of drug from pleural space.[216, 217]

Subcostal block of abdominal wall for laparotomy

This is an extremely easy, quick and useful block for all types of laparotomy, to enhance relaxation and give postoperative pain relief. *See* Chapter 22.

Splanchnic analgesia; coeliac plexus block

Anatomy[218]

Semilunar or coeliac plexus. Two in number, one on each side of the midline, lying on the aorta and the crura of the diaphragm just above the pancreas, at the level of the 1st lumbar vertebra between the adrenal glands and behind the stomach and lesser sac. The renal vessels are inferior to the plexus, and the vessels to the adrenals often pass through it. They are connected with each other and with their associated ganglia (superior mesenteric and inferior mesenteric, etc.) by a network of nerve fibres around the coeliac artery. These fibres are postganglionic fibres of the greater and lesser splanchnic nerves. From this mass of retroperitoneal nerve tissue, fibres pass with the arteries to the abdominal viscera. These plexuses also receive branches from the right vagus and the phrenic nerves. The semilunar or coeliac ganglia with the aorticorenal and superior mesenteric ganglia together make up the solar or epigastric plexus.

Afferent fibres from the abdominal viscera, both sympathetic and parasympathetic (vagus), pass through the coeliac ganglia. Afferent fibres from the pelvic viscera, travelling through the nervi erigentes (S2–S4) do not.

Greater splanchnic nerve (the superior thoracic splanchnic nerve). Like the lesser and the lowest splanchnic, is composed of pre-ganglionic fibres, which are, in effect, elongated white rami. The majority of its fibres are myelinated. It rises from the union of four or five roots coming from the thoracic sympathetic ganglia, which receive white rami from the 5th to the 10th thoracic nerves, sometimes higher. The nerve enters the abdomen through the crus of the diaphragm on each side, with the lesser and lowest splanchnic nerves, and enters the corresponding semilunar ganglion. It mainly contains visceral afferent fibres. Within the abdomen the nerve lies between the diaphragm and the adrenal gland on each side.

Lesser splanchnic nerve (the middle thoracic splanchnic nerve). This arises from the lower thoracic ganglia of the sympathetic cord, connected with the 10th and 11th thoracic nerves. It enters the corresponding aorticorenal ganglion.

Lowest splanchnic nerve (the inferior thoracic splanchnic nerve). This arises from the last thoracic ganglion and enters the renal plexus and the posterior renal ganglion.

The lumbar splanchnic nerves. Are presumably blocked when the coeliac plexus is blocked, by spreading of solution. The 1st lumbar splanchnic nerve arises from the 1st lumbar ganglion; the 2nd from the 2nd and 3rd ganglia (they join the coeliac plexus): the 3rd from the 2nd, 3rd and 4th ganglia; the 4th from the 4th and 5th ganglia. The last two join the superior hypogastric plexus.

The hypogastric nerve (presacral nerves). Extends from the 3rd lumbar vertebra to the 1st sacral where it ends by dividing into the right and left hypogastric nerves or plexuses. It lies in front of the lower part of the abdominal aorta, behind the peritoneum.

The superior hypogastric plexus

Formerly known as the presacral nerve. It is retroperitoneal, lying on the body of the fifth lumbar vertebra. It receives fibres from the sympathetic trunk via lumbar ganglia 3 and 4; fibres known as the intermesenteric plexus coming from the coeliac, mesenteric and pararenal plexuses; and parasympathetic fibres. From it are derived fibres supplying, via the inferior mesenteric artery the transverse, descending and sigmoid colon; the inferior hypogastric nerves to the rectum and ureters, which contain both sympathetic and parasympathetic elements.

The inferior hypogastric plexus

A collection of ganglia and nerve fibres where preganglionic sympathetic fibres synapse. It receives fibres from the inferior hypogastric nerves, together with parasympathetic fibres and supplies the viscera of the female pelvis (except the ovaries). Its sympathetic element provides sensory and motor fibres to the urinary and anal sphincters; the parasympathetic fibres are motor to the bladder and rectum. These fibres travel with blood vessels.

Many of these structures are damaged in pelvic operations. Division of the superior hypogastric plexus (presacral neurectomy) is used in the treatment of dysmenorrhoea.[219]

Afferent pathways from upper abdominal viscera

These visceral afferents travel from sensory nerve endings in the walls of the viscera, mesentery, etc. via the splanchnic nerves and enter the cord with the white rami of the lower seven thoracic nerves (and sometimes higher), having their cell stations in the posterior root ganglia of these nerves. Afferent impulses also travel up in the vagi and the phrenics.

Visceral afferent fibres, travelling with the sympathetic, enter the cord at the following levels: stomach, T6–10; small gut, T9–10; large gut to middle of transverse colon T11–L1; distal colon, L1–2; liver and biliary tract T7–9; pancreas T6–10; kidney and ureter T10–L2; bladder and prostate T11–12; testis and ovary T10–11; uterus T10–11.

Nerve supply to adrenal glands

Preganglionic fibres do not synapse in coeliac or other pre-aortic plexuses, but pass directly to end around chromaffin cells of the medulla. In addition to the lesser splanchnic, fibres go to the adrenals from the 10th thoracic to 2nd lumbar nerves.

Technique of splanchnic block

Splanchnic block can be performed before laparotomy (Wendling) or during laparotomy from the front (Braun), or before laparotomy from behind (Kappis). The Braun technique is usually performed by the surgeon.

1. *Braun's method.*[220] With the abdomen opened, the liver is gently retracted upwards and the stomach is drawn to the left. The anterior aspect of the body of the 1st lumbar vertebra is located medial to the lesser curvature of the stomach; the aorta is retracted laterally and the long Braun needle is inserted down to the bone and 50 ml of solution injected (e.g. 0.5% lignocaine).

2. *Kappis's method.* Described by Max Kappis (1881–1938) in 1914.[221] The patient is in the spinal position, sitting or lying prone. The 4th interspace is located, lying on or before the intercristal line; by counting upward, the spine of the 1st lumbar vertebra is identified. Weals are raised four finger-breadths from this spine, one in each side of the midline. The weals must be below the 12th rib.

A long needle is inserted at an angle of 45° to the median plane through this weal with its bevel facing inwards. It is directed slightly upwards and inserted until it makes contact with the body of the 1st lumbar vertebra. It is then partly withdrawn and its point directed more laterally until its bevel is felt to glance past the lateral aspect of the body of the vertebra. The needle is then advanced a further 1 cm and, after a most careful aspiration test, 20–40 ml of solution are injected. The average distance between the skin and the plexus is 7–10 cm. If blood is aspirated into the syringe, the needle point may be in the vena cava or the aorta and must be moved until it is free of these vessels. Bilateral block is probably unnecessary. The technique has been modified.[222] Fluoroscopy aids accurate placement of the needle. Computer-aided tomography-guided coeliac plexus block has been described,[223] and insertion of the needle at the level of L2 has been advocated.[225]

The usual strengths of solution employed are prilocaine, 0.5%; lignocaine, 0.5%; amethocaine, 1 in 2000 to 1 in 4000. Adrenaline should be added.

Splanchnic block causes a profound fall in blood pressure, which can be partially controlled by an intravenous infusion of fluid or by ephedrine or one of its congeners, should it be considered necessary. It produces analgesia of the abdominal viscera, with the exception of the pelvic viscera, i.e. the sigmoid colon, rectum, bladder and reproductive organs. The bowel becomes contracted and ribbon-like. The patient must be particularly well premedicated, intravenous narcotic analgesic being given until the mental state is calm. The surgeon must be light-handed, especially when the peritoneal cavity is being explored, because its lateral walls are not rendered insensitive either by the splanchnic block or the abdominal field block (but by posterior intercostal block).

Therapeutically, splanchnic block is useful in the treatment of carcinoma of the pancreas and acute pancreatitis (perhaps because it relaxes the sphincter of Oddi). It causes a greater blood supply to be diverted to the pancreas. If these conditions are found at laparotomy, splanchnic block with phenol has much to recommend it.[226] The block may be repeated if desirable. It has also been used in the terminal stages of upper abdominal cancer to relieve pain. Alcohol in saline, 50%, preceded by local analgesic solution, has been employed.[227] Paraplegia has followed this block.[228]

Abdominal field block

Described in 1905.[229]

Anatomy

The superficial fascia in the upper abdomen is a single fatty layer, but from a point midway between the umbilicus and the pubis two layers are described, the deep layer (fascia of Antonius Scarpa; 1747–1832) and the superficial layer (fascia of Petrus Camper; 1722–1789).

Camper's fascia passes over the inguinal ligament and is continuous with the superficial fascia of the thigh. It is continued over the penis, spermatic cord and scrotum where it helps to form the dartos muscle. In the female it is continued into the labia majora.

Scarpa's fascia is tougher. It blends with the deep fascia of the thigh and, like Camper's fascia, is continued over the penis and helps to form the dartos. From the scrotum it becomes continuous with Colles's fascia (1811) over the perineum. There is no deep fascia covering the abdomen.

External oblique. The largest and most superficial of the muscles of the anterior abdominal wall. The aponeurosis is attached below to the anterior superior spine and to the pubic crest and tubercle; it thus forms the inguinal ligament. In the midline it forms the linea alba, which runs from the symphysis pubis to the xiphisternum. The subcutaneous or external inguinal ring is an opening in the aponeurosis.

The fibres of the external oblique pass downwards and inwards, like those of the external intercostal muscles.

Internal oblique. This is a thinner layer than the above.

The fibres of this muscle run upwards and inwards.

Transversus abdominis. The fibres of the muscle run transversely. Between it and the external oblique run the lower intercostal, iliohypogastric and ilio-inguinal nerves. Below the level of the iliac crest the fibres of these three muscles are aponeurotic and run downwards and medially.

Rectus abdominis. Each muscle *arises* from the crest of the pubis and from the ligaments in front of the symphysis. *Inserted* into the anterior aspects of the 5th, 6th and 7th costal cartilages and into the xiphisternum.

Three tendinous intersections cross the muscle and are firmly attached to the anterior layer of its sheath, but not to the posterior layer. One is at the level of the xiphisternum, one at the umbilicus and the third one midway between.

The rectus sheath contains, in addition to the rectus and pyramidalis muscles, the superior and inferior epigastric vessels and the terminations of the lower six intercostal nerves and vessels. The nerves pierce the lateral margin of the sheath and run in relation to its posterior wall, before they enter the substance of the muscle.

Pyramidalis. A small muscle on each side, within the rectus sheath. It is well developed in marsupial mammals and serves to strengthen the linea alba.

The abdominal muscles are supplied by the anterior rami of the lower six thoracic nerves and by the iliohypogastric and ilio-inguinal nerves.

They are accessory muscles of expiration and help to compress the abdominal viscera, as in defaecation, straining, coughing, etc. They are not muscles of normal inspiration.

Transversalis fascia. A thin membrane, continuous with the iliac and pelvic fascia. In the inguinal region it is stronger and thicker than elsewhere and through it, at the abdominal inguinal (internal inguinal) ring, passes the spermatic cord or the round ligament.

Sensory nerve supply of abdominal wall. The anterior primary rami of the lower six thoracic nerves, via the intercostal nerves. The skin in the region of the nipple is supplied by the 5th thoracic nerve. Skin in the epigastrium is supplied by the 7th nerve. Skin in the region of the umbilicus is supplied by the 10th nerve. Skin midway between the umbilicus and the pubis is supplied by the 12th nerve. Skin of the groin is supplied by the iliohypogastric nerve (L1).

Intercostal nerves and the last thoracic nerve pass under the costal margin between the slips of the diaphragm and run forwards between the internal oblique and the transversus abdominis before they pierce the lateral margin of the rectus sheath. After lying behind the rectus muscle, they pierce its substance and supply it, and end as anterior cutaneous nerves.

Vessels of the abdominal wall. The only vessels likely to be injured by the anaesthetist are the superior and inferior epigastric arteries and veins. The superior artery is the termination of the internal mammary and enters the rectus sheath posterior to the 7th costal cartilage. The inferior epigastric artery arises from the external iliac artery and enters the rectus sheath behind the arcuate line of Douglas.

Surface markings. The xiphoid is on a level with the body of T9. The subcostal plane is at L3. The highest part of the iliac crest is on a level with L4 or the L4–L5 interspace.

Technique of abdominal field block

In all operations performed under field block analgesia it is necessary to infiltrate the line of incision both subcutaneously and intradermally. The injections should be commenced 15–20 min before the incision is to be made.

Weals are raised: (1) at the tip of the xiphisternum opposite the body of T9; (2) one on each side at the 9th costal cartilage, where the rectus muscle crosses it; (3) one on each side at the lateral margin of the rectus, just above the umbilicus; and (4) one on each side at the lateral margin of the rectus, below the umbilicus if the incision is to be prolonged.

Through weals 2, 3 and 4 a needle is inserted perpendicularly until it meets the resistance of the rectus sheath. If the patient is conscious he will experience pain when the anterior layer of the rectus sheath is pierced. The needle is advanced a further 0.5 cm and 5 ml of solution is injected into the sheath. After withdrawal into the subcutaneous tissue, the needle is inclined upwards and downwards so that more solution is deposited into the rectus sheath. It is important to remember the positions of the tendinous intersection so that solution is injected between each pair to ensure even distribution of the analgesic drug. Posterior to the muscle, these intersections do not impede the spread of solution. After completion of the deep injections the weals are joined together along the lateral margin of the rectus by lines of subcutaneous injection. Similarly weal 1 is joined to each weal 2 along the costal margin. A total of 50–100 ml of solution is used (e.g. 0.5% lignocaine).

A costo-iliac block gives a wider zone of analgesia and relaxation than the rectus-sheath block outlined below, but is more difficult to carry out successfully. Weals are raised on each side along the costal margin and vertically downward to the iliac crest. Solution is injected, from needles passed through these weals, into the subcutaneous and muscular layers of the abdominal wall, remembering that laterally the intercostal nerves lie between the transversalis and internal oblique. The weals are joined together by subcutaneous infiltration, as described for rectus-sheath block. In muscular subjects, in addition, solution can be injected into the rectus sheath. The volume of solution required is 15–200 ml.

Rectus-sheath block (Carl Ludwig Schleich, 1859–1922)[230] is an excellent method of producing muscular relaxation when combined with a light general anaesthetic, and if the incision is to be midline or paramedian it is usual to do both sides. Perforation of the peritoneum should be avoided, but in the absence of peritonitis or adhesions no serious harm is likely to result. The anterior layer of the rectus sheath is detected by the needle throughout its whole extent, but the posterior layer only for about 7.5 cm above and below the umbilicus. Solution is injected posterior to the muscle so that the intercostal nerves supplying it, together with the zone of skin medial to its outer border, are blocked. If the abdomen shows the scar of a previous operation, abdominal field block may be difficult and undesirable, and intercostal block or paravertebral block may be indicated if the operation is to be performed under local analgesia.

Intermittent injection through a small plastic catheter in each sheath can be used to produce good postoperative analgesia.

Abdominal field block renders the abdominal wall and its underlying parietal peritoneum insensitive. To block pain impulses from the viscera, and posterolateral parietal peritoneum, either light general anaesthesia or a splanchnic block and posterior intercostal block is required.

Regional analgesia for intra-abdominal surgery, requiring multiple punctures and near-toxic doses of local analgesic drugs, finds little favour today although Hans Finsterer (1876–1954), leading surgeon from Vienna, considered it to be the best method of pain relief for gastric surgery in his time (1923).[231]

Ilioinguinal block for repair of inguinal hernia

Anatomy

The inguinal canal is 4 cm long and extends from the internal inguinal ring laterally to the external inguinal ring medially. It lies above the inner half of the inguinal ligament.

The internal or abdominal ring is just above the midpoint of the inguinal ligament; it is an opening in the transversalis fascia and just medial to it is the inferior epigastric artery.

The subcutaneous or external ring lies above and lateral to the pubic crest. It is an opening in the external oblique, and through it passes the spermatic cord in the male and the round ligament in the female. They lie lateral to the pubic spine.

The walls of the inguinal canal are:

1. Anteriorly: external oblique; internal oblique in its lateral third.
2. Posteriorly: fascia transversalis in its whole length; conjoint tendon or falx inguinalis in its inner two-thirds; reflected part of the inguinal ligament in its inner third; the femoral vessels.
3. The floor: inguinal ligament.
4. The roof: arching fibres of the conjoint tendon of the transversus abdominis and the internal oblique.

The contents of the inguinal canal are the ilio-inguinal nerve and the spermatic cord (or the round ligament of the uterus). The spermatic cord comprises the internal and external spermatic arteries and the artery to the vas deferens, the pampiniform plexus of veins, the lymphatic vessels, the autonomic nerve-fibres and the vas deferens in the male.

Indirect inguinal hernia. All inguinal hernias are protrusions through the fascia transversalis. An indirect hernia protrudes through the deep inguinal ring, descends into the cord and receives a covering from the external spermatic fascia, cremesteric muscle and internal spermatic fascia (from the fascia transversalis).

Direct inguinal hernia. This protrudes through the fascia transversalis in the more medial part of osterior wall of the canal through the triangle of Hesselbach (1759–1816),[232] the boundaries of which are: lateral, the inferior or deep epigastric artery; medial, the outer border of the rectus; and inferior, the inguinal ligament.

Nerve supply. The nerve supply of the inguinal region is from the last two thoracic and the first two lumbar nerves via the iliohypogastric, the ilio-inguinal and the genitofemoral.

The last two thoracic nerves run downwards and inwards, just above the anterior superior iliac spine, between the internal oblique and transversus muscles. They end by piercing the rectus sheath.

The iliohypogastric and ilio-inguinal nerves come from the first lumbar root. They are inferior to the last two thoracic nerves and curve round the body just above the iliac crest, gradually piercing the muscles and ending superficially; the ilio-inguinal nerve traverses the inguinal canal, lying anterior to the spermatic cord, and becomes superficial through the external ring and supplies the skin of the scrotum. The iliohypogastric nerve, after running between the internal oblique and the transversus abdominis, pierces the internal oblique just above the anterior superior iliac spine and supplies the skin over the pubis.

The genitofemoral nerve comes from the 1st and 2nd lumbar nerves and divides into a genital and a femoral branch. The former enters the inguinal canal from behind through the internal ring.

Indications

1. In slim, elderly, poor-risk patients, to avoid the risks of general anaesthesia or the possible risks of hypotension associated with intra- or extradural analgesia. Used routinely by some surgeons.[233]
2. To reduce the risks of aspiration of intestinal contents in cases of strangulation, by having a fully awake patient. (Bowel resection usually requires other methods of pain relief).
3. For day-stay surgery.[234]
4. For postoperative pain relief.

Contra-indications to using the technique on its own

Obesity, lack of co-operation by the surgeon and nervousness of the patient.

Technique

Three weals are made as follows: (1) a finger-breadth internal to the anterior superior iliac spine; (2) over the spine of the pubis; and (3) 1.5 cm above the midpoint of the inguinal ligament.

Through weal 1 a larger needle is introduced vertically backwards until it is felt to pierce the aponeurosis of the external oblique with a slight click.[235] After aspiration, 20–30 ml of solution are injected so that both the ilio-inguinal and iliohypogastric nerves are surrounded. At this point a needle introduced perpendicularly to the skin will not pierce the peritoneum. Solution is injected in all layers including that small area of tissue between the weal and the anterior superior spine.

Through weal 2 a larger needle injects solution in the intradermal and subcutaneous layers in the direction of the umbilicus. This blocks nerve branches overlapping from the opposite side.

Through weal 3 a needle is inserted perpendicularly to the skin until it pierces the aponeurosis of the external oblique. At this level about 20 ml of solution is injected so that the genital branch of the genitofemoral nerve is blocked.[236]

Intradermal and subcutaneous infiltration along the line of the incision may be necessary to get perfect analgesia; in addition, infiltration of the periosteum near the pubic tubercle and Astley Cooper's ligament, the conjoint tendon and the lateral border of the rectus abdominis muscle should be performed in cases of direct inguinal hernia.[237]

The use of 0.5% solution of prilocaine with adrenaline allows a generous volume of relatively non-toxic local analgesic solution to be employed. Otherwise 0.25% bupivacaine or 0.5% lignocaine, both with adrenaline, are suitable. Dose of bupivacaine should not exceed 2 mg/kg. Mixing the analgesic with dextran 70 or 150 has been used to prolong local analgesic effect.[238]

If the hernia is strangulated or irreducible, deeper layers should be injected by the surgeon, under vision, as he goes along.

The patient may complain of temporary discomfort when the neck of the sac is under tension; this can often be relieved by infiltration of local analgesic solution around the neck. Infiltration analgesia is a perfectly acceptable method of pain relief in elective inguinal and femoral hernias and patients require less postoperative analgesia and vomit less than after general anaesthesia.[233,234]

In these operations, the surgeon often gives his own injections.[239] Following his experience with 100 000 operations under local analgesia, using the Shouldice surgical technique, Glasgow[240] advises first weight reduction. Then premedication sodium pentobarbitone, 200–250 mg by mouth, 1.5 h before operation, then pethidine 50–75 mg i.m. Procaine 2% solution (for those over 70, 1–1.5%) without adrenaline; total volume 150 ml (a big dose); 80–100 ml subcutaneously with a further 10–20 ml beneath the external oblique aponeurosis, with a similar volume round the internal ring, avoiding the inferior epigastric vessels.

Advantages of regional analgesia: avoids the risks of general anaesthesia; makes the surgeon gentle; patient can cough during the operation if required; surgeon uses less tension in his sutures; patient can walk off the table and be treated as a day-stay case; catheterization is eliminated; and a quicker turn-round of cases.

Systemic absorption of local analgesic is measurable.[241]

Ilio-inguinal block is helpful for postoperative analgesia.[242]

Field block for repair of femoral hernia

Anatomy

A femoral hernia passes through the femoral canal and the saphenous opening or fossa ovalis, an opening in the deep fascia of the thigh, 3.8 cm (1.5 in) below and 3.8 cm (1.5 in) lateral to the pubic tubercle.

The femoral canal is the most medial of three compartments, the most lateral containing the femoral artery and the intermediate one the femoral vein. The femoral canal is 1 to 2 cm long, and at its mouth is the femoral ring.

The femoral ring is bounded in front by the inguinal ligament and behind by the pectineus, laterally by the femoral vein, and medially by the lacunar ligament of Gimbernat (1734–1790). Astley Cooper's (1768–1841) ligament is a backward extension of the lacunar ligament, along the pelvic brim (iliopectineal line) for 1.5 cm. The ring contains the femoral septum or fatty pad.

The coverings of a femoral hernia are, from within outwards: the fat from the femoral septum, the prolongation of the fascia transversalis forming the anterior wall of the femoral sheath, and the cribriform fascia of the fossa ovalis.

Technique

The technique is similar to that for repair of inguinal hernia, with the addition that the lump in the thigh is surrounded by subcutaneous and intradermal weals.

Paravertebral block from T10 to L3 may also be carried out; it is a suitable procedure for operation on strangulated inguinal and femoral herniae.

Iliac crest block

A weal is raised 4 cm from the anterior superior iliac spine on a line joining this spine to the xiphisternum. A needle is inserted laterally, first just beneath the skin and then deeper until the ilium is touched. Solution is injected so that it anaesthetizes the 12th thoracic, iliohypogastric and ilio-inguinal nerves as they lie between the internal oblique and the transversus abdominis muscles.

Field block for appendicectomy

This can be useful in interval cases, but is seldom successful in operation for acute appendicitis.

Two weals are raised, one just above and behind the anterior superior iliac spine, the second below the costal margin at the tip of the 10th rib on the right side. The tissues between the skin and peritoneum in this line are infiltrated, and subcutaneous infiltration is made between the two weals and downwards between the lower weal and the iliac bone. Thus the 10th, 11th and 12th thoracic nerves are blocked, together with the ilio-inguinal and iliohypogastric.

Splanchnic block and bilateral somatic block are usually necessary, except in the very simplest operations on thin subjects.

Field block for operations on the anal canal

A weal is made on each side of the anus and 2.5 cm away from it. From these weals a subcutaneous rhomboidal zone of infiltration is made, using 20 ml of 0.5% bupivacaine and adrenaline. Deep injections are now made from the infiltrated zone into each quadrant, 5 ml into each with a finger in the rectum preventing perforation of the mucous membrane. The nerve to the external anal sphincter is the perineal branch of the 4th sacral nerve. The operation can be done satisfactorily with the patient in the prone position with the pelvis raised, and heavy premedication should be employed, e.g. pethidine and promethazine 50 mg of each i.m. with diazepam i.v.[243]

Penile block; field block for circumcision

Anatomy

The sensory nerves of the penis are derived from the terminal branches of the internal pudendal nerves. The dorsal nerves of the penis travel beneath the pubic bone, one on each side of the midline, lying against the dorsal surface of the corpus cavernosum. The skin at the base of the organ is supplied by the ilio-inguinal and perhaps the genitofemoral nerves. In addition, the posterior scrotal branches of the perineal nerves run para-urethrally to the ventral surface and fraenum, so four nerves have to be blocked.

Technique

An intradermal and subcutaneous ring weal is raised around the base of the penis; the subcutaneous infiltration should precede the intradermal. The dorsal nerve is next blocked on each side by injecting 5 ml of solution into the dorsum of the organ just below but not deep to the symphysis so that the needle point lies against the corpus cavernosum. If the needle pierces the corpus cavernosum, pain is experienced. For the ventral injection of the para-urethral branches, the penis should be pulled upwards and 2 ml of solution injected near the base of the organ into the groove formed by the corpora cavernosa and the corpus spongiosum. Infiltration of 5 ml of 1% lignocaine or 0.5% bupivacaine into each dorsal nerve provides good postoperative analgesia.[244] In infants, smaller volumes are used. Postoperative pain can be relieved by repeated penile block in awake patients, even in children, without undue discomfort.[245]

Adrenaline must not be used because necrosis of tissue results, as the arteries of the penis are end-arteries.

Care must be taken not to cause haematoma formation as this may contribute to gangrene of skin; subpubic injection must be avoided.[246]

Pain following circumcision under general anaesthesia can be relieved by sacral extradural analgesia or by infiltrating each dorsal nerve at the root of the penis[247] with 1–3 ml of local analgesic solution, e.g. 0.5% bupivacaine, without adrenaline. This is a satisfactory alternative to extradural sacral lock, with fewer complications.[248] Lignocaine spray or gel, applied topically gives useful relief.

Nerve block at the upper part of the thigh

Figs. 24.5–24.8.

Anatomy of lumbar plexus

The ventral rami of the lumbar nerves each receive a grey ramus communicans from a lumbar ganglion, while the 1st and 2nd lumbar nerves are also connected with the trunk by a white ramus.

They form the lumbar plexus lying in the psoas major, anterior to the transverse process of the lumbar vertebrae. A branch from the 4th unites with the 5th nerve to form the lumbosacral trunk which joins the sacral plexus.

The branches of the lumbar plexus are:

The iliohypogastric nerve from L1. It leaves the psoas major, crosses the quadratus lumborum, perforates the transversus abdominis and then divides into lateral and anterior cutaneous branches. Its lateral cutaneous branch supplies the skin on the anterior part of the gluteal region after piercing the

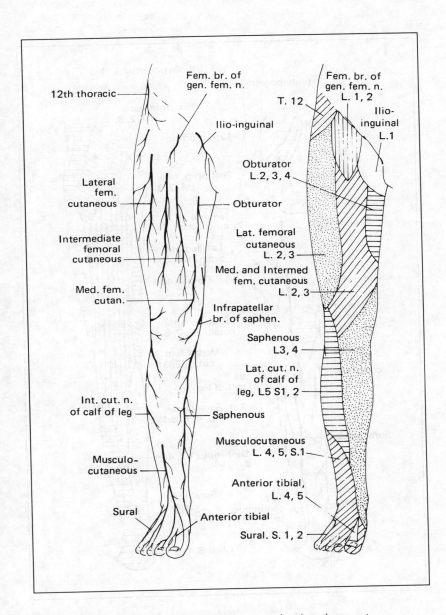

Figure 24.5 The cutaneous nerves of the right lower extremity. Anterior aspect

Figure 24.6 The segmental distribution of the cutaneous nerves of the right lower extremity. Anterior aspect

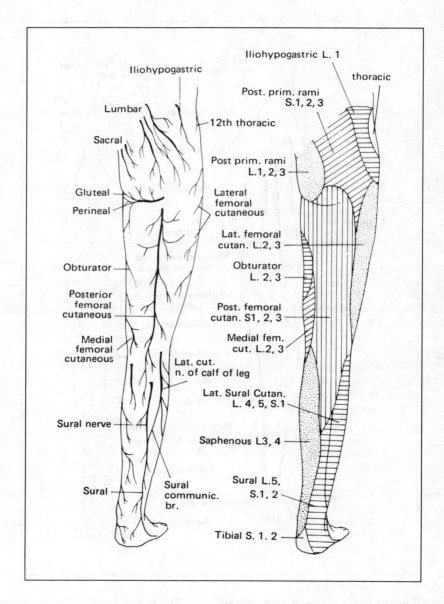

Figure 24.7 The cutaneous nerves of the right lower extremity. Posterior aspect

Figure 24.8 The segmental distribution of the cutaneous nerves of the right lower extremity. Posterior aspect. (*Fig. 5–8 after 'Gray's Anatomy' by kind permission.*)

internal and external oblique muscles 5 cm behind the anterior superior iliac spine and just above the iliac crest, while the terminal part of the nerve supplies the skin over the pubic bone after piercing the aponeurosis of the external oblique, 2 cm medial to the anterior superior iliac spine. It does not divide into anterior and posterior branches. Block after operation reduces pain.

The ilio-inguinal nerve from L1. This accompanies the iliohypogastric nerve, in its early course, lying just inferior to it in close relationship to the iliac crest. About 2 cm anterior and just below the anterior superior spine, it pierces the internal oblique and runs medially behind the aponeurosis of the external oblique. It then passes with the spermatic cord through the inguinal canal and supplies the skin of the upper and medial part of the thigh and the adjacent skin covering the external genitals. It has no lateral cutaneous branch, unlike the iliohypogastric nerve, and in the inguinal canal is sensory.

The genitofemoral nerve from L1 and L2. Its genital branch supplies the skin of the scrotum or labium majus, and the cremaster muscle. Its femoral branch supplies an area of skin on the middle of the anterior surface of the upper part of the thigh.

The lateral cutaneous nerve of the thigh (lateral femoral cutaneous) from L2 and L3 (posterior divisions). It supplies the skin of the anterolateral aspect of the thigh as far as the knee anteriorly, but laterally not quite so low after passing behind the inguinal ligament and the sartorius muscle, just medial and slightly inferior to the anterior superior iliac spine.

The femoral nerve from L2, L3 and L4 (posterior divisions). It emerges from the psoas major, passes between it and the iliacus and enters the thigh behind the inguinal ligament and just lateral to the femoral artery, from which it is here separated by a slip of the psoas major. It has anterior and posterior divisions, the latter giving rise to the saphenous nerve and the medial and intermediate cutaneous nerves of the thigh. The femoral nerve supplies the hip joint and knee joint, the skin of the anterior part of the thigh and the anteromedial part of the leg. It is motor to the quadriceps femoris, the sartorius and the pectineus.

The obturator nerve from L2, L3 and L4 (anterior divisions). It emerges from the medial border of the psoas muscle where it is a posterior relation of the external iliac vessels. After running forwards on the lateral wall of the pelvis it pierces the obturator canal, the nerve divides into anterior and posterior branches; the former supplies the adductor longus and brevis and the gracilis, with a branch going to the hip joint; the posterior branch supplies the adductor magnus and the hip joint. It supplies an area of skin on the medial aspect of the thigh and sends a small branch to the knee joint. *An accessory obturator nerve* is present in about 25% of people and runs a variable course across the superior pubic ramus and not via the obturator foramen; it comes from L3 and L4 (anterior divisions).

Anatomy of sacral plexus

The anterior primary rami of the five sacral and the coccygeal nerves each receive a grey ramus from the sympathetic trunk. From the 2nd, 3rd and 4th sacral nerves white rami (visceral afferent) join the pelvic plexuses, the sacral outflow of the autonomic nervous system or pelvic splanchnic nerves.

The sacral and pudendal plexuses are composed of the lumbosacral trunk (L4 and L5) and the ventral rami of the upper four sacral nerves. They lie on the posterior wall of the pelvic cavity between the piriformis and the pelvic fascia and have in front the ureter, internal iliac vessels, and the sigmoid colon on the left.

The following branches are given off:

The posterior cutaneous nerve of the thigh (S1–S3) supplies the skin of the lower part of the gluteal region, the perineum and the back of the thigh and leg.

The great sciatic nerve (L4 and L5; S1–S3) supplies the skin at the back of the leg and sole of the foot, after dividing into tibial and common peroneal nerves usually at the upper extremity of the popliteal fossa. It leaves the pelvis through the greater sciatic foramen, lying between the piriformis and the superior gemellus muscles, and occupies the space between the ischial tuberosity and the greater trochanter. After splitting into: (1) the tibial nerve, which gives origin to the sural and divides near the ankle into the medial and lateral branches; and (2) the common peroneal, from which originate the deep and superficial peroneal nerves. (The tibial is synonymous with the medial popliteal and posterior tibial, and the common peroneal is synonymous with the lateral popliteal, and from it arise the deep peroneal or anterior tibial and the superficial peroneal or musculocutaneous nerves.)

The perforating cutaneous nerve (S2 and S3) supplies the skin over the medial and lower parts of the gluteus maximus.

The pudendal nerve leaves the pelvis through the greater sciatic foramen, crosses the ischial spine medial to the pudendal vessels and goes through the lesser sciatic foramen. With the pudendal vessels it passes upwards and forwards along the lateral wall of the ischiorectal fossa, in Alcock's canal, a sheath of the obturator fascia. It gives off: (1) the inferior rectal nerve supplying the external anal sphincter and the skin around the anus; (2) the perineal nerve supplying the skin of the scrotum or labium majus and small branches to muscles; (3) the dorsal nerve of the penis or clitoris; (4) the medial and lateral posterior scrotal (or labial) nerves; and (5) visceral branches supplying the rectum and bladder. From the 2nd, 3rd and 4th sacral nerves. They communicate with the sympathetic pelvic plexuses. (Sometimes called the pelvic splanchnic nerves of Gaskell, homologous with the white rami communicantes of the thoracic and upper lumbar nerves.) The levator ani and the coccygeus, and also the external anal sphincter, are supplied by the 4th sacral nerve.

Technique of femoral nerve block

A weal is raised a finger-breadth to the outer side of the femoral artery, just below the inguinal ligament. A needle is inserted for 3–4 cm so that the pulsations of the artery are transferred to the needle and 20 ml of 2% lignocaine is injected. The nerve lies beneath the deep fascia. Femoral nerve block, following injection of solution lateral and deep to the femoral artery, greatly reduces pain, following fractured neck of the femur during movement in adults and children.[249]

Sciatic and femoral nerve blocks in combination are useful in operations on the leg and foot from a point 5 cm below the patella.[250] Operations on or above the knee require, in addition, lateral femoral cutaneous and obturator block, the latter being difficult. Manipulations of the lower half of the femur can, however, be carried out under sciatic and femoral block.

Nerve to quadratus femoris. This branch of the femoral nerve supplies the hip joint. To block it the patient is placed in the prone position with leg externally rotated. A line is drawn with a skin pencil joining the posterior superior iliac spine and the sacrococcygeal joint. The junction of the middle and lower thirds is marked. A weal is raised 5 cm posterior to the greater trochanter on a level with the lower end of the sacrum and a 14-cm 16G needle inserted at 45° to the horizontal towards the point previously marked until it hits bone. The needle point is worked medially 1–2 cm while 20 ml of solution are deposited along the flat surface of the body of the ischium. Useful for relief of pain in the hip joint and to allow gentle physiotherapy in patients with osteoarthritis.

Regional hip blockade

Regional hip blockade involves injection into the region of the nerve to the quadratus femoris and the obturator nerve, with the aim of ameliorating the severe pain due to osteoarthritis of the hip joint.[251] Some workers have found the block of doubtful value.[252] Some pain relief follows the injection into the hip joint of 10 ml of 0.5% bupivacaine.[253]

Inguinal perivascular block[254]

Injection of 25–40 ml of solution into the region of the femoral nerve, after eliciting paraesthesia, from just below the inguinal ligament, will block the femoral, obturator and lateral femoral cutaneous nerves (the 'three-in-one block'). Useful together with sciatic block for analgesia of the leg.

Saphenous nerve block

This is the terminal branch of the femoral nerve and becomes subcutaneous immediately below the sartorius muscle at the medial side of the knee joint; it accompanies the long saphenous vein to the medial malleolus. It can be blocked by a subcutaneous injection of 10–15 ml of local analgesic solution in the close vicinity of the vein just below the knee joint, taking care to avoid intravenous injection. For long saphenous vein stripping under regional analgesia *see* Bromage et al.[255]

Technique of block of lateral cutaneous nerve of thigh[256]

A weal is raised one finger-breadth below and medial to the anterior superior spine of the ilium. A needle is inserted perpendicularly to the skin and 1% lignocaine is injected between the skin and the iliac bone and along the pelvic brim for two finger-breadths internally to the anterior superior spine; 10–15 ml of solution is used. The nerve lies deep to the fascia lata of the thigh.

When associated with femoral block, adequate analgesia is produced for taking skin grafts from the front of the thigh. Alternatively, infiltration analgesia of the skin of the front of the thigh can be performed, using intradermal and subcutaneous injections to cover the desired area.

Technique of obturator block

The obturator nerves arise from the 2nd, 3rd and 4th lumbar nerves. Block is required for operations involving the knee joint, the medial aspect of the thigh, and may be necessary to make application of an arterial tourniquet above the knee tolerable.

The anterior and posterior divisions of the nerve are blocked as they lie in the obturator canal below the superior ramus of the pubis, between the pectineus and the obturator externus. The following techniques can be used:

1. The patient lies supine with leg slightly abducted. A skin mark is made halfway between the pubic tubercle and femoral artery, 2–3 cm below the inguinal ligament. The pubic ramus is palpated here and a disposable 18G spinal needle inserted to strike the bone. The needle is then slightly withdrawn and turned through 90° to a point about 2 cm below the superior ramus and parallel to the shaft of the femur. The needle is now advanced into the obturator foramen by a forward movement of 4–5 cm. After aspiration tests, and provided there is no resistance to injection, 10 ml of solution is injected.

2. A skin weal is raised just below the midpoint of the superior pubic ramus and a 5-cm needle introduced perpendicular to the plane of the obturator foramen and advanced just below the ramus for 1.5 cm. Paraesthesiae should be elicited after the injection of 5 ml of 1.5% lignocaine solution.

3. A weal is raised 1 cm below and lateral to the pubic tubercle and through it a 5-cm needle is thrust backwards until it strikes bones; as it is withdrawn, 10 ml of solution are injected. An 8-cm needle is now inserted in the track of the first one and moved gently laterally until its point enters the obturator foramen where 10 ml of solution is injected. An additional similar volume is finally injected as the needle is withdrawn.[257] Successful block is shown by weakness when the patient attempts to adduct the leg.

Block of the above nerves (other than the saphenous, included in femoral block), together with the sciatic, will produce analgesia of the lower extremity below the level of the symphysis pubis. It can also be used for the treatment of pain in the region of the hip joint or of adductor spasm. The position of the needle point can be checked radiographically or by electrical stimulation (0.5 mA rheobase) using a Teflon-covered needle.[258] Eases the pain during transport.

For nailing, etc. of a fractured neck of fractured femur, the line of incision is infiltrated down to the bone with 0.5% lignocaine or 1 in 2000 amethocaine. Solution is injected between the ends of the fractured neck from above the great trochanter and from a point just external to the pulsating femoral artery.

For arthroscopy of the knee, femoral and lateral femoral cutaneous nerve block has been recommended.[259] Intradural spinal analgesia also gives good results and is used in day-stay surgery.[260]

Doppler localization of the popliteal artery combined with nerve localization with a peripheral nerve stimulator facilitates knee-block by reducing discomfort and increasing efficacy.[261]

Lumbar plexus block[262] (psoas compartment block)

A single injection of solution or serial injections through a catheter introduced via a needle from a weal 5 cm lateral to the upper border of the 4th lumbar vertebra. A 15-cm needle is inserted perpendicularly to the skin until contact with the transverse process is made. It is then partially withdrawn and glided over the transverse process. The injection is made until loss of resistance is felt, and thereafter 40 ml of 0.25% bupivacaine solution with adrenaline 1 in 200 000 are placed within the psoas compartment. This is said to be safe and is recommended for surgery of the hip, including arthroplasty together with light general anaesthesia.[263] This is a useful block in the management of fractured femur before, during and after operation and during transport.

Technique of sciatic nerve block[264]

Posterior approaches. Patient lies on sound side with hip slightly flexed. Methods:

  1. A line connecting the sacral hiatus with the most prominent part of the greater trochanter is drawn and a weal raised at its midpoint. A 21G spinal needle is inserted at right angles to the skin and down to touch the bone at the back of the acetabulum. Through it 10–15 ml of local analgesic is injected[265]

  2. A line is traced between the upper extremity of the great trochanter and the posterior superior iliac spine. From midpoint of this line a perpendicular is dropped 3–5 cm long, and at its end a weal is raised and a needle introduced at right angles to the skin plane until it reaches the ischial spine, 5–7.5 cm from the skin surface. The nerve lies on this area of bone so that paraesthesiae must be elicited before the needle strikes bone; 10–15 ml of 2% lignocaine is then injected. Intraneural injection is undesirable.

  3. A surface marking is the junction of the medial third with the lateral two-thirds of a line joining the ischial tuberosity to the greater femoral trochanter – the needle being inserted at right angles to the skin surface until paraesthesiae are felt by the patient.

  4. A guide to the position of the nerve is the midpoint of a line joining the posterior superior iliac spine to the ischial tuberosity.

The block is useful for reduction of fractures around the ankle, combined if necessary with a saphenous nerve block just below the knee joint as it accompanies the long saphenous vein. It can be used together with femoral block for ligation of varicose veins on the front of the leg. An alternative for operations below the knee is injection into the region of the tibial and common peroneal nerves in the popliteal fossa, and the saphenous nerve adjacent to the knee. Efficacy is enhanced by the use of a peripheral nerve stimulator.[266]

It also causes almost complete vasoconstrictor paralysis of the foot and is better, safer and less painful than lumbar sympathetic block for this purpose. A rise in skin temperature starts in 10 min and is maximal in 20–30 min. Sciatic nerve block gives analgesia of the whole foot with the exception of an area of skin over the medial malleolus supplied by the saphenous branch of the femoral nerve. The pain caused by gangrene of the foot can be relieved by continuous sciatic nerve block in which a catheter is inserted into the neurovascular sheath by the posterior approach.[267]

Anterior Approach.[268] This may be useful when the patient cannot be easily moved from the supine position and when intervention on the foot or lower leg is required. Other nerve blocks in the leg may be combined with it. The needle passes between the sartorius laterally and the rectus femoris medially and reaches the sciatic nerve below the lesser trochanter.

For technique of lateral approach with the patient supine *see* Dalens B., Tanguy A. and Vanneuville G. *Anesth. Analg.* 1990, **70**, 131.

Pudendal nerve block

See Chapter 22 Obstetrics.

Ankle block

A subcutaneous and intradermal weal is raised circumferentially around the ankle just above the medial malleolus.

The deep peroneal (anterior tibial; S1 and S2) is blocked by inserting a needle midway between the most prominent points of the medial and lateral malleoli, on the circular line of infiltration in front of the ankle joint. It is directed medially towards the anterior border of the medial malleolus and solution is injected between the bone and the skin; paraesthesia should be elicited if possible. Instead of blocking this nerve at the ankle, its parent trunk, the common peroneal nerve, can be blocked at the neck of the fibula where it can be rolled under the finger – the only palpable nerve in the leg. It supplies the skin on adjacent sides of the first and second toes, dorsal aspect. The amount of solution used should be 10–15 ml.

The superficial peroneal (musculocutaneous, S1 and S2), also a branch from the common peroneal nerve, can be blocked immediately above the ankle joint by a subcutaneous weal extending from the front of the tibia to the lateral malleolus. It supplies the dorsum of the foot (with the exception of the small area innervated by the tibial nerve).

The sural nerve (L5; S1 and S2). Formed with branches from the tibial and common peroneal nerves and descends with the short saphenous vein below and posterior to the lateral malleolus to supply the outer part of the foot and heel. It is blocked by subcutaneous infiltration between the tendo Achilles and the prominence of the lateral malleolus, using 5–10 ml of solution.

The saphenous nerve (L3 and L4). This is the terminal branch of the femoral nerve and accompanies the long saphenous vein anterior to the medial malleolus where it can be blocked by the injection of 10 ml of local analgesic solution. It supplies an area of skin just below and above the media malleolus.

The tibial nerve (S1 and S2) passes behind the medial malleolus to divide into medial and lateral plantar nerves after giving off the medial calcaneal branch. With the patient in the prone position it is blocked by 10 ml of solution introduced through a point on the circular weal just internal to the tendo Achilles, deep to the flexor retinaculum near the palpable posterior tibial artery. It is easiest with the patient lying prone. The needle is inserted forwards and slightly outwards towards the posterior aspect of the tibia, near which the solution is injected.

After waiting 10 min, ankle block is suitable for operation on the foot. Tibial block is useful for testing vasodilatation of the foot.

Following infiltration of any peripheral nerve, vasomotor paralysis over the area of anaesthetized skin occurs.

Block for hallux valgus

A weal is raised near the proximal end of the first intermetatarsal space, superior surface, and, from this, solution is injected between the two layers of skin, dorsal and plantar, as far forwards as the web between the toes. More solution is injected between the dorsal skin and the first metatarsal bone. A second weal medial to the first one, on the internal aspect of the metatarsal, is raised, and injection made between it and the bone between the plantar skin and the bone. A 10–15 min pause is made before the operation is commenced. From 30 to 50 ml of solution are used (e.g. 1 to 1.5% lignocaine).

Local analgesia of foot[269]

Sole of foot

Supplied by the medial (L4 and L5) and lateral (S1 and S2) branches of the tibial nerve (plantar from sciatic), supplying the media and lateral anterior part of the sole; the sural nerve supplying the posterior and lateral part of the sole and heel; and the tibial nerve (S1 and S2) supplying the medial part of the heel. The plantar surface of the heel is supplied by calcaneal branches of the tibial nerve, but not by the sural nerve.[270]

Tibial nerve block. See above under Ankle block.

Dorsum of foot

Supplied by medial terminal branch of deep peroneal nerve (the adjacent sides of the first and second toes). The sural innervates the lateral side of the fifth toe, the superficial peroneal supplies the remainder. Midtarsal block for surgery of the forefoot (*see* Sharrock N. E. et al. *Br. J. Anaesth.* 1986, **58**, 37).

Medial side of foot

Supplied by saphenous nerve from the femoral nerve. Also from the medial plantar branch of the tibial nerve.

Lateral side of foot

Supplied by sural nerve from the tibial and common peroneal, which goes to fifth toe and lateral side of foot.

Ring block of toe

Lignocaine plain, 1.5 ml of 2% solution, is injected into each side of the proximal phalanx near its base. Injection from dorsal aspect with small amount of solution across from side to side. After an interval of 7–10 min, the operation, e.g. removal of toe nail, can commence.[271]

(*See also* Robertson J. F. R. and Muckart D. J. J. *J. R. Coll. Surg. Edinb.* 1985, **30**, 237.)

Local analgesia for reduction of closed fractures

After localizing the exact site of fracture by means of X-rays, a weal is raised near the fracture and a needle introduced into the haematoma between the broken bone ends. Aspiration of old blood confirms the position and must be obtained; injection is then made of 1.5 or 2% lignocaine without adrenaline. For Colles' fracture[272] the amount required is 15–20 ml; injection should be made from the extensor aspect of the wrist and, in addition, a few millilitres should infiltrate the ulnar styloid. The method is easier, quicker and does not carry the possible risks of intravenous local analgesia; although pain relief is superior with the latter.[273] For Pott's fracture, 10–20 ml of solution with hyaluronidase can be used; for fractured femur, 20–30 ml. These are high doses so the possibility of toxic signs must be borne in mind. Cases of recent fracture are the most suitable for this method of reduction, especially fractures of the metatarsal or metacarpal bones. Good results are claimed for the addition of 1000 units of hyaluronidase to each 20 ml of solution. With lignocaine, analgesia lasts 2–3 h and comes on after 10 min. This technique does not produce complete pain relief but may be employed when dealing with mass casualities or when anaesthetists are not available.

Topical analgesia for gastroscopy, fibreoptic endoscopy and oesophagoscopy

Cocaine was first used for oesophagoscopy by Stoerk and Von Hacker in 1887.

Fibreoptic endoscopes employ very fine bundles of glass fibres, which carry images around corners, an invention patented by J. L. Baird of the UK in 1927; developed by H. H. Hopkins of Reading University.[274] Gastro-intestinal endoscopy developed following pioneering work by Hirschowitz in 1958.[275]

Sedation and supplementation of regional analgesia

Purposes:

1. To allay anxiety – opioids or benzodiazepines.
2. To control restlessness – opioids and benzodiazepines, or propofol infusion.
3. Extra analgesia for less-than-perfect blocks, e.g. opioids,[276] NSAIDS, Piroxicam,[277] or nitrous oxide (sedanalgesia or relative analgesia).[278] Also for where pain is already severe, e.g. fractures. Low-dose ketamine is an excellent extra analgesic.[279] Note that opioids may produce problems as well as prevent them, i.e. nausea, vomiting, bradycardia, hypotension, respiratory depression, bronchospasm, and prevention of paraesthesia while searching for a nerve.[280]

4. To prevent vasovagal faints during the procedure.[281]

These sedatives may be given as premedication, as boluses or infusions. Propofol has the advantage of rapid recovery.[282]

Sedation is chosen with care or omitted in obstetric regional blocks. Children require more sedation, including light anaesthesia.

Dangers of intravenous sedation in regional blockade include undetected (even fatal) respiratory insufficiency. Pulse oximetry is required as a monitor.[283]

Relaxing music may be played through headphones, or the anaesthetist may give reassuring conversation.

Personality traits as measured by e.g. the Eysenck personality inventory, influence the tolerance and future compliance with gastro-intestinal endoscopy. Drugs producing amnesia make repeat examinations more acceptable.[284] The following drugs have been suggested: lorazepam, 2.5–5mg, 90 min before pharyngeal analgesia, then Diazemuls 10–60 mg before endoscopy.[285] Flunitrazepam,[286] midazolam 0.1 mg/kg i.v.,[287] pentazocine and Buscopan may also have their indications.

After administration of the sedative of choice the patient is given a tablet of amethocaine (60 mg) or lignocaine to suck. Too much atropine may make this difficult. Additional intravenous diazepam may be necessary, 5 mg i.v. each minute until ptosis or dysarthria occurs. In cirrhotic patients, diazepam may result in hepatic coma. Chlormethiazole (Heminevrin) may be used instead in hypotensive patients.[288] The gums, tongue, palate and pharynx are now sprayed with 4% lignocaine, 4% cocaine, 1% amethocaine or some other suitable analgesic solution. He can be given amethocaine hydrochloride 2% to gargle, or Xylocaine Viscous to swallow, a 2% solution in a mucilage base, very pleasantly flavoured. In active bleeding, topical analgesia increases the risk of aspiration.[289]

Gargling with 4% lignocaine makes the passage of the small fibreoptic endoscope tolerable in over 90% of patients, without premedication or intravenous sedatives.[290]

Many operators have now discarded the use of local analgesia prior to fibreoptic gastroscopy, relying on the use of intravenous sedative and/or analgesic drugs alone.

Topical analgesia for bronchoscopy

Flexible fibreoptic bronchoscope introduced in 1968.[291]

The gums, tongue, palate and pharynx are sprayed as for oesophagoscopy on two occasions, a few minutes apart. After a short interval, the piriform fossae and the terminal branches of the internal laryngeal nerve beneath its mucosa are made analgesic by application of swabs soaked in the solution (with excess of it removed), applied on a curved applicator or with Krause's laryngeal forceps. After this has been done, and after spraying the epiglottis and the cords, a swab is gently introduced into the glottis and held there for a short while, so that its analgesic solution completes the block of the superior laryngeal nerve endings.

In addition, the trachea must be anaesthetized by:

1. The transtracheal method of Canuyt (1920),[292] which consists in inserting a hypodermic needle through the middle line of the neck into the trachea. The needle should be 3–4 cm long so that if breakage occurs, which is usually near the hub, the remains of the shaft can be easily removed. Aspiration of air proves its presence in the trachea. An injection of 2–3 ml of 4% lignocaine or cocaine is now made after a deep expiration and the patient told not to cough until the solution has trickled down the trachea into the bronchi. Insertion of the needle can be preceded by 100–150 mg of thiopentone. Complications are: (1) infection; (2) a broken needle; (3) surgical emphysema; and (4) haemorrhage.

2. By instillation from a laryngeal syringe, holding the tongue forward, using an indirect laryngeal mirror if thought necessary. A 10% lignocaine aerosol spray is available and enables a measured (10-mg) dose of drug to be given with each 'squirt'. Deep penetration into the bronchial tree can be achieved.

Such topical solutions should not be used on inflamed or traumatized surfaces.

Regional analgesia is probably safer than general anaesthesia for those examinations where there is copious sputum, airway obstruction or when the general condition of the patient is poor. It enables the movements of the vocal cords to be seen.

As an aid to comfortable endoscopy under local analgesia, the concurrent use of divided doses of a narcotic analgesic, neurolept agent or diazepam given intravenously is beneficial.

After topical laryngeal analgesia, instruction must be given to the patient not to eat or drink for at least 3 h, i.e. until function of the sentinel of the larynx has returned.

Topical analgesia of the urethra

Technique

A useful preparation is Xylocaine Gel, a 1–2% preparation put up in 30-ml tubes with carboxymethylcellulose. The maximum dose should probably not exceed 10 ml, i.e. 100–200 mg of lignocaine. The plastic nozzle supplied by the makers of the preparation is used to squeeze the jelly into the urethra. A clamp is applied to the penis and the paste gently massaged into the posterior urethra. After an interval of 10–15 min instrumentation can begin. It is sometimes helpful to pass a small catheter into the urethra connected to the plastic nozzle, so as to deposit gel in the posterior urethra. The gel is also useful for postoperative comfort after general anaesthesia.

Topical analgesia of the peritoneal cavity

Lignocaine, 0.5%, prilocaine, 0.5%, or procaine, 0.5–1%, is used. Volume 200 ml. This is poured into the peritoneal cavity and the peritoneal edges are drawn together. After 5–8 min the solution is sucked out. Results: slackening of the peritoneum, contraction of the bowel and absence of reflex response from visceral trauma. Toxic reactions are said to be rare. Good results are not seen in cases of peritonitis or where the bowel is grossly distended.

(For good illustrations showing some of the techniques described in this and the next chapter the reader is referred to the following books: *Illustrated Handbook of Local Anaesthesia* (Ericksson E. ed.), 2nd ed. London: Lloyd-Luke, 1980; Cousins M. J. and Bridenbaugh P. O. *Neural Blockade in Clinical Anaesthesia and the Management of Pain.* 2nd edn. Philadelphia: Lippincott, 1988; Lee J. A., Atkinson R. S. and Watt M. J. *Macintosh's Lumbar Puncture and Spinal Analgesia,* 5th ed. Edinburgh: Churchill Livingstone, 1985; Scott D. B. et al. (ed.) *Regional Anaesthesia: 1884–1984,* Sondertalje, Production ICM AB. 1984.

References

1. *See also* Raj P. Nolte H. and Stanton-Hicks M. *Illustrated Manual of Regional Anesthesia.* Berlin: Springer-Verlag, 1989; Cousins J. and Bridenbaugh P. *Clinical Anesthesia and Management of Pain,* 2nd ed., Philadelphia, Lippincott, 1988.
2. Koller C. *Klin. Mbl. Augen.* 1884, **22**, 60; *Wien. Med. Wochenschr.* 1884, **34**, 1276, 1309 (translated and reprinted in 'Classical File', *Surv. Anesthesiol.* 1963, **7**, 74); *Lancet* 1884, **2**, 990.
3. Richardson B. W. *Med. Times. Gaz.* 1866, **1**, 115.
4. Redard P. Vera. *Xth. Int. Med. Cong.* 1890, **5**, 14, Abstract 71.
5. Schleich K. L. *Verh. Dtsch. Ges. Chir.* 1892, **21**, 121; *Gesellsch, f. Chir. 1892,* **21**, 121; *Therap. Monats.* 1894, **8**, 429; *Schmerzlöse Operationen.* Berlin: Springer, 1894.
6. Reclus P. *Gaz. Hebd. Med. (Paris),* 1890, 106; *La Cocaine en Chirurgie.* Paris, Masson. 1895.
7. Halsted W. S. *NY Med. J.* 1885, **42**, 294; Hall R. J. *NY Med. J.* 1884, **40**, 463.
8. Vinci G. *Berlin Klin. Wochenschr.* 1896, **27**.
9. Barker A. E. *Lancet* 1899, **1**, 282.
10. Braun H. *Arch. Klin. Chir.* 1902, **69**, 541.
11. Abel J. J. *Johns Hopkins Hosp. Bull.* 1897, **8**, 151.
12. Crile G. W. *Cleveland Med. J. 1897,* **11**, 355.
13. Fourneau E. (1872–1949), *Bull. Soc. Pharmacol.* 1904, **10**, 141.
14. Einhorn A. *Münch. Med. Wochenschr.* 1899, **46**, 1218.
15. Braun H. *Dtsch. Med. Wochenschr.* 1905, **31**, 1667.
16. Eisleb O. et al. *Arch. Exp. Path. u. Phar.* 1931, **160**, 53.
17. Uhlmann T. *Narkose und Anaes.* 1929, **6**, 168.
18. Gordh T. *Anaesthesia* 1949, **4**, 4.
19. Redman A. In: *Hollander Schneidermühl's 'Handbuch des Zahnartz'.* Heilmittellehre, 1890, 149.
20. Rynd F. *Dublin Med. Press* 1845, **13**, 167; *Dublin J. Med. Sci.* 1861, **32**, 13.
21. Wood A. *Edin. Med. Surg. J.* 1855, **82**, 265.
22. Cushing H. W. *Ann. Surg.* 1902, **36**, 321.
23. *See also* Ritchie J. M. *Br. J. Anaesth.* 1975, **47**, 191; de Jong R. *Local Anesthetics.* 2nd ed. Springfield, Ill.: Thomas, 1977.
24. *See also* Hiele B. *J. Gen. Physiol.* 1977, **69**, 497.
25. Bromage P. R. et al. *Br. J. Anaesth.* 1967, **39**, 197.
26. Appleyard J. N. et al. *Br. J. Anaesth.* 1974, **46**, 530.

27. Branch R. A. et al. *J. Pharmacol. Exp. Ther.* 1973, **184**, 515; Munson, E. S. et. al. *Anesthesiology* 1975, **42**, 471; Burney R. G. and Di Fazio C. A. *Anesth. Analg. (Cleve.)* 1976, **55**, 322.
28. Braid D. P. *Br. J. Anaesth.* 1964, **36**, 742.
29. Braid D. P. and Scott D. B. *Br. J. Anaesth.* 1965, **37**, 394; Tucker G. T. et al. *Anesthesiology* 1965, **37**, 277.
30. Pagden D. et al. *Anesth. Analg. (Cleve.)* 1986, **65**, 1063.
31. Editorial, *Anesthesiology* 1979, **51**, 285.
32. Albright G. A. *Anesthesiology* 1979, **51**, 285.
33. Scott D. B. *Br. J. Anaesth.* 1984, **56**, 437.
34. Noble D. S. and Pierce G. F. M. *Lancet* 1961, **2**, 1436.
35. Moore D. C. *Regional Block.* 4th ed. Springfield, Ill.: Thomas, 1965.
36. Brown D. T. et al. *Br. J. Anaesth.* 1981, **53**, 435; Fisher M. McD. and Pennington J. C. *Br. J. Anaesth.* 1982, **54**, 893; Reynolds F. *Br. J. Anaesth.* 1982, **54**, 901.
37. Nagel J. F. and Fuscaldo J. T. *JAMA* 1977, **237**, 1594.
38. Sturrock J. E. and Nunn J. F. *Br. J. Anaesth.* 1979, **51**, 273.
39. Bromage P. R. et al. *Br. J. Anaesth.* 1967, **39**, 197; Catchlove R. F. H. *Br. J. Anaesth.* 1973, **45**, 471; Soderman M. and Duke P. C. *Can. Anaesth. Soc. J.* 1983, **30**, S. 71; Bokesch P. M. et al. *Anesth. Analg. (Cleve.)* 1987, **66**, 9.
40. Cook J. H. *Ann. R. Coll. Surg. Engl.* 1987, **69**, 3. Owen H., Galloway D. J. and Mitchell K. G. *Ann. R. Coll. Surg. Engl.* 1985, **67**, 114; Pybus P. K. *Ann. R. Coll. Surg. Engl.* 1988, **70**, 260; Foate J. A., Owen H. and McLean C. F. *Ann. R. Coll. Surg. Engl.* 1989, **71**, 72.
41. Chapman G. M. *Anaesthesia* 1972, **27**, 185.
42. Pearman T. *J. Laryngol. Otol.* 1979, **93**, 1191.
43. Van Essen E. J. and Ploeger E. J. *Anaesthesia* 1981, **36**, 713.
44. Niemann A. *Justus Liebig's Annals of Chemistry* 1860, **114**, 213.
45. Von Ottingen W. F. *Ann. Med. Hist.* 1933, ns., **5**, 275; Moréno y Maiz T. *Thèse de Paris*, 1868, **91**.
46. von Anrep B. *Arch. Physiol.* 1880, **21**, 38.
47. Musto D. F. *JAMA* 1968, **204**, 27.
48. Koller C. *Wiener Med. Blatt.* 1884, **7**, 1352.
49. Koller C. *JAMA* 1928, **90**, 1742; 1941, **117**, 1284; Koller-Becker H. *Psychoanal. Q.* 1963, **32**, 309; Gay G. B. et al. *Anesth. Analg. (Cleve.)* 1976, **55**, 582, Sigmund Freud, *Cocain Papers* (Byck R. ed.). New York: Stonehill, 1974; Gay G. B. et al. *Anesth. Analg. (Cleve)* 1976, **55**, 582.
50. Halsted W. S. *NY Med. J.* 1885, **42**, 294.
51. von Oettingen W. F. *Ann. Med. Hist.* 1933, ns., **5**, 275; Olch P. D. *Anesthesiology* 1975, **42**, 479.
52. Willstatter R. *Münch. Med. Wochenschr.* 1924, **71**, 849.
53. Withkin J. M. et al. *Life Sci.* 1989, **44**, 1289.
54. Derlet R. W., Albertson T. E. *Am. J. Emerg. Med.* 1989, **7**, 464.
55. Delikan A. E. et al. *Anaesth. Intensive Care* 1978, **6**, 328.
56. Choy-Kwong M., Lipton R. B. *Neurology* 1989, **39**, 425.
57. *Martindale: The Extra Pharmacopoeia* (Wade A. ed.), 27th ed. London: Pharmaceutical Press, 1977, 960, 974; Annotation, *Br. Med. J.* 1979, **1**, 971.
58. Cousins M. J. and Mather L. E. *Anaesth. Intensive Care* 1980, **6**, 270.
59. Ansbro F. P. et al. *Anesth. Analg. Curr. Res.* 1953, **32**, 73.
60. Allen P. R. and Johnson R. W. *Anaesthesia* 1979, **34**, 874; Reisner L. S. et al. *Anesth. Analg. (Cleve.)* 1980, **59**, 452.
61. Wang B. C. and Hillman D. E. *Anesth. Analg. (Cleve.)* 1984, **63**, 445.
62. Lofgren N. *Xylocaine.* Stockholm: Haeggstroms, 1948; *Archiv. Kemi Mineral Geol.* 1946, **18**, 22A.
63. Gordh T. *Anaesthesia* 1949, **4**, 4 (reprinted in 'Classical File', *Surv. Anesthesiol.* 1977, **21**, 314).
64. Forrest J. A. et al. *Br. Med. J.* 1977, **1**, 1384.

65. Katz J. D. and Krich L. B. *Can. Anaesth. Soc. J.* 1976, **23**, 285.
66. Bromage P. R. *Acta Anaesth. Scand.* 1965, **16**, Suppl. 55; Cousins M. J. and Bromage P. R. *Br. J. Anaesth.* 1971, **43**, 1149; Cole C. P. et al. *Anesthesiology* 1985, **62**, 348; Sukhani R. et al. *Anesthesiology* 1985, **63**, A209.
67. Soderman M. and Duke P. C. *Can. Anaesth. Soc. J.* 1983, **30**, S. 71; Bokesch P. M. et al. *Anesth. Analg. (Cleve.)* 1987, **66**, 9.
68. Af Ekenstam B. et al. *Br. J. Anaesth.* 1956, **28**, 503.
69. Dhuner K. G. et al. *Acta Chir. Scand.* 1956, **112**, 350.
70. Jorfeldt L. et al. *Acta Anaesth. Scand.* 1968, **12**, 153.
71. Af Ekenstam B. et al. *Acta Chem. Scand.* 1957, **11**, 1183.
72. Telivuo L. *Ann. Chir. Gynaecol. Fenn.* 1963, **52**, 513. *See also* Watt M. J. et al. *Anaesthesia* 1968, **23**, 2, 331; 1970, **25**, 24.
73. Marx G. *Anesthesiology* 1984, **60**, 3; Rosen M. A. et al. *Anesth. Analg. (Cleve.)* 1985, **64**, 1039.
74. Reynolds F. *Br. J. Anaesth.* 1971, **43**, 33.
75. Adams H. J. et al. *J. Pharm. Sci.* 1972, **61**, 1829.
76. Scott D. B. et al. *Br. J. Anesth.* 1975, **47**, 56; Lund P. C. et al. *Br. J. Anaesth.* 1975, **47**, 313.
77. Lofgren N. and Tegner C. *Acta Chem. Scand.* 1960, **14**, 486.
78. Wiedling S. *Acta Pharmacol. Toxicol. (Copenh.)* 1960, **17**, 233.
79. Eriksson E. and Gordh T. *Acta Anaesthesiol. Scand.* 1959, Suppl. 2, 81.
80. Bardoczky G. I. et al. *Acta Anaesthesiol. Scand.* 1990, **34**, 162.
81. Nilsson A. et al. *Br. J. Anaesth.* 1990, **64**, 72.
82. Wildsmith J. A. W. et al. *Anaesthesia* 1979, **34**, 919.
83. Armstrong P., Brockway M. and Wildsmith J. A. W. *Anaesthesia* 1990, **45**, 11.
84. Meischer K. *Helv. Chim. Acta* 1932, **15**, 163; Uhlmann T. *Narkose u. Anaesth.* 1929, **2**, 168.
85. Christensen C. *Acta Anaesth. Scand.* 1990, **34**, 165.
86. Whitehead E., Arrigoni B. and Bannister J. *Br. J. Anaesth.* 1990, **64**, 67; Akerman B et al. *Acta Anaesthesiol. Scand.* 1988, **32**, 571; Thonpson G. E. et al. *Reg. Anaesth.* 1989, **14**, 6S; Scott D. B. et al. *Anesth. Analg.* 1989, **69**, 563; Brockway M. S. et al. *Br. J. Anaesth.* 1991, **66**, 31–37.
87. Haynes D. H. and Kirkpatrick A. *Anesthesiology* 1985, **63**, 430.
88. Braun H. *Münch. Med. Wochenschr.* 1903, **50**, 352; *Lokalanaestesie*, 4, Auflage, Leipzig: Barth Verlag, 163.
89. Astrom A. *Acta Physiol. Scand.* 1964, **60**, 30.
90. Matteo R. S. et al. *Anesthesiology* 1962, **23**, 360, 597.
91. Montgomery M. B. et al. *Anesth. Analg.* 1973, **52**, 827; Raj P. P. et al. *Anesth. Analg.* 1973, **52**, 897; Zeh D. W. et al. 1978, **57**, 13; Ford D. J. et al. *Anesth. Analg. (Cleve.)* 1984, **63**, 925.
92. Smith D. C. and Miah H. *Anesthesiology* 1985, **60**, 569.
93. Boulton T. B. *Anaesthesia* 1967, **22**, 101.
94. Gunawardene R. D. and Davenport H. T. *Anaesthesia* 1990, **45**, 52.
95. Scott D. B. et al. *Br. J. Anaesth.* 1976, **48**, 899.
96. Cook J. H. *Ann. R. Coll. Surg.* 1987, **69**, 4.
97. Morris R. W. and Whish D. K. M. *Anaesth. Intensive Care* 1984, **12**, 113.
98. French A. J. and Patel Y. U. *Lancet* 1980, **2**, 482.
99. Fry R. A. and Henderson J. *Anaesthesia* 1990, **45**, 14.
100. Hill J. N. et al. *Anesthesiology* 1983, **59**, 144.
101. Macht S. D. et al. *Surg. Gynecol. Obstet.* 1978, **146**, 87.
102. Greenfield Sluder (1865–1928), originator of guillotine tonsillectomy in 1911.
103. Barton R. P. E. and Gray R. F. E. *J. Laryngol. Otol.* 1979, **93**, 1201.
104. Moffett A. J. *Anaesthesia* 1947, **2**, 31.
105. Curtiss E. S. *Lancet* 1952, **1**, 989.
106. Macintosh R. R. and Ostlere M. *Local Analgesia, Head and Neck* 2nd ed. Edinburgh: Livingstone, 1967.
107. Bodman R. I. and Boyes-Korkis F. *Br. Med. J.* 1960, **2**, 1956.

108. Sowray J. H. *SAAD Digest* 1980, **4**, 128.
109. Blaxter P. L. and Britten M. J. A. *Br. Med. J.* 1967, **1**, 681.
110. Curley R. K. et al. *Br. Dent. J.* 1987, **162**, 113.
111. Takahashi T. and Dohi S. *Br. J. Anaesth.* 1983, **55**, 333.
112. Mushin W. W. and Macintosh R. R. *Proc. R. Soc. Med.* 1945, **38**, 308.
113. Gaskill J. R. and Gillies D. R. *Arch. Otolaryngol.* 1966, **84**, 654; Gaskill J. R. *Arch. Otolaryngol.* 1967, **86**, 697; Coghlan C. J. *Anesth. Analg. Curr. Res.* 1966, **45**, 290; Young T. M. *Anaesthesia* 1976, **31**, 570.
114. Cooper M. and Watson R. L. *Anesthesiology* 1975, **43**, 377; Isaac P. A. et al. *Anaesthesia* 1990, **45**, 46.
115. Ramamurthy S. et al. *Anesth. Analg. (Cleve.)* 1978, **57**, 591.
116. *See* Moore D. C. *Stellate Ganglion Block*. Springfield. Ill.: Thomas, 1954.
117. Leriche R. and Fontaine R. *Presse Méd.* 1934, **41**, 849 (reprinted in 'Classical File', *Surv. Anesthesiol.* 1973, **17**, 297); *Rev. Chir.* 1936, **74**, 751.
118. Kuntz A. *The Autonomic Nervous System*, 3rd ed. Philadelphia: Lea and Febiger, 1945.
119. Winnie A. P. *Plexus Anesthesia* Vol. 1, Edinburgh: Churchill Livingstone, 1983, 43.
120. Valman H. B. et al. *Br. Med. J.* 1977, **1**, 1065; Boscoe M. J. et al. *Anaesthesia* 1983, **38**, 669; Bateman D. N. et al. *Anaesthesia* 1984, **39**, 71; Robertson D. B. *Anaesthesia* 1984, **39**, 603.
121. Cook T. G. et al. *Anesthesiology* 1981, **54**, 421.
122. Dyson F. H. et al. *Br. Med. J.* 1985, **291**, 31.
123. Harding S. F. et al. *Br Med. J.* 1986, **292**, 1428.
124. Moore D. C. *Stellate Ganglion Block*, Springfield, Ill. : Thomas, 1954, 83.
125. Apgar, Virginia, *Anesth. Analg. Curr. Res.* 1948, **27**, 49.
126. Goinard P. *Acad. di. Chir.* 1936, 258.
127. Smith D. W. *Am. J. Surg.* 1951, **82**, 344.
128. Horner J. F. *Klin. Mbl. Augenheilk.* 1869, **7**, 193. It was described by Horner, a Swiss ophthalmologist (1831–1886), in 1869, having been previously noted by Claude Bernard in 1862 and by François Pourfois du petit in 1727; and by Jonathan Hutchinson in 1866 (Hutchinson J. *Illustrations in Clinical Surgery*. London: Churchill, 1878, Vol. 1, 203).
129. Benzon H. T. et al. *Anesth. Analg. (Cleve.)* 1985, **64**, 415.
130. Whitehunt L. et al. *J. Bone Joint Surg.* 1977, **A4**, 541.
131. Zee R. F. Y. *Anaesth. Intensive Care* 1977, **5**, 76.
132. McCallum M. I. and Glynn C. G. *Anaesthesia* 1986, **41**, 850.
133. Rovenstine E. A. and Papper E. M. *Am. J. Surg.* 1948, **75**, 713; Montgomery W. and Cousins M. J. *Br. J. Anaesth.* 1972, **44**, 383.
134. Barton S. and Williams J. D. *Arch. Otolaryngol.* 1971, **93**, 186.
135. Wertheim H. M. and Rovenstine E. A. *Anesthesiology* 1941, **2**, 541; Milougky J. and Rovenstine E. A. *Anesthesiology* 1948, **9**, 76.
136. Matas R. *Johns Hopkins Hosp. Bull.* 1925, **2**, 8.
137. Crile G. W. *Cleveland Med. J.* 1897, **2**, 355.
138. Hirschel G. *Münch. Med. Wochenschr.* 1911, **58**, 1555.
139. Kulenkampff D. *Dtsch. Med. Wochenschr.* 1912, **38**, 1878.
140. Patrick J. *Br. J. Surg.* 1940, **27**, 734.
141. Macintosh R. R. and Mushin W. W. *Local Anaesthesia: Brachial Plexus*, 4th ed. Oxford: Blackwell, 1967. (1st ed. 1943.)
142. Winnie A. P. *Plexus Anesthesia*. Vol. 1, Edinburgh: Churchill Livingstone, 1983.
143. Reding M. *Presse Med.* 1921, **29**, 294.
144. Thompson G. E. and Rorie D. K. *Anesthesiology* 1983, **59**, 117.
145. La Grange P. et al. *Br. J. Anaesth.* 1978. **50**, 965.
146. Yasuda I. et al. *Br. J. Anaesth.* 1980, **52**, 409.
147. Randalls B. *Anaesthesia* 1990, **45**, 143.
148. Knoblanche G. E. *Anaesth. Intensive Care* 1979. **7**, 346.
149. Sibson F. (1814–1876), *Trans. Prov. Med. Surg. Assoc.* 1844, **12**, 307.
150. Moraitis K. *Anaesthesia* 1977, **32**, 161.

151. Mulley K. *Beitr. z. Clin. Chirurg.* 1919, **114**, 666; Etienne J. (1925), *see* Vidal-Lopez F. *Anesth. Analg. (Cleve)* 1977, **56**, 486; Winnie A. P. *Anesth. Analg. (Cleve)* 1970, **49**, 455; Ward M. E. *Anaesthesia* 1974, **29**, 147; Winnie A. P. *Surg. Clin. North Am.* 1975, **55**, 874; Vester-Andersen T. et al. *Acta Anaesthesiol. Scand.* 1981, **35**, 81.

152. Labat G. *Br. J. Anaesth.* 1927, **4**, 174; Livingstone E. M. and Wertheim H. *JAMA* 1927, **88**, 1464.

153. Winnie A. P. *Anesth. Analg. (Cleve.)* 1970, **49**, 455; Mathews P. J. and Hughes T. J. *Anaesthesia* 1983, **38**, 813.

154. Miranda D. R. *Br. J. Anaesth.* 1977, **49**, 722.

155. Barutell C. et al. *Anaesthesia* 1980, **35**, 365.

156. Huang K. C. et al. *Anaesth. Intensive Care* 1986. **14**, 87.

157. Edde R. R. et al. *Anaesth. Analg. (Cleve.)* 1977, **54**, 446.

158. Lim E. K. *Anaesth. Intensive Care* 1979, **7**, 53.

159. Lim E. K. *Anaesthesia* 1979, **34**, 370.

160. Brockway M. S. and Wildsmith J. A. W. *Br. J. Anaesth.* 1990, **64**, 224.

161. Labat G. *Br. J. Anaesth.* 1926, **4**, 174.

162. Burnham R. J. *Anesthesiology* 1958, **19**, 281.

163. Eather K. F. *Anesthesiology* 1958, **19**, 683.

164. Hirschel G. *Münch. Med. Wochenschr.* 1911, **58**, 1555 (translated and reprinted in *Surv. Anesthesiol.* 1963, **7**, 281).

165. Parris M. R. and Chambers W. A. *Br. J. Anaesth.* 1986, **58**, 297.

166. Toumineu M. K. et al. *Anaesthesia* 1987, **42**, 20.

167. Rosenblatt R. et al. *Anesthesiology* 1979, **51**, 565; Winnie A. P. *Surg. Clin. North Am.* 1975, **55**, 861.

168. Boures J. B. *Anaesthesia* 1984, **39**, 1250.

169. Dixon J. M. and Crofts T. J. *J. R. Coll. Surg. Edinb.* 1983, **28**, 292.

170. Bier A. *Arch. Klin. Chir.* 1908, **86**, 1007 (translated and reprinted in 'Classical File', *Surv. Anesthesiol.* 1967, **11**, 294).

171. Holmes C. M. *Lancet* 1963, **1**, 245

172. Riha J. *Anaesthesist* 1962, **11**, 230.

173. Johann Friedrich von Esmarch (1832–1908), professor of surgery in University of Kiel (when August Bier gave his first spinal block in 1898). Esmarch became, by marriage, uncle of Kaiser Wilhelm II of Germany (*Samml. Klin. Vortr.* 1873, **58**, 373).

174. Rhys-Davies N. and Stotter A. T. *Ann. R. Coll. Surg. Engl.* 1985, **67**, 193.

175. Finlay H. *Anaesthesia* 1977, **32**, 357.

176. Davies J. A. H. et al. *Anaesthesia* 1984, **39**, 416.

177. Schmitt H. et al. *Acta Anaes. Scand.* 1990, **34**, 104.

178. Armstrong P., Brockway M. and Wildsmith J. A. W. *Anaesthesia* 1990, **45**, 11.

179. Vaughan R. S. et al. *Ann. R. Coll. Surg. Engl.* 1985, **67**, 309.

180. Tucker G. T. and Boas R. A. *Anesthesiology* 1971, **34**, 538.

181. Wallace W. A. et al. *Hosp. Update.* 1978, **17**, 999; Davis J. A. H. and Walford A. J. *Acta Anaesthesiol. Scand.* 1986, **30**; 145; Valli H. and Rosenberg P. H. *Anaesthesia* 1986, **41**, 1196; Nusbaum L. M. and Hamelberg W. *Anesthesiology* 1986, **64**, 91; Turner P. L. et al. *Aust. N. Z. J. Surg.* 1986, **56**, 153.

182. Ryding F. N. *Anaesthesia* 1981, **36**, 969.

183. Hannington-Kiff J. G. *Lancet* 1984, **1**, 2019. *See also* Kepes E. R. et al. *Reg. Anaesth.* 1982, **7**, 92.

184. Goyanes J. *Rev. Clin. Madr* 1912, **8**, 401.

185. Van Niekerk J. P. de V. and Coetzee T. *Lancet*, 1965, **1**, 1353.

186. Bradfield W. J. D. *Br. J. Surg.* 1963, **50**, 495.

187. Sellheim H. *Verh. Dtsch. Ges. Gyn. Anaesth.* 1907, **59**, 149.

188. Läwen A. *Münch. Med. Wochenschr.* 1911, **58**, 1390.

189. Kappis M. *Zentbl. Chir.* 1912, **39**, 249.

190. Macintosh R. R. and Bryce-Smith R. *Local Analgesia: Abdominal Surgery*. 2nd ed. Edinburgh: Livingstone, 1962.

191. Eason M. J. and Wyatt R. *Anaesthesia* 1979, **34**, 638.
192. Adson A. W. et al. *Surg. Gynecol. Obstet.* 1929, **48**, 577.
193. Leriche R. and Fontaine R. *Presse Méd.* 1934, **2**, 1843 (translated and reprinted in 'Classical File', *Surv. Anesthesiol.* 1974, **18**, 430).
194. Mandl F. *Paravertebral Block.* New York: Grune & Stratton, 1947.
195. Sanderson C. J. *Ann. R. Coll. Surg. Engl.* 1981, **63**, 420; Correspondence, *Ann. R. Coll. Surg. Engl.* 1982, **64**, 135; Duncan J. A. T. *Today's Anaesthetist* 1986, **1**, No. 2, 4.
196. Mandl F. *Paravertebral Block.* London: Heinemann (Medical Books) Ltd., 1928 (translated into English, 1947); Parke F. W. and Chalmers J. A. *J. Obstet. Gynaecol. Br. Commonw.* 1957, **64**, 420.
197. Bryce-Smith R. *Anaesthesia* 1951, **6**, 159; 1955, **10**, 173.
198. McCollum P. T. and Spence V. A. *Br. J. Anaesth.* 1985, **57**, 1146.
199. Lofström B. *Illustrated Handbook of Local Anaesthesia* (Eriksson E. ed.). 2nd ed. London: Lloyd-Luke, 1979.
200. Nunn J. F. and Slavin G. *Br. J. Anaesth.* 1980, **52**, 253; Cronin K. D. and Davies M. J. *Anaesth. Intensive Care* 1976, **4**, 259.
201. Sellheim H. *Verh. Dtsch. Ges. Gynäk.* 1906, 176.
202. Moore D. C. *Br. J. Anaesth.* 1975, **47**, 284.
203. Surg M. R. J. and Bingham R. M. *Anaesthesia* 1986, **41**, 401.
204. James N. R. Regional Anaesthesia for abdominal Surgery, London: Churchill, 1943.
205. Cronin K. D. et al. *Anaesth. Intensive Care* 1976, **4**, 259.
206. Ross W. N. et al. *Br. J. Surg.* 1987, **74**, 63; Baxter A. D. et al. *Br. J. Anaesth.* 1987, **59**, 162.
207. Katz J. et al. *Anesthesiology* 1979, **51**, 233; Orr I. A. et al. *Ann. R. Coll. Surg. Engl.* 1983, **65**, 366.
208. Shretting P. *Br. J. Anaesth.* 1981, **53**, 527; Moore D. C. *Br. J. Anaesth.* 1981, **53**, 1235.
209. Moore D. C. and Bridenbaugh L. D. *Anesth. Analg. Curr. Res.* 1962, **41**, 1.
210. Reiestad F. and Stromskag J. E. *Reg. Anesth.* 1986, **11**, 89.
211. Vadeboncoeur T. R. et al. *Anesthesiology* 1989, **71**, 339; Blake D. W. et al. *Anaesth. Intensive Care* 1989, **17**, 269; Lee A. et al. *Anaesthesia* 1990, **46**, 1028.
212. Lee A. et al. *Anaesthesia* 1991, **45**, 1028; Frenette L. et al. *Can. J. Anaesth.* 1991, **38**, 71; Scott P. V. *Br. J. Anaesth.* 1991, **66**, 131.
213. Scheinin B. et al. *Acta Anaesth. Scand.* 1989, **33**, 156.
214. Ahlburg P. et al. *Acta Anaesthesiol. Scand.* 1990, **34**, 156.
215. McIlvaine W. B. et al. *Anesthesiology* 1988, **69**, 261.
216. Miserocchi G. et al. *J. Appl. Physiol.* 1984, **56**, 526.
217. Kambam J. R. et al. *Can. J. Anaesth.* 1989, **36**, 106.
218. Nauss L. A. et al. *Anesthesiology* 1979, **51**, Suppl. 237; Ward E. M. et al. *Anesth. Analg. (Cleve.)* 1979, **58**, 465.
219. Lavelle J. J. *J. Irish Coll. Phys. Surg.* 1983, **12**, 101.
220. Braun H. *Beitr. Klin. Chir.* 1919, **115**, 161; Braun H. *Die Lokal Anaesthesie.* Leipzig, 1905, 311; Kappis, K. M. *Bruns. Beitr. Klin. Chirg.* 1919, **115**, 161.
221. Kappis M. *Zentbl. Chir.* 1920, **47**, 98; *Dtsch. Med. Wochenschr.* 1920, **40**, 535; *Klin. Wochenschr.* 1923, **2**, 1441.
222. Reid W. et al. *Br. J. Surg.* 1970, **57**, 45.
223. Filshie J. et al. *Anaesthesia* 1983, **38**, 498.
224. *Br. J. Anaesth.* 1990, **64**, 125.
225. Umeda S. and Hashida T. *Abs. 8th World Cong. Anaesth.* Manila, 1984, **1**, 90.
226. Gardner A. M. H. and Soloman G. *Ann. R. Coll. Surg. Engl.* 1984, **66**, 498.
227. Jones N. et al. *Ann. R. Coll. Surg. Engl.* 1977, **59**, 46.
228. Cherry D. A. and Lamberty J. *Anaesth. Intensive Care* 1984, **12**, 59.
229. Braun H. *Die Lokal Anaesthesie.* Leipzig. 1905, 311.
230. Schleich C. L. *Schmerzlöse Operationen.* Berlin: Springer, 1899, 240.
231. Mayerhofer O. In: *Regional Anaesthesia (1884–1984)* Scott D. B. et al. ed. Production ICM AB. Sodertalje, 1984.
232. Hesselbach F. C. *Anatomisch-chirurgische Abhandlung.* Würzburg: Baumgartner, 1806.

233. Alexander-Williams J. and Keithley M. R. B. *Ann. R. Coll. Surg. Engl.* 1979, **61**, 251.
234. Glassow F. *Ann. R. Coll. Surg. Engl.* 1976, **58**, 133; Flanagan L. and Bascom J. V. *Surg. Gynecol. Obstet.* 1981, **153**, 557.
235. Bainton A. *Anaesthesia* 1982, **37**, 696.
236. Macintosh R. R. and Bryce-Smith R. *Local Analgesia: Abdominal Surgery.* 2nd ed. Edinburgh: Livingstone, 1962, 70; Glassow F. *Ann. R. Coll. Surg. Engl.* 1976, **58**, 133.
237. Magbagbeola J. A. O. *Br. J. Anaesth.* 1970, **42**, 184.
238. Armstrong D. N. and Kingsnorth A. N. *Ann. R. Coll. Surg.* 1986, **68**, 207.
239. Glassow F. *Ann. R. Coll. Surg. Engl.* 1976, **58**, 133.
240. Glassow F. *Ann. Surg.* 1976, **58**, 134; Glassow F. *Ann. R. Coll. Surg. Engl.* 1984, **66**, 382.
241. Hayse-Gregson P. B., Achola K. J. and Smith G. *Anaesthesia* 1990, **45**, 7
242. Tverskoy M. et al. *Anesth. Analg.* 1990, **70**, 29.
243. Feeley M. et al. *J. Irish Coll. Phys. Surg.* 1974, **3**, 83.
244. Bacon A. L. C. *Anaesth. Intensive Care* 1977, **5**, 63; White J. et al. *Br. Med. J.* 1983, **266**, 1934; Yeoman P. M. et al. *Anaesthesia* 1983, **38**, 862.
245. Muir J. G. *Anaesthnesia* 1985, **40**, 1021.
246. Sara C. A. and Lowry C. J. *Anaesth. Intensive Care* 1985, **13**, 79.
247. Soliman M. G. and Trembley N. A. *Anesth. Analg. (Cleve.)* 1978, **57**, 495; Goldberg P. J. *J. Urol.* 1981, **126**, 337.
248. Yeoman P. M. et al. *Anaesthesia* 1983, **38**, 862.
249. Berry F. R. *Anaesthesia* 1977, **32**, 576; Khoo S. T. and Brown T. C. K. *Anaesth. Intensive Care* 1984, **11**, 40; Grossbard G. D. and Love B. R. T. *Aust. N. Z. J. Surg.* 1979, **49**, 592.
250. Gjessing J. and Harley N. *Anaesthesia* 1969, **24**, 213.
251. James C. D. T. and Little T. F. *Anaesthesia* 1976, **31**, 1060.
252. Coates D. P. et al. *Anaesthesia* 1983, **38**, 588.
253. Casale F. F. and Thomas T. L. *Anaesthesia* 1983, **38**, 1090.
254. Winnie A. P. et al. *Anesth. Analg.* 1973, **52**, 989; Winnie A. P. *Surg. Clin. North. Am.* 1975, **55**, 881.
255. Taylor R. W. et al. *Ann. R. Coll. Surg. Engl.* 1981, **63**, 207.
256. Brown T. C. K. and Dickens D. R. V. *Anaesth. Intensive Care* 1986, **14**, 126.
257. Loftström B. *Illustrated Handbook of Local Anaesthesia* 2nd ed. London: Lloyd-Luke, 1979, 106.
258. Magora F. et al. *Br. J. Anaesth.* 1969, **41**, 695.
259. Patel N. *Reg. Anaesth.* 1985, **10**, 40.
260. Atkinson R. S. and Lee J. A. *Anaesthesia* 1985, **40**, 1059.
261. Wedel D. J. et al. *Reg. Anaesth.* 1985, **10**, 48.
262. Chayen D. et al. *Anesthesiology* 1976, **45**, 95; Brands E. et al. *Anaesth. Intensive Care* 1978, **6**, 256.
263. Odoom J. A. et al. *Anaesthesia* 1986, **41**, 155.
264. Dalens B., Tanguy A. and Vanneuville G. *Anesth. Analg.* 1990, **70**, 131.
265. Bryce-Smith R. *Postgrad. Med. J.* 1966, **42**, 367; Bryce-Smith R. In: *Practical Regional 1 Analgesia* (Lee J. A. and Bryce-Smith R. ed.). Amsterdam: Excerpta Medica, 1976, 70.
266. Kempthorne P. M. and Brown T. C. K. *Anaesth. Intensive Care* 1984, **12**, 14.
267. Smith B. E. et al. *Anaesthesia* 1984, **39**, 155.
268. Beck G. P. *Anesthesiology* 1963, **24**, 222; Winnie A. P. *Surg. Clin. North Am.* 1975, **45**, 887.
269. *See also* Schurman D. J. *Anesthesiology* 1976, **44**, 348.
270. Bradshaw E. G. and Earlam C. M. *Br. Med. J.* 1982, **285**, 977.
271. Orr C. M. E. et al. *Hosp. Update* 1977, **3**, 465.
272. Dinley R. J. and Micjelinakis E. *Injury* 1972–73, **4**, 345; Cobb A. G. and Houghton G. R. *Br. Med. J.* 1985, **291**, 1683; Cobb A. G. *Br. J. Emerg. Med.* **1**, 9.
273. Cobb A. G. and Houghton G. R. *Br. Med. J.* 1985, **291**, 1683.
274. Hopkins H. H. and Kapany N. S. *Nature* 1954, **173**, 39.
275. Hirschowitz B. I. et al. *Gastroenterology* 1958, **35**, 50.
276. Kennedy W. F. In *Neural Blockade in Clinical Anaesthesia and Management of Pain.* Cousins M. J. and Bridenbaugh P. C. Philadelphia: Lippincott, 1980.

277. Charlton J. E. In *Principles and practice of Regional Anaesthesia* (Wildsmith J. A. W. and Armitage E. N. ed.) Edinburgh: Churchill Livingstone, 1987.
278. Edmunds D. H. and Rosen M. *Anaesthesia* 1984, **39**, 138.
279. Austin T. R. *Anaesthesia* 1980, **35**, 391.
280. Nimmo W. S. In *Practical Regional Anaesthesia* (Henderson J. J. and Nimmo W. S. ed.) Oxford: Blackwell Scientific, 1983: 82.
281. McClure J. H. et al. *Brit. J. Anaesth.* 1983, **55**, 1089.
282. MacKenzie N. and Grant I. S. *Anaesthesia.* 1987, **42**, 3; Wilson E. et al. *Anaesthesia* 1988, **43**, Suppl., 93.
283. Caplan R. A. et al. *Anesthesiology* 1988, **68**, 5.
284. Webberley M. J. and Cuschieri A. *Br. Med. J.* 1982, **285**, 260.
285. Jones R. *Br. Med. J.* 1982, **285**, 512.
286. Vatashki H. et al. *J. R. Soc. Med.* 1982, **75**, 627.
287. Al-Khudhairi D. et al. *Anaesthesia* 1982, **37**, 1002; Kauar P. et al. *Ann. R. Coll. Surg. Engl.* 1984, **66**, 283; Brophy T. et al. *Anaesth. Intensive Care* 1982, **10**, 344.
288. Galizia E. J. et al. *Br. J. Anaesth.* 1975, **47**, 402.
289. Hoare A. M. *Br. J. Hosp. Med.* 1980, **23**, 347.
290. Beavis A. K. et al. *Br. Med. J.* 1979, **1**, 1387.
291. Ikeda S. et al. *Keio J. Med.* 1968, **17**, 1.
292. Allen H. A. et al. *Anesth. Analg. Curr. Res.* 1956, **35**, 386.

Chapter 25

Spinal analgesia: intradural and extradural

INTRADURAL SPINAL ANALGESIA

History

Cerebrospinal fluid discovered by Domenico Cotugno (1736–1822) in 1764;[1] its circulation described by F. Magendie in 1825, who named it.[2]

Cocaine isolated from *Erythroxylon coca* in 1860 by Niemann and Lossen; its analgesic properties described by Schroff in 1862 and von Anrep in 1880.[3] Introduced into medicine as local analgesic for ophthalmology by Carl Koller (1858–1944) encouraged by Sigmund Freud (1856–1939) in 1884.

First spinal analgesia by J. Leonard Corning (1855–1923), New York neurologist, in 1885.[4] He accidentally pierced the dura while experimenting with cocaine on the spinal nerves of a dog. Later he deliberately repeated the intradural injection, called it spinal anaesthesia and suggested it might be used in surgery. "Be the destiny of this observation what it may, it has seemed to me, on the whole, worth recording." This failed to influence his contemporaries. Wrote first book on local analgesia, 1886.[5]

Lumbar puncture standardized as a simple clinical procedure by Heinrich Irenaeus Quincke (1842–1922) of Kiel[6] in Germany in 1891 and by Essex Wynter (1860–1945) in England in the same year.[7]

First planned spinal analgesia for surgery in man performed by August Bier (1861–1949) on 16 August 1898, in Kiel when he injected 3 ml of 0.5% cocaine solution into a 34-year-old labourer.[8] After using it on 6 patients, he and his assistant each injected cocaine into the other's theca. Advised it for operations on legs, but gave it up owing to toxicity of cocaine. Tuffier[9] (1857–1929) and Sicard (1872–1929) in Paris soon afterwards extended its scope to include the external genitals and the abdomen. Frederick Dudley Tait (1862–1918) and Guido E. Caglieri (1871–1951)[10] of San Francisco, and also Rudolf Matas (1860–1957) of New Orleans,[11] were its first users in the US in 1899, their works being published in the following year.

Adrenaline used to increase duration and reduce toxicity of spinal analgesia in 1903.[12]

Stovaine synthesized by Fourneau (French, *fourneau,* stove) (1872–1949) in 1904,[13] used first in spinal analgesia in 1904 by Henri Chaput (1857–1904),[14] and novocaine (procaine) described by Einhorn (1856–1917) in Munich the following year.[15] It was used in spinal analgesia soon after its discovery.[16]

Alfred E. Barker (1850–1916) of London, the leading pioneer of spinal analgesia in Britain, was the first to realize (in 1906–7) the importance of the curves of the vertebral canal and the use of gravity in control of level of analgesia.[17] He introduced heavy Stovaine solutions in 1907 in Britain. Other early users of spinal analgesia in the UK were Robert Jones, the Liverpool orthopaedic surgeon,[18] Dean, of the London Hospital[19] and Tyrrell Gray in children.[20] Babcock of Philadelphia first to use light solution, his formula containing Stovaine, alcohol, lactic acid, strychnine, etc.[21]

Spinal analgesia little used until Gaston Labat's work in 1921.[22] He urged use of neocaine (procaine) crystals dissolved in cerebrospinal fluid, together with barbotage and early Trendelenburg position. Then came George Pitkin, pupil of Babcock, with his light (spinocain) and heavy (duracaine), solutions and his use of the fine-bore, short-bevel needle (1927).[23]

Chen and Schmidt introduced ephedrine in 1923,[24] and Ocherblad and Dillon[25] and Rudolf and Graham[26] used it to maintain the blood pressure in spinal analgesia in 1927. The associated hypotension was first thought to be due to anterior abdominal wall paralysis causing decreased intrathoracic pressure during inspiration.[27] Later it was suggested that the cause was paralysis of the vasoconstrictor nerves supplying the splanchnic and other vessels.[28] Gaston Labat insisted that the hypotension itself was not so important as the cerebral ischaemia it might cause, unless a head down tilt was maintained.

Spinal analgesia was used for surgery of the head, neck and thorax by Jonnesco in 1909[29] and Koster, the Brooklyn surgeon, in 1928.[30]

Miescher discovered the analgesic properties of Percaine (nupercaine) in 1929; it was used in hyperbaric solution by Keyes and McLelland of New York in 1930,[31] and Howard Jones of London published his technique, using hypobaric solution, in 1930,[32] Kirschner of Heidelberg in 1932,[33] and Sebrechts of Bruges in 1934.[34]

Etherington Wilson's work appeared in 1934,[35] and Walter Lemmon's first account of continuous spinal analgesia was published in 1940[36] (although, Dean, of the London Hospital had described this technique as early as 1907[37]).

Lincoln Fleetwood Sise (1874–1942) of Boston in the US popularized amethocaine (tetracaine),[38] which was synthesized by Eisleb in 1928.[39] Bupivacaine was first used for intradural block in 1966.[40]

In the UK intradural spinal analgesia was for many years under a cloud, partly because of the tendency to litigation should complications follow, such as the Woolley and Roe case in which paraplegia followed spinal analgesia in two patients on the same day, and was thought to be due to contamination of the analgesic solution by phenol, which had entered the ampoules through minute cracks in the glass.[41] The articles 'The Grave Spinal Cord Paralyses Caused by Spinal Analgesia' by Foster Kennedy[42] and 'Neurological Complications after Spinal Anaesthesia,[43] also had an important effect on the consensus of opinion. They stimulated Dripps (1911–1974) and Vandam[44] to write their article entitled 'The Long-term Follow-up of Patients who received 10 098 Spinal Analgesics: Failure to Discover Major Neurological Sequelae'.

In recent years there has been a steady increase in the popularity of spinal block for surgery. In the UK, bupivacaine is now the analgesic drug readily available for intradural injection and it is used as the 0.5% solution, plain or with added glucose to render the solution hyperbaric. Experience shows that the technique is safe in expert hands and is to be preferred to general anaesthesia for certain operations and in certain groups of patients. At the same time there is greater understanding of the effects of the injected solution in terms of both physiological and potential toxic effects. For example, a reassessment of the Wooley and Roe case[45] shows that it is unlikely that phenol was the cause of postoperative paralysis. Therapeutic injection of phenol for chronic pain does not give rise to the same clinical picture. A much more likely explanation is that the apparatus used was sterilized by boiling in a sterilizer that had been contaminated with acid substances used to prevent scale formation.

Anatomy

The vertebrae

The vertebral column consists of 7 cervical, 12 thoracic, 5 lumbar, 5 sacral and 4 or 5 coccygeal vertebrae. The sacral and coccygeal vertebrae are fused in adult life.

Vertebral column

This has four curves, of which the thoracic and sacral are primary and are concave anteriorly; therefore, when the spine is fully flexed, the cervical and lumbar curves are obliterated. In the supine position the 3rd lumbar vertebra marks the highest point of the lumbar curve, whereas the 5th thoracic is the lowest point of the dorsal curve. Kyphosis, lordosis, scoliosis and hypertrophic arthritis of the spine may upset the curves and make lumbar puncture difficult.

The direction of the spinous processes determines the direction in which the spinal needle must be inserted. The spinous processes of the cervical, the first two thoracic, and the last four lumbar vertebrae are all practically horizontal and are therefore opposite the bodies of their respective vertebra. The other spinous processes are inclined downwards, their tips being opposite the bodies of the vertebrae next below; exception, the tip of the first lumbar is opposite the intervertebral disk. The 5th lumbar spine overhangs the lumbosacral interspace.

Some useful surface markings

The vertebra prominens (spine of C7) is easily palpable. The tip of the spine of T3 is opposite the roots of the spines of the scapula, with the arms at the sides of the body.

The tip of the spine of T7 is opposite the inferior angle of the scapula, with the arms to the sides.

The highest points of the iliac crests are usually on a line crossing the spine of L4 or the L4–L5 interspace.

The dimples overlying the posterior superior iliac spines are on a line crossing the second, posterior sacral foramina and at this level the dural sac in the adult usually ends. The lower end of the spinal cord terminates at the level of the upper border of the body of L2.

The intervertebral discs

At least one-quarter of the length of the vertebral column is made up of these discs, each of which consists of an outer cover, the annulus fibrosus, enclosing a core of gelatinous material, the nucleus pulposus. The discs give flexibility to the column and act as shock-absorbers. The annulus may rupture, usually posteriorly, so causing pressure on nerve roots. Such a prolapsed disc has been described following a lumbar puncture.

The vertebral canal

Bounded in front by bodies of the vertebrae and intervertebral discs; posteriorly by the laminae, ligamenta flava and the arch, which bears spinous processes, and by ligaments between them called the interspinous; laterally by pedicles and laminae. Size and shape vary, but is larger in cervical and lumbar regions.

Contents. (1) Roots of spinal nerves; (2) spinal membranes with their enclosed cord and cerebrospinal fluid; and (3) structures – vessels, fat and areolar tissue of extradural (epidural) space. The narrowest part is between T4 and T9.

Stenosis of the vertebral canal may cause cord compression after central neural blockade.[46] This may be intensified should there be extradural haemorrhage.[47]

The vertebral ligaments bounding the canal

1. Supraspinous ligament. Passes longitudinally over tips of spinous processes from C7 to the sacrum.

2. Interspinous ligaments. Joining spinous processes together. Cyst formation in the interspinous ligament may result in a false positive sign of entry into the intradural space.

3. Ligamenta flava. Running from lamina to lamina, composed of yellow elastic fibres. Half of the substance of the posterior wall of the vertebral canal is composed of the bony laminae, half by the ligamenta flava. They become progressively thicker from above downwards.

4. Posterior longitudinal ligament. Within the vertebral canal on posterior surfaces of bodies of vertebrae, from which it is separated by the basivertebral veins.

5. Anterior longitudinal ligament. Runs along the front of the vertebral bodies to which, as also to the intervertebral discs, it is adherent.

Midline spinal puncture pierces the first three of these. In lateral approach only ligamenta flava are encountered.

The spinal cord

The elongated part of the central nervous system, which occupies upper two-thirds of vertebral canal and is 45 cm long. Extent is from upper border of atlas to upper border of 2nd lumbar vertebra, and lower still in infants. At its rostral end, continuous with medulla oblongata; below, ends in conus medullaris, from apex of which filum terminale descends as far as the coccyx. In fetal life length of cord corresponds with that of vertebral canal, but the canal grows more rapidly than the cord. Thus nerve roots, which pass out transversely in early fetal life, come to be more and more oblique in direction, so that in adult life lumbar and sacral nerves descend almost vertically to meet their foramina, and are known as the cauda equina. They are bathed in cerebrospinal fluid and will be affected by local analgesic solution injected in the lumbar area. The point of a lumbar puncture needle may touch one or more nerve roots but is unlikely to injure them if the injection is given below the level of the upper border of L2 where the cord ends.

The spinal cord is ensheathed by three membranes from without inwards.

Dura mater. The spinal dura mater represents only the inner or meningeal layer of the cerebral dura mater; the outer, or endosteal layer, being represented by the periosteum lining the vertebral canal, which is separated from the spinal dura by the extradural space. It is connected by fibrous slips to the posterior longitudinal ligament, especially near the lower end of the vertebral canal. The dural sheaths of the spinal nerves fuse with the connective tissue in, or slightly lateral to, the intervertebral foramina. A strong fibrous layer forms a tubular sheath attached above to margins of foramen magnum, and ending below at lower border of second sacral vertebra. This does not prevent solutions of local analgesic from passing into the cranial cavity when excessive doses are injected. Main fibres are longitudinal, so the lumbar puncture needle should be introduced with its bevel separating rather than dividing these fibres.

Arachnoid. This is a thin transparent sheath closely applied to the dura. It surrounds the cranial and spinal nerves as far as their points of exit from the skull and the vertebral canal.

Pia mater. This is separated from the arachnoid by the subarachnoid space filled with cerebrospinal fluid. Here local analgesic drugs are injected in spinal analgesia. The pia closely invests the cord and sends delicate septa into its substance. From each lateral surface of the pia mater a fibrous band, the denticulate ligament, projects into the subarachnoid space, and is attached by a series of pointed processes to the dura as far down as the first lumbar nerve. A posterior midline septum, the septum posticum has been described.[48] This may give rise to unilateral analgesia.[49] The pia mater ends as a prolongation, the filum terminale, which pierces the distal end of the dural sac and is attached to the periosteum of the coccyx. Although in some ways the intradural space is like the glass spine modelled for Barker (1907), being filled with fluid and the spinal cord, it is also broken up by nerve roots, the denticulate ligaments and fine trabeculae, which attach the arachnoid to the pia mater. These may cause obstruction to the free flow of analgesic solution by forming baffles, with uneven distribution and occasional unexpected effects.

There are two enlargements of the cord, one in the cervical, the other in the lumbar region, corresponding to the origins of the nerves of the arms and legs.

Spinal segments

The cord is divided into segments by the pairs of spinal nerves, which arise from it. These pairs are 31 in number and are as follows: (*a*) 8 cervical; (*b*) 12 thoracic; (*c*) 5 lumbar; (*d*) 5 sacral; and (*e*) 1 coccygeal.

The nerve roots within the dura have no epineural sheaths and are therefore easily affected by doses of analgesic drugs brought into contact with them. The cord is not transversely blocked by spinal analgesia, but it is probable that there may be some block of the longitudinal columns by penetration of the drug.[50]

Spinal nerves

Anterior root is efferent and motor.

Sympathetic preganglionic axons arise from cells in the intermediolateral horn of the spinal cord from T1 to L2 inclusive. Blockade of these fibres influences the response of some of the endocrine glands to surgical stress.

Posterior root is larger than anterior. All the afferent impulses from the whole body, including viscera, pass into the posterior roots (largely sensory).

Each posterior root has a ganglion and conveys fibres of: (1) pain; (2) tactile; (3) thermal sensation; (4) deep or muscle sensation from bones, joints, tendons, etc.; (5) afferents from the viscera (accompanying sympathetic); and (6) vasodilator fibres.

Pain and temperature fibres enter the posterior horn where they end around cells in the grey matter; fibres then cross to the contralateral side within three segments and ascend in the lateral spinothalamic tract to the thalamus. Tactile impulses ascend in the ventral spinothalamic tract to the thalamus. Deep or muscle sensory impulses ascend in the posterior columns and spinocerebellar tracts. Vibration impulses ascend in the posterior columns.

The anterior and posterior roots each with its covering of pia – arachnoid and dura cross the extradural space and unite in the intervertebral foramina to form the main spinal nerve trunks, which soon divide into anterior and posterior primary divisions – mixed nerves. These are blocked only secondarily in spinal analgesia; it is block of the nerve roots that gives the effect. There is evidence, however, that analgesic drugs after subarachnoid injection can soak along the nerve trunk for as much as 2 cm beyond the intervertebral foramen. Analgesic drugs affect autonomic, sensory and motor fibres in that order, and fibres which block easily hold the drug longest; thus sensory block lasts longer than motor and usually ascends two segments higher up the cord than motor block.

Segmental levels (Fig. 25.1). Perineum, S1–S4; Inguinal region, L1; Umbilicus, T10; Subcostal arch, T6–T8; Nipple line, T4 and T5; Second intercostal space, T2; Clavicle, C3–C4.

The skin above the nipple line has a double innervation from C3 and C4 and from T2, T3 and T4, so even with a successful block to C8 there will be some sensation above the nipple line. The success of a block to T1 is proved by the inability of the patient to hold a sheet of paper between the fingers (innervation of interossei, C8 and T1).

Segmental Levels of Spinal Reflexes. Epigastric, T7 and T8; Abdominal, T9 and T12; Cremasteric, L1 and L2; Plantar, S1 and S2; Knee jerk, L2–L4; Ankle jerk, S1 and S2: Anal sphincter and wink reflexes, S4–S5.

Movement of joints. Hip flexion L1–L3; extension, L5, S1. Knee flexion L5, S1; extension L2–L3. Ankle flexion L4–L5; extension S1–S2.

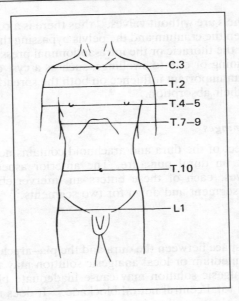

Figure 25.1 Segmental levels

Blood supply to spinal cord

The posterior spinal arteries, two on each side, branch from the posterior inferior cerebellar arteries at the level of the foramen magnum. They supply the posterior columns of the cord.

The anterior spinal artery, a single vessel lying in the substance of the pia mater overlying the anterior median fissure, arises at the level of the foramen magnum from the junction of a small branch from each vertebral artery. It receives communications from the intercostal, lumbar and other small arteries. It supplies the lateral and the anterior columns, three-quarters of the substance of the cord. Thrombosis of this artery causes the anterior spinal artery syndrome in which there is paralysis sparing the posterior columns (joint, position, touch and vibration sense). Communicating branches at the level of T1 and T11 are larger than the others and help to supply the enlargements of the cord (the arteries of Adamkiewicz).[51] The artery at T11 supplies the cord both upwards and downwards; that at T1 only downwards from this level. There are thus three vascular areas in the cord with no anastomosis between them.[52] Normal intra-arterial capillary pressure is 30–35 mmHg. Deprivation of blood supply for 2–3 min may result in infarction of the cord.[53] (*See also* Dommisse G. F. *Arteries and Veins of the Human Spinal Cord from Birth*. Edinburgh: Churchill Livingstone, 1976.)

The extradural veins

These largely form a plexus, most dense in the anterolateral part of the extradural space. They receive blood from the cord and the vertebral canal with its contents and communicate with both the intracranial sinuses and the tributaries of the inferior vena cava and the azygos system. The main longitudinal channels are without valves,[54] thus there is a continuous vascular connection between the cranium and the pelvis bypassing the vena cava. They dilate when either the thoracic or the intra-abdominal pressure is increased as by coughing, straining or due to swellings, such as a cyst or uterus at term. These veins have an important influence on both the spread of local analgesic solutions and on their absorption.

Nerve supply of meninges

The posterior aspect of the dura and arachnoid contains no nerve fibres and so no pain is felt on dural puncture. The anterior aspect is supplied by sinovertebral nerves; each of these enters an intervertebral foramen and passes up for one segment and down for two segments.[55]

The subdural space

This is a potential space between the dura and the pia–arachnoid into which a catheter, contrast medium or local analgesic solution may track.[56] Injection into it of local analgesic solution may cause inadequate block, abnormally high block or even total central neural blockade.[57] It does not communicate with the subarachnoid space but is in free communication with the lymph spaces of the nerves.

The extradural (epidural) space

(*See below* under Extradural block)

The subarachnoid space

This is between the arachnoid and the pia mater and in the lumbar region it occupies more than half the anterior-posterior diameter of the vertebral canal. Communicates with the ventricular system at the base of the brain.

The contents of the space are the spinal nerve roots, the denticulate ligaments, a spongy reticulum of fibres connecting the pia to the arachnoid, the cerebrospinal fluid and the larger vessels.

The cerebrospinal fluid
(*see* Chapter 21)

Its specific gravity averages 1004.5.[58]

Physiology of central neural blockade

Zone of differential block

SENSORY

In intradural block sympathetic fibres are blocked two to three segments higher than sensory fibres. In extradural block the relationship is complex. Some sympathetic afferent fibres escape the block, and when reflex response is high, as in the young anxious patient, considerable sympathetic function may persist.[59] Sympathetic block will be greater when more concentrated solutions are used or when adrenaline is added, as this has a similar effect.[60]

MOTOR

In intradural block, the difference between sensory and motor block is slight (two segments). In extradural block, the difference in levels is greater,[61] depending very much on the nature of the local analgesic solution.[62]

Spinal analgesia will control hyper-reflexia in patients with chronic spinal cord injury.[63]

Nervous system

Order of blocking nerve fibres. (1) Autonomic preganglionic B fibres; (2) temperature fibres – cold before warm; (3) pin-prick fibres; (4) fibres conveying pain greater than pin-prick; (5) touch fibres; (6) deep pressure fibres; (7) somatic motor-fibres; and (8) fibres conveying vibratory sense and proprioceptive impulses.

During recovery, return of sensibility in the reverse order was assumed, but it has been suggested that sympathetic activity returns before sensation.[64] It has been asserted[65] and denied[66] that the cells of the posterior horn of the spinal cord are anaesthetized during both intra- and extradural block.

Spinal analgesia may also exacerbate pain in patients who have severe pain in a limb, e.g. sciatica.[67] In spinal analgesia, entirely adequate for surgery of a lower limb, a patient may complain of pain due to the tourniquet. A concentration of a solution of local analgesic drug may give excellent analgesia for ordinary sensation, conveyed by small nerve fibres, but may not be adequate to block transmission in larger fibres transmitting pressure-pain sensation. An increased concentration will avoid this. Another explanation of bizarre pains occurring during otherwise adequate low spinal analgesia may be that some pain fibres pass with sympathetic nerves to reach the cord at a higher level.[68]

Local analgesic drugs act mainly on the nerve roots leaving the cord, although some drug molecules reach its substance.[69] This depends on: (1) accessibility; diffusion across the pia; the spaces of Virchow-Robin; the arachnoid villi;[70] (2) lipid solubility; and (3) tissue blood flow. Drug molecules are removed from the intradural space[71] by absorption into blood vessels in the pia mater and by movement into the cord substance.

Drugs are removed from the extradural space via the extradural veins; their molecules can also pass through the dura in both directions. Such movement depends on: (1) molecular weight; (2) molecular shape; (3) liposolubility; and (4) the degree of ionization of the molecule. This movement is more important than may be obvious because the dura, although 0.3 mm in thickness in the lumbar area presents a total surface area up to the T10 level of the order of 70 cm^2.[72]

Cardiovascular system

There are six different ways in which intra- and extradural spinal block can influence the cardiovascular system: (1) vasodilatation of resistance and capacitance vessels; (2) block of cardiac efferent sympathetic fibres from T1 and T4 resulting in loss of chronotropic and inotropic drive and fall in cardiac output; (3) the atrial or Bainbridge reflex causing bradycardia; (4) the operation of Marey's law causing tachycardia; (5) depression of vascular smooth muscle and β-adrenergic blockade of myocardium with fall in cardiac output, following systemic absorption of the local analgesic drug (in some circumstances moderate levels of plasma lignocaine may be associated with increased cardiac output, arterial pressure and heart rate, but this is probably a central mechanism dependent upon an intact autonomic system);[73] and (6) adrenaline effect (if used) following absorption, resulting in β-stimulation and associated rise in cardiac output and reduction in peripheral resistance. The overall effect is likely to be a greater fall in mean arterial pressure than if adrenaline had not been used.[74]

Block not extending above T4 is not always associated with fall of blood pressure in fit young adults[75] although the elderly may suffer significant hypotension when moderate volumes are injected into the epidural space.[76] Hypotension is also likely in the debilitated or hypovolaemic subject, and very rarely this may lead to cardiac arrest. When there is cardiac decompensation, removal of sympathetic tone may be dangerous.

Blood pressure fall is usually seen in the first 20 min after injection. Hypotension is seldom a cause for anxiety if the peripheral pulses are easily palpable. Administration of inotropic and chronotropic drugs may cause an increase in the oxygen requirements of cardiac muscle as well as in the oxygen supply. Corrective measures may be considered if arterial pressure falls more than one-third below its pre-operative level.[77]

Slowing of the heart rate is caused if any of the anterior roots carrying sympathetic cardiac-accelerator fibres are blocked, as may happen in high spinals above T4–T5. A further cause of slow pulse rate is the lowering of blood pressure in the right atrium consequent on diminished venous return (Bainbridge (1874–1921) effect).[78] On the other hand, *tachycardia* during spinal analgesia may result from the operation of Mareys (1830–1904) law[79] (a pulse of low tension is fast). Bradycardia is the more frequent effect.

THEORIES OF CAUSATION OF FALL IN BLOOD PRESSURE

1. Diminished cardiac output consequent on reduction of venous return to heart, and lack of muscular propulsive force on veins.

2. Dilatation of post-arteriolar capillaries and small venules due to paralysis of vasoconstrictors. It is seen in entire vascular area, somatic and visceral, where anterior roots are paralysed, together with their sympathetic vasoconstrictor fibres. Compensatory vasoconstriction takes place in areas not anaesthetized, via carotid sinus reflexes. In high spinal blocks, majority of vasoconstrictor fibres, including those to arm (T2–T10), are paralysed, hence low blood pressure. As a concentration of solution less than that required to cause muscular relaxation or analgesia will produce sympathetic block, vasoconstrictor paralysis is often complete even if sensory block is only up as high, say, as T8. The warm, dry arm with dilated veins is often seen in cases of high spinal analgesia. Total peripheral resistance decreases by only 18% following complete sympathetic block in healthy young adults.[80]

3. Paralysis of sympathetic nerve supply to the heart (T1–T4). Bradycardia may give rise to fall in cardiac output.

4. Paralysis of sympathetic nerve supply to adrenal glands (splanchnic nerves), with consequent catecholamine depletion.

5. Absorption of drug into circulation. This is much more likely to be a cause of hypotension after extradural than after intradural analgesia because of the larger amount of analgesic drug injected.

6. Ischaemia and hypoxia of vital centres.

7. Hypovolaemia, if present, may give rise to severe falls in blood pressure if central neural blockade is employed.

8. Compression of the great vessels within the abdomen by the pregnant uterus, abdominal tumours or abdominal packs may cause severe hypotension in the presence of central neural blockade.

TREATMENT OF LOWERED BLOOD PRESSURE (IF THOUGHT TO BE NECESSARY)

Intravenous fluid; oxygen inhalation; injection of pressor drug, e.g. ephedrine 3–6 mg i.v.;[81] elevation of the legs. When there is bradycardia, atropine 0.2 mg alone will often elevate blood pressure.[82] Some anaesthetists use vasopressors prophylactically in high blocks and other cases judged to be doubtful risks.

Electrolyte or colloid solutions used to treat hypotension are successful in a large proportion of cases in amounts up to 2 litres and may be given as a preload.

The vasoconstrictor reflex produced by haemorrhage is abolished by spinal block, in proportion to the height of the block, so that the patient is unable to protect himself against this stress. Early volume replacement is necessary.

Respiratory system

The phrenic nerve supplying the diaphragm rises from the anterior roots of C3, C4 and C5, and should not be encroached on in spinal analgesia, but phrenic paralysis can occur. Apnoea may be due to medullary ischaemia or to a toxic effect of the drug – in extradural blocks. During spinal analgesia, breathing becomes quiet and tranquil. This is due not only to motor blockade, but also to deafferentation with reduction of sensory input to the respiratory centre. Lowered arterial and venous tone also lessens the work of the heart and tends to relieve any pre-existing pulmonary congestion. The ventilation–perfusion relationship during extradural block is not greatly altered and the effect on respiratory function is relatively small with no evidence of change in FRC or V/Q ratio. The pulmonary gas exchange is preserved. The effect of block is largely on the cardiovascular system.[83] Vital capacity and forced expiratory volume may be reduced, especially in cigarette smokers.[84] Intercostal paralysis is compensated for by increased descent of the diaphragm, which is made easier by the lax abdominal walls. This is not accompanied by hypoxia and hypercapnia[85] although the ability to cough forcibly to expel secretions is impaired. Although resulting respiratory function is little affected by spinal analgesia there is less reserve.[86] Obesity is associated with reduced inspiratory capacity. If there is any effect on the phrenic roots, patient cannot talk, but can whisper. Such a condition requires oxygen immediately. Oxygen therapy is beneficial in high block because it decreases heart rate and cardiac output and increases total peripheral resistance, and when a block is accompanied by general anaesthesia.[87] Breathing is quiet and in obstructive airways disease there is some reflex bronchodilatation from stimulation of pressor receptors in the aorticocarotid sinuses by hypotension.[88] There is decreased pulmonary blood volume and pulmonary arterial blood pressure from reduced venous return to the right heart.

After upper abdominal surgery[89] but not following lower abdominal procedures,[90] respiratory function is better if the pain of the operation is relieved by extradural block, rather than by centrally acting analgesics. There is less reduction of FRC and consequent physiological shunting which may arise from airways closure.

The patient may stop breathing so that respiratory support by IPPV and, if necessary, tracheal intubation may be required. Causes may be: (1) inadequate medullary blood flow due to inadequate cardiac output – a serious situation demanding immediate cardiorespiratory support; (2) total spinal analgesia with denervation of all the respiratory muscles. True phrenic paralysis is uncommon because the motor roots are large and the analgesic solution is likely to be weak when it reaches the cervical region; (3) massive epidural spread; (4) accidental subdural injection.[91] A small volume of solution may travel to an unexpectedly high level in this potential space; (5) toxic effects of the local analgesic drug; and (6) injection of narcotic analgesic drug (*see below*).

Gastro-intestinal system

Preganglionic sympathetic fibres from T5 to L1 are inhibitory to gut. No effect on the oesophagus, the innervation of which is vagal. The small gut is contracted as the sympathetic inhibitory impulses are removed, the vagus being all-powerful. Sphincters are relaxed and peristalsis is active although not more frequent. Pressure within the bowel lumen is increased.[92] Handling of the small bowel by the surgeon may cause it to dilate, as may the injection of atropine before operation. Nausea and vomiting due to the hypotension may occur and usually come on in waves lasting a minute or so and then passing away spontaneously. The spleen enlarges two or three times in high block, when its sympathetic efferent fibres (splanchnic nerves) are paralysed. Stimuli arising in the upper abdomen may ascend along the unblocked vagi and perhaps the phrenics, and cause discomfort if the patient is conscious. Para-oesophageal infiltration of local analgesic solution may prevent this by blocking vagal afferents. Colonic blood supply and oxygen availability are increased in animals following spinal analgesia[93] perhaps an important factor in the prevention of anastomotic breakdown following gut resection.

THEORIES OF CAUSATION OF NAUSEA AND VOMITING

(1) Hypotension, correction using a pressor drug may relieve nausea; (2) increased peristalsis; (3) traction on nerve endings and plexuses, especially via vagus; (4) presence of bile in stomach due to relaxation of pyloric and bile-duct sphincters; (5) narcotic analgesics (premedication); (6) psychological factors; and (7) hypoxia. Gastric emptying time is quicker when

extradural block is employed for postoperative pain relief than when narcotic analgesics are used.[94]

TREATMENT OF COMPLICATIONS

This consists in attending to the hypotension and hypoxia, if present; intravenous atropine; deep breathing through the mouth; reassurance and attention to general comfort; anti-emetics; supplementary intravenous anaesthesia with thiopentone and nitrous oxide–oxygen, or a volatile agent, etc., if the condition persists or if the surgeon's work is being affected. Full general anaesthesia may be required.

The liver

There are no specific effects of significance. The degree of hypotension that compromises liver function is not known. Liver disease may interfere with the metabolism of local analgesic drugs.

Endocrine system

The usual increase of antidiuretic hormone during surgery is suppressed.[95] Spinal block delays adrenal response to trauma, whereas operations under general anaesthesia cause a rise in the blood steroids.[96] The rise in blood cortisol levels associated with surgery performed under general anaesthesia may be less marked if afferent impulses are blocked by spinal analgesia. There is, however, no difference when the surgery is major and involving the abdomen or thorax,[97] and in any case there is no difference in the postoperative period once the effects of the block are discontinued.

Spinal block suppresses the hyperglycaemic response to surgery[98] and stress and so is useful in diabetic patients but this does not extend into the postoperative period.[99] The response to insulin is augmented and the anaesthetist should be aware of the possibility of hypoglycaemia. Infused glucose is well utilized.[100] Extradural block prevents lymphopenia and granulocytosis after operation, thus inhibiting the metabolic endocrine response to surgery and preventing immunodepression.[101]

Stress responses

Regional analgesia that blocks afferent impulses plays an important part in avoiding stress responses to surgery. With single-dose blocks the effect is likely to be transitory so that the most effective method is probably continuous extradural block, although even this is not very effective following upper abdominal operations, being better in lower laparotomies. This may be because some afferent pathways (e.g. vagus) remain unblocked.[102]

Genito-urinary system

Sympathetic supply to kidneys from T11 to L1, via the lowest splanchnic nerves.

Any effects on renal function are due to hypotension. Autoregulation of renal blood flow is impaired if mean arterial pressure falls below about 50 mmHg. These changes are transient and disappear when blood pressure rises again. Sphincters of bladder not relaxed, so soiling of table by urine is not seen, and tone of ureters not greatly altered. The penis is often engorged and flaccid due to paralysis of the nervi erigentes (S2 and S3); this is a useful positive sign of successful block. Post-spinal retention of urine may be moderately prolonged as L2 and L3 contain small autonomic fibres and their paralysis lasts longer than that of the larger sensory and motor fibres. During prolonged blockade of the lumbar and sacral segments, the bladder must be palpated so that catheterization can be employed when necessary. Spermatorrhoea is sometimes seen.

The tone of the uterus is not greatly altered after spinal analgesia in pregnancy so that block is not contra-indicated. In late pregnancy smaller doses of analgesic solution are required. Tone of uterus increased in third stage of labour. Block up to T11 is needed for painless labour. *(See* Chapter 22.)

Body temperature

Vasodilatation favours heat loss; absence of sweating favours hyperpyrexia in hot environments. Catecholamine secretion is depressed, hence less heat is produced by metabolism. There is evidence that the extradural space is a temperature sensitive zone, whereas the intradural space is not. Cold solutions injected into the former may induce shivering:[103] (1) because the large veins act as heat exchangers; (2) as a result of the sensory input; and (3) possibly because of the existence of thermal sensors.

Factors influencing height of analgesia in intradural block

1. DOSE OF DRUG INJECTED

Probably the most important single factor.[104] Nerve tissue absorbs local analgesic drugs as blotting-paper absorbs ink; a limited amount of nerve tissue can only absorb so much drug, the surplus being available for convection or absorption into the bloodstream. The greater the dosage and concentration, the higher is the block likely to spread, and the longer will its effect last.

2. VOLUME OF FLUID INJECTED

Recent work suggests that this is much less important than was once thought. Increasing the volume of a fixed concentration of analgesic solution is synonymous with increase in the dose of drug injected. If a fixed amount is given in varying volumes, the spread may be identical.[105]

3. SPECIFIC GRAVITY OF SOLUTION

Baricity. This is the weight of one substance compared with the weight of another substance at the same temperature. Analgesic solutions for intradural injection may be hypo-, iso- or hyperbaric in relation to cerebrospinal fluid (sp.gr. 1004.5 at 37°C).

Plain solutions of local analgesic drugs are likely to be iso- or slightly hypobaric. Addition of glucose between 5 and 8% makes the solution hyperbaric. When the injection is made with the patient in the lateral position the resulting height of segmental block is likely to extend a few segments higher when hyperbaric solution is used in place of plain solution in the same dosage and volume.[106] This may make all the difference between success and failure in spinal analgesia for abdominal surgery.

(*See also*, Brown D. T. et al. *Br. J. Anaesth.* 1980, **52**, 589; Wildsmith J. A. W. et al. *Br. J. Anaesth.* 1981, **53**, 273; Chambers W. A., Edstrom H. H. and Scott D. B. *Br. J. Anaesth.* 1981, **53**, 279; Cummings G. C. et al. *Br. J. Anaesth.* 1984, **56**, 573; Moller I. W., Fernando A. and Edstrom H. H. *Br. J. Anaesth.* 1984, **56**, 1191; Lee A. et al. *Br. J. Anaesth.* 1988, **61**, 135.)

4. POSITION OF PATIENT DURING INJECTION

If the patient sits during the injection and for a short time afterwards, heavy solutions tend to fall, especially if injected slowly, and hypobaric solutions to rise.[107] After injection in the lateral position with the patient turned supine immediately afterwards, the bolus of analgesic solution, if it is hyperbaric, will tend to move either cephalad or caudad, the direction being controlled by the cephalad or caudad inclination of the vertebral canal, which can be influenced by the tilt of the table. The lowest point of the thoracic curve is at the level of T5 and spread above this level is limited unless a very steep head-down tilt is adopted. Further cephalad spread can be inhibited by elevating the head and shoulders of the patient on pillows. A so-called 'brake action' occurs because an analgesic drug becomes fixed to nerve tissue and the concentration in solution becomes less as distance increases from the site of injection.[108]

5. POSTURE OF PATIENT AFTER INJECTION

Whatever the position of the patient within a few minutes of the injection, the effect tends to spread in the same manner. Therefore, injection in the sitting position followed by adoption of the supine state is associated with cephalad spread.[109] If the patient remains on the side, curves of spine are without effect, and specific gravity of solution partially controls side of analgesia, although a predominantly unilateral block soon becomes bilateral.

Positioning of the patient in head-up or head-down tilt will have its major effect on spread of a hyperbaric solution within the first ten minutes following injection. With head-down tilt the lowest point of the thoracic curvature will occur at about T5 level and this will tend to limit upward spread especially if a pillow is placed beneath the shoulders. To limit spread as much as possible to the perineal area the patient should be kept sitting for at least 10 min. Posture has little effect when plain solutions are used.

6. CHOICE OF INTERSPACE

This has only a very marginal effect, but a higher interspace may be chosen when a high block is desired and a lower one for low segmental blocks.

7. PATIENT FACTORS

These include old age (higher segmental block likely for a given dose), height (the effect is marginal), pregnancy (as this progresses the volume of cerebrospinal fluid in the spinal section is decreased and a given dose is likely to spread higher and in a less predictable way)[110]

Factors not influencing height of analgesia in intradural block

These include patient weight, sex, barbotage, speed of injection, composition of cerebrospinal fluid, the circulation of cerebrospinal fluid, the addition of vasoconstrictor drug to the solution, and the direction of the bevel of the standard needle (although not of the Whitacre needle).[111]

The spread of local analgesic solutions within the cerebrospinal fluid has been the subject of much study, but it is often difficult to compare results where conditions are not identical. The reader is referred to some of the reviews published.[112]

Duration of analgesia

Depends on the drug used and the dose administered. The upper end of an abdominal incision regains sensation before the lower end. Addition of adrenaline prolongs the duration of action of amethocaine but not of bupivacaine. These drugs are removed from the intradural space by blood vessels in the pia mater and cord, a process related to lipid solubility. The epidural space has greater vascularity and transfer of analgesic drug to the bloodstream is likely to result in significant plasma levels.

Drugs used to produce intradural spinal analgesia

(For pharmacology, *see* Chapter 24.)

Bupivacaine

Bupivacaine 0.5% is the preferred strength. Higher concentrations result in greater variability of spread[113] and are seldom necessary. In 1% solution, the drug precipitates when mixed with CSF. Hyperbaric solutions are likely to result in block a few segments higher than when plain solutions are used. Dose up to 4 ml of 0.5% solution; this should be reduced in the elderly. *(See also* Tuominen M. *Acta Anaesthesiol. Scand* 1991, **35**, 1.)

Lignocaine hydrochloride, BP

For spinal analgesia has been used in strengths of 2% plain or 5% with dextrose 3.0 and 7.5%.

Other agents

Prilocaine. A 5% solution in 5% dextrose (sp. gr. 1022). Rapid onset of action.

Amethocaine. A 1% solution. Can be combined with dextrose solution to make it hyperbaric or with distilled water to make it hypobaric.[114] The maximal intrathecal dose is 20 mg.

Procaine. The crystals are dissolved in cerebrospinal fluid to make a 5% solution. Analgesia lasts from 40 to 80 min. When a catheter is in place increments may be used to titrate patient needs and prolong effect.

Cinchocaine. A well-tried agent; no longer manufactured.

Mepivacaine. Satisfactory for surgical operations not exceeding 1 h. The 4% solution contains 10% glucose and is hyperbaric.

Vasoconstrictors

Adrenaline (0.2 ml of 1–1000 solution) or phenylephrine (0.5 ml of 1% solution), added to amethocaine prolongs both sensory and motor blockade.[115] Adrenaline added to hyperbaric solutions of bupivacaine[116] or lignocaine[117] does not have this prolongation effect. Vasoconstrictors are seldom used in the intradural space in the UK for fear of compromising the blood supply of the cord, while in addition, the development of catheter technique has made the need for prolonged intradural block by single injection uncommon.

Preliminary medication

Inadequate premedication during spinal analgesia shows callous unconcern for the patient. It may also wreck the smoothness of an otherwise correct technical procedure. Patients who come to the theatre in an anxious state of mind should be helped by further intravenous doses of a suitable sedative or narcotic analgesic.

Many anaesthetists prefer to give premedication such as morphine, 10 mg, with hyoscine, 0.4 mg; agents such as diazepam, midazolam and the neuroleptics are alternatives. An analgesic drug often helps the patient to tolerate the procedure and may be given intravenously before its commencement. Ketamine 0.5 mg/kg has been given when positioning causes pain, as in fractured hip. An intravenous drip should be set up and a preload of crystalloid or colloid given, up to 1 l in fit patients.

Armamentarium

Sterilization is most important and the whole pack should be sterilized by gamma radiation or autoclaved. Disposable sets are available. The lumbar puncture needle should have a short bevel and be as fine as the anaesthetist can with confidence insert through the ligaments. A 25 G needle is commonly employed passed through an introducer, which is prepositioned in the interspinous ligament. In young subjects a 29 G needle has been advocated[118] In young patients there is a greater chance of post-spinal headache, while the ligaments are not likely to be calcified.

Technique of lumbar puncture for intradural block

The lumbar puncture must be done in a good light on a table that can be tilted. Pain can be minimized by the infiltration of local analgesic solution into the subcutaneous and deeper tissues, especially, during the paramedian approach, near the lamina.

Lumbar puncture is contra-indicated in patients with papilloedema or cerebral oedema, especially as the result of tumours in the posterior fossa, for fear of producing a cerebellar pressure cone. Unilateral space-occupying lesions may result in herniation through the tentorial hiatus. It is contra-indicated in suspected spontaneous subarachnoid haemorrhage, unless a CT scan has been performed.[119] Relative contra-indications include blood dyscrasias and those patients on full *anticoagulant therapy*. Skin sepsis and marked spinal deformity are also contra-indications.

Puncture in lateral position

Midline approach. The patient should be supported by a nurse and positioned with back at edge of table and parallel to it, knees flexed on to abdomen, head brought down to knees, and hips and shoulders *vertical to the table* to avoid rotation of the vertebral column. Sudden movement is to be avoided. In the obese the median crease sags downwards sometimes as much as 2.5 cm, so the point of the needle should be inserted above the crease in these cases.

The line joining the highest points of the iliac crests crosses either the spine of the 4th lumbar vertebra or the interspace between L4 and L5. Precise identification of the lumbar spines may be impossible, but this does not matter so long as the first lumbar interspace (and those above this level) are avoided. When the chosen interspace is located the intradermal needle is inserted after careful palpation, midway between the two spines, and a small weal of analgesic solution is raised. A small incision is made in the skin with a large skin needle to prevent a tough skin from grasping the spinal needle tightly and to prevent a core of skin being carried into the intra- or extradural space with the lumbar puncture needle.[120] A Sise or a Rowbotham introducer can be inserted as a cannula through which to introduce a fine spinal needle. A 19 G Butterfly needle can also be used as an introducer for a 25 G spinal needle.[121] The needle is then slowly pushed forwards *parallel to the floor* and at right angles to the back, with its bevel in the plane to separate and not to divide the longitudinal fibres of the dura.[122] If bone is met, it is necessary to withdraw and slightly alter direction either upwards or downwards.

Paramedian approach. A needle is inserted 1.5 cm from the midline directly opposite the centre of the interspace, and the needle is inserted at an angle of 25° to the midline. With this approach, flexion of the back is not so important. It is said to cause minimal pain because tough ligaments are avoided and the sense of touch and needle control are more accurate. Sometimes it is successful when attempts using median approach have failed.

Some advantages of the paramedian approach: (1) the inter- and supraspinous ligaments, sometimes bony hard, are not penetrated, so possibly less backache; (2) the lamina, if touched by the needle, indicates the depth of the extradural space if a marked needle is used; and (3) flexion of the back is not as important as with the median approach; this may be beneficial in late pregnancy.

Puncture in prone position – lumbosacral approach. A weal is raised 1 cm medial and 1 cm inferior to the lowermost prominence of the posterior superior iliac spine. The patient lies prone with a pillow under the hips. A 12-cm needle is inserted at an angle of 55° aiming for the midline at the L5–S1 junction. The ligamentum flavum and the dura are punctured in the usual way. A useful approach in arthritic and obese patients.[123] This approach may also be used for lumbar extradural blocks.

Puncture in the sitting position

Many workers find this easier than the lateral. Patient is placed across the table with the feet resting comfortably on a stool; the spine should be flexed with chin pressed on to sternum. Flexion of the spine rather than flexion of the hips is the aim. It is convenient when block of the sacral roots by hyperbaric solutions is to be done, although this latter block can be done equally well if the puncture is made with the patient in the lateral position, provided that the caudal end of the patient is tipped downwards and the patient placed supine after withdrawal of the needle.

Puncture in the lumbar region requires no after-treatment other than a dab with antiseptic to the skin. Infection seldom occurs in the skin and subcutaneous tissues.

If the needle touches a root of the cauda equina the patient will complain of pain, probably in the leg; usually no harm results from this, but if injection of the drug causes pain the position of the needle should be slightly altered. Such events should be documented. It shows that the needle point is within the vertebral canal and has pierced the ligamentum flavum. If failure results from puncture in one interspace, it can often be made successfully if an adjacent interspace is used.

Injection of the analgesic drug

The prepared solution is drawn up in correct amount into a suitably graduated syringe. It is beneficial to rinse out the syringe first with some of the solution, which is later discarded. To prevent particulate matter from being injected and causing neurological complications, injection into both the intra- and extradural spaces can be made from a syringe fitted with an appropriate filter, pore size 0.22 μm.[124] During injection, occasional aspiration of a small quantity of CSF confirms that all of the solution reaches the subarachnoid space. The needle should remain *in situ* for a few seconds after injection to prevent leak of analgesic solution through the dural puncture hole.

It is advisable to place the patient in the required position without delay so that fixation of the drug does not occur before the desired spread has taken place. For almost any work inside the abdominal cavity analgesia should reach to the subcostal arch (T6–T8). Upper abdominal procedures require block to T4–T5. The cough test is useful in estimating height of block. The patient is asked to cough: the relaxed part of the abdomen bulges out, and any segment not relaxed remains firm and rigid. Disappearance of the knee-jerks shows block at least up to L2, of the ankle-jerk, block of the sacral segments.

Specimen dosage

Doses quoted in the following section are for guidance only. All experienced workers in this field have found the spread of solutions within the intradural space capricious, so that exact levels of analgesia following injection of a given dose cannot always be forecast. In the UK the most commonly available solution is 0.5% bupivacaine, either plain or hyperbaric by addition of 8% glucose. Hyperbaric solutions are likely to spread a few segments higher than plain solutions unless the patient is kept for some minutes in a head-up position.

Sacral block (piles, anal fissure, etc.). Patient sitting or lying lateral with definite caudad tilt; injection of 1 to 1.5 ml of a heavy solution slowly, so that it trickles into the bottom of the subarachnoid space. After 1 min patient can lie supine, as the solution spreads to block the sacral nerves.

Endoscopic work on the prostate and bladder requires block of to the level of T10. As above, patient sitting or in lateral position, injection of 2 to 2.5 ml.

Operations on the lower limbs and hernia operations require block to T10 and a similar technique will suffice. For lower abdominal operations, incision below umbilicus, analgesia to T7 is required. Patient in lateral position, perhaps with slight head-down tilt. Inject 3 ml.

For upper abdominal surgery analgesia must reach T4. This includes colonic surgery. Injection of 4 ml is recommended using head-down tilt immediately after injection and raising the head and shoulders to limit cephalad spread. Afferent stimuli may still pass up vagal fibres. Para-oesophageal block of the vagus may help, as may sedative and analgesic drugs, but light general anaesthesia with tracheal intubation gives the best results. Some workers prefer central neural bockade to relaxant methods because the former is associated with an ischaemic field, gut retraction and good relaxation with adequate spontaneous respiration.

Total spinal analgesia

This was used by Le Filliatre in 1921[125] and by Koster in 1928[126] and was reintroduced by Griffiths and Gillies of Edinburgh[127] as a method of providing the surgeon with an almost bloodless operation field. The technique causes block of all the vasoconstrictors (T1–L2) together with analgesia and relaxation. Now of historic interest only.

Serial or continuous spinal (intradural) analgesia

First described by Dean, of the London Hospital, in 1907.[128] Reintroduced by Lemmon, a Philadelphia surgeon, in 1940.[129] The method was very useful when either the scope or the duration of the operation was uncertain. It enabled minimal dosage to be given without fear of inadequate analgesia, and so was desirable in the aged, the very young and the physically handicapped.

In ill patients, a short-acting agent such as procaine hydrochloride 5%, dissolved either in CSF or 5% glucose solution, is useful.[130] Tuohy[131] designed his lumbar puncture needle for the introduction of a catheter into the intradural space.

In more recent times, a 32 G catheter has been developed.[132] It may be inserted via a 26 G spinal needle and a length of 3 cm left in the intradural space. Increments of 1 to 2 ml plain bupivacaine have been used.[133] There may be problems threading such a fine catheter until the skill has been acquired.[134] One obvious application is in Caesarian section where the extent of spread of solution is capricious.[135] It may also be indicated when the general condition of the patient demands careful control of the height of the block, e.g. in arterial surgery.[136] Microcatheters may also have a place in the administration of narcotic drugs (*see* Chapter 22, Obstetrics).

Conduct of the analgesia

Nausea and vomiting may sometimes be controlled by correction of acute hypotension, but can necessitate sedation or even general anaesthesia, or deep mouth-breathing. If analgesia ascends high up the body, consciousness may be lost, as afferent impulses reaching the cortex become fewer and fewer. Apparatus for general anaesthesia and for oxygen therapy should be at hand, as also should suitable intravenous fluids and pressor drugs. *There must always be an i.v infusion.* It is the duty of the anaesthetist to exercise constant vigilance of the circulation and respiration. Blood pressure estimations should be frequent, particularly during the first half hour following injection, a time when sudden and precipitous falls can occur. The awake patient should be made comfortable on the table.

Difficulties and complications during the operation

The following troublesome symptoms and signs may occur: (1) nausea; (2) vomiting; (3) headache; (4) precordial discomfort; (5) paraesthesiae in the limbs; (6) difficulty in phonation; (7) hypotension; (8) restlessness; (9) inability to cough effectively; and (10) hiccups.

Broken needles and catheters

If a needle breaks, the proximal part and the stylet should, if possible, be left in place to serve as a guide to the distal part. If the proximal part has already been removed, another needle is thrust along the track of the first one for purposes of localization. Removal should be attempted at once. With patient prone, a portable X-ray with image intensifier may be helpful.[137] Should a catheter break, it should be noted and the neurosurgeon informed. It is seldom justified to carry out exploration.

The intradural spinal that does not take

Usual cause is failure to inject all of the analgesic solution in the proper part of the subarachnoid space. May be due to difficulty with lumbar puncture;

displacement of needle point, after successful puncture, movement, etc. It is usually necessary to proceed to general anaesthesia.

Treatment of collapse during spinal analgesia (intradural and extradural)

Turn patient on to back (except in patients in advanced pregnancy or with large abdominal tumours, which may cause pressure on the vena cava and interfere with venous return to the heart – in these cases a bolster placed under the right flank may relieve pressure on the vessel). Tilt the patient head-down. The lungs must be inflated with oxygen, the legs elevated, intravenous fluids infused, and cardiac massage instituted if there is no evidence of cardiac action. A pressor drug (e.g. ephedrine) will be required.

The causes of collapse in spinal analgesia are: (1) lowering of blood pressure to point where coronary arteries are not adequately perfused; (2) hypoxia of vital centres; (3) progressive upward paralysis of respiratory mechanism – should not cause hypoxia as IPPV will carry the patient on until the paralysis wears off; and (4) occasional toxic absorption of drugs injected in extradural block.

Sequelae

Headache[138]

A patient with a postlumbar puncture headache should not be discharged from hospital. It occurs in up to 20% of patients[139] and up to 75% of patients when a large size (e.g. a Tuohy) needle penetrates the dura;[140] much less when fine needles are employed. Onset in first three postoperative days. Usually worse when the patient sits or stands. Often occipital and associated with pain and stiffness in neck; may be vertical or frontal, can cause pain in the orbit.[141] Headaches occur after simple lumbar puncture. The incidence of postlumbar puncture headache in medical wards was estimated at 30%.[142] Sicard first suggested in 1902 that cause might be leakage of CSF into epidural space.[143] The average loss is about 10 ml/h[144] and healing, according to radio-isotope myelography, may take 3 weeks.[145] Air travel, soon after dural puncture, may cause a recurrence of headache.[146] Headache may last days, weeks or months, but usually 1–2 weeks. Loss of up to 10 ml of fluid during lumbar puncture probably has no effect on subsequent headaches. Dural tap has brought to light unsuspected arteriovenous malformations, with delayed neurological signs.[147]

Puncture with an unflexed back may reduce the incidence of headaches as the dural hole is not stretched open.

Theories of causation.

1. Low CSF pressure. The commonest cause is loss of CSF when a hole has been made in the dura either deliberately or accidently. The rate of leakage of CSF exceeds its rate of formation, and this results in changes in the hydrodynamics of the fluid, with loss of cushioning of the brain and pressure or traction on vessels and sensitive brain structures, basal dura, tentorium, etc. In cases of traumatic leakage of CSF, the choroid plexus can form 500 ml/day.

2. High CSF pressure – a response to meningeal irritation. This is the mechanism of headache caused by chemical or bacterial invasion. Quecken-

stedt's test eases pain if applied to patients with low-pressure headache; makes it worse in those with high-pressure headache.[148]

Diagnosis. A postspinal headache is probably caused by the method of analgesia if: (*a*) it is different from any headache previously experienced by the patient; (*b*) it is initiated or made worse by adoption of the sitting or erect posture; (*c*) it has occipital and nuchal components; and (*d*) it is relieved by abdominal compression, which raises the venous pressure.

Treatment. This is prophylactic and combative. *Prophylactic:* (*a*) the elimination of neurotic and unsuitable patients before operation, including those with a history[149] of frequent severe headaches; (*b*) needle gauge in deliberate spinal tap. The smaller the needle gauge the lower the incidence of headache, but the greater the difficulty in its insertion. Fine needles are best inserted through a larger needle that has been advanced into the interspinous ligament; (*c*) the needle point is important. The Whitacre needle has a pencil point and separates rather than tears the fibres and has an orifice not at the tip[150] and in a reavaluation of its use is found to reduce the incidence of headache.[151] The Sprotte needle[152] differs from the Whitacre in the shape and size of the orifice, which is also not at the needle tip, is also effective in reducing the incidence of headache;[153] (*d*) a blunt needle is less likely to penetrate the dura than a sharp one, when attempting extradural block. A larger needle also makes it easier to appreciate the loss of resistance. Both these factors are present when the Tuohy needle with Huber point is used; and (*e*) prevention of dehydration.

Low pressure headache is ameliorated by analgesics. Straining and coughing are predisposing factors.

Treatment of established headache depends on CSF pressure; if this is thought to be low the following measures may help: (*a*) frequent long drinks; (*b*) a tight abdominal binder;[154] (*c*) a continuous drip of Hartmann's solution, via a catheter in the lumbar extradural space, for 24 h;[155] injection of normal saline, 25–50 ml, into the extradural space; (*d*) injection of 10–20 ml of autologous blood into the extradural space, to form a blood patch for sealing the dural puncture; blood patch, using 20 ml had a 92% success rate in 244 cases of postspinal headache.[156] This is occasionally followed by minor neurological changes.[157] Failure of a blood patch to ease headache may be due to incorrect position of the injection or to too small a volume of blood; (*e*) oxygen inhalations may do good while carbon dioxide increases the cerebral blood flow;[158] and (*f*) simple analgesics.

Backache

Probably not much more common after spinal than after general anaesthesia. A small pillow under the lumbar region reduces incidence of postoperative backache irrespective of method of anaesthesia. Damage to intervertebral disc by the needle has been reported.

Retention of urine

No more common after spinal than after general anaesthesia. Usually yields to carbachol, 0.5–1 mg i.m., repeated if necessary, or neostigmine, 0.5 mg i.m. Very occasionally prolonged retention due to spasm of vesical sphincter consequent on spinal analgesia is seen.

Meningitis

Usually due to faulty asepsis, but can occur with a seemingly flawless technique.[159] Aseptic meningitis has been reported.[160] Contamination with chemical antiseptics, starch powder from gloves,[161] detergents, concentration of the drug and variations in pH have all been blamed. The need remains for careful adherence to aseptic technique when blocks are carried out[162]

Paralysis of 6th cranial nerve

Palsy of external rectus causing diplopia. First reported in 1907.[163] Onset commonly between 5th and 11th postoperative days and associated with headache. May be delayed for three weeks. Simple lumbar puncture without injection of analgesic solution can cause it. Has been said to occur in about 1 in 300 cases of spinal analgesia. Paralysis is never complete and is a different entity from the total paralysis associated with such conditions as skull fracture.

Causes. (1) Mechanical, due to upset of hydrodynamics of CSF pressure causing stretching of the abducens nerve. As the 6th nerve runs forwards from the posterior margin of the pons it is crossed by either the anterior inferior cerebellar or the internal auditory artery, or by both, so that if slight displacement of the cerebellum occurs, these arteries are stretched and, being fixed below to the basilar artery, may cut into the nerve like a tight band; (2) inflammatory, low-grade meningitis; and (3) toxic, due to specific action of drug used acting on an unstable binocular vision mechanism, phylogenetically a recently acquired one; a similar condition is seen in acute alcoholic intoxication.

When severe headache occurs, steps must at once be taken to prevent diplopia. The patient must be sent back to bed and rehydrated both orally and parenterally. The antidiuretic hormone in posterior pituitary extract may be useful.

While the condition persists, dark glasses should be worn, with the outer one-third of glass of affected eye made opaque. About 50% of cases recover within a month. If after 2 years spontaneous recovery of function has not occurred, operative cure may be considered. About 25% of the cases show bilateral nerve involvement.

Paralysis of every cranial nerve except the 1st, 9th and 10th has been reported after spinal analgesia, and transient deafness or tinnitus is not uncommon. Diplopia has been reported following general anaesthesia and after the use of relaxants and may then persist for some time.[164]

Other neurological lesions

Permanent neurological sequelae first reported by Koenig in 1906. Transient lesions of cauda equina causing abnormalities of leg reflexes, incontinence of faeces, retention of urine, loss of sexual function, sensory loss in lumbosacral distribution and temporary paralysis of peroneal nerve. Most of these clear up spontaneously.[165] Radiculitis, ascending myelitis, transient transverse myelitis,[166] adhesive arachnoiditis paraplegia,[42] meningo-encephalitis and bulbar involvement have all been reported. Their cause is not fully understood nor is it always due to the method of pain relief.[167] It may well be the result of the drug injected. Distinguished neurologists have blamed the local analgesic drug,[168] and the low pH of a large volume of injected solution has also been blamed. Haematoma formation may cause trouble due to pressure on the cord.[169] Severe back pain with paraplegia requires emergency neurological examination and, if necessary, surgical exploration. Ischaemia of the cord due to severe hypotension, or the use of local vasoconstrictors, may be causal. Electromyographic studies enable lesions of the lower motor neurone type due to spinal analgesia to be differentiated from other neurological and myopathic conditions.[170] In the dog, severe hypotension and/or the intravenous infusion of large volumes of non-colloid solutions, poor in electrolytes (e.g. 5% dextrose solution), tend to increase the incidence of neurological signs.[171] An extradural abscess following several spinal blocks, without causing either sensory or motor impairment, only localized pain, in a diabetic patient with an infected leg, has been reported.[172] Spinal stenosis may be responsible for neurological sequelae.[173]

Anterior spinal artery syndrome.[174] A lower motor neuron paralysis (paraplegia) without involvement of the posterior columns of the spinal cord, subserving joint position sense, touch and vibration sensibility. It has followed spinal analgesia.[175]

A constricting pachymeningitis may develop some time after intradural block. Horner's syndrome has been reported following extradural sacral block in obstetric patients.[176] Phantom limb pain after amputation may be caused by intradural block and may be so severe as to require general anaesthesia for its relief.[177] Intracerebral haematoma formation causing hemiparesis, coincident with a lumbar puncture with a 19 G needle, in a previously fit patient, has been reported.[178] Pruritus following intradural block, in patients with peripheral neuropathy has been seen.[179] The addition of sodium metabisulphite as an anti-oxidant, to solutions for intradural injection (e.g. chloroprocaine) may cause neurological damage.[180] Spinal stroke can occur independently of central neural blockade. An infarcted cord does not recover.[181]

Conditions that may cause signs and symptoms referable to the central nervous system in any postoperative patient may include: vascular, neoplastic, infective or viral disease, myopathies, neuropathies, and operative trauma, e.g. due to the position of the patient on the table, retractors, etc. Careful clinical and electromyographic investigation is always necessary. Prolonged block following extradural injection of 1% etidocaine has been reported.[182] Subdural haematoma with delayed neurological signs, ending in death, has also occurred.[183]

Neurological complications following spinal analgesia are not necessarily due to the method,[167, 184] because such complications following surgical operations may be seen in patients who have have had general anaesthesia.[185] Epidermoid spinal tumours have been reported.[186] Lumbar canal stenosis can result in compression of nervous structures.[187]

THE CHOICE BETWEEN SPINAL INTRA- AND EXTRADURAL ANALGESIA AND GENERAL ANAESTHESIA

Advantages of spinal analgesia

Obviates the need for deep anaesthesia, profound muscle relaxant drug dosage and preserves spontaneous respiration; cheap, ideal for fit patients who object to being put to sleep, lessens risk of vomiting causing pulmonary aspiration in patients with full stomach, quiet relaxed abdomen together with small contracted intestines helps surgeon; intubation is unnecessary; upset of body chemistry minimal; intestinal function returns early; and wound bleeding reduced.

Intradural block can be said to have the following advantages over extradural: (1) it is easier; (2) it is quicker; (3) it requires less skill and experience; (4) it provides slightly better relaxation of the abdomen; (5) it gives better control over the height of the block; and (6) the danger of toxic signs due to the drug are negligible.

Disadvantages of spinal analgesia

Spinal analgesia may cause hypotension in some patients; the incidence of postoperative headache; may take some time to induce; and motor paralysis may persist into the postoperative period. Some patients prefer to be asleep during surgery.

Indications for spinal analgesia (intradural and extradural)

These vary greatly with different surgeons and anaesthetists.

Useful when muscle relaxants are contra-indicated, or when it is thought advantageous to preserve spontaneous respiration. Patients with chronic respiratory disease often do well with central neural blockade as tracheal intubation may be avoided. Following the insertion of a catheter into the extradural space, postoperative pain can be relieved by repeated injections of either opioids or local analgesics, without interfering too much with respiratory function. Some patients fear loss of consciousness and prefer to remain awake. Acute cases, including obstetric patientts, with a full stomach are at less risk of inhalation of stomach contents under spinal than with general anaesthesia. Some patients with compromised hepatorenal function may do well with central neural blockade.[188] Skilled workers may meet fewer difficulties with central neural blockade than with general anaesthesia in the morbidly obese patient, using a thoracic blockade.[189]

Examples of procedures particularly suited to spinal methods are: amputations; hip surgery,[190] when blood loss and postoperative thrombophlebitis are reduced;[191] transurethral endoscopy with resection of prostate gland or bladder tumour; colectomy;[192] hysterectomy and vaginal repair; haemorrhoidectomy; and in operative obstetrics.[193] Useful whenever a bloodless field is desirable, or when a contracted bowel (not seen with muscle relaxants) is advantageous. In surgery of the colon, central neural blockade may improve vascularity at the site of anastomosis; reversal of relaxants, which could be harmful, is unnecessary.[194] For vascular surgery, the use of central neural blockade is controversial. Combined intra- and extradural injection may be performed using a 25 or 26 G needle inserted through a Tuohy needle (than which it must be 1 cm longer). This may give rapid onset of analgesia followed by an extradural catheter. In hip surgery, epidural block is associated with a smaller incidence deep vein thrombosis than general anaesthesia.[195] The changes produced in the cardiovascular system under low block are usually small, unlike those caused by a block to a higher level. Low spinal analgesia may often be indicated in poor-risk cases instead of general anaesthesia.

Contra-indications to intra- and extradural block

Should not, without a good reason, be used on unwilling or unco-operative patients, including young children. Often unwise in the following groups without careful consideration:

1. Cardiovascular. Severe shock; hypovolaemia; dehydration; hypotension below 80–90 mmHg systolic; gross hypertension; patients unable to do reasonable physical work because of obesity; senility; myocardial degeneration; toxaemia; severe ischaemic heart disease, especially with history of recent infarction, because of the dangers of hypotension; and cerebral atheroma. In any patient with a fixed cardiac output (severe valvular stenosis, heart block, medication with β-blocking drugs, etc.) and therefore unable to respond to dilatation of the vascular bed, sudden blood loss, etc. Hypertensive patients whose hypertension is uncontrolled medically are more at risk than those whose blood pressure is controlled when given extradural block. They need careful monitoring.[196]

2. Mechanical. Spinal analgesia, properly performed, is safe for obese patients and for those with obstructive lung disease.[197] Patients with a splinted diaphragm that interferes with breathing, such as hydramnios, large ovarian and uterine tumours, e.g. pregnancy; ascites, omental obesity. Dangers to be considered include hypoxia due to respiratory inadequacy and aortocaval compression by the tumour mass. Lateral tilt, oxygen and IPPV should be used when indicated. Dosage should be reduced in such patients.

3. Respiratory. Patients who are breathless from any cause; they may become hypoxic, especially if level of analgesia is high. On the other hand, patients with emphysema or bronchospasm often do surprisingly well after spinal blocks.

4. Abnormalities of the central nervous system. Spinal analgesia should not be given to a patient with an abnormality of the central nervous system, whether it be congenital or acquired, infective or degenerative, active or inactive or healed unless the indications are compelling, although this view has been contested by experienced workers.[198] Any subsequent symptoms may be blamed on the spinal. Patients who are chronic sufferers from headaches will in all probability get a headache of moderate severity after operation following intradural block. If it is suspected on the history (headache, vomiting, blurred vision) or the physical signs (papilloedema, bradycardia, drowsiness) that the patient has an expanding cerebral lesion, a tumour, cyst or abscess, which may, if the intracranial pressure is suddenly altered, cause obstruction to the cerebrospinal fluid or blood circulation (the pressure cone), intradural block is absolutely contra-indicated.

5. *Gastrointestinal perforations.* Contraction of the gut adds to the soiling of the peritoneum in these cases.

6. *Genito-urinary.* Patients who may have an enlarged prostate (which is not the reason for the surgical procedure). Bladder difficulty may be complained of after operation and blamed on the method of pain relief. In renal failure, the low blood pressure associated with spinal analgesia may result in temporary oliguria, which may compromise renal function.

7. *Cases with deformed backs.* Because of difficulty in the performance of lumbar puncture.

8. *Skin sepsis.* In lumbar region.

9. *Neurological operations.* In operations for lesions of the spinal cord or cauda equina, on medicolegal grounds. Many anaesthetists, however, favour the use of extradural block for laminectomy for prolapsed disc with the patient on his side during operation. (Thorne T. C. and Watt M. J. personal communication.)

10. *Patients with disorder of blood clotting and those on anticoagulants or aspirin.* The precise risk in undertaking lumbar puncture in these patients is unknown. To be considered are: (1) patients on anticoagulant or thrombolytic therapy before operation; (2) patients receiving low dose heparin; (3) patients on low dose aspirin therapy; (4) those requiring perioperative anticoagulants; and (5) those who will need anticoagulants after operation. The risk is difficult to quantify and each patient must be treated individually. Where central neural blockade is thought to be in the interest of the patient an experienced operator is likely to cause less trauma than a beginner. In the case of heparin, the maximum systemic concentration is likely to be within 2 h of subcutaneous administration[199] and it is probably wise to avoid instituting a block within 4 to 6 h of heparin administration. The bleeding time may be an important test and should be not more than 10 min. Lumbar puncture may be dangerous if the thrombotest value is less than 10% at the time of the procedure.[200] It should be remembered that extradural haematoma can occur spontaneously.

(*See also* Macdonald R. *Br. J. Anaesth.* 1991, **66**, 1; Wildsmith J. A. W. and McClure J. H. *Anaesthesia* 1991, **46**, 613.)

11. *In cases of dehydration.* These are bad risks and a much smaller dose of drug than usual is required. A catheter technique may be advisable.

Spinal intradural analgesia in children

Advocated by Tyrrell Gray in 1909,[201] but seldom used today. Risk of circulatory depression minimal because of elasticity of their cardiovascular systems. Puncture should be in the L4–L5 interspace because cord extends lower in children than in adults.

(*See also* Abajian J. C. et al. *Anesth. Analg.* 1984, **63**, 359; Harnik E. V. et al. *Anesthesiology* 1986, **64**, 95; Correspondence, *Anesthesiology* 1986, **65**, 559.)

Spinal intradural analgesia in pregnancy

Spinal and extradural block for surgery in pregnancy do not materially increase the uterine tone and do not harm the fetus. *(See* Chapter 22.)

(There are few aspects of intradural block that are not fully and clearly discussed in the classic treatise by Peere C. Lund In: *Principles and Practice of Spinal Anesthesia.* Springfield, Ill.: Thomas, 1971. *See also* Lee J. A. et al. *Sir Robert Macintosh's Lumbar Puncture and Spinal Analgesia.* 5th ed. Edinburgh: Churchill Livingstone, 1985.)

EXTRADURAL (EPIDURAL) BLOCK

Definition

Blockage of nerve roots outside the dura. A method giving reflex flaccidity of muscles, analgesia, a degree of hypotension and consequent ischaemia secondary to sympathetic blockade while allowing spontaneous respiration to continue relatively unimpaired. May be used for: (1) the relief of pain during and/or following surgical operations; (2) the relief of pain during labour; (3) the reduction of bleeding by producing hypotension during surgery; and (4) to supplement light general anaesthesia and so suppressing the transmission of afferent impulses and hormonal and autonomic responses to surgery.[202] It will provide relaxation of the abdomen without the use of myoneural blocking agents.

History

Introduced by Corning, and used in dogs by Cathelin[203] and Sicard (1872–1929)[204] in 1901, and in man, tentatively, by Kappis[205] and by Bleeck and Strauss,[206] and applied in clinical surgery by Pages[207] in 1921 and by Doliotti[208] and Aburel[209] in 1931. Popularized in Britain by Massey Dawkins.[210] Curbelo of Cuba was the first worker to insert a catheter into the extradural space in 1949.[211] (*See also* Little D. M. *Surv. Anesthesiol.* 1981, **25**, 340.)

Anatomy of the extradural space

The spinal dura mater represents the meningeal layer of the dura mater of the brain; the periosteum lining the vertebral canal represents the outer layer of the cerebral dura. Between the spinal dura and the vertebral canal is the extradural (epidural, peridural) space. Its average diameter is 0.5 cm and it is widest in the midline posteriorly in the lumbar region.

Its boundaries are: superiorly the foramen magnum and inferiorly the sacrococcygeal membrane; posteriorly the anterior surfaces of the laminae and their connecting ligaments, the roots of the vertebral spines and the ligamenta flava, anteriorly the posterior longitudinal ligament covering the vertebral bodies and the discs; and laterally the pedicles and intervertebral foramina. The interspinous ligaments and the ligamenta flava, dense gristly tissue, are important in locating the extradural space.

The contents include the dural sac and the spinal nerve roots, the extradural plexus of veins and the spinal arteries, lymphatics and fat. The veins become distended when the patient strains or coughs, i.e. during bouts of increased intrathoracic or intra-abdominal pressure. The veins form a network that runs in four main trunks along the space. They communicate with venous rings at each vertebral level, with the basivertebral veins on the posterior aspect of each vertebral body, and with the ascending and deep cervical, intercostal, iliolumbar and lateral sacral veins. These veins have no valves and constitute the valveless vertebral venous plexus of Batson.[212] They connect the pelvic veins below with the intracranial veins above, so that air or local analgesic solution injected into one of them may ascend straight to the brain. They drain into the inferior vena cava via the azygos vein, so that when there is obstruction to vena caval flow, as with large abdominal tumours, advanced pregnancy, etc., they become distended. They form an alternative venous pathway to the caval system.

There are 58 intervertebral foramina and the degree of their patency is an important factor in controlling the height of analgesic a given volume of analgesic solution will produce. They tend to be more permeable in the young than in the old, so that a given volume of solution tends to cause a higher block in the old than in the young. The shape of the space is triangular with the apex dorsomedial. A dorsomedial fold of dura mater occasionally divides the space into a ventral and two dorsomedial compartments, which do not always communicate freely with each other. Such abnormalities may explain patchy analgesia or inadvertent dural puncture when the midline approach is used.[213] Reports of cases of unilateral extradural block support the existence of a dorsomedial septum.[214]

The dura mater is attached to the margins of the foramen magnum, but this does not prevent the passage of analgesic drug into the cranial cavity. It is also attached to the 2nd and 3rd cervical vertebrae and to the posterior longitudinal ligament. It ends at the lower border of the 2nd sacral vertebra, a point corresponding in level with the posterior superior iliac spines. Prolongations of the dura surround the spinal nerve roots and fuse with the epineurium of the complete spinal nerves, as they traverse the intervertebral foramina. Extradural block includes blocking of the sympathetic fibres travelling with the anterior or ventral roots, which soon become the white rami. Usual distance between skin and extradural space 4–5 cm.[215] For topography of the lumbar epidural space, *see* Husemeyer R. P. and White D. C. *Anaesthesia* 1980, **35**, 7.

Causes of negative pressure in extradural space

There is a negative pressure in the extradural space in only about 80% of patients.[216]

Possible causes: (1) dimpling of dura by needle;[217] (2) transfer of negative pressure from thorax via paravertebral spaces (especially in the thoracic region),[218] (3) full flexion of the back;[219] (4) the initial bulge forwards of the yellow ligament in front of the advancing needle, followed by its rapid return to the resting position once the needle has perforated the ligament;[220] and (5) one cause of the negative pressure is the redistribution of CSF in the intradural space, which creates a pressure between the dura and the walls of the vertebral canal. This is greater in the recumbent than in the vertical position.[221]

Negative pressure in extradural space is not the same at all levels and in the sacral canal it is absent. It may be lower in the thoracic region than in the lumbar part of the space.

This negative extradural pressure may account for the leakage of CSF into the extradural space after lumbar puncture, contributing to headache.

Caval compression from large intra-abdominal tumours can cause extradural venous distension. A rise in pressure may favour spread of local analgesic solution.[222] The pressure may be positive in labour.[223] Injection of a small volume of fluid is likely to increase both the extradural and the CSF pressure.[224]

Site of action

When a solution of a local analgesic is injected into the extradural space it may exert its effect: (1) on the nerve roots in the extradural space; (2) on the nerve roots in the paravertebral spaces after they have shed their dural sheaths;[225] (3) on the nerve roots in the intradural or subarachnoid space after inward diffusion of the drug across the dura;[226] and (4) diffusion into the subperineural and subpial spaces from the so-called 'ink-cuff' zone[227] where the anterior and posterior nerve roots fuse. Analgesic drug may eventually pass centripetally and reach the substance of the cord and diffuse out from this into the CSF, where its concentration is significant.[228] Injected solution can thus spread up and down the space, especially in the elderly; laterally into the paravertebral space, especially in the young, although this has been questioned; and centripetally into the neuraxis along the subepineural (subperineural) spaces.[229]

The following fibres are blocked: (1) anterior nerve roots; (2) posterior nerve roots and their ganglia; (3) mixed spinal nerves; (4) white and grey rami communicantes; (5) visceral afferents accompanying sympathetic fibres; and (6) certain descending pathways in the spinal cord.[230]

Factors influencing spread of solution: (1) the volume of solution injected; (2) the age of the patient, the old requiring less than the young – the largest dose is required at about the age of 19; (3) the force of injection – fast injection spreads the solution thinly over a wide area and may give an incomplete but extensive zone of analgesia; (4) the amount of drug used; (5) the level at which an injection is given;[231] (6) gravity – a head-down tilt aids cephalad diffusion of the solution and vice versa; (7) the length of the vertebral column; (8) full-term pregnancy or abdominal tumours – one-third to one-half normal doses required; (9) concentration of local analgesic solution – a given volume of a high concentration will spread further than an equal volume of a lower concentration; and (10) in diabetes and in occlusive arterial disease less solution is required, although in the latter condition, this has been questioned.[232] *The height of analgesia produced by a given volume of solution is one of the great uncertainties of anaesthesia.* Four segments on each side of the point of injection are said to be affected by the extradural injections of 10–15 ml of analgesic solution.

Combined intra- and extradural block in the same patient has been described, using either two needles, one intra- and the other extradural[233] or inserting a long needle into the intradural space through a wider needle in the extradural space.[234]

Local analgesic solutions used

Lignocaine 1–2%, which has a rapid onset in about 10 min and gives good relaxation. Duration of effect 1.5–2 h – depending on strength of solution employed; 0.5% solution gives good sensory without motor block. 1.5% solution gives good motor block. In very muscular patients, 2% solution may produce more intense muscular relaxation. Lignocaine and bupivacaine can be given in a mixture.[235]

Bupivacaine (Marcain) is a long-acting drug, which has been used in 0.5% concentration with or without adrenaline, giving analgesia for up to 8 h.[236] Volumes in excess of 20 ml need to be given with care. Motor block is not quite so intense as that produced by 1.5% lignocaine. In obstetrics, 0.25–0.375% solutions are popular. For surgical operations, 0.75% has been advocated.[237] Continuous administration using a syringe pump is safer if plama concentration is monitored because toxic sequelae have been reported.[238]

Ropivacaine hydrochloride is similar to bupivacaine in terms of speed of onset and duration, but ropivacaine is slightly less potent, has a slightly shorter duration of action and causes less motor block.[239] It has been used in concentrations between 0.5 and 1%.

Amethocaine hydrochloride can be added to lignocaine solution, e.g. 50 mg added to 50 ml giving a 0.1% strength. It increases the duration of analgesia by about 50% and gives good motor block.

Prilocaine. Strengths of 1.5, 2 and 3%, with adrenaline 1–200 000, have been recommended. It is a little less toxic than lignocaine. Doses in excess of 600 mg may cause cyanosis from methaemoglobinaemia.

Etidocaine[240] 1 or 1.5% solution. Results in greater motor block than bupivacaine.

Chloroprocaine hydrochloride.[241] Used mainly in the USA as 2–3% solution. Short latency and duration of activity (about 45 min), its effects ceasing suddenly.

Adrenaline. This may be added in the usual strength, i.e. 0.1 ml of the 1 in 1000 solution in 20 ml of local analgesic solution (making 1 in 200000). By preventing absorption of the analgesic drug it may cause more intense blockade of nerve fibres and hence greater sympathetic blockade.[230] Some workers omit adrenaline because they fear the combined effect of hypotension and vasoconstriction on the nerve tissue. It may also be omitted in the presence of thyrotoxicosis, in those receiving tricyclic antidepressant drugs and in labour. The acidity of local analgesic solutions is increased when adrenaline is contained in commercial solutions from about pH 6 to 3. If used, adrenaline is better added freshly.

Potentiation of local analgesic solutions

By raising the alkalinity of solution. Combination of local analgesic bases with CO_2 to form bicarbonate salts, which have a pH of about 6.5. The free base is rapidly liberated in the tissues due to buffering and the liberated CO_2 diffuses, causing a fall in the intracellular pH in the vicinity, so that the local analgesic base is brought close to the nerve membrane in higher concentration for combination with the receptors.[242] These salts are said to combine low toxicity, rapid onset and sensory and motor block of intense degree.[243] Carbonated salts of lignocaine, prilocaine and bupivacaine have been prepared, but are not commercially available in the UK.

Methods of location of the extradural space

Before any block is attempted, an open vein must be guaranteed (by indwelling cannula, drip, etc.). No block must be attempted without this supremely important precaution. The extradural space may be entered from the midline or laterally, with the patient either on the side or sitting. *For midline approach* great care must be taken to insert the needle in the sagittal plane to minimize injury to extradural veins. Selection of the needle depends on individual preference, but the Tuohy is chosen when a catheter is to be inserted. The greater the gauge of the needle the easier it is to appreciate loss of resistance, but the greater the hole if an inadvertant dural puncture occurs. The Tuohy needle is less likely to puncture the dura than a sharper pointed needle. The needle should be suitably marked to enable the depth of the point to be instantly recognized[244] (Fig. 25.2). Full flexion of the spine should be employed for the insertion of the needle into the ligamentum flavum, but this position stretches the dura and makes it more liable to be punctured. The back should therefore be slightly deflexed as the needle is advanced towards the space from the ligamentum flavum. The level from which the block is made is not very important and any easily palpable interspace below L1/L2 should be chosen. The depth of the extradural space has been measured by ultrasound.[245]

For the lateral or paramedian approach a weal is raised 1 cm from the midline opposite the lower edge of the spinous process.[246] The needle is then inserted at right angles to the back until the body lamina is touched and the depth of this noted. The needle is next withdrawn as far as the muscle sheath and reinserted at an angle of 10° upwards and 10° medially. When the needle

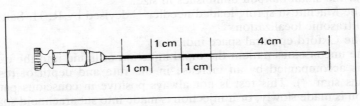

Figure 25.2 The Lee marked needle (*Medical & Industrial Equipment*).

lies at the depth of the laminae, the stylet is withdrawn and the loss of resistance test applied. Useful for mid-thoracic approach.

Both the midline and the lateral entry into the space may be performed with the patient in the sitting position, and this may be the easier way in obese and in some arthritic cases, and also for thoracic puncture, using a negative-pressure method.

An easily palpable interspace should be selected, if possible a high one above L3 for a high block and a lower space for a low block.

Injection in the *thoracic region* is more difficult and is best avoided between T4 and T9. The patient should either be sitting up and a negative pressure test employed or the loss of resistance test used. Injection between T10 and L1 causes little difficulty and is similar to injection between L2 and L5, although the extradural space is shallower. In the midthoracic region, the needle should be inserted at an angle of 40°. Care must be taken not to damage the cord. The angulation, however, renders accidental dural puncture unlikely, since the Tuohy needle tends to 'toboggan' along the dura. The paramedian approach is useful in the thoracic region (*see below*). The prone position, with lumbar elevation by an inflatable rubber pillow beneath the lower abdomen, has been successfully used for gaining access to the extradural space.[247] The beginner can be taught the 'feel' of the extradural puncture in the post-mortem room.[248]

The following points suggest that the needle is in the extradural space:

1. Sudden lack of resistance to advancing needle as it leaves the dense ligamentum flavum.

2. Sudden ease of injection of a little air or liquid from a freely running syringe attached to a needle. If the point is in the ligamentum flavum, the plunger rebounds; if it is in the space, it can be pushed in easily (Sicard and Forestier, 1921;[249] Dogliotti, 1931[208]). A false-positive test may result if the needle point enters a small cyst in the yellow ligament.[250] If air is used care must be taken not to inject too much in case nerve roots are shielded from the analgesic solution by a bubble.[251]

3. Withdrawal of hanging drop of saline on hub of needle. Gutiérrez's sign;[252] useful in the thoracic region but unreliable in the lumbar. Negative pressure in the extradural space described in 1926.[253]

4. Movement of bubble on Odom's indicator,[219] (a glass tube with fine bore containing saline and an air bubble), which can be attached to hub of spinal needle.

5. Macintosh's extradural space indicator is a small rubber balloon attached to an adaptor, which is connected to the needle when it lies in the interspinous ligament. With a fine hypodermic needle, air is injected into the thick rubber of the neck of the balloon, and when the extradural space is entered, the small balloon diminishes in size.[254]

6. The Macintosh spring-loaded needle,[255] devised by R. H. Salt.[256]

7. Ultrasonic localization.[257]

8. The Oxford epidural space indicator.[258]

In the unconscious patient the rapid injection of liquid into the extradural space is accompanied by an increase in the rate and depth of respiration (Durrans sign[259]). This test is not always positive in conscious patients, if injection is made slowly, or if injection is made into subarachnoid space. The injection of 5 ml of distilled water will cause some discomfort to the patient if it is placed in the extradural space – an additional help in localization (Lund). All of the solution injected by even experienced anaesthetists, after a positive loss of resistance test, does not always enter the extradural space.[260] In very difficult cases, or where accuracy is imperative (e.g. in pain therapy), X-ray control may be advisable.

Injection must only commence when position of needle point is certain.

Test dose. An initial injection (following aspiration test) of either 1 ml of hyperbaric lignocaine with adrenaline[261] or 2 ml of 0.5% bupivacaine with adrenaline[262] is made and if in 5 min there is no evidence of intradural block, e.g. inability to move the feet, or tachycardia from possible intravenous injection of adrenaline, the main injection can be made.[263] A volume of 1.5 ml has also been recommended.[264] It has been suggested that 5% lignocaine is more satisfactory than 0.5% plain bupivacaine (which may spread too high and take too long).[265] Many workers of experience omit this test dose. It is more logical when used under stable conditions following insertion and secure fixation of an extradural catheter. There are advantages in injecting the total dose in four aliquots to reduce toxic effects; such a procedure does not influence the eventual height of the block, at least in Caesarean section.[266]

The patient is then turned on the back with slight head-down tilt.

Procedure if dura is pierced. Although dural puncture is usually due to lack of delicacy in technique, it may result from congenital narrowing of the vertebral canal.[267] (This spinal stenosis has caused intermittent claudication of the cauda equina.) The choice is as follows: (1) leave needle in theca so that it occludes the dural puncture and attempt to locate the extradural space from a higher or lower level. Withdraw first needle after injection of local analgesic solution through the second needle into the extradural space; (2) convert the block into an intradural (subarachnoid) one; or (3) abandon the method and use general anaesthesia.

Cerebrospinal fluid dripping from the needle can be differentiated from local analgesic solution by: (1) difference in temperature; (2) testing for glucose and protein on urine-testing paper strips; and (3) allowing a few drops to fall onto thiopentone solution, when local analgesic solution causes turbidity (pH of thiopentone is 10; of analgesic solution, about 5).[268]

A filter is often used to prevent injection of foreign material into the extradural space. The presence of a filter does, however, make aspiration tests difficult.[269]

Thoracic extradural block

Used mainly for the relief of postoperative pain as it is possible to block thoracic roots selectively while sparing the lumbar and sacral roots. The ideal puncture site for thoracic operations is T2–T6; for the upper abdomen, T6–T8; the paramedian approach is recommended. A skin weal is placed just lateral to the spinous process at the inferior aspect of the interspace and the needle directed 10° medially and 45° cephalad. After identification of the space and the usual aspiration test, a test dose may be injected, followed by the insertion of an extradural catheter. Puncture of the theca is less likely than in the lumbar region because of the angulation of the needle and the tendency of the Huber point to 'toboggan' over the dura mater. The dose of solution may vary from 3 to 5 ml of 1.5% lignocaine or 0.5% bupivacaine for a block of 2–4 segments, or up to 10–15 ml when a greater zone of analgesia is required as in abdominal surgery. A constant infusion of 0.125% bupivacaine at 10–15 ml/h has been used for postoperative analgesia.

(*See also* Bromage P. R. *Epidural Analgesia*. Philadelphia: Saunders, 1978; Carron H. et al. *Regional Anesthesia*. Orlando, Florida: Grune & Stratton, 1984.)

Cervical extradural block

Used for the management of intractable pain and by some enthusiasts, for thyroidectomy and for carotid endarterectomy. The concentration of solution should be such as to provide sensory block without motor block of the phrenic nerves, e.g. lignocaine 1% or bupivacaine 0.25%. For the injection the patient sits with the head and neck flexed forward. The C7–T1 interspace (vertebra prominens) is identified and a skin weal made over it in the midline. By the median approach the extradural needle is advanced slowly, inclined at an angle of 30° cephalad. The hanging drop method of localizing the space has been recommended as the negative pressure in the extradural space is likely to be greatest in this situation. Variations with respiration may be noticed if a second drop is placed in the correctly placed needle, while a deep inspiration will usually pull this drop into the needle. Usual dose is 6–8 ml of solution for neck analgesia. Technically, it is easy, although potentially very harmful, should the cord be pithed. None-the-less, experienced workers advocate it. The extradural space is relatively superficial and the yellow ligament thin.

Assessment of successful blockade

Onset of complete analgesia may require 10–20 min and can be checked by: (1) disappearance of anal tone (S4–S5); (2) disappearance of knee-jerks (L2–L4), Westphal's sign 1875; (3) disappearance of tone of abdominal muscles (T8–L1); (4) disappearance of ankle-jerk (S1–S2); (5) the existence and extent of skin analgesia, tested with an ether swab, needle, or ice cube; and (6) absence of muscle tone is shown by weakness or abolition of movement of the hips, knees and ankles.

The maximal concentration of lignocaine in the bloodstream after extradural block occurs, on average, 18 min after injection, and after a shorter period if adrenaline is not used.[270]

Delayed extension of the block (and even delayed apnoea) may be due to medial spread of the local analgesic solution in nerve trunks from the extradural space into the spinal cord itself (intraneural spread). Delay may be as long as 40 min.

Absorption into the intraneural spaces and centripetal spread is said to occur from the region of the junction of the anterior and posterior nerve roots.[271]

Injection of local analgesic solution into the extradural space may cause temporary headache and vertigo. Absorption of drug from this situation or its direct intravascular injection may result in disorientation, psychic abnormalities and twitching or convulsions. The last should be treated by intravenous barbiturate, suxamethonium or diazepam and hyperventilation with oxygen.

Continuous extradural analgesia

Greater control over duration and extent of analgesia can be gained if instead of a single injection of solution, repeated injections are made through a plastic catheter introduced into the extradural space. The plastic catheter, made of nylon or polyvinyl chloride, with markings at 5-cm intervals from the tip,[272] is passed through a larger needle, e.g. Tuohy,[273] the slightly angulated tip of which is accurately placed in the extradural space. The angle at the tip carries the catheter either up or down within the space according to the direction of its opening. This needle, although rather large in bore (16–18 G), is relatively easy to insert and many workers use it routinely,[274] even for 'one-shot' injections. The catheter, however, does not always travel in the desired direction. Many workers give the first dose through the needle before the catheter is introduced. Kinking of the catheter within the hub of the spinal needle can be avoided by partly filling the lumen of the hub by the sawn-off nozzle of a plastic syringe.[275]

The insertion of a catheter into the extradural space is especially useful: (1) when the extent of the operation is uncertain; (2) when the duration is uncertain; (3) when the time of commencement is uncertain – the catheter can be put in at leisure and the injection given when necessary; (4) in handicapped patients, to enable small doses to be given and later increased; (5) for postoperative pain relief, especially in patients with chronic bronchitis. Supplemental doses should be one-half to two-thirds of the original dose and great care taken to prevent the introduction of infection by various methods including the Millipore bacterial filter. The catheter should not be inserted more than 5 cm into the extradural space. The catheter should be firmly fixed to the back so as to avoid kinking and its proximal end taken to the pillow from which serial injections can be given; and (6) in obstetrics.

Volumes of solution of 1.5% lignocaine required (for epidural block). For suprapubic prostatectomy, 10–20 ml; for vaginal and perineal repair, 20–35 ml; for herniae, appendicectomies, etc. 20–30 ml of solution are required; for hysterectomies, etc. 25–35 ml; and for upper abdominal operations, 35–40 ml. For *Caesarean section,* 15–25 ml, taking care to control the blood pressure.

Those workers who regard the mass of solute as more important than the volume of solution in judging dosage suggest that 35 mg per spinal segment to be blocked at age 20, decreasing to 15 mg per segment at age 80, when using solutions between 2 and 5%, is a suitable guide. Adrenaline is added (1–200 000) to the lignocaine solution.

Prilocaine 1.5–2% in dosage a little less than that for lignocaine.

Volumes of bupivacaine for extradural block. Onset of analgesia and duration of block is longer than when lignocaine is used. The addition of adrenaline increases the duration only marginally. Maximum safe dose 2 mg/kg (25–30 ml 0.5% solution in the average adult); 0.75% solution gives a slightly more profound effect and 0.25% solution is useful for postoperative pain relief. Average dose for lower laparotomy 15–25 ml of 0.5% solution, for upper laparotomy, 30 ml.

Indications for extradural block

1. In upper abdominal operations. A block to T4 or T5 is required and this obtunds all afferent impulses from upper abdominal viscera. It does not block those conveyed up the vagus or phrenic nerves and so reflex disturbances, hiccups, nausea and retching, and laryngeal spasm (Brewer-Luckhardt reflex) may cause trouble. The method is suitable in fit young patients. By introducing the catheter from the thoracic region through a Tuohy needle at an angle of 40°, much smaller volumes of solution are required, e.g. 16–22 ml. Greater control is obtained if a tracheal tube is passed before or after the extradural injection, and this allows unimpeded spontaneous respiration of inhalation agents.

2. In lower abdominal operations. The method is seen at its best advantage in these cases. Muscular relaxation, contracted bowels and wound ischaemia with adequate spontaneous respiration combine to give excellent conditions for surgery.

3. In hernia repairs. An excellent method.

4. In operations on the lower limbs. Extradural block gives excellent results in relatively fit patients and has been recommended (as has intradural block),[276] for total hip replacement, fractured neck of femur, and for arthroplasty of the hip in elderly patients.[277]

5. Operations on the vertebral column. In laminectomies the injection of a full dose of solution produces wound ischaemia that many surgeons find most welcome. Experienced workers employ volumes up to 40 ml of 1.5% lignocaine with adrenaline in fit patients.[278]

6. Obstetric analgesia (*see* Chapter 22). If a catheter is inserted, analgesia can be limited to the lower thoracic and upper lumbar segments for the first stage of labour and extended by tilting the vertebral column to the sacral segments for the second stage. It may also be useful to relieve the distress of delayed dilatation of the cervix. Initial dose 6–7 ml of bupivacaine (0.25–0.5%).

7. For postoperative pain relief. (*See* Chapter 26.)

8. Has been used in infants and young children.[279]

Management of the patient during extradural block

The general effects are similar to those described in the section on spinal analgesia. Management of the patient on the operating table is the same as in intradural block (*see above*).

The blood pressure is likely to be higher in a conscious than in an unconscious patient. Most anaesthetists have their patients sedated under light general anaesthesia. Breathing during extradural block is generally quieter and easier than under general anaesthesia, probably consequent upon deafferentiation. Controlled ventilation is relatively easily superimposed if desired. There may be a reflex bronchodilatation initiated by baroreceptors stimulated by low blood pressure, in the aorticocarotid sinuses, or it may be due to relative ischaemia of the mucosae of the bronchi consequent on the low blood pressure in their supplying vessels, the bronchial arteries. During high extradural block the respiratory minute volume, the tidal volume, blood-gas estimations and the vital capacity are not greatly altered.

Complications

1. Inadequate block: this must be covered by some convenient form of general anaesthesia. Unilateral block can occur; its cause is obscure. Occasionally, one or more nerve roots remain unblocked.

2. Hypotension and cardiovascular depression: this should be dealt with *secundum artem* – posture, pressor drugs, intravenous infusions, atropine in the presence of severe bradycardia, and oxygen.

3. Hypopnoea: this will need careful attention to the airway and may call for assisted respiration. It may progress to frank apnoea, which need not be due to either total spinal or extradural block, but to medullary depression from the local analgesic drug. It may take up to 45 min to become established. It usually lasts about 1 h and need not interrupt the operation providing respiration is controlled or assisted.

4. Nausea and vomiting: this can be managed by control of hypotension, if present, or by the institution of general anaesthesia.

5. Total central neurological blockade (total spinal analgesia): the possibility of this must always be present in the mind of the anaesthetist performing an extradural block. Whereas it usually comes on soon after the injection, it may be delayed for 30–45 min.[280] If this has occurred the patient is likely to show, within 3 min of injection of the analgesic drug: (*a*) marked hypotension; (*b*) apnoea; (*c*) dilated pupils; and (*d*) loss of consciousness. There is grave danger of death from asphyxia. *Management:* turn patient into the supine position (but not in labour), ventilate the lungs, elevate legs, inject a pressor drug into the open vein and give intravenous fluid. This will in most cases rescue the patient. Later, a tracheal tube can be passed and IPPV instituted. The operation can in most cases proceed and breathing will probably recommence within the hour. Unpleasant sequelae are unlikely.

6. Toxicity due to the injected drug: may result from accidental intravascular injection or by absorption from the extradural space. The signs are disorientation, going on to twitching, convulsions and perhaps apnoea.[281] These usually come on soon after injection but may be delayed. Management consists of injecting a barbiturate (e.g. thiopentone, 150 mg) into the open vein (to find a vein of a violently convulsing patient may be impossible); diazepam may also have a place; the administration of oxygen by IPPV; and protection of the patient's teeth and tongue from the trauma of the fits, which are usually self-limiting.

7. Prolonged analgesia: 60 h of analgesia have been reported, following the extradural injection of 18 ml of 0.5% bupivacaine (without adrenaline).[282]

8. Horner's syndrome:[283] recovery may be delayed.[284]

9. High block: possibly due to subdural injection.[285] Subdural migration of an extradural verified by X-rays, has been described.

10. Epiduro-cutaneous fistula: successfully treated by a blood patch.[286]

11. Unexplained pain during injection.[287]

12. Trigeminal nerve palsy: following lumbar extradural analgesia.[288]

Advantages claimed for the method as against intradural analgesia are: (1) less danger of neurological sequelae; (2) absence of postoperative headache, and (3) ability to have prolonged postoperative analgesia when a catheter technique is emoloyed.

Advantages, as compared with general anaesthesia: (1) protection of the patient from stress responses of the operation, although the benefits of this are not proved; (2) maintenance of spontaneous respiration; (3) provision, by one injection, of analgesia, of relaxation, ischaemia and contracted bowels; (4) suitable in certain patients with asthma, bronchitis or emphysema; and (5) can be employed in patients who are not suitable for muscle relaxants.

Disadvantages are: (1) difficulty of being sure of position of needle point, with risk of subarachnoid injection of a large volume of solution; (2) time taken over the block; and (3) time taken before onset of analgesia.

Contra-indications

These are similar to those set out above for intradural block. Those with large abdominal tumours, arteriosclerosis and diabetes need special care. Any form of shock is a strong contra-indication.

Sequelae

1. Paraplegia[289] – a rare occurrence. May be due to infarction of the cord or stenosis of the vertebral canal or extradural spinal cord tumour.[290] Intracranial complications e.g. subdural haematoma.[291] In a reported series of 50 000 blocks, 2 patients developed paraplegia, 1 of whom had metastatic carcinoma.[292] Sometimes the cause remains obscure.

2. Anterior spinal artery syndrome.[293] Paraplegia not involving the posterior column of the cord, so that joint position sense, and touch and vibration sense are spared. This was first described in 1909 by Miller.[294] An extremely uncommon occurrence.

3. Intra-ocular haemorrhage has been reported after the rapid injection of 30 ml.[295] This may raise the CSF pressure with resulting subhyaloid bleeding.

4. Occasional backache caused by the needle.

5. Extradural abscess,[296] which may take up to 16 days to develop, may be metastatic. Extradural haematoma has been reported in a patient, 3 days after delivery who received neither extradural block nor anticoagulants.[297] Extradural abscess must be drained immediately after diagnosis, otherwise paraplegia may result.[298]

It is interesting that up to 20 ml of thiopentone[299] and 160 ml of parenteral nutritional solution[300] have been accidentally injected into the extradural space, both without harm. Accidental injection of 5 ml ether led to pain followed by temporary paraplegia with full recovery in 4 h.[301]

Neurological sequelae following extradural block are not necessarily due to the method of analgesia.

Therapeutic use of extradural injections

(1) Postoperative pain relief and for prevention chest complications. Insertion of an extradural catheter into the upper thoracic region will allow injection of local analgesic or narcotic drugs; (2) in the management of closed chest injuries; (3) in eclampsia; (4) to control chronic pain due to cancer; (5) in acute occlusive vascular conditions; (6) in obstetrics for pain relief; (7) in the treatment of post-spinal headache; and (8) in the treatment of the lumbar-sciatic syndrome.

Extradural sacral block (caudal block)

This method of analgesia was introduced by Cathelin[302] and Sicard[303] (1872–1929) of Paris in 1901 but neither employed it for operations. It was used by Schlimpert in 1910,[304] and in obstetrics by Stoeckel[305] in 1909, who was the first to report painless vaginal delivery following injection of the then recently discovered procaine into the extradural space, and by Läwen,[306] who potentiated his solution by the addition of sodium bicarbonate. Arthur Läwen placed extradural block via the sacral route on a firm foundation when he made use of the observation of Gross[307] that procaine acts more effectively in an alkaline medium.[308] Hingson in the US was a pioneer and proponent of the method.[309] Has been used in animals, especially in cattle, since 1925. Very suitable for block of the sacral and lumbar nerves. For higher block the lumbar approach to the extradural space is preferable as less solution will thereby be used.

Anatomy of sacrum

A large triangular bone formed by the fusion of the five sacral vertebrae, articulating above with the 5th lumbar vertebra and below with the coccyx.

Posterior surface is convex and down its middle line runs the median sacral crest with its three or four rudimentary spinous processes. The laminae of the 5th and sometimes of the 4th sacral vertebrae fail to fuse in the midline; the deficiency thus formed is known as the sacral hiatus. The tubercles representing the inferior articular processes of the 5th sacral vertebra are prolonged downwards as the sacral cornua. These cornua, with the rudimentary spine of the 4th vertebra above, bound the sacral hiatus. Four posterior sacral foramina correspond with the anterior foramina. Each transmits a sacral nerve posterior ramus and communicates with the sacral canal.

Apex is directed downwards and articulates with the coccyx.

Coccyx represents four rudimentary vertebrae – sometimes three or five.

Sacral canal is a prismatic cavity running through the length of the bone and following its curves. Superiorly it is triangular on section and is continuous with the lumbar vertebral canal. Its lower extremity is the sacral hiatus, closed by the posterior sacrococcygeal membrane. Fibrous strands sometimes occur in the canal and divide the extradural space into compartments. These may account for some cases of failure to produce uniform analgesia. Its anterior wall is formed by fusion of the bodies of the sacral vertebrae; its posterior wall, by fusion of the laminae. On each lateral wall of the canal, four foramina are present, which divide in the form of a Y into anterior and posterior sacral foramina. The contents of the sacral canal are: (1) the dural sac, which ends at the lower border of the second sacral vertebra, on a line joining the posterior superior iliac spines. The pia mater is continued as the filum terminale; (2) the sacral nerves and the coccygeal nerve, with their dorsal root ganglia; (3) a venous plexus formed by the lower end of the internal vertebral plexus. These vessels are more numerous anteriorly than posteriorly and so the needle point should be kept as far posteriorly as possible; and (4) areolar and fatty tissue – more dense in males than in females.

Each sacral nerve is provided with a thick sheath from the dura.

The sacral hiatus is a triangular opening, caused by failure of the 5th (and sometimes of the 4th) laminar arch to fuse, with apex upwards formed by the 4th sacral spine, and a sacral cornu on each side below and laterally. (But this is so in only 35% of sacra.[310]) It is covered over by the sacrococcygeal membrane, which is pierced by the coccygeal and 5th sacral nerves. It is superior to the sacrococcygeal junction, usually about 3.5–5 cm from the tip of the coccyx and directly beneath the upper limit of the intergluteal cleft.

Anatomical abnormalities of the sacrum are not uncommon. They include: (1) upward and downward displacement of the hiatus; (2) pronounced narrowing or partial obliteration of the sacral canal, making needle insertion difficult; (3) ossification of the sacrococcygeal membrane; (4) absence of the bony posterior wall of the sacral canal, due to failure of laminae to fuse; and (5) dural extension to the level of S.3 – S.4 in 2% of patients, quoted by Louis,[311] or even to the sacrococcygeal membrane itself.[312]

The average capacity of the sacral canal is 34 ml in males and 32 ml in females. Its average length is 10–15 cm.

When a local analgesic solution is injected into the sacral canal it ascends upwards in the extradural space for a distance proportional to the volume of solution, the force of injection, the amount of leakage through the eight sacral foramina and the consistency of the connective tissue in the space. Whereas the first two are controllable, the last are not, so precise placement of the solution is impossible and sometimes leads to unexpected results.

Technique of injection

Careful antiseptic preparation of the skin is essential. An intravenous cannula is inserted. The patient lies in the prone position with hips slightly flexed over two pillows. To prevent tensing of the gluteal muscles the patient should be asked to abduct the legs and turn toes in. Other positions are the lateral, Sims position, knee – chest and knee – elbow. After cleaning and towelling, the tip of the coccyx is identified and the triangular sacral hiatus palpated about 3.5–5 cm above it. The hiatus must be clearly palpated. Its anatomy is not constant; sometimes it is larger, sometimes smaller, than normal. It is difficult to feel in obese patients.

A weal is raised over the hiatus, with a fine intradermal needle using no more than 2 drops of solution, as oedema obscures the landmarks. A 5-cm needle, No. 1, is inserted through the sacrococcygeal membrane so that it makes an angle of about 20° with the line drawn at right angles to the skin surface. Once through the membrane the needle is depressed a further 45° towards the intergluteal cleft and advanced into the sacral canal for 2–3 cm keeping in the midline. The point must not ascend higher than the line joining the posterior superior iliac spines because the dura, which ends at this level, may be pierced. Occasionally the dural sac extends lower down than the level of the second piece of the sacrum. The mean distance between the apex of the hiatus and the dural sac is 4.5 cm.

After aspiration tests for blood and CSF have been proved negative, a test dose can be injected if thought necessary. Should *blood* flow through the needle, its position must be altered. Should *cerebrospinal fluid* appear, the method of analgesia must be abandoned and intradural injection substituted in suitable cases, the proper amount of drug being introduced into the theca through the sacral needle.

Five minutes after the test injection, movement of the toes, if present, indicates an intradural block has not resulted and the needle point is not in the theca; further injection can then be commenced. When the needle is correctly placed, injection is easy, no great force being required to depress the plunger of the syringe. Should the needle be *posterior to the canal*, a tumour is raised over the sacrum as the injection proceeds. Injection of a few millilitres of air will produce surgical emphysema with its crepitus. If the needle point comes to lie *between periosteum and bone* the force needed for injection will be great – a sure sign of an incorrect position.

Drugs

Lignocaine 1–2% or bupivacaine 0.25–0.5% solution with or without adrenaline are excellent, giving a rapid onset and a profound degree of analgesia.

Dosage. Level of analgesia is governed by: (1) quantity of solution; (2) speed of injection; (3) gravity; and (4) age and height of patient. Poor-risk cases require a smaller dose.

Low block, i.e. up to L2–L4, for operations on anus, rectum, perineum or urethra, circumcision, vaginal plastics, etc.: up to 30 ml. In 10 min analgesia develops and will last 1–2 h; 15–20 ml of solution are sufficient for the average case of haemorrhoids or anal fissure.

Toxic reactions to the drugs used are sometimes seen, because dosage is fairly large. Injection of the drug into the venous plexus may also be a cause of this. An occasional twitch requires no treatment, but convulsions should be combated with intravenous suxamethonium or thiopentone, together with IPPV with oxygen. Collapse due to cardiovascular depression consequent on reduction of the blood pressure is treated on the usual lines by elevating the lower limbs, giving a plasma-volume expander, giving oxygen and injecting a pressor drug if required. Too rapid a rate of injection may cause transient unconsciousness.[313]

The extent of analgesia is not by any means related only to the volume of solution injected, but also to the volume that leaks through the sacral foramina and the intervertebral foramina and to the degree of the lumbosacral angle. The best control of the height of analgesia is obtained by the use of the continuous technique via a catheter.

Indications. (1) Haemorrhoidectomy and other perianal operations; (2)

forceps delivery in obstetrics; (3) operations on the lower limbs and transurethral operations, e.g. lignocaine 6 mg/kg of 2% solution or bupivacaine 2 mg/kg of 0.5% solution, both with adrenaline. The extradural injection of large volumes of procaine, e.g. 50 ml of 0.5% solution or other agents, is extensively used for the relief of skeletal pain.

Sacral extradural block in infants and children

First described in 1933.[314]

Advantages

Excellent postoperative analgesia is obtained. Dose of bupivacaine 0.25%, 0.5 ml/kg. Popular for postoperative analgesia in children, e.g. after circumcision and orchidopexy. Useful in adults undergoing haemorroidectomy, urological or vaginal procedures, usually combined with light general anaesthesia.

Disadvantages

(1) Length of time taken for development of analgesia; (2) lack of accurate control of height of analgesia; (3) muscular relaxation not maximal in mid and high blocks, although it is excellent in low blocks; (4) technical difficulty, if anatomy abnormal; (5) risk of inadvertent subarachnoid injection, if dura extends downwards; (6) hypotension and possible signs of drug toxicity; and (7) it produces complete flaccidity of the anal sphincters, a condition unpopular with some surgeons doing operations for fistula-in-ano.

EXTRADURAL AND INTRADURAL NARCOTIC ANALGESICS

The identification of opiate receptors in the central nervous system[315] and the isolation of endorphins led to an interest in the production of analgesia by spinal application of narcotic analgesics. Intrathecal narcotics have been used in animals[316] and in man.[317] The first reports of clinical use of extradural narcotic analgesics came from Jerusalem[318] and it was shown that pethidine was soon transferred from the extradural space to the CSF.

Extradural narcotic analgesics

These have been administered in the treatment of intractable pain,[318] postoperative pain,[319] trauma,[320] ischaemic pain[321] and obstetrics.[322]

Pharmacokinetics and pharmacodynamics

Analgesic drug injected into the extradural space has to pass through the dura into the intradural space to reach the substance of the cord, the greatest concentration of opioid receptors being in lamina 2 (substantia gelatinosa) and lamina 5 of the cord.

The dura presents a substantial barrier to drug diffusion. The concentration gradient may be several hundred fold.[323] In the lumbar region the dura is about 0.3 mm thick and it becomes thicker in the cephalad direction. Factors affecting drug movement include molecular weight, molecular shape, solubility in fat and the concentration.[324] Fentanyl has a relatively high permeability.

Human studies are difficult[325] but animal work[326] shows that following extradural injection of morphine, the concentration in lumbar CSF can peak at high levels after 2 h. There is a considerable concentration gradient in the CSF with very low concentrations near the fourth ventricle. Activities such as coughing can, however, disturb the equilibrium, allowing much higher concentrations to reach the brain.[327] The volume in which the drug is dissolved is also probably important.[328]

Systemic absorption also takes place from the extradural space. The plasma profile resembles that following intramuscular injection,[329] although peak blood levels tend to be lower. Systemic absorption contributes to analgesia and also decreases the concentration gradient across the dura. Some of the drug also diffuses into extradural fat to form a depot.

Addition of adrenaline to the injected solution is likely to enhance both analgesia and side-effects.[330] The danger of respiratory depression is greater when a patient has recently received an intramuscular injection of a narcotic analgesic drug.[331]

Clinical use. Although it may be more logical to inject local analgesic solution directly into the intradural space and hence near to the cord itself, extradural placement allows the use of repeated doses via a catheter. The correct positioning may be validated by injection of local analgesic solution. The segmental level of injection should be as near to the cord segment where analgesia is desired as possible. This is higher than would be required when local analgesic drugs are used. Narcotic analgesic drug without preservative is used, although the shelf-life of morphine is then only 1 week. A 0.1% morphine hydrochloride solution (1 mg/ml) in 10% glucose may be prepared in the pharmacy. The desired dose, 2–4 mg morphine, is then made up to 10 ml by addition of isotonic saline.

The onset of analgesia can be expected in 20–30 min and the duration of effect may vary between 4 and 36 h. Arterial pressure, heart rate and respiratory rate should be monitored, although cardiovascular stability is the rule. Posture is not important in relation to spread of analgesic effect. Other analgesics that have been used include pethidine,[323] fentanyl,[332] methadone,[333] buprenorphine, lofentanil,[334] and sufentanil.[335] Fentanyl has been given by infusion.[332] Ketamine 4 mg in 10 ml of 5% dextrose in water injected into the extradural space provides potent analgesia postoperatively, without side-effects.[336] Extradural opiates do not directly influence the metabolic response to surgery, but decrease the cortisol response postoperatively, secondary to improved analgesia.[337]

Advantages. (1) Reduced dosage compared to intramuscular injection; (2) good and prolonged analgesia without depression of consciousness, skin numbness or motor block; (3) cardiovascular stability due to lack of sympathetic block; and (4) absence of constipation.

Complications.[338] (1) Severe respiratory depression, sometimes delayed, can occur;[339] (2) itching, particularly in the area supplied by the 5th cranial nerve; (3) some nausea and dizziness has been reported; (4) urinary retention may occur[340] but is difficult to assess. Urinary retention after extradural morphine may be relieved or prevented by 4 oral doses of phenoxybenzamine 10 mg given before and after surgery;[341] and (5) may cause temporary inability to ejaculate in males.[340]

Extradural opioid injection is now widely employed in the management of postoperative pain, although patients are best nursed in an intensive care or high dependency unit so that continuous observation is possible, with instant correction of respiratory depression, perhaps by the use of naloxone. This reverses the respiratory depression without diminishing analgesia, but its duration of action is less than that of the extradural opioid, so that continuous observation is still necessary.

Choice of drug. Some drug doses that have been recommended for extradural injection for pain relief include: morphine, 2–4 mg; diamorphine, 0.1 mg/kg; methadone, 5–6 mg (top-up dose 4 mg); fentanyl, 1.5 µg/kg (bolus), infusion, 0.5 µg/kg/h; buprenorphine, 0.3 mg; lofentanil 5 µg, and pethidine 25 mg. The dose is commonly dissolved in 10 ml, sometimes in 20 ml saline. Other agents have been used, e.g. midazolam.[342] Morphine has been used in many studies perhaps because it is regarded as the standard for reference, but since most other narcotic analgesics are more lipophilic than morphine, it might be more logical to use another agent. If less of the drug is dissolved in cord lipid, more may remain free to diffuse rostrally to cause respiratory depression.

Intradural narcotic analgesics

Intradural injection has been used in the management of various types of pain.[343] Morphine 1.5 mg has been used successfully in labour.[344] However, there is no doubt that intrathecal narcotics are associated with a much higher incidence of severe respiratory depression than when the drugs are given extradurally, and apnoea has been described many hours later.[345] Close observation of patients is therefore required and naloxone should be available for immediate use in case of respiratory depression.[346] It reverses respiratory depression without loss of analgesia. The danger is less if hyperbaric solutions are used and head-up tilt maintained and can probably be disregarded when elective IPPV is carried out postoperatively. Drug doses for intradural injection, morphine 0.5–1 mg.

(*See also* Bullingham R. E. S. et al. In: *Recent Advances in Anaesthesia and Analgesia—14* (Atkinson R. S. and Hewer C. L. ed.) London: Churchill Livingstone, 1982; Symposium 'Opioid Receptors'; *Br. Med. Bull.* 1983, **39**, January; Cousins M. J. and Mather L. E. *Anesthesiology* 1984, **61**, 276; Lee J. A. et al. *Sir Robert Macintosh's Lumbar Puncture and Spinal Analgesia* 5th ed. Edinburgh: Churchill Livingstone, 1985.)

References

1. Viets H. R. *Bull. Hist. Med.* 1935, **3**, 701.
2. Magendie F. *J. Physiol. Exp. Path.* 1827, **7**, 66.
3. von Anrep B. *Arch. Physiol.* 1880, **21**, 38.
4. Corning J. L. *NY Med. J.* 1885, **42**, 483 (reprinted in 'Classical File', *Surv. Anesthesiol.* 1960, **4**, 332); *Med. Rec. (NY)* 1888, **33**, 291.
5. Corning J. L. *Local Anesthesia.* New York: Appleton. 1886; *See also* Little D. M. 'Classical File', *Surv. Anesthesiol.* 1979, **23**, 271.
6. Quincke H. I. *Berl. Klin. Wochenschr.* 1891, **28**, 930; *Verh. Kongr. Inn. Med.* 1891, **10**, 321.
7. Wynter W. E. *Lancet* 1891, **1**, 981.
8. Bier A. *Dtsch. Z. Chir.* 1899, **51**, 361 (translated and reprinted in 'Classical File', *Surv. Anesthesiol.* 1962, **6**, 352).
9. Tuffier T. *C. R. Soc. Biol. (Paris)* 1899, **51**, 882.
10. Tait F. D. and Caglieri G. E. *JAMA* 1900, **35**, 6.
11. Matas R. *Phil. Med. J.* 1900, **6**, 882.
12. Donitz A. *Münch. Med. Wochenschr.* 1903, **50**, 1452; Bier A. *Verh. Dtsch. Ges. Chir.* 1905, **34**, 115.
13. Fourneau E. *Bull. Soc. Pharmacol. (Paris)* 1904, **10**, 141.
14. Chaput H. *Bull. Soc. Chir. (Paris)* 1904, n.s., **30**, 835.
15. Einhorn A. *Ditsch. Med. Wochenschr.* 1905, **31**, 1668.
16. Heineke H. and Läwen A. *Dtsch. Z. Chir.* 1905, **80**, 192; Braun H. *Dtsch. Med. Wochenschr.* 1905, **31**, 1667.
17. Barker A. E. *Lond. Clin. J.* 1906 **28**, 4; *Br. Med. J.* 1907, **1**, 665; 1908, **1**, 244; **2**, 453; Lee J. A. *Anaesthesia* 1979, **34**, 885.
18. Brownlee A. *Practitioner* 1911, February, p. 214.
19. Dean H. P. *Br. Med. J.* 1906, **1**, 1086; Akhtar M. *Anaesthesia* 1972, **27**, 330.
20. Gray H. T. *Lancet* 1909, **2**, 913.
21. Babcock W. W. *NY J. Med.* 1914, **50**, 637.
22. Labat G. *Ann. Surg.* 1921, **74**, 673.
23. Pitkin G. P. *J. Med. Soc. NJ.* 1927, **24**, 425; *Am. J. Surg.* 1928, **5**, 537.
24. Chen K. K. and Schmidt C. F. *J. Pharmacol. Exp. Ther.* 1924, **24**, 331; *JAMA* 1926. **87**, 836.
25. Ocherblad N. F. and Dillon T. G. *JAMA* 1927, **88**, 1135.
26. Rudolf R. D. and Graham J. D. *Am. J. Med. Sci.* 1927, **173**, 399.
27. Gray H. T. and Parsons L. *Q. J. Med.* 1912, **5**, 339.
28. Smith G. S. and Porter W. T. *Am. J. Physiol.* 1915, **38**, 108.
29. Jonnesco T. *Br. Med. J.* 1909, **2**, 1396 (reprinted in 'Classical File', *Surv. Anesthesiol.* 1978, **22**, 301).
30. Koster H. *Am. J. Surg.* 1928, **5**, 554 (reprinted in 'Classical File', *Surv. Anesthesiol.* 1968, **12**, 306).
31. Keyes E. L. and McLelland A. M. *Am. J. Surg.* 1930, **9**, 1; *JAMA* 1931, **96**, 2085.
32. Jones H. W. *Br. J. Anaesth.* 1930, **7**, 146.
33. Kirschner M. *Surg. Gynecol. Obstet.* 1932, **55**, 317.
34. Sebrechts J. *Br. J. Anaesth.* 1934, **12**, 4.
35. Wilson W. E. *Br. J. Anaesth.* 1934, **11**, 43.
36. Lemmon W. T. *Ann. Surg.* 1940, **111**, 141.
37. Dean H. P. *Br. Med. J.* 1907, **2**, 870.
38. Sise L. F. *Surg. Clin. North Am.* 1935, **15**, 1501 (reprinted in 'Classical File', *Surv. Anesthesiol.* 1957, **1**, 266).
39. Eisleb O. *Arch. Exp. Path. Pharmak.* 1931, **160**, 53.
40. Ekblom L. and Widman B. *Acta Anaesthesiol. Scand.* 1966, Suppl. 23, 419.
41. Cope R. W. *Anaesthesia* 1954, **9**, 249; *Br. J. Anaesth.* 1954, **26**, 233.

42. Foster Kennedy G. et al. *Surg. Gynecol. Obstet.* 1950, **91**, 385 (reprinted in 'Classical File', *Surv. Anesthesiol.* 1964, **8**, 273).
43. Thorsen G. *Acta Surg. Scand.* 1947, Suppl. 95, 121.
44. Dripps R. D. and Vandam L. D. *JAMA* 1954, **156**, 1486 (reprinted in *Surv. Anesthesiol.* 1970, **14**, 308).
45. Hutter C. D. D. *Anaesthesia* 1990, **45**, 859.
46. Critchley E. M. R. *Br. Med. J.* 1982, **284**, 1588.
47. Newman B. *Anaesthesia* 1983, **38**, 350.
48. Key E. A. H. and Retzius M. G. *Studien in der Anatomie des Nervensystems.* Stockholm: Samson and Wallin, 1875.
49. Jenkins J. G. *J. R. Soc. Med.* 1986, **79**, 110.
50. Shantha T. R. and Evans J. A. *Anesthesiology* 1972, **37**, 543.
51. Adamkiewicz A. *Sber. Akad. Wiss. Wien. Abt. II*, 1882, **85**, 101.
52. Djindjian R. *Proc. R. Soc. Med.* 1970, **63**, 181.
53. Dommisse G. F. *Ann. R. Coll. Surg.* 1980, **62**, 369.
54. Batson O. *Ann. Surg.* 1940, **112**, 138; Dommisse G. F. *Arteries and Veins of the Human Spinal Cord from Birth.* Edinburgh: Churchill Livingstone, 1976.
55. Edgar M. A. and Nundy S. J. *J. Neurol. Neurosurg. Psychiatry* 1966, **29**, 530.
56. Sechzer P. H. *Anesthesiology* 1963, **24**, 869; Cohen C. A. and Kallos T. *Anesthesiology* 1972, **37**, 352; Boys J. E. and Norman P. F. *Br. J. Anaesth.* 1975, **47**, 1111.
57. Boys J. E. and Norman P. F. *Br. J. Anaesth.* 1975, **47**, 1111; Mehta M. and Maher R. *Anaesthesia* 1977, **32**, 760; Reynolds F. and Speedy H. M. *Anaesthesia* 1990, **45**, 120.
58. Bryce-Smith R. *Proc. R. Soc. Med.* 1976, **69**, 75.
59. Bromage P. R. *Epidural Analgesia.* Philadelphia: Saunders, 1978.
60. Consino M. J. and Wright C. J. *Surg. Gynecol. Obstet.* 1971, **133**, 59.
61. Walts L. F. et al. *Anesthesiology* 1964, **25**, 634; Freund F. et al. *Anesthesiology* 1967, **28**, 834.
62. Rosenberg P. H. and Heinonen E. *Br. J. Anaesth.* 1983, **55**, 163.
63. Barker I. et al. *Anaesthesia* 1985, **40**, 533.
64. Roe C. F. and Cohn F. L. *Surg. Gynecol. Obstet.* 1973, **136**, 265.
65. Urban B. J. *Anesthesiology* 1973, **39**, 496.
66. Forbes A. R. and Roisen M. F. *Anesthesiology* 1978, **48**, 440.
67. Harrison, Gwendolen *Anaesthesia* 1951, **6**, 115; Leatherdale R. A. *Anaesthesia* 1956. **11**, 249.
68. de Jong R. H. and Cullen S. C. *Anesthesiology* 1963, **24**, 628.
69. Bromage P. R. et al. *Science* 1963, **140**, 392; Moller I. W. et al. *Acta Anaesthesiol. Scand.* 1982, **26**, 58; Traynor C. et al. *Br. J. Anaesth.* 1982, **54**, 319.
70. Shantha T. J. and Evans J. A. *Anesthesiology.* 1972, **37**, 543.
71. Greene N. M. *Anesth. Analg. (Cleve.)* 1983, **62**, 1013.
72. Moore R. A. et al. *Br. J. Anaesth.* 1982, **54**, 1117.
73. McWhirter W. R. et al. *Anesthesiology* 1973. **39**, 398.
74. Bonica J. J. et al. *Acta Anaesthesiol. Scand.* 1966, Suppl. 23, 429.
75. Bonica J. J. and Berges P. V. *Anesthesiology* 1970, **33**, 619.
76. Dohi S. et al. *Anesthesiology* 1979, **50**, 319.
77. Greene N. M. *Reg. Anaesth.* 1982, **7**, 55.
78. Bainbridge F. A. J. *Physiol.* 1914, **48**, 332; 1915, **50**, 65.
79. Marey E. J. *C. R. Acad. Sci. (Paris)* 1861, **53**, 95.
80. Sansetta S. M. et al. *Circulation* 1952, **6**, 559.
81. Klingstrom P. *Acta Anaesthesiol. Scand.* 1960, suppl. 4.
82. Germann P. A. S. et al. *Anaesth. Intensive Care* 1979, **7**, 229.
83. Cundh R. et al. *Acta Anaesthesiol. Scand.* 1984, **27**, 410.
84. Aldrete J. A. et al. *Anesth. Analg. (Cleve.)* 1973, **52**, 809.
85. Moir D. D. *Br. J. Anaesth.* 1963, **35**, 3; Moir D. D. and Mone J. G. *Br. J. Anaesth.* 1964, **36**, 480; Askrog V. F. et al. *Surg. Gynecol. Obstet.* 1964, **119**, 563; de Jong R. H. *JAMA*

1965, **191**, 698; Ward R. J. et al. *JAMA* 1965, **191**, 275; Wishart H. Y. *Anaesthesia* 1971, **26**, 37; James M. L. and Fisher A. *Anaesthesia* 1969, **24**, 511.

86. Takasaki M. and Takasaki T. *Br. J. Anaesth.* 1980, **52**, 1271.
87. James M. L. and Fisher A. *Anaesthesia* 1969, **24**, 511.
88. Bromage P. R. *Anaesthesia* 1956, **11**, 139.
89. Spence A. A. and Smith G. *Br. J. Anaesth.* 1971, **43**, 144.
90. Drummond G. B. and Littlewood D. G. *Br. J. Anaesth.* 1977, **49**, 999.
91. Boys J. E. and Norman P. F. *Br. J. Anaesth.* 1975, **47**, 1111; Mehta M. and Maher R. *Anaesthesia* 1977, **32**, 760.
92. Eckenhoff J. E. and Cannard T. H. *Anesthesiology* 1960, **21**, 96.
93. Aitkenhead A. R. et al. *Br. J. Anaesth.* 1980, **52**, 1071.
94. Nimmo W. S. et al. *Br. J. Anaesth.* 1978, **50**, 559.
95. Bonnet F. et al. *Br. J. Anaesth.* 1982, **54**, 29.
96. Kehlet. H. *Reg. Anaesth.* 1982, **7**, 538.
97. Bromage P. R. *Surg. Gynecol. Obstet.* 1971, **132**, 1051; Lines J. G. *Br. J. Anaesth.* 1971, **43**, 1136.
98. Traynor C. et al. *Br. J. Anaesth.* 1982, **54**, 319.
99. Oyoma T. and Matsuki A. *Br. J. Anaesth.* 1970, **42**, 723; Moller I. W. et al. *Acta Anaesthesiol. Scand.* 1982, **58**; Traynor C. et al. *Br. J. Anaesth.* 1982, **54**, 319; Buckley F. P. et al. *Br. J. Anaesth.* 1982, **54**, 325.
100. Houghton A. et al. *Br. J. Anaesth.* 1978, **50**, 495.
101. Rem J. et al. *Lancet* 1980, **1**, 283.
102. Kehlet H. *Clin. Anesthesiol.* 1984, **2**, 315.
103. Walmsley A. J. et al. *Br. J. Anaesth.* 1986, **58**, 1130; Walmsley A. J. et al. *Anesth. Analg. (Cleve.)* 1986, **65**, S. 164; Crawford J. S. *Anaesthesia* 1986, **41**, 765.
104. Sheskey M. C. et al. *Anesth. Analg.* 1983, **62**, 931
105. Wildsmith J. A. W. et al. *Br. J. Anaesth.* 1981, **53**, 1103.
106. Sinclair C. J. et al. *Br. J. Anaesth.* 1982, **54**, 497.
107. Taivainen T. et al. *Br. J. Anaesth* 1990, **65**, 234
108. Bryce-Smith R. *Proc. R. Soc. Med.* 1976, **69**, 75.
109. Mitchell R. W. D. et al. *Br. J. Anaesth.* 1988, **61**, 139; Povey A. M. R. et al. *Acta Anaesthesiol. Scand.* 1987, **31**, 616.
110. Bridenbaugh P. O. and Greene N. M. In: *Neural Blockade in Clinical Anaesthesia and Management of Pain* (Cousins M. J. and Brindenbaugh P. O., Ed.) 2nd ed. Philadelphia: Lippincott, 1988.
111. Neigh J. L., Kane P. B. and Smith T. C. *Anesth. Analg.* 1970, **49**, 912.
112. Greene N. M. *Anesth. Analg.* 1985, **64**, 715; Lee J. A., Atkinson R. S. and Watt M. J. *Sir Robert Machintosh's Lumbar Puncture and Spinal Analgesia* 5th ed. Edinburgh: Churchill Livingstone, 1985; Atkinson R. S. In: *Recent Advances in Anaesthesia and Analgesia – 15* (Atkinson R. S. and Adams A. P. ed.) Edinburgh: Churchill Livingstone, 1985; Stienstra R. and Greene N. M. *Regional Anesthesia* 1991, **16**, 1.
113. Chambers W. A. et al. *Br. J. Anaesth.* 1982, **54**, 75.
114. Lund P. C. and Cameron J. D. *Anesthesiology* 1945, **6**, 565.
115. Armstrong I. R. et al. *Anesth. Analg. (Cleve.)* 1983, **62**, 793; Concepcion M. et al. *Anesth. Analg. (Cleve.)* 1984, **63**, 134.
116. Chambers W. A. et al. *Br. J. Anaesth.* 1982, **54**, 230P; Chambers W. A. et al. *Anesth. Analg. (Cleve.)* 1982, **61**, 49.
117. Chambers W. A. et al. *Anesth. Analg. (Cleve.)* 1981, **60**, 417.
118. Dahl J. B. et. al. *Br. J. Anaesth.* 1990, **64**, 178; Flatter A. et al. *Br. J. Anaesth.* 1990, **65**, 294.
119. Dufy G. P. *Br. Med. J.* 1982, **285**, 1163.
120. Charlebois P. A. *Can. Anaesth. Soc. J.* 1966, **13**, 585.
121. Ariaraj S. J. P. *Anaesthesia* 1981, **36**, 72.
122. Norris M. et al. *Anesthesiology,* 1989, **70**, 729.

123. Taylor J. A. *J. Urol.* 1940, **43**, 561 (reprinted in 'Classical File', *Surv. Anesthesiol.* 1969, **13**, 325); Surks S. N. and Wood P. *Anesthesiology* 1951, **12**, 239.
124. Crawford J. S. et al. *Br. J. Anaesth.* 1975, **47**, 807.
125. Le Filliatre G. *Précis de Rachianesthésiegénérale.* Paris: Libraire Le François, 1921.
126. Koster H. *Am. J. Surg.* 1928, **5**, 554 (reprinted in 'Classical File', *Surv. Anesthesiol.* 1968, **12**, 306).
127. Griffiths H. W. C. and Gillies J. *Anaesthesia* 1948, **3**, 134 (reprinted in 'Classical File', *Surv. Anesthesiol.* 1980, **24**, 342).
128. Dean H. P. *Br. Med. J.* 1907, **2**, 870; Akhtar M. *Anaesthesia* 1972, **27**, 330.
129. Lemmon W. T. *Ann. Surg.* 1940, **111**, 141.
130. Lee J. A. *Lancet* 1943, **2**, 156.
131. Tuohy E. B. *Surg. Clin. North Am.* 1945, **111**, 141 (reprinted in 'Classical File', *Surv. Anesthesiol.* 1971, **15**, 310).
132. Hurley R. J. and Lambert D. *Reg. Anesth.* 1987, **12**, 54.
133. Kestin I. G. *Br. J. Anaesth.* 1990, **65**, 280P.
134. Kestin I. G. et al. *Br. J. Anaesth.* 1991, **66**, 232; Kestin I. G. and Goodman N. W. *Anaesthesia* 1991, **46**, 93.
135. Kestin I. G. *Br. J. Anaesth.* 1991, **66**, 596.
136. Morrison L. M. M. et al. *Anaesthesia* 1991, **46**, 576.
137. Eng. M. and Zorotovitch R. A. *Anesthesiology* 1977, **46**, 147; Maxon L. H. *Spinal Anesthesia.* Philadelphia: Lippincott, 1938, 172; Lahey F. H. *JAMA* 1929, **93**, 518.
138. Fink B. R. *Anesth. Analg.* 1990, **71**, 208.
139. Phillips O. C. et al. *Anesthesiology* 1969, **30**, 284; Abouleish E. et al. *Anesth. Analg. (Cleve.)* 1975, **54**, 459; Flaatten H. et al. *Anaesthesia* 1987, **42**, 202.
140. Croft J. B. et al. *Anesth. Analg. (Cleve.)* 1973, **52**, 228.
141. Kumar C. M. and Dennison B. *Anaesthesia* 1986, **41**, 556.
142. Gibb W. R. G. and Wen P. *Br. Med. J.* 1984, **289**, 530.
143. Sicard A. *Le Liquide céphalo-rachidien.* Paris: Masson, 1902.
144. Franksson C. and Gordh T. *Acta Chir. Scand.* 1946, **94**, 443.
145. Liebermann L. R. et al. *Neurology* 1971, **21**, 925.
146. Vacanti J. J. *Anesthesiology* 1972, **37**, 358; Mulroy M. F. *Anesthesiology* 1979, **51**, 479.
147. Wark R. J. *Anaesthesia* 1977, **32**, 336.
148. Queckenstedt H. *Dtsch. Z. Nerv. Heilk.* 1916, **55**, 325.
149. Greene B. A. *Anesthesiology* 1950, **11**, 464.
150. Hart J. R. and Whitacre R. J. *JAMA* 1951, **147**, 657.
151. Thomas T. A. and Noble H. A. *Anaesthesia* 1990, **45**, 459.
152. Sprotte G. *Reg. Anaesth.* 1987, **10**, 104.
153. Cesarini M. et al. *Anaesthesia* 1990, **45**, 656.
154. Mosavy S. H. and Shafei M. *Anaesthesia* 1975, **30**, 807.
155. Crawford J. S. *Br. J. Anaesth.* 1972, **44**, 598.
156. Crawford J. S. *Anaesth. Intensive Care* 1983, **11**, 384.
157. Rainbird A. and Pfitzner J. *Anaesthesia* 1983, **38**, 481.
158. Sikh S. S. and Agawal G. *Anaesthesia* 1974, **29**, 297.
159. Roberts S. P. and Petts H. V. *Anaesthesia* 1990, **45**, 377; Lee J. J. and Parry H. *Br. J. Anaesth.* 1991, **66**, 383.
160. Seigne T. D. *Anaesthesia* 1970, **25**, 402; Phillips O. C. *Anesth. Analg.* 1970, **25**, 402.
161. Dunkley B. and Lewis T. T. *Br. Med. J.* 1977, **2**, 1391.
162. Lowberry E. J. L. et al. In: *Control of Hospital Infection – A Practical Handbook.* London Chapman and Hall, 1981.
163. Venua E. *Wien. Klin. Wochenschr.* 1907, **20**, 566.
164. Norman J. E. *Anaesthesia* 1955. **10**, 87.
165. Ballin N. C. *Anaesthesia* 1981, **36**, 952; Sarate G. S. *Can. Anaesth. Soc. J.* 1981, **28**, 283.
166. Birkhahn H. J. and Rosenberg B. *Anaesthesia* 1977, **32**, 680.
167. Lee J. A. *Anaesthesia* 1967, **22**, 342; Neumark J. et al. *Anesthesiology* 1980, **52**, 518; Schremer E. et al. *Anaesthesia* 1983, **38**, 226.

168. Walsh F. M. R. *Lancet* 1956, **1**, 859.
169. Scott D. B. *Br. Med. J.* 1982, **285**, 1048.
170. Marinacci A. A. *JAMA* 1959, **168**, 1337; *Bull. Los Angeles Neurol. Soc.* 1960, **25**, 170; Marinacci A. A. and Courville C. B. *JAMA* 1958, **168**, 1337.
171. Funkquist B. *Acta Anaesthesiol. Scand.* 1967, **11**, 237.
172. Beaudoin M. G. and Klein L. *Anaesth. Intensive Care* 1984. **12**, 163.
173. Yates D. A. H. *J. R. Soc. Med.* 1981, **74**, 334.
174. Lancet 1958, **2**, 515; Wells C. E. C. *Proc. R. Soc. Med.* 1966, **59**, 790.
175. Annotation, *Lancet* 1967 **2**, 143, Bryce Smith R. In: *Recent Advances in Anaesthesia and Analgesia – 11* (Hewer C. L. ed.), Edinburgh: Churchill Livingstone, 1972, 260.
176. Clayton K. I. *Anaesthesia* 1983, **38**, 583.
177. MacKenzie N. *Anaesthesia* 1983, **38**, 886.
178. Wedel D. J. and Mulroy M. F. *Anesthesiology* 1983, **59**, 475.
179. Cashman J. N. *Anaesthesia* 1984, **39**, 248.
180. Wang. B. C. et al. *Reg. Anesth.* 1982, **7**, 85.
181. Silver J. R. and Buxton J. H. *Brain* 1974, **97** (III) 539; Annotation, *Lancet* 1974, **2**, 1299.
182. Ramachandran S. et al. *Anesth. Analg. (Cleve.)* 1978, **57**, 361.
183. Edelman J. D. and Wingard D. W. *Anesthesiology* 1980, **52**, 166.
184. Leatherdale R. A. L. *Anaesthesia* 1959, **14**, 274; Wark H. J. *Anaesthesia.* 1977, **32**, 336.
185. Hewer C. L. and Lee J. A. *Recent Advances in Anaesthesia and Analgesia*, 8th ed. London: Churchill, 1957, 133; Lett Z. *Br. J. Anaesth.* 1964, **36**, 266; Current Comment, *Anesthesiology* 1948, **9**, 439; Newbery J. M. *Anaesthesia.* 1977, **32**, 78.
186. Rifaat M. *J. Neurosurg.* 1973, **38**, 366; Shaywitz B. A. *J. Pediatr.* 1972, **80**, 638; Batnitzky S. et al. *Lancet* 1977, **1**, 635.
187. Hawkes C. H. and Roberts G. M. *Br. J. Hosp. Med.* 1980, **23**, 498.
188. Runciman W. B. et al. *Br. J. Anaesth.* 1984, **56**, 1247.
189. Buckley F. P. et al. *Anaesthesia* 1983, **38**, 840.
190. Sculco T. P. et al. *J. Bone. Joint Surg.* 1975, **57A**, 173; Loudon J. R. et al. *Br. Med. J.* 1978, **1**, 1550.
191. Thorburn J. et al. *Br. J. Anaesth.* 1980, **52**, 1117; McDonogh A. J. and Cranney B. S. *Anaesth. Intensive Care* 1984, **12**, 364.
192. Aitkenhead A. R. et al. *Br. J. Anaesth.* 1980, **52**, 1071.
193. Crawford J. S. *Br. J. Anaesth.* 1970, **51**, 531.
194. Aitkenhead A. R. et al. *Br. J. Anaesth.* 1978, **50**, 177.
195. Davis F. M. and Quince M. *Br. Med. J.* 1980, **281**, 1528; Thorburn J. et al. *Br. J. Anaesth.* 1980, **52**, 1117.
196. Dagnino J. and Prys-Roberts C. *Br. J. Anaesth.* 1984, **56**, 1065.
197. Bonica J. J. *Surv. Anesthesiol.* 1970, **14**, Annotation, p. 270.
198. Crawford J. S. et al. *Anaesthesia* 1981, **36**, 821.
199. Cooke E. D. et al. *N. Engl. J. Med.* 1976, **294**, 1066.
200. Odoom J. A. *Anaesthesia* 1984, **39**, 602.
201. Gray H. T. *Lancet* 1909, **2**, 913; 1910, **1**, 1611.
202. Germann P. A. S. et al. *Anaesth. Intensive Care* 1979, **7**, 229.
203. Cathelin F. *C. R. Soc. Biol. (Paris)* 1901, **53**, 452.
204. Sicard J.-A. *C. R. Soc. Biol. (Paris)* 1901, **53**, 396.
205. Kappis M. *Münch. Med. Wochenschr.* 1912.
206. Bleeck and Strauss *Zeit. Geburtsch. Gynek.* 1912, **2**, 72.
207. Pagés-Miravé F. *Revta Sanid. Milit. (Madrid)* 1921, **11**, 351 (translated and reprinted in 'Classical File', *Surv. Anesthesiol.* 1961, **5**, 326).
208. Dogliotti A. M. *Zbl. Chir.* 1931, **58**, 3141.
209. Aburel E. *Bull. Soc. d'Obstet. Gynaecol. (Paris)* 1931, **20**, 85.
210. Dawkins C. J. M. *Proc. R. Soc. Med.* 1945, **38**, 299.
211. Curbelo M. M. *Anesth. Analg. Curr. Res.* 1949, **28**, 13.
212. Batson O. V. *Ann. Surg.* 1940, **112**, 138; *Am. J. Roentgenol*, 1942, **48**, 715.
213. Husemeyer R. P. and White D. C. *Anaesthesia* 1980, **35**, 7.

214. Nunn G. and Mackinnon R. P. G. *Anaesthesia* 1986, **41**, 439.
215. Harrison G. R. and Clowes N. W. B. *Anaesthesia* 1985, **40**, 685.
216. Dawkins C. J. M. and Steel G. C. *Anaesthesia* 1971, **26**, 41.
217. Janzen E. J. *Dtsch. Z. NervHeilk.* 1926, **94**, 280; Aitkenhead A. R. et al. *Anaesthesia* 1979, **34**, 14.
218. Macintosh R. R. and Mushin W. W. *Anaesthesia* 1947, **2**, 100.
219. Odom C. B. *Am. J. Surg.* 1936, **34**, 547.
220. Zazur E. *Anaesthesia* 1984, **39**, 1101.
221. Andrade P. *Br. J. Anaesth.* 1983, **55**, 85.
222. Usubiaga J. E. et al. *Br. J. Anaesth.* 1967, **39**, 612.
223. Galbert M. W. and Marx G. F. *Anesthesiology* 1974, **40**, 499.
224. Shah J. L. *Anaesthesia* 1981, **36**, 627.
225. Flowers C. E. *Anaesthesia* 1954, **9**, 146.
226. Usubiaga J. E. et al. *Anesthesiology* 1964, **25**, 752.
227. Brierly J. B. *J. Neurol. Psychiatry* 1950, **13**, 203.
228. Shantha T. R. and Evans J. A. *Anesthesiology* 1972, **37**, 543.
229. Bromage P. R. *Br. J. Anaesth.* 1974, **46**, 504.
230. Bromage P. R. *Epidural Analgesia.* Philadelphia: Saunders, 1978.
231. Sharrock N. E. et al. *Br. J. Anaesth.* 1984, **56**, 285.
232. Sharrock N. E. *Anesthesiology* 1977, **47**, 307; Grundy E. M. et al. *Br. J. Anaesth.* 1978, **50**, 805.
233. Brownridge P. *Anaesthesia* 1981, **36**, 70.
234. Forster S. J. *Anaesthesia* 1983, **38**, 72.
235. Magee D. A. et al. *Can. Anaesth. Soc. J.* 1983, **30**, 174.
236. Watt M. J. et al. *Anaesthesia* 1968, **23**, 2, 311; 1970, **25**, 24; Ekblom L. and Widman B. *Acta Anaesthesiol. Scand.* 1966, Suppl. 21, 33.
237. Moore D. C. et al. *Anesth. Analg. (Cleve.)* 1978, **57**, 42.
238. Dunne N. M. and Kox W. J. *Br. J. Anaesth.* 1991, **66**, 617
239. Akerman B. et al. *Acta Anaesthesiol Scand.* 1988, **32**, 571; Thonpson G. E. et al. *Reg. Analg.* 1989, **14**, 6S; Whitehead E. et al. *Br. J. Anaesth.* 1990, **64**, 67; Scott D. B. et al. *Anesth. Analg.* 1989, **69**, 563; Brockway M. S. et al. *Br. J. Anaesth.* 1991, **66**, 31
240. Abdel-Salem A. R. et al. *Br. J. Anaesth.* 1975, **47**, 1081; Galindo A. et al. *Br. J. Anaesth.* 1975, **47**, 41; Stanton-Hicks M. et al. *Anesthesiology* 1975, **42**, 398; Buckley F. P. et al. *Br. J. Anaesth.* 1978, **50**, 171.
241. Ravindran R. S. et al. *Anesth. Analg. (Cleve.)* 1980, **59**, 477, Editorial. *Anesth. Analg. (Cleve.)* 1980, **59**, 401.
242. Schulte-Steinberg O. et al. *Anaesthesia* 1970, **25**, 191.
243. Bromage P. R. *Acta Anaesthesiol. Scand.* 1965, Suppl. 16, 55; Bromage P. R. et al. *Br. J. Anaesth.* 1967, **39**, 179; Bromage P. R. *Epidural Analgesia.* Philadelphia: Saunders, 1978, 82, 314.
244. Lee J. A. *Anaesthesia* 1960, **15**, 186.
245. Currie J. M. *Br. J. Anaesth.* 1984, **56**, 345.
246. Bonica J. J. *Principles and Practice of Obstetrical Anesthesia and Analgesia.* Philadelphia: Davis, 1967; Lee J. A. et al. ed. *Sir Robert Macintosh's Lumbar Puncture and Spinal Analgesia,* 5th ed. Edinburgh: Churchill Livingstone, 1985.
247. Mustafa K. et al. *Anesthesiology* 1983, **58**, 464.
248. Duffy B. *Anaesth. Intensive Care* 1982, **10**, 373.
249. Sicard J. A. and Forrestier J. *Rev. Neurol.* 1921, **28**, 1264.
250. Sharrock N. E. *Br. J. Anaesth.* 1979, **51**, 253.
251. Valentine S. J. et al. *Br. J. Anaesth.* 1991, **66**, 224.
252. Gutièrrez A. *Rev. Cirg. B. Aires* 1932, **12**, 665; 1933, **13**, 255.
253. Jansen E. *Dtsch. Z. NervHeilk.* 1926, **94**, 280.
254. Macintosh R. R. *Anaesthesia* 1950, **5**, 98.
255. Macintosh R. R. *Br. Med. J.* 1953, **1**, 398.
256. Salt R. H. *Anaesthesia* 1963, **18**, 404.

257. Cork R. C. et al. *Anesthesiology* 1980, **52**, 513.
258. Evans J. M. *Lancet* 1982, **2**, 1432.
259. Durrans S. F. *Anaesthesia* 1947, **2**, 106.
260. Mehta M. and Salmon N. *Anaesthesia* 1985, **40**, 1009
261. Moore D. C. and Batra M. S. *Anesthesiology* 1982, **57**, 141
262. Peters G. C. *Anaesthesia* 1983, **38**, 72.
263. *See also* Prince G. and MacGregor D. *Anaesthesia* 1986, **41**, 1240; McKeown D. W. et al. *Anaesthesia* 1986, **41**, 1262.
264. Kumar C. M. et al. *Anaesthesia* 1985, **40**, 1023
265. Mallaiah S. *Anaesthesia* 1986, **41**, 334.
266. Batra M. S. and Bridenbaugh L. D. *Reg. Anesth.* 1985, **10**, 32.
267. Ehni G. *Proc. Staff Meet. Mayo Clin.* 1975, **50**, 327; Verbiest H. *J. Bone Joint Surg.* 1954, **34b**, 230; *Clin. Neurol.* 1973, **20**, 204; Sullivan M. *Br. J. Hosp. Med.* 1976, **15**, 25.
268. Catterberg J. *Anesthesiology* 1977, **46**, 309.
269. Charlton G. A. and Lawes E. G. *Anaesthesia* 1991, **46**, 573.
270. Bromage P. R. and Robson G. *Anaesthesia* 1961, **16**, 461.
271. Shantha T. R. and Evans J. A. *Anesthesiology* 1972, **37**, 543.
272. Lee J. A. *Anaesthesia* 1962, **17**, 248.
273. Tuohy E. B. *JAMA* 1945, **128**, 262.
274. Bromage P. R. *Epidural Analgesia.* Philadelphia: Saunders, 1978, 465. Keane P. W. *Anaesthesia* 1983, **38**, 701.
275. Ruston F. G. *Can. Anaesth. Soc. J.* 1954, **1**, 37; 1964, **11**, 12.
276. Thorburn J. et al. *Br. J. Anaesth.* 1980, **52**, 11 17.
277. Hole A. *Acta Anaesthesiol. Scand.* 1980, **24**, 279; Modig J. et al. *Acta Anaesth. Scand.* 1980, **24**, 3005.
278. Thorne T. C. and Watt M. J. personal communications; Seovill W. B. *Surg. Neurol.* 1977, **7**, 163.
279. Dalens B. et al. *Anesth. Analg. (Cleve.)* 1986, **65**, 1060; Desparmet J. *Anaesthesia* 1986, **41**, 338.
280. Woerth S. D. et al. *Anesthesiology* 1977, **47**, 380.
281. Scott D. B. *Br. J. Anaesth.* 1981, **53**, 553.
282. Pathy G. V. and Rosen M. *Br. J. Anaesth.* 1975, **47**, 520.
283. Evans J. M. et al. *Anaesthesia* 1975, **30**, 774.
284. Hertz R. et al. *Anesth. Analg. Curr. Res.* 1980, **59**, 299.
285. Brindle-Smith G. et al. *Anaesthesia* 1984, **39**, 355; Pearson R. M. G. *Anaesthesia* 1984, **39**, 262, 460.
286. Longmire S. and Joyce T. H. *Anesthesiology* 1984, **39**, 1115.
287. Edwards G. M. and Sprigge J. *Anaesthesia* 1984, **38**, 194.
288. Shigematsu L. et al. *Anesth. Analg. (Cleve.)* 1985, **64**, 653.
289. Urquhart-Hay D. *Anaesthesia* 1969, **24**, 461; Harrison P. D. *Anaesthesia* 1975, **30**, 778; Ballin N. C. *Anaesthesia* 1981, **36**, 952.
290. Hirlekar G. *Anaesthesia* 1980, **35**, 363.
291. Eerola M. et al. *Acta Anaesthesiol. Scand.* 1981, **25**, 115.
292. Hillmann K. *Can. Anaesth. Soc. J.* 1965, **12**, 4.
293. Annotation, *Lancet* 1958, **2**, 515; Davies A. et al. *Br. Med. J.* 1958, **2**, 654.
294. Miller J. *Nerv. Ment. Dis.* 1909, **36**, 601.
295. Kelman H. *Am. J. Surg.* 1944, **64**, 183; Clark C. J. and Whitwell J. *Br. Med. J.* 1961, **2**, 1612.
296. Chaudhari L. S. et al. *Anaesthesia* 1978, **33**, 722; Loarie D. J. and Fairley H. B. *Anesth. Analg. Curr. Res.* 1978, **57**, 351.
297. Crawford J. S. *Br. J. Anaesth.* 1975, **47**, 412.
298. Male C. G. and Martin R. *Lancet* 1973, **1**, 609.
299. Cay D. L. *Anaesth. Intensive Care* 1984, **12**, 61.
300. Patel P. C. et al. *Anaesthesia* 1984, **39**, 383.
301. Mappes A. and Schaer H. M. *Anaesthesia* 1991, **46**, 435.

302. Cathelin F. *C. R. Soc. Biol. (Paris)* 1901, **53**, 452.
303. Sicard J. A. *C. R. Soc. Biol. (Paris)* 1901, **53**, 396 (both Cathelin's and Sicard's papers are translated and reprinted in 'Classical File'. *Surv. Anesthesiol.* 1979, **23**, 271).
304. Schlimpert H. and Schneider K. *Münch. Med.* Wochenschr. 1910, **57**, 2561.
305. Stoeckel W. *Zbl. Gynäk.* 1909, **31**, 1.
306. Läwen A. *Zbl. Chir.* 1910, **37**, 708; *Dtsch. Z. Chir.* 1910, **108**, 1; Läwen A. and von Gaza W. *Dtsch. Z. Chir.* 1911, **111**, 289.
307. Gros O. *Arch. Exp. Pathol. Pharmac.* 1910, **63**, 80.
308. Läwen A. and von Gaza A. *Dtsch. Zahnarztl. Chir.* 1911, **111**, 289.
309. Hingson R. A. and Southworth J. L. *Am. J. Surg.* 1942, **58**, 92; Hingson R. A. and Edwards W. B. *Anesth. Analg. Curr. Res.* 1942, **21**, 301; *JAMA* 1943, **121**, 252.
310. Trotter M. and Letterman G. S. *Surg. Gynecol. Obstet.* 1944, **78**, 418.
311. Nolte H. and Farrar M. D. *Anaesthesia* 1984, **39**, 1142.
312. Meyer R. J. *Anaesthesia* 1984, **39**, 610.
313. Semple A. J. and Bissett W. I. K. *Anaesthesia* 1985, **40**, 380.
314. Campbell M. F. *Am. J. Urol.* 1933, **30**, 245.
315. Snyder S. H. *N. Engl. J. Med.* 1977, **296**, 266; Pert C. B. and Snyder S. H. *Science* 1973, **179**, 1011.
316. Yaksh T. L. and Rudy T. A. *J. Pharmacol. Exp. Ther.* 1977, **202**, 411; Yaksh T. L. and Rudy T. A. *Pain* 1978, **4**, 299; Yaksh T. L. and Rudy T. A. *Science* 1976, **192**, 1357.
317. Wang J. K. *Ann. Anaesth. Franc.* 1978, **19**, 371; Wang J. K. et al. *Anesthesiology* 1979, **50**, 149.
318. Behar M. et al. *Lancet* 1979, **1**, 527; Howard R. P. et al. *Anaesthesia* 1981, **36**, 51.
319. Graham J. L. et al. *Anaesthesia* 1980, **35**, 158; Bromage P. R. et al. *Anesth. Analg. (Cleve.)* 1980, **59**, 473; Gjessing J. and Tomlin P. J. *Anaesthesia* 1981, **36**, 268; Boskovski N. et al. *Anaesthesia* 1981, **36**, 67; McClure J. H. et al. *Lancet* 1980, **1**, 975.
320. Johnson J. R. and McCaughey W. *Anaesthesia* 1980, **35**, 155.
321. Clemensen S. E. et al. *Br. Med. J.* 1987, **294**, 475.
322. Perriss B. W. *Lancet* 1979, **2**, 422; Perriss B. W. *Anaesthesia* 1980, **35**, 380.
323. Cousins M. J. et al. *Lancet* 1979, **1**, 1141.
324. Moore R. A. et al. *Br. J. Anaesth.* 1982, **54**, 1117.
325. Jorgensen B. C. et al. *Anesthesiology* 1981, **55**, 714.
326. Strube P. J. et al. *Br. J. Anaesth.* 1985, **56**, 921.
327. Kafer E. R. et al. *Anesthesiology* 1983, **58**, 418.
328. Chrabasik J. et al. *Lancet* 1984, **1**, 793.
329. Wedel S. J. and Ritter R. R. *Anesthesiology* 1981, **54**, 210.
330. Bromage P. R. et al. *Anesthesiology* 1983, **58**, 510.
331. Magora F. et al. *Br. J. Anaesth.* 1980, **52**, 247.
332. Bailey P. W. and Smith B. E. *Anaesthesia* 1980, **35**, 1002; Welchew E. A. and Thornton J. A. *Anaesthesia* 1982, **37**, 309; Welchew E. A. *Anaesthesia* 1983, **38**, 1037; Lam A. M. et al. *Can. Anaesth. Soc. J.* 1983, **30**, 578; Lomessy A. et al. *Anesthesiology* 1984, **61**, 466; Ahuja B. R. and Strunin L. *Anaesthesia* 1985, **40**, 949.
333. Welch D. B. and Hrynaszkiewicz A. *Anaesthesia* 1981, **36**, 1051; Nyoka M. et al. *Br. Med. J.* 1986, **293**, 1347.
334. Bilsback P. et al. *Br. J. Anaesth.* 1985, **57**, 943.
335. Donadoni R. et al. *Anaesthesia* 1985, **40**, 634.
336. Islas J. A. et al. *Anesth. Analg. (Cleve.)* 1985, **64**, 1161.
337. Normandale J. P. et al. *Anaesthesia* 1985, **40**, 748.
338. Reiz S. and Westberg M. *Lancet* 1980, **2**, 203; Boas R. A. *Anaesth. Intensive Care* 1980, **8**, 377.
339. Glynn C. J. et al. *Lancet* 1979, **2**, 356; Liolios A. and Andersen F. H. *Lancet* 1979, **2**, 357; Scott D. B. and McClure J. *Lancet* 1979, **1**, 1410; Sidi A. et al. *Anaesthesia* 1981, **36**, 1044.
340. Torda T. A. et al. *Br. J. Anaesth.* 1980, **52**, 939.
341. Evron S. et al. *Br. Med. J.* 1984, **288**, 190.
342. Niv D. et al. *Br. J. Anaesth.* 1983, **55**, 541.

343. Samil K. et al. *Lancet* 1979, **1**, 1142; Samil K. et al. *Anesthesiology* 1979, **50**, 149.
344. Scott P. V. et al. *Br. Med. J.* 1980, **281**, 351.
345. Daines G. K. et al. *Anesthesiology* 1980, **52**, 280; Davies G. K. *Anaesthesia* 1980, **35**, 1080.
346. Jones R. D. M. and Jones J. G. *Br. Med. J.* 1980, **281**, 645; Gjessing J. and Tomlin P. J. *Anaesthesia* 1981, **36**, 268.

Section 5
PAIN MANAGEMENT

Chapter 26

Acute pain

(*See also* Warfield R. *Manual of Pain Management*. Philadelphia: Lippincott, 1991.)

There are a few differences between acute and chronic pains.

REDUCTION OF POSTOPERATIVE PAIN

Two main problems exist in this area[1] (*see also* Chapter 9, on intraoperative analgesia).

1. Management of pain on return to consciousness. Since the introduction of postoperative observation recovery wards into European anaesthesia 30 years ago, this situation has been well managed. The dose of an analgesic required to prevent pain is only a fraction of that required to control it once it has become severe.

2. Management of the return of pain when the first postoperative dose of analgesic has worn off. At this point the patient may suffer unless the surgical team is careful to maintain appropriate prescriptions, and the nurses deliver the analgesics prescribed before pain breaks through. Several approaches have been made to solve this problem: (*a*) intermittent injections of opioids, to be given at the discretion of the nurse; (*b*) the use of continuous i.v. or subcutaneous infusion of opioids; (*c*) patient-controlled analgesia; (*d*) the use of long-acting regional blocks where appropriate; and (*e*) the use of the very long-acting opioids, e.g. methadone, dextromoramide, which give up to 12 h of analgesia especially useful at night. (If the first dose fails to control pain rapidly, it may be reinforced with one intravenous dose of a fast-acting opioid, e.g. pethidine.)

An 'Acute Pain Service' can teach, encourage and oversee the delivery of analgesia. It involves surgeons, physicians, pharmacists, anaesthetists and nurses. The relief of postoperative pain can be badly managed, simply by neglect.[2] Failure can occur at the point of writing prescriptions and at the point of delivery of analgesia by nurses. Experience with 'Pain Teams' has heightened awareness, but the risk is that the whole of the pain (and fluid and other) management of the hospital may be transferred by default to the team by those surgeons and nurses who previously looked after it. Thus, pain team activity may need to be mainly advisory in continuing effective analgesia and developing even more efficient methods by nurses, surgeons, etc. Perfect pain relief is often not attainable in practice, and sometimes not even desirable, since pain is a protective mechanism and the experience of pain on excessive movement may persuade the patient to take proper rest after surgery or trauma. 'Pain-free at rest' is a reasonable aim.

Pain relief is necessary for both humanitarian and therapeutic reasons. Pain causes peripheral vasoconstriction, and reduces FRC and sputum clearance. Many patients in human trials get pain relief from inert placebos.

Severity of acute surgical pain depends on: (1) the site of operation (in a report of a large series of operations, postoperative analgesia was required in 74% of thoracic cases; 63% of upper abdominal cases; 51% of lower abdominal cases; 23% of body-wall operations);[3] (2) age; (3) sex; (4) premedication employed; (5) anaesthetic agents used; (6) psychological factors; and (7) diurnal factors – time of day. Often worse in the evening.

Abdominal and thoracic wounds result in grunting, inefficient respiration with the production of hypoxia. Areas of spontaneous atelectasis may arise with regional underventilation, perfusion inequality and shunting of venous blood. FRC is reduced. The normal periodic deep breaths are inhibited by pain so that its relief undoubtedly aids respiration.

Pain scoring

A simple code is:
1. Comfortable (awake or asleep).
2. Slight pain – only elicited by close questioning.
3. Moderate pain – bothering the patient but often controllable by lying still. The patient will either be asking for analgesia or gladly receive it if offered.
4. Severe pain – dominating the consciousness and calling out for urgent relief.

Many research pain scoring systems exist, e.g. analogue, reflex and descriptive scales.

Many opioids are also sedatives (highly desirable in some situations), and sedation scores may be recorded, e.g. awake/asleep/respond to vocal commands/respond to touch/respond to painful stimuli/no response/severe respiratory depression (rate < 3 breaths per min).

Methods of pain relief

This is managed by analgesics, regional blocks, removal of cause of pain (e.g. distended bladder) and other methods, e.g. hypnosis, acupuncture.

1. Simple analgesics. For example non-steroidal anti-inflammatory drugs. A suppository, diclofenac 100 mg, or aspirin 1 g are effective.[4] Aspirin reduces platelet stickiness, the antithrombotic activity being thought due to its effect on thromboxane A2 synthesis together with the reduction of the formation of prostacyclin. It works peripherally. It is not recommended for children because of the rare risk of Reye's syndrome. Paracetamol is an active metabolite of phenacetin. It works centrally; it is analgesic and antipyretic, although not anti-inflammatory. It inhibits prostaglandin synthesis within the central nervous system. It does not cause gastric irritation and is relatively non-toxic in therapeutic doses, but 5 g may be enough to cause centrilobular hepatic necrosis. Aspirin and paracetamol form an effective mixture.

2. *Other non-steroid anti-inflammatory drugs (NSAIDs).*[5] For example diflunisal (Dolobid), 500 mg twice daily, especially in bone pain; indomethacin (Indocid), 100 mg oral or per rectum; naproxen (twice daily); piroxicam, 40 mg 'once daily', but initially may need to be given six-hourly for postoperative pain – dispersible tablets are available; tenoxicam 20 mg, diclofenac 100 mg, given orally, i. m., i.v. or as a suppository during the operation. Intramuscular diclofenac may be very painful for a long time.

NSAIDs are 99% bound to plasma albumin and metabolized by the liver. Some are given as inactive 'pro-drugs' which are converted to active drugs in the liver, e.g. sulindac, fenbufen.

NSAIDS should be avoided in severe renal failure, which the propionic acid derivatives worsen reversibly (severe renal toxicity is rare), in severe hepatic failure (they may prolong the bleeding time), in fluid retention (which they increase) and in peptic ulceration (which they may cause, especially the longer-acting ones in the elderly). Blood dyscrasias are rare (except phenylbutazone). They may worsen ulcerative colitis.

They may usefully be combined with paracetamol.

NSAIDs:
1. Modify the nociceptive responses caused by bradykinin.
2. Inhibit synthesis of prostaglandin E.
3. Have direct analgesic effect on the higher centres.
4. Reduce stickiness of blood platelets.
5. May cause hypothrombinaemia in large doses.
6. Lower body temperature in pyrexia, in low dosage.
7. Lower blood sugar in low dosage; reverse effect in high dosage.
8. May cause acid-base imbalance and acidosis.
9. Produce a background level of analgesia, lasting through the first postoperative day, equal in intensity to a reasonable dose of opioid. This background can then be built upon by opioid administration to produce a far higher level of analgesia, without a high level of side-effects.

Indomethacin can be given per rectum for postoperative pain relief[6] and indoprofen has also been recommended.[7] Indomethacin can also be given i.v. for pain relief after operation.[8] Diclofenac is versatile and can be given orally, i.m.[9] or as a suppository during the operation.[10]

3. *Opioids. See below for details.*

Patient-controlled analgesia (PCA).[11] The patient presses a button on an infusing device, resulting in a small i.v. or epidural bolus injection of opioid, e.g. 1–2 mg morphine, rapidly relieving pain. A 'lockout' control, e.g. 3–5 min for morphine, prevents excessively frequent demands and risk of overdose or abuse by previously unrecognized addicts. The total quantity of opioid received by the patient is said to be sometimes less than when the drug is given on an i.m. 'as necessary' basis. A one-way Y-connector enables use with i.v. infusions. Antireflux valves are recommended to prevent reflux delivery of drug into gravity fed infusion tubing in the event of an occlusion.

These valves may store a large bolus of drug, or impede the i.v. infusion.[12] The use of background additional opioid infusion is controversial, with risk of excessive sedation in some patients in the first 12 h, removal of some of the control from the patient, and need for reprogramming in the middle of the night. Pre-operative pain counselling (at least one day before operation) by the pain nurse is helpful. Syringe size and drug concentration are chosen to allow 48–60 h use from the initial filling.

There is a risk of theft of the drug in the PCA infusor, and of tampering with the PCA device. The quality of analgesia is normally good, and allows for wide inter-patient variation. Care is required in ensuring the correct concentration of opioid of the syringe in the infusor. Any opioid analgesic may be used.

This method reduces the falls of oxygen saturation seen with intermittent i.m. boluses.[13] A portable, disposable PCA system is available.

Pain control, respiration and sedation are monitored. Epidural PCA with lipophilic opioids may be improved by addition of local analgesics.

The advantages welcomed by patients include[14] not having to bother nurses who are too busy with other things; rapid pain relief; self control of their own pain; exact titration of dose; and lack of i.m. injections. Some worry about overdose, addiction, lack of personal contact with nurses and machine dysfunction, and can be reassured.

PCA is also useful in children over 5 years,[15] obstetrics, in acute medical diseases, e.g. angina, and malignant pain. Parent controlled analgesia and spouse controlled analgesia have been described.[16]

4. *Regional local analgesic blockade, including epidural infusion analgesia.*[17] (*See* Chapters 24 and 25.) This avoids the side-effects of the opioids, etc., can be applied to an area of the body no larger than the source of pain, and can give supremely good analgesia. Prolonged action is possible with insertion of microcatheters to the site of the block, and top-ups of analgesic. Particular postoperative care is needed when epidural opioids have been given.[18]

5. *Codeine phosphate, BP.* (Codeine is derived from the Greek name for 'poppy-head'.) Dose 15–60 mg as analgesic, antitussive and antidiarrhoeal agent.

This is methyl morphine and together with morphine and papaverine forms the chief alkaloidal derivative of opium. It was isolated in 1832 by Pierre Jean Robiquet (1780–1840).[19] It depresses respiration less, and causes less constipation and vomiting than morphine. Its analgesic effect is one-tenth that of morphine. Non-sedating, non-addictive and excreted unchanged by the kidneys; it may release histamine in children.[20]

6. *Dihydrocodeine tartrate (DF118).* Dose 0.5–1.0 mg/kg 4–6 hourly, oral, i.m. or i.v. Analgesic, constipating, and antitussive. May cause nausea, dysphoria and vertigo. It releases histamine.

7. *Blockade of pain afferents by regional techniques,*[21] For example postoperative high extradural analgesia,[22] intercostal nerve block,[23] and subcutaneous bupivacaine after herniorrhaphy.[24] A continuous lignocaine drip (2 mg/min) has been used with success and absence of signs of toxicity.[25]

8. *Inhalation of analgesic gases and vapours,* For example nitrous oxide and oxygen.

9. *Transcutaneous electrostimulation.*[26]

10. *Cryoanalgesia.* Of individual nerves.[27]
See also RCS and College of Anaesthetists commission on postoperative pain, 1990.

Opioids

Are commonly used and very effective. They can be arranged in a long series depending on their affinities for endorphin receptors, ranging from pure agonists (morphine, pethidine, diamorphine, methadone), through partial agonists (buprenorphine) and partial antagonists (pentazocine, nalorphine, levallorphan), to the pure antagonists (naloxone).

Opioids also influence the emotional aspects of pain, such as anxiety and fear, as well as reducing the actual pain threshold, so making intolerable pain, tolerable. They act on specific opiate receptors in the brain and spinal cord. Enkephalins (the natural neurotransmitters) are present in the brain and in the gastro-intestinal tract; they may be formed in the adrenal medulla. They are like natural opioids. Beta-endorphin is a potent opioid, more stable and potent than the enkephalins.[28]

Problems with opioids

1. Nausea and vomiting in up to 50% of cases.
2. Respiratory depression.
3. Considerable variation of individual response (up to 10-fold) making it difficult to predict the correct dose. In those resistant to opioids, simply increasing the dose above the normal range, is usually adequate. Opioid premedication helps predict individual sensitivity or resistance to these drugs.
4. Bradycardia with short-acting opioids.
5. Relatively slow onset of analgesia. Intravenous alfentanil and pethidine are fastest (1–2 min); papaveretum and fentanyl may take 15–20 min to produce analgesia (respiratory depression has a faster onset).
6. Addiction in susceptible individuals. (More likely in those who prescribe them, than in those who have their pain treated by them.) Tachyphylaxis in the more chronic situation, and occasional hallucinations with prolonged administration.
7. Antagonism of their analgesia by other commonly-used drugs, e.g. for neuromuscular relaxation reversal.

Some of the problems of opioids can be reduced, and analgesia potentiated, by pretreatment with oral clonidine, a partial α_2 adrenoceptor agonist, 50–150 µg, orally, i.v., i.m., or epidurally. For epidural use *see* Motsch J. et al. *Anesthesiology* 1990, **73**, 1067; Vercauteren M. et al. *Anaesthesia* 1990, **45**, 531; Eisenach J. C. et al. *Anesthesiology* 1989, **71**, 640.

Oral opioids[29]

Morphine and diamorphine, given in water or chloroform water without any additions, give good analgesia; with diamorphine the analgesia comes on quicker but is of shorter duration. An anti-emetic may be needed should the patient require more than 20 mg of morphine. A tablet of morphine containing 10 mg of base, placed and kept between the upper lip and the upper gum will control pain as efficiently as the same dose given intramuscularly. (*See also* Bell M. D. D. et al. *Lancet* 1985, **1**, 71).

Opioids by injection

Morphine 10 mg, diamorphine 5 mg, pethidine 100 mg or buprenorphine 0.3 mg can be given intramuscularly. Infants, neonates, the elderly and the unfit are more susceptible to respiratory depression. Children and young adults are often quite resistant.

A continuous intravenous infusion of morphine or other narcotic analgesic can be given until pain is relieved, and then the dose titrated against the pain. Infusions of fentanyl efficiently relieve postoperative pain.[30] Such infusions need not be followed by either psychological dependence or physical sequelae[31] (*see also* patient-controlled analgesia, the Cardiff Palliator[32] and the Janssen on-demand infusion of dilute fentanyl[33]). Infusions give good pain relief at a lower dosage than intramuscular injection.

Efficient postoperative pain relief can be provided by a continuous subcutaneous infusion powered by a syringe pump. A simple regime is: after recovery from anaesthesia, good analgesia is secured by intravenous morphine, up to 0.2 mg/kg and subcutaneous infusion is then started; average dose rate 0.8 mg/kg/24 h. The infusion site may be easily changed by the nurses. In addition, either the infusion pump may have a bolus boost facility, or a 'as necessary' prescription for i.m. morphine (0.1–0.2 mg/kg) available for extra pain (dressings, turning) or to regain pain control.[35] Continuous subcutaneous pethidine for routine postoperative analgesia (2 mg/h) after a loading dose, has proved successful and reasonably free from side-effects.[36]

It has been reported that the opioid requirements of patients receiving high doses of corticosteroids is less than normal in the control of postoperative pain.[37]

It is important that whatever regime is used, for the majority of patients, that it can be administered by the ordinary nurse on the ordinary ward, without constant intervention by doctors.

The sale of opium was unrestricted in the UK until the Pharmacy Act of 1868.

Extradural injections of narcotic analgesics

(*See* Chapter 25). One of the problems here is that the lipophilic opioids are only slightly more potent by this route than when given systemically, unless they are mixed with local analgesics.

Pharmacology of individual opioids

MORPHINE

(From the Greek, Morpheus, god of dreams, son of Somnos, god of sleep). There is large inter-patient variability with morphine.

Opium is derived from the Greek word for 'juice'. Has been in use as opium for over 2000 years and is still the best available analgesic (first used by

Table 26.1. Narcotic analgesics (with equivalent adult doses in mg)

Alkaloids of opium
  Morphine (10)
  Codeine (30)
  Papaveretum (20)

Semisynthetic alkaloids
  Diamorphine (5)
  Dihydrocodeine (DF 118) (50)
  Dihydromorphinone (Dilaudid) (2)

Synthetic agents
  Benzomorphinans and morphinans
  Pentazocine (Fortral, Talwin) (30)

Piperidine derivatives
  Pethidine (Mepiridine, Demerol) (100)
  Phenoperidine (Operidine) (2)
  Fentanyl (Sublimaze) (0.05–0.2)
  Alfentanil (Rapifen) (0.25–0.5)
  Sufentanil (0.005–0.01)
  Lofentanil (0.005)

Diphenylheptane derivatives
  Methadone (Physeptone) (10)
  Dextromoramide (Palfium) (5)

Mixed agonist/antagonists
  Pentazocine (30)
  Buprenorphine (0.3)
  Butorphanol (2)

Theophrastus in the third century B.C.). "Among the remedies which it has pleased Almighty God to give to man to relieve his sufferings, none is so universal and so efficacious as opium" – Thomas Sydenham (1627–1682), London physician, 1680, who introduced tincture of opium (laudanum) into England. Opium comes from the dried latex from unripe capsules of the poppy head.

Morphine isolated from opium by F. W. A. Sertürner (1783–1841) of Paderborn in 1806.[38] Morphine salts are not destroyed by boiling.

It was used before anaesthesia to prevent anxiety by Bruno of Turin in 1850,[34] and by the Munich surgeon J. N. von Nussbaum (1829–1890) to reduce the amount of anaesthetic needed, in 1864.[39] In 1869, Claude Bernard (1813–1878), professor of physiology at the Sorbonne, used morphine in animals before anaesthesia[40] and this led some of his pupils (e.g. Guibert[41] of St Brieuc) to use it clinically in an effort to reduce the amount of chloroform needed to ensure deep anaesthesia.[42] (*See also* report in *Medical Times, London,*[43] and Aubert of Lyons.[44])

As the combination of morphine and anaesthesia caused hypoventilation resulting in a rigid abdomen, it failed to become a popular method, although in intracranial surgery, Sir Victor Horsley (1857–1916) pioneer neurosurgeon, used it to reduce bleeding in 1886.[45]

The somewhat mutually antagonistic effects of morphine and atropine were pointed out by Benjamin Bell,[46] by John Harley[47] and by the French physiologist, Brown Sequard (1817–1894), Claude Bernard's successor in Paris. The report of the Second Hyderabad Chloroform Commission in 1889–1890 recommended the use of morphine before chloroform as an aid to anaesthesia, not to reduce anxiety. Chloralhydrate given to produce sleep and sedation before operation in 1874 by Forné. Chemical structure determined in 1925 and was synthesized by Gates and Tschudi (1952).[48] One of over 25 alkaloids. (Alkaloid = like alkali, a term first used by K. F. W. Meissner (1792–1853) of Halle, Germany.) Contained in opium *(Papaver somniferum)*, but only morphine, codeine and papaverine have wide clinical use. Concentration of morphine in opium is 9-17%.

Summary of actions of morphine.

1, *Central nervous system.* (a) Depresses awareness, anxiety, pain sensation and respiration; (b) stimulates vomiting centre; secretion of antidiuretic hormone; Edinger–Westphal nucleus causing small pupils; hallucinations occur rarely, as with other opioids.

2. Smooth muscle. (a) Depresses vascular tone and peristalsis; and (b) stimulates bronchoconstriction, bowel sphincters, biliary spasm, Fallopian spasm, and erectores pilorum.

3. Addiction. Both psychological and physical. Patients may develop both tolerance (or tachyphylaxis) and dependence (or addiction). In addicts, withdrawal symptoms come on in about 8 h after the last dose and are very distressing. They include agitation, severe abdominal cramps, diarrhoea and lacrimation ('cold turkey'). Relieved by further doses of morphine or methadone;

4. Other. Stimulates secretion of catecholamines, depresses metabolism, releases histamine (short-acting opioids induce bradycardia). Naloxone antagonizes its analgesia as well as most side-effects. Note the relative lack of effects on the vascular system, even in large doses (but infants may become hypotensive on 1 mg/kg morphine). It is a good analgesic and poor relaxer of smooth muscle. (Papaverine is a poor analgesic but a good relaxant of smooth muscle.)

Central Nervous System. It is analgesic, sedative, anxiolytic, euphoric, addictive, a respiratory depressant, and causes nausea and vomiting. More effective against dull, continuous, visceral, than against sharp, intermittent pain. Very rarely, restlessness and delirium follow its injection (as in the horse and cat) and dysphoria follows. The intracranial pressure is increased because of the raised Pco_2.

Effect on the Eye. Miosis by central action, via the oculomotor nerve, stimulating the Edinger–Westphal nucleus. Atropine can counteract this miosis. Intra-ocular tension reduced in both normal and glaucomatous eyes.

Respiratory System. The response of the respiratory centre to $Paco_2$ is diminished, with 50% depression of the $Paco_2$ response curve at plasma levels of 100 μg/l. (Postoperative analgesia at 12–25 μg/l.)[49] (*See* Figure 26.1.)

Respiratory rate, rather than tidal volume, decreased. Arterial and alveolar Pco_2 not usually much raised. Respiratory depression is difficult to define or measure clinically, and the respiratory rate is often used, by default (< 5 breaths per minute). Breathing may become periodic (Cheyne–Stokes)[50] or irregular (Biot). Bronchoconstriction occurs, worse in asthmatic patients. Maximal respiratory depression comes on 30 min after intramuscular injection, sooner after i.v. injection. Depresses the cough reflex.

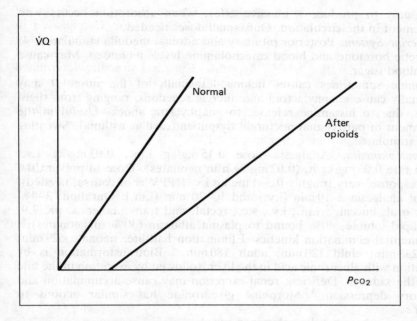

Figure 26.1 Effect of opioids on respiratory response to CO_2.

Gastrointestinal Tract. Morphine constricts the sphincters of the gut and reduces peristalsis, more so when given i.m. than when given orally.[51]

Nausea and vomiting are due to central stimulation. This is seen most strongly with the allied drug, apomorphine. Vomiting after morphine depends partly on the movements of the body and the position of the patient; it sensitizes the vomiting centre to vestibular movements. Ambulation after morphine will cause more nausea than quiet bed-rest. Anti-emetics can control this nausea, some more effectively than others. About a third of postoperative patients will feel sick after opioids, women much more so than males.

Morphine contracts the sphincter of Oddi, raising the pressure in the bile ducts, and rarely causing severe pain. Atropine does not fully antagonize this action, but glyceryl trinitrate, nalorphine, levallorphan, adrenaline, aminophylline and amyl nitrite do.

Urinary Tract. The tone and peristalsis of the ureters and other smooth muscle, e.g. of the hollow viscera, bladder sphincter, fallopian tubes, etc., are increased, an action antagonized by atropine. The tone of the vesical sphincter is increased and may hinder micturition, a common postoperative problem. Urinary output decreased due to stimulation of secretion of antidiuretic hormone.

Little relaxation of uterus during labour. Crosses placental barrier and depresses fetal respiration.

Cardiovascular System. Mild vasodilatation in clinical doses, bradycardia sometimes seen. Patients in shock should be given their morphine intravenously, so that it does not accumulate unabsorbed in the ischaemic tissues, only to produce a massive effect when absorption occurs with improvement in the circulation. Only small doses needed.

Endocrine System. Posterior pituitary and adrenal medulla stimulated, so antidiuretic hormone and blood catecholamine levels increased. May cause rise in blood sugar.

Morphine sometimes causes itching, especially of the nose. It may occasionally cause anaphylactoid and allergic reactions, ranging from slight syncope, due to histamine release, to anaphylactic shock. Useful in the management of paroxysmal nocturnal dyspnoea (cardiac asthma). Sweating may be stimulated.

Pharmacokinetics. Analgesia dose 0.15 mg/kg i.m., 0.03 mg/kg i.v., infusion rate 0.03 mg/kg/h, (0.02 mg/kg/h in neonates). Dose to prevent the 'stress response' very roughly 0.5–1 mg/kg i.v. (IPPV is of course, needed). Onset of analgesia 3–10 min (i.v.) and 10–20 min (i.m.). Duration: 3–4 h. Routes: oral, buccal,[52] i.m., i.v., s.c., rectal, and transcutaneous. pK 7.9, poorly lipid-soluble, 40% bound to plasma albumin (30% in neonates).[53] Triexponential elimination kinetics. Elimination half-life: neonate 629 min; infant 233 min; child 120 min; adult 180 min.[54] Biotransformation is by conjugation with glucuronic acid in the liver, followed by excretion in the bile and by the kidneys. Deficient renal excretion may cause accumulation and respiratory depression.[55] Morphine glycuronide has similar actions to morphine.

It appears in breast milk, saliva and sweat.

It is very useful in premedication and postoperative pain control.

Special care is necessary. (1) in infants under 6 months, the aged, feeble and debilitated; and (2) in patients with a raised Pco_2, suprarenal insufficiency, myasthenia, myotonia, hypothyroidism, asthma, raised intracranial pressure, respiratory depression, hepatic failure, renal failure, acute alcoholism, diverticulitis and labour.

Morphine kills by causing respiratory arrest.

DIAMORPHINE HYDROCHLORIDE, BP (HEROIN)

This is the diacetyl ester of morphine and is the most likely of the opium derivatives to become a drug of addiction, because of the euphoria it creates. Introduced into medicine in 1898 by H. Dreser (1860–1924). In the US and in Australia its use is proscribed. Should be freshly prepared from powder. It depresses the respiratory centre and the cough reflex more than morphine and is twice as efficient as an analgesic. Diamorphine 5 mg has a quicker onset of activity and fewer emetic sequelae than morphine 10 mg. An excellent postoperative analgesic although its effect does not last as long as that of morphine. In coronary occlusion, 5 mg i.v. cause little cardiovascular depression or vomiting, if given slowly. Useful by mouth in the treatment of chronic pain in doses up to 30 mg,[56] and as an epidural opioid.

Excretion is chiefly by the kidneys after conversion to morphine in the body.

Dose 2.5–5 mg. Onset. i.v. 5 mins; i.m. 10 mins.

PAPAVERETUM, BPC (*Omnopon, Pantopon, Alopon, Opoidine*)

Introduced in 1909 by Sahli[57] (1856–1933) of Berne. It is a mixture of purified opium alkaloids in the proportion found in nature, as follows: anhydrous morphine 47.5–52.2%, anhydrous codeine 2.5–5%, noscapine 16–22%, papaverine 2.5–7%.[58] Clinically 20 mg papaveretum equals 13.3 mg morphine sulphate. There is no evidence that papaveretum causes fewer unpleasant side-effects than morphine. Dosage, 10–20 mg. Onset, 20 min. Duration 2–4 h. Premedication in children: 0.2–0.4 mg/kg. (*See also* Chapter 22, Paediatrics.) The Committee on Safety of Medicines has proscribed its use in females of child-bearing potential in the UK because of its noscapine content. A formulation without noscapine is available.

PAPAVERINE, BP

Isolated by Georg Franz Merck (1825–1895) of Darmstadt in 1848 from opium.[59] Does not suppress intestinal peristalsis. Relieves spasm in arteries. Has almost no central effects. Dose up to 30 mg i.v. or i.a., very slowly; orally, 120–250 mg.

PETHIDINE HYDROCHLORIDE, BP (*Demerol,* meperidine hydrochloride USP, isonipecaine, *Dolatin, Dolantal, Dolosal, Pantalgin*)

The hydrochloride of the ethyl ester of 1-methyl-4-phenyl-piperidine-4-carboxylic acid. Dose: 0.5 mg/kg i.v., 1.5 mg/kg i.m. Onset, rapid, 2–5 min. Duration, 2 h.

Pharmacodynamics.

1. Analgesic. Relieves most types of pain, especially those associated with plain muscle spasm. Depresses respiratory centre and cough reflex. Is also a local analgesic. No effect on ciliary body or iris. Raises the CSF pressure. Can cause addiction.

2. Has a direct papaverine-like effect on the smooth muscle of the bronchioles, intestine, ureters and arteries. Will often relieve bronchospasm. Vasodilation may be unwelcome in trauma cases and uncontrolled hypertensives.

3. Has an atropine-like effect on cholinergic nerve-endings.

4. May release histamine from tissues.

5. Side-effects may include sweating, hypotension, vertigo and limb tingling. Postoperative nausea is similar to that following morphine, but comes on earlier. These are worse after intravenous than after intramuscular injection. Like morphine, pethidine may cause hypotension if the head of the patient is raised, or with sudden movement. Because of its circulatory depressant effects it is probably not the ideal drug for the relief of pain in myocardial infarction. Phenobarbitone enhances the production of toxic metabolites of pethidine. These two drugs should not be given together.[60]

Pharmacokinetics. Routes of administration same as morphine; 64% plasma protein bound. Pethidine is metabolized at the rate of 17%/h. The biological half-life is 3–4 h in man.[61] 80% hydrolysed in liver. About 5–10% is excreted unchanged by the kidneys. One metabolite, norpethidine, may cause convulsions or hallucinations if pethidine is given in large doses or with mono-amine oxidase inhibitors.

Pethidine in labour. See Chapter 22, Obstetrics.

Precautions. The administration of pethidine to patients receiving mono-amine oxidase inhibitors may cause severe reactions and even death.

There is restlessness, hypertension, convulsions and coma with absent tendon jerks and an extensor plantar response; hypotension may also be seen. The reaction is said to be due to interference with the microsomes in liver cells which detoxicate pethidine. Treatment is supportive, and with 25 mg prednisolone or chlorpromazine.

PHENOPERIDINE (*Operidine*) (*See* Chapter 9)

FENTANYL (*Sublimaze, Fentanest, Lepantal*) (*See* Chapter 9).

ALFENTANIL (*Rapifen*) (*See* Chapter 9).

SUFENTANIL (*See Chapter 9*).

LOFENTANIL

Twenty times more potent than fentanyl, and 6000 times more than morphine. Long duration of action attributed to persistent occupation of receptor sites.

PENTAZOCINE (*Fortral, Talwin*)

A narcotic agonist/antagonist analgesic derived from benzmorphinan. Dose, 30 mg, onset 20 min, routes oral and i.m. Respiratory depression is dose-related but has a ceiling effect. Non-addictive and not euphoric. Raises rather than lowers blood pressure and the dextro-isomer has a positive inotropic effect on the myocardium (β-receptor stimulation).[62] Does not influence pupil size or intra-ocular tension. Crosses the placental barrier less easily than pethidine.[63] A very weak narcotic antagonist, one-fiftieth the activity of nalorphine. Hallucinations may follow its use but may be controlled by nalorphine[64] or diazepam.

DEXTROPROPOXYPHENE

May cause dependence and, taken with alcohol, respiratory depression. Distalgesic is made up of 32.5 mg with paracetamol 325 mg. Overdose will result in liver toxicity and respiratory depression.

DEXTROMORAMIDE ACID TARTRATE, BP (*Palfium*)

A morphine-like analgesic but twice as potent. Dose, 5 mg tablet or 5–10 mg by intramuscular injection. Relatively non-soporific. Can be given by mouth.

METHADONE HYDROCHLORIDE, BP (*Physeptone, Amidone, Dolophine, Miadone, Adanon, Butalgin*)

This is a powerful analgesic, with a half-life 40 to 90 h. (Duration of action extends with subsequent doses.) Dose, 0.1 mg/kg i.m. or 0.05 mg/kg i.v. Onset: i.v. 1 min; i.m. 5 min. Causes less sedation and has a more prolonged action than morphine (half life 4–90 h, increasing with subsequent doses).

Absorption from fatty sites (e.g. s.c. and epidural) is very slow. Has been used to wean addicts from morphine and for chronic pain. (*See also* Bullingham, R. E. S. *Br. J. Hosp. Med.* 1981, **5**, 59; and Gourlay G. K. et al. *Anaesth. Intensive Care*, 1981, **9**, 183.)

Long-acting analgesics methadone and dextromoramide are invaluable in acute and chronic pain control where there is delay in delivering top-up doses when pain returns after i.m. injection (a common problem). The sustained duration of analgesia greatly reduces the frequency of those painful intervals before the next dose is given.

BUPRENORPHINE (*Temgesic*)

A powerful, long-acting synthetic thebaine derivative, with agonist/antagonist properties. Dose, 0.2–1 mg; routes, sublingual, i.m., i.v., epidural; duration of action up to 10 h.[65] A single dose may therefore last through the night hours, which is important in postoperative analgesia.[66] Buprenorphine may accentuate urinary obstruction.[67] A dose of 0.3 mg relieves the pain of ureteral colic.[68] It has different disposition in patients with renal impairment.[69] Only partly reversed by naloxone but because of its agonist/antagonist properties, respiratory depression shows a 'ceiling effect' and apnoea, or even a respiratory rate below 4/min, is very unlikely to occur.

NALBUPHINE HYDROCHLORIDE (*Nubain*)

Has been used for perioperative analgesia. Has less effect on delay of coordinated bowel motility than morphine.[70] Dose, 10–20 mg. Not likely to cause bronchoconstriction in asthmatics. Suggested for military 'buddy' use as it does not obscure signs of head injury.

MEPTAZINOL (*Meptid*)

Used for perioperative analgesia. Dose, by mouth 200 mg, repeated. Intramuscularly, 75–100 mg.

The Misuse of Drugs Act, 1971

Schedule 1 drugs

No records need be kept or entries made in a register of controlled drugs. LSD and cannabis.

Schedule 2

Listed drugs: Class A. Opium, morphine, diamorphine, fentanyl, cocaine, methadone, pethidine, dextromoramide, dipipanone, oxycodone, phenazocine, phencyclidine, amphetamines and quinol barbitone.

Records of Schedule 2 drugs must be kept in a special register and signed in the doctor's own handwriting.

A sister or acting sister for the time being in charge of a theatre may, when acting in her capacity as such, supply any drug in Schedule 2 to any person who may lawfully have that drug in his possession provided that the drug is used in that theatre in accordance with the prescription of a doctor or dentist. A record of administration should be made in the patient's case notes.

Schedule 3 (minor stimulants, buprenorphine)

No need for records in the register. Buprenorphine stored in safe custody.

Schedule 4 (benzodiazepines)

No safe custody requirements.

Schedule 5 (codeine, pholcodeine, etc.)

No safe custody or register.

Specific narcotic antagonists

These are usually the *n*-allyl derivatives of narcotic analgesics. The more potent the narcotic, the smaller the dose of its allyl derivative necessary to antagonize narcotic-induced respiratory depression. They have high receptor affinity and low receptor activity. They do not lead to addiction. They may cause signs of withdrawal in narcotic addicts. Probable mode of action is competition at receptor sites on cell surfaces. The antagonists counteract the analgesia produced by morphine, pethidine and oxymorphone although less so with morphine.

Specific antagonism to narcotics was first described in 1915 by Pohl.[71]

NALOXONE (*Narcan*)

This is *n*-allyl noroxymorphone and is derived from the potent oxymorphone. It was synthesized in 1972.[72] It also antagonizes the respiratory depression caused by pentazocine and dextropropoxyphene. Duration of effect, 1 h; may be less than the narcotic it is designed to antagonize, so that repeat dosage may be necessary. It relaxes spasm of the sphincter of Oddi induced by narcotic analgesics. With careful titration of dosage, analgesia is not reversed. Can be used in the treatment of opioid-induced respiratory depression and in midwifery to reverse fetal respiratory depression due to opiates. It also prevents the impairment of psychomotor performance due to low levels of alcohol.[73] Naloxone reverses respiratory depression but not the analgesia of intrathecal morphine.[74] Naloxone may raise blood pressure in septic shock, suggesting that endorphins may contribute to this hypotension.[75] Naloxone has caused acute pulmonary oedema in a previously fit patient, so it is to be used with care.[76] Has also caused dysrhythmia and even sudden death.[77] Can be given i.m. for a more prolonged effect.

Pharmacokinetics. Half-life 20 min. Metabolized in the liver. Dose, 0.1–0.4 mg i.v. repeated. In neonates 0.01 mg/kg.

LEVALLORPHAN TARTRATE, BP, USP (*Lorfan*)

It is the *n*-allyl derivative of laevomorphinan (laevo-dromoran) to which it bears a similar relationship as does nalorphine to morphine. Levallorphan was synthesized in 1950 by Schneider and Hellerbach[78] and used as an antidote to respiratory depression by Fromherz and Pellmond two years later.[79]

Suggested dosage to reverse respiratory depression: 0.5–1 mg, i.v. repeated at 3–5 min intervals, or, in neonates, 0.25–0.5 mg into the umbilical vein. Pethilorfan contains pethidine and levallorphan 100 to 1.25 (80:1).

Opioid overdose[80]

Coma, respiratory depression, hypoxia, acidosis, muscle compression (from deep sedation) all leading to rhabdomyolysis and acute renal failure. Pulmonary oedema (non-cardiogenic), cerebral oedema, convulsions, aspiration pneumonia also occur. Treatment is by immediate reversal with naloxone and by organ support, e.g. oxygenation/IPPV.

References

1. Dahl J. B., et al. *Br. J. Anaesth.* 1990, **64**, 178.
2. Cartwright P. D. *Ann. R. Coll. Surg.* 1985, **67**, 13. .
3. Loan W. B. and Dundee J. W. *Practitioner* 1967, **198**, 759.
4. Canto J. et al. *Acta Anaesthiol. Scand.* 1981, **25**, 25.
5. Orme M. *Prescribers Journal* 1990, **30**, 95.
6. Keenan D. J. M. et al. *Br. Med. J.* 1984, **288**, 240.
7. Rigamonti G. et al. *Br. J. Anaesth.* 1983, **55**, 513.
8. Mattila M. A. H. et al. *Br. Med. J.* 1983, **287**, 1026.
9. Buchanan J. M. and Halshaw J. *Ann. R. Coll. Surg.* 1988, **70**, 286.
10. Hodsman N. B. A. et al. *Anaesthesia* 1987, **42**, 1005.
11. Ferrante F. M., Ostheimer G. W. and Covino B. G. *Patient-controlled analgesia.* Oxford: Blackwell Scientific, 1990.
12. Kluger M. T. and Owen H. *Anaesthesia* 1991, **45**, 1059.
13. Wheatley R. G. et al. *Br. J. Anaesth* 1990, **64**, 267.
14. Kluger M. T. and Owen H. *Anaesthesia* 1991, **45**, 1072.
15. Lawrie S. C. et al. *Anaesthesia* 1991, **45**, 1074.
16. Wakerlin G. and Larson C. P. *Anaesth. Analg.* 1990, **70**, 119.
17. Wildsmith J. A. W. and McClure J. H. *Conduction blockade for postoperative analgesia* London: Edward Arnold, 1991.
18. Ross N. L. *Anesthesiology* 1990, **72**, 212; Ready B. L. and Edwards W. T. *Anesthesiology* 1990, **72**, 213.
19. Robiquet P. J. *Analls Chim. Phys.* 1832, **51**, 225.
20. Shanahan E. C. et al. *Anaesthesia* 1983, **38**, 40.
21. Edmonds-Seal J. et al. *J. R. Soc. Med.* 1980, **73**, 111.
22. Spence A. A. and Smith G. *Anaesthesia* 1979, **34**, 320
23. Nunn J. F. and Slavin G. *Br. J. Anaesth.* 1980, **52**, 253.
24. Hashemi K. and Middleton M. D. *Ann. R. Coll. Surg.* 1983, **65**, 38.
25. Cassuto J. et al. *Anesth. Analg. (Cleve.)* 1985, **64**, 971.
26. Baker S. B. C. et al. *Can. Anaesth. Soc. J.* 1980, **27**, 150.
27. Wood G. J. et al. *Anaesthesia* 1981, **36**, 603; Evans P. J. D. et al. *Br. J. Anaesth*, 1981, **53**, 1121.
28. *See* Editorial, *Br. Med. J.* 1984, **288**, 259.
29. Gordon A. *Physician* 1988, **7**, 33; Hillier E. H. *Br. Med. J.* 1983, **287**, 701.
30. Nimmo W. S. and Todd J. G. *Br. J. Anaesth.* 1985, **57**, 250.
31. Morgan R. J. M. *Anaesthesia* 1983, **38**, 492.
32. Chakravarty K. et al. *Br. Med. J.* 1979, **2**, 895.

33. White D. C. et al. *Br. Med. J.* 1979, **2**, 116.
34. Quoted by Dogliotti A. M. *Anesthesia*. Chicago: S. B. Debom, 1939, 20.
35. Goudie T. A. et al. *Anaesthesia* 1985, **40**, 1086.
36. Davenport H. T. et al. *Ann. R. Coll. Surg.* 1985, **67**, 379.
37. Korman B. and McKay R. J. *Anesth. Intensive Care* 1985, **13**, 395.
38. Sertürner F. W. A. *J. Pharm. fürAertze und Apoth. Chem.* Leipzig 1806, **14**, 47.
39. von Nussbaum J. N. *Med. Times, Lond.* 1865, 259.
40. Bernard C. *Bull Gen. de Thérap.* 1868, **77**, 241; Annotation, *Lancet* 1969, **2**, 789; Lee J. A. *Anaesthesia* 1978, **33**, 733.
41. Guibert C. R. *Acad. Sci. Paris* 1872, **74**, 815.
42. Labbé C. and Goujon E. *C. R. Acad. Sci. Paris* 1870, **74**, 815.
43. *Med. Times, Lond.* 1872, **1**, 359.
44. Aubert P. *C. R. Soc. Biol. Paris* 1883, **5**, 242.
45. Horsley V. *Br. Med. J.* 1886, **2**, 670.
46. Bell B. *Edin. Med. J.* 1858–1859, n.s. **4**, 1.
47. Harley J. *Br. Med. J.* 1874, **2**, 518.
48. Gates M. and Tschudi G. *J. Am. Chem. Soc.* 1952, **74**, 1109.
49. Lynn A. M. and Slattery J. T. *Anesthesiology*, 1987, **66**, 136.
50. Cheyne J. (1777–1836) *Dubl. Hosp. Rep.* 1818, **2**, 216 and Stokes Wm. (1804–1878) *The Diseases of the Heart and Aorta*. Dublin: Hodge & Smith, 1854.
51. Park G. R. *Anaesthesia* 1984, **39**, 645.
52. Manara, A. R. et al. *Br. J. Anaesth.* 1989, **62**, 498.
53. Kupferberg H. J. and Way E. L. *J. Pharm. Exp. Ther.* 1963, **141**, 105; Koren G. et al. *J. Pediatr.* 1985 **107**, 963.
54. Aitkenhead A. R. et al. *Br. J. Anaes.* 1984, **56**, 813.
55. McQuay H. and Moore A. *Lancet* 1984, **2**, 284.
56. Twycross R. G. *Br. Med. J.* 1975, **4**, 212.
57. Sahli H. *Ther. Mh. (Halbruch.) 1909*, **23**, 1.
58. *Martindale: The Extra Pharmacpoeia* (Wade A. ed.) 1977, 27th ed. London: The Pharmaceutical Press, 976.
59. Merck G. F. *Ann. Phys. Chem. (Leipzig)* 1848, **66**, 125.
60. Stambough J. E. et al. *Lancet* 1977, **1**, 398.
61. Mather L. E. et al. *Clin. Pharmacol. Ther.* 1975, **17**, 21.
62. Appleyard T. N. *Proc. R. Soc. Med.* 1975, **68**, 770.
63. Moore J. et al. *Br. J. Anaesth.* 1973, **45** (Suppl.), 798.
64. Jago R. H. et al. *Anaesthesia* 1977. **32**, 904.
65. Kay B. *Br. J. Anaesth.* 1978, **50**, 605.
66. McQuay H. J. et al. *Br. J. Anaesth.* 1980, **52**, 1013.
67. Murray K. *Br. Med. J.* 1983, **286**, 761.
68. Finlay I. G. et al. *Br. Med. J.* 1982, **284**, 1830.
69. Hand C. W. et al. *Br. J. Anaesth.* 1990, **64**, 276; Bullingham R. E. S. et al. *Anaesthesia* 1984, **39**, 329; Derbyshire D. R. et al. *Anaesthesia* 1984, **39**, 324.
70. Shah M. et al. *Br. J. Anaesth.* 1984. **56**, 1235.
71. Pohl J. *Z. Exp. Path Ther.* 1915, **17**, 370.
72. Blumberg H. and Drayton H. D. In: *Naloxone and Related Compounds* (Kossterlitz H. W. et al. ed.) London: Macmillan, 1972.
73. Jeffcote W. C. et al. *Lancet* 1979. **2**, 688.
74. Jones R. D. M. and Jones J. A. *Br. Med. J.* 1980, **2**, 646.
75. Peters W. P. et al. *Lancet* 1981, **1**, 529; Annotation, *Lancet* 1981, **1**, 538.
76. Taff R. H. *Anesthesiology* 1983, **59**, 576.
77. Dhamce M. S. and Ghandi S. K. *Anaesthesia* 1982, **37**, 342.
78. Schneider O. and Hellerbach J. *Helv. Chem. Acta* 1950, **33**, 1437.
79. Fromherz K. and Pellmond B. *Experientia* 1952, **8**, 394.
80. Conti G. Teboul J. L. and Gasparetto A. In: *Update in Intensive Care and Emergency Medicine 10*, Vincent J-L. Berlin: Springer-Verlag, 199.

Chapter 27

Non-acute pain[1]

Both acute and chronic pain require careful and coordinated management. The anaesthetic service is involved in both. For acute pain, *see* Chapter 26.

Algology is the specialty of chronic pain relief. 'Pain is an unpleasant experience that is associated with tissue damage, described in terms of tissue damage, or both.' It consists of the sensation of pain, together with the patient's psychological response to it, both of which need attention.[2] For history *see* Roll R. J. *J. R. Soc. Med.* 1982, **75**, 812; Bonica J. J. *Clin. Anaesthesiol.* 1985, **3**, 1. The patient with intractable pain requires careful evaluation, diagnosis and sympathetic understanding. The patient should know that the doctor will welcome him back for further treatment (but every pain clinic has 'failures', which receive scant attention in publications). Audit is undertaken.[3]

Organization of a pain clinic[4]

A clinic requires outpatient room, an interested and dedicated consultant in charge, a secretary, operating theatre sessions, a drug cupboard, data storage, ECG, EMG, skin thermometers, nerve stimulator, cryoprobe, muscle strength assessment equipment, full resuscitation equipment, a wide range of diagnostic tools, if possible with an image intensifier (and a back door for the staff to escape, if necessary).

Three levels of provision have been described, minimal, average and comprehensive. The multidisciplinary approach has been advocated, for example, while it is important to have primary referrals from family doctors, many of these patients will need an exact diagnosis to be made by hospital colleagues before treatment is attempted.

The patient should, if possible, see the same members of staff at each visit. Semiotic skills have a high pofile, as there is evidence that good communications will speed recovery. The patients can be encouraged to write a list of questions before coming to the somewhat awe-inspiring domain of the hospital. (*See also* Edwards M. H. *Br. J. Surg.* 1990, **77**, 463.)

Assessment of pain[5]

This is a subjective evaluation of the patient's feelings, except in a few areas, where a measurably severe pain, e.g. various pressures of a sphygmomanometer cuff, with resulting pain levels, is compared with the original pain before and after treatment.

Type – e.g. central or peripheral. This may only become clear after treatment has started.

Cause of the pain – e.g. inflammatory, muscle spasm, colic, malignant, hysterical or somatization disorder.

Duration – How long has it existed? Has it changed? The pain clinic is unlikely to be able to help those who have had pain for a very long time.

Location – Is it focal or diffuse? Superficial, deep, neurological, psychological? Is it false? i.e. a habit reference to some previous site of pain? (30% of cancer patients have two or more pains, about half have no pain.) The site of origin of a pain may move from the periphery to the spinal cord or even to the brain stem.

Quality – Is it aching, crushing, tight, lancinating, vice-like, sharp, throbbing, burning, pressing, colicky, stabbing, pricking, constricting, jaggy, variable? Cancer pain is different from postoperative wound pain.

Intensity measurement – The patient is asked to complete a linear analogue scale (0 = no pain, 10 = terrible pain) or categorical scale (no pain – just noticeable – weak – mild – moderate – strong – severe – excruciating).

Modifying factors – Can the pain be relieved by non-drug treatment, e.g. food, hot water bottle, exercise, posture, reclining/walking, rest.

Time relations – Variation from day to day, hour to hour (e.g. migraine in the early morning). Presence of a basic background with exacerbations. Is it likely to get better on its own, or worse?[6]

Response to a test dose of a drug.

Physiological effects – e.g. nausea and vomiting, dysuria, diarrhoea. Do these need treatment in their own right?

Habits – interference with work or sleep, physiological functions, tolerance of others, relationships (including doctor/patient).

Mental changes – depression (early morning wakening, lowered morning mood, miserable face, weight loss, apathy, guilt); anxiety, guilt, fear, tension, aggression, obsession, introversion, hypochondriasis, hysteria? (These will need to be treated in their own right.) What is the home situation like? Have there been mental changes only since the pain started or did they exist previously? Has the patient previous experiences of success or failure in pain control? The help of an enthusiastic psychologist is an enormous asset to a pain clinic.

The emotional content and intensity of the patient's language are noted for future comparison (the existence of denial, anger, depression, acceptance, and the extent to which emotional conditioning is contributing to the pain).[7] Also demeanour, facial expression, posture, gait, and a full physical examination.

Has the patient got 'total pain'? i.e. pain + hopelessness/anxiety + fear of impending death?

Cancer pain is often continuous, at the same location (which enlarges progressively), and is preoccupying and demoralizing.

A pain map may be drawn.

Further investigations – urine and blood analysis (untreated intractable pain from malignant disease produces a metabolic alkalosis related to the severity of the pain), ESR, coagulogram, ECG, perhaps EEG, EMG, appropriate X-rays and endoscopy.

Reassessment

Reassessment is made regularly to determine whether there is good control or poor control of pain, bearing in mind that pain relief is not usually an instant cure, because old pains reappear and new pains may develop. Partial relief may enable the patient to regain control. Pain is often not the only form of suffering for the patient. It is especially difficult to achieve relief in the depressed, anxious, and those whose pain is worsened by activity.

The patient and appropriate relatives should participate fully in decisions about timing and type of treatment. Informed consent is obtained.

Approach to Treatment of Non-acute Pain[8]

Each individual aspect of treatment is used as part of a comprehensive multimodular therapeutic strategy. Enabling the patient to get a good night's sleep has high priority. This may be helped by giving the patient his own (small) supply of analgesic on his bedside table at night (a form of oral 'patient-controlled analgesia'!).

19% of hospital cancer patients and 29% of home cancer patients have severe pain[9] (about 5–10% of all deaths). About half of all cancer patients will have significant pain in the course of the disease and in about half of these it may be severe, requiring specific treatment. In addition there are all the non-malignant pains, e.g. backache, in a community. The overwhelming majority are 'surgical' cases.

For pain treatment in children, *see* Tyler D. C. and Krane E. J. ed. *Pediatric Pain*. New York: Raven Press, 1990.

Notes on drugs used for intractable pain

Anthranilic acids – mefenamic and flufenamic (500 mg daily). Not gastric irritants, but may cause diarrhoea.

Aspirin – (max dose 3 g daily). Especially good for metastatic bone pain. Gastric irritant, faecal blood loss may occur, controlled by cimetidine 300 mg or ranitidine 150 mg, without affecting plasma salicylate levels. Very rarely associated with Reye's Syndrome in children, under 12 years and perhaps in teenagers.

Aspav – Aspirin 500 mg/papaveretum 10 mg, an exceptionally useful and powerful oral analgesic, with few side-effects.

Buprenorphine – strong, long-acting agonist/antagonist. May be given sublingually, 0.2 mg. (onset in 0.5–1 h, peak effect in 2 h). Some patients are excessively sensitive (confusion and dysphoria) or excessively resistant to this drug. May cause vomiting. Semi-controlled.

Butorphanol – strong agonist/antagonist.[10]

Carbamazepine – good for trigeminal neuralgia, glossopharyngeal neuralgia, migraine, and lightening pains of tabes. May cause aplastic anaemia, leucopenia and liver damage in prolonged use.

Clonidine – useful for migraine, 50 μg twice daily and in spinal pain. (Can be given epidurally.) Used in Gilles de la Tourette syndrome.

Clonazepam – adult dose 1 mg, at night. Anticonvulsant, useful co-analgesic. Potentiates the analgesic effects of opioids and local analgesics.

Chlorpromazine – 25–50 mg, anti-emetic, antidepressive, potentiates analgesics, reduces responsiveness of CNS. May produce subcutaneous oedema with other antidepressants. May cause parkinsonism.

Codeine – 30 mg. Slightly stronger than aspirin, antitussive, antidiarrhoeal. Has caused cardiac arrest when given i.v. Its lack of respiratory depression makes it a favourite in neurosurgery.

Dextromoramide – 5–10 mg orally or rectally. Rapid onset, good for 'breakthrough pain'.

Dextropropoxyphene – 65 mg q.d.s. Equal strength to codeine; oral route only; may cause euphoria.

Diamorphine – 5 mg. Euphoric, soluble in very small volumes. Advantage over morphine, is that it causes less nausea and vomiting.

Diazepam – 5–10 mg. Central muscular relaxation, good with minor analgesics, may be useful at night, not as potent as phenothiazines.

Diclofenac – oral 25–100 mg, i.m. 25 mg, rectal suppository 100 mg, very versatile, convenient and effective NSAID.

Diflunisal (Dolobid) – duration of action 10 h. Similar to aspirin.

Dihydrocodeine – 30–60 mg. For moderate to severe pain, good when combined with aspirin or paracetamol.

Dipipanone – 25–50 mg. Similar to methadone.

Ethoheptazine – 75–150 mg t.d.s. For moderate pain. Antispasmodic.

Indomethacin – up to 150 mg/day. Gastric irritant; can be given rectally as suppositories, 100 mg. Very cheap.

Ketanserin[11] – a 5HT blocker for peripheral vascular disease.

Meptazinol – adult, 200 mg orally; 100 mg i.m. or i.v.; duration 2–7 h; little respiratory depression (useful in neurosurgery); may cause vomiting.

Local analgesics – infused intravenously in sub-toxic doses.

Methadone – 5–10 mg orally. Long acting, very strong analgesic, less sedating, less nauseating than morphine, good for weaning morphine addicts. Plasma half-life 15 h, increases after 2–3 days therapy. The plasma concentration plateau is reached only after 1–3 weeks. Cimetidine inhibits its metabolism. Rifampicin speeds up its metabolism.

Methyl salicylate – absorbed through the skin, for athletic strains.

Morphine (see Chapter 26) – best given orally, twice daily as MST,[12] or by subcutaneous infusion in chronic pain,[13] also i.m., i.v., epidurally and intrathecally. Some pains are not morphine-sensitive, regardless of dose or route. Oral, rectal/parenteral potency ratio is 1–3.[14] Problems – constipation (50%); sedation; nausea and vomiting; respiratory depression; itching; addiction/tachyphylaxis. Anti-emetics and laxatives likely to be required.

Nalbuphine – 10–20 mg. Medium to strong analgesic, and mild sedative.[15] Useful in military situations, because of its relative lack of respiratory depression, lack of addiction, and it does not confuse the assessment of head injury. Safer for asthmatics.

Nefopam – 15 mg. Peak effect at 2 h, ceiling effect at 20–30 mg, side-effects include insomnia, dry mouth, nausea, nervousness, light-headedness, vomiting, blurred vision, tachycardia, sweating, urinary retention, enhanced motor neurone activity, anticholinergic effects.

Oxycodone – 10 mg. Less addictive and sedating than morphine. Long acting when given as the pectinate. Can be given rectally, 30 mg. Very cheap.

Paracetamol – centrally acting prostaglandin inhibitor. Ceiling effect at adult dose of 1 g every 6 h. Overdose effect is severe hepatic damage (protected by methionine and acetyl cysteine). Analgesic effect enhanced by combination with many other analgesics, e.g. propoxyphene, aspirin.

Papaveretum – a basic opiate analgesic (*see* Chapter 17).

Pericyazine – 25 mg t.d.s. (more at night). Effective phenothiazine tranquillizer.

Pentazocine – moderate analgesic with marked dysphoria.

Pethidine – up to 100 mg. Good antispasmodic for gut and uterus. Dysphoric, may cause hypotension, tachycardia and dryness of mouth. Reacts with mono-amine oxidase inhibitors giving hypertension, or coma and hypotension.

Phenazocine – a μ-receptor agonist, which can be given sublingually.

Phenoperidine – 1–2 mg. Strong analgesic and respiratory depressant, low incidence of vomiting. Duration 1–2 h.

Propoxyphene (*Dextropropoxyphene*) – effect builds up with each dose, and its metabolite is even longer acting. As an occasional drug it is unpredictable. In overdose it causes respiratory depression and acute heart failure. Often mixed with paracetamol for extra efficacy.

Tricyclic antidepressants – antidepressive, analgesic, hypnotic, in moderate pain, potentiate other analgesics, antagonize guanethidine, potentiate adrenaline, may produce oedema with phenothiazines (*see* chlorpromazine, above).

See also Benedetti C., Chapman C. R. and Giron G. ed. *Opioid Analgesia*. New York: Raven Press, 1990.

Methods of pain relief[16]

1. Analgesics

Classically divided into mild and strong, the stronger ones having more side-effects. (Doxapram, 1 mg/kg, or small doses of naloxone reverse respiratory depression without influencing analgesia.)

With any analgesic, there is a ceiling dose, above which there is no more analgesia, only more side-effects. Then progression to more powerful analgesics is needed. Some pains are untouched by morphine, but respond to other analgesics. The longer-acting analgesics, e.g. diflunisal and methadone produce a smoother result, especially at night.

2. Co-analgesics

Antidepressants, e.g. amitryptilene,[17] potentiate analgesics by stimulating the descending modulating pathways, elevate mood, and may relax muscle spasm. Particularly useful for enabling sleep. They are not always helpful, may have unpleasant side-effects in high dose (dry mouth, blurred vision, urinary retention, constipation and diaphoresis) and their withdrawal may lead to depression. The patient is informed that these drugs are not being prescribed for depression. *Anxiolytic drugs,* e.g. benzodiazepines, have a role for controlling agitation and producing sleep at night. *Antispasmodic drugs,* e.g. baclofen and orphenadrine. *Clonidine* (by mouth, potentiates and prolongs the action of analgesics and local anaesthetics). *Antiepileptic drugs,* e.g. sodium valproate, carbamazepine. (The patient is informed that he is not an epileptic.)

3. Hyperstimulation analgesia[18]

This includes cupping, transcutaneous electric nerve stimulation (TENS),[19] acupuncture, needling and ice massage. A brief, intense stimulation encourages the central biasing mechanism to inhibit chronic pain, which the brain or spinal cord has remembered and repeated long after the initial injury had healed.[20]

4. Occupational therapy/psychotherapy

Unsuitable for patients with a major language barrier, severe deafness, dementia, severe cardiac failure or cognitive deficit. This type of therapy is particularly appropriate for the 'learned pain syndrome' (*see below*), and in overcoming self-perpetuating inactivity caused by pain and the fear that activity will cause harm especially in the elderly and depressed. Such inactivity causes insomnia, muscle loss, bone decalcification, hypercalcuria, joint fibrosis, reduced lung function, altered eating habits, constipation, and obesity or cachexia.

5. Nerve blockade (sensory, autonomic or motor)[21]

For diagnostic, prognostic, prophylactic and therapeutic purposes. For diagnosis, differential subarachnoid block is sometimes employed. Isotonic saline is injected. A short response indicates a placebo effect. A prolonged response indicates that the pain was psychogenic. A response to 0.25% procaine suggests sympathetic pain; a response to 0.5% procaine suggests a sensory problem; and a response to 1% procaine suggests a motor problem. In the course of time after a phenol block, the C fibres may make new connections, producing various abnormal shunts, e.g. afferent input via anterior roots, and reappearance of the pain. Unfortunately, when the pain reappears, it is often worse, and resistant to any treatment (perhaps due to development of neuromas at the site of the block?). For technique of various blocks *see below* and Chapters 24 and 25 . Extradural block with catheter is most suitable for short-term pain relief.[22] Long-term implantation can be employed using tunnelling techniques. Nerve blockade is less used now.

6. Hypnosis

This is a state of altered consciousness characterized by heightened suggestibility, narrowed awareness, selective wakefulness, and restricted attentiveness. About 10–15% of adults are not susceptible. Children are the most susceptible and adults over 55 years the least susceptible. A trance is usually brought about by repetitive auditory, visual or tactile stimuli. The aim is a reduction of sensory intake to one or two monotonous stimuli.[23] Sedative drugs may help. The advantage of hypnosis is that there is no danger of the toxic side-effects of drugs. However, it is difficult and time-consuming, and not suitable for every patient. The contra-indications are: (1) refusal of the patient; (2) psychiatric illness; and (3) absence of quiet surroundings. Naloxone does not abolish analgesia produced by hypnosis (Needham, J. personal communication). (*See also* Merskey H. *Postgrad. Med. J.* 1971, **47**, 572.)

7. Deafferentation drugs

E.g. carbamazepine, clonazepam, sodium valproate, L-tryptophan. Helpful where nerve blocks have failed to relieve pain.

8. Central nervous stimulation, and destructive procedures.[24]

E.g. percutaneous cordotomy, used for unilateral pains (see below). The tracts may regenerate in about 2 years. Epidural dorsal column stimulators with induction loop are often dramatically successful (See below).

Agents used for nerve block

1. Local analgesics. Their effect is often prolonged, perhaps by closing the 'gate' at spinal level.

2. Phenol 5% in glycerin[25] 0.5–1 ml. Duration, 1 week–3 months. Patients should be warned about the effects of motor block from this agent. This solution is hyperbaric and is used for intradural posterior root block with the patient lying semi-supine with the appropriate segment at the lowest point.

3. Chlorocresol 2% in glycerin.[26] 0.5–1 ml intradurally. Duration, weeks to months.

4. Absolute alcohol.[27] 0.5–1 ml. Onset, in days, duration months or years. This is hypobaric, and for intradural block the affected segment is placed uppermost with the patient in the semi-prone position. Nerve stimulation can be used to accurately localize the injection.[28] Injection is very painful and so should be preceded by local analgesia. Arachnoiditis is a complication. Has been used via the trans-sphenoidal approach to destroy the pituitary for metastatic bone pain,[29] when X-ray control in two planes and washout check for sphenoidal sinus infection is required.

5. Intradural ice-cold saline.[30] Selectively blocks C fibres, lasting for weeks, but the injection is very painful. Spinal barbotage[31] is used in a similar way.

6. Cryoprobe block, percutaneously.[32] Duration, 6–10 weeks block, including pituitary ablation.[33] Post-cryoprobe neuritis and dysaesthesia are very rare.

7. Opioids[34] (*intradural or extradural*). *See also* Chapter 25. Should be free of preservatives.[35] Act on the substantia gelatinosa of the posterior horn of the spinal cord.[36] Extradural opioids act partly by systemic absorption, and in the case of water-soluble agents, e.g. morphine, by cephalad spread in the CSF.

Prolonged spinal opioids may be given by catheter and syringe pump or PCA. A subcutaneous injection port can be implanted, with the catheter brought subcutaneously round the body wall to the front. An aseptic protocol is followed for injections.

Complications – non-segmental pruritus, nausea, vomiting, retention of urine, and, uncommonly, respiratory depression (onset up to 24 h after block, especially by water-soluble opioids). Extradural opioid sedation and respiratory depression is reversible by naloxone.

8. *Ammonium salts.* These are reputed to have a lower incidence of neuritis.

2   9. *Guanethidine* intravenously or intra-arterially for sympathetic block and for diabetic neuropathy.

Placebo blocks are used for weaning patients off spinal blocks, and training patients to cope with pain.

Nocebo blocks are where complaints of bodily impairments follow nerve blockade, not fitting any known pattern of anatomical or physiological effect, sometimes seen in patients with disability settlements pending.[37] One source of failure of intradural nerve blocks is the existence of afferent fibres in the anterior roots.[38] Another is 'central pain', which may be treated by deafferentation drugs (*see above*).

Notes on various intractable pains

Amputation pains

1. *Phantom limb pain.* (*See below.*)
2. *Stump pain.* Injection of trigger points or TENS therapy.
3. *Brachial plexus avulsion injury.* TENS may help. Radiofrequency cervical block has been used. The patient may request amputation, but this is of no help.

Anaesthesia dolorosa

Pain in the desensitized face.[39] Deafferentation treatment (*see above*).

Anal pain

Involves spinal segments S2–S5 (or supratentorial. Proctalgia fugax may occur.

Angina

Differential diagnosis from: (1) costal cartilage pain; (2) oesophageal reflux spasm; (3) left mammary pain due to anxiety; (4) neuralgias; (5) mediastinitis; (6) pericarditis; and (7) gastric pain.

Management. (Chronic) glyceryl trinitrate, calcium antagonists (e.g. verapamil 360 mg daily, diltiazem 360 mg daily), β-blockers, left stellate ganglion block and trigger point injection.

Arthritic pain

Probably the commonest form of pain in the population.[40]

Atypical facial pain

Typically maxillary, in a middle-aged female, unresponsive to trigeminal nerve block. Sphenopalatine block and deafferentation (*see above*).

Back pain[41]

Treat bad posture, poor muscle tone, obesity, gynaecological pathology, or pancreatitis as appropriate. Bed rest, analgesics required. In selected cases, facet nerve blocks and cryotherapy are effective. Chemical sympathectomy may help for referred buttock and leg pains.

Muscle, disc and ligament strain backache – good prognosis indicators are lack of obesity, lack of smoking, lack of previous low back pain, job satisfaction, jobs that do not involve strenuous twisting during lifting, motivation to keep fit (e.g. 15 min exercises per day), excellent coping skills, low pain behaviour, well-documented pathology. Diagnostic features are fractures, spondylolisthesis, and tumours. Myelogram, CT scans and MRI are highly diagnostic (over 90% accurate). Moderate to major analgesics, diazepam, physiotherapy, improvement of job satisfaction and correction of obesity are a starting point in treatment. Those with acute sciatica radiating below the knee may benefit from an initial 7-day bed rest. If pain still persists, extradural steroid injection is indicated (and for acute intervertebral disc pathology). Methylprednisolone 80 mg (or 50 mg of triamcinolone) in lignocaine or bupivacaine, has an onset in some days, and may need repeating two or three times. A short general anaesthetic is often required for the injection. Myofascial syndrome and interlaminar joint problems may require localized injections. Substance P is reduced in saliva of patients with chronic back syndromes.[42]

Cancer pain in the back – analgesics, radiotherapy, neurolytic blocks.

Postmyodil arachnoiditis – prevention is better than cure.

Ankylosing spondylitis – posture control; radiotherapy has been used. The biggest problem in this area is postlaminectomy pain.

Bladder pain

Involves spinal segments S2–S4.

Breast pain

A common presenting symptom. Response to treatment graded using the Cardiff Breast Score. 1 = no residual pain; 2 = some residual pain, which the patient considers bearable; 3 = substantial residual pain; and 4 = no response.[43]

Carcinomatosis bone pain

Analgesics, aminoglutethimide, tamoxifen, cyproterone, consider hypophysectomy. Aspirin and non-steroidal anti-inflammatory drugs (NSAIDs) are specific, and may reduce the rate of tumour growth.

Causalgia[44]

Regional sympathetic blockade; tranquillizers to control emotional crises. Epidural block may be required.[45]

Central pain

(1) Post-stroke, thalamic in origin (self-limiting, but pituitary alcohol injection has been used). (2) Residual pain, in a patient whose peripheral source of pain has been controlled, e.g. rendered numb by nerve block, deafferentation (*see above*).

Cluster headache

(*See* Migrainous neuralgia, below).

Diabetic neuropathy

Guanethidine block may help. (*See* Sympathetic block below.)

Gallbladder pain

Pethidine, splanchnic (coeliac plexus) block if surgery is not appropriate.

Geniculate neuralgia

Analgesia, divide nervus intermedius.

Giant-cell arteritis

Corticosteroids.

Glossopharyngeal neuralgia

(*See* Chapter 24).

Headache

An almost universal cause of pain, due to many causes, e.g. tension, migraine, craniomandibular stomatognathic disorders, accommodation problems, menstruation, etc.

Herpes zoster neuralgia

The vesicles come out on the 3rd–5th day of infection with varicella virus. Mainly a disease of the elderly. Early and completely adequate analgesia is important in preventing post-herpetic neuralgia. Extradural block and steroids, perhaps repeated, nerve blocks, repeated, sympathetic blocks.[46]

Acyclovir, 800 mg qds, for 7 days can be given up to 3 months after the disappearance of the rash of herpes zoster.[47]

(*See also* postherpetic neuralgia.)

Hyperaesthesia[48]

Octreotide, a longer acting analogue of somatostatin, administered topically with DMSO as a penetrant, has controlled the symptoms.

Hysterical pain[49]

Ischaemic pain

Alcoholic night-caps, α-blockers, sympathectomy, surgery.

Learned pain syndrome

(Chronic intractable benign pain syndrome).[50]

There is:
1. Dramatization of complaints, the descriptions of which have a high emotional content.
2. Disuse – self-perpetuating prolonged physical inactivity.
3. Drug misuse – need for multiple or frequently changed prescriptions.
4. Dependency – helplessness and parasitism on others.
5. Disability – need for social security handouts and litigation awards.
Exact diagnosis is not wanted because of a desire for the reward factors of chronic illness, e.g. discharge from military service.

Treatment by behaviour modification.[51] The behaviour to be modified is first defined from as many sources as possible (to avoid bias), e.g. (1) Pavlovian or conditioned behaviour – the sight of a bottle of tablets or alcohol leads to unnecessary consumption; (2) social modelling, where the patient reacts as he thinks others expect him to – for better or worse depending on the model chosen; and (3) helplessness, where the patient feels that he is the victim of disease, at the mercy of an inevitable fate.

The basic tenets of behaviour modification are: (1) removal of the conditioning stimulus (e.g. a bottle), focusing the patient's attention away from the pain, and replacing it by rewards for the target behaviour; (2) correction of unhelpful antecedents, e.g. muscle tension, overwork, bad posture, idleness; (3) setting positive goals for progress, e.g. in the area of physical activity; (4) reinforcement of new healthy habits and attitudes, e.g. sleep, posture, drug-taking, with emphasis on *self*-improvement, i.e. it is the patient's responsibility to get well; (5) return to suitable work at a graded pace; and (6) sorting out unsatisfactory relationships.

Measurement of progress is necessary, e.g. using biofeedback techniques such as EMG levels in migraine and low back pain. The fully informed support of close relatives is crucial.

Lyme disease

Spirochaetal disease named after the town of origin. Intense pain requiring opioids, myocarditis occurs 6 weeks after initial attack, with AV block. Treated by penicillin, tetracycline, ceftriaxone. Anaesthesia is postponed until remission.[52]

Migraine[53]

Diagnosis – can be difficult, especially in the major cases of migrainous hemiplegia, migrainous aphasia, and migrainous coma (where the diagnosis is often retrospective).

Treatment – possibly avoid starvation and tyramine-containing foods (chocolate, cheese, red wine). Counselling and minor tranquillizers useful. Ergotamine, 0.25 mg s.c. or i.m., or 0.5 mg orally, sumatriptan 6 mg s.c. for the acute attack, with metoclopramide 10 mg i.m. Clonidine and methysergide are used for prophylaxis. Acupuncture has been tried.[54] Simple measures like keeping the hands warm and deliberately relaxing muscle tension are encouraged.

Migrainous neuralgia

Often unilateral in eye and cheek, occurring in the early hours of the morning, in the middle-aged male. 'Like a hot needle going into the eye'. Builds up over 5 min, lasts 1 h. Has autonomic features, e.g. epiphora, conjunctival injection, orbital oedema, ptosis, miosis, nasal stuffiness. Precipitated by alcohol. Sphenopalatine and stellate ganglion blocks may help. Ergotamine 1 mg bd and pizotifen 0.5 mg bd are used.

Myofascial pain (muscular rheumatism; myalgia; myositis; fibrositis; fibromyositis)

'Trigger points' are identified.[55] They are sometimes palpable, extremely sensitive, produce intense sharp pain and muscle spasm on needling or pressure, may occur anywhere (especially back and pectoral girdle), and are sometimes related to surgical scars. Histologically they show oedema and accumulation of mast cells. Infiltration with 5–10 ml of 0.25% bupivacaine often removes the original pain that sensitized the trigger point.

Neck pain

When originating in the neck, is usually due to muscle spasms and responds to analgesics and physiotherapy. When the pain radiates outside the neck, it probably arises from meninges or spondylosis. Muscle tension headache is not often relieved by tranquillisers, but acupuncture may help.[56]

Nerve entrapment

There is burning, tingling or shooting pain, tenderness, weakness, muscle wasting, or loss of sensation. Treatment is surgical, with or without repeated local analgesic injections. Radiotherapy may help if the nerve is trapped by tumour.

Occipital pain

Usually due to nerve root pain from the neck, responding to cervical collar wearing, nerve block, manipulation, or surgery. May also be due to a form of migraine.

Painful scars

Classically the wound has been healed for several weeks. Local or regional blocks are required, perhaps repeated, with surgical excision of neuroma if present.

Pancreatic pain

Involves dermatomes T6–T12 and when malignant, with limited life expectancy, may require splanchnic or coeliac ganglion block. Under general anaesthesia, needles are inserted bilaterally, preferably under image intensifier control and the effect tested with local analgesic. Absolute alcohol is then injected in divided doses. Resultant postural hypotension lasting from minutes to weeks may be controlled by elastic stockings. Extradural block, especially with opioids, is satisfactory for acute and chronic pancreatitis. Intrapleural block has a place.[57]

Phantom limb

(1) Local analgesic block of nerves to the phantom limb, but not spinal block, which may make the pain worse; (2) TENS; (3) infiltration of trigger points in trunk and opposite limb (*see above*); (4) sympathectomy; and (5) cordotomy in the worst cases.

Posthemiplegic dystrophy/postsympathetic dystrophy/post-traumatic dystrophy

Intravenous regional sympathetic blockade may relieve superficial but not deep pain.

Postherpetic neuralgia[58]

(Prevention, *see* herpetic neuralgia.) Mainly seen in the elderly. Onset as the scabs separate or up to 4 weeks later, with background soreness and episodic sharp stabbing pain, and even transverse myelitis with temporary paralysis. Triggered by touching, draughts, or emotions. May last many years, but when resolved, is soon forgotten. Treatment is by analgesics, skin vibrators, TENS, local anaesthetic creams, local analgesic subcutaneous injections, nerve and extradural blocks (occasional permanent relief). Intradural alcohol and phenol is often disappointing. Neurosurgery for head and neck neuralgia, or anterolateral cordotomy, is reserved for the worst cases, and is often disappointing. Steroids (extradural or systemic) and idoxuridine have been recommended.[59] Sodium valproate and amitriptyline may help at night. The painful area may recede with time. Acyclovir cream and injections have been tried with varying success. Postherpetic neuralgia is frequently permanent and incurable, especially if it has been present for 2–3 months before presenting at the clinic.

Raynaud's disease

Treatment includes avoidance of cold, i.v. regional sympathetic blockade (*see below*) and sympathectomy.

Reflex dystrophy

E.g. shoulder-hand syndrome in myocardial ischaemia. Regional sympathetic blockade may help.[60]

Recurrent pain

That pain which recurs after a previous successful nerve block, and is often resistant to treatment.[61]

Renal pain

Involves dermatomes T11–L2.

Sympathetic dystrophy

(*See* Postsympathetic dystrophy, above). A guanethidine sympathetic block on 4–5 occasions may be sufficient.

Temporomandibular joint pain

May be due to arthritis or masseter spasm (bruxism). The latter is usually unilateral, may radiate in any direction, or may trigger trigeminal neuralgia and migraine. It is relieved by local analgesic injection into the masseter, dental attention to occlusion, and wearing better fitting new dentures.

Tennis elbow and various other joint pains

Bupivacaine and steroid injection, under anaesthesia, if necessary.

Trigeminal neuralgia[62]

Aetiology unknown (except rarely due to local vascular disease and in multiple sclerosis). Most often in the maxillary division, rarely mandibular, and very rarely ophthalmic. Intermittent unilateral pain, with or without twitches, usually in an elderly patient, with relapse and remissions (weeks or months). Worse in the mornings. An infraorbital trigger zone is especially common. There is no sensory loss except in postherpetic trigeminal neuralgia. The patient may be so disabled as to be dehydrated. Treatment is by carbamazepine, 100 mg–1 g daily, phenytoin, clonazepam, valproate,[63] local analgesic blocks of trigger points. Trigeminal ganglion block (thermocoagulation or neurolytic)[64] or surgical extirpation should be considered early. Some patients develop postoperative 'anaesthesia dolorosa' which is resistant to treatment.

Percutaneous cordotomy[65]

Technique originally introduced by Mullan (Chicago) in 1963 using a strontium needle. Later modified by Rosomoff who used radiofrequency current to create a high cervical lesion. Lin and Polakoff have developed an anterior approach for percutaneous lower cervical cordotomy. These techniques are effective and may replace open cordotomy. However, a bilateral high cervical lesion can cause damage to the respiratory outflow fibres with the risk of death when the patient goes to sleep and relies on the involuntary mechanism. Radiological control is used for accurate placement of the needle.[66] Has been reported as giving good results in 64% of patients.[67]

Dorsal column stimulation

By an implanted epidural electrode attached to a subcutaneous implanted receiver. The patient operates the transmitter power and frequency.[68] Anterolateral tracts, thalamic and internal capsule have also been similarly stimulated.

Sympathetic block

Sympathetic dysfunction can cause symptoms due to vasospasm, the production of pain and alteration of function, so that therapy is directed to vasodilatation, relief of pain and restoration of function. Pain due to central nervous system lesions can be treated with either sympathetic blocks or intravenous guanethidine.[69]

Vasomotor block may be performed at any of five levels: (1) peripheral nerve block, e.g. the ulnar nerve, causing vasodilatation of the skin of the little finger; (2) the sympathetic ganglia, e.g. the stellate or the 2nd and 3rd lumbar ganglia, causing release of vasomotor tone in the upper and lower limbs; (3) the vascular smooth muscle using intravenous guanethidine[70] for reflex sympathetic dystrophies and arterial insufficiency;[71] (4) extradural block; and (5) subarachnoid block. The last two are examples of preganglionic block and must extend in the case of the lower limb to the 10th thoracic segment so as to paralyse all the preganglionic fibres going to the limb.

Indications for chemical sympathectomy block[72]

Painful limbs due to vascular disease. Raynaud's (1834–1881) phenomena;[73] vasospasm associated with lesions of the spinal cord, e.g. poliomyelitis and some cases of pyramidal disease; arteriosclerosis and thrombophlebitis obliterans; chronic ulceration of the extremities; embolism of major vessels; thrombophlebitis; erythromelalgia (Weir Mitchell, 1878); and after intra-arterial thiopentone injection. Peripheral arterial disease. This may be: (1)

vasospastic; (2) vasospastic and organic (Buerger); or (3) degenerative organic (arteriosclerosis). Increased blood supply to the limb is shown by: (1) increased surface temperature; (2) increased oscillations shown by an oscillometer; and (3) increased function, e.g. later onset of claudication.[74]

Conditions due to idiopathic and post-traumatic pain of limbs. Causalgia;[71] amputation stump neuralgias; and Sudeck's atrophy.[75]

Unclassified conditions of the limbs. Hyperhidrosis; after embolectomy; and in the posthyperaemic stage of the immersion foot syndrome.

Abdominal disease. Pancreatitis (bilateral block of T6–12) and splanchnic block;[76] inoperable carcinoma (coeliac plexus/splanchnic block);[77] and eclampsia (*see* Chapter 22).

Coeliac plexus block. Blocked by 25 ml of 50% alcohol inserted via posterior, transaortic[78] or anterior[79] approach, with or without a catheter for 5 days treatment.[80] (For review, *see* Petriccione di Vadi P. and Wedley J. R. *Pain Clinic* 1990, **3**, 223.)

The pain associated with neurolytic sympathetic block can be prevented by first giving a segmental extradural block using 2–3 ml 2% lignocaine at L2/L3.[81]

Post sympathectomy neuralgia may be due to partial sympathectomy and be removed by a repeat sympathectomy.[82]

'Escape' of sympathetic drive from stellate ganglion block may be stopped by upper thoracic paravertebral blocks.

Intravenous regional sympathetic block (arms or legs)[71, 83, 84]

Advantages. Few complications, still works after excision of stellate ganglion, etc.

Disadvantages. Effects of tourniquet and risk of effects of release of the agent into the general circulation.

Precautions. The following should be available: resuscitation facilities, a tilting table, a reliable tourniquet at 100 mmHg above the patient's systolic pressure, and an i.v. cannula in place, in both the limb to be treated and another limb.

Procedure. Average dose is guanethidine 10–20 mg with 500 units heparin in 25 ml saline for the arm (double for the leg). Duration of treatment 5–10 min. Tourniquet released for 30 s then reinflated for 5 min before removal. Effects assessed 30 min after release.

Other techniques

Transnasal destruction of the pituitary with alcohol, under X-ray control, in certain forms of carcinomatosis.[85] Percutaneous vibration or electrical stimulation[86] has a 30–50% success rate in postherpetic neuralgia.[87] Portable stimulators are available. Acupuncture in the affected dermatome is under assessment.[88] Rubbing counter-irritants into the overlying skin is traditional treatment. Cryoprobe application to the spinal cord at open operation has been described, and also to the painful area[84] (e.g. the perineum[89]).

These techniques give results that tend to be poor when employed by the occasional anaesthetist. However, keen, dedicated workers who are willing and able to devote time and attention to acquiring experience in their performance, tell a different tale.

(*See also* Mehta M. *Recent Advances in Anaesthesia and Analgesia* – 14 (Atkinson R. S. and Hewer C. L. ed.) Edinburgh: Churchill Livingstone, 1982.)

Acupuncture

Acupuncture[90] for pain relief goes back 4000 years, but its use in anaesthesia dates from 1958.[91] The idea is that the 'vital life force' (chi) flows in 'meridians' in the body, being disturbed in disease. The location of the disturbed meridian is found by 'pulse diagnosis' and insertion of a needle to stimulate one of over 1000 'acupuncture points' corrects the disturbance, leading to analgesia. Opinions differ widely about the right points for needle insertion.

Acupuncture may be acceptable for chronic pain not amenable to conventional forms of therapy.[92] Acupuncture points are points of low skin resistance, detected by neurometers, which measure current flow at 6 V, e.g. Ta-ch'ang yu is 3.6 cm from the midline of the back at the L4–L5 interspace. Ch'êng-san is between the heads of the gastrocnemius and Jen Chung is in the middle of the philtrum.

Stimulation. May be electrical (12 V, 100–200 µA, 3–10 Hz for 30 min at 2–3-day intervals) or manual (twirling of needles) or thermal (burning of moxa tufts on the skin or a hot probe at 80°C).

Naloxone inhibits the analgesic effects of acupuncture[93] (suggesting that endorphin release may be one of the mechanisms) but not the autonomic effects.[94] Controlled studies have shown acupuncture to have a marked pain relieving effect.[95] Stimulation is continued until Te Chi is developed, i.e. a sensation of numbness, heat, tingling and distension at the needle site. Traumatic sympathetic dystrophy has been successfully treated by electro-acupuncture.[96] Complications include haematomas, infection (including AIDS), pneumothorax and serum hepatitis.[97] Care with the sterility of acupuncture needles is most important. Perichondritis of the pinna has been reported.[98]

(For history of acupuncture, *see* Loh S. T. *Anaesth. Intensive Care* 1980, **8**, 373.)

References

1. Wall P. D. and Melzack R. ed. *Textbook of Pain*. Churchill Livingstone, 1989; Warfield R. *Manual of Pain Management*. Philadelphia: Lippincott, 1991; Abram J. et al. *The Pain Clinic Manual*. Philadelphia: Lippincott, 1990.
2. Wall P. D. and Melzack R. *Textbook of Pain*. 2nd. ed. Edinburgh: Churchill Livingstone, 1989; Glynn C. J. *Br. Med. J.* 1986, **292**, 222.
3. Nash T, *Pain Clinic* 1990, **3**, 203.
4. Annotation, *Lancet* 1982, **1**, 486; Rolls R. J. R. *J. R. Soc. Med.* 1982, **75**, 151, 818.

5. Aronoff G. N. et al. *Pain* 1983, **16**, 1; Bromm B. ed. *Pain Measurement in Man.* Amsterdam: Elsevier, 1984; Foley K. M. *Clin. Oncol.* 1984, **3**, 17; Smith G. and Covino B. G. *Acute Pain.* London: Butterworth 1985.
6. McQuay H. J. and Dickenson A. H. *Anaesthesia* 1990, **45**, 101.
7. Pilowsky I. *Clin. Anesthesiol.* 1985, **3**, 143.
8. Twycross R. G. and Lack S. A. *Therapeutics in Terminal Cancer.* London: Pitman, 1983; Twycross R. G. *J. R. Coll. Phys.* 1984, **18**, 32.
9. Parkes C. M. *J. R. Coll. Gen. Pract.* 1978, **28**, 19.
10. Heel R. C. et al. *Drugs* 1978, **16**, 473.
11. Knoght C. L. *Front. Pain* 1990, **2**, 6.
12. Walsh T. D. *Pain* 1984, **18**, 1; Gordon A. *Physician* 1988, **7**, 33.
13. Oliver D. J. *Br. Med. J.* 1983, **287**, 1218.
14. Aherne G. W. et al. *Br. J. Clin. Pharmacol.* 1979, **8**, 577.
15. Lewis J. R. *JAMA* 1980, **243**, 1465.
16. Mehta M. In: *Recent Advances in Anaesthesia and Analgesia – 14* (Atkinson R. S. and Hewer C. L. ed.) Edinburgh: Churchill Livingstone, 1982.
17. Livingston M. *Prescribers J.* 1990, **30**, 139.
18. Melzack R. *Clin. Anesthesiol.* 1985, **3**, 81.
19. Navarathnam R. G. et al. *Anaesth. Intensive Care* 1984, **12**, 345; *Advances in Pain Research and Therapy*, Vol. 2. New York: Raven Press, 1984, 509.
20. Melzack R. and Wall P. D. *The Challenge of Pain.* Harmondsworth: Penguin Books, 1982.
21. Bonica J. J. In: *Textbook of Pain* (Wall P. D. and Melzack R. ed.) Edinburgh: Churchill Livingstone; 1984, Sect. 3B. No. 1; Cytovic R. *Nerve Block for Common Pain.* Berlin: Springer-Verlag, 1990
22. Forrest J. B. *Can. Anaesth. Soc. J.* 1978, **25**, 218; Perkins H. M. and Hanlon P. R. *Arch. Surg.* 1978, **113**, 253.
23. Pilowsky I. In: *The Therapy of Pain* (Swerdlow M. ed.) Lancaster: MTP Press, 1981.
24. Editorial *J. R. Soc. Med.* 1983, **76**, 905.
25. Maher R. M. *Lancet* 1955, **1**, 18; Nathan P. W. and Scott T. G. *Lancet* 1958, **1**, 76.
26. Maher R. M. *Lancet* 1963, **1**, 965; Swerdlow M. *Anaesthesia* 1973, **28**, 297.
27. Dogliotti A. M. *Presse méd.* 1931, **39**, 1249.
28. Loubser P. G. *Anesth. Analg.* 1990, **70**, 119.
29. Moricca G. In: *Advances in Neurology* (Bonica J. J. ed.) No. 4. Liverpool: Raven Books, 1974; Corssen G. et al. *Anesth. Analg. (Cleve.)* 1977, **56**, 414; Cook P. R. et al. *Anaesthesia* 1984, **39**, 540.
30. Hitchcock E. *Lancet* 1967, **1**, 1133.
31. Lloyd J.W. et al. *Lancet* 1972, **1**, 354; Lloyd J. W. *Proc. R. Soc. Med.* 1973, **66**, 540.
32. Evans P. J. D. *Anaesthesia* 1981, **36**, 1003.
33. Duthrie A. *Anaesthesia* 1983, **38**, 448, 495.
34. Behar M. et al. *Lancet* 1979, **1**, 527.
35. Mathews E. *Lancet* 1979, **1**, 1724.
36. Snyder R. H. *Sci. Am.* 1977, **236**, 44.
37. Parris W. C. V. *Clin. Anesthesiol.* 1985, **3**, 93.
38. Coggeshall R. E. *Physiol. Rev.* 1980, **6**, 716.
39. Sweet W. H. and Wespic J. G. *J. Neurosurg.* 1974, **40**, 143.
40. Valkenberg H. *Gerontology* 1988, **34**, suppl.1, 2.
41. Chaturvedi S. K. et al. *Pain* 1984, **19**, 87; Nachemson A. and Bogduk N. *Front. Pain* 1990, **2**, 8.
42. Parris W. C. V. et al. *Anesth. Analg.* 1990, **70**, 63.
43. Gateley C. A. and Mansell R. E. *Pain Clinic* 1990, **3**, 207.
44. Richards R. L. *Arch. Neurol.* 1967, **16**, 339.
45. Cicala R. S., Jones J. W. and Westbrook L. L. *Anesth. Analg.* 1990, **70**, 218.
46. Lipton S. *Br. Med. J.* 1984, **289**, 98.
47. Morton P. and Thompson A. N. *N. Z. Med. J.* 1989, **102**, 93.
48. Ellis W. V. *Pain Clinic* 1990, **3**, 239.

49. Hughes A. M. *Front. Pain* 1990, **2**, 1.
50. Brena S. F. and Chapman S. L. *Postgrad. Med.* 1981, **69**, 53; Tyrer S. P. *Br. Med. J.* 1986, **292**, 1.
51. Chapman S. L. *Clin. Anesthesiol.* 1985, **3**, 111.
52. Bateman D. E. *Hosp. Update* 1990, **16**, 677.
53. Whitty C. W. M. et al. *Lancet* 1966, **1**, 856.
54. Marcus P. *J. R. Soc. Med.* 1983, **76**, 983.
55. Travell J. G. and Simons D. G. *Myofascial Pain and Dysfunction, the Trigger Point Mancl.* Baltimore: Williams and Wilkins, 1983.
56. Carlsson J. et al. *Pain Clinic* 1990, **3**, 229.
57. Ahlburg P. et al. *Acta Anaesth. Scand.* 1990, **34**, 156
58. Raftery H. *Front. Pain* 1990, **2**, 5.
59. Lipton S. *Br. Med. J.* 1984, **298**, 98.
60. Cronin K. D. and Kirsner R. D. *Anaesthesia* 1982, **37**, 848.
61. McQuay H. J. and Dickenson A. H. *Anaesthesia* 1990, **45**, 101.
62. Fromm G. H. et al. *Front. Pain.* 1990, **2**, 7.
63. Swerdlow M. and Cundill J. G. *Anaesthesia* 1982, **37**, 1129.
64. Jefferson A. L. *J. Neurol. Neurosurg. Psychiatry* 1963, **26**, 345.
65. Lipton S. In: *Textbook of Pain* (Wall P. D. and Melzack R. ed.) Edinburgh: Churchill Livingstone, 1984, Sect. 3B. No. 1.
66. Lipton S. *Clin. Oncol.* 1984, **3**, 195.
67. Lahuer J. et al. *Ann. R. Coll. Surg. Engl.* 1985, **67**, 41.
68. Nashold B. and Friedman H. *J. Neurosurg.* 1972, **36**, 590.
69. Loh L. et al. *Br. Med. J.* 1981, **1**, 1026.
70. Holland A. J. C. et al. *Can Anaesth. Soc. J.* 1977, **24**, 597.
71. Hannington-Kiff J. C. *Br. Med. J.* 1979, **2**, 367; Kepes E. R. et al. *Reg. Anaesth.* 1982, **7**, 52.
72. Walker P. M. et al. *Surg. Gynecol. Obstet.* 1978, **146**, 741, New Sydenham Soc., 1888, 150.
73. Bridenbaugh D. L. et al *JAMA* 1964, **190**, 369.
74. Feldman S. A. and Yeung M. L. *Anaesthesia* 1975, **30**, 174; Fyfe T. and Quin R. O. *Br. J. Surg.* 1975, **62**, 68.
75. Sudeck P. H. M. *Arch. f. Klin. Chir.* 1900, **62**, 147.
76. Kune G. A. et al. *Med. J. Aust.* 1975, **2**, 789; Thompson G. F. et al. *Anesth. Analg. (Cleve.)* 1977, **56**, 1.
77. Jones J. and Gough D. *Ann. R. Coll. Surg.* 1977, **59**, 46; Thompson G. E. and Moore D. C. *Anesth. Analg. (Cleve.)* 1977, **56**, 1.
78. Ischia S. et al. *Pain* 1983, **16**, 333.
79. Motero Malamata A. et al. *Pain* 1988, **34**, 285.
80. Wald Oboussier G. et al. *Reg. Anaes.* 1987, **10**, 27.
81. Morris R. W. and Loong E. D. *Anaesth. Intensive Care* 1984, **12**, 177.
82. Campbell N. N. *Pain Clinic* 1990, **3**, 243.
83. Hannington. Kiff J. G. In: *Textbook of Pain* (Wall P. D. and Melzack R. ed.) Edinburgh: Churchill Livingstone; 1984, Sect. 3B, No. 1.
84. Barnard D. *Ann. R. Coll. Surg. Engl.* 1980, **62**, 180.
85. Williams N. E. *Ann. R. Coll. Surg. Engl.* 1980, **62**, 263.
86. Pike P. M. H. *Anaesthesia* 1978, **33**, 165.
87. Nathan P. W. and Wall P. D. *Br. Med. J.* 1974, **3**, 645.
88. Lipton S. *Proc. R. Soc. Med.* 1974, **67**, 731.
89. Evans P. J. D. et al. *J. R. Soc. Med.* 1981, **74**, 805.
90. Mehta M. In: *Recent Advances in Anaesthesia and Analgesia – 14* (Atkinson R. S. and Hewer C. L. ed.) Edinburgh: Churchill Livingstone, 1982.
91. *Acupuncture Anaesthesia.* Peking: Foreign Language Press, 1973; Diamond E. G. *JAMA* 1971, **218**, 1558.
92. Yamaichi N. *Can. Anaesth. Soc. J.* 1976, **23**, 196.
93. Mayer D. J. et al. *Brain Res.* 1977, **124**, 523.
94. Lee D. C. *Can. Anaesth. Soc. J.* 1979, **26**, 410; Pomeranz B. *New Scientist* 1977, **73**, 12.

95. Edelist G. et al. *Can. Anaesth. Soc. J.* 1976, **23**, 303. Chan C. S. and Chow S. P. *Br. J. Anaesth.* 1981, **53**, 899.
96. Chan C. S. and Chow S. P. *Brit. J. Anaes.* 1981, **53**, 899.
97. Carron H. et al. *JAMA* 1974, **228**, 1552; Bonica J. J. *JAMA* 1974, **228**, 1544.
98. Warwick-Brown N. P. and Richards A. E. S. *Br. Med. J.* 1985, **291**, 450.

Section 6
CARDIORESPIRATORY INTENSIVE CARE

Chapter 28

The intensive therapy unit[1]

History of intensive care

An intensive therapy unit was opened in Copenhagen in 1953 by Björn Ibsen; the first to be run by anaesthetists. *See also* Hilberman M. *Crit. Care Med.* 1975, **3**, 159 and Symposium on Critical Care, *Anesthesiology* 1977, **47** (August).

Intensive therapy consists of the care of patients who are deemed to be recoverable[2] but who need continuous supervision and who need, or are likely to need, specialized techniques by experienced skilled personnel.[3]

Intensive therapy units provide for the management of the critically ill patient who requires facilities greater than those available in the traditional ward. They provide additional space, staff and equipment. The vital functions of the body can be continuously observed and when necessary supported promptly and efficiently.

Admission criteria should be worked out.[4] Certain broad groups may be defined: (1) patients requiring the use of an artificial machine to support a vital system until the primary disease of the system is cured (e.g. ventilator, renal dialysis); (2) patients requiring continuous monitoring (e.g. certain cases of cardiac infarction); (3) certain patients with severe metabolic or electrolyte disorders; (4) those who require heavy or specialized nursing (e.g. difficult tracheostomy, the comatose patient); and (5) a place of safety for patients at risk of lethal complications.

Patients should not be admitted to an intensive therapy unit unless a definite therapeutic advantage for the patient is to be gained. The number of beds set aside for this purpose has been stated to be 1% of the acute bed complement of a hospital,[3] but the need for a unit in every hospital is now being questioned. Many patients require only short-term management and could be treated satisfactorily in a High Dependency Unit. The anaesthetist has a major role to play in the management of patients in the Intensive Therapy Unit because of: (1) special knowledge of ventilatory and resuscitation problems; (2) wide knowledge of medical and surgical conditions; and (3) commitment to continuous communication with colleagues, nurses, patients and relatives, i.e. liaison. Intensive therapy is multi-disciplinary, but in the UK anaesthetists play the major role.

Prediction of survival is an important aspect of the intensivist's work. The Apache (Acute Physiology And Chronic Health Evaluation) scoring system has international recognition.[5] Apache II is a later modification.[6]

See also Bion J. In: *Recent Advances in Anaesthesia and Analgesia – 17* (Atkinson R. S. and Adams A. P. ed.) Edinburgh: Churchill Livingstone, 1991.

Design of the unit[7]

A unit of 6–8 beds is an economic size (a 4-bed area and 2 side wards). Wall-mounted monitoring boxes are useful. The plan should be as flexible as possible to allow for future changes. Mobile partitions are useful. About 18–28 m^2 floor space should be allowed for each bed. Piped oxygen, suction, adequate light, a wash-basin, fresh-air inlet pipe, exhaust pipe, sealable waste-disposal facilities and 8 electric sockets[9] per bed should be provided. The danger of cross-infection is a particular hazard.[10] Division into cubicles and the wearing of gowns and masks by the staff help to reduce this. Adequate storage space for equipment must be provided, and a small laboratory is advantageous.

Staff facilities will occupy a space equal to the patient space. So will the storage area. A high staff/patient ratio is important.[11]

Stress in the intensive care unit

Psychological aspects require consideration.[12] Outside window views, radio, television and occupational therapy are vital factors for some patients. Diurnal rhythm of patients is maintained by modifying the regime at night: (1) reduction of light to minimal adequate intensity; (2) reduction of disturbance due to recording, to the safe minimum; (3) silence as far as possible; (4) sedation[13] is increased at night if possible; and (5) artificial feeding is 'cyclical' when possible.

Effects of stress include psychosis, exacerbated by cimetidine,[13] hallucinations, acute peptic ulceration (largely prevented by early enteral nutrition)[14] and reduced immunocompetence. Prophylactic measures include sedation, antacids, cimetidine 200 mg i.v. t.d.s., clomipramine 25 mg t.d.s. and prevention of awareness in paralysed patients. The critical environmental temperature for adults is 21°C and for infants 24°C.

Cross-infection

Any organism may be involved, bacteria[15] (especially *Pseudomonas aeruginosa*),[16] fungi,[17] viruses, e.g. AIDS.[18] Reduced by careful hygiene, handling of fomites, and hand cleansing of staff when moving between patients.

Intensive care of the neonate and infants

Special Care Baby Units are usually under the care of paediatricians because of the highly specialized nature of their care. Some important considerations are:

1. Temperature. The neonate is liable to heat loss and care should be taken not to expose the baby unnecessarily. A mattress with coils for circulation of warm water or an incubator is useful. Note that a stockinet cap is valuable since the head has a larger proportion of body-surface area than in the case of the adult. The normal neonate makes use of the metabolic activity of the brown fat to maintain body temperature. Small or premature babies, or babies who have suffered from intrauterine malnutrition, may have a lack of brown fat and so are at a disadvantage in the heat losing environment. Hyperthermia is also a risk.[19]

2. Feeding. This must be considered under the heading of water, electrolytes and calories. Dehydration can lead to fever, acidaemia, shock and brain damage. The normal weight loss in the first two days of life may be taken as 44 g/day/kg birth weight – about half as urine and faeces, and about half as insensible fluid loss. The small or premature baby is liable to severe hypoglycaemia if unfed, and this may be severe enough to produce brain damage or death. Hypernatraemia is also a risk and 1/5 normal saline is usually the strongest salt solution that should be given for maintenance infusion.

3. Acidaemia. If present this should be corrected before surgery. Arterial sampling is avoided if possible. If it is essential, the greatest care is taken with the arteries.

4. Oxygen. This is important in that although hypoxaemia may be dangerous, administration of high concentrations of oxygen may result in retrolental fibroplasia. Arterial oxygen tension can be measured, sampling being undertaken from umbilical artery catheters. Hypoxaemia results in inhibition of the brown-fat metabolism (*see above*). Assisted respiration may be necessary.

5. Cross-infection. One hazard particular to the neonate is that the cord stump can act as a culture medium for pathogenic organisms. This can be reduced by the use of a Polybactrin spray to the cord stump daily. *Pseudomonas pyocyanea* is a hazard and polymyxin methane sulphonate may be given as a protection. In babies on respirators it can be instilled into the trachea.

6. IPPV. E.g. in respiratory distress syndrome. The small size of the patient calls for specially designed small tracheal tubes (e.g. Jackson Rees), ventilators, light-weight small connections, fine suction catheters, all difficult in an incubator. Measurement of tidal volume is equally difficult, as is arterial sampling for blood-gas estimation. To prevent damage to the lungs from attempted spontaneous respiration during IPPV, muscle relaxant drugs have been recommended.[20] Special ventilators have been designed.[21]

7. *The Haemorrhagic shock and encephalopathy syndrome.* Has been described.[22]

Mobile intensive care[23]

For history of mobile medical emergency units, *see* Drouet N. *Br. Med. J.* 1982, **284**, 1924; Park G. R. and Johnson S. *Anaesthesia* 1982, **37**, 1204.

Specially designed and equipped ambulances and helicopters have been used[24] to provide a resuscitation and ambulance service outside the hospital. They are equipped to a high level for intubation of the trachea, IPPV, monitoring and ventricular defibrillation. Foot-operated aspirators are carried. In some areas a mobile coronary care service has been provided, in conjunction with education of the public in first-aid resuscitation. Radio-communication and facilities for ECG telemetry may be available. An anaesthetist may go with the team. For portable lung ventilators, *see* Gray A. J. G. *Br. J. Hosp. Med.* 1981, **25**, 173; Marsh R. H. K. and Ledingham I. McA. *Br. J. Hosp. Med.* 1981, **25**, 377.

Transport of sick and injured children, *see* Owen H. and Duncan A. W. *Anaesth. Intensive Care* 1983, **11**, 113. Airway management in transfer of the unconscious patient *see* Robinson N. and Macleod K. G. H. *Ann. R. Coll. Surg. Engl.* 1983, **63**, 372. Ambulance equipment, *see* Woollam H. M. *Br. J. Hosp. Med.* 1982, **27**, 538.

High dependency units

These units are strongly advocated as being the best place for the medical and nursing care of patients who need more facilities than are usually available in the general ward, but are not sick enough to require intensive therapy. They have a place in progressive patient care, particularly as it affects the postoperative patient. Facilities that are likely to be needed include: management of severe postoperative pain, including the supervision of extradural catheters; those with problems of fluid and electrolyte balance, including the care of central venous lines; those requiring frequent observations; and the need for short-term IPPV.

References

1. Hinds C. J. *Intensive Care.* Baillière Tindall, 1987; Rippe J. M. et al. *Intensive Care Medicine.* Boston: Little Brown, 1985; Oh T. E. *Intensive Care Manual.* Australia: Butterworth, 1985.
2. Champion H. R. *Crit. Care Med.* 1982, **10**, 552.
3. BMA Planning Unit Report No. 1, *Intensive Care,* November 1967.
4. Telpick R. et al. *Anesth. Analg. (Cleve.)* 1983, **62**, 572.
5. Knaus W. A. et al. *Crit. Care Med.* 1981, **9**, 591; Le Gall J. R. et al. *Crit. Care Med.* 1982, **10**, 575; Keene A. R. and Cullen D. J. *Crit. Care Med.* 1983, **11**, 1.
6. Knaus W. A. et al. *Crit. Care Med.* 1985, **10**, 818.
7. Robinson J. S. *Br. J. Anaesth.* 1966, **38**, 132; Sherwood Jones E. *Postgrad. Med. J.* 1967, **43**, 339; BMA Planning Unit Report No. 1 *Intensive Care,* November 1967.

8. Ryan D. W. et al. *Br. Med. J.* 1982, **285**, 1634.
9. *Hospital Building Note, Intensive Therapy Unit*, No. 27, 1970, London: HMSO.
10. Seal D. V. and Strangeways J. M. *Anaesth. Intensive Care* 1981, **19**, 260.
11. Gribbens R. E. and Marshall R. E. *Crit. Care Med.* 1982, **10**, 865; Phillips G. D. et al. *Anaesth. Intensive Care* 1983, **11**, 118.
12. Fuller B. F. and Foster G. M. *Heart Lung* 1982, **11**, 457.
13. Cerra F. B. *Ann. Surg.* 1982, **196**, 565.
14. Pringleton S. and Hadzima S. K. *Crit. Care Med.* 1983, **11**, 13.
15. Muder R. R. et al. *JAMA* 1983, **249**, 3184.
16. Freeman R. and McPeake P. K. *Thorax* 1982, **37**, 732.
17. Craven P. C. et al. *Ann. Intern. Med.* 1983, **98**, 160.
18. Davis K. C. et al. *Ann. Intern. Med.* 1983, **98**, 284.
19. David P. and Mughal R. *J. R. Soc. Med.* 1985, **77**, 721.
20. Pollitzer M. J. et al. *Lancet* 1981, **1**, 346.
21. Hall M. W. and Peevy K. J. *Crit. Care Med.* 1983, **11**, 26.
22. Levin M. et al. *Lancet* 1983, **2**, 64.
23. Park G. R. et al. *Br. J. Anaesth.* 1982, **54**, 1081.
24. Cruikshank A. D. N. *Anaesthesia* 1981, **36**, 427; Kee S. et al., Care of the Critically Ill, 1989, **5**, 200; Ramage C. et al. *Br. J. Hosp. Med.* 1990, **43**, 147; Bion J. F. et al. *Br. Med. J.* 1988, **296**, 170, Kee S. S. et al. *J. Roy. Soc. Med.* 1992, **85**, 29; Martin T. E. *J. Roy. Soc. Med.* 1992, **85**, 32.

Chapter 29

Cardiovascular failure

The term 'shock' is applied to a pathological state of diverse aetiology in which tissue blood flow is inadequate to support their metabolic needs. For resuscitation, *see* Chapter 31.

History

'Shock' was used in its current sense in 1832 by Thomas A. Latta, of Leith, Scotland,[1] who used an intravenous infusion of salt solution to treat cholera in 1831–2. More than 150 years earlier, Sir Christopher Wren (1632–1723) gave a dog an intravenous infusion using a quill and bladder, the first intravenous syringe.[2]

Theories of causation have included: (1) vasomotor collapse or vasodilatation (G. W. Crile (1865–1943) in 1899); (2) vasoconstriction (Malcolm, 1905); (3) carbon dioxide depletion, acapnic theory (Yandell Henderson (1873–1944), Yale physiologist, 1909);[3] (4) increased capillary permeability and hypovolaemia due to toxic substances liberated in the injured area (W. B. Cannon (1871–1945), Boston physiologist, and Sir W. M. Bayliss (1860–1924), London physiologist, 1919); (5) fluid loss at site of injury (Alfred Blalock (1899–1964), 1930); (6) vasoconstriction due to hypovolaemia (Freeman, 1933); (7) contribution of left ventricular failure (C. J. Wiggers (1893–1963), of Cleveland, 1947); and (8) bacteraemia.

The first scientific investigation into shock took place during the First World War.

Causes

The causes of shock can be divided into peripheral and cardiogenic. It is worsened by cold, pain and rough movement of the patient.

Peripheral circulation

1. Hypovolaemia. Haemorrhage is commonest; other causes of fluid depletion include burns, inadequate intake, gut losses (*see below*). A loss of

1 l of blood (normal adult blood volume = 5 l) is usually well compensated by splanchnic and cutaneous vasoconstriction. Blood pressure is maintained until 30% of blood volume is lost, but the increase in sympathetic activity shows itself with increased heart and respiratory rates, postural hypotension, increased pulse pressure, cold, pale, clammy skin, thirst and sodium and water retention. CVP and cardiac output fall. Further loss of up to 40% causes a progressive fall in BP. Haematocrit is a poor guide to blood loss in the early stage. The elderly and dysautonomic have poor compensatory responses.

If intravenous fluids are not given, the patient may:

(*a*) Restore blood volume and cardiac output, resulting in anaemia. Pre-capillary vasoconstriction causes a shift of fluid from the ECF to the vascular space. Rapid blood or fluid transfusion at this stage may overload the circulation. Packed red cells should be given slowly.

(b) Fail to rehydrate, and the compensatory mechanisms become harmful. The gut mucosa loses its integrity and releases endotoxins; phagocytes and clotting mechanisms are activated; post-capillary vasoconstriction will tend to shrink the blood volume further by transfer of fluid into the ECF.

Fluid balance. The normal adult has a daily water turnover of 2600 ml (*intake:* 1100 ml in food, 1500 ml as drink; *output:* 1500 ml urine, 100 ml in faeces, 400 ml from the lungs and 600 ml via the skin). Minimum daily urine volume needed for excretory products is 500 ml, with its sp.gr. up to 1032 and osmolality 1400 mosmol/l. There is a tendency to run young patients too dry perioperatively, and the old too wet.

Fluid losses are increased in hot climates (insensible loss may exceed 2000 ml/day); also by diarrhoea, vomiting, paralytic ileus and intestinal fistulae. Clinical signs of dehydration such as thirst (especially with water depletion), loss of skin elasticity and sunken eyes occur when 6% of body water has been lost, and in severe dehydration 10% may have been lost. Abnormal fluid and electrolyte losses should be replaced in addition to normal fluid requirements.

Table 29.1 Composition and volume of normal gut secretions

	Na	K	Cl	Volume
		mmol/l		*ml/day*
Saliva		Depends on volume		1500
Stomach (acid)	50	10	110	2500
Small intestine	120	10	110	1000
Bile	130	10	100	500
Pancreatic juice (alkaline)	130	10	60	1500
Recent ileostomy	130	10	120	1000
Established ileostomy	50	3	20	700

2. *Septicaemia.* Especially Gram-negative (e.g. *E. coli*), but also *Strep. pneumoniae* and other organisms, can cause intense peripheral vasoconstriction due not only to circulating catecholamines and angiotensin, but also to local prostaglandins, leukotrienes and thromboxane A_2. Despite this, overall systemic vascular resistance is usually low, indicating gross maldistribution of

the microcirculation. Disseminated intravascular coagulation may also occur. Oxygen extraction by tissues can no longer increase as capillary blood flow falls, and the use of oxygen becomes dependent on its supply by the arterial blood. Tissue hypoxia and acidosis further impair function of vital organs (liver, kidneys, lungs, heart, brain). Fat or amniotic fluid embolism can produce a similar picture. This can all develop over just a few hours. *See* Chapter 33.

3. *Anaphylaxis.*[4] (Opposite of prophylaxis meaning 'to be on guard'. A neologism coined by C. R. Richet, Nobel prize winner 1913.) Classically, a reaction to foreign protein. Onset usually within a few minutes of exposure. Characterized by pruritus, urticaria, flushing, oedema, dyspnoea, wheezing, cyanosis, nausea and vomiting and hypotension. There may be a massive loss of intravascular volume and deranged tissue perfusion.

4. *Endocrine.* Acute adrenal cortical deficiency.

5. *Neurogenic.* Operative trauma or injuries may cause temporary circulatory derangement due to sudden afferent stimulation, e.g. disarticulation of the hip joint, dilatation of a pregnant cervix uteri, traction on the spermatic cord, acute inversion of the uterus, traction on the gall-bladder or cardiac end of the stomach. These reflexes are dramatic in the hyper-reflexia after spinal cord injuries. Head injuries and subarachnoid haemorrhage can cause prolonged sympathetic discharge.

6. *Subjection to massive G forces.* Sudden deceleration in aerospace and motor-racing accidents, or sudden acceleration, e.g. in bomb blasts, without other injury may lead to cessation of circulation and respiration. Resolves spontaneously after a few minutes' resuscitation.

The heart (cardiogenic shock)

Pump failure due to ischaemia, cardiomyopathy, dysrythmias, trauma to the heart, tamponade, valve disruption, after cardiopulmonary bypass, pulmonary vascular obstruction, massive air embolism, metabolic causes (hypoxia, anaemia, acidosis, electrolyte disorders, hypothermia, toxins and drugs). In acute infarction, cardiogenic shock is likely if more than 40% of the ventricles is infarcted, less if there is an acute ventricular septal defect or papillary muscle rupture.

Consequences of impaired tissue perfusion

Impaired organ function

Brain: restlessness, confusion, hypoxic brain damage.

Heart: impaired coronary perfusion, myocardial dysfunction and even infarction. This will lead to a further decline in cardiac output and a downward spiral in the patient's condition.

Kidneys: acute tubular necrosis, impaired ability to concentrate urine and excrete nitrogenous waste and many drugs. Urine flow is a useful guide to adequacy of renal perfusion in the acute phase. Patients particularly at risk include those with septicaemia, muscle trauma, abdominal aortic surgery, acute liver failure and burns.

Lungs: intrapulmonary shunting, adult respiratory distress syndrome.
Liver: jaundice, bleeding diathesis, altered drug metabolism.

Metabolic

Hypermetabolism. Increased secretion of adrenaline, ACTH, corticosteroids, aldosterone and vasopressin. Reduced secretion of insulin. Hyperglycaemia. Retention of salt and water. Rise in serum potassium if too much is given when urine flow is reduced. Catabolism of body protein and increased urinary nitrogen excretion. Inhibition of the 5'-deiodinase that converts thyroxine to triiodothyronine, resulting in a fall in plasma T_3.

Rise of blood lactate and pyruvate, and a metabolic acidosis.[5] Use of excess lactate production to indicate tissue hypoxia was introduced by W. E. Huckabee.[6] Lactate and lactate/pyruvate ratio is of only limited value in the assessment of most shocked patients.

Disseminated intravascular coagulation may occur. Decreased oxygen consumption and a fall in body temperature occur late.

Management

Although some specific causes of shock demand specific treatments (e.g. overt bleeding, perforated viscus, papillary muscle rupture), it is most commonly a matter of correcting the physiological derangements of hypovolaemia, cardiogenic shock or septicaemia.

1. Assessment

Clinical examination: skin perfusion; pulse and blood pressure; jugular venous pressure; auscultation of lungs and heart; higher brain functions and conscious level; and urine output.

Instrumental: skin-core temperature gradient; acid-base status; pulse oximetry; transcutaneous Po_2; chest radiograph; central venous pressure; ECG; pulmonary artery wedge pressure; mixed venous saturation; cardiac output measurement; systemic vascular resistance; assessment of myocardial function by echocardiography or radionuclides; and oxygen consumption.

2. Treatment

GENERAL

Hypoxaemia and electrolyte and acid-base disturbances should be corrected along with treatment directed at the cardiovascular system. Oxygen therapy, IPPV, and perhaps PEEP to correct intrapulmonary shunting, may be vital. Pain relief by intravenous opioids should be used if indicated, but requirements are not often high and respiratory depression must be avoided. Selective decontamination of the gut may reduce the risk of endotoxaemia in patients with particularly poor tissue perfusion.[7]

MAINTENANCE OF CIRCULATING VOLUME

Arrest haemorrhage. Elevate legs 15–20°. The head-down position is not recommended as it may actually lower cerebral perfusion pressure, risk cerebral oedema, retinal detachment and brachial plexus damage, and make nursing care more difficult. Pneumatic antishock trousers[8] have been used to maintain central blood volume. Thirst may be more distressing in haemorrhagic shock than pain, but is better relieved by mouthwashes and intravenous fluid than by drinks, if operation is pending.

Intravenous fluids.[9] Replacement of all blood lost is not essential as haematocrits of 30–35% are well tolerated and may even benefit tissue perfusion. Crystalloids are cheap, do not cause anaphylaxis, are less likely to cause serious volume overload and may be appropriate if the ECF is depleted. They can be warmed in a microwave oven (2 min at full power will raise 1 l of Hartmann's solution to about 45°C).[10] Colloids need be given in smaller volume (perhaps a third that for crystalloids), expand the intravascular space and so are appropriate for the haemodynamic measurements that are used, and do not leak into the pulmonary interstitium (unless the capillaries are leaky).

Table 29.2 Composition of intravenous crystalloid fluids

	Constituents	g/dl	Na	K	Cl	Lactate
				mmol/l		
Normal saline	NaCl	0.9	154	–	154	–
Ringer lactate	NaCl	0.6	102	–	102	–
(Hartmann's solution)	Na lactate	0.31	29	–	–	29
	KCl	0.03	–	4	4	–
	CaCl$_2$	0.02	–	–	4	–
Total			131	4	110	29
Glucose 5%	Glucose	5	–	–	–	–
Plasma (for comparison)			140	5	103	–

A mixture of crystalloid and colloid, with blood when needed to maintain the haematocrit above 30–35%, is often used. CVP and pulmonary wedge pressure monitoring is useful. Hypertonic saline solutions may have a place in field use.

If there is fluid overload, excess fluid may be withdrawn from the vascular space by venesection (or more space created by vasodilator therapy). Fluid may be taken from the ECF by diuretics (frusemide 20–100 mg) or, if they are insufficient or if renal function is inadequate, by arteriovenous haemofiltration or pump-assisted veno-venous haemofiltration.

MAINTENANCE OF CARDIAC OUTPUT

1. Correct heart rate and rhythm. Too high or too low a rate will reduce cardiac output, especially in heart disease. Use atropine, sympathomimetics, pacing, and anti-dysrhythmics as needed.

2. Correct preload (venous pressures). The change in cardiac output to small fluid challenges (200 ml) will allow construction of primitive ventricular function curves (cardiac output against atrial pressure) and thus choice of best atrial pressures. It is useless to give inotropic drugs before adequate fluid replacement.

3. Improve myocardial contractility and correct the systemic vascular resistance (*see below* for drugs used).

4. Maximize oxygen intake. Consider further the balance between myocardial oxygen supply and demand. Supply is a function of arterial oxygen content (Pao_2 and haemoglobin), coronary vascular resistance, perfusion pressure (diastolic pressure minus LVEDP), and perfusion time (length of diastole). Demand depends on afterload (mean arterial pressure), heart rate and contractility.

5. Consider the intra-aortic balloon pump; cardiopulmonary bypass with membrane oxygenator; and transplantation.

6. Work is in progress on drugs such as synthetic prostaglandins (epoprostenol, 5 ng/kg/min, pre-capillary vasodilator and inhibitor of platelet aggregation); cyclo-oxygenase inhibitors (NSAIDs) and oxpentifylline (a xanthine that inhibits the production of tumour necrosis factor from macrophages). These act on the microcirculation and may improve the distribution of perfusion in the tissues.[11]

Vasoactive drugs used in shock

Catecholamines

Prolonged use, especially in the failing heart, may cause tolerance due to down-regulation of β-receptors.[12]

Dopamine. Naturally-occurring biological precursor of noradrenaline, and a neurotransmitter in the brain stem and substantia nigra. Peripherally, it acts on dopaminergic, β_1 and α_1 receptors at low, medium and high doses respectively. Dopaminergic DA_1 receptors stimulate adenyl cyclase and cause vasodilatation of renal and mesenteric beds, and are antagonized by butyrophenones, phenothiazines, and metoclopramide. Stimulation of the prejunctional DA_2 receptors on sympathetic nerve endings inhibits the release of noradrenaline.

Probably the most widely-used inotrope in the intensive care unit, because its renal effects are particularly valuable. Presented as 200 mg in 5 ml, and diluted before use in 5% glucose, normal saline or Hartmann's to 400–1600 μg/ml, or stronger if using a syringe pump. Inactivated by alkalis, and incompatible with bicarbonate solutions. At a dose of 2–5 μg/kg/min it is used to dilate renal vessels, increase renal blood flow, urine output, and sodium excretion. At 5–15 μg/kg/min it also stimulates cardiac β_1-receptors to improve cardiac contractility. Cardiac output and blood pressure increase. Cardiac rate is affected much less. This effect is blocked by β-antagonists. At high doses of 15–25 μg/kg/min α_1-adrenergic vasoconstriction predominates, which can be lessened by vasodilators. This vasoconstriction increases myocardial oxygen demand, and any tachycardia reduces supply. Side-effects depend on dose, and include nausea and vomiting, headache, angina and dysrhythmias.

Dobutamine. Synthetic derivative of dopamine with strong cardiac β_1 and weak β_2 stimulant activity. As with dopamine it affects contractility more than rate. It has relatively weak α_1 agonist activity, and no specific effect on dopaminergic receptors in the renal vessels or elsewhere. A relatively pure cardiac stimulant. Presented as 250 mg in 20 ml. Dilute with 5% glucose or normal saline to 0.5–1.0 mg/ml for infusion, stronger if using a syringe pump. Incompatible with bicarbonate. Dose range, 2.5–10 μg/kg/min.

Dopexamine. Synthetic dopamine analogue. Its main effect is as a β_2 agonist,[13] dilating skeletal muscle and splanchnic vessels, although it also acts as a mild dopaminergic agonist with one-third the potency of dopamine, and a weak indirect cardiac β_1 agonist. It has no α effects. So it both vasodilates and also acts as an inotrope, with little change in myocardial oxygen consumption. Increases renal blood flow. Causes tachycardia but few dysrhythmias. Presented as 50 mg in 5 ml. Dilute with 5% glucose or normal saline to 0.4–0.8 mg/ml for infusion. Incompatible with bicarbonate. Half-life 6–11 min. Dose 0.5–6.0 μg/kg/min.

Isoprenaline (Isoproterenol, USP). Powerful synthetic β_1 and β_2-adrenergic stimulant, with little α effect. Causes peripheral vasodilatation, with inotropic and chronotropic effects. Also a bronchodilator. 1–5 mg is diluted in 500 ml 5% glucose and infused at 0.5–10 μg/min or given in small boluses (10 μg). May be used orally as 30 mg tablets in heart block. Less used now as tachycardia and dysrhythmias may be troublesome.

Noradrenaline. The neurotransmitter of post-ganglionic sympathetic fibres. Mainly an α_1 agonist, but also has β_2 stimulant properties, especially at lower doses. Produces vasoconstriction, baroreceptor reflex slowing of the heart, and some inotropic stimulation. Coronary blood flow is usually increased. Dose range, 5–20 μg/min. Used to counteract excessive vasodilatation by other drugs.

Adrenaline. Stimulates all the adrenergic receptors. At lower doses the β_2 effect predominates causing vasodilatation, at higher doses the α_1 effect causes constriction. Renal vessels constrict, coronaries generally dilate. The β_1 cardiac effects are inotropic, chronotropic, improved conduction and a lowered threshold for ventricular dysrhythmias. Dose range, 2–30 μg/min.

Phosphodiesterase inhibitors

Little tolerance is seen, unlike with catecholamines. They increase cyclic AMP levels in cardiac and vascular smooth muscle, and have inotropic, vasodilator, venodilator and little chronotropic activity. The vasodilatation allows an increase in cardiac output with no increase in myocardial oxygen consumption. Also a pulmonary vasodilator. Dysrhythmias have not been troublesome. Long half-life. Useful addition to catecholamine therapy. Have been used as a 'bridge' to cardiac transplantation.[14]

Enoximone may be given orally or intravenously. The solution is incompatible with glucose and is diluted with normal saline to 2.5 mg/ml. Dose 0.5–1.0 mg/kg initially, up to 3 mg/kg every 3–6 h, or by infusion 5–20 μg/kg/min. Half-life 6 h, and the liver produces an active sulphoxide metabolite.

Milrinone is excreted largely by the kidneys. It is given intravenously diluted with either dextrose or saline to 0.2 mg/ml, loading dose 25–50 μg/kg and then an infusion at 0.25–0.75 μg/kg/min. Half-life 2 h.

Vasodilators

Pure arterial dilators such as *hydralazine* (5–20 mg i.v.) and *nifedipine* are little used in intensive care. *Phentolamine* (1–10 mg i.v.), a pure α_1 and α_2 blocker, is used in acute hypertensive crises, e.g. phaeochromocytoma. Its α_2 blockade causes some cardiac stimulation.

Pure venodilators such as the *nitrates* and *glyceryl trinitrate* (nitroglycerin, GTN) reduce filling pressures, increase coronary perfusion, improve myocardial oxygen supply and may be a pharmacological alternative to venesection. They also dilate coronary vessels. The action of GTN only lasts about 10 min. It is diluted and infused at 10–200 µg/min. Loses potency in contact with PVC containers.

A mixed arterial and venous dilator such as *sodium nitroprusside* reduces the high systemic vascular resistance seen in cardiogenic shock, and reduces myocardial oxygen demand while augmenting supply. If the drop in blood pressure is excessive, an inotrope may be added. Nitroprusside has a very brief action, 2–3 min, and so is ideal for precise control of blood pressure for limited periods. Dose range 0.3–6.0 µg/kg/min. Each molecule of nitroprusside contains five cyanide radicals, which are released during its metabolism. Although the metabolism of cyanide may be enhanced by administering sodium thiosulphate 75 mg/kg i.v., it is better to limit the dose of nitroprusside to 1.5 mg/kg or 10 µg/kg/min. The development of a metabolic acidosis is one sign of cyanide toxicity.

Other drugs

Glucagon. Stimulates adenyl cyclase and can be useful as an inotrope, especially after cardiopulmonary bypass or in the presence of large doses of β-blockers.

Digoxin.[15] Inhibits Na^+/K^+ ATP-ase in cell membranes. Inotrope, but also increases systemic vascular resistance. Delays A-V conduction, making it suitable for controlling a fast ventricular rate in atrial fibrillation. Although inotropic in patients in heart failure even if in sinus rhythm,[16] the difference between therapeutic and toxic levels is small and it finds little place in the intensive care unit. Dose for rapid digitalization is 1.0–1.5 mg over the first 24 h. Maintenance dose 0.0625 to 0.5 mg/day depending on renal function. Therapeutic range of plasma levels: 1.0–2.6 nmol/l (0.8–2.0 ng/ml).

Combinations. Detailed haemodynamic monitoring is needed to get the best out of these drugs. Combinations are often effective. An inotrope such as dobutamine may increase myocardial oxygen demand, which is lessened by the addition of a vasodilator. Pulmonary vasodilators (isoprenaline, nitroprusside) may be accompanied by unacceptable systemic hypotension, and simultaneous vasoconstrictor (noradrenaline) would be helpful.

ACUTE MYOCARDIAL INFARCTION[17]

Patients with acute infarction are usually admitted immediately to a coronary care unit, although the complexity of monitoring required varies. Dysrhythmias and heart failure may supervene abruptly and resuscitation equipment is kept immediately at hand. Although the ECG is monitored continuously, haemodynamic monitoring such as blood pressure, CVP, wedge pressure, cardiac output, blood gases and urine output is at a level appropriate to the patient's actual or expected needs.

Management

1. *Pain relief:* intravenous opiates, often diamorphine, and Entonox.
2. *Oxygen:* by face-mask or nasal prongs.
3. *Drugs that modify clotting:* immediate aspirin (150 mg orally) improves survival. Thrombolytic therapy[18] (e.g. streptokinase 1.5 MU in 1 h) has an additive effect if given within 24 h of the onset of symptoms, but is most effective if given within 6 h. Neurosurgery, head injury or CVA within the preceding 2 months are contra-indications to thrombolysis. Relative contra-indications include surgery in the last 10 days, severe hypertension and external cardiac massage. The place of anticoagulants is not established. Thrombolysis is preferable to coronary angioplasty.
4. *Other drugs:* low dose *nitrates*, e.g. GTN 5 µg/min or isosorbide dinitrate 1 mg/hour, as coronary vasodilators; β-*blockers*, e.g. atenolol 5–10 mg i.v. then 50 mg 12-hourly orally, may limit infarct size or reduce chance of cardiac rupture; low-dose *heparin* 5000 units s.c. 12-hourly to prevent deep venous thrombosis; oral *diltiazem*, 60 mg 8-hourly.
5. *Dysrhythmias.* Common immediately after infarction, and not necessarily related to the size of the infarct. Often occur with the reperfusion after thrombolysis. The treatment of occasional ventricular ectopics, even if R-on-T, is of no proven benefit. Most anti-dysrhythmic drugs are myocardial depressants. Correct any hypokalaemia, and ventricular tachycardia is treated with lignocaine, 100 mg i.v. followed by 1–4 mg/h, or by synchronized DC shock if immediately life-threatening. Supraventricular tachycardia may need DC shock, verapamil 5–10 mg or digitalization. The latter will also reduce a fast ventricular rate in atrial fibrillation, although β-blockers, amiodarone 5 mg/kg, flecainide 1–2 mg/kg have also been successful. Sinus bradycardia is common after inferior infarction and may be treated by atropine, 0.3–2.0 mg, isoprenaline or transvenous pacing.
6. *Cardiogenic shock:* treated as detailed above. If the cause is massive infarction, these patients have a poor prognosis. However, urgent coronary angioplasty may be of value, and has been safely performed under general anaesthesia.[19] Coronary artery bypass graft may be considered if this is not successful. A surgically correctable cause of the pump failure should be sought, such as papillary muscle rupture (mitral regurgitation), acute ventricular septal defect, left ventricular aneurysm or cardiac rupture.

Patients with continuing ischaemia (on stress test or with angina), poor left ventricular function, or ventricular dysrhythmias are considered at high risk after infarction. They may be offered early angiography with a view to coronary artery surgery.

References

1. Latta J. A. *Lancet* 1832, **1**, 274 (reprinted in 'Classical File' *Surv. Anesthesiol.* 1970, **14**, 563).
2. Wren C. *Phil. Trans. R. Soc.* 1665, **1**, 128.
3. Henderson Y. *Am. J. Physiol.* 1908, **21**, 126.
4. Portier P. and Richet C. R. *C. R. Séanc. Soc. Biol.* 1902, **54**, 170; Richet C. R. *Anaphylaxis.* Engl. transl. Liverpool University Press, 1913, 2; Levy J. H. *Anaphylactic Reactions in Anaesthesia and Intensive Care.* London: Butterworth, 1986.
5. Root W. S. et al. *Am. J. Physiol.* 1947, **149**, 52.
6. Huckabee W. E. *J. Clin. Invest.* 1958, **37**, 264.
7. Ledingham I. McA. et al. *Lancet* 1988, **1**, 785.
8. Abraham E. *Crit. Care Med.* 1982, **10**, 754.
9. Hillman K. In: *Recent Advances in Anaesthesia and Analgesia – 16* (Atkinson R. S. and Adams A. P. ed.) Edinburgh: Churchill Livingstone, 1989, 105.
10. Thomas D. V. *Anesth. Analg.* 1987, **66**, 283.
11. Kong K-L. et al. In: *Intensive Care: Developments and Controversies* (Dobb G. J. ed.) *Clin. Anaesthesiol.* 1990, **4**(2), 305.
12. Brodde O.-E. et al. *Eur. Heart J.* 1989, **10**, (Suppl. B), 38.
13. Stephan H. et al. *Br. J. Anaesth.* 1990, **65**, 380.
14. Watson D. M. et al. *Anaesthesia* 1991, **46**, 285.
15. Withering W. M. (1741–1799) *An Account of the Foxglove and some of its Medical Uses.* Birmingham, 1785.
16. Smith T. W. *N. Engl. J. Med.* 1988, **318**, 358.
17. Donovan K. D. and Hockings B. E. In: *Intensive Care: Developments and Controversies* (Dobb G. J. ed.) *Clin. Anaesthesiol.* 1990, **4**(2), 383; Thomas P. and Sheridan D. *Prescribers' J.* 1990, **30**, 4.
18. Petch M. C. *Br. Med. J.* 1990, **300**, 483.
19. deBruijn N. P. et al. *Anesth. Analg.* 1989, **68**, 201.

Chapter 30

Respiratory failure

Respiratory failure is a common indication for admission to an intensive therapy unit. Defined by Campbell[1] as a state present in a patient at rest, breathing air at sea level if, because of impaired respiratory function, the arterial Po_2 is below 60 mmHg or the Pco_2 is above 49 mmHg.[2] (Artificial ventilation of the lungs is dealt with in Chapter 12; intubation of the trachea in Chapter 11.)

Causes of failure to maintain normal blood-gas homeostasis[3]

(1) Respiratory depression, either central or neuromuscular; (2) respiratory obstruction; (3) pulmonary failure, including chronic bronchitis, acute bronchiolitis, emphysema, fibrosis, asthma, ARDS, pneumothorax, pneumonia and pulmonary oedema; (4) cardiac failure; (5) upper abdominal surgery. (*a*) a restrictive syndrome immediately after operation, with 60% reduced FEV_1 and FVC; it recovers in a week or so; (*b*) change in pattern of breathing, i.e. rapid and shallow, persisting even after complete pain relief with opioids;[4] (*c*) decrease of FRC by 500 ml starting during operation, maximal at 24 h and resolving in a week;[5] and (*d*) diaphragmatic dysfunction;[6] (6) thoracic surgery (atelectasis and diaphragmatic dysfunction);[7] (7) phrenic nerve and other injuries after cardiac surgery;[8] (8) acidosis; (9) hypermetabolism, e.g. hyperpyrexia, thyroid crisis; and (10) respiratory muscle dysfunction is, in practice, a common precipitating cause of respiratory failure.

For mechanisms of lung injury and non-pulmonary causes of respiratory failure, *see* ARDS below.

Signs of respiratory failure

Restlessness, fatigue, sweating, cyanosis, (falls of Spo_2, low Pao_2/Fio_2 ratio), tachycardia, ectopic beats, dyspnoea, tachypnoea, use of accessory muscles of respiration, facial anxiety patterns and tracheal tug. Reduction of number of words per breath.

Assessment of respiratory failure

(1) Respiratory rate, depth, paradox, pattern; auscultation of chest; (2) cough and sputum; (3) respiratory volumes. Patient's FVC (below 2 l surgery is a problem; below 1.5 l they cannot cough; below 1 l/min they may need respiratory assistance; below 0.8 l cannot sleep; below 150 ml/min need continuous IPPV); (4) blood-gas analysis and pulmonary diffusion gradient; (5) pulse and pulsus paradoxus, blood pressure, CVP and ECG; (6) chest X-ray; (7) pulmonary shunt estimation; (8) APACHE II score; and (9) echocardiography for evaluation of heart failure in patients presenting with respiratory failure.

Management of respiratory failure

This depends on the severity of the failure. It includes:

1. Prevention of postoperative respiratory failure by the use of thoracic extradural analgesia.[9]

2. General respiratory care, education of the patient, nursing expertise, physiotherapy, monitoring of signs, blood gases, X-rays, bacteriology, hydration of the patient, and humidification of inspired air. Specific drug administration, including antibiotics, bronchodilators, diuretics and cardiac stimulants.

3. Oxygen therapy (*see below*) plus pressure support.

4. Mechanical ventilation of the lungs (IPPV).[10] The time for intervention may be judged on clinical grounds, such as fatigue, pulmonary measurements (e.g. inadequate tidal volume or blood-gas estimation as when the Pao_2 is lower than the $Paco_2$ even when breathing oxygen-enriched mixtures). The wave-forms, pressures and frequencies of the machine must be tailored to the particular needs of the patient. Fio_2 is set to maintain Pao_2 at 14 kpa (100 mmHg) and is normally 25–40%. If IPPV with 50% oxygen fails to correct hypoxaemia, PEEP may be tried. Reduction of oxygen consumption by induced hypothermia to 34°C.[11] When on IPPV the inspired gases should be humidified and the patient sedated (whether relaxants are required or not). Tracheostomy may be performed after 5 days of oral or nasal intubation. Facilities may exist for this operation to be performed in the intensive therapy unit.

5. Respiratory stimulants, e.g. Doxapram infusion, 1–5 mg/min or almitrine.[12]

6. Diaphragmatic pacing.[15]

7. Lung transplantation has to be considered.

8. Other measures, e.g. plasmapheresis in Guillan-Barré syndrome.[16]

9. Nursing care of patient on artificial ventilation. In addition to care of the tracheostomy (*see below*): (*a*) the patient should never be left unattended; and (*b*) in case of mechanical failure, alternative means of ventilation must be available and understood by the nursing attendants.

Wider management of the patient

1. *Fluid balance and calorie intake.* Generally speaking, the intake (via gastric tube) should be above 2 l of fluid and 2000 calories/day. For information about parenteral and tube feeding, *see* Chapter 34.

2. *Infection*. The relapse may have been precipitated by an infection. Chest infections may occur unless prophylactic measures are taken. Suction catheters should be sterile and used on one occasion only before resterilization. Antibiotic cover is advisable.[17] Patients should be turned at regular intervals (2-hourly) and physiotherapy three or four times daily helps to prevent atelectasis. Visitors may be required to wear gowns and masks.

3. *Pressure areas*. These require careful nursing attention.

4. *Sedation and pain relief*. This may be required: (*a*) to help the patient to become accommodated to artificial ventilation, particularly in the early stages; and (*b*) to ensure adequate rest at night.

5. *Neuromuscular blockade with relaxants*. Now less popular because of respiratory muscle atrophy over periods of a week or more, making weaning more difficult, and risk to paralysed patient if the ventilator fails.

6. *Communication*. The conscious patient must be given bell, mirror, pencil and paper.

7. *Eyes*. If the muscles of the eyelids are paralysed corneal abrasions may occur unless protective measures are taken.

8. *Bladder and bowels*. Function may become automatic in the unconscious or immobilized patient. Manual removal of faeces sometimes requiring sacral extradural blocks and manual compression or catheterization of the bladder may be necessary.

9. *Monitoring*. Blood pressure, pulse, tidal volume, respiratory rate, blood-gas estimation, blood-sugar, chest radiographs and bacteriology of trachea and pharynx (the incidence of nosocomial pneumonia is less when non-acid-reducing drugs are used for ulcer prophylaxis, e.g. sucralfate). Pulse oximeters are very useful. Mixed venous oxygen saturation is a determinant of arterial oxygenation in COAD (COPD)[18] and may need monitoring.

10. *Psychological aspects*. Special arrangements must be made to enable patients to read newspapers and books, watch television, etc. Windows, calendars and clocks help to keep the patient orientated as do visits by close relatives.

Various modes of artificial ventilation

(1) IPPV; (2) NEEP; (3) CPAP[13] (pressure support ventilation[14]); and (4) PEEP, *see* Chapter 12.

Computerized control of ventilatory support using loop-feedback management from vital monitored functions is feasible.

Common indications for IPPV

1. Chronic respiratory failure, either for an acute exacerbation, or postoperatively.

2. Oncology. Immunosuppressed patients with opportunistic infections may be referred for IPPV and antibiotic therapy, with reverse barrier nursing. Their thrombocytopenia is often such that they require platelet transfusion even for insertion of central venous lines. The pulmonary problem may be a very fast-growing tumour, infection, superinfection, cardiac failure, or due to toxic effects of drugs. Early lung biopsy is frequently very helpful.

3. Post cardiopulmonary bypass patients (*see* Chapter 22).

4. Neurosurgery, a 48-h period of elective ventilation in the patient with raised intracranial pressure (ICP). ICP monitoring is common and is reduced as necessary by lowering $Paco_2$, infusing a diuretic such as mannitol or frusemide. Patients with poor cranial pressure compliance, while responding well at first, sometimes show a decreasing response to these therapeutic measures. Sedation is maintained with fentanyl and propofol, monitored with cerebral function monitor.

Complications of long-term IPPV

(1) Tracheal tube enters right main bronchus; (2) tracheal tube becomes blocked by kink, sputum, occlusion of tracheal end by wall of trachea; (3) failure or disconnection of mechanical ventilator; (4) pressure ulceration of mouth or nose, vocal cords or trachea; (5) lung infection and septicaemia due to sputum retention and chest infection from inadequate humidification and bacterial contamination. Lung abscess. Atelectasis in a patient on IPPV is an emergency; (6) hypotension due to CO_2 wash-out and raised intrathoracic pressure; (7) difficulties in communication; (8) psychological disturbances, including hallucinations; (9) surgical emphysema and pneumothorax; (10) water and sodium retention with pulmonary oedema (not reduced by PEEP) and systemic oedema (worsened by PEEP); (11) rarely, tracheal stenosis;[19] (12) subpleural air cysts.[20]

In the ITU, nasotracheal is preferable to orotracheal intubation,[21] although neither is free from complications.[22] To change a nasotracheal tube, a long bougie may be passed down it and the tube withdrawn, leaving the bougie as a guide for the new tube.

For complications of PEEP, HFPPV and CPAP, *see* Chapter 12.

Weaning from a ventilator

It is usually easier to put a patient on a ventilator than to take him off it. Weaning may take anything from minutes to weeks.

Indications: (1) the patient can cough; (2) the chest compliance is good; (3) oxygen exchange is good, the Pao_2 being normal while the patient is ventilated with 25% oxygen; (4) chest infection and other pathology has been substantially cleared; and (5) muscle power, especially respiratory muscles, and nutrition are as normal as possible (i.e. there is no abdominal paradox within spontaneous respiration and the vital capacity is one litre or more). Allowing the patient to breathe against the ventilator, within limits, during prolonged IPPV, will tend to keep the respiratory muscles in reasonable condition.

IMV and SIMV (*see* Chapter 12). Analgesics, muscle relaxants and sedatives are stopped. The $Paco_2$ is allowed to rise to normal or above. The patient is instructed and encouraged to breathe; then, during the morning, the ventilator is switched to IMV. The patient is watched for signs of respiratory distress, sweating, struggling, cyanosis or exhaustion. If these appear the ventilator is returned to complete IPPV. A trial period of up to an hour, repeated later, or prolonged as necessary is a good start. If PEEP was required during IPPV, then CPAP is likely to be required during weaning. Arterial blood-gas monitoring and A-aDo$_2$ measurements are useful. Various ventilators employ triggered ventilation (which is varied progressively) or mandatory minute volume (MMV) (*see* Chapter 12), especially valuable where experienced nursing is in short supply.

Extubation of the trachea may follow 24 h adequate spontaneous ventilation, provided there is reasonable brainstem function, or earlier if the patient is intolerant of the tube.

Rehabilitating and weaning the ventilator-dependent patient can be difficult.

Tracheostomy[23]

History[24]

Performed by Pedro Virgili (1699–1776) of Cadiz for the relief of quinsy. George Martine (1702–1741)[25] was the first to employ it in a case of diphtheria in Britain. Heister (1683–1758) introduced the term 'tracheotomy' in place of 'bronchotomy' in 1718 and this gave place to 'tracheostomy' at the suggestion of Negus (1887–1974) of London in 1938 (*see* Wath J. M. *Br. J. Surg.* 1963, **50**, 954). Employed to relieve laryngeal diphtheria by Brettonneau (1778–1862) in 1818 (which was its chief use for the next 120 years),[26] and in the treatment of poliomyelitis in 1943.

Types of tube

1. The King's College Hospital pattern silver tube. Size 32 or 34 for men. Size 28 for women. Later a valved tube can be inserted, which enables the patient to speak.
2. Cuffed plastic tracheostomy tube. Low-pressure cuffs are preferable to high-pressure cuffs as they cause less damage. Other types that have been advocated include double cuffs, solid cuffs and automatic inflating cuffs.
3. Fenestrated tube for speaking.

Laryngostomy

Easier to perform than tracheostomy and need not result in postoperative laryngeal obstruction.[27]

Minitracheostomy

Can be rapidly performed using a set designed for the purpose. Useful in life-saving situations. The initial stab incision should enter the trachea, otherwise, great force may be needed to penetrate it. A needle introducer with guide-wire and dilators is available. Not an easy technique where there is swelling of the neck. Is also frequently used for short-term tracheobronchial toilet.

Needle tracheostomy

In extremis, e.g. after failed intubation, the insertion of an intravenous cannula No. 12 (internal diameter 2.3 mm, length 7 cm) into the trachea, above or below the cricoid, will provide oxygenation if connected to a source of oxygen or even air from a reservoir bag or Ambu bag. A minute volume of 3–4 l can be provided while over-inflation (which is unlikely due to oxygen leak through the larynx) can be prevented by a vent controlled by a finger, on the tubing. Such cannulae and connectors should be readily available in all operating suites and trauma centres.

There is a danger of transmission of HIV-infection from infected patients to personnel during these tracheostomies because of inoculation of sputum spray.

Complications of tracheostomy

1. Early complications. Include: haemorrhage; displacement or obstruction of the tube; difficult insertion or reinsertion of the tube; injury to the trachea, tracheitis, crust formation; respiratory complications; and surgical emphysema and pneumothorax.

2. Infection. May arise from: (*a*) contamination during tracheal suction. Aseptic 'no-touch' methods, with the use of disposable gloves, help to minimize this; (*b*) The wound itself is liable to become infected. Hourly spraying with polybactrin aerosol is helpful, and so is application of nystatin; and (*c*) the humidifier. Can be prevented by raising the temperature of the water to 60°C (140°F) so that pasteurization occurs. Despite all measures, tracheostomy wounds may become infected.

3. Tracheal ulceration. Erosions of the tracheal mucous membrane are not uncommon. In some cases, ulceration has produced exposure of the tracheal rings, secondary haemorrhage from erosion of a major vessel, and even ulceration into the oesophagus.

4. Tracheal dilatation. Mechanism not fully understood.

5. Tracheal stenosis. The Björk flap[28] is unlikely to be associated with stenosis.[29] It involves making a circular opening in the trachea at the level of the third tracheal ring the size of the proposed tube, the edges being sutured to the skin. Symptoms do not occur unless the tracheal diameter is 60% reduced. Stridor indicates a diameter of 6 mm or less. It may occur: (*a*) in the subglottic region; (*b*) at stoma level; (*c*) at the level of the cuff; or (*d*) below the tube. Commonest sites are at cuff and stoma sites. Symptoms may not arise until late, usually after the patient has left hospital. In severe cases, definitive treatment by resection of the stenosed area with primary suture is required. Dilatation usually affords temporary benefit only.

Soft-cuff or floppy-cuff tracheal tubes overcome the problem of pressure ulceration of the trachea to a large extent. The position of the curve of a tracheostomy tube should be checked by lateral soft-tissue X-ray of the neck.

6. Cardiovascular collapse. In the shocked patient whose circulation has been boosted by high Pa_{CO_2}. When normal ventilation returns, the true severity of existing shock is revealed.

Humidification

In 1h of IPPV with dry gases, 20 ml of water are lost from the lungs.

Methods of humidification

1. A container of warm water in the airstream. Tubing between humidifier and patient should be lagged to prevent condensation. A water trap placed between expired gases and a volume meter helps to prevent false readings caused by condensation. Colonization by bacteria has proved to be a major disadvantage, but it can be prevented if chlorhexidine is added to the water and the temperature of the water maintained at 60°C (140°F) so that a process of pasteurization occurs. This type of humidifier is 90-100% efficient.
2. Nebulizers are used to produce a supersaturated mist. (*a*) Gas-driven nebulizers. Droplets from 5 to 20 μm; and (*b*) spinning-disc humidifiers. Water is drawn from a reservoir by an Archimedean screw to impinge on the surface of a rapidly rotating disc that flings water to produce a wide range of droplet sizes. Over 100% efficient.
3. Ultrasonic humidifiers. Water drops on to a vibrating plate and is broken up into particles of 1–2 μm size. Over 100% efficient.
4. Condenser humidifiers ('artificial or Swedish nose'). Layers of wire gauze may be interposed between the tracheostomy tube and the external air. Dead space can be as low as 17 ml. May offer some resistance to respiration. Not suitable for use in small children. Can also act as reservoirs of infection. To prevent this they should be changed 3-hourly. 70% efficient.
5. A simple method is to insert a fine needle through the wall of the tracheal tube and infuse water at a rate of 4 drops/min using a standard transfusion set.

Whatever method of humidification is used it is important to make sure that the patient is adequately hydrated.

Nursing care of patient with tracheostomy

The following points are important:
1. All conscious patients should have a bell, pencil and paper, and mirror at hand.
2. The inner tube of a silver tracheostomy tube should be cleaned at regular (4-hourly) intervals.
3. The cuff of a cuffed tube may be deflated at regular intervals and reinflated with just enough air to make an airtight seal. The pharynx should be sucked out before, and the trachea after, carrying out such a manoeuvre. Many workers now prefer to inflate the cuff carefully and then leave it with pressure unchanged until it is time to remove the tube.
4. Use a humidifier to prevent crusting. Maintain hydration.
5. The trachea should be sucked out when indicated with aseptic no-touch technique.
6. Sterile dressing to tracheostomy wound daily, using no-touch technique.

Permanent IPPV

A tracheostomy tube, if used, is uncuffed. Such intubation may of course be unnecessary if an 'iron lung' or rocking bed is used. Tunnicliffe jackets or cuirasses may also be employed.

For polio, or nocturnal ventilation at home in the very long term, e.g. using a cuirass ventilator. This may reverse the hypersomnolence, polycythaemia, and pulmonary hypertension seen in chronic severe respiratory failure. Some permanent ventilation units exist.

Specific pulmonary conditions

Acute exacerbations of chronic bronchitis and emphysema

An acute infection may precipitate acute respiratory failure. Arterial oxygen tension falls and arterial carbon dioxide tension rises. Respiration is maintained by the hypoxic drive via the aortic and carotid body reflexes in the very severe case. Further depression of respiration occurs and a state of carbon dioxide narcosis results. In other circumstances, long-term oxygen therapy has been given in the home. Oxygen must, however, be administered to relieve hypoxia and respiration maintained. This may be achieved by:

1. The use of controlled concentrations of oxygen. Hypoxic hypoxia is always very responsive to the Po_2 of the inspired air. Raising this from normal 20 to 26 kpa (28% O_2) has a very significant effect.

2. Sedatives and hypnotics should be avoided.

3. Full humidification of inspired gases is important, perhaps with nebulized medication (antibiotics, sputum solvents, etc.)

4. Regular and vigorous chest physiotherapy, although a session of therapy may temporarily increase the hypoxia.

5. Respiratory stimulants (e.g. doxapram) may be useful in marginal cases. It should be given slowly.

6. IPPV via tracheal tube. First used in the treatment of respiratory failure in 1952. (Lassen H. C. A. *Lancet* 1953, **1**, 37.) This is indicated if: (*a*) tidal volume is inadequate; (*b*) $Paco_2$ exceeds Pao_2; and (*c*) patient is becoming exhausted and cannot effectively cough or clear secretions.

It is unwise to provide mechanical ventilation for patients with terminal emphysema in the absence of a clearly remediable pathology. Bronchoscopy can be useful in identifying the causative organism.

Status asthmaticus

Status asthmaticus can be defined as a severe and prolonged episode of bronchospasm, causing distress to the patient, and not relieved by conventional therapy.

TREATMENT

1. Oxygen. The aim should be to maintain arterial oxygen tension above 7.5 kPa (50 mmHg). As hypercapnia may be present in late stages and the chemoreceptor drive lost, oxygen must be given with care, in controlled concentrations. Sedatives are not given unless the patient is on IPPV.

2. *Drugs*. Aminophylline and theophylline (first used in the treatment of bronchial constriction in 1937)[30] are given intravenously or per rectum, improving the contractile properties of the diaphragm, causing bronchodilatation and stimulating respiration. Isoprenaline or salbutamol are useful as an aerosol inhalation. Salbutamol may be given intravenously (100–300 µg) or orally (2–4 mg, three times daily, maximum 8 mg). Terbutaline has a longer duration of action. Dose: 0.25 mg s.c. or slow i.v.; 0.25 mg by inhalation; oral, 5 mg 8-hourly.

3. *Fluid replacement*. To correct dehydration. The deficit may be great and should be corrected with normal saline using CVP monitoring.

4. *Lignocaine*. Spray to laryngeal mucosa; deep anaesthesia with halothane[31] or ether and oxygen may be required.

5. *IPPV*. Indications: (*a*) exhaustion apnoea; (*b*) pneumothorax (after insertion of chest drain), pneumomediastinum; (*c*) deteriorating general condition, reduced consciousness, oliguria, acidosis, peripheral circulatory failure, rising pulse, dysrhythmias; (*d*) pulsus paradoxus greater than 40; (*e*) Pao_2 less than 9 kPa (60 mmHg); $Paco_2$ more than 9 kPa (60 mmHg); (*f*) night. Many deaths from asthma occur soon after midnight. The serum potassium should be above 3 mmol/l and a pneumothorax, if present, should be drained. Sodium bicarbonate is rarely needed. The trachea is sprayed with lignocaine prior to insertion of the tracheal tube. The ventilator is timed to start inspiration when the expiratory wheeze (auscultated) ceases. Inspiration is usually short; expiration, long; (*g*) antacids and a nasogastric tube are frequently required; and (*h*) ECMO or ICMO *in extremis*.

6. *Corticosteroids*. The effect may not be seen for 12 h. These should be given, often in massive dosage, especially when the patient is already on long-term steroid therapy.

7. *Antibiotics*. Unless the precipitating factor is obviously allergic or psychological, it is wise to give a bactericidal antibiotic.

8. *Ketamine infusion*.

Legionnaires disease[32]

Caused by a virulent mycobacterium, *Legionella pneumophila*; causes severe pneumonia often requiring oxygen therapy and IPPV. The organism multiplies in warm water and has airborne spread, especially via air-conditioning systems. Cross-infection is common and severe epidemics occur. The organism is frequently sensitive to erythromycin.

Adult Respiratory Distress Syndrome (ARDS)

A term first used by Ashbaugh.[33]

CAUSES

These include massive (especially unfiltered) blood transfusion, sepsis (*see* Chapter 33), polytrauma (*see* Chapter 32) (injury scores over 2.5 are a strong risk for ARDS), fat embolism, pulmonary micro-embolism, cardiopulmonary bypass, pancreatitis, ulcerative colitis, peritonitis, barbiturate overdose and prolonged severe hypotension. Some authorities also include drowning and direct lung injuries (prolonged pulmonary oedema, including neurogenic, crushed chest, radiation, burns, explosions, smoke, gas or acid inhalation, immunosuppression, pulmonary oxygen toxicity,[34] anaphylactic reactions and prolonged IPPV). The commonest cause is sepsis. Two types have been described: (*a*) cardiac,[35] responds to diuretics; and (*b*) non-cardiac ARDS[36] or 'permeability pulmonary oedema', the one described here. ARDS also occurs in children.[37]

SYMPTOMS

Progressive respiratory distress with decreased lung compliance and increased work of breathing; resistant hypoxaemia, tachypnoea (> 20 rpm). Chest X-ray shows diffuse alveolar infiltration. In addition, there is often multiple organ failure (*see* Chapter 33).

DIAGNOSIS

Early stage, dyspnoea and tachypnoea existing with or following the above conditions. Later, diffuse patchy clouding in chest X-ray, increasing dyspnoea and hypoxia. Later still, circulatory instability, hypotension, deepening cyanosis, loss of consciousness, moribundity and finally cardiac arrest. Swan–Ganz catheterization is useful in diagnosis and progress monitoring.

PATHOPHYSIOLOGY[38]

Mechanisms of injury in ARDS. The cytokines (leucotrienes IL-1, IL-2, and IL-6, possibly derived from activated ('angry') macrophages) initiate the complement cascade and produce a tissue procoagulant factor. Prostaglandins 'E', tumour necrosis factor (TNF), platelet activating factor and thromboxanes (A_2) are then implicated in the appearance of oxygen radicals and eicosanoids, which specifically damage the inter-alveolar capillary endothelium. This leads to endothelial dehiscence, leakage, increased extravascular lung water, abnormal platelet deposition, white cell plugging, and microvascular thromboses. Increased alveolar dead space, impaired diffusion, ventilation/perfusion inequality and micro-shunting (the major factor) follow (with hypoventilation due to decreased compliance and muscle weakness), reducing oxygen delivery to the blood. The effect of this is worsened by lowered $P\bar{v}o_2$.[39] Alveolar oedema and hyaline membrane appear.

Pulmonary thromboxane-A_2 production may cause pulmonary vasoconstriction, resulting in right ventricular failure and high CVP and PAP. The lung does not exchange gases very well, but it can recover function.

A generalized disease process, often producing multisystem organ failure, of which lung failure (ARDS) is the commonest and earliest. Useful markers of the process are temperature, white cell count, Pao_2/Fio_2 gradient, myeloperoxidase, elastase, $C5_a$, serotonin (*see also* Chapter 33). Fibrosis occurs early in this process, and regresses with later resolution of the disease. Pulmonary endothelial permeability can be measured.[40]

The secondary consequences of severe hypoxia during ARDS are to worsen failure in other organs (*see* Chapter 33).

TREATMENT

1. Correction of the primary cause if possible, especially correction of sepsis.

2. Humidified oxygen therapy up to Fio_2 40% to maintain Pao_2.

3. IPPV, if necessary; the indications being: a respiratory rate greater than 35/min, vital capacity less than 10 ml/kg, A-aPo_2 gradient of 7 kPa on air or 40 kPa on pure oxygen, $Paco_2$ greater than 7 kPa, V_D/V_T greater than 60%, right to left shunt greater than 15%. PEEP[41] is likely to be of value and is adjusted to keep Pao_2 greater than 7 kPa with Fio_2 less than 50% if possible. The resulting reduction of cardiac output reversed by dobutamine and other inotropes. However, raising the cardiac output may also raise the shunt fraction. Ventilator settings are important to maximize gas transport and minimize pulmonary barotrauma.

4. Sedation, paralysis and hypothermia to reduce oxygen demand.

5. Plasma colloid osmotic pressure is maintained by keeping the serum albumin above 30 g/l.

6. Reduction of pulmonary vascular resistance by: (*a*) pulmonary vasodilators, nitroprusside and α-blockade; (*b*) ibuprofen 400 mg to antagonize thromboxane A_2; and (*c*) prostacyclin treatment may have a place.

7. Extracorporeal membrane oxygenation (ECMO) and ICMO[42] will buy time but not cure. The carbon dioxide membrane lung (CDML) has been used in this condition in an effort to rest the lung, with a little success.[42]

8. The patient is turned every half hour.

9. Prevention of failure of other organs, e.g. kidney (*see* Chapter 33).

Specific treatment. Specific monoclonal antibodies offer hope of genuine reduction of mortality of this condition. *See* Chapter 33.

PROGNOSIS

Predictors of survival are:

1. Younger age.
2. Shorter time on ventilator.
3. Shorter time in ICU.
4. Pao_2/Fio_2 ratio at admission > 300.
5. Serum lactate at admission < 2.5 mEq/L.
6. Serum bilirubin after 1 wk < 7 mg/dl.
7. Serum creatinine < 200 mEq/l.
8. A smaller number of organs failing at the same time. Concurrent renal failure carries a bad prognosis.

The mortality of established ARDS is about 90% without special treatment; about 40% with treatment. Additional failure of other organs in the body, e.g. kidney, increases mortality considerably. The survivors show reduced pulmonary function for a long time.

Other conditions which may require IPPV

AIDS (Acquired Immune Deficiency Syndrome)[43]

The indications for intensive therapy in AIDS include life support of a promptly reversible complication, and to allow time for affairs to be settled, family visits, etc. The average survival may be extendable to 6 months in the case of *Pneumocystis carinii* pneumonia (PCP) or about 18 months in the case of Kaposi's sarcoma. PCP is by far the commonest complication and may respond to trimethoprim, sulphamethoxazole or pentamidine, giving a survival rate of 30–50% from the first attack and about half this from the second attack. Sputum for bacteriological analysis is obtained by hypertonic saline sputum induction and has a high yield for *P. carinii*, but bronchoscopy and even lung biopsy may be required. PCP shows a dry, granular appearance on chest X-ray. Many AIDS patients also have oral candidiasis. A few have open TB. Those AIDS patients with CNS complications are not usually presented for intensive therapy. The HIV is usually killed by 1% glutaraldehyde for 30 min or 5% hypochlorite for 5 min (good for cleaning surfaces). (*See also Guidance for Staff treating Patients with AIDS*, London: DHSS, 1986.)

Poliomyelitis

This may be spinal, bulbar or bulbospinal. Patients with bulbar poliomyelitis can breathe but cannot maintain the integrity of their upper air passages. The semi-prone head-down position together with suction will prevent soiling of the bronchial tree. Bulbospinal poliomyelitis is the dangerous type as it is a combination of the first two above.

The tracheostomy and cuffed tube technique provide for suction of the airways, protection of the airways from soiling and an easy route for IPPV. (*See also* Permanent IPPV.)

Polyneuropathy

E.g. Guillain-Barré syndrome (*see* Chapter 20).

Tetanus

There may be pharyngeal and laryngeal insufficiency due to spastic, not flaccid, muscles. Mild cases have been treated with sedatives (e.g. diazepam). When reasonable doses fail to control convulsions, muscle relaxants and IPPV must be considered, often through a tracheostomy, although tracheal narrowing may occur later. Tetanus may be accompanied by overactivity of the sympathetic nervous system, shown by wild fluctuations in heart rate and arterial pressure. These changes may be aggravated by tracheal suction. For these *autonomic storms* β-blockade and calcium antagonists are used to protect the heart; atropine controls salivation and α-blockade controls the blood pressure.[44] Tracheal suction in curarized patients on artificial ventilation may result in marked rises in arterial and central venous pressure.

Myasthenia gravis

Cases may require IPPV and careful supervision over a long period of time. (For details of management, *see* Chapter 20.)

Status epilepticus

Muscle paralysis and IPPV are sometimes required and diazepam or a thiopentone[45] drip has been used.[46] EEG and cerebral function monitor are used to monitor fits in the paralysed patient.

Management of rabies encephalitis

In the present state of knowledge, the aim should be to provide full supportive therapy in the hope that immunoglobulins and immunization at the time of diagnosis might allow recovery. This will include IPPV, and cardiovascular support with appropriate sedation. Muscle spasms are controlled by muscle relaxant drugs; intubation will prevent pulmonary soiling; loss of vasomotor tone may result in the need for vasopressors (e.g. dopamine). Brainstem death is likely to supervene. Monitoring may include direct arterial pressure, arterial oxygen tension, Swan–Ganz catheterization, and use of the cerebral function monitor.

Barrier nursing should be carried out and the number of medical and nursing attendants kept to a minimum. Those in direct contact with the patient or the patient's ventilator, should receive active immunization.

(*See also DHSS Memorandum on Rabies.* London: HMSO, 1977; Editorial, *Br. Med. J.* 1975, **3**, 721; Cohen S. L. et al. *Br. Med. J.* 1976, **1**, 1041; Cundy J. M. *Anaesthesia* 1980, **35**, 35.)

Respiratory problems in children[47]

Respiratory problems in infants (*see also* Chapter 22)

Special factors to be considered include: (1) restricted vital capacity; (2) increased right-to-left shunt; (3) increased closing volume; (4) narrow airways; (5) pulmonary and neurological developmental immaturity; (6) susceptibility to infection; (7) specific abnormalities, e.g. pulmonary dysplasia with high pulmonary vascular resistance, congenital cardiac lesions, respiratory distress syndrome; (8) diazepam increases pulmonary vascular resistance in infants; tolazoline, 1–2 mg/kg, reduces it; (9) considerable adrenergic activity leading to early severe hyperglycaemia, exhaustion of glycogen followed by severe hypoglycaemia; and (10) inspiratory stridor suggests obstruction above larynx, expiratory stridor, below.

Indications for IPPV in Infants

(1) Clinical (in the words of Sir William Osler (1849–1919): "Don't touch the patient; note first what you see"): tachypnoea, tachycardia, facial distress, indrawing of the ribs, tracheal tug, use of accessory muscles of respiration, and irregular gasping and exhaustion. (2) Biochemical: Pao_2 less than 8 kPa (60 mmHg). (3) Prophylactic: i.e. strong likelihood of failure. (4) Post-cardiac surgery.

Acute epiglottitis

This is an acute inflammatory condition, which may cause respiratory obstruction and is a danger to life. The history is short, usually a matter of looks toxic; often prefers to sit up with the neck extended. If viewed with a spatula or laryngoscope the epiglottis is seen to be red and oedematous. The causal agent is often *Haemophilus influenzae* and this organism can be grown from the pharynx and sometimes the bloodstream. There are general signs of fever and toxicity. Suspicion of this condition demands urgent admission to hospital. The tongue frequently protrudes, the stridor is often inspiratory. Age range mostly 2–6 years. The leucocyte count is usually less than 10 000.

As soon as the condition is diagnosed, steps must be taken to ensure the adequacy of the airway. The child is not left alone, laid flat, or sent to the X-ray department. The mouth and tongue are not manipulated. Crying can precipitate laryngeal obstruction in acute epiglottitis.[48] Where the necessary facilities are to hand, tracheal intubation by a skilled anaesthetist can be performed. This should be accomplished in the operating-theatre environment with facilities for immediate tracheostomy available (in other circumstances, tracheostomy may be preferred). The child is given an oxygen/halothane induction by a skilled anaesthetist. The tracheal tube should be small enough to allow a slight leak. An i.v. cannula may be inserted after the child is asleep. A nasogastric tube may be passed. Humidified oxygen-enriched air is breathed, usually spontaneously. Diazepam, 0.1 mg/kg, or morphine, 0.1 mg/kg, or chloral hydrate, 30 mg/kg, may be used for sedation following intubation. Some advocate an oral tube changed later to a nasotracheal tube for comfort and fixation.

Once the airway is secured, the child will usually sleep, but sedatives can be given if necessary. The tube should stay in position for 24–36 h after the commencement of antibiotic treatment to allow resolution of the condition. Antibiotics, e.g. ampicillin or chloramphenicol[49] are given, and hydrocortisone may help to reduce oedema.[49] Hydrocortisone cream may be smeared on the tracheal tube. Oxygen-helium mixtures have been used.[50]

Pulmonary oedema may follow relief of acute infective upper airway obstruction and may require IPPV and PEEP.[51]

Supraglottitis has been described.[52]

Suggested protocol for management of children suspected of suffering from acute epiglottitis, *see* Baines D. B. et al. *Anaesth. Intensive Care* 1985, **13**, 25.

Fulminating acute epiglottitis and supra-epiglottitis is becoming more frequent in adults and may progress rapidly from sore throat and dysphagia to salivation and stridor, with pyrexia and leucocytosis.[52] Acute respiratory distress is less common at presentation in adults (8%) than in children.[53] In adults there may be time for lateral soft tissue X-rays of the neck,[54] helpful in 75–95%, CAT scan,[55] or fibreoptic laryngoscopy.[56] Pharyngeal culture is normally negative.[57] Parenteral amoxycillin, with or without chloramphenicol, or cephalosporins is the treatment.

Acute laryngotracheitis

Acute infection is often viral in origin, with superimposed bacterial infection. Obstruction occurs due to oedema and exudate, and is most likely in the immediate subglottic region in the 1–2 year age group. Tracheal intubation and gentle suction may be necessary. Tracheostomy is to be avoided if possible. The child may develop acute pulmonary oedema.

Reye's syndrome

Acute non-inflammatory encephalopathy with microvesicular fatty infiltration of the liver confirmed by biopsy or suggested by liver function test results (aspartate transaminase, alanine transaminase, blood ammonia) greater than three times normal. Incidence 80 cases/year in UK. Average age 15 months. Prognosis – 43% survived intact, 41% died, 12% neurologically damaged.[58]

(*See also* Brown T. C. K. in: *Current Opinion in Anaesthesiology*, 1990, **3**, 325; Hatch D. J. in: *Recent Advances in Anaesthesia and Analgesia* – 15 (Atkinson R. S. and Adams A. P. ed.) Edinburgh: Churchill Livingstone, 1985.

Septicaemia

See Chapter 33.

Poisoning

Buy time for recovery by life support of respiratory and other organ function. For self-poisoning, psychiatric advice is an important part of the follow-up.

Acute carbon monoxide poisoning (*see* Chapter 32).

Transport of respiratory failure patients requires oxygen, facilities for IPPV, pulse oximetry and capnography in addition to ECG and arterial pressure.

Obstructive sleep apnoea may be treated conservatively by analeptics, doxapram or surgically by palatoplasty. Such patients are worse after anaesthesia and when receiving postoperative opioids.

Oxygen therapy[59]

Modern oxygen therapy initiated in 1917 by J. S. Haldane (1860–1936).[60] The first satisfactory measurement of blood oxygen content performed in 1924.[61]

The fundamental aim of oxygen therapy is to restore the tissue oxygen tension towards normal. A partial pressure of at least 1.3 kPa is required at the cellular mitochondria.[62] Oxygen therapy is most valuable when the blood oxygen tension is low (hypoxic hypoxia). In anaemic and stagnant hypoxia it does not greatly increase the amount of oxygen carried by haemoglobin, although the rise in dissolved oxygen in the plasma is significant. It is doubtful whether histotoxic hypoxia is benefited by oxygen therapy.

SOME RELEVANT PHYSIOLOGICAL DATA

Oxygen content of air 20.93%. Oxygen content of expired air 16.3%. Oxygen content of alveolar air 14.2%. Partial pressure of oxygen in air 21 kPa (160 mmHg). Partial pressure of oxygen in alveolar air 13.3 kPa (104 mmHg). Partial pressure of oxygen in venous blood 5.3 kPa (40 mmHg). Solubility of oxygen in plasma 0.3 ml/dl/100 mmHg. Oxygen capacity of haemoglobin 1.34 ml/g Hb. Oxygen capacity of arterial blood 19.8 vol%. Oxygen saturation of arterial blood 97%. Oxygen tension of arterial blood 13 kPa (100 mmHg).

Oxygen flux

The amount of oxygen flowing in the blood can be calculated as follows: 100 ml of blood contains 19.8 ml of oxygen when fully oxygenated. If the cardiac output is 5 l/min, then the oxygen available (oxygen flux) to the body is $19.8 \times 50 = 990$ ml/min. Normal oxygen consumption is 250 ml/min. There is thus a large reserve. In severe exercise, cardiac output increases to 20 l/min. Demands in excess of the oxygen flux build up a temporary oxygen debt, by anaerobic metabolism. For oxygen monitoring and pulse oximetry,[63, 64] *see* Chapter 18.

Oxygen flux (oxygen delivery) is a determinant of the outcome of severe sepsis (*see* Chapter 33).

Oxygen flux to individual organs (e.g. brain) also merits consideration.

Types of oxygen lack

"Oxygen lack not only stops the machine, but wrecks the machinery" (J. S. Haldane).

Cyanosis may be detected by trained observers when the reduced Hb is only 1.5 g/dl, although for many people, detection is only possible at 5 g/l ($Pa_{O_2} = 8$ kPa, 55 mmHg).[65]

Reduced utilization of oxygen by tissues may be of the following types – the first three were described by Joseph Barcroft,[66] the fourth by Peters and van Slyke[67] (1883–1971) (1931).

1. Hypoxic hypoxia. The arterial Po_2 is low. It occurs whenever oxygen is prevented from reaching the pulmonary capillaries.

Diffusion hypoxia may occur during recovery from nitrous oxide anaesthesia. Air containing nitrogen enters the alveoli. This results in a reduction of concentration of oxygen since there is also a large concentration of nitrous oxide present. The remedy is to give pure oxygen at the end of, and after anaesthesia.[68]

Alveolar oxygen tension is also reduced when the concentration of carbon dioxide in alveolar gas is increased. Pa_{O_2} and Pa_{CO_2} are linked by the *alveolar air equation:*

$$Pa_{O_2} = Pi_{O_2} - \frac{Pa_{CO_2}}{R}$$

R is the respiratory exchange ratio (usually 0.8). The equation can also be written:

$$Pa_{O_2} = Pi_{O_2} - 1.25 \times Pa_{CO_2}.$$

The relationship between Pa_{O_2} and Pa_{CO_2} is linear, and the line will be shifted if Pi_{O_2} is changed.

2. Anaemic hypoxia. Oxygen-carrying capacity of blood is reduced in proportion to degree of anaemia, although the oxygen tension is normal.

3. Stagnant hypoxia.[69] Two types: (*a*) low cardiac output; and (*b*) local, due to partial or complete vascular occlusion.

4. Histotoxic or cytotoxic hypoxia. Occurs when tissues are unable to utilize the normal supply of oxygen brought to them; seen in cyanide poisoning.

The effects of oxygen lack

For physiological effects of oxygen lack at altitude, *see* Mills F. J. and Harding R. M. *Br. Med. J.* 1983, **286**, 1269. Commercial aircraft are pressurized to between 5000 and 7000 ft (1524–2134 m).

1. The respiratory system. Hyperpnoea is due to reflex stimulation of respiratory centre by chemoreceptors in aortic and carotid bodies, which react to the lowered oxygen tension. The respiratory centre becomes less sensitive to carbon dioxide with increasing hypoxia. Dyspnoea and hyperpnoea are not necessarily indications for oxygen therapy, as both may be seen without hypoxia, just as hypoxia can occur without these symptoms.

2. The cardiovascular system. Coronary systemic and cerebral vasodilatation, with large decreases in afterload, increased cardiac output, stroke volume and tachycardia. Arterial pressure falls in simple hypoxia, but rises if hypercapnia coexists. Effects similar in the anaesthetized and conscious subject. In severe hypoxia, cardiovascular collapse occurs. The ECG: T wave becomes inverted or decreased and there is slowing of conduction and a lengthening of the PR interval. Capillaries lose their tone and their walls allow the leakage of fluid and cells into the tissues. Pulmonary vasoconstriction occurs.

3. The central nervous system. In healthy young men, the oxygen utilization of the brain is 3.3 ml per 100 g of brain/min or about one-fifth of the body's total oxygen consumption. The nervous tissue is more susceptible to oxygen deficiency than any tissue in the body. The blood flow to the brain is increased, an effect also produced by the raised carbon dioxide tension, which is often concurrent. Later, oedema of the brain results from capillary damage. The CSF pressure is increased. Hypotension greatly magnifies the brain-damaging effect of hypoxia. The patient is first restless, then aggressive, then in coma.

4. Kidney. Renal failure.

The effects of inhalation of 100 per cent oxygen[70]

Carbon dioxide. As reduced haemoglobin aids in the transport of carbon dioxide, inhalation of 100% oxygen, by lessening the amount of reduced haemoglobin, interferes with the transport of carbon dioxide, especially if the gas is given at a raised pressure.

Respiration. This is often slightly depressed at first, owing to the removal of the peripheral chemoreceptor stimulation.

Circulation. There is decrease in the pulse rate, as a result of the chemoreceptor effect. Slight increase in diastolic blood pressure. Blood vessels directly constricted (reflexly, via chemoreceptors, dilated), former effect predominating. Cerebral vessels constrict, coronary vessels also constrict, but pulmonary artery dilates, constricting in hypoxia. Very prolonged administration of oxygen may interfere with red-cell formation.

Table 30.1 Results of inhalation of pure oxygen

	Breathing air O_2 21 kPa (159 mmHg)	Breathing 100% oxygen O_2 101 kPa (7600 mmHg)
Alveolar air		
Oxygen tension	13.3 kPa (104 mmHg)	90 kpa (675 mmHg)
Arterial blood		
Oxygen tension	13 kpa (100 mmHg)	85 kPa (637 mmHg)
Oxygen saturation	97%	100%
Oxygen combined with haemoglobin	19.5 ml%	20.1 ml%
Oxygen in solution in plasma	0.3 ml%	1.9 ml%
Total oxygen content	19.8 ml%	22.0 ml%
Mixed venous blood		
Oxygen tension	5.3 kPa (40 mmHg)	7 kPa (52 mmHg)
Oxygen saturation	75%	85%
Oxygen combined with haemoglobin	15.07 ml%	17.19 ml%
Oxygen in solution in plasma	0.12 ml%	0.16 ml%
Total oxygen content	15.19 ml%	17.35 ml%

Arterial blood contains an additional 2.2 vol%, a rise of more than 10% after inhalation of pure oxygen. This represents about 100 ml O_2 transported to the tissues per min or about one-fifth of requirements. Fluorocarbon (Fluosol DA 20%) carries 0.75 ml/ml at 110 kPa[71] (i.e. 7.5 ml/100 ml at FIO_2 100%).

Adverse effects of high oxygen concentrations

In a few patients with chronic bronchitic respiratory failure, respiration is driven by hypoxic drive from peripheral chemoreceptors. Full correction of hypoxia thus reduces repiratory drive, with a rise in arterial PCO_2. CO_2 narcosis may develop with loss of consciousness and ultimately death. The risk of this chain of events is said to be greater when arterial PCO_2 is already above 10 kpa.

Controlled oxygen therapy is required to give enough oxygen to reduce hypoxia, but not enough to remove the respiratory drive. The characteristics of the dissociation curve for haemoglobin are such that a relatively small rise in oxygen tension will result in a relatively large increase in saturation (and oxygen flux) in the middle part of the curve. PaO_2 estimations aid therapy. 'Pink puffers' may be benefited by oxygen.[72]

Intermittent oxygen therapy is particularly dangerous since the increased alveolar CO_2 concentration which may then occur results in an even lower O_2 concentration when the patient breathes air. (*See* the alveolar air equation).

Should oxygen administration, carefully regulated, fail to correct hypoxia without depressing respiration, then IPPV becomes necessary.

Following hypoxia. The oxygen paradox was first described by Ruff and Strughold in 1939. Has subsequently been re-examined by Latham.[73] It is a temporary blackout due to the sudden administration of a high oxygen atmosphere, seen in airmen. If the gas is first inhaled at normal tensions, and later gradually increased, ill effects are not seen.

Retrolental fibroplasia. (There are other causes of this condition.) Neonatal PaO_2 should be kept between 6.5 and 13 kPa by adjusting inspired concentration. Danger exists when PaO_2 remains high for a significant period of time and inspired oxygen concentration should not normally exceed 40%. Doubt has been cast on the relationship of the administration of a high oxygen atmosphere to neonates and retrolental fibroplasia.[74]

Cerebral Oxygen toxicity. Acute oxygen poisoning is manifest as convulsions, the Paul Bert effect.[75] These are similar in nature to idiopathic epilepsy, and do not occur except under hyperbaric conditions (3 atmospheres). The causes have not been fully elucidated, although the incidence appears to be related to an increased cerebral Po_2.

Chronic pulmonary toxicity.[76] May occur when concentrations over 60% are inhaled for prolonged periods at atmospheric pressure. Perhaps due to inactivation of surfactant and damage to pulmonary epithelium. Untoward effects reported[77] include substernal distress, reduction in vital capacity, paraesthesiae, joint pains, anorexia, nausea, contracted visual fields, vomiting, bronchitis and atelectasis, and mental changes.

Chest X-ray changes take the form of bilateral patchy opacities spreading to the whole of the lung fields, with increase of alveolar-arterial Po_2 difference, so that despite high inspired oxygen, Pao_2 may be low. The mechanism of such lung damage by oxygen is uncertain. Suggested effects are: (1) airways closure leading to atelectasis in the absence of nitrogen; and (2) loss of surfactant. It may nevertheless be justified to administer high concentrations of oxygen when Pao_2 cannot be raised to acceptable levels by any other means.

Whereas in a healthy person inspiration of 100% oxygen may be harmful if continued for more than a few hours, 40% can be inhaled indefinitely, with impunity. The crucial level may be the arterial Po_2. Free oxygen radicals are proposed as the causative factor in alveolar damage in these circumstances, by inactivating the antiprotease α_1-antitrypsin of alveolar cells. Leucocytes activated by complement then flood the area giving the typical picture of leucoaggregates and intra-alveolar haemorrhage and exudation.

(*See also* Karsner H. T. *J. Exp. Med.* 1916, **23**, 149 (reprinted in 'Classical File', *Surv. Anesthesiol.* 1972, **16**, 495); Poulton E. C. *Aerospace Med.* 1974, **45**, 482.)

Indications for oxygen therapy

The relief of all forms of hypoxia other than histotoxic. Cardiac output is just as important as arterial oxygen content, in oxygen flux.

1. Cyanosis. Shunts, intracardiac or intrapulmonary, are the only types of hypoxaemia not completely corrected by the inhalation of 100% oxygen.

2. Following major operations,[78] chest wounds or rib fractures. The 35% Ventimask is satisfactory. Regional analgesia lessens hypoxia.[79]

3. In shock, severe haemorrhage and coronary occlusion. The central feature of shock is diminished cardiac output leading to reduction in cellular oxygenation. In shock there is an increase in physiological dead space and a compensatory hyperventilation. Reduction of this hyperventilation by airway obstruction, chest injuries, drugs, etc. may be dangerous. Oxygen administration may prevent this.

4. To decompress distended bowels, reduce surgical emphysema, pneumothorax and air embolism. The gas imprisoned in these cases is 70% nitrogen. Prolonged inhalation of 100% oxygen reduces the nitrogen tension

in the blood, so that the molecules of gas in the tissues diffuse into the blood and are carried away.

5. When metabolic rate is raised, e.g. in thyroid crisis, hyperthermia and shivering, because in these conditions the demand for oxygen is increased.

6. In carbon monoxide poisoning.

7. In the treatment of pneumatosis coli.[80]

8. Preoxygenation before induction of anaesthesia.

9. Chronic respiratory failure treated with domiciliary long-term oxygen therapy (LTOT) usually from an oxygen concentrator. Applied to patients with an FEV_1 less than 1.5 l or $Paco_2$ less than 7.3 kPa (55 mmHg.), especially those with peripheral oedema.[81] For prescribing an oxygen concentrator, *see* Drug Tariff, 1990, Appendix 7. Commercial oxygen is pure enough for inhalation and is much cheaper than medicinal oxygen. Oxygen therapy presents a definite fire hazard.

Inspired oxygen concentration and Pao_2 should be considered together. It is sometimes possible to predict the change in Pao_2 that will occur with changes in FIo_2. Measurement of cardiac output is valuable in conjunction with Pao_2. Or Pvo_2 can be measured directly.

Techniques of administration

The first method of oxygen administration was from a glass funnel held some distance from the face. The first to advocate a closely fitting face-mask was Leonard Hill.[82] Modern oxygen therapy requires separate devices for administering oxygen in high and low concentration.

Oxygen-administration devices can be classified into:[83] (1) fixed-performance system – patient independent; (*a*) high air flow oxygen enrichment (HAFOE) – Ventimasks; (*b*) lower flow – anaesthetic circuits; and (2) variable performance system – patient dependent; (*a*) without rebreathing – catheters and cannulae; (*b*) with rebreathing – MC, Polymask. The former group supply the predetermined oxygen concentration irrespective of the patient's ventilatory parameters. The latter group vary in their performance according to the patient's inspiratory flow-rate and duration of the expiratory pause.

Reservoirs. Use of a reservoir prevents wastage of oxygen but may allow rebreathing with low flows. The T-piece system can be used, the degree of air dilution or rebreathing being determined by flow-rates, tidal volumes and the volume of the expiratory limb. The majority of commercial face-masks may be considered as modifications of the T-piece system, the mask dead space being equivalent to the expiratory limb of the T.

TYPES OF DELIVERY SYSTEM

1. The MC (Mary Catterall) oronasal masks.[84] A plastic cone mask with padded foam to encourage a good fit to the face. A flow of 6 l/min oxygen provides an FIo_2 of about 60%, but there is significant dead space at low flows.

2. Harris mask. Made from stiff semi-translucent plastic with small dead-space volume. FIo_2 approaches 60% with a flow of 6 l/min.

3. Ventimask. An HAFOE device (*see above*). Oxygen is entrained in air on the Venturi principle to provide a concentration of 24, 28 and 35%. The oxygen flow-rates are written on the mask. There is no apparatus dead space. The Venturi[85] method is useful for providing controlled oxygen concentration, such as is required in the treatment of chronic lung disease. It has been shown that the oxygen concentration in the trachea may be up to 5% less than that delivered from the Ventimask, probably due to the addition of water vapour, also when peak flow exceeds the 32 l/min supplied by the 35% mask. The holes in the side of the mask are for breathing out.

4. *Edinburgh mask*. This is a semi-rigid mask designed to give controlled oxygen at low concentrations. At 1 l/min the F_{IO_2} is 25–29%; at 2 l/min 31–35%; at 3 l/min 33–39%.

5. *A nasal catheter*. First used by Arbuthnot Lane in 1907. Accidental rupture of the stomach has been reported following oxygen therapy by nasopharyngeal catheter.[86] A T-piece dipping into 25 cm of water in a vessel is a safety factor and acts as a blow-off if the tip of the catheter slips into the oesophagus.

6. *Plastic nasal 'spectacle' cannulae*.

7. *BLB mask* (Boothby, Lovelace and Bulbulian, 1938).[87] The oronasal and the nasal types.

8. *The portable oxygen apparatus*. E.g. the B.O.C. Portogen.

9. *An oxygen chamber or tent*. This is best for babies and young children, and when prolonged administration is necessary. To enable real benefit to be obtained from a tent, it must be flushed with 10 l/min of oxygen and maintained with a flow of 8 l/min. It gives lower levels of oxygen concentration than the various masks and spectacles.

10. *IPPV. see above*.

Oxygen therapy should be controlled by serial estimations of F_{IO_2} and P_{aO_2} when carried out over a period of days, to prevent use of unnecessarily high concentrations with risk of lung damage. Positive end-expiratory pressure may be advantageous when high inspired concentrations fail to correct arterial hypoxaemia. Pulse oximetry is useful for finding the minimum oxygen required.

Oxygen concentrators

These produce oxygen (94% pure) from room air by the absorption of atmospheric nitrogen on Zeolite (Greek – to seethe) crystals (an aluminosilicate). Two or more absorption tanks are used alternately in each machine, one producing oxygen and the other being purged of nitrogen ready for its next cycle. The smallest machines produce 3 l/min, at a cost of about 3.7 pence/l, slightly more than liquid oxygen and two-thirds of the price of cylinder oxygen.[88] It is possible to provide the needs of a general by oxygen concentrators. Also has uses in underdeveloped countries and for military situations.

Hyperbaric oxygen

Breathing air, 100 ml of plasma will dissolve 0.3 ml of oxygen. For each 13 kpa (100 mmHg) of oxygen tension 0.3 vol% oxygen is dissolved in the plasma. Breathing 100% oxygen, 100 ml of plasma will thus dissolve 2.1 ml of oxygen. Breathing 100% oxygen at 2 atmospheres, 100 ml of plasma will dissolve

4.2 ml of oxygen. Breathing 100% oxygen at 3 atmospheres, 100 ml of plasma will dissolve 6.5 ml of oxygen.

An efficient and rapid method of restoring cellular oxygenation is to give the gas under pressure. At 2 atmospheres pressure, although the oxygen carried as oxyhaemoglobin will only increase by 1 vol%, the gas carried in solution in the plasma rises from 0.3 to 4.2 vol%. The pressure gradient is greatly increased between the arterial and the hypoxic tissue tension and this allows an increased rate of oxygen transport from blood to cells.

Vascular resistance is increased during hyperbaric oxygenation, especially in the brain and pulmonary circulation.

Oxygen at high pressure can be given from a pressure chamber into which patient and attendants enter. The patient then receives oxygen from an ordinary mask and cylinder. A pressure of 2 atmospheres is generally employed.

Decompression is accompanied by a sharp fall in temperature with mist formation due to condensation. This may be uncomfortable for patients and staff. Otherwise the hyperbaric oxygen bed can be used. This consists of a steel chamber with perspex dome in which the patient lies at an oxygen pressure of 2.5 atmospheres. Rate of compression and decompression is controlled from an adjacent console.

Hyperbaric oxygen in medical conditions

(1) In treatment of carbon-monoxide poisoning; (2) in the treatment of infections by anaerobic organisms, e.g. gas gangrene. The growth of aerobic organisms may also be inhibited; (3) in incipient gangrene and frostbite; (4) for topical application in the treatment of pressure-sores and skin ulcers; (5) in purpura fulminans; (6) in burns; (7) acute trauma; (8) in acute ischaemic vasculitis; and (9) acute and chronic sepsis, resistant to orthodox treatment.

Elimination of carbon dioxide

During hyperbaric oxygenation, haemoglobin remains fully saturated, even in the venous blood. The buffering capacity of the blood is not increased by the presence of desaturated haemoglobin. Carbon dioxide is therefore transported in venous blood at a higher cost in terms of Pco_2. Arteriovenous difference in Pco_2 may double. The rise in venous and tissue Pco_2 occurs also at the respiratory centre to give an increase in ventilation. The fall in arterial Pco_2 that results compensates in part for the raised tissue Pco_2 and is probably partly responsible for the cerebral vasoconstriction that occurs with hyperbaric oxygen.

The finding of a significant rise in Pco_2 of the blood during exercise in the hyperbaric chamber has little to do with the above. It is due rather to the increased density of the inhaled gas mixture, and occurs with both air and oxygen under pressure. The resistance to gas flow is such that there is an increase in the work of breathing. The body adapts by lowering alveolar ventilation and allowing a higher Pco_2.

Dangers of hyperbaric oxygen

These include: (1) risk of fires and explosions; (2) 'bends', unless nitrogen has been eliminated; (3) acute oxygen toxicity[89] and convulsions; (4) avascular necrosis of bone; (5) barotrauma ear discomfort; and (6) inflammation of the lungs (Lorraine-Smith effect).

References.

1. Campbell E. M. J. *Br. Med. J.* 1965, **1**, 1451.
2. *See also* MacNee W. *J. R. Soc. Med.* 1985, **78**, 61.
3. Nunn J. F. *Applied Respiratory Physiology* 3rd ed. London: Butterworth, 1987.
4. Clergue F. et al. *Anesthesiology* 1984, **61**, 677.
5. Ali J. et al. *Am. J. Surg.* 1974, **128**, 276.
6. Road J. D. et al. *J. Appl. Physiol.* 1984, **57**, 576.
7. Maeda H. et al. *Am. Rev. Respir. Dis.* 1988, **137**, 678.
8. Wilcox P. et al. *Chest* 1988, 93, 693.
9. Mankikian B. et al. *Anesthesiology* 1988, **68**, 379.
10. Hubmayr R. D., Abel M. D. and Rehder K. *Crit. Care Med.* 1990, **18**, 103.
11. Sherwood Jones E. *Essential Intensive Care.* Lancaster: MTP Press, 1978.
12. *Br. J. Anaesth.* 1990, **64**, 256; Gaudy J. H., Sicard, J. F. and Gateau O. *Acta Anaesthesiol. Scand.* 1990, **34**, 95.
13. Gregg R. W. et al. *Crit. Care Med.* 1990, **18**, 21.
14. Wong D. H., Stemmer E. A. and Gordon A. *Crit. Care Med.* 1990, **18**, 114.
15. Lozewicz S. et al. *Br. Med. J.* 1981, **282**, 1015.
16. Hart G. K. *Intensive Care World* 1990, **7**, 21.
17. Darrell J. H. and Uttley A. H. C. *Br. J. Anaesth.* 1976, **48**, 13.
18. Mithoefer J. C. et al. *Am. Rev. Respir. Dis.* 1978, **117**, 259.
19. Flowers M. W. and Edmondson R. S. *Br. Med. J.* 1980, **1**, 303.
20. Albelda S. M. *Am. Rev. Respir. Dis.* 1983, **127**, 360.
21. Slavin G. et al. *Br. Med. J.* 1982. **285**, 931.
22. Pippin L. K. and Bowes J. B. *Anaesthesia* 1983, **38**, 791.
23. *See also* Atkinson R. S. et al. *Handbook of Intensive Care.* London: Chapman & Hall, 1981, 58.
24. McCelland I. M. A. *Progress in Anaesthesiology.* Amsterdam: Excerpta Medica, 1970, 195.
25. Martine G. *Phil. Trans. R. Soc.* 1730, **36**, 448.
26. Brettonneau P. F. *New Sydenham Soc. (Lond.)* 1859.
27. Hardy R. H. *Accidents and Emergencies.* 2nd ed. Oxford: Oxford University Press, 1978.
28. Björk V. O. *J. Thorac. Cardiovasc. Surg.* 1960, **39**, 179.
29. Magregor I. A. and Neill R. S. *Anaesthesia* 1984, **39**, 718.
30. Hermann G. and Aynesworth M. *J. Lab. Clin. Med.* 1937, **23**, 1244.
31. Raine J. M. *Br. Med. J.* 1981, **1**, 520.
32. Muder R. R. *JAMA* 1983, **249**, 3184
33. Ashbaugh D. G. and Bigelow D. B. *Lancet* 1967, **2**, 319.
34. Klein J. *Anesth. Analg.* 1990, **70**, 195.
35. Wagner P. D. et al. *Clin. Res.* 1976, **24**, 110A.
36. Danzker D. R. et al. *Am. Rev. Respir. Dis.* 1979, **120**, 1039.
37. Pfenninger et al. *J. Paediatr.* 1982, **101**, 352.
38. Nunn J. F. *Applied Respiratory Physiology* 3rd ed. London: Butterworth, 1987.
39. West J. B. *Am. Rev. Respir. Dis.* 1977, **116**, 919.
40. Basran G. S. and Hardy J. G. *J. Thorac. Imag.* 1988, **3**, 28.
41. Viquerat C. E. *Chest* 1983, **83**, 509.
42. Hickling K. G. *Anaesth. Intensive Care* 1986, **14**, 46.
43. Kunkel S. E. and Warner M. A. *Anaesthesiology* 1987, **66**, 195.
44. Domenighetti G. M. et al. *Br. Med. J.* 1984, **288**, 1483.
45. Partinen M. et al. *Br. Med. J.* 1981, **1**, 520.
46. Chin L. S. et al. *Anaesth. Intensive Care* 1979, **7**, 50.

47. Hatch D. J. In: *Recent Advances in Anaesthesia and Analgesia – 15* (Atkinson R. S. and Adams A. P. ed.) Edinburgh: Churchill Livingstone, 1985.
48. Tarnow-Mordi W. O. and Berill A. M. *Br. Med. J.* 1985, **290**, 629.
49. Warner J. A. and Findley W. E. I. *Anaesthesia* 1985, **40**, 348.
50. Duncan P. G. *Can. Anaesth. Soc. J.* 1979, **26**, 206.
51. Barin E. S. et al. *Anaesth. Intensive Care* 1986, **14**, 54.
52. Yardley T. H. *Br. Med. J.* 1985, **290**, 861.
53. Fontanarosa P. B. et al. *J. Emerg. Med.* 1989, **17**(3), 223.
54. Baxter F. J. and Dunn G. L. *Can. J. Anaes.* 1989, **35**, 428.
55. Walden C. A. and Rogers L. F. *J. Comput. Assist. Tomogr.* 1989, **13**, 883.
56. Cox G. J. et al. *Ann. R. Coll. Surg.* 1988, **70**, 361; Baker A. S. and Eavey R. D. *N. Eng. J. Med.* 1986, **314**, 1185.
57. Stanley R. E. and Lliang T. S. *J. Laryngol. Otol.* 1988, **102**, 1017.
58. Report, *Br. Med. J.* 1985, **291**, 329.
59. Scurr C. and Feldman S. A. (ed.) *Scientific Foundations of Anaesthesia* 4th ed. London: Heinemann, 1988; Herrick I. A., Champion L. K. and Froese A. B. *Can. J. Anaesth.* 1990, **37**, 69.
60. Haldane J. S. *Br. Med. J.* 1917, **1**, 181.
61. Van Slyke D. D. and Neill J. M. *J. Biolog. Chem.* 1924, **61**, 523.
62. Flenley D. C. *Lancet* 1967, **1**, 270.
63. Hanning C. D. *Br. J. Anaesth.* 1985, **57**, 359.
64. Nunn J. F. *Anaesthesia* 1987, **42**, iv.
65. Kelman G. R. and Nunn J. F. *Lancet* 1966 **1**, 1400.
66. Barcroft J. *Lancet* 1920, **2**, 485. (1872–1947) (1920).
67. Peters J. P. and van Slyke D. D. *Quantitative Clinical Chemistry*. Baltimore: Williams and Wilkins, 1932, Vol. 2, 579.
68. Fink B. R. *Anesthesiology* 1955, **16**, 511.
69. Barcroft J. *Nature* 1920, **106**, 125.
70. Herrick I. A., Champion L. K. and Froese A. B. *Can. J. Anaesth.* 1990, **37**, 69.
71. Faithfull N. S. *Anaesthesia* 1987, **42**, 234.
72. Woodcock A. A. et al. *Lancet* 1981, **1**, 907.
73. Latham F. *Lancet* 1951, **1**, 77.
74. Flynn J. T. *Anesthesiology* 1984, **60**, 397.
75. Bert, Paul, *La Pression Barométrique*. Paris, 1878.
76. Klein J. *Anesth. Analg.* 1990, **70**, 195.
77. Barach A. L. *Ann. Intern. Med.* 1938, **12**, 454.
78. Fiaccadori E. et al. *Crit. Care Med.* 1989, **17**, 1286.
79. Catley D. M. et al. *Anesthesiology* 1985, **63**, 20.
80. Watson R. D. S. *Br. Med. J.* 1976, **1**, 199.
81. *Drug Ther. Bull.* 1990, **28**, 99.
82. Hill L. *Br. Med. J.* 1912, **1**, 71.
83. Leigh J. M. *Anaesthesia* 1971, **25**, 210.
84. Catterall M. et al. *Lancet* 1967, **1**, 415.
85. 'Venturi and Bernoulli' *Lancet* 1983, **1**, 183
86. Fenton E. N. S. *Br. J. Anaesth.* 1956, **28**, 220, Walstad P. M. and Conklin W. S. *N. Engl. J. Med.* 1961, **264**, 1201.
87. Series of papers, *Proc. Staff Meet. Mayo Clin.* 1938, **13**, 641.
88. *Drug Ther. Bull.* 1982, **20**, 65; Harris C. E. and Simpson P. J. *Anaesthesia* 1985, **40**, 1206; Carter J. A. et al. *Anaesthesia* 1985, **40**, 560
89. Klein J. *Anesth. Analg.* 1990, **70**, 195.

Chapter 31

Resucitation

History[1]

Expired air ventilation has been used throughout history in an effort to revive the apparently dead.[2] Tracheostomy was performed in the twelfth and thirteenth centuries in the treatment of drowned persons. Paracelsus (1493–1541) is usually credited with the introduction of the bellows to ventilate the lungs.

Modern history of resuscitation begins in the middle of the eighteenth century. This was a period when a wave of humanitarianism spread through Europe. A Society for the Recovery of Drowned Persons was founded in Amsterdam in 1767. In Britain the Humane Society, later the Royal Humane Society, was established by William Hawes in 1771. Classic early contributions to the literature include those of John Hunter (1718–1783)[3] in 1776, Kite[4] in 1788 and Herholdt and Rafn.[5]

Artificial ventilation of the lungs was advocated by Marshall Hall (1790–1857)[6] in 1856, the discoverer of reflex action, who described a method of rotating the patient's body combined with pressure on the back to aid expiration. Silvester (1818–1902)[7] described his method in 1858, and Holger Nielsen[8] published details of a new technique in 1932. In the same year Eve (1871–1952) introduced the tilting board method.[9] Artificial respiration by direct laryngeal intubation with a modified O'Dwyer's tube was performed by Rudolph Matas of New Orleans in 1902.[10] In the past four decades positive-pressure ventilation applied to the upper airways has displaced these methods.[11] First use of IPPV in respiratory paralysis by Lassen of Copenhagen in 1952.[12]

Reports of deaths during anaesthesia, in the years following 1846, led to interest in the study of cardiac arrest. The first successful internal cardiac massage was probably performed in Norway in 1901[13] and by Beck in 1947.[14] The first in Britain was reported by Starling (1866–1927)[15] in 1902. Beck[16] successfully defibrillated the human heart in 1937. First external defibrillation of the human heart in 1956.[17] External cardiac compression became popular following the work of Kouwenhoven and others in 1960.[18] Teaching aids in resuscitation are valuable.[19] First successful cardiopulmonary resuscitation outside the operating theatre by Beck in 1956.[20]

Cardiac arrest

Cessation of the heart beat occurs in two entirely different forms: (1) cardiac asystole; and (2) ventricular fibrillation. They can change one to the other, either spontaneously or as a result of treatment.

Asystole. No complex on the ECG.

Ventricular fibrillation. First described by MacWilliam (1857–1937),[21] of Aberdeen. There is a fine or coarse irregular uncoordinated twitching of the heart-muscle fibres. Metabolism continues at about the normal rate. During fibrillation blood pressures of 20–30 mmHg have been observed, but this is due to residual vascular tone and there is no flow of blood.

Causes of cardiac arrest

1. Cardiac disease. Certain forms of cardiac disease are particularly prone to sudden arrest: (*a*) where there is a danger of acute circulatory obstruction (atrial myxoma or ball-valve thrombus with change of posture); (*b*) in fixed output states (tight valvular stenosis, constrictive pericarditis, severe pulmonary hypertension, cardiac tamponade); (*c*) cardiac myopathies; (*d*) myocardial ischaemia; and (*e*) acute myocarditis.

2. Haemorrhage. Massive haemorrhage may cause cardiac arrest due to a fall in coronary perfusion pressure. There is also the danger of hyperkalaemia in massive transfusions of stored blood.

3. Hypoxia. Hypoxia results in: (*a*) tachycardia and rise of blood pressure (sympathetic stimulation) leading to bradycardia, heart block and asystole; (*b*) serum potassium may rise by 50% in 5 min; and (*c*) potentiation of the depressant effects of drugs. The end-result is usually cardiac asystole.

4. Fainting. This may be fatal if the patient is prevented from assuming the horizontal position. There is a danger of this during anaesthesia (e.g. in the dental chair) and in the postoperative period if the patient is sat up in bed.

5. Electrocution.

6. Drowning.

7. Electrolyte changes. Administration of *potassium* ions leads to loss of conductivity, contractility and a decreased threshold to vagal stimulation. Eventually, if given slowly, the heart action ceases in diastole. If given quickly, causes ventricular fibrillation. *Calcium* administration leads to increased contractility, prolongation of systole, shortening of diastole and eventual cardiac arrest in systole. The ratio of potassium to calcium in the blood is important. Rise of serum potassium occurs in anuria, dehydration, diabetic acidosis, drowning in fresh water, extensive tissue breakdown, in transfusion of stored blood, and in hypoxia. Intravenous iron and mercurial diuretics have caused cardiac arrest.

8. Effect of drugs. Has occurred during administration of all anaesthetic agents including the use of local and spinal techniques. Anaesthetic drugs may exert an effect on the heart in a variety of ways: (*a*) direct myocardial depression (specific impairment of contraction of the muscle fibres); (*b*) vagotonic effect; (*c*) sympathetic stimulation; (*d*) increased excitability of ventricular muscle; (*e*) hypotension, especially in patients with inability to increase cardiac output (severe valvular stenosis, heart block, constrictive pericarditis); (*f*) hypoxia as a result of respiratory depression; and (*g*) hypercapnia associated with respiratory depression.

9. *Hypercapnia*. Results in: (*a*) increase of circulating catecholamines; (*b*) increase of serum potassium level; and (*c*) prolongation of the period of asystole induced by vagal stimulation.

In a healthy patient, moderate hypercapnia is well tolerated in the absence of hypoxia.

Sudden hypocapnia after a period of hypercapnia is associated with severe dysrhythmias and even ventricular fibrillation in dogs, the Brown and Miller effect.[22]

In asphyxia there is both hypoxia and hypercapnia.

10. *Hypothermia*.

11. *Acute hypotension*. For example, after central neural blockade.

12. *Cardiac catheterization and angio-cardiography*. Ventricular fibrillation may occur, most likely when the tip of the catheter is in the right ventricle.

13. *Vagal reflex mechanisms*. Sources of stimuli that may provoke bradycardia or asystole include the rectum, uterus and cervix, glottis, bronchial tree, bladder and urethra, mesentery, the carotid sinus, heart, biliary tract, traction on extraocular muscles (especially the medial rectus) and testis. Atropine may prevent them.

14. *Circulating catecholamines*. The heart is more sensitive to adrenaline in the presence of anaesthetic drugs, especially chloroform, cyclopropane, halothane, trichloroethylene and in the presence of myocardial hypoxia. A rise in the blood catecholamine level occurs with injection of adrenaline, anxiety, adrenal tumours and after haemorrhage. Fenfluramine (for obesity) acts as a catecholamine. Discontinuation for 1 week before anaesthesia, has been recommended.[23]

15. *Air embolism and pulmonary embolism*. See Chapter 14.

Diagnosis of cardiac arrest

1. *The pulse*. Inability to palpate any arterial pulsation. It is sometimes impossible to feel a peripheral pulse in the obese, vasoconstricted or shocked patient, even though a circulation to the brain is obviously maintained, since other vital functions are present. Continuous monitoring of the pulse is valuable in rapid diagnosis. The electrocardiogram is useful if it has been giving a continuous record and in the differential diagnosis between asystole and ventricular fibrillation. But normal tracings do not necessarily imply that the circulation is effective. Femoral and carotid pulses are the easiest to feel.

2. *Auscultation of the heart*. Absence of heart sounds.

3. *The pupils*. The pupils dilate, but they may be dilated due to hypoxia, drugs, etc. The intensely constricted pupil (e.g. after morphine) may not dilate at once in cases of arrest. During resuscitation the pupils should be examined frequently. Diminution in size is a most valuable and sensitive sign of effective treatment. If the pupils become smaller within 3 min of the arrest the prognosis is good.

4. *Absence of bleeding*. Venous bleeding may occur and should not be confused with arterial bleeding, which is absent.

5. *Respiration*. Blood flow to the respiratory centres ceases and respiratory arrest occurs, which may be preceded by some irregular gasps, 1–3 min after the cardiac arrest.

6. *Ophthalmoscopy*. The veins of the fundus show segmentation of the blood column.

7. *General appearance of the patient*. Cyanosis occurs and there are no signs of a circulation. In other cases pallor is present.

The effects of cardiac arrest on the brain

1. Unconsciousness supervenes in about 15 s.
2. EEG changes occur in 4 s and the tracing is flat within 20–30 s.
3. The Po_2 of cerebral blood falls to 2.5 kPa at the time consciousness is lost. Tissue $Pflo_2$ falls to zero within 1 min.
4. Histological changes.[24] Diffuse neuronal damage is not restricted to any particular vascular territory of the brain. Petechial haemorrhages also occur. Brain damage may be diffuse or focal. The mildest structural damage is selective neuronal necrosis, but with more severe hypoxia neuroglial cells are also affected and areas of infarction may arise.

Barbiturates were formerly thought to aid brain resuscitation after hypoxia[25] but this has been questioned.[26]

Cardiopulmonary rescuscitation (CPR)[27]

The person who should treat cardiac arrest is the person immediately available. There are two vital factors that must be accomplished quickly if adequate cerebral circulation is to be restored: *pulmonary ventilation* and *cardiac compression*.

Procedure recommended:[28] The Revised Recommendations of the Resuscitation Council suggest: AIRWAY. If the patient is unresponsive make sure the airway is clear. BREATHING. If there is no breathing, institute artificial respiration, by mouth to mouth or bag and mask, with oxygen if available. CIRCULATION. If there is no palpable pulse start cardiac compression. At the same time call for HELP. This should include defibrillator, apparatus for maintaining the airway, oxygen and the emergency kit as well as the cardiac arrest team. An ECG monitor should be attached as soon as possible. A large vein should be cannulated.

If the ECG shows *ventricular fibrillation* the following sequence is recommended: (*a*) defibrillation 200 J repeated; (*b*) then if needed 360 J; (*c*) then try adrenaline 1 mg i.v.; (*d*) then defibrillation 360 J; (*e*) then lignocaine 100 mg i.v.; and (*f*) then repeated defibrillation 360 J. If there is a poor result consider: different paddle positions, a different defibrillator and other antiarrythmic drugs.

If the ECG shows *electro-mechanical dissociation* adrenaline 1 mg is given i.v. The diagnosis of hypovolaemia, pneumothorax, tamponade and pulmonary embolus must be excluded. Administration of calcium chloride, 10 ml of 10% solution should be considered, especially if there is hyperkalaemia, hypocalcaemia or the previous administration of calcium antagonists.

If the ECG shows apparent *asystole*: if ventricular fibrillation can be excluded, adrenaline 1 mg i.v. and atropine 2 mg i.v. may be given and pacing considered if P waves or other electrical activity is present. If ventricular fibrillation cannot be excluded there should be three attempts at cardioversion (200, 200, 360 J) first. After any drug is given CPR should be continued for up to 2 min and should not be interrupted for more than 10 s. Should it prove imposible to establish an intravenous line, consider giving double doses of adrenaline, lignocaine or atropine via an endotracheal tube. When resuscitation is prolonged adrenaline 1 mg i.v. is recommended every 5 min. This is an attempt to maintain cerebral and myocardial perfusion pressure. Sodium bicarbonate is now less fashionable, but 50 mmol (50 ml of 8.4%) may be given provided carbon dioxide is eliminated by artificial ventilation and may be monitored by blood gas results.

Post resuscitation care will include measurements of arterial blood gases and electrolytes, and chest X-ray. The patient will be monitored and nursed in an intensive care environment.

Clinical signs of cerebral hypoxia. These may follow either an acute hypoxic episode after cardiac standstill or a prolonged period of suboxygenation. Recovery may occur after the episode and the patient may regain consciousness after resuscitation, but may relapse into coma later. Respiration is gasping and stertorous and may be accompanied by a tracheal tug. There may be sweating, hyperpyrexia, dilated pupils and a coarse nystagmus. There may be restlessness, rigidity, choreo-athetosis or fits and twitching. These may progress to deepening coma, periodic breathing, tachycardia and death.

Treatment. The following measures may be required. Dehydration with use of hypertonic intravenous fluids to reduce cerebral oedema. Dexamethasone. Reduction of body temperature by surface cooling, if raised; there is doubt whether hypothermia is useful in the absence of hyperpyrexia. Elevation of the head. Support of the circulation, physiotherapy, antibiotics, tracheostomy and IPPV to maintain $Paco_2$ of 3.5 kPa (25 mmHg).

Prediction of awakening after cardiac arrest

A reasonably accurate prognosis can be made,[29] based on the following variables: the arrest was witnessed; resuscitation was started immediately; the first observed ECG was asystole; spontaneous eye movements were present; pupil light reflex was present; corneal reflex was present; the heart responded in less than 2.5 min by reasonable pulse and arterial pressure; normothermia; and arterial blood gases rapidly returned to normal.

Drowning (the immersion incident)[30]

About 700 fatalities from drowning occur in the UK every year, about a quarter in the sea. There are pathophysiological differences between fresh and salt water drowning, although these are largely of academic interest since survivors who reach hospital need similar therapeutic measures in both situations.

Fresh water

Due to the difference in osmotic pressure, water passes rapidly from the lungs to the general circulation. There may be a 50% increase in circulatory volume within 3 min. This results in haemolysis, and ventricular fibrillation, resistant to treatment, which occurs at an early stage. The heart is submitted to hypoxia, overfilling, potassium excess and sodium deficit. The clinical features can be demonstrated readily in animals, but there is evidence that the haemodilution is much less in man, and it is possible that some other factor may be operative. The prognosis is poor.

Salt water

The osmotic effect is exerted in the opposite direction. Fluid passes out from the circulation into the alveoli to produce pulmonary oedema. In practice, fresh and salt water drowning are clinically very similar.

Vagal inhibition

Death from vagal inhibition can occur without entrance of fluid into the lungs. Or vagal inhibition may prevent fluid entering the lungs for several minutes. Prompt resuscitation is likely to be successful in this type of case.

Other effects

Drowning is likely to be complicated by: (1) hypothermia (see also Chapter 14); (2) acute pulmonary oedema; (3) respiratory distress syndrome; (4) pulmonary infection; and (5) cerebral oedema (not a common complication).[31]

Monitoring

Temperature, blood pressure, pulse, blood-gases, chest auscultation, venous filling, CVP, and even intracranial pressure and cerebral perfusion pressure.[32]

Treatment

Speed is vital. Experiments in Denmark on cadavers suggest that the lungs cannot be emptied by posture, and that regurgitation from the stomach does not occur except with inflation pressures greater than 25 cmH$_2$O. Treatment should consist of: (1) very quick efforts to clear the mouth and pharynx of debris and efforts to drain the lungs in salt water drowning; (2) artificial ventilation, mouth-to-mouth, mouth-to-nose or by means of an apparatus, if possible while the subject is still in the water; (3) external cardiac compression; (4) administration of pure oxygen as soon as practicable and transfer to hospital; (5) treatment of hypothermia, if present, by rapid rewarming in water at 37°C and intravenous glucose and steroid administration; (6) tracheal intubation and IPPV if indicated; (7) chest X-ray, blood and urine analysis, blood-gas estimation and intensive therapy as indicated; (8) 1 l of quadruple strength human albumin solution infused rapidly i.v.; and (9) don't give up easily.

Prognosis

Better after immersion in salt water than in fresh water. Recovery unlikely if the lungs have been flooded with fresh water for a period of over 2 min owing to the rapid circulatory changes with irreversible ventricular fibrillation. Hypothermia may, however, exert a protective effect, and when a cold subject is rescued from the water, resuscitation should always be attempted, even when no sign of life is apparent. Survival can occur after 18 min cardiac arrest.[33] Severe near-drowning is defined as requiring cardiopulmonary resuscitation in hospital. Survival of this is around 14%.[31]

See also Baskett P. J. F. *Br. J. Anaesth*. 1992, **69**, 182. For training, *see* Bristow A. et al. *Resuscitation and Training*. London: Farrand Press, 1990.

References

1. *See also* Hawkins L. H. *Br. J. Hosp. Med*. 1970, **4**, 495; *History of Resuscitation*, Little D. M. 'Classical File', *Surv. Anesthesiol*. 1981, **25**, 415; ABC of resuscitation, *Br. Med. J*. 1986, **292**, 1002, 1123, 1257 and 1316; McLellan I. *Anaesthesia* 1981, **36**, 307; Wilkinson D. J. In: 'A History of Anaesthesia' (Atkinson R. S. and Boulton T. B. ed.) London: Royal Society of Medicine, 1989, 348; and Huston K. G. *ibid*, 352.
2. Holy Bible, 2 Kings iv. 34–35.
3. Hunter J. *Phil. Trans*. 1776, **66**, 412.
4. Kite C. *An Essay on the Recovery of the Apparently Dead*. London: Dilly, 1788.
5. Herholdt J. D. and Rafn C. G. *Life Saving Measures for Drowning Persons*. Copenhagen, 1796 (Reprinted by Scandinavian Society of Anaesthesiologists, 1960, Aarhus).
6. Marshal Hall M. *Lancet* 1856, **1**, 229; Ellis R. *Lancet* 1868, **2**, 538.
7. Silvester H. R. *Br. Med. J*. 1858, **2**, 576.
8. Nielsen H. *Ugeskr. Laeg*. 1932, **94**, 1201.
9. Eve F. C. *Lancet* 1932, **2**, 995.
10. Matas R. *Am. Med*. 1902, **3**, 97 (reprinted in 'Classical File', *Surv. Anesthesiol*. 1978, **22**, 401.
11. Safar P. *JAMA* 1958, **167**, 335.
12. Lassen H. C. A. *Lancet* 1953, **1**, 37.
13. Keen W. W. *Ther. Gaz*. 1904, **28**, 217.
14. Beck C. S. et al. *JAMA* 1947, **135**, 985.
15. Starling E. A. *Lancet* 1902, **2**, 1397 (reprinted in 'Classical File', *Surv. Anesthesiol*. 1975, **19**, 497).
16. Beck C. S. and Mautz F. R. *Ann. Surg*. 1937, **106**, 525.
17. Zoll P. M. and Paul M. H. *Circulation* 1956, **14**, 745.
18. Kouwenhoven W. B. et al. *JAMA* 1960, **173**, 1064.
19. Woolam C. H. M. *Br. J. Clin. Equip*. 1979, **4**, 182; Eaton J. M. *Br. J. Hosp. Med*. 1984, **31**, 67.
20. Beck C. S. et al. *JAMA* 1956, **161**, 434.
21. MacWilliam J. A. *J. Physiol. Lond*. 1887, **8**, 291; *Br. Med. J*. 1889, **1**, 6.
22. Brown F. B. and Miller F. *Am. J. Physiol*. 1952, **169**, 56.
23. Bennett J. A. and Eltringham R. J. *Anaesthesia* 1977, **32**, 8.
24. Adams J. H. *Br. J. Anaesth*. 1975, **47**, 121.
25. Rockoff M. A. and Shapiro H. M. *Anesthesiology* 1978, **49**, 385.
26. Gisvold S. E. et al. *Anesthesiology* 1984, **60**, 88.
27. *See also* Report of Joint Cardiology Committee. *Br. J. Hosp. Med*. 1985, **53**, 477; and Br. Med. J. 1989, **299**, 446.

28. Chamberlain D. *Br. Med. J.* 1989, **299**, 446; Wendon J. and Bihari D. J. In: *Recent Advances in Anaesthesia and Analgesia – 17* (Atkinson R. S. and Adams A. P.) Edinburgh: Churchill Livingstone, 1991.
29. Longstreth W. T. et al. *N. Engl. J. Med.* 1983, **308**, 1378.
30. Orlowski P. *Crit. Care Med.* 1978, **6**, 94; Conn A. W. et al. *Can. Anaesth. Soc. J. 1978*, **25**, 259; Golden F. S. *Br. J. Hosp. Med.* 1980, **23**, 371.
31. Oakes D. D. *J. Trauma* 1982, **22**, 544.
32. Nussbaum E. and Galant S. P. *J. Pediatr.* 1983, **102**, 215.
33. Singh S. V. *J. R. Soc. Med.* 1980, **73**, 292.

Chapter 32

Trauma and multiple injuries[1]

The involvement of the anaesthetist in trauma varies widely from continent to continent, and even from centre to centre in a locality. Much of this involvement depends on personal enthusiasm and remuneration. It is therefore difficult to transpose models from one place to another, and this chapter offers the description of features that have worked in some places. Some trauma units are run by anaesthetists, whereas in others they may only be called specifically for providing anaesthesia.

Management of advanced trauma[2]

Organization at the site of small and major accidents

1. Initial reporting of a disaster to local emergency services.[3] (a) General: site, area, extent of damage to existing structures; and (b) medical: number of dead, number of injured, nature of injuries.

2. First-aid treatment of multiple trauma at the accident site.[4] Some of those severely injured in accidents die from respiratory obstruction, so it is essential to establish a clear airway and adequate oxygenation as a first priority in the unconscious subject. (*Airway, Breathing* and *Circulation* are the three primary priorities.) This includes placing these patients on their side in anticipation of the first vomit (with the greatest care until it can be proved that the spinal column is not injured). Urgent tracheal intubation may be required, in addition pain relief and experienced triage. Disasters have been categorized for scale.[5] Triage includes: Primary survey: categorizing victims for priority and type of evacuation, e.g. the 6-category triage, which includes priority 1 life-threatening but saveable; priority 2 serious injury but stable and can wait a little; priority 3 non-walking wounded; priority 4 walking wounded; priority 5 life-threatening but unsaveable (e.g. high velocity head injury); and priority 6 dead:

Other history and examination protocols for priority 1 and 2 patients include a fall of more than 20 feet; a pedestrian or cyclist hit by a motor vehicle, ejection from vehicle, death of passenger in same vehicle; vehicular impact at >20 mph; physiological parameters in adults include systolic pressure <90 mmHg, pulse >120 bpm, and respiratory rate >30 or <10/min; persistent unconsciousness; suspected cervical spine injury;

penetrating injury of abdomen or thorax, flail chest (the chest and abdomen should be exposed at this initial survey); fractures of more than 2 long bones; and burns > 15% or of face or airway.

3. 'Category' triage with scoring systems:

	Value	Code	Score
A. Respiratory rate	10–24	4	
	25–35	3	
	> 36	2	
	1–9	1	
	0	0	A = ………
B. Respiratory effort	normal/retractive	1	
	none	0	B = ………
C. Systolic pressure	> 90	4	
	70–89	3	
	50–69	2	
	0–49	1	
	0	0	C = ………
D. Capillary refill	normal	2	
	delayed	1	
	none	0	D = ………

E. Glasgow Coma Score

Eye opening		TOTAL CGS SCORE		
spontaneous	4		14–15	5
to voice	3		11–13	4
to pain	2		8–10	3
none	1		5–7	2
			3–4	1

Verbal response		
orientated	5	
confused	4	E = ………
inappropriate words	3	
incomprehensible	2	
none	1	

Motor response	
obeys commands	6
localizes pain	5
withdrawal on pain	4
flexion on pain	3
extension on pain	2
none	1

TRAUMA SCORE = A+B+C+D+E

Survival is about 99% for a score of 16 – walking wounded: priority 3
90% for a score of 12 – treat and transport: priority 2
50% for a score of 8 – treat and transport: priority 1
10% for a score of 4 – treat and transport: immediate priority 1

Figure 32.1 Trauma score (trauma index)[6] assessment of general physiological stability

Revised trauma score is based on the systolic pressure, respiratory rate and Glasgow Coma Scale. It is inaccurate in the phase of physiological compensation ('Golden Hour').

Assessment of injury priority in children is always a problem and they tend to get high priority.

Shock index (SI)[7] is the pulse rate divided by the systolic pressure and relates to haemorrhage, being about 0.5 with no blood loss to 1.5 in major blood loss. Mortality was 40% with SI >1.2 and 20% at <1.2.

SI is inversely related to left ventricular stroke work. It fails to take account of other, especially painful injuries.

Triss scoring[8] (*See* trauma score above.)

Abbreviated injury scale (AIS).[9]

Direction of evacuation: The victims are dispersed to as many hospitals in the area as possible to avoid overloading any one. The most easily accessible hospital may not be the nearest one. Hospitals may have to be set up in refugee camps.

Timing of evacuation: A complex equation, e.g. where high priority wounded will take long to extricate (e.g. train crashes), walking wounded may be moved first. Protection of casualties from the elements is important.

Cardiopulmonary cerebral resuscitation (CPCR) and life supporting first aid (LSFA)

1. *Basic Trauma Life Support (BTLS).*

   (*a*) Airway – extend head, open and clear mouth, lift jaw, insert airway or intubate, etc.

   (*b*) Breathing – mouth to mouth, manual bag-mask, or ventilator. Oxygen if available.

   (*c*) Circulation – pressure control of external haemorrhage, elevate legs (or MAST pants), cardiac massage.

2. *Advanced Trauma Life Support (ATLS), Advanced Cardiac Life Support (ACLS).*

   (*a*) Drugs and i.v fluids.

   (*b*) ECG monitoring.

   (*c*) Defibrillation if indicated.

3. *Prolonged Life Support (PLS).*

   (*a*) Measurement of trauma score.

   (*b*) Cerebral resuscitation.

   (*c*) Intensive care organ support.

Head injured patients, especially children, have cervical support (collar, sandbags, Hines splint, etc.) until proof of cervical stability.[10]

Field equipment

Box, bag or rucksac. Intravenous fluids, of value even days after the event,[11] crystalloids, colloids, and include group-compatible blood if ready-grouped donors are available, i.e. 'blood on the hoof.' Cannulas, bandages, support splints, etc. Airways and tracheal tubes, larygoscopes, self-inflating ventilation bags. Drugs: analgesics, opioids,[12] especially nalbuphine 20–30 mg in spring-loaded self-administration syringes (and naloxone to differentiate opioid stupor from head injury coma), ketamine with midazolam.[13] Entonox, sublingual buprenorphine, atropine, ephedrine, local analgesics; syringes, needles. Triservice apparatus and foot-operated sucker for the field hospital. Oxygen, portable oxygen concentrator,[14] with thiopentone, etomidate, halothane, tricloroethylene, vecuronium. Sterilizing system for tracheal tubes, etc.

A TIVA technique has been described;[15] midazolam 5 mg, ketamine 200 mg, vecuronium 12 mg in 50 ml saline, infused at 0.5 ml/kg/h. The mixture is stable for at least 24 h and finds special application in a theatre closed down against chemical weapon attack.

Organization in the accident reception centre

The *major accident plan* is activated. The appointed 'controllers' (medical, theatres, nursing, administrative, and triage officer) are informed, and all resident staff alerted, including medical records staff, porters, mortuary technician, and chaplains. Each reports to the control room for identity and action cards. Non-resident staff are informed by private telephone (i.e. not via the hospital switchboard). If the accident site calls for a mobile team (surgeon, anaesthetist, house officer, nurses) these pick up clothing and equipment and are dispatched. Each staff member has a designated and defined job.

Disaster equipment is packaged and labelled ready for use. Resuscitation is a highly valuable skill.[16] Ketamine has a place in anaesthetic management of painful treatments, at the site, or in the accident department, when more usual methods are overwhelmed by numbers or unavailable for other reasons. Clinical monitoring assumes greater importance, but genuinely portable instrumental monitoring can be helpful.

Secondary triage is undertaken. Takeover of other hospital areas and facilities is planned and agreed in advance (the emergency medicine 'buffer ward' is useful in accidents of small numbers. Ventilation facilities in the Intensive Care Unit are planned to be expandable in equipment personnel and space.

Head injury is common and should always be considered. Treatment of treatable head injury (especially an adequate supply of oxygenated blood flow) takes priority over most other considerations.

A simple scheme for remembering priorities is:

1. *Airway* – is it clear?
2. *Breathing* – is it adequate?
3. *Circulation* – nearly always improved by setting up an infusion immediately, and by stopping haemorrhage by simple pressure.

Most patients are reasonably stable for the first hour after injury, and their vital organs will regain function if resuscitation is instituted in this period ('the Golden Hour'). After this time, decompensation and organ failure is progressively more common. Patients intoxicated with alcohol[17] are more likely to have full stomachs, brain injuries, inhaled vomit, and hypotension.[18]

Analgesia is important. In war injuries, infusion of pentazocine relieves pain efficiently, but in the presence of hypotension or respiratory depression, ketamine is superior.[19] Self- or 'buddy'-injected morphine, or, more recently, nalbuphine is used at military trauma sites. Surprisingly, opioids have not been found to obscure signs of head injury in these situations, but the problem of 'pooling' in the muscle of shocked patients still exists, with massive release during resuscitation.

ARDS and MSOF may develop within hours or days. Whether it does or not is partly dependent on whether sepsis can be prevented. In military, high velocity and explosive injuries, special techniques are used, since this type of trauma will disperse bacteria far into normal-looking tissue planes. Exteriorization of damaged areas of bowel, and wide amputation of limbs may be necessary for this. Maximization of oxygen delivery is also important.[20]

Breaking bad news to relatives requires skill and sensitivity,[21] and the help of hospital chaplains.

Chest injuries[22]

Respiration is embarrassed should bleeding occur into the airway or into the pleural cavity. Blood clot, saliva, stomach content and other debris may be inhaled to produce suffocation. The flail chest embarrasses physiological ventilatory exchange as some degree of paradoxical respiration occurs. Pain from fractured ribs may also prevent proper excursion of the diaphragm and thoracic cage. Pain relief without respiratory depression is thus important. Up to a quarter of these patients require IPPV, one-fifth are severely shocked and about a third will have other (especially head) injuries. In major thoracic injury the first priority is to treat hypoxia and hypovolaemia. In some cases, IPPV will be required[22] and subsequent chest infection is common in these patients.

Other thoracic injuries that may require treatment include haemothorax (which requires drainage), pneumothorax (requiring intercostal tube to waterseal), chylothorax, direct lung trauma, diaphragmatic rupture, or injury to heart and great vessels. Bronchial tears may give rise to large leaks requiring negative pressure to intercostal drains. They usually heal in time. If air enters the mediastinum the whole body may become bloated with surgical emphysema. (Thoracic stabbing is a particularly difficult problem, often requiring emergency surgery.) Early CVP measurement is helpful in detecting concealed haemorrhage and cardiac tamponade.

Crush injury of the chest

This may cause painful breathing or subsequent hypoxia and cardiorespiratory embarrassment. Injury (and operation) to the chest wall is likely to interfere with the patient's ability to rid the tracheobronchial tree of secretions. Pulmonary contusion is common.

To help the patient to breathe and cough, extradural block via an indwelling catheter in the thoracic region is invaluable. Intercostal and interpleural[23] block may also be helpful. A patent airway must be maintained using suction, endotracheal intubation or tracheostomy. The control of paradoxical movements of the chest wall may be managed by IPPV. Surgical fixation using Rush nails has also been advocated in suitable cases as the patient becomes mobile in a shorter time.

Cardiac injury may coexist and has been diagnosed by single photon-emission computed tomography.[24] For outcome of chest injury, *see* Moore P. C. et al. *Anaesth. Intensive Care* 1985, **13**, 362.

Head injuries[25]

(*See also* Chapter 22, Neurosurgery).

Responsible for two-thirds of trauma deaths in hospital, up to half ITU occupancy, and a third of scans.

Pathophysiology. Primary injury results from impact; secondary injury from bleeding in the brain, and oedematous swelling of undamaged brain after impact; and tertiary injury from compression due to oedema around a haematoma or pressure from outside, e.g. subdural haematoma.[26]

Monitoring. Clinical, instrumental, e.g. cerebral function monitor, (twin scalp electrodes, amplitude normally $5-15\mu V$) and intracranial pressure monitoring.

It is vital that proper oxygenation of the brain is maintained. Primary efforts should therefore be directed to maintenance of the airway and adequate pulmonary ventilation, arrest of any serious haemorrhage and maintenance of an adequate blood circulation. The brain may be damaged by contusion, haemorrhage, local or global ischaemia, with diffuse axonal injury,[27] hypoxia (low Pao_2), very low $Paco_2$ or very low BP, hyperthermia, alkalosis, oedema due to fluid overload or embolism. Blood loss from scalp wounds can be significant, so that transfusion is required. Uncomplicated head injury should not prevent the treatment of abdominal injuries, compound limb fractures or haemothorax, although faciomaxillary fractures can usually be left to a later date. Astrocytes and endothelial cells appear to protect against cerebral oedema, and these cells may be spared, even when ischaemia has damaged neurones. Hyperglycaemia (and hypoglycaemia) increases the infarction associated with ischaemia, especially with brain lactate levels above 16 mmol/kg.[28]

Middle meningeal haemorrhage

This is the most frequent serious remediable head injury and requires urgent operation.

The most important physical signs are: (1) progressive deterioration of consciousness; (2) progressive dilatation of a previously normal pupil; (3) progressive bradycardia, perhaps with a rising systolic blood pressure; (4) progressive weakness of the face, arm and even leg on the side opposite to the injury; and (5) apnoea, which carries the gravest prognosis, even when instantly remedied by IPPV.

Management of head injuries[29]

1. First aid, airway management and avoiding delays in treament. Lateral position in anticipation of vomiting, control of haemorrhage, speedy hospitalization, with neck support (and in some centres, intubation and IPPV).

2. Clinical diagnosis of injuries (*see above*) – is the head injury localized or diffuse? Glasgow coma scale[30] recording is established and an agreed flow chart commenced. Skull, cervical spine and chest X-rays may be taken.[31]

Other injuries are treated, especially haemorrhage. CVP measurements may be needed (in many head injuries, the neck is also damaged, and not suitable for inserting CVP lines). Note that muscle relaxants and sedatives in head injury make the clinical diagnosis of other injuries more difficult, and extra use may have to be made of scans.

3. Reduction of raised intracranial pressure by intubation, IPPV, etc. Prevention of coughing and vomiting is an important component of this. Mannitol may be needed, producing at least part of its effect by reducing blood viscosity and thereby increasing cerebral blood flow without dilating cerebral vessels. The value of steroids is in doubt. Hyperventilation is advocated in the management of head injuries. The cerebral vasoconstriction, which results in normal brain tissue from hypocapnia, may lead to increased blood supply to the damaged areas.[45]

4. Evaluation of extent of injury, by CT scan,[32] NMR, isotope scans, etc.

5. Control of clinical or subclinical fits, as shown on the EEG, by barbiturates or benzodiazepines. Sedation reduces the ICP, provided that pulmonary ventilation is maintained. Propofol is useful for sedation and control of seizures[33] but there is a risk of reducing arterial pressure.

6. Monitoring of cerebral function within the controlled neurosurgical environment, by intracranial pressure, using the moving diaphragm with fibreoptic light system, and compliance (and ICP waveform analysis), EEG and cerebral function monitoring, brainstem auditory evoked potentials (BSAEP), spinal evoked potentials, cerebral blood flow, cerebral oxygen consumption ($CMRO_2$) – normally 3–4 ml/100 g/min, cerebral arteriovenous oxygen difference (A-JDO_2) – normally 6–7 vol%, phosphorus spectroscopy, positron emission tomography, etc. The cerebral function monitor should produce a waveform between 5–15 µV. A fall below 5 µV may indicate reduced cerebral perfusion, and the need for inotropes.

7. Brain protection.[34] This includes: (*a*) speed of resuscitation; (*b*) use of adrenaline to raise perfusion pressure. Cerebral blood flow is often below 20% of normal during cardiac massage,[35] unless adrenaline is used to raise arterial pressure. Adrenaline does not appear to raise $CMRO_2$; (*c*) moderate hypothermia; (but care is needed to maintain insulin levels and thus glucose supply); (*d*) Thiopentone (once discredited[36] but now revived), provided that the blood pressure and cerebral blood flow can be maintained during its use, e.g. by adrenaline, dobutamine etc. (*e*) calcium channel blockers, e.g. nimodipine and N-type presynaptic calcium channel blockers;[37] (*f*) 21-aminosteroid lipid peroxidase inhibitor, U-74 006F;[38] and (*g*) lignocaine, phenytoin, etomidate, prostacyclin, naloxone, ATP, magnesium chloride, plasmapheresis and cardiopulmonary bypass have all been tried.

8. Prevention of rises of ICP caused by phenoperidine, reversal of benzodiazepine sedation by flumazenil and chest physiotherapy.

9. Managing the reperfusion phenomenon by antagonizing oxygen radicals and tissue damage mediators, e.g. with indomethacin 30 mg/kg/hr. *See also* Chapter 33.

10. General intensive care. Early enteral feeding, H_2 blockers, and antacids prevent gastric ulceration.[39] Cholecystitis may complicate head injuries,[40] as may pulmonary damage, due to increased alveolar cholesterol.[41]

Concurrent hypoxia due to pulmonary problems adversely influences the outcome, as does the existence of sepsis, even as trivial as paranasal sinusitis.

Calcium channel blockers may improve cerebral blood flow in the head-injured patient.[42] The long-term effects of head injury can seldom be assessed at the time of admission to the intensive therapy unit. In general the younger the patient the better is the prognosis. Recovery may be complete or partial. Social and personality problems may arise subsequently.

    11. Transfer to neurosurgical units.

Transportation of neurosurgical patients[43]

    1. The airway is secured by tracheal intubation, or facilities are carried for this if the patient is conscious. Oxygen and a self-inflating bag are kept alongside the patient.[44] Intubated patients are normally paralysed and ventilated during transport.

    2. One or two intravenous cannulae are in place before leaving. A pressure infusor will be required because of the limited head-room for elevation of the fluid container.

    3. Recording blood pressure, pulse oximetry and pulse rate is very difficult. Occasional stops may be necessary. The ECG is monitored continuously.

    4. The doctor and nurse are advised to take travel sickness pills.

    5. The following drugs should be carried: atropine, barbiturate, e.g. thiopentone, suxamethonium, ephedrine, dexamethasone and diuretics. CPR equipment must be to hand.

Prognosis

Prognosis after head injury is related to CSF enzyme levels. A CPK level > 150 units/l and LDHi > 150 units/l both carry a bad prognosis.[46] Of those patients in coma for 6 h or more, mortality is up to 40%. In patients more than 40 years old, mortality is up to 70%.[47]

Most head injuries are in the low risk category (mortality $= 10\%$) and respond to the conventional care outlined above. In the severe head injury group, the problem is how to avoid inappropriate treatment. Prognostic decisions can be made in about half the head injury cases on arrival at hospital, and the patients and relatives may be informed of their rights to a living will and powers of attorney for health decisions (in the USA).

Brainstem death[48]

First described clinically in 1959.[49]

For this diagnosis *all* the following signs must be present, in addition to a clear diagnosis of the underlying condition, for at least 12 h: pupils have no response to light; oculovestibular reflex absent[50] (there should be no wax in the ear; the 'doll's-eye reflex' does not mean that there is brain death; corneal reflex absent; gag reflex absent; carinal reflex absent; no response to pain inflicted on head; and no spontaneous respiration for 4 min[51] in the absence of hypothermia, and anoxia, with an adequate (> 6.6 kPa) $Paco_2$ provided that no drugs which affect these reflexes persist in the body. PEEP is useful here.[52] EEG confirmation is useful but opinions vary concerning its necessity. Such a diagnosis is made by two doctors independently. It should be noted that spinal reflexes may persist after brain death.

(*See also* Annotation, *Br. Med. J.* 1982, **285**, 1487; Pallis C. *Br. Med. J.* 1983, **286**, 123; Editorial, Jennett B. *Br. J. Anaesth.* 1981, **53**, 111; Pallis C. (ed.) *ABC of Brain Stem Death*. London: BMA, 1985.)

Spinal column injuries

The utmost care is necessary during transport and movement.[53]

Early management

Should tracheal intubation be necessary to procure a patent airway, the production of muscle relaxation with suxamethonium may remove the protective splinting provided by the support muscles allowing subluxation and cord damage.[54] This is prevented by stiff cervical collars (e.g. Philadelphia), some of which have opening front flaps for cricoid pressure. The most dangerous neck movement is flexion. The Bullard laryngoscope has been designed for this situation. Emergency cricothyrotomy may be needed.

(*See also* Swain A et al. *Br. Med. J.* 1985, **291**, 1558.)

Abdominal injuries

All penetrating wounds of the abdomen require laparotomy. The signs of intra-abdominal trauma may be misleading in the presence of other injuries, but an accurate diagnosis should not be necessary in making the decision to perform laparotomy. CAT scanning is useful but may waste valuable time.

Blood transfusion

This will often be required where there are multiple injuries. An estimate of blood loss from fractures can be made as follows: humerus 500–1000 ml; radius and ulna, 500 ml; pelvis, over 3000 ml; femur, 500–2000 ml; and tibia and fibula, 500–1000 ml.[55] Monitoring of central venous pressure is routine in these cases, and a blood volume estimation carried out later as a check on the adequacy of replacement. Estimated or measured blood loss of 20% of blood volume is an indication for transfusion (*see* Chapter 17).

Fat embolism

This was first described in man by Friedrich Albert Zenker (1825–1898) in 1862,[56] was first diagnosed clinically by von Bergmann (1836–1907) in 1873,[57] and may be wrongly diagnosed as shock. Due to escape of droplets of fat into the circulation, and their deposition in the lungs, brain or skin. Often associated with fractures of lower-limb bones. Onset of symptoms may rapidly follow the injury or may be delayed for 2 or 3 days.

Pulmonary signs and symptoms include dyspnoea, pallor, cyanosis, pyrexia and frothy sputum. Bilateral shadowing is seen in chest X-rays. Fat globules may be seen in sputum and urine.

Cerebral changes (really signs of cerebral hypoxia) usually seen in the first 24 h after operation or injury, with pyrexia, and there may be restlessness, leading to coma, convulsions and paralysis; deep coma carries a bad prognosis; fat emboli may sometimes be seen in the retinal vessels with an ophthalmoscope.

Skin signs are likely to be a purpuric eruption with petechiae over the upper chest, neck and conjunctivae and are seen on the second or third day.

Metabolic signs. Hypoxaemia, acidosis, hypocalcaemia, anaemia and thrombocytopenia.

The lung manifestations are the most common and constitute the major threat to life. Pao_2 is often low, despite high inspired oxygen concentration due to ventilation/perfusion imbalance. If the patient's respiratory exchange can be maintained, the prognosis is good.

Treatment

All therapeutic measures depend upon proper respiratory management. Blood gas estimation is important, especially monitoring of Pao_2. IPPV is often necessary, and where Pao_2 cannot be satisfactorily maintained despite high inspired oxygen concentration, a positive pressure in the expiratory phase may be helpful. Steroids are useful in the first 24 h but harmful thereafter.

Fulminant fat embolism syndrome. Onset within a few hours of the injury or operation with rapid progress to a fatal conclusion.[58]

It has been said that collapse in the second hour after operation is likely to be due to shock; in the second day, to fat embolism; in the second week, to pulmonary embolism.

Anaesthesia for the injured patient

There is emphasis on the attainment of supranormal values of cardiac index (e.g. $> 4.5 \, l/min/m^2$) and oxygen delivery (e.g. $> 600 \, ml/min/m^2$) as therapeutic goals in trauma patients, as with other high-risk cases.[20] In practice this means IPPV, the use of inotropes such as dobutamine, vasodilators such as sodium nitroprusside, energetic intravenous replacement of losses, and the maintenance of renal function, started as soon after trauma as possible. Pre-operative pulse rate is not usually helpful in assessing blood volume. The military or other outdoor patient, e.g. mountaineer, is likely to be moderately to severely dehydrated, especially in hot climates. A large crystalloid infusion is appropriate here as preanaesthetic resuscitation, in addition to colloid or blood replacement of haemorrhage losses. 'Hidden' haemorhage is often present. Such patients may also be dehydrated from burns exudation.

Operations in chemical/biological warfare isolation theatres presents special problems of anaesthetic pollution, poor lighting (pulse oximetry is invaluable), lack of temperature control (for the staff as well as the patient) and air conditioning, water supply, and facilities for clearing up of spilt blood and other waste (sand is useful for this). A total intravenous technique is useful, using the triservice equipment for added oxygenation and IPPV.

Maintaining tissue perfusion is an important part of the resuscitation and anaesthesia of these patients.[59] It should be remembered that there is altered (usually reduced) drug clearance after trauma.[60]

Later rehabilitation – includes the psychiatric management of Post Traumatic Stress Disorder.[61] Later fat embolism is a risk.[62]

Burns[63]

In the military situation, burns and limb injuries form the largest group of patients. (For anaesthesia, *See* Chapter 22.) Chemical warfare burns with mustard gas. Initial assessment of burns patients includes fluid needs, extent of burn (extent, and depth of skin burn, and respiratory injury); need for pain relief; incipient sepsis; chemical injury (e.g. CO, cyanide, chlorine, phosgene); other physical injury.

The rule of 9s and Lund and Browder charts are used to assess percentage burn. Blood is taken for cross-matching. Evidence of other medical conditions is actively sought, e.g. epilepsy, stroke, diabetes, overdose, child abuse.

Clinical assessment of respiratory injury

(Mortality 50%.)

Is there upper airways obstruction. (Usually due to dry heat.) Coughing, soot in nostrils or sputum, pulmonary oedema, cyanosis, dyspnoea, tachypnoea, stridor, hoarseness, and swelling of lips, tongue, pharynx or larynx? (Tracheal intubation should not be undertaken without very good indication, but when indicated should be done immediately under local analgesia.)

Is there lower airway injury due to chemical burn (HCN, Cl_2, phosgene) or later ARDS? Expiratory ronchi are heard. Even in the absence of respiratory burn, hypoxia may occur due to fluid shifts and ARDS (*see* Chapter 31).

Is there carbon monoxide (CO) poisoning? (The 'cherry red' colour is unreliable for diagnosis.) Greater than 15% HbCO is significant and requires ECG monitoring. The HbCO level is not a very good guide to severity, as in severe hypoxia, it often falls. (*See* Carbon monoxide poisoning, below.) In circumferential thoracic burn, is escharotomy indicated?

Instrumental assessment of respiratory injury

Immediate PFR, blood gases, blood carboxyhaemoglobin expressed as % concentration (cyanide levels are also increased in those with raised carboxyhaemoglobin, PCV, urea and electrolytes), ECG (high incidence of silent ischaemia in CO poisoning), and chest X-ray.

Invasive monitoring is avoided if possible to prevent spread of infection.

Early management of the burns patient:

1. Pain relief for partial-thickness burns by i.v. opioids or Entonox.
2. Oxygen inhalation, with high humidification; this reduces the half life of HbCO to 3 h, and improves oxygen delivery to the tissues. HbCO estimation repeated after 4 h.
3. Intravenous fluid replacement is of greatest importance in first 48 h. Initially 500 ml is normal saline, then colloid (e.g. 5% albumin in saline).

$$\text{Volume (ml) required in first 4 h} = \frac{\text{Wt in kg} \times \% \text{ burn}}{2}$$

If only crystalloid is used, volume $=$ wt in kg $\times$ % burn

CVP monitoring indicated in the elderly and those arriving after long delays. After first 4 h, intravenous fluids judged by hourly microhaematocrit (target 35%) until stable. In war or disaster situations, a mixture of Hartmann's solution and gelatin solution has been used.[64]

4. Catheterization of the bladder to assess urine flow and osmolality (target flow 0.5 ml/kg/h may take a day or so to achieve because of high ADH levels). Initial urine osmolality may be high (900 mOsmol), unless high output renal failure occurs (300 mOsmol). Samples are sent for protein and 'casts'. Black urine indicates myoglobinuria. Renal failure is common.

5. If intubation is needed for severe upper airway obstruction, it is done immediately under local analgesia with possible fibreoptic laryngoscope help. Cuff pressure is rechecked hourly and the patient kept sitting if possible to reduce pulmonary oedema. Apnoeic, acidotic patients are of course intubated immediately, and may well have cyanide poisoning, requiring dicobalt edetate and sodium thiosulphate.

6. 'Burns encephalopathy' is looked for: hyperpyrexia, irritability, vomiting, twitching, coma amd hyponatraemia.

Later management

(1) No prophylactic antibiotics are given, but infections are treated as they arise. Aminoglycosides, ticarcillin, azlocillin are commonly used; (2) ARDS (*see* Chapter 30); (3) DVT (60% incidence) and PE (5% incidence) are treated; (4) blood transfusion often needed; and (5) nutritional care needed if burn > 15% in adults or 10% in children, because of (*a*) reduced intake; (*b*) increased calorie need and nitrogen loss; and (*c*) diarrhoea and vomiting caused by enteral feeds. Protein requirement $= 1\,$g/kg $+ 2\,$g/% burn area. Calorie requirement $= 20\,$kcal/kg $+ 50\,$kcal/% burn area. Metabolic needs may be reduced by preventing hyperpyrexia and adequate analgesia. A weight loss of 10% is common, and is monitored.

The rise in metabolic rate following burns is greater than after other forms of trauma. There is loss of body heat, disturbance of the vasoconstrictor mechanism, and a reset of the hypothalamic thermostat, all made worse by pain and apprehension. There is a rise in plasma catecholamines, cortisol and glucagon. Hyperglycaemia is common and there is probably enhanced degradation of insulin. Energy requirement may be as high as 17 MJ/24 h

(4000 Kcal). Palatable food is best but will often need to be supplemented by enteral tube feeding and sometimes parenteral nutrition if alimentary function is disturbed. During anaesthesia, hypermetabolism is reflected in the need for increased alveolar ventilation. *See also* Chapter 34.

Clinical pharmacology in burns

1. Aminoglycoside losses are increased, so higher doses required for adequate blood levels.
2. Cimetidine losses are increased, partly due to decreased protein binding from hypoproteinaemia.
3. Benzodiazepines (normally highly protein bound) have more free drug available and may be initially more potent. They are however, distributed into a larger volume than usual.
4. Suxamethonium causes hyperkalaemia due to increased numbers of extrajunctional receptors.
5. Resistance to nondepolarizing relaxants, ED_{95} is doubled (peak effect 2 weeks after burn), possibly due to increased number of neuromuscular junction receptors.

Prognosis

If % burn + age in years = > 100, prognosis is very poor. As a very rough guide, of those patients hospitalized 6 weeks after a burn, mortality is around 20%; of those hospitalized 3 months after a burn, mortality is around 50%. (*See also* Brown J. and Ward D. J. *Br. J. Hosp. Med.* 1984, **31**, 360; Brown J. In: *Recent Advances in Anaesthesia and Analgesia* – 15. (Atkinson R. S. and Adams A. P. ed.) Edinburgh: Churchill Livingstone, 1985; Martyn J. *Anesthesiology* 1986, **65**, 67.)

Prognosis scoring in critically ill patients

These tests should show correct prediction of mortality, and be useful for inter-unit comparisons and multicentre trials. (*See* Willatts S. M. *Bailliere's Clin. Anaesthesiol.* 1990, **4**, 253.)

Acute physiology score (APS) based on 34 physiological measurements.[22]

Simplified acute physiology score (SAPS) based on 13 physiological measurements.[65]

Acute physiology and chronic health evaluation (APACHE).[66]

APACHE II[67] and III are a development of this, based on *general health*, severe organ insufficiency or immunocompromised state (5 points for nonoperative or emergency postoperative cases, and 2 points for elective postoperative cases). Organ failure defined as proven cirrhosis, portal hypertension or hepatic failure: cardiovascular – NYHA class IV; respiratory - severe exercise restriction, unable to climb stairs, respirator dependency, pulmonary hypertension > 40 mmHg; chronic renal dialysis; immunocompromised by drugs, radiotherapy, or advanced disease e.g. leukaemia, lymphoma, AIDS.

Age points: < 44 years $= 0$; $45–54 = 2$; $55–64 = 3$; $65–74 = 5$; $> 75 = 6$.
Worst value of 12 physiological measurements during the first 24 h after admission. These are:

1. Rectal temperature points, °C: $> 41 = 4$; $> 39 = 3$; $> 38.5 = 1$; $36–38.4 = 0$; $34–35.9 = 1$; $32–33.9 = 2$; $30–31.9 = 3$; and $< 29.9 = 4$.
2. Mean arterial pressure, mmHg: $> 160 = 4$; $130–159 = 3$; $110–129 = 2$; $70–109 = 0$; $50–69 = 2$; $40–54 = 3$; and $< 49 = 4$.
3. Heart rate, bpm: $> 180 = 4$; $140–179 = 3$; $110–139 = 2$; $70–109 = 0$; $55–69 = 2$; $40–54 = 3$; and $< 39 = 4$.
4. Respiratory rate, bpm: $> 50 = 4$; $35–49 = 3$; $25–34 = 1$; $12–24 = 0$; $10–11 = 1$; $6–9 = 2$; and $< 5 = 4$.
5. Oxygenation points. $AaDO_2$ on FIO_2 > 0.5, KPa: $> 66.8 = 4$; $46.7–66.7 = 3$; and $26.7–46.5 = 2$; Pao_2 on FIO_2 < 0.5, KPa: $8.1–8.3 = 1$; $7.3–8 = 3$; and $< 7.3 = 4$.
6. Arterial pH points: $> 7.7 = 4$; $7.6–7.69 = 3$; $7.5–7.59 = 1$; $7.33–7.49 = 0$; $7.25–7.32 = 2$; $7.15–7.24 = 3$; and $< 7.15 = 4$.
7. Serum Na^+ (mmol/l), points: $> 180 = 4$; $160–179 = 3$; $155-159 = 2$; $150–154 = 1$; $130–149 = 0$; $120–129 = 2$; $111–119 = 3$; and $< 110 = 4$.
8. Serum K^+ (mmol/l) points: $> 7 = 4$; $6–6.9 = 3$; $5.5–5.9 = 1$; $3.5–5.4 = 0$; $3–3.4 = 1$; $2.5–2.9 = 2$; and $< 2.5 = 4$.
9. Serum creatinine (mmol/l) (points are doubled for *acute renal failure*): $> 300 = 4$.
10. Haematocrit.
11. White cell count.
12. Glasgow Coma Score.[30] (Rating $= 15$ – actual GCS).
Each parameter is scored from 0 (normal) to $+4$ (abnormally high or low).

A total score of 10 relates to a mortality of about 10%.
A total score of 20 relates to a mortality of about 20%.
A total score of 30 relates to a mortality of about 40%.
A total score of 35 relates to a mortality of about 75%.
A total score of 40 relates to a mortality of about 90%.
A total score of 55 relates to a mortality of about 100%.

APACHE III allows for developments of the patient's condition while in the ITU, and decision-making about stopping active treatment.[68]
Therapeutic Intervention Scoring System (TISS).[69] This is based on treatments given to patients during illness. It is valuable in assessing costings but is of little help in comparisons between units.
Mortality Prediction Modelling (MPM).[70] Systolic pressure, level of consciousness, type of admission, prior CPR, age, and presence of cancer and presence of infection, are noted at admission and after 24 h. The admission figures show a higher prediction of outcome.
The Burn Index.[71]
Injury Severity Scoring System (ISS) is based on the type and extent of injury in the various anatomical regions.[72]

INTENSIVE THERAPY UNIT	APACHE SCORING SHEET						NAME:			
POINTS >	4		3		2		1		0	SUM
TEMP °C	>41	<29.9	39-40.9	30-31.9		32-33.9	38.5-38.9	34-35.9	36-38.4	
MEAN S.B.P.	>160	<49	130-159		110-129	50-69			70-109	
HEART RATE	>180	<39	140-179	40-54	110-139	55-69			70-109	
RESP. RATE	>50	<5	35-49			6-9	25-34	10-11	12-24	
FiO2 >0.5 A-aDO2	>68.8		46.7-68.7		26.7-46.6					
FiO2 <0.5 PaO2		<7.3	7.3-8.0					8.1-8.3		
ART.pH	>7.7	<7.15	7.6-7.69	7.15-7.24		7.25-7.32	7.5-7.59		7.33-7.49	
SERUM Na+	>180	<110	160-179	111-119	155-159	120-129	150-154		130-149	
SERUM K+	>7.0	<2.5	6-6.9			2.5-2.9	5.5-5.9	3.0-3.4	3.5-5.4	
SERUM CREATININE	>301		169-300		125-168		<53		54-124	
PCV	>60	<20			50-59.9	20-29.9	46-49.9		30-45.9	
WBC	>40	<1			20-39.9	1-2.9	15-19.9		3-14.9	

AGE RANGE	>75	65-74	55-64	45-54	<45
AGE POINTS	6	5	3	2	0

GLASGOW COMA SCALE

BEST EYE RESPONSE -----> 1-4 POINTS
BEST MOTOR RESPONSE ---> 1-5 POINTS
BEST VERBAL RESPONSE --> 1-6 POINTS

TOTAL [ ]   15 MINUS TOTAL

CHRONIC HEALTH SCORE
CIRRHOSIS OR PORTAL HYPERTENSION
CARDIOVASCULAR STATUS NYHA CLASS IV
SEVERE CHRONIC RESPIRATORY DISEASE
RENAL DIALYSIS PATIENTS
IMMUNOSUPPRESSION DUE TO DISEASE/DRUGS/THERAPY

NO ------------>SCORE 0
YES—ELECTIVE POST-OP?
⌐YES------->SCORE 2
└NO-------->SCORE 5

SCORING DOCTOR	SIGNATURE	DATE	TOTAL APACHE SCORE ____ PTS.

Figure 32.2 A typical APACHE scoring sheet

Paediatric trauma

Head is larger in paediatric patients, therefore, more likelihood of head and neck injuries. There is faster loss of body heat, which means active warming needs to be started earlier.

Hypothermia[73]

1. Assessment – Is the patient alive or dead? If there is respiration and a palpable or auscable pulse, resuscitation is started.
2. Treatment – external rewarming in horizontal position at a temperature tolerable by the rescuers elbow. Extracorporeal circulation rewarming is highly effective.[74]
3. Minimal interference with the patient. Intubation and adrenaline are avoided, as is unnecessary cardiac massage.
4. Prognosis may be revealed by serum potassium (average 14.5 mmol/l in non-survivors of avalanches).[75]
5. Factors other than simple exposure need attention, e.g. trauma, assault, drowning, stroke, myxoedema, etc.[76]

Management of major disasters: organizational aspects

1. The anaesthetist is already involved with designated 'disaster' responsibilities in the hospital setting (*see above*).
2. The anaesthetist has a contribution in assessment for triage and resuscitation at the site of physical disasters.
3. Familiarity with acute pulmonary injury, cardiotoxicity and nerve blockade enable a valuable anaesthetic contribution at major chemical disasters.[77] 'Porton liners' may be used where chemical disasters and physical trauma coexist.[78]
4. The intensive care unit sends the MICU to the site, and in expectation of being overwhelmed by major casualties, extends its borders to prearranged areas and unpacks its disaster equipment, which includes beds, documentation, monitors (unsophisticated but practical), ventilators, suckers, intravenous therapy, syringe drivers, etc. Regular reassessment of patients and rest periods and refreshment for staff are given priority. Ready prepared standing orders for investigations, intravenous therapy and ventilator settings are used.

A list of pre-trained volunteers (e.g. ex-members of the ITU nursing staff who live locally) is used to extend the staff. It is helpful if they can be paid. All staff may expect to perform tasks beyond their normal experience, but it is recognized that in these areas they will not perform as efficiently as their own specialties.

Some notes on the early management of ingestion of poisons

1. Decontamination of the gastrointesinal tract. Traditional gastric lavage is of value within one hour after ingestion, and if the poison is highly toxic. It has little value after this interval, or if the patient has already vomited. It carries the risk of encouraging gastric contents into the small bowel, or the lungs if the patient has no airway reflexes. Emetics, e.g. ipecacuanha syrup 30 ml in adults, apomorphine injection, have value if the ingested pills are too large to pass through a lavage tube, or are known not to adsorb on to charcoal, e.g. iron. The benefits of early lavage and emesis normally outweigh the possible complications (mechanical damage to oesophagus, stomach, mediastinum, pericardium, pleura). Activated charcoal (dose 1g/kg), is given as a 10–25% slurry. Each gram is said to have $1000 \, m^2$ of surface area and increases drug clearance from gut lumen, blood, and conjugated metabolites being excreted in the bile by an average of 70%. It is valuable for salicylates, phenobarbitone, tetracyclines, paracetamol, theophylline, cimetidine, β-blockers and paraquat. It is avoided in cases of abdominal trauma. Purgation by polyethylene glycol solution, or other 'bowel preparations' acts by powerful intestinal hurry, and has been used for removal of drug bags from the guts of smugglers. Rarely, gastric endoscopy may be required for removal of physically large poisons.

2. *Agricultural and military poisons*. Organophosphates, e.g. EPN, trichlorophon, malathion, fenthion, respond well to early (within 3 h) direct haemoperfusion. Each charcoal column is used for its full length, i.e. about 12 h. Symptomatic relief is gained by atropine or glycopyrronium. Blood levels of the poisons can be calculated from pharmacodynamic graphs of decay vs. time. Paraquat ingestion may be treated by adsorbents such as activated charcoal and kaolin preparations. Paraquat has a large volume of distribution, and the prolonged haemoperfusion used to clear it may be complicated by thrombocytopenia in up to half the cases. Specific antidotes include chlorpromazine, a highly pulmophilic, lipophilic drug that inhibits pulmonary uptake and efflux of paraquat, vitamins C and B_2, niacin and clofibrate.

3. *Mushroom poisoning*. In addition to specific knowledge of mycology, various general principles are helpful.

(a) Diarrhoea and vomiting are a common feature in the first 18h. These should be encouraged (*see above*). Activated charcoal is given in repeated dosage.

(b) If the patient is conscious, pictures of poisonous fungi may be recognized, e.g. *Amanita phalloides*, which guide specific therapy and prognosis.

(c) Blood, gastric juice and urine are taken for toxin analysis. A serum transaminase level of 1000–5000 is suggestive of amatoxin poisoning and carries a poor prognosis.

(d) Aggressive fluid replacement, electrolyte correction and forced diuresis.

(e) Fresh frozen plasma may be needed, and penicillamine is considered.

(f) Respiratory support if encephalopathy appears.

(g) Hepatic and renal failure are a feature in 1–10 days after poisoning and require support.

(h) Plasma exchange has been disappointing.

4. *Carbon monoxide (CO) poisoning*.

(a) Early and rapid removal of CO from the body by good ventilation, IPPV if necessary. 85% of the CO is in the haemoglobin, 15% in myoglobin.

(*b*) Oxygen is the primary therapy in this condition, particularly for protection of the brain. Brain damage is both time and dose related, with early alteration of mental status, and a late neuropsychiatric syndrome with evidence of basal ganglion damage. As well as blocking oxygen delivery (flux), CO poisons cytochrome a3. Oxygen therapy reduces tissue hypoxia, reduces the half-life of CO to less than 30 min, restores phosphocreatine and ATP production, restores glucose utilization, reduces succinate levels to normal and reduces the lactate/pyruvate ratio.

(*c*) Blood samples are taken for HbCO. The absorption spectum peaks at 590–610 nM. (HbCO of 15% requires full monitoring; 30% means severe hypoxia with Pvo_2 levels of 2 kPa or less, lactic acidosis, and is an indication for hyperbaric oxygen therapy.) Pulse oximetry is affected by HbCO, giving readings around 85%.

(*d*) Poor prognosis is associated with delay in treatment of over 2 h, age over 40 years, metabolic acidosis, coma, cardiac ischaemia, and cerebral abnormalities on CT scan.

References

1. *See also* Stoddart J. C. In: *Recent Advances in Anaesthesia and Analgesia* (Atkinson R. S. and Adams A. P. ed.) Edinburgh: Churchill Livingstone, 1989; Skinner D., Driscoll P. and Earlam R. ed.) *ABC of Major Trauma*. London: British Medical Association, 1991; Baskett P. J. F. and Weller R. M. *Medicine for Disasters*. Bristol: John Wright, 1989; Editorial, *Br J Anaesth* 1990, **64**, 139.
2. Anderson I. D. et al. *Br. Med. J.* 1988, **296**, 1305.
3. Emergency care in natural disasters: view of an international seminar. *WHO Chronicle*, 1980, **34**, 96.
4. Mather S. J. and Edbrooke D. L. *Prehospital Emergency Care*. Bristol: Wright, 1985.
5. Rutherford W. H. and de Boer J. *Injury* 1983, **15**, 10–13.
6. Champion H. R. et al. *J. Trauma* 1989, **29**, 623.
7. Little R. A. *J. Trauma* 1989, **29**, 903.
8. Boyd C. R. et al. *J. Trauma* 1989, **27**, 370.
9. Baker S. P. et al. *J. Trauma* 1974, **14**, 187.
10. Crosby E. T. and Lui A. *Can. J. Anaesth.* 1990, **37**, 77.
11. Safar P. J. *Wld. Assoc. Emerg. Disaster Med.* 1986, **14**, 34.
12. Davidson T. J. and Cotev S. *Ann. R. Coll. Surg. Engl.* 1975, **56**, 304.
13. Jowitt M. D. and Knight R. J. *Anaesthesia* 1983, **38**, 776.
14. Hall L. W., Kellagher R. E. B. and Fleet K. J. *Anaesthesia* 1986, **41**, 516.
15. Restall J. and Knight R. J. In: *Medicine for Disasters* (Baskett P. J. F. and Weller R. M. ed.) Oxford: Butterworths, 1988.
16. Baskett P. J. F. (ed.) *Resuscitation Handbook*. London: Gower Medical, 1989.
17. Yates D. W. et al. *J. R. Soc. Med.* 1987, **80**, 486.
18. Swan K. et al. *J. Trauma* 1977, **17**, 215.
19. Bion J. F. *Anaesthesia* 1984, **39**, 560.
20. Shoemaker W. C. et al. *Chest* 1988, **94**, 1176.
21. ABC of Major Trauma, *Br. Med. J.* 1990, **301**, 1145.
22. McCoy J. A. and Azim E. *Anaesthesia* 1976, **31**, 532; Jette N. T. and Barasch P. G. *Anaesthesia* 1977, **32**, 475.
23. Lee A. et al. *Anaesthesia* 1991, **45**, 1028.
24. Holness R. and Waxman K. *Crit. Care Med.* 1990, **18**, 1.

25. Hunter A. R. *Neurosurgical Anaesthesia* 2nd ed. Oxford: Blackwell, 1976; Horton J. M. *Anaesthesia* 1975, **30**, 212. *Br. J. Anaesth.* 1976, **48**, 767.
26. Seelig J. M. et al. *N. Eng. J. Med.* 1981, **304**, 1511.
27. Genarrelli T. A. et al. *Ann. Neurol.* 1982, **12**, 564; Adams J. H. *Ann. Neurol.* 1982, **12**, 557.
28. Plum F. *Neurology (NY)* 1983, **33**, 222.
29. Teesdale G. et al. *Br. Med. J.* 1982, **285**, 1695; Michenfelder J. D. *J. Irish Coll. Phys. Surg.* 1983, **12**, 154; Mendelow A. D. *Hosp. Update.* 1990, **16**, 195.
30. Teasdale G. and Gentleman D. *Scott. Med. J.* 1982, **27**, 7; Teasdale G. *Br. J. Anaesth.* 1976, **48**, 761; Teasdale G. and Jennett W. B. *Lancet* 1974, **2**, 81; Jennett W. B. and Teasdale G. *The Management of Head Injuries* 3rd ed. Philadelphia: Davis, 1980.
31. Royal College of Radiologists, *Lancet* 1983, **1**, 115.
32. Vicario S. et al. *Ann. Emerg. Med.* 1982, **11**, 475.
33. Mackenzie S. J. et al. *Anaesthesia* 1991, **45**, 1043.
34. McDowell D. G. *Br. J. Anaesth.* 1985, **57**, 1.
35. Symon L, *Br. J. Anaesth.* 1985, **57**, 34.
36. Abramson M. S. et al. *N. Eng. J. Med.* 1986, **314**, 397.
37. Steen P. A. et al. *Anesthesiology,* 1985, **62**, 406.
38. Means E. D., Braughler J. M. and Hall E. D. In: *Update in Intensive Care and Emergency Medicine* (Vincent J.-L. ed.) 1990, Berlin: Springer Verlag.
39. Gudeman S. K. *Neurosurgery* 1983, **12**, 175.
40. Branch C. L. et al. *Neurosurgery* 1983, **12**, 98.
41. Crittenden D. J. *J. Trauma* 1982, **22**, 766; Popp A. *J. J. Neurosurg.* 1982, **57**, 784; Weiner F. et al. *Crit. Care Med.* 1983, **11**, 132.
42. Harris R. J. *Stroke* 1982, **13**, 759.
43. Gentleman D. and Jennett B. *Lancet* 1981, **2**, 853; Brydon J. S. and Jennett B. *Br. Med. J.* 1983, **286**, 1791.
44. For portable lung ventilators, *see* Gray A. J. G. *Br. J. Hosp. Med.* 1981, **25**, 144.
45. McDowall D. G. In: *Recent Advances in Anaesthesia and Analgesia – 12* (Hewer C. L. and Atkinson R. S. ed.). Edinburgh: Churchill Livingstone, 1976.
46. Hans P. et al. *Acta Anaesthesiol. Belg.* 1984, **35**, 79.
47. Levati A. et al. *J. Neurosurg.* 1982, **57**, 779.
48. Conference of the Royal Colleges and Faculties, *Br. Med. J.* 1976, **2**, 1187; Report of Ad hoc Committee of the Harvard Medical School. *JAMA* 1977, **237**, 982; Searle J. and Collins C. *Lancet* 1980, **1**, 641; Jennett B. *Br. J. Anaesth.* 1981, **53**, 1, 111.
49. Mollaret P. and Goulon M. *Rev. Neurol.* 1959, **101**, 3.
50. Klug N. *J. Neurol.* 1982, **227**, 219.
51. Pallis C. *Br. Med. J.* 1982, **285**, 1487.
52. Perel A. et al. *Intensive Care Med.* 1983, **9**, 25.
53. ABC of spinal cord injuries, *Brit. Med. J.* 1986, **292**, 743.
54. Crosby E. T. and Lui A. *Can. J. Anaesth.* 1990, **37**, 77.
55. Wilson J. N. *Proc. R. Soc. Med.* 1967, **60**, 951.
56. Zenker F. A. *Beiträge zur Anatomie der Lungen.* Dresden: G. Shonfeld's Buchhandlung, 1862.
57. Von Bergmann E. *Berl. Med. Wochensch.* 1873, **10**, 385.
58. Hagley S. R. *Anaesth. Intensive Care* 1983, **11**, 162.
59. Tremper K. K. *Crit. Care Med.* 1989, **17**, 1362.
60. Shikuma L. R. et al. *Crit. Care Med.* 1990, **18**, 37.
61. *J. R. Soc. Med.* 1991, **84**, 2.
62. Fabian T. C. et al. *Crit. Care Med.* 1990, **18**, 42.
63. Robertson C. and Fenton O. *Br. Med. J.* 1990, **301**, 282.
64. Williams J. G. et al. *Br. Med. J.* 1983, **286**, 775.
65. LeGall J. R. et al. *Crit. Care Med.* 1984, **12**, 975.
66. Knaus W. A. et al. *Crit. Care Med.* 1981, **9**, 591.
67. Knaus W. A. et al. *Crit. Care Med.* 1985, **13**, 124.
68. Zimmerman J. E. *Crit. Care Med.* 1989, **17**, s169.

69. Keene A. R. and Cullen D. J. *Crit. Care Med.* 1983, **11**, 1.
70. Teres D. et al. *Crit. Care Med.* 1987, **15**, 86; Lemeshow S. et. al. *Crit. Care Med.* 1988, **16**, 470.
71. Feller I. et al. *JAMA* 1980, **244**, 2074.
72. Baker S. P. et al. *J. Trauma* 1974, **14**, 187.
73. Keatinge W. R. *Br. Med. J.* 1991, **302**, 3–4.
74. Spittgerber F. H. et al. *Am. J. Surg.* 1986, **52**, 407.
75. Schaller M. D. et al. *JAMA,* 1990, **264**, 1842.
76. Slater D. N. *Br. Med. J.* 1988, **296**, 1643.
77. Editorial, *Br. Med. J.* 1991, **302**, 61; Thanabalasingham T. et al. *Br. Med. J.* 1991, **302**, 101.
78. Chambers D. et al. *Br. Med. J.* 1991, **302**, 68.

Chapter 33

Sepsis and the septic syndrome[1]

Incidence of sepsis is high in the ITU, compared with other types of unit, e.g. coronary care. Approximately 25% of patients entering an ITU are already infected, and a further 25% of patients become infected in the ITU, due to cross-infection with virulent organisms, reduction of immunocompetence, or both. Septic shock develops in 40% of cases of sepsis.[2]

Classification. Sepsis includes localized infections, bacteraemia, septicaemia, septic shock and 'multi-system organ failure'. There is a variable use of these terms by different authorities, which has led to some confusion. The more precise the protocols of studies in this area, the better. It should be noted that 'septic shock' can be non-infective! Septic syndrome is characterized by fever (> 38.5°C) or hypothermia (< 35.5°C), tachycardia (> 90 bpm), tachypnoea (> 20 rpm), and organ failure with oliguria (< 0.5 mls/kg/h), hypoxia (< 10 kPa).

Aetiology

1. Self-infection with gut organisms in cases of abdominal disease, surgery, and also gut ischaemia in trauma and haemorrhage, mediated at least partly by the renin-angiotensin system.[3]

2. Iatrogenic infection via prostheses, indwelling urinary catheters, vascular access catheters, nasogastric tubes and probes.

3. Alteration of lung flora due to IPPV.

4. Alteration of gut organisms due to H_2 antagonists and to enteral nutrition.

5. Primary sepsis due to abscess, burns, cellulitis.

Presentation and diagnosis

Pneumonia and bacteraemia are the commonest presentations. Pyrexia is common but not universal. The patient is in a hyperdynamic, hypermetabolic state. Hypoxia and arterial hypotension (systolic < 90 mmHg) may be the heralds of ARDS due to sepsis. Septic shock may present as acute renal failure (ARF), or multi-system organ failure (MSOF). Organs commonly affected by such failure include the heart, the alimentary tract, the liver, the pancreas, the brain, muscle, blood clotting system and bone marrow; in fact every system of the body.

Useful markers of the process are temperature, white cell count, myeloperoxidase (> 200 ng/ml), elastase, $C5_a$, serotonin and Limulus coagulation assay for endotoxin.[4] Fibrosis in the affected organs occurs early in this process, and regresses with later resolution of the disease. (Note that MSOF also occurs after haemorrhage, major trauma, cardiac arrest, acute pancreatitis and major surgery. *See also* ARDS in Chapter 30.)

Identification and elimination of the source of sepsis, and bacteriological control by antibiotics are central to the management of this condition.

Micropathophysiology[5] of septic shock

Surgery, trauma, severe infections, burns and self-infection from gut lead to endotoxinaemia,[6] usually gram negative, e.g. *E. coli* endotoxinaemia, but occasionally gram positive. Activated ('angry') macrophages[7] produce the cytokines: leucotrienes IL 1 (endogenous pyrogen), IL 2, and IL 6.[8] Prostaglandins, tumour necrosis factor (TNF, a 10–20 kD protein) and thromboxanes are then implicated in the appearance of oxygen radicals and eicosanoids (e.g. PGE_2, 6-keto-PGF_1, TXB_2), which specifically damage the capillary endothelium of the target organs mentioned above. This leads to endothelial dehiscence, leakage, pericapillary oedema, abnormal platelet deposition, white cell plugging, and microvascular thromboses. The process finally results in microscopic tissue hypoxia, localized lactic acidosis, hyperosmolarity, disequilibrium of cations, and necrosis, starting in the cells furthest from the capillaries. Reperfusion may only produce further white-cell mediated endothelial injury with development of more oxygen radicals from the incoming oxygen. Lipoperoxidation has been linked to vitamin E deficiency.[9] Septic plasma suppresses superoxide anion synthesis by normal homologous polymorphonuclear leukocytes.[10]

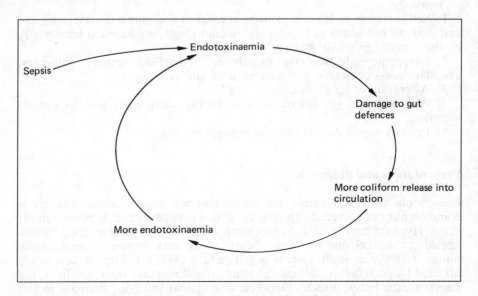

Figure 33.1 A cycle of progressive damage causing endotoxinaemia.

Release of endorphins and arachidonic acid metabolites occurs.[11] *Endothelins* have also been implicated.[12]

Normal granulocyte cellular defence mechanisms (phagocytosis, margination and plugging microhaemorrhages) are important in the recovery from sepsis.

Oxygen transport is reduced because of anaemia, cardiac failure and ARDS,[13] but some haemodilution is beneficial by reducing demand for cardiac work and restoring perfusion in damaged capillaries. Calcium homeostasis is disturbed.[14] There is alteration of regional blood flow, with opening of arteriovenous anastomoses, depriving the capillaries of blood, leading to higher venous oxygen saturation (Svo_2), tissue hypoxia and increased lactate levels.

Specific organs

The lung. Microthromboses, increase in extravascular lung water, micro- and macro-atelectasis. Resistant hypoxia ($Pao_2 < 10\,kPa$, 75 mmHg) and respiratory alkalosis develop. *See* Chapter 30.

Cardiovascular alterations in sepsis.[15] Normal or raised cardiac output, ($> 3.5\,l/m^2/min$ is important for survival[16]); tachycardia (> 90 bpm), left and right ventricular dilation, reduction of left and right ventricular ejection fraction with abnormal movements of the interventricular septum, normal coronary flow;[17] low SVR (< 800 dynes/sec.cm^{-5}); decreased myocardial contractility[18] (responsive to inotropes, and possibly due to TXA_2[19]). These effects possibly due to IL 2. Survivors have more ventricular dilation, and maintain stroke volume by better use of the Starling effect. Non-survivors show a right and downward shift of the Starling curve, but some have high cardiac outputs up to the moment of death.[20] Coexistence of coronary artery disease is a bad prognostic indicator and goes with lower cardiac outputs.[21] Systemic vascular resistance remains low in both groups, but pulmonary vascular resistance is high,[22] an effect which is worsened by adrenaline and improved by moderate doses of dopamine. Circulating catecholamines are raised, and clinically the cardiac output often responds well to administered dopamine, dobutamine or dopexamine, in spite of desensitization of beta-adrenergic receptors in heart and lymphocytes.[23] Endotoxic peripheral blood pooling is as important as cardiac failure.[24] Cardiac calcium regulation is abnormal.[25] Myocardial Na-K pump is also abnormal, affecting the Na-Ca pump.[26]

Endocarditis of natural or prosthetic valves gives resistant cardiac failure, murmurs, and septic emboli.[27]

Vascular alterations in sepsis include peripheral pooling, opening of arteriovenous anastomoses, and generalized capillary blockage and failure.

The reliability of right atrial pressure monitoring to assess left ventricular preload in critically ill septic patients has been questioned,[28] because of the high pulmonary vascular resistances involved.

The liver (and drug pharmacokinetics). The liver takes part in the generalized endothelial injury, perhaps mediated by the Kupffer cells. Liver dysfunction appears within hours of onset of sepsis.[29] The result is that pharmacokinetics and pharmacodynamics of most drugs is abnormal, and that 'normal' knowledge of the action of drugs does not necessarily apply in sepsis.[30]

The kidneys. Renal failure is common and severely worsens the prognosis.

The gut. Dysfunction can be the cause or the result of sepsis, or both. A vicious circle develops, starting with endotoxinaemia, leading to damage to the gut wall defences, leading to leakage into the circulation of organisms and endotoxins, leading to more endotoxinaemia. Selective decontamination of the gut has been partly succesful in reducing this problem.

The pancreas. A diabetic-type glucose tolerance due to resistance to insulin, with decreased ability to transport and oxidize glucose in the cells. Pancreatitis also occurs.

The immune system. Cell-mediated immunocompetence[31] (WBC > 12 000 µl or < 3000/µl). Fever generated by IL 1 (> 39°C), or hypothermia (< 35°C). Nosocomial pulmonary infections are common, especially in the intubated patients.[32]

The brain. Septic encephalopathy due to: (1) direct CNS infection; (2) inadequate cerebral perfusion as a result of critical illness; (3) toxaemia;[33] (4) deranged brain aromatic and branched-chain amino acid transport;[34] (5) secondary to liver failure,[35] with raised aromatic amino acids and methionine. (6) part of the generalized pathophysiology.[36] (7) due to abnormal neurotransmitter levels,[37] especially initially reduced noradrenaline and dopamine (later reversed), increased serotonin, and false transmitters; and (8) metabolic and electrolyte disturbances.[38]

Muscle. Reduction of power, micronecrosis, lactic acid production. Rhabdomyolysis and myoglobin release may cause the myonephropathic-metabolic syndrome.[39]

Skin. Multivariate rash. A bad prognostic sign.

Metabolism. Metabolic acidosis (base deficit > 5 mEq/l), resistant hyperglycaemia.

Blood. Clotting abnormalities due to DIC, and acute anaemia due to marrow depression.

Prevention

Prevention of cross-infection is crucial, as the critically ill patient may be immunocompromised,[40] and over half ventilated patients have gram negative oropharyngeal colonization due to reduced mucosal fibronectin.[41] Topical, non-absorbable antibiotics (e.g. polymyxin B & E, tobramycin, amphotericin B, povidone iodine)[42] are used in *selective decontamination of the gut*, although influence on infection rates is disappointing. Maintaining gastric acidity is important in preventing bacterial colonization of the upper gut, and if anti-peptic ulcer treatment is used, agents which do not severely raise pH are used, e.g. sucralfate. Dopexamine 1–5 µg/kg/min may be used to maintain gut mucosa oxygenation and integrity.

Treatment[43]

This should begin after taking blood cultures, but usually before complete diagnostic criteria are available.

   1. Support of vital organs, *see below*.

2. Active diagnosis of sepsis, blood culture, searching for pus (usually apparent in previously normal patients, but not in the immunocompromised[44]). A 'second look' laparotomy may be needed. Fungal infections must be borne in mind.

3. Active control of sepsis such as aggressive bactericidal antibiotics (preferably specific to identified organisms), e.g. vancomycin 2 g/day, flucloxacillin 4 g/day, third generation cephalosporin, rifampicin, and attainment of adequate plasma levels is emphasised;[45] percutaneous drainage of pus.

Removal of *in-vivo* foreign bodies (if proved to be the cause of resistant sepsis), e.g. CVP catheters, orthopaedic prostheses, vascular grafts. Gut decontamination.

4. Maximizing oxygen delivery (Do_2) by active resuscitation. There is emphasis on the attainment of supranormal values of cardiac index (e.g. $> 4.5 \, l/min/m^2$) and oxygen delivery (e.g. $> 600 \, ml/min/m^2$) as therapeutic goals in sepsis,[46] $\dot{V}o_2$ is dependent on Do_2 below a certain critical level, and in sepsis this critical level is much higher.[47] (*See* Fig 33.2). Oxygen consumption in sepsis is pathologically supply-dependent.

IPPV is used to maximize lung function, inotropes to maximize cardiac function, and vasodilators to (hopefully) maximize capillary function.

In sepsis there is reduction of vasomotor tone, reactive hyperaemia is not seen, and autoregulation is poor. Abnormal extraction of oxygen from blood is due to (*a*) loss of capillary reserve by microembolization and leucocyte plugging; (*b*) altered vascular reactivity to endothelial relaxing and

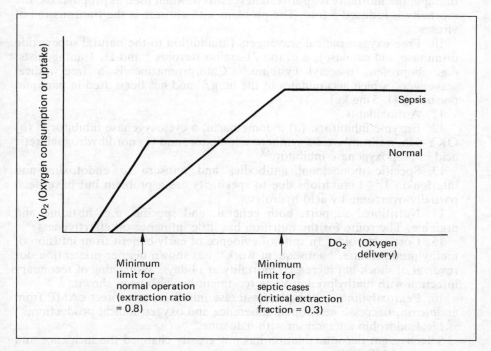

Figure 33.2 Relationship between oxygen delivery and oxygen consumption.

contracting factors; (c) interstitial oedema; and (d) microvascular maldistribution of blood flow related to demand.

In practice, maximizing oxygen delivery means the use of inotropes such as
dobutamine, 5–10 µg/kg/min; dopexamine 5–10 µg/kg/min;[48] vasodilators
such as sodium nitroprusside; and energetic intravenous replacement of
losses, although careful monitoring is needed as response to crystalloids is
abnormal.[49] A reasonable target PAWP is 15 mmHg.[44] It is often easy to
overshoot this figure because of abnormally high pulmonary vascular
resistance.[15] Prostaglandins have been used, *see above*.[50] ECMO and ICMO
may be needed.

Induction of cardiovascular stability is the primary step in reversing septic
pathophysiology, by eliminating flow-dependent oxygen consumption and
lactic acidosis. It implies intensive monitoring.

5. Encouraging increases in oxygen uptake, or consumption, ($\dot{V}o_2$) by
hypoxic tissues, with full metabolic support, e.g. glucose, insulin, electrolytes, parenteral nutrition.

6. The maintenance of renal function (dopamine 5–10 µg/kg/min,
frusemide 50 mg, possible mannitol challenge) which is started as soon as
possible. Dialysis is often required.

7. Blood replacement to correct anaemia. A reasonable target Hb is
100 g/l.

8. Reversal of coagulation defects by cryoprecipitate, anti tissue factor
and anti thrombin III.

9. Immunomodulatory therapy using immune antisera.[51] When used as
therapy, the mortality is approximately halved; when used as prophylaxis, the
mortality is reduced 5-fold. The problem with antisera is the transmission of
viruses.

10. Free oxygen radical scavengers (in addition to the natural superoxide
dismutase and catalase), e.g. the 21-amino steroids[52] and IL 1 antagonists,
e.g. ibuprofen, n-acetyl cysteine.[53] Chlorpromazine is a free radical
scavenger[54] which accumulates in the lung,[55] and has been used in paraquat
poisoning (1–5 mg/kg).

11. Antioxidants

12. Enzyme inhibitors: (a) indomethacin, a cycloxygenase inhibitor;[56] (b)
OKY-046, a thromboxane synthetase inhibitor; and (c) nordihydroguaiaretic
acid, a 5-lipoxygenase inhibitor.[57]

13. Specific monoclonal antibodies and antisera to endotoxins and
interleukin 1.[58] Limitations due to specificity are a problem but have been
partially overcome by acid hydrolysis.[59]

14. Nutritional support, both general, and specific, e.g. histidine and
arginine. The route for the nutrition has little influence on effectiveness.[60]

15. Corticosteroids? In spite of evidence of early benefit from infusion of
methylprednisolone,[61] subsequent work[62] has shown neither prevention nor
reversal of shock but increased mortality at 14 days. Worsening of secondary
infection with methylprednisolone treatment has also been shown.[63]

16. Pentoxifylline, a phosphodiesterase inhibitor, to protect cAMP from
endotoxin, decrease neutrophil adherence and oxygen radical production.[64]

17. Endorphin antagonism with naloxone.[65]

Selective gut decontamination has not greatly changed the incidence and
outcome of MSOF.[66]

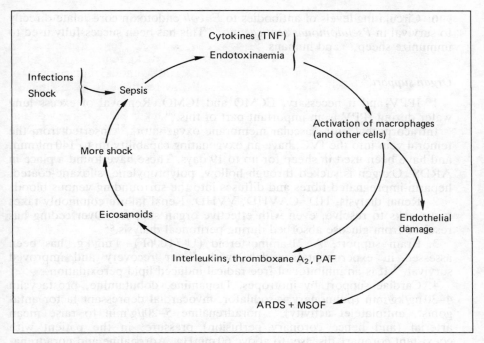

Figure 33.3 A possible sequence in septic shock.

Prognosis

(Mortality still 50–90%). This depends on

1. The presence or absence of shock (hypotension/hypoperfusion)[67]
2. The number of vital organs involved (1 organ – 50% mortality; 3 organs, 90%).[68]
3. The duration of the disease before and during treatment.
4. The adequacy of oxygen supply during the crisis.

Clinical bad prognosis markers include[69] greater tachycardia, cardiac output increases (or falls to 'normal' levels[70]), falls of SVR (< 500 dynes/sec.cm^{-5}), refractory hypotension, Pao_2/Fio_2 gradient (< 10 kPa/ 100%), longer duration of disease, older age of patient (> 65 years) previous steroid or cytotoxic therapy, previous uraemia or cardiac failure.[71]

APACHE II and III scores of 20 or more reflect these bad prognostic signs. (*See* Chapter 32).

Biochemical prognosis indicators include:

1. Subtherapeutic levels of antibiotics[72] carry a very bad prognosis.
2. Admission TSH levels below 0.6 iu/l associated with a nearly 90% mortality rate, while TSH above 3 iu/l with less than 10% mortality.
3. Higher lactic acid levels higher (but with some overlap) in non-survivors.[73]
4. Angiotensin converting enzyme blood levels correlate directly with severity of ARDS.[74]
5. Plasma fibronectin levels are inversely related to clinical severity of septic shock.[75]

6. Circulating levels of antibodies to *E. coli* endotoxin core relate directly to survival in *Pseudomonas septicaemia*.[76] This has been successfully used to immunize sheep,[77] and humans.[78]

Organ support[79]

1. IPPV and if necessary, ECMO and ICMO. Removal of excess lung water during IPPV is an important part of this.[80]

Intracorporeal, intravascular membrane oxygenators,[81] inserted from the femoral vein into the IVC, have an oxygenating capability up to 140 ml/min, and have been used in sheep for up to 19 days. These have found a place in ARDS. Oxygen is sucked through hollow, polypropylene, siloxane-coated, heparin-impregnated fibres and diffuses into the surrounding venous blood.

2. Renal dialysis, HD, CAVHD, VVHD. Renal failure commonly takes two weeks to resolve, even with effective organ support. Overfeeding has resulted from glucose absorbed during peritoneal dialysis.[82]

3. Brain support. A 21-aminosteroid (U-74006F), 1 mg/kg, has been assessed in experimental models, with faster recovery and improved survival.[83] It is an inhibitor of free radical induced lipid peroxidation.

4. Cardiac support by inotropes. Dopamine, dobutamine, prostacyclin 4–30 ng/kg/min (pulmonary vasodilator, myocardial depressant factor antagonist, antiplatelet activity),[84] noradrenaline 5–20µg/min to raise mean arterial (and hence coronary perfusion) pressure, in the patient with coexistent coronary disease, to above 60 mmHg. Adrenaline and noradrenaline may, in high doses, damage the myocardium and contribute adversely to high pulmonary vascular resistance.[15] Alternative agents for inadequate response to catecholamines include digoxin,[85] amrinone plus a vasoconstrictor,[86] enoximone and milrinone.

5. Liver. Amino acid support may help and is related to plasma cholesterol levels.[87]

6. Bone marrow depression may call for blood and platelet transfusions.

7. Muscle. Muscle wasting due to decreases in muscle protein synthesis. This is partly due to decreased amino acid substrate (*See* Chapter 34), partly to disuse, and partly to the effect of hormones. Treatment includes amino acid therapy (high intensity infusions), which is anabolic, as is insulin and steady β-2 adrenergic infusions (e.g. salbutamol), with increase in muscle mass, RNA content and strength.

8. Electrolyte support and correction of hypocalcaemia and hypoproteinaemia.

Toxic shock syndrome[88]

Initially reported in children,[89] and later due to tampons in menstruation.[90] Diagnosed by the following criteria:

1. Temperature > 38.9°C.
2. Erythematous rash, desquamating 2 weeks later.
3. Shock, hypotension (< 90 mmHg), peripheral circulatory failure.
4. At least 3 system organ failure (including mucous membrane ulceration).

5. Culture of toxin-producing *S. aureus* from ulcers/wound/nasopharynx.
6. Rise in TSST-1 antibody titre.
Exotoxin 1, IL-1 and TNF are involved.[91]

Some particularly difficult specific forms of sepsis

1. Infective endocarditis.[92] Diagnosis: cardiac murmur, failure, fever, embolism, anaemia, high ESR, rash, renal failure. Caused by *Streptococci* (70%) and faecal oganisms in the elderly, *Staphlococci* in postoperative cases and addicts, candida, etc.

Blood culture is performed (negative in 20%) and minimal bactericidal concentrations established. Treatment by penicillin, gentamicin, vancomycin, teicoplanin. Surgery may be required.

Prophylaxis: amoxycillin, clindamycin, erythromycin, vancomycin, gentamycin (especially urology and gut surgery.)

2. Meningitis.

3. Systemic candidiasis.

4. Burns sepsis. Influenced by: (*a*) topical therapy, flamazine, early skin application; (*b*) regular change of dressings; and (*c*) strict aseptic technique.

Signs: pyrexia, cellulitis, lymphangitis, septic episodes with organ dysfunction, hypotension/hypoxia/oliguria/peripheral shutdown (*see above*). Some burns bacteraemias are 'silent' i.e. apyrexial. *See also* Chapter 32.

Prevention of cross-infection in the intensive therapy unit

1. Staff and visitors change outer clothing on entering the unit.
2. Washing of hands between cases (handbasin at each bedstation); use of sterile gloves for specific procedures, e.g. tracheal suction.
3. Keeping the environment dry.
4. Adequate space for each bed (300 sq. ft).
5. Regular cleaning of floor and walls (e.g. with phenol solution).
6. Isolation rooms for severely infectious patients.
7. No changes of ventilator during a period of IPPV.
8. Bacterial filters used on ventilator circuits.
9. Use of disposable equipment.
10. Careful direction of room ventilation air flows.

References

1. Civetta W. et al. *Critical Care* 1988, Philadelphia: Lippincott, 1988.
2. Kreger B. E. W., et al. *Am J. Med.* 1980, **68**, 344.
3. Bailey R. W., Ann. Surg. 1986, **203**, 590.
4. Tesh V. L. and Morrison D. C. *J. Immunol.* 1988, **141**, 3523.
5. Stoelting R. K. *Pharmacology and Physiology in Anesthetic Practice* 2nd Ed. Philadelphia: Lippincott, 1991.
6. Van Deventer S. J. H. et al. *Lancet* 1988, **2**, 605.
7. Mege J. L. and Matrin C. *Crit. Care Med.* 1989, **17**, 1247.

8. Debets J. M. H. et al. *Crit. Care Med.* 1989, **17**, 489.
9. Richard C. et al. *Crit. Care Med.* 1990, **18**, 4.
10. Zimmerman J. J., Millard J. R. and Farrin-Rusk C. *Crit. Care Med.* 1989, **17**, 1241.
11. Vadas P. et al. *Crit. Care Med.* 1988, **16**, 1. Distler W. and Beck L. *Endorphins in Reproduction and Stress.* Berlin: Springer Verlag, 1990.
12. Nayler W. G. *The Endothelins.* Springer Verlag, 1990.
13. Wendt M. and Lawin P. *Oxygen Transport in the Critically Ill Patient.* Berlin: Springer Verlag, 1990.
14. McDonough K. H. *Circ. Shock* 1988, **25**, 291.
15. Raper R. F. and Fisher M. McD. *Clin. Anaesth.* 1990, **4**, 333.
16. Parker M. M. et al. *Crit Care Med.* 1987, **15**, 923.
17. Cunnion R. E. et al. *Circulation* 1986, **73**, 637
18. Artucio H., Digenio A. and Pereyra M. *Crit. Care Med.* 1989, **17**, 323.
19. Matiesson M. et al. *Surg. Gynecol. Obstet.* 1983, **157**, 500.
20. Parker M. M. et al. *Crit Care Med.* 1987, **15**, 923.
21. Raper R. F. and Sibbald W. J. *Chest* 1988, **94**, 507.
22. Sibbald W. J. et al. *Chest* 1978, **73**, 583.
23. Silverman H. J. et al. *Am. Rev. Resp. Dis.* 1989, **135**, 351.
24. D'Orio V. and Wahlen C. et al. *Crit. Care Med.* 1989, **17**, 1314.
25. McDonough K. H. et al. *Circ. Shock* 1985, **17**, 1.
26. Liu M. S. and Xuan Y. T. *Am. J. Physiol.* 1986, **251**, R1078.
27. Gnann J. W. and Cobbs C. G. In: *Principles and Practice of Infectious Diseases* (Mandell G. L., Douglas R. G. and Bennett J. E. ed.) 2nd Ed New York: Wiley, 1985.
28. Knobel E. and Akamine N. et al. *Crit. Care Med.* 1989, **17**, 1344.
29. Chaudry J. H. *Arch. Surg.* 1982, **117**, 151.
30. Runciman W. B., Myburgh J. A. and Upton R. N. *Clin. Anaesth.* 1990, **4**, 271.
31. McCabe W. R. *N. Engl. J. Med.* 1973, **288**, 21.
32. Hemmer M. *Clin. Anaesth.* 1990, **4**, 475.
33. Mela L. *Prog. Clin. Biol. Res.* 1981, **62**, 15.
34. Jeppsson B. et al. *Am. J. Surg.* 1981, **141**, 136.
35. Freund H. R. et al. *Ann. Surg.* 1987, **188**, 123.
36. Moyer E. D. et al. *J. Trauma* 1981, **21**, 263.
37. Freund H. R. et al. *Arch. Surg.* 1986, **121**, 209.
38. Plum F. and Posner B. *The diagnosis of stupor and coma* 3rd. ed. Philadelphia: Davies, 1980.
39. Haimovici H. *Surgery* 1979, **85**, 461.
40. Weinstein R. A. *Ann Intern Med* 1989, **110**, 853.
41. Wenzel R. P. *Eur. J. Clin. Microbiol. Infect. Dis.* 1989, **8**, 56.
42. Brun-Buisson C. *Ann. Int. Med.* 1989, **110**, 873.
43. Zimmerman J. J. *Crit. Care Med.* 1990, **18**, 118.
44. Ognibene F. B. et al. *Chest* 1988, **93**, 903.
45. Moore R. D. *J. Infect. Dis.* 1984, **149**, 443.
46. Shoemaker W. C. et al. *Chest* 1988, **94**, 1176.
47. Kaufman B. S. et al. *Chest* 1984, **85**, 336.
48. Colardyn F. C. et al. *Crit. Care Med.* 1989, **17**, 999.
49. Weisel R. D. et al. *Am. J. Surg.* 1977, **133**, 512.
50. Holcroft J. W. et al. *Ann. Surg.* 1986, **203**, 371.
51. Ziegler E. J. et al. *N. Eng. J. Med.* 1982, **307**, 1225; Lachman E., Pitsoe S. B. and Gaffin S. L. *Lancet* 1984, **1**, 981; Baumgartner J. D. et al. *Lancet* 1985, **ii**, 59.
52. Natale J. E. et al. *Stroke* 1988 **19**, 1371.
53. Bernard G. R. et al. *J. Clin. Invest.* 1984, **73**, 1772.
54. Cohen H. J. *Blood* 1980, **56**, 23.
55. Syrota A. *J. Nucl. Med.* 1981, **22**, 145.
56. Yen M. H. and Lee S. H. *Europ. J. Pharmacol.* 1987, **144**, 369.
57. Cotev S. et al. In: *Update in Intensive Care and Emergency Medicine – 10.* (Vincent J-L. ed.) Berlin: Springer Verlag, 1990.

58. Baumgartner J. D. et al. *Lancet* 1985, **ii**, 59; Anon, *Pharm. J.* 1990, **244**, 724.
59. Pollack M. et al. *J. Infect. Dis.* 1989, **159**, 168.
60. Cerra B. et al. *Surgery* 1988, **104**, 727.
61. Sprung C. L. et al. *N. Eng. J. Med.* 1984, **311**, 1137.
62. Bone R. C. et al *N. Eng. J. Med.* 1987, **317**, 653.
63. Veterans Administration Systemic Sepsis Cooperative Study Group, *New Eng. J. Med.* 1987, **317**, 659.
64. Mandell G. L. *Am. Rev. Resp. Dis.* 1988, **138**, 1103.
65. Holaday J. W. and Faden J. I. *Nature* 1978, **275**, 450; Hackshaw K. V., Parker G. A. and Roberts J. W. *Crit. Care Med.* 1990, **18**, 47.
66. Kever A. H. J. et al. *Crit. Care Med.* 1988, **16**, 1087.
67. Goldfarb R. D. et al. *Am. J. Physiol.* 1983, **244**, H370.
68. National Heart Lung and Blood Institute Collaborative Study, Washington DC 1979.
69. Parker M. M. et al. *Crit Care Med.* 1987, **15**, 923.
70. Abraham E. et al. *Crit. Care Med.* 1983, **11**, 799.
71. Kreger B. E. W. et al. *Am J. Med.* 1980, **68**, 344.
72. Moore R. D. *J. Infect. Dis.* 1984, **149**, 443.
73. Winslow E. J. et al. *Am. J. Med.* 1973, **54**, 421.
74. Fourrier F. et al. *Chest* 1985, **87** 191.
75. O'Connel M. T. et al. *Crit Care Med* 1984, **12**, 479.
76. Pollack M. et al. *J. Clin. Invest.* 1984, **72**, 1874.
77. Girotti M. J. et al. *J. Appl. Physiol.* 1984, **56**, 582.
78. Ziegler E. J. et al. *N. Eng. J. Med.* 1982, **307**, 1225; Lachman E., Pitsoe S. B. and Gaffin S. L. *Lancet* 1984, **1**, 981.
79. Schlag G., Redl H. and Siegel J. H. *Shock, Sepsis and Organ Failure,* Berlin: Springer Verlag, 1990.
80. Sosnowski N. W. et al. *Brit. Med. J.* 1990, **301**, 303.
81. Mortensen J. D. and Barry G. *Int. J. Artif. Org.* 1989, **12**, 384.
82. Manji N. et al. *Crit. Care Med.* 1990, **18**, 29.
83. Means E. D. et al. *Update in Intensive Care and Emergency Medicine – 10* (Vincent J-L. ed.) Berlin: Springer Verlag, 1990.
84. Chernow B. and Roth B. L. In: *Perspectives on Sepsis and Septic Shock.* (Sibbald W. J. and Sprung C. ed.) Washington: *Soc. Crit. Care Med.* 178.
85. Nasraway S. A. et al. *Chest* 1989, **95**, 612.
86. Vincent J-L. et al. *Circ. shock* 1988, **25**, 75
87. Chiarla C. et al. *Crit. Care Med.* 1990, **18**, 32.
88. Hanafiah S. R. and Chong S. K. F. *J. R. Soc. Med* 1991, **84**, 48.
89. Todd J. et al. *Lancet* 1978, **ii**, 1116.
90. Davis J. P. et al *N. Eng. J. Med.* 1980, **303**, 1429.
91. Parsonnet J. *Rev. Infect. Dis.* 1989, **II**, S8.
92. Oakley C. M. *Prescibers J.* 1990, **30**, 152.

Chapter 34

Nutrition

Nutritional requirements

The daily basal requirements are shown in Table 34.1.

Table 34.1 Typical daily nutritional requirements

	Requirement per kg body weight	Requirement for 70 kg man
Water	25–35 ml	1500–2500 ml
Protein	1 g	70 g (4 kcal or 17 kJ per g)
Carbohydrate	2 g	140 g (4 kcal or 17 kJ per g)
Fat	1–2 g	140 g (9 kcal or 38 kJ per g)
Calories	30 kcal (125 kJ)	2100 kcal (8750 kJ)

The proportion of fat and carbohydrate is very variable. Minerals, vitamins and some trace elements are also necessary. Alcohol provides 7 kcal (29 kJ) per g.

The calorie requirement of an acutely-ill patient is highly variable. Indirect calorimetry,[1] i.e. measuring oxygen consumption, may help, but such a patient will need about 30–35 kcal/kg/day. This can be increased in various situations as follows: 6% per °C temperature rise;[2] 10% for elective operative stress; 25% for a long-bone fracture; 30% for peritonitis; 50% for multiple injuries or major sepsis; area of any burns (25% if < 20%, 75% if 20–40%, 100% if > 40%).

Indications for artificial feeding include: (1) major surgery, trauma, burns, sepsis; (2) any cause of gastro-intestinal failure; (3) preoperative malnutrition; (4) severe anorexia nervosa; (5) coma; and (6) some patients with kidney or liver failure, where their usual dietary restrictions apply with equal importance to enteral and parenteral nutrition.

Assessment of nutritional status[3]

1. *Simple measurements:* body weight; mid-triceps skin-fold thickness (indicates fat stores) should be more than 10 mm in men and 13 mm in

women; mid-arm muscle circumference (indicates muscle mass), which is mid-arm circumference minus (π × triceps skin-fold thickness), and should be more than 23 cm in men and 22 cm in women. These are subject to errors if oedema is present.

2. *Biochemical estimates of protein lack:* serum albumin; transport proteins with a rapid turnover, e.g. transferrin, thyroxine-binding pre-albumin, retinol-binding protein; ratio of urinary creatinine to patient's height. Note that there is normally a turnover of some 100 g of protein per day.

3. *Tests of immunity:* lymphocyte count, suppression of cell-mediated delayed hypersensitivity, e.g. skin reactions to mumps, streptokinase, Candida. Of limited value.

Enteral feeding[4]

When the patient cannot take oral food, but has a functioning gut, enteral feeding with a liquid diet is more effective and less hazardous than intravenous nutrition. Although a normal gastric tube can be used, a 1 mm ID plastic tube, with a stylet to stiffen it for insertion, is more comfortable, causes less trauma to the oesophagus and stomach, and may be left in place for up to a month. It can be placed in the stomach or duodenum, but may be misplaced into the lungs.[5] The position is checked by X-ray or endoscopy. The feed is given continuously from a reservoir, controlled by a clamp or pump. The tube is too small for puréed hospital food, and commercial preparations are simple, safe, sterile and not too expensive.

The protein sources used are casein, milk or soya. The degree of protein hydrolysis varies. Vegetable oils are used as sources of fat, and starch or corn syrup for carbohydrate. The latter usually provides over half the calories. Most feeds have about 1 kcal (4.2 kJ) per ml. Clinifeed, Isocal and Ensure are widely used. Clinifeed ISO has 260 g of carbohydrate, 56 g of protein, 82 g of fat and 2000 kcal (8400 kJ) per 2000 ml. It provides the usually-recommended 200 kcal (840 kJ) of non-protein calories per gram of nitrogen (1 g nitrogen is equivalent to 6.25 g protein). Vitamins, minerals and trace elements are included; it is low in sodium and the osmolality is 270 mosmol/kg. Vivonex and Flexical have a high proportion of elemental, pre-digested nutrients. Such feeds have a higher osmolality, which can cause diarrhoea, and the indications for them are uncertain.

Some nutrients such as glutamine, short-chain fatty acids and polyunsaturated fatty acids may be trophic to the gut and be of particular benefit to septic patients.[6]

Complications[7]

1. *Of the tube:* trauma and ulceration of nose, pharynx and gut mucosa; sinusitis (if nasal); misplacement in the lungs; regurgitation and aspiration, reflux can be reduced by nursing the patient 10° head up.

2. *Gastro-intestinal:* change of gut flora, vomiting and diarrhoea. The latter is common and may be due to infection of the feed, antibiotics, lactose intolerance or high osmotic pressure of feed. The feed should be slowed,

diluted with water or changed. Loperamide 2 mg, up to 16 mg daily, or codeine phosphate 30 mg, up to 180 mg daily, are useful.

3. Metabolic: Fluid balance and electrolyte abnormalities; hyperglycaemia; folate deficiency.

Parenteral feeding[8]

Intravenous nutrition, used when feeding via the gut is not possible. May be total (TPN) or supplement partial oral or tube feeds. Maintains the patient until the gut failure is corrected, and is usually started after a few days' starvation, or when prolonged feeding difficulties are expected, e.g. major abdominal surgery. Nitrogen loss in a moderately catabolic patient will exceed 15 g/day, and can be easily measured as urinary urea, adding any proteinuria or rise in total body urea:

$$\text{Nitrogen loss (g/day)} =$$

$$\text{daily urinary urea} \; \frac{\text{grams}}{2} \; \text{or} \; \frac{\text{mmol}}{30}$$

$$+ \text{daily urinary protein excretion} \; \frac{\text{grams}}{6.25}$$

$$+ \text{body wt. (kg)} \times \text{daily rise in blood urea} \; \frac{\text{mg/dl}}{360} \; \text{or} \; \frac{\text{mmol/l}}{60}$$

$$(1 \text{ g urea} = 17 \text{ mmol urea} = 0.47 \text{ g nitrogen})$$

15 g of nitrogen loss represents the breakdown of 94 g of protein, or 450 g of muscle. 200 kcal (840 kJ) of non-protein calories per gram of nitrogen should be given, although this may have to be reduced to 150 kcal (630 kJ) per gram nitrogen in the sickest patient. If glucose is the only non-protein energy source, protein anabolism is not optimal, and CO_2 production is higher, putting a strain on patients with poor respiratory reserve. Non-protein energy is best provided equally from glucose and fat.[9]

Carbohydrate

Body stores of carbohydrate are limited, the average adult having only 5 g of blood glucose and 100 g of liver glycogen. Adequate carbohydrate is needed to allow fat utilization without ketosis, the minimum for this being 400 kcal (1.7 MJ) of carbohydrate energy per day, although normally at least 50% of the administered calories are from glucose. Fructose, sorbitol, ethanol, xylitol have all been used as alternative carbohydrate energy sources in the past but offer no advantage over glucose, and indeed can cause metabolic problems, such as lactic acidosis or an osmotic diuresis.

Glucose provides 4.0 kcal (17 kJ) per gram. One litre of isotonic (5%) solution provides only 200 kcal (840 kJ), so concentrated solutions are needed to give enough calories without over-hydration. 25% glucose supplies 250 g glucose and 1000 kcal (4 MJ) per litre. 25% or 50% are commonly used, and these solutions need a central vein. The metabolic response to surgery or trauma includes impaired glucose tolerance, but insulin does not often need to be given if less than 500 g glucose is given per day. If needed it may be given i.v. by infusion, normally about 1 unit per 4 g glucose infused, keeping the blood glucose below 12 mmol/l.

Fat

Provides 9.0 kcal (38 kJ) per gram. Advantages include iso-osmolarity and neutral pH (can be given into a peripheral vein). No losses occur in faeces or urine. Fat is provided as a 10% or 20% soya oil emulsion, with particle diameters 0.2–1.0 μm, much the same as a chylomicron. The surfactant is egg phospholipid and glycerol is added to make the solution isotonic. 500 ml of 20% emulsion provides 1000 kcal (4.2 MJ). Provides the essential fatty acids. Well utilized in all patients. The fasting patient's spun plasma may be examined each day for excessive milkiness (which calls for a reduction in fat intake). This is more likely in liver insufficiency, acute pancreatitis, uraemia and septicaemia. Occasional side-effects are shivering, flushing and fever.

Protein

Given as a mixture of essential and non-essential crystalline amino acids in the physiological laevo-rotatory form. Solutions with higher proportions of branched-chain amino acids (valine, leucine, isoleucine) have no advantage in most patients. Most solutions have nitrogen contents ranging from 9–18 g/l, are hyperosmolar and have a pH around 5.6. Some however have 5 g nitrogen per litre, an osmolality of only 370 mosmol/kg and so can be given peripherally. There is no point in giving more than 24 g of amino acid nitrogen per day, as it then cannot be handled by the liver. A typical dose in most clinical situations would be 0.2–0.25 g nitrogen/kg/day. The electrolyte composition varies, some are nearly electrolyte-free. Extra electrolytes may be added by the pharmacy.

Additives

These are conveniently provided by commercial additive preparations.
   Electrolytes. Daily requirements very variable with the clinical situation, but approximately: sodium 100 mmol and potassium 60 mmol (or 6 mmol/g nitrogen, more if febrile); phosphate 40 mmol, less if in renal failure and more if very catabolic, should not be mixed with calcium or magnesium for injection; calcium 5–15 mmol; magnesium 10 mmol or 1 mmol/g nitrogen. Chloride is also present in most additives.
   Vitamins. Their importance was first pointed out by F. Gowland Hopkins (1861–1947) of Cambridge in 1912 for which he received the Nobel Prize in 1929.[10] Daily requirements:[11] thiamine (B$_1$) 3 mg: riboflavine (B$_2$) 3.6 mg; pyridoxine (B$_6$) 4 mg; nicotinamide 40 mg; vitamin B$_{12}$ 5 μg; biotin 60 μg; pantothenic acid 15 mg; folic acid 0.4 mg; vitamin A 1 mg; vitamin C (ascorbic acid) 100 mg; vitamin D 200 IU; vitamin E 10 mg; vitamin K 150 μg. The B vitamins degrade when exposed to light.

Trace elements. Daily requirements:[12] iron 20 μmol; zinc 100 μmol, more if very catabolic; copper 20 μmol; manganese 5 μmol; chromium 0.2 μmol; selenium 0.4 μmol; molybdenum 0.2 μmol; fluorine 50 μmol; iodine 1 μmol.

Management

A central venous catheter is needed for most TPN solutions, inserted under aseptic conditions, preferably placed through a subcutaneous tunnel (for insertion, *see* Chapter 17) and used for nothing else. If a multi-lumen catheter is used, one lumen should be reserved only for TPN. Some lower osmolality solutions (lipids, and low nitrogen amino acid solutions) may be given through a peripheral vein using a fine-bore silicone catheter.[13] TPN is generally managed by a multi-disciplinary team including a nurse and pharmacist,[14] and can be carried out at home for patients with e.g. Crohn's disease. The desired mixture is made up in pharmacy, presented in a 3-litre bag and infused over 24 hours with a controlled volumetric pump. Albumin or red cells should be given to patients with hypoproteinaemia or anaemia. Albumin may be ineffective at correcting the plasma level.

Complications of parenteral feeding[8]

These can largely be prevented by adequate biochemical monitoring.

1. Glucose metabolism. Hyperglycaemia, due to excess hypertonic glucose or insufficient insulin. Ketoacidosis may occur. May progress to hyperosmolar syndrome (facial flushing, lethargy, coma) with a poor prognosis. Hypercapnia may occur with too much glucose.

2. Amino acid metabolism. Patients in acute renal failure will have to be dialysed or have haemofiltration more frequently due to pre-renal uraemia. Patients with hepatic encephalopathy may benefit from a higher proportion of branched chain amino acids. Metabolic acidosis may be due to excessive chloride in some amino acid solutions.

3. Fats. The sicker patients may be less able to metabolize fat. Essential fatty acid deficiency.

4. Water and electrolytes. Circulatory overload, excess water and hyponatraemia relatively common. Electrolyte deficiencies include potassium, calcium (tetany and muscle spasm), phosphate (weakness, metabolic bone disease resembling osteomalacia, left-shift oxygen dissociation curve), magnesium (tetany, weakness, tremor, dysrhythmias).

5. Vitamin and trace element deficiencies. Thiamine deficiency for even one month may produce cardiac failure from acute beri-beri. Lack of vitamin B_{12} or folate causes anaemia, and lack of vitamin K causes clotting defects. Zinc deficiency causes acrodermatitis enteropathica (crusty skin lesions around the mouth, nostrils and sites of trauma), chronic infections and diarrhoea. Copper deficiency causes anaemia, osteoporosis, leucopenia and reduced red cell superoxide dismutase.

6. Catheter sites.[15] Infection, thrombophlebitis, complications of central venous cannulation (pneumothorax, damage to arteries and nerves, etc).

7. Miscellaneous. Cholestasis may occur, possibly due to overgrowth of intestinal bacteria. It has been prevented by metronidazole, suggesting anaerobic infection.[16]

References

1. Bursztein S. et al. *Am. J. Clin. Nutr.* 1989, **50**, 227.
2. Vermeij C. G. et al. *Crit. Care Med.* 1989, **17**, 623.
3. Goodinson S. M. and Dickerson J. W. T. In: *Nutrition in the Clinical Management of Disease.* (Dickerson J. W. T. and Lee H. A. ed.) 2nd ed. London: Edward Arnold, 1988, 456.
4. Dobb G. J. In: *Intensive Care: Developments and Controversies.* (Dobb G. J. ed.) *Clin. Anaesthesiol.* 1990, **4**(2), 531.
5. Harris M. R. and Huseby J. S. *Crit. Care Med.* 1989, **17**, 917.
6. Grimble G. et al. *Intensive Ther. Clin. Monit.* 1989, **10**, 51.
7. Bastow M. D. *Gut* 1986, **27**, 51.
8. Lee H. A. In: *Nutrition in the Clinical Management of Disease.* (Dickerson J. W. T. and Lee H. A. ed.) 2nd ed. London: Edward Arnold, 1988, 496.
9. MacFie J. et al. *Gastroenterology* 1981, **80**, 103; Roulet M. et al. *Clin. Nutr.* 1983, **2**, 97.
10. Hopkins F. G. *J. Physiol. (Lond.)* 1912, **44**, 425.
11. American Medical Association. *J. Parent. Ent. Nutr.* 1979, **3**, 258; Shenkin A. *Proc. Nutr. Soc.* 1986, **45**, 383.
12. American Medical Association. *JAMA* 1979, **241**, 2051; Shenkin A. et al. *Clin. Nutr.* 1986, **5**, 91; Shenkin A. *Intensive Ther. Clin. Monit.* 1987, **8**, 38.
13. Jaeger H. J. et al. *Clin. Nutr.* 1990, **9** (Suppl.1), P115.
14. In adults: Nehme A. E. *JAMA* 1980, **243**, 1906; In children: Puntis J. W. L. and Booth I. W. *Intensive Ther. Clin. Monit.* 1990, **11**, 132. For a survey of UK hospitals, *see* Payne-James J. et al. *Health Trends* 1990, **22**, 9.
15. McIntyre A. S. et al. *J. Roy. Soc. Med.* 1990, **83**, 371.
16. Capron J-P. et al. *Lancet* 1983, **1**, 446.

Section 7
HISTORY

Chapter 35

History of anaesthesia

The development of anaesthesia since its introduction in 1846 has been erratic, long periods of stagnation being occasionally broken by improvements and advances. For the history of pain relief in surgery before 1846 *see A History of Anaesthesia* (Atkinson R. S. and Boulton T. B.) London: Royal Society of Medicine, 1989.

Anaesthesia as we know it today was first used by W. T. G. Morton of Boston in the US who gave ether at the Massachusetts General Hospital on 16 October 1846 to Gilbert Abbott. C. W. Long of Georgia had given the same agent several times 4 years previously[1] but failed to report his work at the time so that this was unknown to Morton. Thus was Henry Hill Hickman's idea that anaesthesia could be produced by the inhalation of gases and vapours, finally vindicated. Horace Wells, a colleague of Morton, had used nitrous oxide for the painless extraction of teeth quite successfully in 1844, but his public demonstration of this practice was a disastrous failure and the gas was temporarily forgotten. The news of Morton's discovery soon spread throughout the civilized world, and on 19 December 1846 Francis Boott, a physician, born and trained in the US but working in London, received news of Morton's discovery[2] and encouraged Mr James Robinson, a dentist to give ether to a Miss Lonsdale for a dental extraction, Mr Robinson acting as dentist and anaesthetist. A commemorative plaque has now been placed on his residence at No. 14, Gower Street, London. (On the same day, Dr Scott operated under ether at the Dumfries and Galloway Infirmary in Scotland.) So successful was this that Boott persuaded Robert Liston, the University of London's professor of surgery, to experiment with the new drug. It was tried out with considerable publicity and brilliant success for the amputation through the thigh of Frederick Churchill's leg at University College Hospital on 21 December 1846.

The technical difficulties associated with the administration of ether were partly overcome by the substitution with chloroform by James Young Simpson, professor of midwifery at Edinburgh University, in the following year. He poured drops of this newer agent on to gauze held near the face of the patient, so avoiding the inhalers that were used for ether.

John Snow, a London physician, was the first to attempt some sort of scientific investigation into the new anaesthetic agents and the methods of their administration, and he devised several pieces of apparatus for delivering to the patient known percentage concentrations of anaesthetic vapour in an attempt to increase their safety. This work was undertaken because of the reports of deaths associated with anaesthesia. Different uses of the drugs and different methods of administration were adopted in different countries. Thus chloroform was used more frequently in Scotland, the greater part of Europe and in the southern states of America, while ether remained the favourite in England and in the northern states of America. There was much controversy as to which was the safer of the two drugs but eventually ether won the day. When in 1858 John Snow, who was England's leading physician anaesthetist, died, his place was taken by J. T. Clover, and partly due to the influence of these two pioneers, the administration of anaesthetics in the UK has always been in the hands of medical men and, as time has passed, in the hands of specialists in the subject.

Meanwhile, nitrous oxide still had its friends in the US, and in 1863 G. Q. Colton, who introduced it to Wells, embarked on a campaign of popularization of the gas. Its disadvantages were difficulty in administration and the asphyxia inseparable from its use. The latter was partly overcome by Edmund Andrews of Chicago who in 1868 gave it with 20% oxygen, and by Paul Bert of Paris who gave it under pressure 10 years later. The first major war in which anaesthetics were used was the Crimean War (1854–1855). It is an interesting fact, however, that even 25 years after Morton introduced the use of ether in surgery, operations were still being performed in the complete absence of any form of anaesthesia, even in European teaching hospitals.[3]

During the next 40–50 years there were few significant changes in anaesthesia, but in the 1920s the pace of progress quickened. In the 1920s, ether and chloroform were the main agents used but ethyl chloride and nitrous oxide were often employed for induction. Simpson's open drop method was the most popular, while the first Boyle machine appeared in 1917. One of the early pioneers was Sir Geoffrey Marshall, who gained experience of anaesthesia while serving in the R.A.M.C. in the First World War. (*See* Boulton T. B., *Survey of Anesthesiology* 1992, **36**, 40.) Before the 1930s the anaesthetist administered one or two volatile agents to produce unconsciousness, muscle relaxation and deafferentation. This gave place to various techniques of so-called balanced anaesthesia and so the amount of toxic drugs to which the patient was exposed was reduced and the hazard of general anaesthesia made less. Among other innovations were the popularization of endotracheal techniques by Ivan W. Magill and E. Stanley Rowbotham, the appearance of bromethol (Avertin), divinyl ether, cyclopropane and trichloroethylene, and the induction of anaesthesia by intravenous barbiturates in the early 1930s. Because of the difficulty of obtaining relaxation of the jaw and larynx with ether, blind nasotracheal intubation became increasingly used. Controlled respiration was used with cyclopropane so that when curare was first tried out by Harold Griffith in Montreal in 1942, the way to deal with hypoventilation and apnoea was well established, and soon intermittent positive-pressure ventilation became routine practice.

Local analgesia made its appearance in 1884 when Carl Koller of Vienna demonstrated the use of cocaine for topical analgesia in the eye. Infiltration and regional block followed from this. Spinal analgesia was first described by August Bier in Kiel in 1898 and extradural block by Fernand Cathelin and

Jean Athanese Sicard in Paris in 1901 and by Fidel Pages of Madrid in 1921 and Achille Mario Dogliotti of Turin in 1931. The two world wars stimulated both surgery and anaesthesia, and following each, the number of doctors who continued their anaesthetic work, learnt under service conditions, into civilian life had a considerable influence on the development of the specialty.

Technical improvements were slowly accompanied by academic recognition, but not always by adequate financial rewards. The first examination for the Diploma in Anaesthetics was held in London in 1935 and the first chair in anaesthetics was created in Oxford,[4] with R. R. Macintosh as professor, 2 years later. Ralph Waters was appointed as the first professor of anaesthesia in a university in the US in 1933. In the UK the recognition of anaesthesia as a specialty with full equality with other medical and surgical specialties was secured in 1948 with the introduction of the National Health Service, and since then anaesthesia has not only kept pace with the rapid advances made in surgery, but has in many instances enabled these advances to be made. In recent decades the scope of the anaesthetist's work has widened and now takes in not only pre-operative assessment and postoperative care, but supervision of intensive therapy units, pain services, and in many cases research and postgraduate education. An enormous development in the use of monitoring equipment, some of it highly sophisticated, has taken place in the last 20 years. Among those workers who remember clinical anaesthesia in the 1930s and early 1940s, few would disagree with the statement that what is known as 'modern anaesthesia' commenced with the introduction of the muscle relaxants. (*See also* Duncum B. *The Development of Inhalation Anaesthesia*. London: Oxford University Press, 1947; and Rupreht J. et al. (ed.) *Anaesthesia: Essays on its History*. Berlin: Springer-Verlag, 1985.)

Following a joint congress of anaesthetists in London in 1951 of which Sir Ivan Magill was President, and a similar meeting in Paris the same year, it was decided to form a Federation of Societies of Anaesthesiologists and the first Congress of the new body was held in Scheveningen in Holland in 1955. Other similar congresses have been held in Toronto (1960), Sao Paulo (1964), London (1968), Kyoto (1972), Mexico City (1976), Hamburg (1980), Manila (1984), Washington (1988) and The Hague (1992). (See also van Lieburg M. J. In: Rupreht J. et al. (ed.) *Anaesthesia: Essays on its History*. Berlin: Springer-Verlag, 1985, 307; Organe G. *ibid.* 309; and Howat, D. D. C. *ibid.* 314.)

Among training courses arranged by the World Health Organization were those of the Anaesthesiology Centre in Copenhagen (1950–1973) and in Manila (under the guidance of Professor Quintin Gomez).[5]

Some outstanding contributors to the science and art of anaesthesia

Joseph Priestley (1733–1804)

Born in Fieldhead near Leeds, the son of a handloom worker, and brought up in a strict Nonconformist Calvinistic atmosphere by an aunt. Educated at Batley Grammar School. Trained as a dissenting minister and took charge of Mill Hill Chapel in Leeds in 1773. He then became a schoolmaster and experimenter in chemistry, physics and electricity. He never gave up the phlogiston theory, unlike Lavoisier who discredited it and who was guillotined during the French Revolution. Next, Priestley spent seven years as librarian and companion to the second Earl of Shelbourne (1737–1805) at Bowood, and isolated or identified 'alkaline air' (NH_3), 'vitriolic acid air' (SO_2), 'dephlogisticated air' (O_2) in 1774, a gas given the name of oxygen by Lavoisier (1743–1797) and produced by heating mercuric oxide with a burning glass; 'dephlogisticated nitrous air' (N_2O) in 1773 and 'Nitrous acid air' (NO_2). (One of his teachers, Mathew Turner of Manchester, described the anaesthetic effects of ether in 1744.[6]) He also discovered methane and the absorption of carbon dioxide (fixed air) by green plants in the presence of sunshine with the formation of oxygen. By subjecting carbon dioxide to pressure in water he discovered 'soda water'. He was elected a Fellow of the Royal Society and became a Doctor of Laws of the University of Edinburgh. From the former institution he received a Copley Medal for a paper on 'The Different Kinds of Air'.[7] His discoveries led Thomas Beddoes (1760–1808) of Bristol to experiment with the therapeutic effects of these 'airs'. In 1780 he went to Birmingham to take charge of a Unitarian congregation, The New Meeting House, and in this city he became a member of the famous Lunar Society, which brought him into contact with Erasmus Darwin (1731–1802), physician and grandfather of Charles (1809–1882), James Watt (1736–1818), scientist and inventor and William Murdoch (1757–1839), engineer and the inventor of gas lighting. He became a close friend of, and correspondent with Benjamin Franklin (1706–1790), American printer, inventor and diplomat. He was an opponent of political discrimination against Dissenters, and on the second anniversary of the fall of the Bastille (14 July 1789) his chapel, home, scientific apparatus, books and manuscripts were looted by a High Tory Royalist mob, forcing him to seek refuge in Hackney, near London. His left-wing political opinions still separated him from his scientific colleagues so that in 1794 he joined his sons in Northumberland, Pennsylvania. Here, he added farming to his other activities and soon became a leader of his new community. He died of oesophageal obstruction in 1804 at the age of 70. A statue to Priestley was unveiled in Birmingham by Thomas Henry Huxley in 1874 to mark the centenary of the discovery of oxygen. Hilaire Belloc (1870–1953), the poet, journalist and historian, was a great-grandson. (*See also* Smith W. D. A. *Under the Influence: A History of Nitrous Oxide and Oxygen Anaesthesia*. London: Macmillan, 1982; and McDowell D. G. *Anaesth. Intensive Care* 1982, **10**, 4.)

Humphry Davy (1778–1829)[8]

Born in Cornwall, the son of a wood carver. Became apprenticed to J. B. Borlase, surgeon, of Penzance, in 1795. At the age of 17 he experimented with nitrous oxide and the effects of its inhalation. In 1798 Davy became superintendent of Thomas Beddoes's (1760–1808) Pneumatic Institute in Clifton, Bristol, for the treatment of pulmonary tuberculosis by inhalation of gases; other gases used were hydrogen, oxygen, 'water gas' and carbon dioxide. Humphry Davy published his book *Researches, Chemical and Philosophical: Chiefly Concerning Nitrous Oxide* (London: J. Johnson, 1800). "On the day when the inflammation was most troublesome, I breathed three large doses of nitrous oxide. The pain always diminished after the first four or five respiration."[9] In this, Davy suggested that nitrous oxide inhalations might be used to relieve the pain of surgical operations and named it 'laughing gas'. A nitrous oxide container was made by James Watt (1736–1819) in 1799 to assist this research.[10] The idea was not pursued by Humphry Davy or anyone else, except for its entertainment value, but his work was known to, and may have influenced, Gardner Quincy Colton (1814–1898) 44 years later. In later life, Davy became famous. He invented the miner's safety lamp, was created a baronet in 1818, and was elected President of the Royal Society in 1820. Among Davy's colleagues at Bristol was Dr Peter Mark Roget, FRS, famed for his *Thesaurus of English Words and Phrases* (1852). Davy prepared nitrous oxide by the method of Berthollet (1785) by heating ammonium nitrate. He was Faraday's teacher and was the first to describe sodium and potassium.

Henry Hill Hickman (1800–1830)[8]

Born 27 January 1800 at Lady Halton, Bromfield, in Shropshire. Medical education received in Edinburgh, but did not graduate there (MRCS, England, 1821). He settled in practice in Ludlow and later in Tenbury Wells in Worcestershire. He married in 1821. While at Shifnal, in Shropshire, his interest in gas therapy was aroused, as the village was the birthplace of Thomas Beddoes. Familiarizing himself with the pioneer work of Davy, Priestley and Michael Faraday (1791–1867), Hickman returned to Ludlow and commenced experiments on animals (controlled asphyxiation) in 1825. He was able to perform surgical operations painlessly on them, by causing them to inhale carbon dioxide. This was the first work on surgical anaesthesia induced by inhaling a gas. His results where published in a paper, 'A Letter on Suspended Animation' (Ironbridge, 1824), when W. T. G. Morton was a child of 5, but attracted no attention from scientific men in England. Even Sir Humphry Davy, who was approached by Hickman's friend, T. A. Knight, FRS,[11] showed no interest. Charles X of France (1752–1827) was appealed to in 1828,[8] and the French Academy of Medicine agreed to investigate Hickman's results, but nothing came of the matter. Baron Dominique Jean Larrey (1766–1842), one of Napoleon's surgeons, however, gave Hickman some encouragement. Hickman died prematurely, aged 29, at Tenbury Wells, and was buried in Bromfield churchyard, Shropshire, where, in 1930, a memorial was erected in the porch by the Anaesthetic Section of the Royal Society of Medicine, unveiled by Sir St Clair Thompson and dedicated by the Bishop of Hereford (*Br. Med. J.* 1930, 12 April). The first allusion to Hickman in recent times was in an article by C. J. S. Thompson in the *Br. Med. J.* 1912, **1**, 843.

Horace Wells (1815–1848)

Born in Hartford, Connecticut. In 1844, on 10 December, Gardner Q. Colton (1814–1898), a travelling lecturer in chemistry, gave a demonstration of the effects of inhaling nitrous oxide at Hartford, Connecticut. Horace Wells, a local dentist, was present and noticed that a young shop assistant, Samuel Cooley, while under the influence of the gas, banged his shin and made it bleed, but stated afterwards that he experienced no pain. Wells persuaded Colton to try the gas during a dental extraction, and on the following day, 11 December 1844, the experiment was carried out with Colton as anaesthetist,

John M. Riggs (1810–1885) as dentist and Wells as patient. It was a big success. "A new era in tooth pulling", according to Wells. Wells learnt from Colton the method of manufacture of nitrous oxide and used it in his dental practice on 15 patients. It was administered from an animal bladder through a wooden tube into the mouth, while the nostrils were compressed. Later he went to Boston to interest a larger audience in his discovery. He demonstrated the method to the students of Harvard Medical School, in the class of Dr John Collins Warren (1778–1856), but the patient complained of pain; the affair was a fiasco and Wells was hissed out of the room as a fraud. Morton and Charles T. Jackson (1805–1880) were present at this operation in January 1845. Wells returned to Hartford and continued to use the gas, but the introduction of ether gradually ousted nitrous oxide. In 1847 Wells published his letter 'A History of the Discovery of the Application of Nitrous Oxide Gas, Ether, and Other Vapours to Surgical Operations' (Hartford, Conn., 1847; *see also* 'Classical File', *Surv. Anesthesiol.* 1958, **2**, 1). In 1847 he opened a dental office in New York City but soon afterwards Wells gave up dentistry, became a chloroform addict, travelled around the country with a troop of performing canaries, and was incarcerated in jail after bespattering a New York prostitute with sulphuric acid, while recovering from self-administered chloroform.[12] He commited suicide by cutting his femoral artery, aged 33.

Colton reintroduced the use of nitrous oxide in dentistry in 1863, at New Haven.

William Thomas Green Morton (1819–1868)[13]

Morton deserves the chief credit for the introduction of ether as an anaesthetic agent, although W. E. Clarke (1818–1878), of Rochester, New York, gave ether for a dental extraction in 1842, and Crawford Williamson Long (1815–1878) removed a tumour from the neck of James M. Venable quite painlessly, in Jefferson County, Georgia, a few months after Clarke's experiment. By the time (1849) that Long reported his work,[14] Morton's fame was well established. In science, the credit for a new discovery belongs to the man who convinces the world, not to the man to whom the idea first occurs. Morton convinced the world of the advantages of ether anaesthesia and the credit for this discovery is his.

Morton, born at Charlton, Worcester County, Massachusetts, started work at the age of 16 in a printing house; later went into business but was a failure. As a young man he suffered the pain of a surgical operation, in Cincinnati. He studied at the Baltimore College of Dental Surgery, set up in practice at Farmington, Connecticut, and later became a pupil and later a partner of Wells, at Hartford. He separated from Wells and, becoming a medical student in Boston at the Harvard Medical School, was present when Wells failed to satisfy the audience as to the efficiency of nitrous oxide. He never qualified in medicine, but received an honorary MD in 1852. Charles T. Jackson (1805–1880),[15] one of Morton's lecturers at Harvard, suggested that ether could be used as a surface analgesic in dentistry. Morton, however, went further; he experimented on dogs to find out the effect of giving ether vapour by inhalation. Impressed with the results, he gave the vapour to Eben

Frost for the removal of a tooth on 30 September 1846. The operation was painless. After gaining further experience, including the administration of 37 anaesthetics for Henry Bigelow, and while still a medical student, Morton gave a demonstration at the Massachusetts General Hospital on 16 October 1846, in what is now the 'Ether Dome', when Dr John Collins Warren (1778–1856) removed a tumour from the jaw of his patient, Gilbert Abbott, a printer and journalist,[16] without producing any pain. This success gained him the support of Warren and also of Henry Jacob Bigelow (1818–1890), surgeon and professor of materia medica. Oliver Wendell Holmes (1809–1897), professor of anatomy and physiology at Harvard Medical School, said:[17] "This priceless gift to humanity went forth from the operating theatre of the Massachusetts General Hospital, and the man to whom the world owes it is Dr T. W. G. Morton." Much wrangling occurred between Morton and Jackson as to who should be given credit for the discovery.[15] Morton three times petitioned the US Congress, and even obtained an interview with the President (Franklin Pierce, 1804–1869), but he was never in his lifetime officially recognized as the pioneer of ether anaesthesia. Time later vindicated his claim. He spent his later years farming at Needham, Massachusetts, and died of cerebral haemorrhage quite suddenly in Central Park, New York City, on 15 July 1868;[18] a disappointed man. The inscription on his tombstone in Mount Auburn Cemetery, Boston, composed by Henry J. Bigelow reads: "Inventor and Revealer of Inhalation Anesthesia: Before Whom, in All Time, Surgery was Agony; By Whom, Pain in Surgery was Averted and Annulled; Since Whom, Science has Control of Pain". His agent, which he tried to patent under the name Letheon, became widely used.

It was given in London and Paris in 1846. Robert Liston (1794–1847) was the first surgeon to operate under ether in England (Liston died of a ruptured aortic aneurysm 1 year after this operation); this was at University College Hospital on 21 December 1846, using Squire's inhaler when he amputated the leg of Frederick Churchill, a 36-year-old butler.[19] The apparatus was designed by Peter Squire, the Queen's chemist and druggist (who in 1804 founded the *Companion to the British Pharmacopoeia*, which later became *Martindale's Extra Pharmacopoeia*) as a modification of Dr Nooth's apparatus for the production of soda water. The actual anaesthetic was given by the designer's nephew, William Squire, a 21-year-old medical student.[20] When the leg had been painlessly amputated Liston said to the large audience: "This Yankee dodge beats mesmerism hollow." It was, however, probably given on 19 December in the Dumfries and Galloway Royal Infirmary by William Scott (1820–1887), surgeon and William Fraser (1819–1863), ship's surgeon[21]. This followed a verbal report of Morton's successful use of the agent, carried by Fraser, who arrived in Liverpool from Boston on 16 December, as medical officer on the steamship *Arcadia*.

The name anaesthesia was suggested by Oliver Wendell Holmes. It also appeared in Bailey's *English Dictionary* in 1751.[22]

Ether became known in England through a letter written by Jacob Bigelow (1786–1865), Henry's (1818–1890) father, to his friend, Dr Boott (1792–1863) an American doctor practising in Gower Street, London,[23] who, with Mr J. Robinson (1813–1861), gave the first ether anaesthetic, a dental case, 2 days before Robert Liston's first use of it. News then spread quickly to all parts of the civilized world.

John Snow (1813–1858)

Born in York, 15 March, 1813, the eldest of 9 children of a farmer. After Morton, the first whole-time anaesthetist. Starting his medical studies in Newcastle, at the age of 14, as apprentice to Mr William Hardcastle, he was one of the eight medical students who entered the Newcastle on Tyne Medical School at its inception in 1832. Snow worked at the Newcastle Infirmary and became interested in the first cholera epidemic at Killingworth Colliery in 1831–1832. In 1833 he left Newcastle and worked for a time at Burnop Field near Newcastle, then at Pateley Bridge in Yorkshire and in 1836 he migrated to London, travelling on foot, and attended lectures at the Hunterian School of Anatomy in Great Windmill Street, founded by William Hunter (1718–1784), elder brother of John Hunter (1728–1792) and also at Westminster Hospital. He became a member of the Royal College of Surgeons of England in 1838 and also passed the examination of he Apothecaries Hall; became MD, London, in 1844, and was appointed lecturer (1844–1849) in forensic medicine at the Aldersgate School of Medicine just before its closure. Settled first at 54 Frith Street, where a commemorative plaque has now been erected[24] and then at 18 Sackville Street in London as a general practitioner. Here he lived for the remainder of his life. He became interested in ether soon after its introduction and quickly perceived that the common method of administration was faulty. To overcome this, he invented an ether inhaler in 1847 and adapted the face-piece of Dr Francis Sibson (1816–1876) of Nottingham. Later he invented his own. He was appointed anaesthetist to out-patients at St George's Hospital, where his first anaesthetics (for dental extraction) were given, and in 1847 was promoted to the in-patient appointment. He also worked with Robert Liston (1794–1847) at University College Hospital and with Sir William Fergusson (1808–1877) at King's College Hospital. His health was poor and he suffered from phthisis and from nephritis, being treated for the kidney disease by Richard Bright (1789–1858). For many years he was a vegetarian and temperance advocate. He experimented with many substances to see if they possessed anaesthetic properties, trying many of them on himself.

Snow rapidly became the leading anaesthetist in London and wrote a book in 1847, *On the Inhalation of Ether in Surgical Operations* (reprinted in the *Br. J. Anaesth.* 1953, **25**, 53 et seq.). He did much useful work on the physiology of anaesthesia, and described five stages or degrees of anaesthesia. He emphasized the importance of knowing how deep to take the anaesthetized patient. He later abandoned ether for chloroform in adults, but was familiar with the dangers of the newer drug, believing it to cause primary cardiac failure consequent on the use of too strong a vapour. To overcome this danger he invented a percentage chloroform inhaler. For anaesthesia during labour, Snow poured a little chloroform on to a folded handkerchief but for surgical operations he preferred the greater accuracy provided by his inhaler. In Scotland, the 'open method' originated by Simpson was the usual method of both types of administration. He gave over 4000 chloroform anaesthetics without a death. In 1853 Snow originated the method of 'chloroform à la reine', when he acted as anaesthetist at the birth of Queen Victoria's (1819–1901) eighth child, Prince Leopold (1853–1884) (later Duke of Albany, who died of haemophilia), at the request of Sir James Clark, on 7 April and in 1857 at the birth of Princess Beatrice (1857–1944) on 17 April. These royal occasions made anaesthesia in midwifery morally respectable. He gave his royal patient 15-minim doses intermittently on a handkerchief, the administration lasting 53 minutes: it met with the Queen's warm approval: "Dr Snow gave that blessed chloroform and the effect was soothing, quieting, and delightful beyond measure." The birth of Leopold George Duncan Albert (1853–1884), later Duke of Albany, finally canonized "that blessed chloroform". Even the names of the Queen's attendants seemed to share the aura of purity which her royal participation had given to the subject: Mrs Lilly and Mrs Innocent the midwives, and of course Dr Snow.[25] Snow introduced amylene as an inhalation anaesthetic in 1856. His income never exceeded £1000 per annum although during the last 10 years of his life he gave an average of 450 anaesthetics a year. His last work, *On Chloroform and Other Anaesthetics*, was published posthumously in 1858, Snow having been seized with paralysis while at work on the manuscript and dying on 11 June 1858.

In his later years he proved that cholera was a water-borne disease, when he ordered the removal of the Broad Street (Golden Square) pump handle in 1854 in London and so terminated the third cholera epidemic (although this particular epidemic had commenced to wane before the actual removal of the handle).[26] The theory of the mode of transmission of cholera was set out in the second edition of his book (first edition 1849, following the epidemic of 1848 in which over 5000 people died), *On the Mode of Communication of Cholera*, 2nd ed. (London: Churchill, 1855). Snow's theories were substantiated by William Budd (1811–1880) ('Malignant Cholera: Its Mode of Propagation, and its Prevention', *Lond. Med. Gaz.* 1849, **44**, 724). It was, however, many years before Snow's views were generally accepted, Max von Pettenkoffer (1818–1901) being a leading anti-contagionist until his suicide in 1901. It is interesting that the cholera vibrio had been described in 1854 by Picini of Florence,[27] 30 years before Koch's paper.[28] Near the site of the pump, in Broadwick Street, a public house has been named 'The John Snow' (although Snow was a teetotaller). Snow's grave in Brompton Cemetery was restored in 1938 by anaesthetists from Britain and the United States. Benjamin Ward Richardson's (1828–1896) (*see Br. J. Anaesth.* 1955, **27**, 517) epitaph reads: "In Brompton Cemetery there was laid to rest, at the age of forty-five, John Snow (1813–1858), exemplary citizen and useful physician. He demonstrated that cholera is communicated by contaminated water; and he made the art of anaesthesia a science." The tombstone was destroyed by bombing in April 1941, but was restored in 1950 and unveiled on 6 July 1951.[29] Three of his case books with a record of his chloroform administrations 1848–1858 are in the possession of the Library of the Royal College of Physicians of London.[30]

(*See also*: 'John Snow; First Anaesthetist', *Bios,* 1936, **7**, 25; Keys T. E. 'John Snow; Anaesthetist', *J. Hist. Med. Allied Sci.* 1946, **1**, 551; *John Snow: Biography*, by Sir Benjamin Ward Richardson, reprinted in the *Br. J. Anaesth.* 1952, **24**, 267; 'Snow on the Water of London', *Mayo Clin. Proc.* 1974, **49**, 480; Lord Cohen of Birkenhead, 'John Snow – the Autumn Loiterer', *Proc. R. Soc. Med.* 1969, **62**, 99; Snow J. *On Narcotism by the Inhalation of Vapours* (facsimile edition), Ellis R. H., ed., *R. Soc. Med.,* London, 1992.

James Young Simpson (1811–1870)[31]

Born at Bathgate, near Edinburgh. Qualified 1830; MD, 1832. Elected to Chair of Midwifery at Edinburgh, 1840, spending £500 on canvassing, etc. Started university career in atmosphere of hostility from his colleagues, but his ability as a lecturer soon attracted large classes of students. Simpson took an interest in a wide range of subjects, including leprosy, puerperal sepsis and hospital design. He put forward the method of haemostasis by acupressure to promote better wound healing. He made many contributions to the literature of archaeology, becoming President of the Society of Antiquaries of Scotland in 1861. He was made one of Her Majesty's Physicians in Scotland in 1847 and was created baronet in 1866. He also received many foreign honours.

He is most famous for the introduction of chloroform in 1847.[32] (Davy, Faraday, Hickman, Wells, Morton, and Koller were all in their twenties when they made their discoveries: Simpson was a veteran of 36.) He was the first to use ether in obstetric practice on 19 January 1847, but wanted to find a better agent. Chloroform was discovered independently by Justus von Liebig (1813–1873), Darmstadt chemist, Soubeiran (1793–1858), Paris pharmacist, and Guthrie (1782–1848), American chemist, in 1831. Jean Baptiste Andre Dumas (1800–1848), Paris pharmacist, gave it its name and wrote the first full description of its physical and chemical properties. In 1847 Flourens showed that it had anaesthetic powers on animals.

David Waldie (1813–1889), a Liverpool chemist, suggested that Simpson should try chloroform as an anaesthetic vapour.[33] Simpson experimented on himself and his assistants, Matthews Duncan (1823–1890) and George Keith, on 4 November 1847 at Simpson's house, 52 Queen Street, Edinburgh. Four days later it was used clinically and a report was read to the Edinburgh Medical and Chirurgical Society on 10 November: 'Notice of a New Anaesthetic Agent as a Substitute for Sulphuric Ether in Surgery and Midwifery'. Simpson was harshly attacked more on moral than on theological grounds[34] (Genesis, ch. 3, verse 16) for using pain relief for women in labour, but following the administration of chloroform to Queen Victoria during the delivery of her eighth child (Prince Leopold) in 1853 by John Snow, the seal of respectability was set on the relief of pain in childbirth by anaesthetics. Although Simpson was the first obstetrician to employ ether for delivery (19 January 1847), he held that chloroform has the following advantages over ether: (1) action more rapid, complete and persistent; (2) smaller quantity required; (3) pleasanter; and (4) cheaper. Chloroform was first given in London at St Bartholomew's Hospital on 20 November 1847 (though it had in fact been used at St Bartholomew's Hospital earlier in the year under the name of 'chloric ether' by Sir William Lawrence (1783–1867) and Holmes Coote at the suggestion of Michael Cudmore Furnell – before Simpson).[35] After the publication of Simpson's works chloroform temporarily displaced ether in most parts of the world. Simpson remained an enthusiastic salesman for chloroform anaesthesia.

From 1845 to his death in 1870, Simpson lived at No. 52 Queen Street, Edinburgh. The dining room has been preserved as 'The Discovery Room' and contains some of Simpson's furniture and possessions.[36] There is a memorial to Sir James Young Simpson in Westminster Abbey. He was buried in the family plot in Warriston Cemetery, Edinburgh.

Joseph T. Clover (1825–1882)

After the death of Snow, Clover became the leading scientific anaesthetic investigator and practical anaesthetist in Britain. He was born in Aylesham, Norfolk, and was educated at the Gray Friar's Priory School in Norwich and at University College Hospital in London (1844). Although it is unlikely[37] that Clover was present in the operating theatre at University College Hospital on 21 December 1846, when Robert Liston (1794–1847) amputated the leg of Frederick Churchill when ether was given by William Squire, a medical student, the first major operation performed under ether anaesthesia in England, he was interested in anaesthesia from its commencement. Joseph Lister (1827–1912) was a fellow student. Became house surgeon to James Syme (1799–1870) and later RMO at University College Hospital and took FRCS in 1850. He was the pioneer of the art of completely and immediately removing from the urinary bladder the calculus fragments produced by lithotrity and invented a bladder aspirator (the forerunner of Bigelow's evacuator (1878)). He also devised 'Clover's crutch', a simple but effective piece of apparatus for maintaining a patient in the lithotomy position. Worked as general practitioner in London (because of poor health) (1853), later specializing in anaesthetics, thereby helping to fill the vacancy created by the early death of John Snow in 1858. Was appointed to staff of University College and Westminster Hospitals, and also worked at the London Dental Hospital. Was for many years the leading anaesthetist in London and attended many famous people, including the ex-Emperor Napoleon III of France (1808–1873) at Chislehurst where he was operated on 3 times, in 1871, the Princess of Wales (later Queen Alexandra), Sir Robert Peel and Miss Florence Nightingale. In 1862 he invented a chloroform inhaler, which enabled percentage mixtures of chloroform and air to be accurately measured and administered. It took the form of a large bag, slung over the back of the anaesthetist, and it contained 4.5% of chloroform vapour in air. Realizing the dangers of chloroform, Clover set to work to make the administration of ether more simple and easy. This he did by inducing anaesthesia with nitrous oxide, later adding ether to the gas.[38] Was co-opted on to Committee of Royal Medical and Chirurgical Society which advised the use of a mixture of chloroform and ether, because of the danger of chloroform alone (1864). In 1868 published a paper 'On the Administration of Nitrous Oxide', *Br. Med. J.* 1868, **2**, 491. In 1877 he described his portable regulating ether inhaler,[39] which did much to make ether more popular at the expense of chloroform. Ombrédanne's inhaler from France was a slightly modified copy, using a pig's bladder instead of a rubber bag[40] (Louis Ombrédanne (French surgeon, 1871–1956). 'L'Anaesthésie par l'Ether', *Gazette des Hospit.* 1908, 1095). Another of Clover's achievements was his teaching that ether could be safely given over long periods with anaesthesia carried to adequate depth. He was never a man of robust constitution and died at the age of 57.[41] Eleven years before his death he was to claim that he had had no deaths in 11 000 administrations, 7000 of them using chloroform.[42] An eponymous lecture is given every two years in his honour, alternately with a similar lecture honouring the name of Frederick Hewitt, at the Royal College of Surgeons in London. He is buried in Brompton Cemetery, London, his grave (No. U 113122) being 200 yards from that of John Snow.[43]

Sir Frederick Hewitt (1857–1916)

Educated at Merchant Taylors' School, Christ's College, Cambridge, and St George's Hospital, London, where he was a distinguished student. Became an anaesthetist as defective eyesight prevented his becoming a consulting physician, and was appointed to Charing Cross Hospital in this capacity in 1884, the National Dental Hospital in 1885, and lecturer on anaesthesia at the London Hospital in 1886. In 1902 became physician anaesthetist to his old teaching hospital, St George's. He emphasized that nitrous oxide anaesthesia is possible without asphyxia and that chloroform is specially dangerous during induction. Hewitt modified Junker's chloroform bottle and redesigned Clover's inhaler, enlarging the bore of the central tube (as suggested by Wilson Smith)[44] and arranging for its rotation within the ether reservoir.[45] He devised a dental prop and also an airway (*Lancet*, 1908, **1**, 490), and wrote a popular textbook (1893) on anaesthesia (*Anaesthetics and their Administration*. London: Griffin), the fifth edition of which appeared in 1922. He strongly advocated better teaching of anaesthetics to medical students. A superb clinical anaesthetist, he was a tireless advocate for greater care to be taken in the administration of anaesthetics and constantly sought to improve conditions under which anaesthetics were given, and to protect the public against their use by unqualified persons. Hewitt invented the first practical machine for giving nitrous oxide and oxygen in fixed proportions in 1887 and the years following.[46] In 1911 he was knighted. Administered an anaesthetic to Edward VII for drainage of an appendix abscess on 27 June 1902,[47] two days before his coronation day (the ceremony took place on 9 August 1902). Sir Frederick Treves (1853–1916) was the surgeon. Hewitt died at Brighton of a gastric neoplasm. His grave lies in Brighton and Preston Cemetery.[48]

Sir William Macewen (1847–1924)

Born in Rothesay in the Isle of Bute, Scotland, on 22 June 1847 youngest of 12 children and son of a sea captain, just 7 months after Simpson's introduction of chloroform. A medical student in the University of Glasgow, he qualified in 1869 and proceeded to the MD degree 3 years later. While the Regius Professor of surgery, Joseph Lister, was developing his system of antiseptic surgery, Macewen became his dresser and this association with the great man had a profound effect on Macewen's subsequent professional development. Following resident appointments in the Royal Infirmary, he was appointed medical superintendent of the Belvedere Fever Hospital, where he had the harrowing experience of treating patients suffering from respiratory obstruction due to laryngeal diphtheria, an experience which led him to his great discovery of oral laryngeal intubation. Leaving the Fever Hospital he went into general practice and became a parochial medical officer but gradually his interests centred on surgery and he obtained appointments at both the Glasgow Royal Infirmary and Western Infirmary, culminating in his nomination to the chair as Regius Professor of surgery in the University of Glasgow in 1877, a post he was to fill with great distinction for the next 15 years. He was invited to become the first professor of surgery at the new Johns Hopkins Hospital in Baltimore, but refused it, the post going to William Stewart Halsted. On the accession of King Edward VII in 1902, he was knighted. Macewen became president of the British Medical Association in 1922 and of the International College of Surgeons when it met in London the following year. A tall, handsome, impressive personality who tolerated fools badly, and went his own way.

His numerous surgical contributions included the diagnosis and treatment of cerebral abscess, surgery of the brain, the spine, chest and bones. He was an early exponent of aseptic surgery in which sterilization of instruments and dressings was carried out by heat.

He was the pioneer of oral and nasal tracheal intubation as an alternative to tracheotomy, performing the manoeuvre by touch in the conscious patient. He first used rubber and gum elastic catheters in the treatment of laryngeal diphtheria, later metal and 'flexometallic tubes' during operations on the base of the tongue and pharynx in 1878.[49] A sponge was packed round the superior laryngeal aperture and chloroform and air administered through the tube, thus protecting the lungs from contamination.

In addition to his great technical advances. Macewen paid constant attention to teaching his students the rudiments of safe anaesthesia, a form of tuition uncommon at that time. He remained a great believer in chloroform anaesthesia. He became a Surgeon Rear-Admiral and Consultant to the Royal Navy in Scotland in 1914.

(*See also* Keys, T. E. *Anesth. Analg. Curr. Res.* 1974, **53**, 537; James C. D. T. *Anaesthesia*, 1974, **29**, 743; Bowman A. K. *The Life and Teaching of Sir William Macewan*. London & Edinburgh: Wm Hodge, 1942; and Wakeley C. (ed.) *Great Teachers of Surgery in the Past*. Bristol: Wright, 1969.)

Carl Koller (1857–1944)

Carl Koller was the first medical man to make use of and to publicize the analgesic properties of cocaine (which had been known for 25 years) to prevent the pain of a surgical operation. This he did in September 1884 in Vienna where he was a 27-year-old trainee ophthalmologist. He was born in 1857 in Schüttenhofen, then in Bohemia, a part of the Austro-Hungarian empire, the son of a Jewish businessman who lacked strict religious convictions. He was educated in Vienna, thought of studying the law, served for two years as a conscript in the imperial army and finally enrolled as a medical student in the University of Vienna. While still an undergraduate he published the results of some highly regarded experimental pathological investigations into the embryology of the mesoderm of the chick. He qualified as a doctor in 1882 at the age of 25 and became a member of the department of ophthalmology in the Allegemeine Krankenhaus whose director was Professor Carl Ferdinand von Arlt (1812–1887).

Koller soon began to share with his professor considerable dissatisfaction with the standard of the anaesthetists and of the conditions of anaesthesia they produced; restlessness during the operation and cough and vomiting afterwards. He began to realize that this problem would only be solved if he could find some drug which, when instilled into the conjunctival sac would abolish pain. With this end in view he tried morphine and other sedative drugs, but of course without success. So the turbulent general anaesthetics continued.

In the summer of 1884, Sigmund Freud (1856–1939) a friend and contemporary who was working in a junior capacity in the neurology department of the hospital and who was later to achieve world fame as the originator of psychoanalysis, was busy investigating what was then a fairly new drug, cocaine, which had reached Europe from South America in the middle 1850s. It was an alkaloid extracted from the bush *Erythroxylon coca*, which grew in Bolivia and Peru and was well known to the local Indians as a euphoriant and stimulant. Freud's studies led him to believe that it might be a remedy for morphine addiction as well as a tonic for his psychoneurotic patients. He wrote a monograph entitled 'Ueber Coca' in August 1884. He knew that it deadened mucous membranes but was not clear as to its effects on muscular contraction, and asked Koller to do some experiments to elucidate the problem. Freud then went on holiday while Koller set to work with cocaine. He started by applying some to his own tongue[50] and was immediately struck, as others had been before him, by its strange power to deaden all sensation. In a flash he realized that this might be the agent he had been looking for to act as a local analgesic in his eye operations. He quickly set about investigating its analgesic effects in the experimental pathology laboratory on animals, then on himself, on his friends and lastly on his patients. He satisfied himself that not only did it work but that it worked extremely well, and lost no time in making his discovery public. He wrote a short preliminary report[50] and asked his friend, Dr Josef Brettauer (1835–1905) from Trieste, to read it for him at the forthcoming meeting of the German Ophthalmological Society to be held in Heidelberg, which Koller himself was not able to attend. Brettauer's paper caused a sensation and this was reinforced when, after a lecture, he gave a clinical demonstration of the use of 2% cocaine solution in the out-patient clinic. The date was 15 September 1884. The following month Koller read two fuller papers before the Imperial Medical Society. Freud, whose interest in surgical anaesthesia was minimal, made no claim to the discovery.

News of the event soon spread throughout Europe and the US and Koller became a notable figure. But not notable enough for him to secure a senior post in the academic department of eye surgery to which he aspired and to which he was reasonably entitled. So he moved off from Vienna and joined the eye clinic in Utrecht where he pursued his postgraduate studies under Professor Frans Cornelius Donders (1818–1889) and his son-in-law, H. Snellen (1834–1908) and where he remained for two years. Koller was, however, a restless and somewhat awkward man and decided to try his luck once more in Vienna, but he found the going hard. His prospects were not enhanced by his involvement in a duel, fought with sabres, against a fellow reserve medical officer because of a personal quarrel. So, although Koller wounded his opponent and won the day, the illegality of duelling placed him in a difficult professional position and had an adverse effect on his advancement. Once again he decided to leave Vienna, this time for New York where he arrived in 1888 and where he spent the remainder of his active life. He soon built up a thriving hospital and private practice and established a solid reputation as a first-class ophthalmic surgeon. He took no further part in the development of local analgesia, leaving that to others. As time passed he achieved something of the fame his discovery as a young man rightly earned for him and he was awarded gold medals, scrolls and commendations from various academic bodies in Europe and America. Some controversy arose about this great discovery, but Carl Koller was its true begetter. He died in 1944 aged 86.[51]

William Stewart Halsted (1852–1922)

For anaesthetists, Halsted's claim to fame is his early experiments with the new local analgesic solutions of cocaine. He originated nerve-block or regional analgesia and showed that a reduction in the circulation of a part of the body, as by an Esmarch bandage, would prolong the effects of local analgesia. He demonstrated that for skin analgesia, intradermal injection – 'the distension method' – was superior to subcutaneous injection.

His ancestors came from Britain in the seventeenth century and he was born into a substantial family in New York City. He was educated at Yale College where his athletic prowess surpassed his academic abilities. Deciding to study medicine, he entered the College of Physicians and Surgeons in New York in 1874 and graduated 3 years later. While a resident at Roosevelt Hospital, New York, in 1878 he became friendly with William H. Welch (1850–1934), later to become the first professor of pathology in the US and the world-famous dean of American medicine. The next 2 years were spent in postgraduate studies in Austria and in Germany, where he visited the clinics of Theodore Billroth (1829–1924) and Anton Woefler (1850–1917) in Vienna, Ernst von Bergmann (1836–1907) in Wurzburg, Carl Thiersch (1822–1895) in Leipzig, Richard von Volkmann (1830–1889) in Halle and J. F. A. von Esmarch (1823–1908) in Kiel, When he returned home he entered surgical practice in New York City. He achieved considerable success and developed into a bold extroverted and original surgeon. Halsted was one of the first to recognize the importance of the discovery of cocaine and, with some of his colleagues, commenced to experiment with the new drug on themselves, not realizing its grave addictive properties. The results of their work were soon published.[52] Halsted was the first surgeon to block the nerves of the face, the brachial plexus, the internal pudendal and posterior tibial nerves. In 1886, his uncontrolled addiction to cocaine led to his admission to a psychiatric hospital. He seems to have exchanged the craving for cocaine for the craving for morphine, possibly as a result of therapy, and remained, off and on, a morphine addict for the rest of his life.

On discharge from hospital his personality was seen to have changed and he now appeared as a slow, meticulous and rather morose man who gave great attention to the smallest detail of what occupied him. He found his way back to Welch's laboratory at the new Johns Hopkins Hospital in Baltimore in 1887 where he aspired to become surgeon-in-chief, but Sir William Macewen (1847–1924) was offered the post (although he never took it up). Eventually in 1889 Halsted was appointed the first professor of surgery in the Johns Hopkins University and chief surgeon to the hospital. During the next 30 years of his life he made his clinic world famous and became one of the founding fathers of twentieth-century surgery, becoming mentor, guide, philosopher and friend to countless young colleagues, over fifty of whom eventually occupied chairs of surgery in American hospitals. His early enthusiasm for regional analgesia waned and in later life he always preferred to operate on unconscious patients. He died following a second operation for gallstones and obstructive jaundice.[53]

Among his contributions to surgery were his radical operation for the removal of the whole breast with its lymphatic drainage for the relief of breast cancer (1890).[54] In 1890 he introduced the use of rubber gloves into surgery, an idea borrowed from his colleague W. H. Welch the pathologist (in an effort to prevent skin irritation from antiseptic solutions affecting the hands of his operating-room sister, who was later to become his wife).

(*See also* MacCallum W. G. *William Stewart Halsted*. Baltimore: The Johns Hopkins Press, 1930; Boise M. 'Halsted as an anesthetist knew him', *Surgery* 1952, **32**, 498; Halsted Centenary Meeting. *Proc. R. Soc. Med.* 1952, **45**, 555; Olch P. D. *Anesthesiology*, 1975, **42**, 479; letter from W. S. Halsted to Sir William Osler in Fulton J. *Harvey Cushing; A Biography*. Oxford: Blackwell, 1946, 142; 'William Stewart Halsted and the Germanic influence on training and education programs in surgery', *Surg. Gynecol. Obstet.* 1978, **147**, 602; *Bull. N. Y. Acad. Med.* 1984, **60**, 176; Matas, Rudolf, *Am. J. Surg.* 1934, **25**, 195, and 362; Matas R. *Bull. Johns Hopkins Hosp*, 1925, **36**, 1; Matas R. *Arch. Surg.* 1925, **10**, 293 and Boulton T. B. 'Classical File' *Surv. Anesthesiol.* 1984, **28**, 150.)

August Karl Gustav Bier (1861–1949)

Bier was born in Helsen in Waldeck in Germany in 1861 and graduated in 1889 at Kiel where he later became assistant to the professor of surgery, von Esmarch. While there he supervised the transition from antiseptic to aseptic techniques in the operating theatres, following the teachings of von Bergmann (1836–1907) and Curt Schimmelbusch (1860–1895) of Berlin. He became familiar with the work of a medical colleague at Kiel, Heinrich Irenaeus Quincke (1842–1922), who established lumbar puncture as a safe investigation in routine neurological examination.[55] In 1898 he gave the first deliberate spinal anaesthetic[56] and to prove his faith in the method allowed his assistant, Dr Hildebrandt, to inject into his own theca 2 ml of 1% cocaine solution. Leaving Kiel, Bier became professor of surgery successively at Griefswald, Bonn, and as successor to Ernst von Bergmann at Berlin, and in the capital he was to spend the greater part of his professional life. In addition to his discovery of spinal analgesia, he invented the method of treating chronic inflammation by the method of passive hyperaemia with Esmarch's (1823–1908) bandage (1892)[57] and pioneered intravenous procaine analgesia (1908)[58] while holding the chair of surgery at Bonn. He was one of the great figures of German surgery, as teacher, lecturer and operator (Hon. FRCS (Eng.), 1913). Introduced the 'tin helmet' into the German army in the First World War. In later life he came to hold unorthodox ideas, advocated physical education, callisthenics, etc. and deviated from the views of his colleagues. He died, aged 88, at Sauer in the German Democratic Republic in 1949.

Heinrich Friedrich Wilhelm Braun (1862–1934)

Braun has been called 'the father of local analgesia' and he coined the term 'conduction anaesthesia'. He was born in Rawitch in Poland in 1862, and although intending to become a musician, he graduated in medicine in 1887 in Dresden, and after a period as assistant to Karl Thiersch (1822–1895) in Leipzig and Richard von Volkmann (1830–1889) in Halle, whose niece he married in 1888, became director of the Deaconess Hospital in Leipzig where his interest in local analgesia was developed, having been stimulated by Max Oberst (1849–1925) of Halle. In 1902 he introduced the use of adrenaline in local analgesic solutions of cocaine,[59] and in 1905 became the pioneer of the new drug procaine.[60] In this year also appeared the first edition of his classic textbook, *Local Anaesthesia;* the eighth edition was published in 1933. He preferred conduction (nerve) block to Schleich's infiltration. Braun was appointed to direct the new hospital at Zwickau in 1906, and here he passed the remainder of his professional life. He introduced dental local analgesia into Germany. He described the anterior approach to the coeliac plexus (anterior splanchnic block) and was the inventor of the Braun splint. He was also interested in general anaesthetics but realized their danger and devised an apparatus for the safe administration of chloroform and ether vapour.[61] Was president of the German Surgical Society in 1924 and retired in 1928 (*see also* Röse W. *Anesteziol. Reanimatol.* 1982, **1**, 3). He died in 1934, aged 72.

Arthur Läwen (1876–1958)

Läwen was born in 1876 in Waldheim in Saxony, and qualified at Leipzig in 1900. He became in Leipzig a pupil of Heinrich Braun and later of Friedrich Trendelenburg (1844–1924) and Erwin Payr (1871–1976) of Griefswald. He held senior posts at Leipzig and Marburg and was appointed professor of surgery at Königsberg in East Prussia where his chief work was done. In 1912 he employed curare to reduce the amount of ether needed for relaxation, in an attempt to reduce the incidence of postoperative pulmonary complications, which were then thought to be due to ether vapour.[62] This work was interrupted by the First World War. Läwen was the first to describe paravertebral conduction anaesthesia, and in 1910 he was the first to show that extradural analgesia was a safe and practical form of pain relief in pelvic and abdominal surgery. For this he used large volumes of 1.5 or 2% procaine solution with sodium bicarbonate, injected through the sacral hiatus.[63] He did a great deal to popularize local analgesia, tracheal intubation and artificial respiration. After 1945 he became a refugee from East Germany, having lost his sons, his possessions and his university chair during the war. He died in 1958, aged 82.

Gaston Labat (1877–1934)

Born in the Seychelles and graduated at Montpellier. Took up the study of medicine at the age of 37 in 1914 after running a successful pharmacy in Mauritius. Became anaesthetist to Victor Pauchet (1869–1936), surgeon to the St Michael Hospital in Paris, and was co-author with Pauchet of the later editions of the latter's book.[64] Was invited to the Mayo Clinic in 1920 and became special lecturer on regional anaesthesia there. Wrote his classic book *Regional Anesthesia: Its Technique and Clinical Application* in 1922. Subsequently became clinical professor of surgery (anaesthesia) at New York University and worked at the Bellevue Hospital. Founded American Society of Regional Anesthesia in 1923. Died in October 1934 in New York. A third (posthumous) edition of his book was published in 1967, edited by J. Adriani, and a fourth in 1985.

His book, outstanding in its time, had a great influence on the development and acceptance of regional analgesia. In 1922 its main readers were surgeons. Only in later years was regional analgesia practised by anaesthetists.

Arthur E. Guedel (1883–1956)

Born in Cambridge City, Indiana, and received his medical education at the Indiana School of Medicine, Indianapolis, qualifying in 1908. Lost three fingers of his right hand, aged 13, but nevertheless became a skilled pianist. Started as a general practitioner/anaesthetist. Lecturer on anaesthesia in the University of Indianapolis (1920–1928), during which time he was a practising anaesthetist in that city. Gave anaesthetics in France during the First World War (1917–1919) and made notes on which his book is based. Later moved to Los Angeles, where he became associate clinical professor of anesthesiology at the University of Southern California School of Medicine. A leading pioneer of American anaesthesia, and like most of his contemporaries in the specialty he was self-taught.

He made many contributions to his chosen specialty, including an early description of the self-administration of nitrous oxide and air for obstetrics and minor surgery;[65] a description of the anaesthetic properties of divinyl ether; reintroduction, with R. M. Waters, of a cuffed tracheal tube,[66] a systemization of the signs of inhalation anaesthesia;[67] a pharyngeal airway;[68] the introduction of controlled respiration using ether, with Treweek;[69] and a classic description of the clinical use of cyclopropane.[70] He received the Hickman Medal from the Royal Society of Medicine in 1941, the first worker outside the UK to do so, and the Distinguished Service Award of the American Society of Anesthesiologists in 1951. There is a Guedel Memorial Anesthesia Centre in San Francisco, together with an eponymous lecture established in his honour by the University of California Medical Center in Los Angeles.

(*See also* Waters R. M. 'Eminent Anaesthetists: A. E. Guedel', *Br. J. Anaesth.* 1952, **24**, 292; Neff, W. B. In: Volpitto P. P. and Vandam L. D. (ed.) *The Genesis of Contemporary American Anesthesiology.* Springfield Ill.: Thomas; Calverley R. K. In: *Anaesthesia: Essays on its History.* (Rupreht J. et al. ed.) Berlin: Springer-Verlag, 1985, 18.)

Henry Edmund Gaskin Boyle (1875–1941)

Born in Barbados and qualified at St Bartholomew's Hospital, London, in 1901, where as a student he was president of the Abernethian Society. Became casualty officer in Bristol and then returned to St Bartholomew's as junior resident anaesthetist, rising in due course to become head of the department. About 1912, became interested in nitrous oxide and oxygen anaesthesia and in 1917 got Coxeter, the instrument maker, to copy James Tayloe Gwathmey's (1855–1943) gas-oxygen machine, which became the first 'Boyle' apparatus.[71] He introduced gas-oxygen into France for use in anaesthetizing wounded soldiers in the First World War and for this received the decoration of OBE. After the war he visited the US and brought back with him Davis's gag,[72] which he introduced to British throat surgeons. He was an early user of Magill's endotracheal techniques and was elected FRCS and DA in 1935; was one of the original pair of examiners for the latter diploma. A founder member of the Association of Anaesthetists of Great Britain and Ireland in 1932.

In 1907 wrote the first edition of his textbook, *Practical Anaesthetics*, the third edition of which was prepared by his junior colleague C. Langton Hewer. Boyle was a 'character' and was universally known as 'Cockie'.

His anaesthetic machine, modified in every particular, is used in most British hospitals today.[73]

(*See also* Hadfield C. F. 'Eminent Anaesthetists: H. E. G. Boyle', *Br. J. Anaesth.* 1950, **22**, 107).

Ralph Milton Waters (1883–1979)

Born in North Bloomfield, Ohio, of Anglo-Scottish descent. Became a student at Western Reserve University in Cleveland in 1903 and after taking an arts degree became MD in 1912. Settled in general practice in Sioux City in Iowa, married and remained there for 5 years. Gradually became interested in anaesthesia and the basic sciences so that by 1916 anaesthesia came to occupy much of his time and he decided to specialize; an unusual step to take at the time. He opened a private clinic as a commercial venture with an operating room and facilities for minor surgery, where he gave the anaesthetics; one of the first 'day-stay' clinics in the US. In 1923, he acquired an anaesthetic practice in Kansas City where he remained for 3 years. He hurt his back, lifting an overweight patient, and as a result had to spend 6 months in a brace. On recovery he visited John S. Lundy (1884–1973), chief anaesthetist at the Mayo Clinic, and on his way home stopped off with friends at Madison. Here he met Chauncey Leake (1896–1978) the pharmacologist, and Erwin Schmidt, professor of surgery, and as a result he was invited in 1927 to take charge of anaesthesia at the new Hospital of the State of Wisconsin at Madison, which opened in 1924. He became in turn assistant professor, associate professor and in 1933 full professor of anaesthesia with clinical charge of anaesthesia in the university hospitals. This was the first such post in the US. He had a long and distinguished career and his clinic became one of the leading centres of anaesthesia in the world. He visited Europe and the UK in 1936 and was awarded the Hickman Medal by the Royal Society of Medicine in London in 1938. He retired in 1949 and was succeeded by Alexander MacKay and then by Sidney Orth in 1952. His pupils included Drs Rovenstine, Gillespie, Hingson, Lucien Morris, Gordh, Apgar, Neff and many others.[74]

His contributions to the growing specialty were numerous and important and he wrote more than a hundred papers. Among the more noteworthy are the following: insistence on proper training programmes for young anaesthetists; encouragement on careful note keeping during anaesthesia by means of 'punch-cards'; the introduction of cyclopropane into anaesthetic practice;[75] the development of the to-and-fro carbon dioxide absorption system;[76] a re-evaluation of chloroform;[77] pioneering use of thiopentone in 1934;[78] endobronchial intubation.[79]

He exercised a great influence on anaesthesia in the US and in the UK during 1930–1950 and trained many anaesthetists who later occupied important posts in universities in the US and in Europe. He was one of the most important founding fathers of anaesthesia as we know it today. He received numerous medals, citations and honours from academic bodies throughout the world and lived to enjoy 30 years of retirement, latterly growing citrus fruit in Florida, where he died in Orlando on 19 December 1979.

Sir Ivan Magill (1888–1986)

Ivan Whiteside Magill was born in Larne, Northern Ireland, then with what is now the Republic, an integral part of the UK. His birth in 1888 took place 42 years after Morton's first use of ether and just two years after the discovery of local analgesia, using cocaine. He attended the local grammar school and then became a medical student at Queen's University, Belfast, qualifying in 1913. He became a house surgeon at the Stanley Hospital in Liverpool and with the outbreak of the 1914–1918 War, joined the RAMC and served with the Irish Guards at the battle of Loos. When peace came again, Magill was posted to the Queen's Hospital in Sidcup, Kent. With a young colleague, Stanley Rowbotham (1890–1979), neither of whom was at that time an experienced anaesthetist, they soon found themselves responsible for giving anaesthetics for reconstructive operations on the face and jaws in wounded soldiers, under the care of Harold Gillies, later to become a world-famous pioneer of plastic surgery. Here after trial and error, they became among the first workers to develop tracheal intubation, initially using two narrow gum-elastic tubes, one afferent and the other efferent, for the insufflation of ether vapour under slight positive pressure, and then employing a single wider bore rubber tube for spontaneous breathing. They were also among the first to develop the technique of nasotracheal intubation by the so-called blind method. These Magill tubes eventually became indispensable to all anaesthetists. While their methods earned for them the support and approval of the surgeons with whom they worked, many other surgeons discouraged the use of intubation partly because of the possibility of tissue damage and partly due to conservatism. It took many years before intubation was accepted into the general employment of anaesthetists. Those who learnt how to perform blind intubation soon realized its great advantages, especially the fact that it would enable a patient to be taken to the level of anaesthesia necessary for a laparotomy very quickly with ether, then the commonly used agent, thus reducing the time for induction. In addition, intubation provided a clear airway, prevented laryngeal spasm and enabled the lungs to be protected against foreign material.

When the work at the unit in Sidcup decreased, Magill decided to devote his professional life to the administration of anaesthetics and was soon elected to the staffs of various hospitals in London. Eventually he chose the Westminster Hospital and the Brompton Hospital for Diseases of the Chest as his main bases, while, in addition, his skill and personality enabled him to acquire a large private practice in London and beyond. He was a man of great practical ingenuity and over the years originated or developed many new pieces of equipment and refinements of technique for the safety of his patients and the convenience of his surgeons. Among these must be mentioned a laryngoscope and laryngeal forceps, and the 'Magill attachment' a simple combination of a breathing tube, reservoir bag and expiratory valve, used for spontaneous respiration, which featured on all anaesthetic machines in the UK for over 50 years. He developed methods of administering anaesthetics in thoracic surgery employing endobronchial tubes and bronchus blockers for the control of pulmonary secretions, and these techniques for the production of one-lung anaesthesia greatly contributed to the development of thoracic surgery in the 1920s and 1930s.

He took a leading part in organizing the Association of Anaesthetists of Great Britain and Ireland in 1932; in instituting an examination for the Diploma in Anaesthetics, the first such examination in 1935; and in persuading the Royal College of Surgeons of England to found a Faculty of Anaesthetists in 1947. His great experience and reputation as a safe and skilled clinical anaesthetist resulted in his being asked to employ his abilities on a large number of very distinguished patients, including many members of the British and other royal families when they required surgical treatment. He received a very large number of honours and medals including a knighthood (the KCVO) awarded personally by the Queen in 1960, the FRCS (Eng.), the honorary FFARCS, the DSc of his old University, the Henry Hill Hickman Medal from the Royal Society of Medicine, and many others. For 50 years he was the doyen of British anaesthetists and his name was known worldwide. Tracheal intubation is the *sine qua non* of safe anaesthesia in many operations and this is largely due to the work of Ivan Magill and his colleague Stanley Rowbotham.

In the 1920s when Ivan Magill's career began, anaesthesia was a little regarded specialty and those who practised it exclusively attracted little esteem from their colleagues. He lived to see it achieve parity with other specialties, a change in which he took a leading part because of his firm character and common sense, pre-eminence in clinical anaesthesia and his international reputation. (*See also* Bowes J. B. and Zorab J. S. M. In: *Anaesthesia: Essays on its History* (Rupreht J. et al. ed.) Berlin: Springer-Verlag, 1985, 13.)

Helmut Weese (1897–1954)

Helmut Weese deserves an honoured place in the history of anaesthesia as the first man to make intravenous induction a safe and practical procedure. He was born in Munich into a family originating from the German part of Poland, and the son of a lecturer in the history of art. When he was nine, the family moved to Berne where his father became a privatdozent at the University. Switzerland had a great influence on his development. He decided to study medicine and attended the Universities of Berne, Zurich and Munich where he qualified. His first post was in internal medicine under von Romberg, and then he changed to pharmacology in 1925 and worked with W. Straub. He did well in the new discipline and in his own turn became privatdozent. He paid particular attention to the study of digitalis, wrote a book on it and as a result, became well known both inside and outside Germany to physicians as well as to pharmacologists. When in 1928, F. Eicholtz who had previously described the effects of bromethol (Avertin) moved to Konigsberg and then to

Heidelberg, Weese followed him as director of pharmacology at the Farbwerk Bayer at Wuppertal-Elberfeld, and as lecturer at the University of Cologne. He was appointed professor there in 1936. Following the debacle of 1945 he took charge, in addition, of the department of pharmacology at Dusseldorf. He was no purely academic scientist and always strove to direct his energies to the relief of his fellow man. In 1931, Kropp and Taub synthesized a new barbiturate, hexobarbitone, later to become known as Evipan. He saw that this might be the long-awaited, short-acting and safe agent for induction of anaesthesia, and at once set about investigating it both in the laboratory and personally in the operating theatre. He was soon able to show that it fulfilled his expectations and in 1932 published his results, thus becoming the undisputed creator of practical clinical modern intravenous anaesthesia. He won recognition at the International Congress of Anesthesia at New York in 1938, during which he was elected an honorary member.

During the Second World War, Weese, who was consultant pharmacologist to the armed forces, investigated the possibility of producing a synthetic plasma volume expander, and as a result, polyvinyl pyrrolidone (Periston, polyvidone) became available and saved many lives. He also devoted time to investigating the application of phenothiazines to clinical anaesthesia, following the stimulus of the Frenchmen, Laborit and Huguenard. With Hans Killian he wrote a book on anaesthesia, *Die Narkose*. Weese practised both anaesthesia and pharmacology and was honoured by members of both specialties. He used his considerable influence to advance the status of anaesthesia in postwar Germany.

He died following a fall from a chair in his laboratory, an unusual event in a man well used to climbing in the high Alps (*see also* Obituary: Killian, Hans. *Der Anaesthesist*, 1954, Band 3; Heft 2. 97. Translation, Dr Heinrich Niehoff).

John Silas Lundy (1894–1973)

Dr Lundy of the Mayo Clinic, Rochester, Minn., had a great influence on our specialty, particularly as the pioneer of the use of thiopentone (Pentothal sodium). He was born in Seattle, Washington, the son of a doctor. He took an arts degree in 1917 and qualified in medicine from the Rush Medical College in Chicago two years later. After serving as a resident in Chicago hospitals he returned to his birthplace and entered general practice. In April 1924 he was invited to become head of the Department of Anesthesiology at the Mayo Clinic and this he directed for the next 28 years although his connection with the Clinic did not end until 1959. He became professor in the Mayo Graduate School of Medicine in 1934 and was one of the founders of the American Board of Anesthesiology. He was a prolific writer, and this together with the worldwide reputation of the Mayo Clinic where he worked, soon carried his name throughout the US and Europe. He established the first laboratory of gross anatomy to be used at the Clinic and this was important for his teaching of the techniques of regional analgesia, which had been stimulated there by Gaston Labat. In 1925 he developed the theory and practice of 'balanced anesthesia'[80] and although Waters of Madison used thiopentone before he did, Lundy used it on 18 June 1934 and continued throughout his professional life to advocate its use. It is largely due to his efforts that intravenous induction spread so widely. In 1942 he opened the first post-anaesthesia observation room in the world at St Mary's Hospital, Rochester. In 1935 he established the first blood bank in the US at Rochester. Dr Lundy was the author of the textbook, *Clinical Anesthesia* published in 1942, one of the first authoritative volumes dealing with the so-called 'modern anaesthesia'. He received many medals, awards and honours from academic bodies throughout the world. He retired first to Chicago and later to Seattle where he continued to practise anaesthesia (*see also* Corssen G. In: (Rupreht J. et al. ed.) *Anaesthesia: Essays on its History*. Berlin: Springer-Verlag, 1985, 42).

Harold Randall Griffith (1896–1985)

On 23 January 1942 Harold Griffith, assisted by his resident Enid Johnson, injected Intocostrin intravenously, a preparation containing curare, to aid muscle relaxation in a 150-lb male patient undergoing interval appendicectomy under cyclopropane anaesthesia at the Homeopathic Hospital (later the Queen Elizabeth Hospital) in Montreal. This was an outstanding event of supreme importance in the development of modern anaesthesia.[81]

Harold Griffith was born near Montreal on 25 July 1894, obtained the BA (Magill) in 1914 and the MD CM in 1922. In this year he also married. The following year he obtained the MD in homeopathic medicine from the Hahnemann Medical College in Philadelphia. Before graduating in medicine he served with distinction as a stretcher-bearer in the Canadian Army and was awarded the Military Medal for bravery in the 1914–1918 war. An interest in anaesthesia developed early in his career and after a time he became chief anaesthetist at the Montreal Homeopathic Hospital where his father had been medical director and his brother, surgeon-in-chief, and here he spent his active professional life until his retirement in 1966. Before the days of relaxants he developed an expertise in tracheal intubation and, along with Dr Ralph Waters of Madison, became a world expert on the use of the then new agent cyclopropane. As anaesthesia advanced he became involved in its academic side and was appointed professor of anaesthesia and chairman of the department at Magill University. He held high office in the International Anesthesia Research Society and was a founder member of the World Federation of Societies of Anesthesiology and president of its first congress held in Holland in 1955 and at its second congress held in Toronto in 1959 he was elected permanent Founder-President.

Dr Griffith was a much loved man of modest disposition who was known to his younger colleagues as 'Uncle Harold'. In later life he received many honours and distinctions including the Hickman Medal from the Royal Society of Medicine in London in 1956, and he was the only non-US citizen to receive the Distinguished Service Award from the American Society of Anesthesiology.

The sample of Intocostrin was handed to him in 1942 by Dr Lewis Wright of the pharmaceutical firm of E. R. Squibb. They were aware of the muscle relaxing 'shock-absorbing' effects of curare when used to control the muscular spasms associated with ECT,[82] while his familiarity with the treatment of respiratory depression by controlled breathing following his very frequent use of cyclopropane, enabled him to deal with the same complication which might be associated with curare, and presented to him no problems.

Harold Griffith died aged 90 of Parkinson's disease on 7 May 1985. (*See also* Griffith H. R. and Johnson E. *Anesthesiology* 1942, **3**, 418; Gillies D. M. M. *Can. Anaesth. Soc. J.* 1985, **32**, 570; 'Classical File' *Surv. Anesthesiol.* 1985, **29**, 358; Seldon T. H. *Anesth. Analg. (Cleve.)* 1986, **65**, 1051.)

Sir Robert Reynolds Macintosh (1897–1989)

Born at Timaru, New Zealand, Robert Macintosh travelled to Britain when the First World War broke out and joined the Royal Flying Corps only to become a prisoner of war. He qualified in medicine from Guy's Hospital in 1924 and after abandoning a career in surgery became a successful dental anaesthetist in London. In 1937 he moved to Oxford to become the first Nuffield Professor of Anaesthetics in the University, the first such chair in Europe. He built up a renowned department in Oxford, undertaking clinical work, teaching and the development of anaesthetic apparatus. He secured the appointment of anaesthetic sisters and nurses, wrote text books noted for their clarity and encouraged the practice of regional analgesia. '*Essentials of General Anaesthesia*', which he wrote with Dr Freda Bannister, was the first anaesthetic book to be published by Blackwell Scientific Publications Ltd, in 1941. Robert Macintosh was first and foremost a clinical anaesthetist and his name became associated with many practical pieces of equipment, the most famous being the Macintosh laryngoscope. He had an enormous and wordwide influence on the evolution of anaesthesia. He travelled to many countries, including the underdeveloped ones, and his work was recognized by the bestowal of honorary degrees from Universities in Argentina, France and Poland. He was made an Honorary Fellow of the Faculties of Anaesthetists in England, Ireland and Australia and an Honorary Doctor of Science in the University of Wales. He was knighted in 1955.

The Corporate Organization of Anaesthesia in Britain[83]

The Society of Anaesthetists was founded in 1893 by J. F. W. M. Silk (1878–1943) of King's College Hospital, and forty anaesthetists joined it. First president, Woodhouse Braine (1837–1907) of Charing Cross Hospital, with Silk as Honorary Secretary and Dudley W. Buxton (1855–1931) of University College Hospital, as Treasurer. Published first volume of *Transactions* in 1898. In 1908 was incorporated into the Anaesthetic Section of the new Royal Society of Medicine. The first society of anaesthetists in the world which had as its object the discussion of problems of anaesthesia and the advancement of the science and art of the subject. The Scottish Society of Anaesthetists dates from 1914.

The Association of Anaesthetists of Great Britain and Ireland was founded in 1932 to perform functions that could not be performed by the Anaesthetic Section of the Royal Society of Medicine. These were (and are): to promote the development and study of anaesthetics and their administration and the recognition of the administration of anaesthetics as a specialized branch of medicine; to co-ordinate the efforts and activities of anaesthetists; to represent anaesthetists and to promote their interests; to promote the establishment of diplomas and degrees in anaesthesia; to encourage and promote co-operation and friendship between anaesthetists; and to do all such lawful things as may be incidental or conducive to the attainment of such objects. The first president was Henry Featherstone (1894–1967) of Birmingham with W. Howard Jones of Charing Cross Hospital as Secretary and Z. Mennell (1876–1959) of St Thomas Hospital, London as Treasurer. At this time there were only fifty specialist anaesthetists in the whole of the UK.[84] (For a description of the 'Arms' of the Association, *see* Boulton T. B. *Anaesthesia*, 1974, **29**, 627.)

The Faculty of Anaesthetists of the Royal College of Surgeons of England was created in 1948 at the request of the Association of Anaesthetists.[85] The Fellowship (FFARCS) was proposed in 1946 and the first examinations held in 1953. A. D. Marston (1891–1962) of Guy's Hospital was the first dean.

The College of Anaesthetists was created in 1989 when a new charter allowed the Faculty of Anaesthetists to evolve to collegiate status. It became The Royal College of Anaesthetists in 1992.

The Faculty of Anaesthetists of the Royal College of Surgeons in Ireland was founded in 1959, the first examination for its fellowship taking place in 1961.

For the history of World Federation of Societies of Anesthesiologists, *see* Griffith H. R. *Anesth. Analg. Curr. Res.* 1963, **42**, 389; *Indian J. Anaesth.* 1970, **18**, 145; Zorab J. *Anaesthesia* 1976, **31**, 285; Boulton T. B. *Anaesthesia* 1976, **31**, 1103.

For the development of anaesthesia in the US, *see* Waters R. M. *J. Hist. Med. Allied Sci.* 1946, **1**, 595; and Eckenhoff J. E. *Anesthesiology* 1978, **49**, 272.

Introduction of anaesthesia into France (by Jobert de Lamballe and J. F. Malgaigne at the Hopital St Louis, Paris), *see* Neveu R. *J. Hist. Med. Allied Sci.* 1946, **1**, 607.

For the development of anaesthesia in the Netherlands, *see* van Wijhe M. '*From Stupefaction to Narcosis*'. Slinger, Alkmaar, Netherlands, 1991.

Introduction of anaesthesia into Germany (by Heyfelder of Erlangen), *see* Frankel W. K. *J. Hist. Med. Allied Sci.* 1946, **1**, 612; Whitacre R. J. and Dumitra J. H. M. *J. Hist. Med. Allied Sci. 1946*, **1**, 618; von Hintzenstern U. In: *A History of Anaesthesia.* (Atkinson R. S. and Boulton T. B. ed.) London: Royal Society of Medicine, 1989, 502. For the early development of anaesthesiology as a specialty in Germany, *see* Schwarz W. In: *A History of Anaesthesia.* (Atkinson R. S. and Boulton T. B. ed.) London: Royal Society of Medicine, 1989, 170.

In Ireland the first anaesthetic was given by John MacDonnell in Dublin at the Richmond hospital.

First anaesthetic in New Zealand (for dental extraction) given by Mr Marriott with Dr J. P. Fitzgerald as surgeon.[86]

First anaesthetic in Australia given by Dr Wm Russ Pugh of Tasmania on 7 June 1847.[87] First anaesthetic in Melbourne on 2nd July 1847 and on 30th September 1847 in South Australia by Kent.[88] For history of the Australian Society of Anaesthetists, *see* Wilson G. C. *Fifty Years.* Glebe, NSW: The Australian Society of Anaesthetists, Flannel Flower Press, 1987. Faculty of anaesthetists of the Royal Australian College of Surgeons founded in 1952; first examination for fellowship in 1956.

For history of anaesthesia in the Republic of S. Africa, *see* Kok O. V. S. *Progress in Anaesthesiol. Proc. 4th World Congress Anaesth.* Amsterdam: Excerpta Medica, 1970, 167.

For the very early history of inhalation anaesthesia in Canada, *see* Matsuki A. *Can. Anaesth. Soc. J.* 1974, **21**, 92.

For anaesthesia in Argentina, *see* Cooper I. *Br. Med. Bull.* 1946, **4**, 147.

For the development of anaesthesia in other countries *see* Rupreht J. et al. (ed.) *Anaesthesia: Essays on its History.* Berlin: Springer-Verlag, 1985. Countries with page numbers – Czechoslovakia, Dworacek B. and Keszler H. 41; Italy, Pantaleoni M. 113; Ecuador, Pinto O. M. 115; Japan, Yamamura H. 165; China, Shieh Yung, 136; Yugoslavia, Darinka Sobin, 139; Nigeria, Sodipo J. O. A. 141; Ukraine (CIS), Treshchinsky A. I. 153; Holland, Vermeulen-Cranch D. 156; Thailand, Tupavong S. 154; Lebanon, Haddad F. S. 60; Spain, Franco A. et al. 48; Hungary, Forgacs I. and Varga P. 45; CIS Damir E. 28. *also*, Atkinson R. S. and Boulton T. B. (ed.) *A History of Anaesthesia.* London: Royal Society of Medicine, 1989; page numbers – Netherlands, Rupreht J. 86; South Africa, Cooper J. L. 147; Hong Kong, Lett Z, 153; Canada, Maltby J. R. 112; California, Calmes S. H. 129.

For documentation of 46 'first anaesthetics' in the world, *see* Secher O. *Acta Anaesthesiol Scand.* 1990, **34**, 55.

For a list of some of the earliest books dealing with anaesthesia, *see* Secher O. *Anaesthesia* 1985, **40**, 385.

Interesting and important dates in the history of medicine and anaesthesia

1516   Curare, South American arrow poison, described by Peter Martyr Angherius.

1518   Foundation of the College of Physicians in London.

1540   Valerius Cordus (1515–1544) synthesized sweet oil of vitriol (ether), possibly aided by Theophratus Bombast von Hohenheim, named Paracelsus (1493–1541).
United Company of Barber Surgeons given Royal Charter by Henry VIII.

1543   Andreas Vesalius (1514–1564) of Basel, Louvain and Padua published his revolutionary book on anatomy, *De Humani Corporis Fabrica*. Professor of surgery and anatomy at Padua, where he replaced moribund mediaeval scholarship by detached scientific observation.
Publication of *The Revolutions of the Heavenly Spheres* by Copernicus.

1628   Wm Harvey (1578–1657) of London (pupil of Galileo (1564–1642) of Padua and contemporary of Francis Bacon (1561–1626), English philosopher, and of Descartes (1596–1660), French philosopher), described the circulation of the blood: *De Motu Cordis*. Frankfurt: Fitzeri.

1662   Robert Boyle (1627–1691) enunciated his law of the relationship of the volume and pressure of a gas.

1665   First intravenous injection of a drug (tincture of opium) into an animal (a dog) by Sir Christopher Wren (1633–1723) and Robert Boyle (1627–1691) using a bladder attached to a sharpened quill. Richard

Lower (1631–1691) transfused blood from one animal to another.

1707 Sir John Floyer (1649–1734) of Lichfield, the first physician to time the pulse during his clinical examination of patients.

1730 August Siegmund Frobenius, a German chemist, living in London, named 'sweet oil of vitriol' ether.

1733 Stephen Hales (1677–1761) inserted tubes into the arteries and veins of animals; the first experiments in direct measurement of blood pressure. (Clark-Kennedy A. E. *Br. Med. J.* 1977, **2**, 1656.)

1742 Anders Celsius (1701–1744) of Sweden described his system of thermometry, which has displaced the 'centigrade' scale.

1751 'Anaesthesia' defined in Bailey's *English Dictionary* as 'a defect of sensation' (Gillies J. quoted by Beecher H. K. *Anesthesiology*, 1968, **29**, 1068).

1754 Carbon dioxide ('fixed air') discovered by J. B. von Helmont (1577–1644), Belgian physician, and isolated by Joseph Black (1728–1799).

1761 Joseph Leopold Auenbrugger (1722–1809) in Vienna described percussion of the chest.

1768 Wm Heberden (1710–1801), of London, described angina of effort (*Med. Trans. Call. Phys. Land.* 1768, **2**, 59).

1771 Discovery of oxygen by Joseph Priestley (1733–1804) and Carl Wilhelm Scheele (1742–1786) of Uppsala, independently.

1772 Priestley discovered nitrous oxide.

1777 Antoine Lavoisier (1743–1794) of Paris, scientist and tax collector, named the 'new air' of Priestley 'oxygen' and demolished the 'phlogiston' theory, which supposed that only substances containing 'phlogiston' would burn and in so doing would lose their 'phlogiston'.

1788 J. A. C. Charles (1746–1823) of France formulated his law of the pressure/temperature relationship of a gas.
Chas. Kite of Gravesend first used tracheal tubes in resuscitation of the drowned.

1794 Thomas Beddoes (1760–1808) founded the Pneumatic Institute in Bristol for the treatment of pulmonary tuberculosis and experimented with the therapeutic inhalation of gases and vapours. Humphry Davy (1773–1829) appointed superintendent in 1798.

1800 Discovery of analgesic properties of nitrous oxide by Davy who named it 'laughing gas'.
Royal College of Surgeons of England given Royal Charter by George III (1738–1820).

1806 Isolation of morphine from opium by Friedrich Wilhelm Adam Serturner (1783–1841), a Paderborn pharmacist.

1807 Baron Larrey (1766–1842) performed painless amputations, using ice, on the battlefield of Preuss Eylan.
Seishu Hanaoka (1760–1835) of Hirayama, Japan used a mixture of alkaloids, mainly scopolamine and atropine ('tsusensan') in Oct. 1807 for the first time, to give pain relief to a 60-year-old woman for the removal of a breast cancer.[89]

1811 Charles Bell (1774–1842) of Edinburgh published his *Idea of a New Anatamy of the Brain* in which he differentiated motor nerves and sensory nerves.

1816   René Laënnec (1781–1826) of Paris invented stethoscope (*stethas* the chest; *skapeein* = to explore).[90] The binaural stethoscope introduced by Camman in 1855.

1818   Michael Faraday (1779–1867) is said to have discovered narcotic action of ether vapour.

1822   Francois Magendie (1783–1855) of Paris proved in humans that while anterior spinal roots are motor, posterior roots are sensory: 'insensible' and 'sensible' nerves.

1824   Henry Hill Hickman (1800–1830) of Ludlow, England carried out operations on animals under carbon dioxide, with freedom from pain, thus establishing the principle of inhalation anaesthesia.

1831   Chloroform discovered independently by von Liebig (1830–1873) in Darmstadt, Germany, Guthrie (1782–1848) in New York and Soubeiran (1793–1858) in France.
        Atropine prepared from *Atropa belladonna*, by Mein a German pharmacist (*Ann. Pharmacie*, 1833, **6**, 67) and by P. L. Geiger (1785–1836) professor of pharmacy of Heidelberg and Hesse.

1832   Thomas Aitchison Latta used intravenous saline in the treatment of circulatory collapse in cholera (not in surgical shock).

1833   Marshall Hall (1790–1857), English physician, introduced the concept of reflex action. Thomas Graham (1805–1869), a Scottish chemist, published *On the Law of the Diffusion of Gases*.

1834   Jean-Baptiste Dumas (1800–1884) in Paris described chemical composition of, and gave name to, chloroform.

1842   Ether given by W. E. Clarke (1818–1878) of Rochester, New York, for dental extraction, and by Crawford W. Long (1815–1878) on 30 March in Jefferson, Georgia (the patient, John Venable).[91]
        Marie Jean Pierre Flourens (1794–1867), Paris physiologist, first isolated respiratory centre in medulla.

1843   Royal Charter given by Queen Victoria (1819–1901) to Royal College of Surgeons of England. Establishment of FRCS (England) diploma.

1844   Horace Wells (1815–1848), dentist, of Hartford, Connecticut, introduced nitrous oxide inhalation to produce anaesthesia during dental extraction. Francis Rynd (1801–1861), surgeon, of Dublin invented hypodermic trocar.

1846   Wm T. G. Morton (1819–1868), Boston dentist, successfully demonstrated the anaesthetic properties of ether, 16 October. The patient was Gilbert Abbott (1825-1855), a not very robust printer/editor, for a congenital vascular malformation of the floor of the mouth and tongue, the surgeon J. C. Warren. The patient remained in hospital for 7 weeks.[92]
        The word 'anaesthesia' was suggested by Oliver Wendell-Holmes (1809–1894), Boston academic and writer, for Morton's 'etherization'. Tooth extracted and ether given by a dentist, Mr Robinson in London, 19 December. Dr Francis Boott (1792–1863) in attendance at 52 Gower Street (now Bonham Carter House, London).[19] (Letters of Boott to *Lancet* reprinted in 'Classical File', *Surv. Anesthesiol.* 1957, **1**, 65).
        First surgical operation performed in England under ether anaesthesia by Robert Liston (1794–1847), 21 December, when Frederick

Churchill underwent amputation through the thigh and William Squire gave the anaesthetic at University College Hospital (North London Hospital).

1847   Marie Jean Pierre Flourens (1794–1867), French physiologist, described anaesthetic properties of chloroform and ethyl chloride vapour in animals. James Y. Simpson (1811–1870) on 8 November introduced chloroform into clinical work, to ease pains of labour in Edinburgh.

John Snow (1813–1858), London practitioner, published his book, *On the Inhalation of Ether in Surgical Operations,* the first scientific description of its clinical uses, physical and pharmacological properties. Deaths from ether reported from Grantham and Colchester.[93]

1848   Hannah Greener, aged 15, died from chloroform administered by Dr Meggison, 28 January – the first recorded case – at Winlayton, Co. Durham, 11 weeks after its introduction into medicine.[94] Johan Heyfelder (1798–1869) of Erlangen first used ethyl chloride in humans and first to use ether in Germany (in 1847).

1849   First anaesthetic death in a London teaching hospital – chloroform – 10 October – St Thomas's Hospital.[95]

1850   Wm Gairdner (1824–1907) of Glasgow differentiated between postoperative pneumonia and pulmonary collapse, the latter due to bronchial obstruction.

1853   John Snow, London physician and anaesthetist, gave chloroform analgesia on 7 April to Queen Victoria (1819–1901) at birth of Prince Leopold (1853–1881) later Duke of Albany, hence *'chloroform' a la reine'.* Sir Charles Locock (1799–1875) was the accoucheur.

Invention of hypodermic syringe and needle by Alexander Wood (1817–1874) of Edinburgh.

1855   Friedrich Gaedicke of Germany isolated cocaine from coca plant. Indirect laryngoscopy described by Manuel Garcia (1805–1906), a Spanish singing teacher working in London.

Foundation of the British Medical Association, which developed from Sir Charles Hastings' Worcester Medical and Surgical Society.

1857   Claude Bernard (1813–1878), physiologist of Paris, showed that curare acts on the myoneural junction.[96]

1858   Publication of John Snow's book *On Chloroform and Other Anaesthetics.* General Medical Council established in the UK to supervise medical registration, education and professional conduct.

1859   First examination for the MRCP (London) held.

Charles Darwin (1809–1882) published *The Origin of Species by Natural Selection.*

1860   Albert Nieman (1834–1861) purified the alkaloid that Gaedicke had isolated from coca leaves. He named it cocaine.

1861   I. P. Semmelweiss (1818–1865) a Hungarian obstetrician, demonstrated in Vienna that puerperal fever is both infectious and contagious.

1862   Thos. Skinner, a Liverpool obstetrician, introduced his domette-covered, wire-framed mask, frequently imitated since (e.g. by Curt Schimmelbusch (1860–1895), of Berlin, in 1890). Clover's chloroform inhaler.

1863   Gardner Quincy Colton (1817–1898) popularized the use of nitrous oxide in dentistry, neglected since Horace Well's discovery in 1844. Louis Pasteur (1822–1895) showed that micro-organisms cause fermentation, which led Lister to his discovery of antisepsis in 1865.

1864   Report of Chloroform Committee of Royal Medical and Chirurgical Society, which confirmed chloroform's position as first favourite although ether was shown to be safer.
Johan Nepomuk von Nussbaum (1829–1890) surgeon of Munich gave morphine pre-operatively to prolong the action of chloroform.

1865   Professor J. Lister (1827–1912) of Glasgow treated by means of carbolic acid the compound fracture of James Greenlees's leg – the birth of antiseptic surgery (12 August) in Glasgow[97]

1867   Ferdinand Edelberg Junker (von Laugegg) (1828–1902), Austrian surgeon working in London described his chloroform insufflation apparatus.

1868   Edmund Andrews (1824–1904) surgeon, of Chicago combined oxygen with nitrous oxide.[98] Thomas Wiltberger Evans (1823–1897), American dentist working in Paris, who had learnt about nitrous oxide administration from Colton in 1867, introduced it to London dentists. In the following year, nitrous oxide was supplied in cylinders in compressed form commercially 4 years before US manufacturers put it on the market. Supplies of nitrous oxide may well have been obtainable in London in 1856 from the Medical Pneumatic Appliance Co. (Barth).
C. A. Wunderlich (1815–1877) of Leipzig published his work on medical thermometry, *Temperature in Diseases: A Manual of Medical Thermometry*. London: New Sydenham Society, 1868. He found fever a disease and left it a symptom (Garrison).

1869   Nasal N_2O inhaler used (independently) by Joseph Thomas Clover (1825–1882) and Alfred Coleman (1828–1902), London dentist.

1870   Gustav Simon (1827–1913) of Heidelberg performed the first nephrectomy.

1871   Friedrich Trendelenburg (1844–1924) surgeon from Rostock, gave anaesthetics via a tracheostomy wound, and used in 1869 a cuffed tracheostomy tube.[99]

1872   Antisalivary effects of atropine described by R. P. H. Heidenhain (1834–1897), Breslau (Wroclaw) physician.
In England, use of ether became much more frequent following the visit of B. Joy Jeffries, an ophthalmic surgeon of Boston, Massachusetts, USA. He 'sold' the American method of ether administration to British surgeons and anaesthetists, a method involving forcing ether on to the patient who was, if necessary, held down during induction. Previously in Britain, chloroform was used almost exclusively.
Pierre-Cyprien Oré (1828–1889) of Bordeaux produced general anaesthesia with intravenous chloral hydrate in animals and 2 years later applied the method in man.[100]
Clover introduced his nitrous oxide–ether sequence at BMA Annual Meeting at Norwich.

1874   Forné, French naval surgeon, gave chloral hydrate by mouth to produce sleep before chloroform anaesthesia.

1875 Richard Caton (1842–1926) of Liverpool demonstrated the presence of electric currents in the brain and so was the pioneer of electroencephalography.

1876 Hyperventilation (which produced hypocapnia) with air shown to have analgesic effects by Bonwill.[101]

1877 Joseph Clover introduced his portable regulating ether inhaler.

1880 W. Macewen (1848–1924), Glasgow surgeon, introduced tracheal intubation by mouth.[102]

1881 Stanislaw Klikovich (1853–1910), of St Petersburg, surgeon, used nitrous oxide and oxygen to ease labour pains (*Arch. Gynaek.* **18**, 81),[103] a technique later employed by Frederick Hewitt in 1887. Frederick Trendelenburg (1844–1924), professor of surgery at Rostock (afterwards at Bonn and Leipzig), introduced the head-down tilt with pelvic elevation, for abdominal surgery.
First successful partial gastrectomy performed by Theodore Billroth (1829–1894) at Allgemeine Krankenhaus on 29 January on Therese Heller, in Vienna.[104] First successful gastro-jejunostomy performed: A. Woelfler (1850–1917).[105]

1882 Synthesis of cyclopropane by August von Freund (1835–1892), Viennese chemist.
Robert Koch (1843–1910), Berlin physician, described the tubercle bacillus.

1884 Koller, Vienna ophthalmologist, demonstrated local analgesic properties of cocaine on the cornea (in a paper read by Joseph Brettauer) (1835–1905) of Trieste, at Ophthalmological Congress at Heidelberg. W. Stewart Halsted (1852–1922) and Richard John Hall, in New York, did the first nerve block with cocaine: the nerve, the mandibular. Rickman J. Godlee (1849–1925), Lister's nephew and biographer performed the first operation for the removal of a cerebral tumour.[106]

1885 J. L. Corning (1855–1923), New York neurologist, produced analgesia by the accidental subarachnoid injection of cocaine.
Medical Defence Union founded in London.

1886 Ernst von Bergmann (1836–1907), Berlin surgeon, introduced heat sterilization, the beginning of aseptic surgery.

1887 Sir Frederick Hewitt (1857–1916), London anaesthetist, invented the first practical gas and oxygen machine.

1888 First Hyderabad Chloroform Commission.

1889 Second Hyderabad Chloroform Commission. Reports stated that chloroform is never a cardiac depressant and that breathing stops before the heart. This is now known to be untrue. Both Commissions were financed by the Nizam of Hyderabad, Mir Mahbad Ali Khan (1866–1911), who was only 3 years old when he became Nizam.

1890 P. Vera Redard of Geneva introduced the ethyl chloride spray for local analgesia.
W. Stewart Halsted (1852–1922), professor of surgery at the Johns Hopkins Hospital, Baltimore, introduced rubber gloves for surgery. Paul Reclus (1847–1914), Paris surgeon, advocated infiltration analgesia with cocaine.

1891 Lumbar puncture demonstrated to be a practical clinical procedure by

H. I. Quincke (1842–1922) of Kiel in Germany and by Essex Wynter (1860–1945), a physician, in England at the Middlesex Hospital.

1892   The term 'Nerve blocking' introduced by Francois-Frank.[107]
Heinrich Braun introduced the term 'conduction anaesthesia'.
Karl Ludwig Schleich (1859–1922) of Berlin introduced infiltration analgesia.

1893   London Society of Anaesthetists founded by F. W. Silk of King's College Hospital, London, with Woodhouse Brain as its first president. Other early presidents were G. Hewlett Bailey (1896–1898); Dudley W. Buxton (1897–1898); F. W. Silk (1899–1900) (*see* Dinnick O. P. *Progress in Anaesthesiology*, Proc. 4th WFSA London, 1970. Amsterdam: Excerpta Medica, 1970). It became the Anaesthetic Section of the Royal Society of Medicine in 1908.

1894   Ernest Amory Codman (1869–1940) and Harvey Cushing (1869–1939) in Baltimore advocated use of anaesthetic record charts. Later, 1901, blood-pressure readings, taken with a Riva-Rocci instrument, were added to these charts. (Scipione Riva-Rocci (1863–1937) of Padua).

1895   X-rays discovered on 8 November by Wilhelm Konrad v. Roentgen (1845–1923) of Würzburg, Nobel prizeman, 1901 (1st award).

1898   August Bier (1861–1949), surgeon of Kiel, induced first successful clinical spinal analgesia.
Theodore Tuffier (1857–1929) of Paris developed and popularized spinal analgesia.
Transactions of the Society of Anaesthetists founded in 1893, published fairly frequently from this date.

1899   Rudolf Matas (1865–1957), New Orleans surgeon, adapted the technique of artificial respiration with bellows (the Fell-O'Dwyer technique) to thoracic surgery.[108]

1900   Karl Landsteiner (1868–1943) of the University of Vienna, later of the Rockefeller Institute, New York City, Nobel prizeman, 1930, described ABO blood groups.

1901   Extradural caudal injection introduced by Sicard (1872–1929) and Cathelin (1873–1945) both of Paris, independently.
First awards of Nobel prizes established by Alfred Bernhard Nobel 1832–96, Swedish chemist and inventor of dynamite.
Franz Kuhn of Kassel published his work on tracheal intubation.[109]

1902   Heinrich Braun (1862–1934), Leipzig surgeon, added adrenaline to cocaine solution to prolong its effect and retard its absorption. A. G. Vernon Harcourt (1832–1919), FRS, reader in chemistry at Christ Church, Oxford, described his chloroform inhaler in which the concentration of vapour could be measured and its volume regulated, e.g. 2% at temperatures between 16 and 18°C.
E. H. Embley, anaesthetist of Melbourne, Australia described death due to vagal inhibition of the heart during chloroform anaesthesia.[110]

1903   Barbitone (Veronal) synthesized by Emil Fischer (1852–1919), Berlin chemist and Nobel prizeman, 1902, and von Mering (1849–1908) of Munich. This was the first barbiturate.
Willhelm Einthoven (1860–1927) of Leiden, Holland, applied the principles of the string galvanometer to ECG recording and for this was awarded the Nobel prize for medicine in 1924.[111]

1904   Ernest Fourneau (1872–1949) of Paris synthesized stovaine.
       Procaine synthesized by Alfred Einhorn (1856–1917), Munich
       chemist.

1905   The first society of anaesthetists founded in the US by G. A. F.
       Erdmann, the Long Island Society of Anesthetists, later (1911)
       combined with a group from Manhattan to form the New York Society
       of Anesthetists; in 1935 the organization became national and in 1936
       was named the American Society of Anesthetists Inc. In 1945 the title
       was changed to the American Society of Anesthesiologists Inc., at the
       suggestion of Paul Wood (1897–1963), New York anaesthetist, the
       name 'anesthesiology' having been coined by Seifert in 1902.
       Procaine used by Heinrich Braun (1862–1934).

1907   Arthur E. Barker (1850–1916), surgeon, of University College
       Hospital, London, made use of the curves of the vertebral column in
       spinal analgesia and introduced hyperbaric solutions. The pioneer of
       spinal analgesia in Britain.[112]
       Foundation of the Royal Society of Medicine in London.
       Chevalier Jackson (1865–1958), of Philadelphia, described his work on
       laryngoscopy.

1908   Massive collapse of the lungs described by Wm Pasteur, English
       physician (1856–1943).[113]
       Louis Ombrédanne (1871–1956), Parisian surgeon, described his
       ether–air inhaler.
       Bier described intravenous procaine local analgesia.
       George Washington Crile (1864–1943), of Cleveland, Ohio, surgeon,
       described his theory of 'anociassociation' (*Am. Surg.* 1908, **47**, 864).
       The Society of Anaesthetists became the Anaesthetic Section of the
       Royal Society of Medicine.

1909   S. J. Meltzer (1851–1920) and J. Auer (1875–1948), of the Rockefeller
       Institute NY used tracheal insufflation anaesthesia in animals.
       First Nobel prize awarded to a surgeon Theodore Kocher of Berne
       (1841–1907) for his work on the treatment of goitre.

1910   C. A. Elsberg (1871–1948), New York surgeon, applied Meltzer and
       Auer's technique to man (tracheal intubation).
       Elmer Ira McKesson (1881–1935) of Toledo, Ohio, anaesthetist and
       inventor, introduced the first on-demand intermittent-flow gas and
       oxygen machine, with percentage calibration of the two gases.[114]
       Arthur Läwen (1876–1958) of Königsberg showed that extradural
       analgesia via the sacral route was a useful and practical method of
       analgesia.

1911   Goodman Levy (1856–1954) proved that chloroform can cause death
       (from ventricular fibrillation) in light anaesthesia.
       A. E. Guedel (1883–1956) working in Indianapolis, reported on the
       technique of self-administration of nitrous oxide in obstetrics.[115]
       Commencement of the National Insurance Act in the UK with its
       'panel' of general practitioners.
       Robert Kelly of Liverpool (1879–1944) was first to use insufflation
       tracheal anaesthesia in England.[116]

1912   Walter Meredith Boothby (1880–1953), of Rochester, Minn. and
       Frederic Jay Cotton (1869–1938), Boston surgeon, introduced a sight

feed gas and oxygen flow-meter.

A. Läwen (1876–1958), Königsberg surgeon, used curare to produce relaxation.

J. B. Herrick (1861–1954), Chicago physician, described the features of acute coronary thrombosis.[117]

1913   Danis was first to describe trans-sacral analgesia. James Tayloe Gwathmey (1865–1944) of New York introduced rectal oil-ether and in the following year published his classic textbook *Anesthesia*. New York: Appleton.

1914   Albert Hustin of Belgium (1882–1907) was first to use citrate in blood transfusion.

Anesthetic supplements to the *American Journal of Surgery* commenced publication, quarterly – the first official regularly published literature devoted to the specialty, edited by Frank Hoeffer McMechan (1879–1939). Terminated in the US 1926.

1915   Use of carbon dioxide absorption in animals by Dennis Jackson of St Louis, later of Cincinnati.[118]

1916   Sir F. E. Shipway (1875–1968) of Guy's Hospital, London, introduced his warm ether insufflation apparatus.[119]

1917   Edmund Boyle (1875–1941) of St Bartholomew's Hospital, London, described his portable N_2O and O_2 apparatus.

Avertin described by Fritz Eicholtz (1889–1968), pharmacologist, of Heidelberg.

1919   The American Association of Anesthetists founded by James T. Gwathmey and Frank McMechan (1879–1939).

1920   Guedel's first paper on signs of anaesthesia. These supplanted Snow's signs. Ivan Whiteside Magill (1888–1986) and E. Stanley Rowbotham of London (1890–1979) developed endotracheal anaesthesia.

1921   Extradural lumbar analgesia described by Pagés (1886–1923) of Spain.

1922   *Current Researches in Anesthesia and Analgesia* appeared in August. Founded and edited by Dr. F. H. McMechan and sponsored by the National Anesthetic Research Society in the US. In 1957 changed its name to *Anesthesia and Analgesia Current Researches;* the first journal to appear regularly in the world exclusively devoted to anaesthesia.

Labat's (1877–1934) *Regional Anesthesia* published.

1923   Carbon dioxide absorption used in man, by Ralph Milton Waters. *British Journal of Anaesthesia* appeared.

1924   Howard Wilcox Haggard (1891–1959) of Yale University published his classic papers on 'The Absorption, Distribution and Elimination of Ether'.[120]

1926   Concept of 'balanced anaesthesia' put forward by J. S. Lundy (1894–1972) of the Mayo Clinic.[121]

Otto Butzengeiger (1885–1968) of Wuppertal-Elberfeld, used tribromethyl alcohol (Avertin).[122]

For the first time there was a section of Anaesthetics at the annual scientific meeting of the British Medical Association.

1927   Ocherblad and Dillon of Kansas City, used ephedrine in spinal analgesia to prevent hypotension.

Pernocton used in Germany by R. Bumm (1899–1942). The first barbiturate routinely used for induction of anaesthesia.

1928 Lucas and Henderson in Toronto proved that cyclopropane had anaesthetic properties.
   I. W. Magill popularized blind nasal intubation.
1929 Alexander Fleming (1881–1955) of St Mary's Hospital, London, Nobel prizeman, 1945, discovered that the mould, *Penicillium notatum*, secreted an anti-staphylococcal substance.[123] This discovery was later developed.[124]
1930 Introduction of circle method of carbon dioxide absorption by Brian Sword (1889–1956) of New Haven, Conn.
1931 Achille Mario D. Dogliotti (1897–1966) of Turin, reintroduced extradural analgesia in Italy, and 4 years later founded the Italian Society of Anaesthetists.
   Foundation of the Liverpool Society of Anaesthetists, the oldest provincial society in the UK.
1932 Helmut Weese (1897–1954), Scharpff and Rheinoff were the first to use hexobarbitone (Evipan)[125] synthesized by Kropp and Taub.
   Christopher Langton Hewer's (1896–1986) *Recent Advances in Anaesthesia* appeared.
   Foundation of the Association of Anaesthetists of Great Britain and Ireland; the first president, Henry Featherstone (1894–1976) of Birmingham.
1933 A. Evarts Graham (1883–1957) of St Louis performed the first successful pneumonectomy for cancer.
   Ralph Waters (1883–1979) appointed professor and chairman of the new Department of Anesthesia in the University of Wisconsin at Madison: the first such appointment in the USA. (Thomas Drysdale Buchanan was appointed clinical professor of Anesthesiology at the College of Physicians and Surgeons of Colombia, New York, a non-university appointment in 1918.)
   Polyethylene (polythene) synthesized by R. O. Gibson and E. W. Fawcett in the UK. Manufacture commenced in 1939 by Imperial Chemical Industries.
1934 Ralph Waters and associates from Madison, Wisconsin, reported on the clinical use of cyclopropane where it was first administered on 9 October 1930.
   J. S. Lundy, anaesthetist of the Mayo Clinic, popularized thiopentone.
   Australian Society of Anaesthetists formed.
1935 Commencement of the intravenous drip.[126]
   An Elberfeld chemist with IG Faben Industrie, Gerhard Domagk, (1895–1967),[127] Nobel prizeman 1939, introduced the first 'sulpha' drug for the control of haemolytic streptococcal infections.
   First examination for DA held. H. E. G. Boyle and C. W. Morris, the first examiners.
1936 Successful treatment of puerperal fever with sulphanilamide, by C. Leonard Colebrook and Méave Kenny.[128]
1937 R. R. Macintosh (1897-1989) appointed Nuffield Professor of Anaesthesia in the University of Oxford, the first chair of anaesthesia in Europe.
   American Board of Anesthesiology established.
   Guedel's *Inhalation Anesthesia* published.

1938   Positive-pressure respirator used in surgery by Crafoord, surgeon (1899–1984) – the spiropulsator of Poul Frenckner (1886–1967), an otorhinolaryngologist of Stockholm.

1939   Pethidine synthesized by Schaumann and Eisleb at Hoechst Farbwerke, Germany.

1940   The journal, *Anesthesiology* first published.
Development of controlled breathing by Guedel and by Michael Nosworthy (1902–1980) of St Thomas' Hospital, London.
Karl Landsteiner (1888–1943) and Alexander Wiener (1906-1976) of the Rockefeller Institute, New York City, isolated the Rh factor in blood.
Preparation of an active and concentrated form of penicillin described.[129]
Penicillin given on 15 October at Colombia-Presbyterian Hospital, New York to a patient by Dr Aaron Alston.

1941   Trichloroethylene advocated by Langton Hewer and Charles Frederick Hadfield (1875–1965).

1942   Harold Randall Griffith (1894–1985) and G. Enid Johnson of Montreal used curare in anaesthesia.

1943   Macintosh described his curved laryngoscope in Oxford.
The first electronic computer was designed in the USA by Eckert and Mauchley to calculate artillery firing tables (electronic numerical integrator and computer – ENIAC). It weighed 30 tons and contained 18 000 thermionic valves. Created at the University of Pennsylvania.

1946   Centenary celebrations of anaesthesia.[130]
The journal *Anaesthesia*, appeared.

1947   First clinical use of lignocaine (Xylocaine) by Torsten Gordh (1907–) of Stockholm.

1948   Faculty of Anaesthetists established by the Council of the Royal College of Surgeons of England; A. D. Marston (1891–1962), of Guy's Hospital, London, the first dean.
First use of hypotensive anaesthesia by H. W. C. Griffiths (1915–1991) and John Gillies (1895–1976) in Edinburgh using high spinal analgesia.
Commencement of the two-part Diploma in Anaesthetic examination.
National Health Insurance started in the UK (July).
Invention of the transistor in the US.

1949   Penta- and hexamethonium described by W. D. M. Paton and Eleanor Zaimis (1915–1983).
Short-acting muscle relaxants described by Daniel Bovet (who was the first to prepare antihistamines) and used clinically 2 years later in Italy and Sweden.
Cortisone used at the Mayo Clinic.[131]

1950   Induced hypothermia in cardiac surgery described by Wilfred Gordon Bigelow, surgeon, and his colleagues from Toronto.
Scandinavian Society of Anaesthetists formed. Their first Congress held in Oslo.

1951   C. W. Suckling of Manchester synthesized halothane.

1952   Faculty of Anaesthetists of the Royal Australasian College of Surgeons founded; D. Renton, the first dean.
First examination for fellowship held in 1956.

Use of IPPV with bag and tracheal tube in Copenhagen polio epidemic.[132]

1953 First examination for Fellowship in Faculty of Anaesthetists of the Royal College of Surgeons of England in London.
First successful open-heart operation performed by John J. Gibbon at Thomas Jefferson Medical School, Philadelphia, using Gibbon extracorporeal bypass apparatus 6 May.

1954 *Canadian Anaesthetists' Society Journal* first published.

1955 Vibierg Olof Björk and Carl Gunnar Engström, surgeons, described IPPV for the treatment of postoperative respiratory failure.
World Federation of Societies of Anaesthesiologists formed.
First Congress in Scheveningen, Holland.

1956 Michael Johnstone of the Manchester Royal Infirmary used halothane clinically.

1957 *Survey of Anesthesiology* and *Acta Anaesthesiologica Scandinavica* first published.

1959 Faculty of Anaesthetists established by the Royal College of Surgeons in Ireland. T. Gilmartin, the first dean.
Neurolept analgesia reported by De Castro and Paul Mundeleer.

1962 First European Congress of Anaesthesiology in Vienna.
First Asian–Australasian Congress of Anaesthesiologists held in Manila.

1966 Ketamine used clinically by Corssen (1916–1990) and Domino in the USA.
Enflurane used by Virtue of Denver and his colleagues.

1970 Intensive Care Society founded in the UK. Society for Critical Care Medicine founded in the US.

1971 Isoflurane first used.

1982 First Meeting of the European Society of Regional Anaesthesia (ESRA) held in Edinburgh.
First International Symposium on the History of Anaesthesia held in Rotterdam.

1988 College of Anaesthetists established in London.

1992 Royal College of Anaesthetists created.

See also Davison M. H. Armstrong, *The Evolution of Anaesthesia*. Altrincham: J. Sherratt and Son, 1965; Duncum, Barbara, *The Development of Inhalation Anaesthesia*. London: Oxford University Press, 1947; Faulconer A. Jr and Keys T. E. *Foundations of Anesthesiology*. Springfield, Ill.: Thomas, 1965; Thomas K. Bryn, *The Development of Anaesthetic Apparatus*. Oxford: Blackwell, 1975; Keys T. E. *The History of Surgical Anesthesia*. New York: Dover Pubs. Inc. 1963; Bryce-Smith R., Mitchell J. V. and Parkhouse J. *The Nuffield Department of Anaesthetics*, 1937–62. London: Oxford University Press, 1963; Smith W. D. A. *Under the Influence: a History of Nitrous Oxide and Oxygen Anaesthesia*. London: Macmillan, 1982; *Genesis of Contemporary American Anesthesia*. Volpitto P. P. and Vandam L. D. (ed.) Springfield, Ill.: Thomas, 1982; *Essays on the first 100 Years of Anaesthesia*, Sykes W. D. Vol. 1 and 2. 1961/2 and Vol. 3 (ed. Ellis R. H.) London & Edinburgh: Churchill Livingstone, 1982; Anaesthesia and analgesia. Centenary of anaesthesia. *Br. Med. Bull.* 1946, **4**, 81; *Bibliography on the History of Anaesthesia*. Secher Ole. Copenhagen: Rigshospitalet, 1984; Secher O.

History of the modern development of the inhalation anaesthetics. *Acta Anaesthesiol. Scand.* 1982, **26**, 269; *Anaesthesia; Essays on its History,* Rupreht J. et al. (ed.) Berlin: Springer-Verlag, 1985; Atkinson R. S. and Boulton T. B. (ed.), *A History of Anaesthesia* London: Royal Society of Medicine, 1989.

References

1. Long C. W. *South Med. Surg. J.* 1849, **5**, 705.
2. Ellis R. H. In: *A History of Anaesthesia* (Atkinson R. S. and Boulton T. B. ed.) London: Royal Society of Medicine, 1989, 69.
3. *Med. Times Lond.* 1868, **2**, 9; and Pernick M. S. *A Calculus of Suffering.* New York: Columbia University Press, 1985.
4. Macintosh R. R. (1897–1989) In: *Anaesthesia: Essays on its History* (Rupreht J. et al. ed.) Berlin: Springer-Verlag, 1985, 352.
5. Secher O. In: *Anaesthesia: Essays on its History* (Rupreht J. et al. ed.) Berlin: Springer-Verlag, 1985, 321.
6. Fuller J. F. *Anesthesiology* 1947, **8**, 464.
7. *See* 'Classical File', *Surv. Anesthesiol.* 1976, **20**, 283.
8. *See also* Cartwright F. F. *The English Pioneers of Anaesthesia.* Bristol: Wright, 1952; and Bryn-Thomas K. *Anaesthesia* 1978, **33**, 903.
9. Excerpts reprinted in *Surv. Anesthesiol.* 1968, **12**, 92; also facsimile reproduction, London: Butterworths, 1972.
10. Cartwright F. F. *Proc. 4th World Cong. Anaesth.* 1968, 203.
11. Reprinted in 'Classical File', *Surv. Anesthesiol.* 1966, **10**, 92.
12. *Boston Med. Surg. J.* 1848, **38**, 25.
13. *See also* MacQuitty B. *The Battle for Oblivion.* London: Harrap, 1969.
14. Long C. W. *South. Med. J.* 1849, n. s, 705 (reprinted in 'Classical File', *Surv. Anesthesiol.* 1960, **4**, 120).
15. Gould A. B. ·In: *Anaesthesia: Essays in its History* (Rupreht J. et al. ed.) Berlin: Springer-Verlag, 1985, 384.
16. Vandam L. D. and Abbott J. A. *N. Engl. J. Med.* 1984, **311**, 991
17. Holmes O. W. *Br. Med. J.* 1902, **2**, 1368.
18. Thomas, K. Bryn, *Anaesthesia* 1968, **23**, 676.
19. Dawkins R. J. Massey, *Anaesthesia* 1947, **2**, 51.
20. Zuck D. *Br. J. Anaesth.* 1978, **50**, 393; Squire W. *Lancet* 1888, **2**, 1220.
21. Baillie T. W. *From Boston to Dumfries.* Dumfries, 1966; and *Br. J. Anaesth.* 1965, **37**, 952.
22. *See* Miller A. H. *Boston Med. Surg. J.* 1927, **197**, 1218; Miller A. H. *Anesthesiology* 1947, **8**, 471 (reprinted in 'Classical File', *Surv. Anesthesiol.* 1972, **16**, 193); *also* Straton J. Br. Med. J. 1972, **3**, 181.
23. Ellis R. H. *Anaesthesia* 1976, **31**, 766; Ellis R. H. *Anaesthesia* 1977, **32**, 1973.
24. Ellis R. H. In: *A History of Anaesthesia* (Atkinson R. S. and Boulton T. B. ed.) London: Royal Society of Medicine, 1989.
25. Longford E. *Victoria,* R. I. London: Weidenfeld and Nicolson, 1964, 234.
26. Winterton W. R. *Hist. Med.* 1980, **8**, 11; Schoenberg B. S. et al. *Mayo Clinic Proc.* 1974, **49**, 680.
27. Picini F. *Osservazioni microscopische e deduction patologische sul cholera asiatica.* Firenze, 1854.
28. Koch R. Ueber die cholera bakterien. *Dtsch. Med. Wochenschr,* 1884, **10**, 725.
29. *Anaesthesia* 1952, **7**, 192.
30. Atkinson R. S. Proc. *4th World Cong. Anaesth. (London),* 1968, 197.
31. *See also* Shepherd J. A. *Simpson and Syme of Edinburgh.* Edinburgh and London: Livingstone, 1969; Simpson, Myrtle, *Simpson the Obstetrician.* London: Gollancz, 1972.

32. Simpson J. Y. *Lond. Med. Gaz.* 1847, n.s., **5**, 934; *Lancet* 1847, **2**, 549 (reprinted in 'Classical File', *Surv. Anesthesiol.* 1961, **5**, 93).
33. Wade D. *The True Story of the Introduction of Chloroform into Anaesthetics.* Edinburgh: Linlithgow, 1870.
34. Farr A. D. *Anaesthesia* 1980, **35**, 896.
35. Sykes W. S. *Essays on the First Hundred Years of Anaesthesia*, Edinburgh and London. Livingstone, 1961, Vol. II, p. 168; Coote H. *Lancet* 1847, **2**, 571.
36. Atkinson R. S. *Simpson and Chloroform.* London: Priory Press, 1973, and Atkinson R. S. *Anaesthesia* 1973, **28**, 302.
37. Thomas K. Bryn, *Anaesthesia* 1971, **27**, 436.
38. Clover J. T. *Br. Med. J.* 1876, **2**, 75 (reprinted in 'Classical File', *Surv. Anesthesiol.* 1964, **8**, 87).
39. Clover J. T. *Br. Med. J.* 1877, **1**, 69, Atkinson R. S. and Bouton T. B. *Anaesthesia* 1977, **32**, 1033.
40. Elliott C. J. R. *Anaesthesia* 1979, **34**, 681, Brown A. G. *Anaesthesia* 1979, **34**, 681, Weisser Ch. *Anaesthesist* 1983, **32**, 52.
41. Lee J. Alfred, *Ann. R. Coll. Surg.* 1960, **26**, 280; Wylie W. D. *Ann. R. Coll. Surg.* 1975, **56**, 171.
42. Clover J. T. *Br. Med. J.* 1871, **2**, 33.
43. *See* Calverley R. In: *Anaesthesia, Essays on its History* (Rupreht J. et al. ed.) Berlin: Springer-Verlag, 1985, 18.
44. Wilson Smith T. *Lancet* 1898, **1**, 1005.
45. Hewitt F. W. *Anaesthetics and their Administration.* London: Macmillan, 1901, 277–8.
46. Hewitt F. W. *Anaesthetics and their Administration.* London: Macmillan, 1901, 209.
47. *See* Edwards G. *Ann. R. Coll. Surg.* 1951, **8**, 233.
48. Binning R. *Anaesthesia* 1978, **33**, 55.
49. Macewen W. *Glas. Med. J.* 1879, **2**, 72; *Br. Med. J.* 1880, **2**, 122; *Lancet* 1980, **2**, 906.
50. Koller C. *Klin. Nbl. Augen.* 1884, **22**, 60; *Wien, Med. Wochenschr.* 1884, **34**, 1276, 1309, (translated in 'Classical File', *Surv. Anesthesiol.* 1965, **9**, 288).
51. *See also* Koller C. *JAMA* 1928, **90**, 1742 and *JAMA* 1941, **117**, 1284; Koller-Becker H. *Psychoanal. Q.* 1963, 32, 509; Liljestrand G. *Acta Physiol. Scand.* 1967, **3** (Suppl. 299), 30; Wyklicky H. and Skopec M. In: *Regional Anaesthesia, 1884–1984* (Scott D. B. et al. ed.) 1984, Sodertalje: Production ICM AB; McAuley J. F. *Br. Dent. J*, 1985, **158**, 339.
52. Hall R. S. *New York Med. J.* 1884, **40**, 643; Halsted W. S. *New York Med. J.* 1885, **42**, 294.
53. Glen F. and Dillon L. D. *Surg. Gynecol. Obstet.* 1980, *151*, 518.
54. Halsted W. S. *Johns Hopkins Hosp. Rep.* 1890, **2**, 255.
55. Quincke H. I. 'Die Lumbalpunktur des Hydrocephalis', *Berlin Klin. Wochenschr.* 1891, **25**, 809.
56. Bier A. *Dt. Z. Chir.* 1899, *51*, 361 (translated in *Surv. Anesthesiol.* 1962, **6**, 352).
57. Bier A. *Zbl. Chir.* 1892, **19**, 57.
58. Bier A. *Verh. Dtsch. Ges. Chir.* 1908, **37**, 204.
59. Braun H. *Arch. Klin. Chir.* 1902, **69**, 541.
60. Braun H. *Dtsch. Med. Wochenschr.* 1905, **31**, 1667.
61. Röse W. In: *Regional Anaesthesia, 1884–1984. Centennial Meeting of Regional Anaesthesia.* (Scott D. B. et al. ed.) Sodertalie: Production ICM AB, 1984.
62. Läwen A. *Beitr. Klin. Chir.* 1912, **80**, 168.
63. Läwen A. *Zbl. Chirurg.* 1910, **37**, 708; *Dtsch. Zeit. Chir.* 1911, **108**, 11.
64. *L'Anaesthésie Régionale* Paris: Doin, 1921; *see also* Macintosh R. R. *Reg. Anaesth.* 1978, **1**, 2 and Lee, J. Alfred, *Reg. Anaesth.* 1985, **10**, 99.
65. Reprinted in 'Classical File', *Surv. Anesthesiol.* 1979, **23**, 340; *Indianap. Med. J.* October 1911
66. Guedel A. E. and Waters R. S. *Curr. Res. Anesth. Analg.* 1928, **7**, 238.
67. *Curr. Res. Anesth. Analg.* May 1920; *Inhalation Anesthesia, A Fundamental Guide.* New York: Macmillan, 1937.
68. Guedel A. E. *JAMA* 1933, **103**, 1862.

69. *Curr. Res. Anesth. Analg.* December 1934.
70. *Anesthesiology, 1940*, **1**, 1.
71. Boyle H. E. G. *Br. Med. J.* 1917, **2**, 653.
72. G. Davis was anaesthetist to Harvey Cushing at the Johns Hopkins Hospital.
73. Watt O. M. *Anaesthesia* 1968, **23**, 103.
74. Morris L. E. In: *Anaesthesia: Essays on its History.* (Rupreht J. ed.) Berlin: Springer-Verlag, 1985, 32; Gordh T. *ibid.* 36.
75. Stiles J. A. et al. *Curr. Res. Anesth. Analg.* 1934, **13**, 56.
76. Waters R. M. *Curr. Res. Anesth. Analg.* 1924, **3**, 20.
77. Waters R. M. (ed.) *Chloroform: A Study after 100 Years.* Madison: University of Wisconsin Press, 1951.
78. Pratt T. W. et al. *Am. J. Surg.* 1936, **31**. 464.
79. Gale J. W. and Waters R. M. *J. Thorac. Surg.* 1932, **1**, 432.
80. Lundy J. S. *Minn. Med.* 1926, **9**, 399.
81. Betcher A. M. *Anesth. Analg. Curr. Res.* 1977, **56**, 303.
82. Bennett A. E. et al. *JAMA* 1940, **114**, 322.
83. Dinnick O. P. *Proc. 4th World Cong. Anaesth. (London.)* 1968, 181.
84. Hunter A. R. *Anaesthesia* 1983, **38**, 1214; Helliwell P. J. *Anaesthesia* 1982, **37**, 394 and 913; Boulton T. B. In: *A History of Anaesthesia* (Atkinson R. S. and Boulton T. B. ed.) London: Royal Society of Medicine, 1989.
85. Atkinson R. S. In: *A History of Anaesthesia* (Atkinson R. S. and Boulton T. B. ed.) London: Royal Society of Medicine, 1989.
86. Newson A. J. *Anaesth. Intensive Care*, 1975, **3**, 204.
87. Wilson G. C. M. *Anaesth. Intensive Care*, 1985, **13**, 71.
88. Wilson G. *Anaesth. Intensive Care.* 1987, **15**, 451; Schurr P. H. *'Benjamin's Son'.* London: Royal Society of Medicine, 1991.
89. Matsuki A. *Anesthesiology* 1970, **33**, 446.
90. Bishop P. J. *J. R. Soc. Med. 1980,* **73**, 448.
91. Young H. *A Surgeon's Autobiography.* New York: Harcourt Brace, 1940, 69.
92. Eavey R. D. N. *N. Engl. J. Med.* 1983, **309**, 990.
93. Nunn R. *Lond. Med. Gaz.* 1847, **39** (4, n.s.), 414; Annotation, *Lancet* 1847, **1**, 340.
94. Snow, *On Chloroform and Other Anaesthetics* (reprinted in *Br. J. Anaesth.* 1955, **27**, 501); 'Classical File', *Surv. Anesthesiol.* 1973, **17**, 381; report of coroner's inquest reprinted in *Surv. Anesthesiol.* 1959, **3**, 137; Annotation, *Lancet*, 1848, **1**, 161 (reprinted in 'Classical File', *Surv. Anesthesiol.* 1959, **3**, Feb).
95. Wylie W. D. *Ann. R. Coll. Surg.* 1975, **56**, 171.
96. Lee J. A. *Anaesthesia* 1978, **33**, 741.
97. *Lancet*, 1867, **1**, 326; **2**, 353.
98. *See* 'Classical File', *Surv. Anesthesiol.* 1963, **7**, 74.
99. *Arch. Klin. Chir.* 1871, **12**, 112.
100. *C. R. Acad. Sci. Paris*, 1874, **515**, 651.
101. *Phil. J. Dent. Science* 1876, **3**, 37 (*see* 'Classical File', *Surv. Anesthesiol.* 1964, **8**, 348).
102. Macewen W. *Br. Med. J.* 1880, **2**, 122.
103. Richards W. et al. *Anaesthesia* 1976, **31**, 933.
104. Billroth T. *Wien. Med. Wochenschr.* 1881, **31**, 161, Obituary, *Surg. Gynecol. Obstet.* 1979, **148**, 252, Mann R. J. *Mayo Clin. Proc.* 1974, **49**, 132.
105. Woelfler A. *Zbl. f. Chirurg.* 1881, **8**, 705.
106. Bennett H. and Godlee R. J. *Lancet* 1884, **2**, 1090.
107. *Arch. Physiol. Normal Path.* 1892, **24**, 562.
108. Matas R. *Ann. Surg.* 1899, **29**, 426.
109. Sweeney B. *Anaesthesia* 1985, **40**, 1000.
110. Reprinted in 'Classical File' *Surv. Anesthesiol.* 1965, **9**, 511, 634, from *Br. Med. J.* 1902, **1**, 817, 885, 951. *See also* Wilson G. C. M. *Anaesth. Intensive Care* 1972, **1**, 9.
111. Einthoven W. *Arch. Ges. Physiol.* 1903, **99**, 472.
112. Lee J. A. *Anaesthesia* 1979, **34**, 885.

113. Lee J. A. *Anaesthesia* 1978, **33**, 362.
114. *Surg. Gynecol. Obstet.* 1911, **13**, 456; *see also* Waters R. M. J. *Hist. Med. Allied Sci.* 1946, **I**, 595.
115. *Indianap. Med. J.* 1911, **14**, 476.
116. *Br. J. Surg.* 1911, **1**, 90.
117. *JAMA* 1912, **59**, 2015.
118. *J. Lab. Clin. Med.* 1915, **1**, 1.
119. *Lancet*, **1**, 70.
120. *J. Biol. Chem.* 1924, **59**, 737; reprinted in 'Classical File', *Surv. Anesthesiol.* 1957, **1**, 629; *see also Anesth. Analg.* 1975, **54**, 654.
121. *Minn. Med.* 1926, **9**, 399.
122. *Dtsch. Med. Wochenschr.* 1927, **53**, 712.
123. Fleming A. *Br. J. Exp. Pathol.* 1929, **10**, 226.
124. Chain E. et al. *Lancet* 1940, **2**, 226.
125. *Dtsch. Med. Wochenschr.* 1932, **2**, 1205.
126. Marriott H. L. and Kekwick A. *Lancet* 1935, **1**, 977.
127. Gerhardt Domagk, *Dtsch. Med. Wochenschr* 1935, **61**, 250.
128. *Lancet* 1936, **1**, 1279.
129. Chain E. B. et al. *Lancet* 1940, **2**, 226.
130. Bourne W. *Anesthesiology* 1948, **9**, 239, 358; *J. Hist. Med. Allied Sci.* 1946, **1**, No. 4, October.
131. Hench P. S. et al. *Proc. Staff Meet. Mayo Clin.* 1949, **24** 181.
132. Lassen H. C. A. *Lancet*, 1953, **1**, 37; Ibsen B. *Proc. R. Soc. Med.* 1954, **47**, 72.

Chapter 36

Agents and techniques no longer in common use

Cyclopropane (C₃H₆)

History[1]

Cyclopropane or trimethylene was first synthesized by August von Freund (1835–1892) of Poland[2] in 1882. Its anaesthetic properties were shown by G. W. H. Lucas and V. E. Henderson, of Toronto, in 1929,[3] and used on a human volunteer by W. Easson Brown, the patient being Professor Henderson.

Properties

Stored in orange cylinders as a liquid at a pressure of 5 bar, no reducing valves being required. Blood-gas partition coefficient 0.46. MAC 9.2%. Very explosive. Not decomposed by soda-lime. No toxic products of metabolism.

Rapid induction, using 30–50% concentration in oxygen. A powerful respiratory depressant. Cardiac output is usually increased with arterial pressure well maintained. Vagotonic and ventricular dysrhythmias may be seen. Deaths. have been reported from ventricular fibrillation. Adrenaline should be avoided when using cyclopropane. Complications can be minimized by preventing hypercapnia. Nausea and vomiting was not uncommon postoperatively. Some anaesthetists found it useful in old, ill and shocked patients. It was also popular for induction in children.

Ether (CH₃.CH₂-O-CH₂.CH₃)

History

Prepared in 1540 by Valerius Cordus (1515–1544), who called it sweet oil of vitriol. Sigmund August Frobensius, the German chemist, physician and botanist from Wittenberg, named it ether.[4] Used clinically for anaesthesia by W. E. Clarke (1818–1878) of Rochester, NY, in January 1842, when Dr Elijah Pope extracted a tooth from a Miss Hobbs,[5] and by Crawford Long (1815–1893) of Jefferson, Georgia, on 3 March 1842,[6] but they did not publish their results until later.[7] Introduced to the profession by W. T. G. Morton of Boston (1819–1868) on 16 October 1846.[8] The operation was for the removal of avascular tumour from just below the mandible; the patient (who gave 'informed consent') was Gilbert Abbott. After the operation he remained in hospital for 7 weeks. The first account of its pharmacological and clinical properties appeared in John Snow's book *On the Inhalation of Ether*, published in 1847. It did not attain much popularity in Britain until B. Joy Jeffries came from the US, advocating the safer ether instead of chloroform in 1872. Two years later Clover introduced his gas-ether sequence.[9] It is still the safest all-purpose anaesthetic. "I hold it therefore to be almost impossible that a death from this agent can occur in the hands of a medical man who is applying it with ordinary intelligence and attention" (John Snow, *On Chloroform and Other Anaesthetics*, 1858). In 1847, at least 25 books were published on its use.

Crawford Long was born in Danielsville, Georgia, 1 Feb. 1815, the son of a state senator. He graduated in 1839 and after working in New York settled with his former tutor, Dr Grant, in Jefferson. Removed a cyst from the neck of James Venables under ether anaesthesia 3 March 1842. A museum built on the site of Long's original office was dedicated in 1957, in Jefferson, Georgia.

Properties

SVP at 20°C is 425 mmHg. Blood/gas partition coefficient 12.0. Slow induction and recovery. MAC 1.92. Flammable in air and explosive in oxygen. Irritant vapour, which can readily induce laryngeal spasm.

Liberates catecholamines and tends to maintain blood pressure. Dysrhythmias are rare. Adrenaline is relatively safe with ether. Respiration first increases, and then decreases as anaesthesia deepens. Bronchial smooth muscle is relaxed. Nausea and vomiting occurs frequently. Skeletal muscle is also relaxed.

Its advantages are: (1) it is relatively non-toxic especially in light planes of anaesthesia; (2) it produces excellent relaxation without severe respiratory depression; (3) respiratory depression with overdosage is not accompanied by cardiac depression, and may be treated with IPPV; (4) the products of its metabolism, alcohol, acetaldehyde and acetic acid, are relatively non-toxic; (5) little tendency to cause dysrhythmias; and (6) a safe anaesthetic in the absence of severe hypoxia. For the unskilled anaesthetist dealing with the unfit patient it has a lot to commend it.

Its disadvantages are: (1) risk of explosion and fire, especially with oxygen or nitrous oxide; (2) mucus secretion from the salivary glands and upper airway; (3) nausea and vomiting postoperatively; and (4) slow induction and recovery. Irritant nature prevent rapid increase in vapour strength.

Light anaesthesia is obtained with an inspired concentration of 3–6%. Muscle relaxation requires up to 13%. For more than a hundred years ether provided safe and efficient anaesthesia worldwide, and during most of that time it was given by the open-drop method on to a gauze mask. Ether 3% in air as from an EMO inhaler, with a muscle relaxant, produces a very safe, economical and acceptable anaesthetic.[10] Explosions have not been described during the administration of ether and air even when diathermy has been used.

Chloroform CHCl₃

History

Its anaesthetic properties were discovered in animals by Jean Pierre Marie Flourens (1794–1867),[11] Paris physiologist, in 1847 before Simpson used it in humans. Used at St Bartholomew's Hospital by Holmes Coote in the spring of 1847,[12] 6 months before Simpson. Introduced to clinical practice and popularized by James Young Simpson and his assistants, James Mathews Duncan (1826–1890) and George Keith, after experimenting on themselves, in Edinburgh in November 1847.[13] Within a few months chloroform superseded ether as the most popular anaesthetic agent. The first reported death due to chloroform was that of Hannah Greener of Winlayton, near Newcastle upon Tyne, little more than two months after its introduction (28 Jan 1848). The anaesthetic was given for a minor operation by Dr Meggison. John Snow gave over 4000 chloroform anaesthetics without a death and, early on, recommended that for safety a concentration of not more than 4% in air should be used. Following 1890, reports of liver damage appeared in the literature (Guthrie, 1894).[14] In 1911, Goodman Levy (1856–1954) showed that death due to ventricular fibrillation might occur in light anaesthesia.[15]

Light chloroform analgesia was given to Queen Victoria by John Snow for birth of her last two children, Prince Leopold (7 May 1853) and Princess Beatrice (14 May 1857).

Properties

SVP at 20°C is 160 mmHg. Blood/gas partition coefficient 8.0. MAC 0.8%. Induction requires about 4%, but prolonged inhalation of 2% vapour may produce respiratory arrest.

The blood pressure gradually falls as with halothane. Sudden cardiac arrest, occurring during light anaesthesia,[16] may be due to ventricular fibrillation (adrenaline is contra-indicated during chloroform anaesthesia) or vagal inhibition. Delayed chloroform liver damage may occur from the first to the third day after anaesthesia. More likely to follow repeated administrations.

Trichloroethylene (CCl₂CHCl)

History

First described in 1864 by E. Fischer (1852–1919), chemist, of Jena,[17] since when it has been used in industry both as a fat solvent and in the dry-cleaning trade. Its poisonous properties have been long recognized,[18] especially its power to produce analgesia in distribution of fifth cranial nerve and relieve trigeminal neuralgia. Relief afforded is probably not a local action but part of a general analgesia. General anaesthetic effects described by Karl B. Lehmann (1858–1940) of Würzburg in 1911[19] and by Dennis Jackson[20] of Cincinnati in 1933. Cecil Striker[21] used it to anaesthetize 300 patients in 1935, but its introduction to clinical anaesthesia was due to Christopher Langton Hewer (1896–1986) of St Bartholomew's Hospital, London, who published case reports in 1941.[22]

Properties

SVP at 20°C is only 60 mmHg. Blood/gas partition coefficient 9.0. MAC 0.2%. Not flammable under clinical conditions. May be decomposed into phosgene ($COCl_2$) and hydrochloric acid at temperatures above 125°C as by the cautery, especially in the presence of oxygen. If used in a closed circuit with soda-lime, toxic products may be formed,[23] the most important being dichloracetylene:

$$C_2HCl_3 + NaOH \rightarrow C_2Cl_2 \text{ (dichloracetylene)} + NaCl + H_2O$$

This is a potent nerve poison and may produce temporary or permanent paralysis of cranial nerves or even death. The V and VII nerves are most commonly involved, but damage to the III, IV, VI, X and XII nerves has been reported.

Induction is relatively slow. Cardiovascular stability is good, although dysrhythmias are seen. The heart is sensitized to the effects of adrenaline. There is tachypnoea, which may be controlled with opiates. Postoperative nausea and vomiting is fairly common. Muscular relaxation is poor.

Trichloroethylene is used mainly either to supplement relaxant/nitrous oxide/oxygen anaesthesia or to produce analgesia. Maintenance concentration is about 0.5%. The same concentration in air produces excellent analgesia in labour.

Its advantages are: (1) good analgesia; (2) relative lack of irritation of upper respiratory tract; (3) non-flammable; (4) does not depress cardiovascular system; (5) does not depress respiration; and (6) vastly less expensive than more modern agents.

Its disadvantages are: (1) tachypnoea; (2) dysrhythmias; (3) no muscle relaxation; (4) postoperative nausea and vomiting; (5) cannot be used with soda-lime; and (6) addiction has been reported.

Methoxyflurane ($CHCl_2.CF_2-O-CH_3$)

First used in clinical anaesthesia by Artusio and Van Poznak in 1960.[24]

Properties

SVP at 20°C is only 23 mmHg. Blood/gas partition coefficient 13. MAC 0.16%. Non-flammable, non-explosive, no reaction with soda-lime.

Slow induction. A good analgesic. For induction 2–3% is used and 0.5–1.0% for maintenance. A significant amount is metabolized, and the metabolites (including fluoride) are excreted in the urine for up to 12 days. Fluoride is toxic to the kidney. High output renal failure may follow methoxyflurane anaesthesia.[25]

Portable anaesthetic apparatus

Open drop administration

Introduced by Sir James Y. Simpson for chloroform in 1847, using a folded handkerchief. The Schimmelbusch (1860–1895, Berlin surgeon and pioneer of aseptic surgery) mask[26] is a modification of Skinner's wire frame of 1862[27] (Liverpool G.P. and obstetrician). Useful for giving chloroform and diethyl ether. G. H. Bellamy Gardner[28] of Charing Cross Hospital was a leading British exponent of the method.

Open drop methods do not deserve the disdain they usually receive. *Advantages are:* (1) cheapness; (2) portability; (3) ease of administration; and (4) minimal dead space. *Disadvantages are:* (1) uneven anaesthesia due to variations in concentration of vapour; (2) risk of fire, except with chloroform and modern agents; (3) wastefulness; (4) pollution of atmosphere; (5) risk of damage to eyes or skin of patient from anaesthetic liquid; and (6) fall in oxygen concentration under the mask (remedied by giving oxygen under the mask via small catheter).

The EMO Inhaler (Epstein–Macintosh–Oxford)[10]

Height 24 cm, diameter 23 cm, weight 6.5 kg when the water compartment is full. Was developed in the Nuffield Department of Anaesthetics in the University of Oxford. It will deliver a predetermined concentration of ether vapour in air, the accuracy of which is greatest at high concentrations and high tidal volumes.[29] Only suitable for plenum use (continuous flow) if the carrier gas is greater than 10 l/min.[30] There is an automatic thermocompensator bellows mechanism. A water compartment of approximately 1200 ml acts as a heat buffer.

It is usually employed as a 'draw-over' apparatus, but if combined with an Oxford Inflating Bellows[31] it can be used for IPPV. Useful apparatus in countries where nitrous oxide is not readily available or when portability is important. Ether and air can be used after thiopentone or halothane induction. For light anaesthesia with spontaneous respiration the ether concentration should gradually increase to 15%, after which it may be reduced to about 7% for maintenance. For controlled respiration with a non-depolarizing muscle relaxant and intubation, IPPV with 12% ether in air reducing to 2–3% is satisfactory.

The Oxford miniature vaporizer[32]

This can be calibrated for halothane or trichloroethylene. Chloroform and methoxyflurane were also used. Capacity 20 ml. Vaporization is from a stainless-steel wick and there is a permanent water jacket to limit temperature changes, although no elaborate thermocompensation mechanism is provided. Can be used (with halothane) to smooth induction with the EMO ether inhaler. Can also be used with the Oxford inflating bellows. Two of these vaporizers are incorporated into the Triservice anaesthetic apparatus that is in military use, *see* Chapter 23.

References

1. Lucas G. W. H. *Anesth. Analg.* 1961, **40**, 15.
2. von Freund A. *Monats. f. Chemie* 1882, **3**, 625.
3. Lucas G. W. H. and Henderson V. E. *Can. Med. Assoc. J.* 1929, **21**, 173.

4. Frobensius J. A. S. *Phil. Trans. R. Soc. Lond.* 1739, **36**, 283.
5. Bigelow H. J. *Am. J. Med. Sci.* 1876, **141**, 164.
6. Jeffereys J. *Lancet* 1872, **2**, 241; *Br. Med. J.* 1872, **2**, 499.
7. Long C. W. *Sth Med. J.* 1849, **5**, 705 (reprinted in 'Classical File', *Surv. Anesthesiol.* 1960, **4**, 120); *JAMA* 1965, **194**, 1008; Cole W. H. J. *Anaesth. Intensive Care* 1974, **2**, 92; Taylor F. C. W. *Long and the Discovery of Ether.* New York: Hoebner, 1928.
8. Bigelow H. J. *Boston Med. Surg. J.* 1846, **35**, 309 (reprinted in 'Classical File', *Surv. Anesthesiol.* 1957, **1**, February); Morton W. T. G. *Remarks on the Proper Mode of Administration of Sulphuric Ether by Inhalation.* Boston: Dutton & Wentworth, 1847.
9. Clover J. T. *Med. Times, Lond.* 1874, **2**, 603; Vandam L. *Anesthesiology* 1980, **52**, 62.
10. Epstein H. G. and Macintosh R. R. *Anaesthesia* 1956, **11**, 83; Farman J. V. *Anaesthesia and the EMO System.* London: English Universities Press, 1973.
11. Flourens M.-J. P. *C. R. Seances Acad. Sci. III* 1847, **24**, 340.
12. Furnell M. C. *Lancet* 1871, **1**, 433; 1877, **1**, 934.
13. Simpson J. Y. *Lond. Med. Gaz.* 1847, **5**, 934; *Lancet* 1847, **2**, 549; reprinted in *Foundations of Anesthesiology* (Faulcolner A. and Keys T. E. ed.) Springfield, Ill.: Thomas, Vol. 1, 463; and also in 'Classical File', *Surv. Anesthesiol.* 1961, **5**, 93. (When Simpson, on being awarded a baronetcy, was looking for a suitable crest, it was suggested that there should be a picture of a 'wee naked bairn' with the motto "Does your mother know you're oot?").
14. Guthrie L. *Lancet* 1894, **1**, 193, 257; 1903, **2**, 10 (reprinted in 'Classical File', *Surv. Anesthesiol.* 1967, **6**, August).
15. Levy A. G. *Chloroform Anaesthesia.* London: Bale Son & Daniellson, 1922; *Proc. R. Soc. Med.* 1914, **7**, 57 (reprinted in 'Classical File' *Surv. Anesthesiol.* 1973, **17**, 477).
16. *Proc. R. Soc. Med.* 1914, **7**, 57 (reprinted in 'Classical File', *Surv. Anesthesiol.* 1973, **17**, 383).
17. Fischer E. *Jena Z. Med. Naturw.* 1864, **1**, 123.
18. Plessner W. *Berl. Klin. Wochenschr.* 1916, **53**, 25.
19. Lehmann K. B. *Arch. Hyg. Berl.* 1911, **74**, 1.
20. Jackson D. E. *Curr. Res. Anesth. Analg.* 1934, **13**, 198.
21. Striker C. et al. *Curr. Res. Anesth. Analg.* 1935, **14**, 68.
22. Hewer C. L. and Hadfield C. F. *Br. Med. J.* 1941, **1**, 924 (reprinted in 'Classical File', *Surv. Anesthesiol.* 1963, **7**, April); Hewer, C. L. *Proc. R. Soc. Med.* 1942, **35**, 463.
23. Morton H. J. V. *Br. Med. J.* 1943, **2**, 838; McAuley J. *Br. Med. J.* 1943, **2**, 713.
24. Artusio J. F. et al. *Anesthesiology* 1960, **21**, 512 (reprinted in 'Classical File', *Surv. Anesthesiol.* 1968, **12**, 196).
25. Paddock R. B. et al. *Anaesthesiology* 1964, **25**, 707; Cransell W. B. et al. *Anaesthesiology* 1966, **27**, 591; Richey J. E. and Smith R. B. *Anaesthesia* 1972, **27**, 9.
26. Schimmelbusch C. *Anleitung Z. aseptischen Wundbehandling.* Berlin: Hirschwald, 1894.
27. Skinner T. *Retrosp. Pract. Med.* 1862, **46**, 185.
28. Bellamy Gardner G. H. *Br. Med. J.* 1907, **2**, 1516; *Br. Med. J.* 1910, **2**, 766.
29. Marsh D. R. G. and Herbert P. *Anaesthesia* 1983, **38**, 575.
30. Schaefer H.-G. and Farman J. V. *Anaesthesia* 1984, **39**, 171.
31. Macintosh R. R. *Br. Med. J.* 1953, **2**, 202.
32. Parkhouse J. *Anaesthesia* 1966, **21**, 498; Schaefer H.-G. and Farman J. V. *Anaesthesia* 1984, **39**, 171.

Appendix

SI Units (Système Internationale d'Unités)

Physical quantity	Name of SI unit	Symbol for SI unit
Length	metre	m
Mass	kilogram	kg
Volume	cubic metre	m^3
Time	second	s
Electric current	ampere	A
Thermodynamic temperature	kelvin	K
Luminous intensity	candela	cd
Amount of substance	mole	mol
Energy	joule	J
Force	newton	N
Power	watt	W
Pressure	pascal	Pa
Electrical charge	coulomb	C
Electric potential difference	volt	V
Electric resistance	ohm	Ω
Electric conductance	siemens	S
Electric capacitance	farad	F
Magnetic flux	weber	Wb
Inductance	henry	H
Magnetic flux density	tesla	T
Luminous flux	lumen	lm
Illumination	lux	lx
Frequency	hertz	Hz

Ampère, André Marie (1775–1836), French mathematician.
Coulomb, Charles Augustin de (1736–1806), French physicist.
Faraday, Michael (1791–1867), English experimental physicist.
Henry, William (1797–1884), English chemist and mathematician.
Hertz, Heinrich (1857–1894), Bavarian physicist.
Joule, James Prescott (1818–1889), English physicist.
Kelvin, William, First Lord Kelvin of Largs (1824–1907), Ulster-Scottish physicist.

Newton, Sir Isaac (1642–1727), English mathematician.
Ohm, Georg Simon (1787–1854), Bavarian physicist and mathematician.
Pascal, Blaise (1623–1662), French philosopher and mathematician.
Siemens, Sir William (1823–1883), German born, naturalized British, inventor and engineer.
Tesla, Nikola (1856–1943), Croatian-American electrical engineer.
Volta, Alessandro (1745–1827), Italian mathematician and physicist.
Watt, James (1736–1819), Scottish mathematical instrument maker and inventor.
Weber, Wilhelm Eduard (1804–1891), German physicist.

Torr: 1 torr is 1 mmHg and equals $1/760$ normal atmospheric pressure. (Toriccelli, Evangelista (1608–1647), Italian physicist and mathematician.) The metric system was adopted in France in January 1840.

Factor	Prefix	Symbol
10^{12}	tera	T
10^9	giga	G
10^6	mega	M
10^3	kilo	k
10^{-1}	deci	d
10^{-2}	centi	c
10^{-3}	milli	m
10^{-6}	micro	μ
10^{-9}	nano	n
10^{-12}	pico	p
10^{-15}	femto	f

Strengths of solutions

0.1% contains 1 mg/ml.
0.5% contains 5 mg/ml.
1% contains 10 mg/ml.

Conversion factors

	SI unit	Old unit	Old to SI	SI to old
Pressures	kPa	mmHg	× 0.1333	× 7.5
		cmH$_2$O	× 0.0981	× 10
		lb/sq in	× 6.894	× 0.145

Blood chemistry

Glucose	mmol/l	mg/100 ml	× 0.0555	× 18
Creatinine	μmol/l	mg/100 ml	× 88.4	× 0.01
Urea	mmol/l	mg/100 ml	× 0.166	× 6.0
Calcium	mmol/l	mg/100 ml	× 0.25	× 4.0

Conversion factors for temperature

Temp. C = (temp. F minus 32) × ⅚.
Temp. F = (temp. C × ⅚) + 32.

Some useful addresses

The Royal College of Anaesthetists, 48–49 Russell Square, London WC1B 4JP.

The Faculty of Anaesthetists of the Royal College of Surgeons in Ireland, St Stephen's Green, Dublin 2.

The Faculty of Anaesthetists, The Royal Australasian College of Surgeons, College of Surgeons Gardens, Spring Street, Melbourne 3000, Australia.

The Faculty of Anaesthetists, The College of Medicine of South Africa, 17 Milner Road, Rondebosch 7700, Republic of South Africa.

The Association of Anaesthetists of Great Britain and Ireland, 9 Bedford Square, London WC1B 3RA.

The Royal Society of Medicine (Section of Anaesthetics), 1 Wimpole Street, London W1M 8AE.

World Federation of Societies of Anesthesiologists, Secretary Professor M. D. Vickers, Heath Park Hospital, Cardiff, UK.

American Society of Anesthesiologists Inc., 515 Busse Highway, Park Ridge, Illinois 60068, USA.

International Anesthesia Research Society, 3645 Warrensville Centre Road, Cleveland, Ohio 44122, USA.

Canadian Anaesthetists Society, 178 St George Street, Toronto, Ontario M5R 2M7, Canada.

Index

Note: In the interests of clarity and conciseness, only those individuals whose biographies appear in Chapter 35 have been included in the index.